The A–Z of Neurological Pra

Guide to Clinical Neurology

C000058667

This is a pocket-sized ready-reference to neurology. Organised from A to Z, the content consists of a series of entries, each one describing in a readable and accessible style an aspect of neurology. This ranges from providing overviews of major groups of diseases (e.g. the dementias) to more detailed coverage of specific disease categories (e.g. Alzheimer's disease). Specific neurological conditions are described according to a very structured template covering the definition of the condition, its clinical features, investigation, pathogenesis and treatment, finishing with a small number of relevant and up-to-date references. In addition, there are hints about differential diagnosis with extensive cross-referencing between entries. This will become an essential resource for those undertaking training in neurology and will be of interest to those with interests closely allied to neurology (e.g. neurosurgery, neurorehabilitation), as well as providing a reference source for generalists looking for a readable synopsis of neurological conditions.

The A–Z of
Neurological
Practice

A Guide to Clinical Neurology

ROGER A. BARKER
Department of Neurology, University of Cambridge, UK

NEIL J. SCOLDING
Institute of Clinical Neurosciences, Bristol, UK

DOMINIC ROWE
University of Sydney, Australia

ANDREW J. LARNER
Walton Centre for Neurology and Neurosurgery, Liverpool, UK

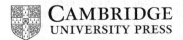
CAMBRIDGE
UNIVERSITY PRESS

PUBLISHED BY THE PRESS SYNDICATE OF THE UNIVERSITY OF CAMBRIDGE
The Pitt Building, Trumpington Street, Cambridge, United Kingdom

CAMBRIDGE UNIVERSITY PRESS
The Edinburgh Building, Cambridge CB2 2RU, UK
40 West 20th Street, New York, NY 10011-4211, USA
477 Williamstown Road, Port Melbourne, VIC 3207, Australia
Ruiz de Alarcón 13, 28014 Madrid, Spain
Dock House, The Waterfront, Cape Town 8001, South Africa

http://www.cambridge.org

First published 2005

Printed in the United Kingdom at the University Press, Cambridge

Typeface Utopia 7.5/11pt.   *System* QuarkXpress®

A catalogue record for this book is available from the British Library

ISBN 0 521 62960 8 paperback

The publisher has used its best endeavours to ensure that the URLs for external
websites referred to in this book are correct and active at the time of going to press.
However, the publisher has no responsibility for the websites and can make no
guarantee that a site will remain live or that the content is or will remain appropriate.

Every effort has been made in preparing this book to provide accurate and up-to-
date information that is in accord with accepted standards and practice at the time of
publication. Nevertheless, the authors, editors and publisher can make no warranties
that the information contained herein is totally free from error, not least because
clinical standards are constantly changing through research and regulation. The
authors, editors and publisher therefore disclaim all liability for direct or consequen-
tial damages resulting from the use of material contained in this book. Readers are
strongly advised to pay careful attention to information provided by the manufac-
turer of any drugs or equipment that they plan to use.

Preface

This book is designed for neurologists in training; which is to say, in light of current recommendations on continuing medical education and lifelong learning, *all* neurologists, whether or not in the earliest years of their career.

Information is presented in a structured (and hopefully succinct) way, following what might be termed a "trickle-down" principle, extending from overviews (e.g. "Dementia: an overview") to specific disease categories (e.g. "Alzheimer's disease"), the latter covered in terms of pathophysiology, clinical features (i.e. information accessed by history-taking and physical examination), investigations, differential diagnosis, treatment and prognosis. A few references are appended to most entries, the unsystematic (quirky?) nature of which may incur the wrath of disciples of the evidence-based movement, but which we have found informative. "Small-print" (i.e. rare) conditions have shorter entries. All sections are fully cross-referenced.

Of course, any attempt to produce a "fully comprehensive" neurological text is doomed to failure for many reasons, and readers may disagree with some of our emphases. Because we have individually published in the fields of neuroscience,[1] neurological signs,[2] and therapeutics,[3] we have not over-emphasised these areas. We have tried to include psychiatric and paediatric disorders that may be seen in adult neurological practice, but accept our limitations in these areas.

[1] Barker RA, Barasi S. *Neuroscience at a Glance.* Oxford: Blackwell Science, 1999.

[2] Larner AJ. *A Dictionary of Neurological Signs: Clinical Neurosemiology.* Dordrecht: Kluwer, 2001.

[3] Scolding NJ (ed.). *Contemporary Treatments in Neurology.* Oxford: Butterworth-Heinemann, 2001.

Aa

■ Abducens nerve palsy – see Cranial nerve disease: VI: Abducens nerve

■ Abetalipoproteinaemia
Bassen–Kornzweig syndrome

Pathophysiology Bassen and Kornzweig first described the association of a progressive ataxic syndrome with fat malabsorption, atypical retinitis pigmentosa and acanthocytosis with a lack of serum betalipoproteins in two siblings of consanguineous parents in the 1950s. Abetalipoproteinaemia is a rare autosomal-recessive condition characterized by the defective assembly and secretion of apolipoprotein B-containing lipoproteins, which are required for secretion of plasma lipoproteins that contain apolipoprotein B. In consequence there are very low plasma concentrations of cholesterol and triglyceride, and of fat-soluble vitamins, especially vitamin E, which produces the clinical features of a peripheral neuropathy, retinitis pigmentosa and cerebellar degeneration. The condition is caused by mutations in the gene coding for microsomal triglyceride transfer protein (MTP) on chromosome 4q22–q24, a protein required for the assembly of lipoproteins which contain apolipoprotein B.

A related condition, hypobetalipoproteinaemia, is inherited in an autosomal-dominant fashion with a defect in the apolipoprotein B gene in some cases, and in the homozygous state may be indistinguishable from abetalipoproteinaemia.

Clinical features: history and examination

- Malabsorption: steatorrhoea, with failure to thrive in children.
- Retinal degeneration: usually before the age of 10 years, with impaired night sight (night blindness = nyctalopia) initially, and progressive retinitis pigmentosa; vitamin A deficiency may be significant. However visual impairment is seldom severe.
- Peripheral neuropathy: a sensorimotor neuropathy with areflexia is often the presenting feature and is usually present by 10–30 years of age; vitamin E deficiency may be making a significant contribution to this.
- Ataxic syndrome: with dysarthria, nystagmus and head titubation. It results from a combination of peripheral neuropathy, spinocerebellar tract degeneration and direct cerebellar damage (i.e. sensory and cerebellar ataxia); vitamin E deficiency may be making a significant contribution to this.
- Dorsal column sensory loss and extensor plantar responses.
- Ophthalmoplegia in later stages.
- Skeletal abnormalities: pes cavus, scoliosis; may be secondary to the peripheral neuropathy.
- Subdural, retroperitoneal haemorrhages; excessive blood loss during surgery (vitamin K deficiency may be significant).

- No autonomic abnormalities, but cardiac involvement with cardiomegaly is found in the late stages of the disease.

Investigations and diagnosis
- Bloods: low ESR; often a mild haemolytic anaemia; acanthocytosis on blood film (but must be fresh to exclude false negatives), usually 50% or more of the red blood cells show acanthocytic morphology; low levels of apolipoprotein B (as demonstrated with immunoelectrophoresis) with very low plasma levels of chylomicrons, very low-, intermediate- and low-density lipoproteins (VLDL, IDL, LDL, respectively). The plasma levels of cholesterol and triglycerides are very low, in the region of 1–2 and 0–1 mmol/l, respectively.

    Low concentrations of fat-soluble vitamins, especially vitamin E.
- Imaging: CT/MRI: no specific abnormalities seen.
- CSF: usually normal.
- Neurophysiology:

    EMG/NCS: peripheral sensorimotor neuropathy (axonal, demyelinating, or mixed).

    Somatosensory evoked potential (SSEP): abnormal posterior column function.

    *B*rainstem *A*uditory *E*voked *P*otential (BSAEP): Brainnormal.

    Visual evoked response (VER): consistent with optic neuropathy.

    ERG: consistent with retinal degeneration.
- Other: malabsorption tests; jejunal biopsy reveals normal villi but the intestinal mucosal cells are vacuolated due to the presence of fat droplets that accumulate within them as they cannot be taken up by the chylomicrons.

Differential diagnosis Friedreich's ataxia.

Vitamin E deficiency secondary to other malabsorption syndrome (e.g. coeliac disease, cystic fibrosis).

Isolated vitamin E deficiency (ataxia with vitamin E deficiency, AVED).

Treatment and prognosis Treatment of the malabsorption syndrome is achieved by substitution and restriction of fat intake (i.e. low fat diet and medium chain triglycerides).

Many of the neurological complications can be prevented by oral administration of vitamin E (1–10 g/day).

Replacement of other fat-soluble vitamins (vitamins A, D and K).

Untreated patients are usually unable to stand or walk by the time they reach adolescence and rarely survive beyond the age of 40 years.

References Hardie RJ. Acanthocytosis and neurological impairment – a review. *Quarterly Journal of Medicine* 1989; **71**: 291–306.

Muller DP. Vitamin E: its role in neurological function. *Postgraduate Medical Journal* 1986; **62**: 107–112.

Rowland LP, Pedley TA. Abetalipoproteinemia. In: Rowland LP (ed.). *Merritt's Textbook of Neurology* (9th edition). Baltimore: Williams & Wilkins, 1995: 594–596.

Other relevant entries Ataxia with vitamin E deficiency; Friedreich's ataxia; Gastrointestinal disease and the nervous system; Hypobetalipoproteinaemia;

Neuroacanthocytosis; Retinitis pigmentosa; Tangier disease; Vitamin deficiencies and the nervous system.

■ Abscess: an overview

An abscess is a focal suppurative process, which may occur within or adjacent to nervous tissue with resultant neurological features, as well as systemic disturbance (pyrexia) from infection.

- Cerebral abscess

    Focal suppuration within brain parenchyma may present with symptoms and signs of a space-occupying lesion: headache, focal signs, impaired level of consciousness, seizures. Fever is not universally present, so its absence should not rule out the diagnosis. Predisposing causes include penetrating head trauma and haematogenous spread (e.g. infective endocarditis), but the commonest cause is spread from contiguous infection, for example in the ear, paranasal sinuses or teeth. Pulmonary fistulae in Osler–Weber–Rendu syndrome (hereditary haemorrhagic telangiectasia) predispose to cerebral abscesses. Fungal infections may also result in cerebral abscess formation (aspergillosis, blastomycosis, coccidioidomycosis, mucormycosis), as may filamentous bacteria (actinomycosis).

- Spinal cord abscess

    Abscess within the spinal cord is extremely rare; symptoms and signs are indistinguishable from epidural abscess.

- Epidural or extradural abscess

    These are located between dura and bone; they may be spinal or, less often, cranial.

    Spinal: Spread of infection is from vertebral osteomyelitis or retroperitoneal, mediastinal, or paraspinal infection. Severe back $+/-$ radicular pain; compressive spinal cord syndrome (myelopathy $+/-$ radiculopathy) may develop (thoracic > lumbar > cervical), often with systemic features of infection.

    Bloods: elevated white blood cell count, ESR.

    Radiology: plain radiographs show narrowing of disc spaces and/or lytic changes.

    MRI: investigation of choice for visualization of abscess.

    CSF: if done, reveals raised white blood cell count (typically <100 cells/µl), raised protein and normal glucose.

    Treatment: surgical decompression with antibiotic cover + send material for culture: _Staphylococcus aureus_ is the commonest organism, but other organisms include streptococci, enterobacteria, _Mycobacterium tuberculosis_, various fungi, and parasites. Prognosis is good if surgical intervention is early.

    Cranial: Almost always associated with an overlying osteomyelitis or local paranasal sinus infection.

The features and management are similar to subdural empyaema.

CSF: pleocytosis (20–100 cells/μl) with normal glucose and protein.

Treatment: with antibiotics; *Staphylococcus aureus* is the commonest organism.

- Subdural abscess/empyaema

These are located between dura and arachnoid. Spinal subdural abscess is clinically indistinguishable from epidural abscess.

References Kaplan K. Brain abscess. *Medical Clinics of North America* 1985; **69**: 345–359.

Mathisen GE, Johnson JP. Brain abscess. *Clinical Infectious Diseases* 1997; **25**: 763–781.

Other relevant entries Discitis; Endocarditis and the nervous system; HIV/AIDS and the nervous system; Infection and the nervous system: an overview; Osler–Weber–Rendu syndrome; Parameningeal infection; Subdural empyaema; Tumours: an overview.

■ Absence epilepsy

Absence seizures may be characterized as:

- Typical

A brief interruption of consciousness with unresponsiveness, with abrupt onset/offset. The attacks may be barely noticeable, without postictal confusion or awareness that an attack has occurred. Such typical absence seizures characterize idiopathic generalized epilepsies such as:

childhood absence epilepsy (CAE; pyknolepsy; "petit mal");

juvenile absence epilepsy (JAE).

EEG typically shows 3-Hz spike and slow-wave abnormalities, which may be elicited by hyperventilation.

Typical absence seizures may also be seen in:

idiopathic generalized epilepsy with absences of early childhood;

perioral myoclonia with absences;

Jeavons syndrome (*q.v.*).

- Atypical

There is a more obvious distancing, "clouding", or "glazing over", possibly with associated automatisms such as lip smacking, as in a complex focal seizure of temporal lobe origin. Activities may continue (*cf.* typical absence), albeit slowly, sometimes with clumsiness or mistakes. Atypical absences may be seen in Lennox–Gastaut syndrome, Dravet syndrome.

Ethosuximide and/or sodium valproate are the treatments of choice for idiopathic generalized absence epilepsies, whereas carbamazepine or lamotrigine is the first choice for complex partial seizures.

Reference Crunelli V, Leresche N. Childhood absence epilepsy: genes, channels, neurons and networks. *Nature Reviews Neuroscience* 2002; **3**: 371–382.
Other relevant entries Dravet syndrome; Epilepsy: an overview; Jeavons syndrome; Lennox–Gastaut syndrome.

▨ Acalculia

Acalculia, or dyscalculia, is an acquired impairment of arithmetical skills. It usually results from damage to the left parietotemporal cortex (angular gyrus, Brodmann areas 39 and 40) and often coexists with the disorders of language such as aphasia, alexia, and agraphia. The Gerstmann syndrome describes the constellation of acalculia, agraphia, finger agnosia, and right–left disorientation.

"Secondary" acalculias, for example resulting from a deficit in space perception, such as neglect, may be distinguished from "primary" acalculia, in which the problem is in comprehending numeration and mathematical principles, which cannot be attributed to defects in other cognitive domains. Such isolated acalculia, in which only certain mathematical operations may be lost whilst others are preserved, may also be known as anarithmetria.

Structural (CT/MRI) or functional (SPECT/PET) brain imaging may help to identify the anatomical substrate of the deficit. Most cases result from cerebrovascular insults, in which case recovery with time is possible.

References Butterworth B. *The Mathematical Brain*. London: Macmillan, 1999.
Denburg NL, Tranel D. Acalculia and disturbances of body schema. In: Heilman KM, Valenstein E (eds). *Clinical Neuropsychology* (4th edition). Oxford: OUP, 2003: 161–184.
McCarthy RA, Warrington EK. *Cognitive Neuropsychology. A Clinical Introduction*. San Diego: Academic, 1990: 262–274.
Other relevant entries Agraphia; Alexia; Alzheimer's disease; Aphasia; Cerebrovascular disease: arterial; Gerstmann syndrome; Tumours: an overview.

▨ Acanthamoeba

Acanthamoeba is one of the free-living amoebae which may cause sporadic (primary amoebic) meningoencephalitis, spreading haematogenously from a cutaneous (skin ulcer) or pulmonary source, particularly in immunocompromised patients. CSF shows pleocytosis; organisms are never cultured from CSF. Bacterial, fungal and tuberculous meningitides enter the differential diagnosis. Treatment with pentamidine is recommended and single abscesses may be surgically removed. Mortality is very high.

Reference Grunnert ML, Cannon GH, Kushner JP. Fulminant amebic meningo-encephalitis due to *Acanthamoeba*. *Neurology* 1981; **31**: 174–177.
Other relevant entries Amoebic infection; Infection and the nervous system: an overview; Naegleria.

■ **Acanthocytosis** – see Neuroacanthocytosis

■ **Accessory nerve palsy** – see Cranial nerve disease: XI: Accessory nerve

■ **Acephalgic migraine** – see Migraine

■ Aceruloplasminaemia

This rare, recessively inherited, disorder, in which ceruloplasmin is absent from the plasma, is clinically similar to Wilson's disease, with cerebellar ataxia, dementia, and involuntary movements, although copper metabolism is normal. Diabetes mellitus may also be present. Iron deposition in the basal ganglia is thought to be the cause. Similar cases from Japan with raised serum ferritin are also reported (ceruloplasmin deficiency with haemosiderosis).

References Logan JL, Harveyson KB, Wisdom GB, Hughes AE, Archbold GPR. Hereditary caeruloplasmin deficiency, dementia and diabetes mellitus. *Quarterly Journal of Medicine* 1994; **87**: 663–670.

Morita H, Ikeda S, Yamamoto K *et al*. Hereditary ceruloplasmin deficiency with hemosiderosis: a clinicopathological study of a Japanese family. *Annals of Neurology* 1995; **37**: 646–656.

Other relevant entries Menkes' disease; Wilson's disease.

■ **Acetylgalactosamine-4-sulphatase deficiency** – see Maroteaux–Lamy disease

■ **Acetylgalactosaminidase deficiency** – see Schindler's disease

■ **Acetylglucosamine phosphotransferase deficiency** – see I-cell disease

■ **Acetylglutamate synthetase deficiency** – see Urea cycle enzyme defects

■ **Acetylneuraminidase deficiency** – see Sialidosis

■ **Achalasia** – see Allgrove's syndrome; Gastrointestinal disease and the nervous system

▪ Achondroplasia
Chondrodystrophy

Pathophysiology Achondroplasia is the commonest form of bone dysplasia, inherited as an autosomal-dominant condition, with an incidence of 1 : 25 000. Failure of normal endochondral bone formation, as a consequence of mutations in the fibroblast growth factor 3 gene, results in diminished vertebral body height and short stature. Such changes may be exacerbated with age due to further flattening and wedging of vertebral bodies, disc prolapse and osteophyte formation. In 20–50% of cases there are neurological complications, including hydrocephalus, foramen magnum abnormalities with cervico-medullary compression, syringomyelia, and spinal canal stenosis with cord or root entrapment. Whilst their management is difficult, surgical decompression should be considered.

Clinical features: history and examination

- Short stature.
- Spinal cord/root compression: can be anywhere but typically in cervico-medullary region (causing progressive paraparesis or quadriparesis) or the cauda equina.
- Skull base compression may result in hydrocephalus, syringomyelia, +/− lower cranial nerve palsies, with myelopathy.
- Respiratory disturbances, including sleep apneoa syndrome.

Investigations and diagnosis *Bloods*: usually normal.

Imaging:

Plain radiography of the spine will demonstrate abnormal development: diminished vertebral body height, small neural arches with thick laminae and short, squat peduncles.

Skull X-rays: may show basilar impression (i.e. elevation in the floor of the posterior fossa).

CT/MRI of brain: may show primary basilar impression with hydrocephalus.

MRI of cord/myelogram: may show compressed spinal cord within a small spinal canal with nerve root entrapment or syringomyelia.

Neurophysiology:

EMG/NCS: often demonstrates degree of radiculopathy.

Somatosensory evoked potential (SSEP): may be useful in the early identification of brainstem and spinal abnormalities.

Neurogenetics: fibroblast growth factor 3 gene mutations.

Treatment and prognosis Surgery for cord or root compression is often difficult due to the extent of the stenosis but seems to be the most successful when done in young patients. However, in some cases decompression is ineffective and the stenosis continues to progress and is ultimately fatal.

> **References** Hamamci N, Hawran S, Biering-Sorensen F. Achondroplasia and spinal cord lesion. Three case reports. *Paraplegia* 1993; **31**: 375–379.
>
> Hecht JT, Butler IJ. Neurologic morbidity associated with achondroplasia. *Journal of Child Neurology* 1990; **5**: 84–97.

Ruiz-Garcia M, Tovar-Baudin A, del Castillo-Ruiz V *et al.* Early detection of neurological manifestations in achondroplasia. *Childs Nervous System* 1997; **13**: 208–213.

Other relevant entries Cauda equina syndrome and conus medullaris disease; Dwarfism; Foramen magnum lesions, Foramen magnum syndrome; Hydrocephalus; Paraparesis: acute management and differential diagnosis; Quadriplegia: an overview; Radiculopathies: an overview; Spinal stenosis; Syringomyelia and syringobulbia.

■ Achromatopsia
Colour blindness

Pathophysiology Achromatopsia is an impairment of colour perception. It is most commonly due to an inherited defect in the photopigments of the retinal cones, resulting in so-called colour blindness. This is an X-linked defect and is thus found principally in men, although occasional cases of inherited colour blindness are reported in women. Achromatopsia may also be seen in cases of optic neuropathy, and with cortical lesions in the occipitoparietal cortex, corresponding to the area described in primates as visual area V4. The standard bedside testing of colour vision uses pseudo-isochromatic (Ishihara) colour plates, which were originally devised for detecting congenital colour blindness. More precise techniques for detecting deficiencies in colour vision are available including the Holmgen wool-sorting test and the Farnsworth-Munsell 100-hue test.

Clinical features: history and examination The deficit in colour vision can be isolated or associated with other defects in visual processing.

- Congenital colour blindness

    Characteristically patients have difficulties distinguishing the red–green plates on testing with the Ishihara pseudo-isochromatic plates (Daltonism). They do not normally complain of any difficulty perceiving colours in their normal life and it is usually only detected because of a family history or on screening.

- Optic neuropathy

    Characteristic of acute optic nerve inflammation and following optic neuropathy. There is an impairment in colour perception which does not follow any particular pattern on the Ishihara plates. It is often the only deficit after an episode of optic neuritis. The loss of colour vision under such circumstances is felt to reflect the selective involvement of the P ganglion cells and visual pathway. Patients rarely complain of any clear loss of colour vision, although may comment that objects seem less brilliant in appearance. There may be an associated reduction in visual acuity in the affected eye.

- Cortical achromatopsia

    This may involve the whole, half, or a quadrant of the visual field. These patients often complain of defects in colour vision, and are severely impaired on both the

Holmgren wool-sorting test and the Farnsworth-Munsell 100-hue test. There are often other neurological deficits as cortical lesions are unlikely to respect the boundaries of area V4, the commonest accompanying feature being a visual field defect.

History taking should include a detailed family history.

Examination may require the following tests, although the latter two are usually administered by neuropsychologists:

Ishihara (pseudo-isochromatic) colour plate testing.

Holmgren wool-sorting test: the patient is required to name or match colours or arrange them in a series according to brightness or saturation.

Farnsworth-Munsell 100-hue test: the patient has to arrange a range of coloured counters in the correct order.

Investigations and diagnosis For congenital colour blindness, no further specific investigation is required.

If an optic neuropathy, optic neuritis or cortical lesion is the likely cause, then the following investigations may be required:

Imaging: MR optic nerve, brain for evidence of demyelination.
Neurophysiology: visual evoked response (VER), ERG.
CSF: if demyelination suspected.

Treatment and prognosis Dependent on cause:
Congenital colour blindness: no change and little disability.
Optic nerve: optic neuritis may recover in early stages, but if impairment is long standing, it is likely to be permanent; some optic neuropathies are progressive.
Cortical achromaptopsia: may improve, for example after cerebrovascular lesion, but it depends on the cause.

Reference Zeki S. A century of cerebral achromatopsia. *Brain* 1990; **113**: 1721–1777.

Other relevant entries Cerebrovascular disease: arterial; Cranial nerve disease: II: Optic nerve; Optic neuritis; Tumours: an overview.

■ Acid lipase deficiency – see Wolman's disease

■ Acid-maltase deficiency
Glycogenosis type II • Pompe's disease

Pathophysiology Acid-maltase deficiency (AMD) is an autosomal-recessive disorder of glycogen storage due to deficiency of the lysosomal enzyme acid α-glucosidase, or acid-maltase, in the central nervous system (CNS) and skeletal muscle. This enzyme does not contribute to the normal control of blood glucose levels, but deficiency leads to massive accumulation of glycogen within lysosomes, with subsequent cell damage and death. The clinical phenotype is variable, with age of onset ranging from infancy to adulthood. More than 50 mutations in the acid α-glucosidase gene on chromosome 17 have been identified; gene deletions lead to more severe disease. There is no curative treatment but supportive therapy can be helpful.

Clinical features: history and examination

- Infantile (Pompe's disease)

    Profound weakness and hypotonia +/− muscle firmness ("woody texture"); paucity of movement; frog-leg posture, normal social interaction.

    Loss of deep tendon reflexes.

    Heart failure due to cardiomyopathy, with cardiomegaly.

    +/− hepatosplenomegaly; macroglossia.

- Late infantile/juvenile (Smith's disease)

    Motor delay

    Progressive myopathy

    +/− organomegaly.

- Adult: (Engel's disease): two peaks, in third to fourth and sixth to seventh decades.

    Progressive myopathy, usually of the legs.

    Respiratory insufficiency may be presenting feature (type II respiratory failure), due to early involvement of respiratory muscles; cardiomyopathy much less prominent than in infantile disease.

    +/− cranial nerve involvement (e.g. bulbar); macroglossia; distal limb involvement.

Investigations and diagnosis *Bloods*: creatine kinase may be raised (usually only modest elevation, approximately three to four times normal) especially in infantile and juvenile forms, but may be normal in adult-onset disease. Acid α-glucosidase levels may be measured in the blood leukocytes, fibroblasts or muscle. Normal leukocyte levels with reduced values in muscle may occur.

Imaging: CXR in infantile/juvenile forms may show globular cardiomegaly.

Neurophysiology: EMG: usually compatible with a myopathy, but variable. Myotonic discharges and neurogenic changes (fibrillations) may be found. Important to examine paraspinal muscles.

Muscle biopsy: characteristically shows increased glycogen within lysosomes and vacuolar change. Increased acid phosphatase may be seen especially in small fibres. Crystalloid inclusions may be seen in mitochondria. Acid α-glucosidase level may be assayed in muscle tissue.

ECG: in juvenile forms shows biventricular hypertrophy, short PR interval and high-amplitude QRS complexes. ECG may also be abnormal in adult-onset disease.

CSF: normal.

Differential diagnosis Juvenile disease may be confused with Duchenne muscular dystrophy. Adult disease may be confused with inflammatory myopathy or limb-girdle muscular dystrophies.

Treatment and prognosis In infantile (Pompe's) disease, progression is relentless with death usually by the age of 2 years. Likewise, in the juvenile form, the disease is fatal within a few months of onset of heart failure.

In the adult disease, prognosis depends on the degree of respiratory involvement. Ventilatory aids such as nocturnal intermittent positive-pressure ventilation may be used to support these patients.

Enzyme replacement therapy remains a hope for the future. There are some reports that the use of high protein, low carbohydrate diets are beneficial in slowing the rate of progression of the disease.

Some reports suggest an increased incidence of cerebral aneurysms in this condition, but the role of screening for these is not defined.

References Felice KJ, Alessi AG, Grunnet AL. Clinical variability in adult-onset acid maltase deficiency: report of affected sibs and a review of the literature. *Medicine (Baltimore)* 1995; **74**: 131–135.

Trend PStJ, Wiles CM, Spencer GT, Morgan Hughes J, Lake BD, Patrick AD. Acid maltase deficiency in adults. *Brain* 1985; **108**: 845–860.

Other relevant entries Duchenne muscular dystrophy; Glycogen-storage disorders: an overview; Lysosomal-storage disorders: an overview; Myopathy: an overview; Respiratory failure.

▣ Acoustic neurinoma, acoustic neuroma – see Vestibular Schwannoma

▣ Acquired immunodeficiency syndrome – see HIV/AIDS and the nervous system

▣ Acrocephalopolysyndactyly – see Acrocephalosyndactyly; Carpenter syndrome

▣ Acrocephalosyndactyly

A number of syndromes, dominantly inherited, are characterized by acrocephalosyndactyly, the combination of tower skull and fusion of digits:

Types I and II: Apert's syndrome
Type III: Saethre–Chotzen syndrome
Type IV: Waardenburg syndrome
Type V: Pfeiffer syndrome.

There is overlap with syndromes classified as acrocephalopolysyndactyly, such as Carpenter syndrome.

> **Other relevant entries** Apert's syndrome; Carpenter syndrome; Craniostenosis; Pfeiffer syndrome; Saethre–Chotzen syndrome; Waardenburg syndrome.

■ Acromegaly

Excessive pituitary gland secretion of growth hormone in adults results in acromegaly (*cf.* gigantism in children). This is a cause of secondary diabetes mellitus, so untreated acromegalics are at risk of all the potential neurological complications of diabetes as well as pituitary tumours. In addition, recognized neurological features of acromegaly include:

- proximal myopathy (acromegalic myopathy);
- thickening of the peripheral nerves +/− peripheral neuropathy (distal paraesthesia, weakness, and areflexia, i.e. slowed nerve conduction velocities);
- carpal tunnel syndrome;
- central sleep apnoea syndrome.

The myopathy may be accompanied by a raised creatine kinase, with myopathic features on EMG and muscle biopsy, with variation in fibre size, type 2 fibre atrophy, and non-specific increase in glycogen and lipofuscin on electon microscopy.

> **References** Khaleeli AA, Levy RD, Edwards RH *et al.* The neuromuscular features of acromegaly: a clinical and pathological study. *Journal of Neurology, Neurosurgery and Psychiatry* 1984; **47**: 1009–1015.
>
> Low PA, McLeod JG, Turtle JR *et al.* Peripheral neuropathy in acromegaly. *Brain* 1974; **97**: 137–152.
>
> Mastaglia FL, Barwick DD, Hall R. Myopathy in acromegaly. *Lancet* 1970; **2**: 907–909.
>
> **Other relevant entries** Carpal tunnel syndrome; Diabetes mellitus and the nervous system; Endocrinology and the nervous system; Gigantism; Myopathy: an overview; Neuropathies: an overview; Pituitary disease; Sleep apnoea syndromes.

■ Actinomycosis

Actinomycosis is caused by various Gram-positive anaerobic or microaerophilic rods (filamentous bacteria) of the genus *Actinomyces*. The commonest clinical manifestation is "lumpy jaw", cervicofacial abscess formation. These may spread to the brain by direct extension or haematogenous spread to cause cerebral abscess(es) and/or acute or chronic non-specific meningitis. Organisms are seldom identified from the CSF, but culture from extraneural sites may be possible. Yellow exudates from cutaneous abscesses contain "sulphur granules". Actinomycosis resembles nocardiosis, although it may occur in immunocompetent patients.

> **Other relevant entries** Abscess: an overview; Meningitis: an overview; Nocardiosis.

▪ Acute confusional state – see Delirium

▪ Acute disseminated encephalomyelitis
Acute haemorrhagic leukoencephalitis • Acute necrotizing haemor-
rhagic encephalomyelitis • Acute post-infectious encephalomyelitis
(APEM) • Hurst's disease

Pathophysiology Acute disseminated encephalomyelitis (ADEM) is a monophasic
illness characterized by a meningitic and encephalomyelitic syndrome, usually
following an infective illness or vaccination, with evidence of widespread
demyelination within the central nervous system (CNS). In its less fulminant form it
may be difficult to distinguish from the first episode of multiple sclerosis (MS): since
abnormalities in CSF, evoked potentials and MRI are similar in both conditions,
continued follow-up may be the only way to make the distinction. ADEM typically
occurs in children and young adults, is uncommon, and has a significant morbidity
and mortality. Treatment with high-dose parenteral steroids is often tried, but is of
unproven benefit.

Clinical features: history and examination ADEM is a clinical syndrome: there are
currently no accepted diagnostic criteria.

Preceding infection: measles, rubella, chickenpox; rarely mumps, influenza,
Mycoplasma pneumoniae.

Preceding vaccination: rabies, smallpox, rarely tetanus antitoxin.

Prodromal phase: fever, malaise, myalgia.

Rapid onset (hours, days) of:

- Encephalopathy: ranging from confusion and somnolence to fits, stupor
  and coma.
- Transverse myelitis: with varying degrees of bladder and bowel
  involvement.
- Focal or multifocal signs and symptoms: for example hemiparesis, optic neuritis
  (often bilateral), ataxia, myoclonus, and choreoathetosis.
- Meningism: with headache, fever, and neck stiffness.

Investigations and diagnosis *Bloods*: usually unhelpful, but leukocytosis is not
uncommon especially in cases of acute necrotizing haemorrhagic encephalomyelitis,
when there is also an elevated ESR.

Imaging: MRI demonstrates multifocal white matter lesions that are often more
symmetric in their distribution, than those found in MS. As with MS the lesions
enhance and persist, but in contrast with MS no new lesions develop beyond the
time the disease typically evolves, which rarely extends beyond 2 weeks. Hence
interval scanning may help differentiate ADEM from MS.

CSF: usually increased protein and cells (lymphocytes) with a normal glucose
concentration. This is most florid with the acute necrotizing haemorrhagic

encephalomyelitis variant when there may be associated red blood cells in the CSF. Oligoclonal bands may be found, but usually do not persist; persistent oligoclonal bands are more suggestive of MS.

Neurophysiology: evoked potentials and EEG may be abnormal depending on extent and distribution of lesions.

Pathology: rarely available. Perivascular inflammation with lymphocytes and mononuclear cells may be seen, with oedema and microglial activation, and disseminated foci of demyelination throughout the brain and spinal cord centred on small- and medium-sized veins (peripheral nervous system spared). In its most severe form (acute haemorrhagic leukoencephalitis, Hurst's disease) there is necrosis of small blood vessels and brain tissue around the vessels; these lesions may coalesce and lead to almost complete haemorrhagic necrosis of whole hemispheres.

Differential diagnosis The major differential diagnosis is between ADEM and the first episode of MS. Other conditions that may enter the differential diagnosis include:

multiple emboli;
viral encephalitis;
granulomatous disease (e.g. sarcoidosis);
vasculitis.

Treatment and prognosis 10–30% mortality rate; in the fulminant haemorrhagic form death may occur in a few days.

50% make a complete recovery.

Recovery usually begins within weeks.

Recurrence may occur: multiphasic disseminated encephalomyelitis (MDEM).

No treatment has been critically evaluated in ADEM, but there is some anecdotal evidence of benefit with intravenous methylprednisolone, intravenous immuno-globulin and plasmapharesis.

The development of more purified vaccines has greatly reduced the incidence of ADEM as a post-vaccinial disorder.

Rate of reclassification of ADEM as MS varies but a recent large retrospective survey found 35% of affected adults were reclassified as MS in 1 year.

References Dale RC, de Sousa C, Chong WK, Cox TCS, Harding B, Neville BGR. Acute disseminated encephalomyelitis, multiphasic disseminated encephalomyelitis and multiple sclerosis in children. *Brain* 2000; **123**: 2407–2422.

Höllinger P, Sturzenegger M, Mathis J, Schroth G, Hess CW. Acute disseminated encephalomyelitis in adults: a reappraisal of clinical, CSF, EEG, and MRI findings. *Journal of Neurology* 2002; **249**: 320–329.

Hynson JL, Kornberg AJ, Coleman LT, Shield L, Harvey AS, Kean MJ. Clinical and neuroradiologic features of acute disseminated encephalomyelitis in children. *Neurology* 2001; **56**: 1308–1312.

John L, Khaleeli AA, Larner AJ. Acute disseminated encephalomyelitis: a riddle wrapped in a mystery inside an enigma. *International Journal of Clinical Practice* 2003; **57**: 235–237.

Kesselring J, Miller DH, Robb SA *et al*. Acute disseminated encephalomyelitis. MRI findings and the distinction from multiple sclerosis. *Brain* 1990; **113**: 291–302.

Schwarz S, Mohr A, Knauth M, Wildemann B, Storch-Hagenlocher B. Acute disseminated encephalomyelitis: a follow-up study of 40 adult patients. *Neurology* 2001; **56**: 1313–1318.

Other relevant entries Clinically isolated syndromes; Demyelinating diseases of the nervous system: an overview; Encephalitis: an overview; Encephalomyelitis: differential diagnosis; Immunosuppressive therapy and diseases of the nervous system, Multiple sclerosis; Sarcoidosis; Vasculitis.

■ Acute idiopathic/inflammatory demyelinating polyneuropathy – see Guillain–Barré syndrome

■ Acute intermittent pophyria – see Porphyria

■ Acute mountain sickness – see Altitude sickness

■ Acute neuropathies – see Neuropathies: an overview

■ Acyl-CoA dehydrogenase deficiency – see Fatty acid oxidation disorders

■ ADCA – see Autosomal-dominant cerebellar ataxia

■ Addison's disease – see Adrenoleukodystrophy; Endocrinology and the nervous system

■ ADEM – see Acute disseminated encephalomyelitis

■ Adhalinopathy – see Sarcoglycanopathy

■ Adie's syndrome, Adie's tonic pupil – see Holmes–Adie syndrome

■ Adiposogenital dystrophy – see Froehlich's syndrome

■ Adrenoleukodystrophy

Adrenomyeloneuropathy • Siemerling–Creutzfeldt disease

Pathophysiology Adrenoleukodystrophy (ALD), the commonest of the peroxisomal disorders, is an X-linked-recessive condition that has a variable clinical phenotype, even within families. The spectrum of disease varies from an aggressive cerebral form of progressive demyelination with deafness, blindness, dementia, spasticity, as well as adrenal insufficiency, to an adult presentation (including carrier females) with a spastic paraparesis and a mild distal polyneuropathy, termed adrenomyeloneuropathy (AMN). X-linked ALD (X-ALD) is due to mutations in a gene encoding a peroxisomal membrane protein ("ALD protein") that belongs to the ATP-binding-cassette (ABC) protein family. This leads to accumulation of very long-chain fatty acids (VLCFA) that characterizes the disease. Dietary treatment with Lorenzo's oil has been tried but with uncertain clinical benefit.

Clinical features: history and examination Heterogeneity of expression is very common in X-ALD, including within families. It affects approximately 1 : 25 000 males.

- Childhood cerebral presentation: age of onset <10 years.

  Progressive personality change and intellectual decline leading to dementia.

  Gait abnormalities that evolve into a spastic quadriparesis.

  At a later stage, hearing and visual impairments develop leading to deafness and blindness.

  Seizures rare.

  Adrenal insufficiency (hypotension, skin pigmentation) is found in >90% of cases but to varying degrees, some clinically overt, some biochemical only. In 70–80% of cases the neurological deficits precede the adrenal insufficiency.

  Pathology is more inflammatory than in other varieties.

- Adolescent cerebral presentation: 10–21 years.

  As for childhood presentation but with a slower or "stuttering" onset. Motor involvement and cortical blindness may be absent.

- AMN: age 28 ± 9 years.

  Progressive spastic paraparesis.

  Mild distal polyneuropathy.

  Adrenal insufficiency.

  Hypogonadism.

  Perhaps 45% develop later cerebral involvement: Psychiatric disturbances, typically schizophreniform psychosis.

  Dementia: late, slowly progressive.

- Adult cerebral: age >21 years.

  Rapidly progressive cerebral disease, as in childhood form, without preceding AMN; dementia may be presenting feature (rare).

- Addison's disease only; no neurological features.

- Asymptomatic: genetic abnormality only, without endocrine or neurological features.

- Female heterozygotes:

    20% have an AMN-like illness of variable severity (mild spastic paraparesis to wheelchair bound); 1–3% develop dementia, behavioural disturbance, or visual failure; 1% develop adrenal failure.

- Neonatal adrenoleukodystrophy:

    Presents at birth, with a mean survival of 3 years. It is distinct from other forms of ALD.

    Profound hypotonia.

    Seizures.

    Abnormal neonatal reflexes.

    During first year there is growth failure with developmental delay, ataxia, spasticity, peripheral neuropathy, deafness, and visual loss.

    No specific dysmorphism (*cf.* Zellweger syndrome); clinical evidence of adrenal insufficiency is rare.

    Occasional hepatic fibrosis without cirrhosis and normal kidneys.

Investigations and diagnosis *Bloods*: Electrolytes, adrenocorticotropin hormone (ACTH) and cortisol: may demonstrate adrenal insufficiency. VLCFAs are raised in serum, white cells or cultured fibroblasts (in particular the C26 to C22 ratio).

Neurogenetics: mutations in an ABC transporter gene; over 500 described.

Imaging: brain CT/MRI shows extensive white matter demyelination, predominantly parieto-occipital, with incomplete sparing of U-fibres; contrast enhancement at the advancing margin of demyelination is characteristic. May be predominantly posterior or anterior in distribution. MR spectroscopy shows reduced N-acetyl aspartate, increased choline.

CSF: variable abnormalities, with occasional raised protein and increased cell counts.

Neurophysiology:

EMG/NCS: demyelinating neuropathy.

Evoked potentials may be abnormal.

Neuropsychology: frontal pattern of deficits may be found; Balint syndrome has also been described.

Tissue: electron microscopy of macrophages in peripheral nerve, conjunctiva, or skin shows trilaminar bodies 7×10 nm (not specific for ALD). In the brain, there is demyelination of central white matter, degeneration of corticospinal tracts and dorsal spinocerebellar tracts.

Differential diagnosis Other leukodystrophies, especially metachromatic leukodystrophy in adults. In adults, other conditions to consider include:

    hereditary spastic paraparesis,

    subacute combined degeneration of the cord,

    multiple sclerosis,

    chronic inflammatory demyelinating polyneuropathy (CIDP) with central demyelination.

Treatment and prognosis Adrenal replacement therapy for adrenal insufficiency.

Symptomatic treatments of spasticity.

Treatment of ALD *per se*:

- Dietary: Lorenzo's oil (a mixture of glycerol trioleate acid and trierucic acid in 4 : 1 ratio) normalizes plasma VLCFA but produces no change in the brain levels or clinical improvement.
- Bone marrow transplantation: of no use in rapidly advancing disease, but may have a place in early disease to arrest, stabilize and maybe even reverse early cerebral disease as measured by MRI and neuropsychology; no current indication in asymptomatic patients.
- Immunosuppressive therapy.
- Gene therapy.

Nearly two-thirds of ALD patients escape the most severe phenotype.

References Dubois-Dalcq M, Feigenbaum V, Aubourg P. The neurobiology of X-linked adrenoleukodystrophy, a demyelinating peroxisomal disorder. *Trends in Neurosciences* 1999; **22**: 4–12.

Larner AJ. Adult-onset dementia with prominent frontal lobe dysfunction in X-linked adrenoleukodystrophy with R152C mutation in ABCD1 gene. *Journal of Neurology* 2003; **250**: 1253–1254.

Moser H. Adrenoleukodystrophy: phenotype, genetics, pathogenesis and therapy. *Brain* 1997; **120**: 1485–1508.

Van Geel BM, Assies J, Wanders RJA, Barth PG. X linked adrenoleukodystrophy: clinical presentation, diagnosis and therapy. *Journal of Neurology, Neurosurgery and Psychiatry* 1997; **63**: 4–14.

Other relevant entries Alexander's disease; Chronic inflammatory demyelinating polyneuropathy; Endocrinology and the nervous system; Hereditary spastic paraparesis; Leukodystrophies: an overview; Metachromatic leukodystrophy; Peroxisomal disorders: an overview; Vitamin B$_{12}$ deficiency; Zellweger syndrome.

■ Adrenomyeloneuropathy – see Adrenoleukodystrophy

■ Agenesis of the corpus callosum

Agenesis of the corpus callosum may occur in isolation, when it may be asymptomatic, or it may occur as a feature in a variety of syndromes including:

Neonatal adrenoleukodystrophy

Aicardi syndrome

Andermann's syndrome

Apert syndrome

Fetal alcohol syndrome

Glutaric aciduria type II

Holoprosencephaly: alobar and semilobar variants

Hurler's syndrome
Leigh's syndrome
Menkes' disease
Naevoid basal cell carcinoma syndrome
Non-ketotic hyperglycinaemia
Pyruvate dehydrogenase (PDH) deficiency
Shapiro syndrome
Trisomies: 8, 11, 13
Zellweger syndrome.

References Aicardi J, Chevrie J-J, Baraton J. Agenesis of the corpus callosum. In: Vinken PJ, Bruyn GW, Klawans HL, Myrianthopoulos NC (eds). *Handbook of Clinical Neurology, Vol. 6 (50): Malformations.* Amsterdam: Elsevier, 1987: 149–173.

Kolodny EH. Agenesis of the corpus callosum: a marker for inherited metabolic disease? *Neurology* 1989; **39**: 847–848.

Other relevant entries See individual entries, including Andermann's syndrome (1).

■ Agnosia

Pathophysiology Agnosia is an acquired failure to recognize or identify stimuli despite ostensibly intact primary sensory functions, intellect and language.

Two kinds of agnosia have been described:
- Apperceptive: a defect of complex (higher order) perceptual processes.
- Associative: intact perception with a defect in giving meaning to the percept: "perception without knowledge".

Clinical features: history and examination Agnosias can occur in any sensory modality; examples include:
- Visual agnosia, and more circumscribed forms such as prosopagnosia (*q.v.*); colour agnosia, a loss of colour knowledge despite intact perception (*cf.* achromatopsia); pure word alexia may also be an agnosic phenomenon.
- Auditory agnosia: inability to recognize either speech or environmental sounds (*cf.* pure word deafness).
- Tactile agnosia: inability to recognize an object by touch, despite being able to describe its feel and shape (*cf.* astereognosis).
- Anosognosia: failure to appreciate the severity of a clinical deficit (e.g. hemiplegia, hemianopia, cortical blindness (Anton's syndrome), cognitive decline).
- Asomatognosia: denial of ownership of a body part (e.g. paretic limb).
- Finger agnosia; inability to identify which finger is touched by an examiner; one component of Gerstmann syndrome, although it may occur in isolation.

Investigations and diagnosis Anatomically, agnosias generally reflect dysfunction at the level of the association (especially posterior parietal) cortex, although they can on occasion result from thalamic pathology. Some may be of localizing value.

Differential diagnosis

Anomias.

Colour agnosia may be confuded with achromatopsia or colour anomia.

Treatment and prognosis No specific treatment known; treatment of underlying pathological process where possible.

References Bauer RM, Demery JA. Agnosia. In: Heilman KM, Valenstein E (eds). *Clinical Neuropsychology* (4th edition). Oxford: OUP, 2003: 236–295.

Farah MJ. *Visual Agnosia: Disorders of Object Recognition and What They Tell Us about Normal Vision*. Cambridge: MIT Press, 1995.

Other relevant entries Achromatopsia; Alexia; Anton's syndrome; Capgras syndrome; Gerstmann syndrome; Landau–Kleffner syndrome; Prosopagnosia.

■ Agraphia

Agraphia or dysgraphia refers to a loss of the ability to write, spontaneously or to dictation. This often occurs in the context of other language problems (aphasia, alexia) with a dominant hemisphere frontoparietal lesion (usually vascular), but also as a consequence of neglect or motor weakness. Pure or isolated agraphia is rare.

Agraphias may be classified neurologically as:

- Pure agraphia: neither alexia nor aphasia present.
- Aphasic agraphia: accompanying an aphasia syndrome.
- Agraphia with alexia ("parietal agraphia").
- Apraxic agraphia: difficulty forming letters and words.
- Spatial agraphia: abnormal placement of letters on page, may be explicable by neglect.

Testing for agraphia requires analysis of both linguistic and motor components, best done by evaluating spontaneous writing, writing to dictation (single words, phrases), and copying (nonsense figures, letters, words, sentences).

Reference Roeltgen DP. Agraphia. In: Heilman KM, Valenstein E (eds). *Clinical Neuropsychology* (4th edition). Oxford: OUP, 2003: 126–145.

Other relevant entries Alexia; Alzheimer's disease; Aphasia; Cerebrovascular disease: arterial; Disconnection syndromes; Tumours: an overview.

■ Agrypnia – see Insomnia; Morvan's syndrome

■ Agyria–pachygyria – see Lissencephaly

■ Aicardi's syndrome

Aicardi's syndrome, first described in 1965, is characterized by chorioretinopathy with retinal lacunae, mental retardation, myoclonic epilepsy, vertebral anomalies, and with imaging evidence of agenesis of the corpus callosum. MRI may also show cortical dysplasia with polymicrogyria, and a "bat-wing" deformity of the third and lateral ventricles. EEG shows a typical asymmetric and asynchronous burst-suppression pattern. The syndrome occurs almost exclusively in females and is thought to be an X-linked-dominant syndrome, linked to a locus at Xp22.

Reference Aicardi J, Lefebvre J, Lerique-Koechlin A. A new syndrome: spasms in flexion, callosal agenesis, ocular abnormalities. *Electroencephalography and Clinical Neurophysiology* 1965; **19**: 609–610.

Other relevant entry Agenesis of the corpus callosum.

■ Aicardi–Goutières syndrome

Aicardi–Goutières syndrome, first described in 1984, is an autosomal-recessive disorder presenting in the first weeks of life and characterized by leukodystrophy with calcification of the basal ganglia and CSF lymphocytosis. Decerebration and death ensue within a few years. The differential diagnosis encompasses other leukodystrophies.

Reference Aicardi J, Goutières F. A progressive familial encephalopathy in infancy with calcifications of the basal ganglia and chronic cerebrospinal fluid lymphocytosis. *Annals of Neurology* 1984; **15**: 49–54.

Other relevant entries Basal ganglia calcification; Leukodystrophies: an overview.

■ AIDS – see HIV/AIDS and the nervous system

■ Akathisia

Pathophysiology Akathisia refers to a sense of restlessness and the feeling of a need to move. Once it had been accepted as a true neurological (rather than psychiatric) condition, it was described in association with idiopathic and postencephalitic parkinsonism, but is now most commonly seen as a side-effect of the major tranquilizing drugs. The movements of akathisia are very variable but often consist of repetitive hand rubbing, crossing and uncrossing of the arms, rocking movements, and marching or pacing about. It can occasionally involve vocalizations. It is distinct from restless leg syndrome in which sensory symptoms are present in the legs at rest and relieved by movement.

Akathisia may be caused by or associated with:

- Drugs
    Acute or delayed complication of neuroleptic treatment.
    Other psychoactive medications including paroxetine.
    Other agents including metoclopramide.
- Idiopathic or postencephalitic parkinsonism
- Unknown pathogenesis: possibly abnormal dopaminergic/catecholaminergic interactions in the striatum +/− spinal cord.

Clinical features: history and examination This is a clinical diagnosis. It is important to exclude other causes of similar symptoms, such as neuropathy, and metabolic causes such as uraemia.

Unpleasant feeling of restlessness in the legs, usually most severe in the calves, and only rarely affecting the arms. Movement (which may be bizarre and complex) often relieves the symptoms temporarily. The severity of akathisia is increased by stress, age and fatigue.

About a third of patients are reported to have periodic leg movements during sleep also, although some may be misdiagnosed cases of restless legs syndrome.

There are often secondary complications such as poor drug compliance and suicidal ideation or behaviour.

Investigations and diagnosis *Bloods*: usually normal, but must exclude diabetes, hepatic failure, uraemia, and anaemia.

Imaging: brain and spinal cord MRI is usually normal.

CSF: usually normal.

Neurophysiology: NCS/EMG usually normal.

Differential diagnosis
Restless legs syndrome.
Tardive dyskinesia.

Treatment and prognosis If possible, the offending drug should be stopped, or the dose lowered, or changed to an alternative medication.

Other agents worth trying for symptomatic relief are:

β-blockers (e.g. propanolol),
anticholinergics,
clonidine,
benzodiazepines.

Other agents that have been tried include opiates, amantadine, buspirone, piracetam, amitriptyline, and dopamine depleters.

References Blaisdell GD. Akathisia: a comprehensive review and treatment summary. *Pharmacopsychiatry* 1994; **27**: 139–146.

Sachdev P. *Akathisia and Restless Legs*. Cambridge: CUP, 1995.

Stacy M, Cardoso F, Jankovic J. Tardive stereotypy and other movement disorders in tardive dyskinesia. *Neurology* 1993; **43**: 937–941.

Other relevant entries Drug-induced movement disorders; Parkinsonian syndromes, parkinsonism; Parkinson's disease; Restless legs syndrome.

■ Albers–Schönberg disease
Osteopetrosis

A condition characterized by increased bone density throughout the skeleton which may occasionally lead to cranial nerve palsies or hydrocephalus.

Other relevant entries Cranial polyneuropathy; Hydrocephalus.

◼ Albinism

Albinism is a genetically determined abnormality of melanin synthesis which may be:
- Ocular: affecting the eyes only.
- Oculocutaneous: affecting skin and eyes.

The ocular features include:

Impaired visual acuity

Nystagmus

Fundus may be blond or totally devoid of pigment.

Albinism may be one feature of the Chédiak–Higashi syndrome (*q.v.*) and of the Hermansky–Pudlak syndrome (albinism with a haemorrhagic diathesis).

Other relevant entries Chédiak–Higashi syndrome; Nystagmus: an overview.

◼ Alcohol and the nervous system: an overview

Pathophysiology Alcohol can have many effects on the central and peripheral nervous system. The pleasurable short-term effects are familiar to most people. However adverse effects of alcohol consumption are common and may be classified as acute or chronic in nature. This distinction relates to the amount and the period of time over which alcohol has been consumed. Many of the chronic complications of alcoholism are due to a combination of the toxic effects of alcohol coupled with the nutritional deficiencies commonly coexisting with excessive alcohol consumption, along with some as yet unidentified genetic predisposition.

Alcohol does not act at specific receptors but does appear to stimulate selectively chloride ion flux through the GABA/barbiturate/benzodiazepine receptor, with a particular anatomical preference for the brainstem.

Damage to the nervous system may possibly result from:
- Direct toxic effects.
- Oxidation to glutaraldehyde.
- Non-oxidative metabolism to fatty acid ethyl esters.
- Malnutrition.

Alcohol-induced pathology differs in different sites:
- Muscle: muscle-fibre damage and myopathy, including an acute necrotizing myopathy after an alcoholic binge.
- Peripheral nerve/optic nerve: axonal loss (peripheral neuropathy; optic atrophy).
- Cerebellum: Purkinje cell loss especially in anterior/superior vermis.
- Cerebral hemispheres: cortical atrophy and possibly cholinergic deafferentation of cortex.
- Brainstem: symmetrical pallor and haemorrhage around the third/fourth ventricles, aqueduct and in the mammillary bodies and medial thalamus (Wernicke–Korsakoff's syndrome, WKS).

Clinical features: history and examination Not everyone who consumes excessive quantities of alcohol develops neurological complications. It is unclear why only certain individuals do, and why they should develop some of the neurological complications but not others.

- Alcohol intoxication

  Dependent on the plasma level of alcohol, although chronic consumption of alcohol leads to tolerance:

  >5.4 mmol/l; mild intoxication: altered mood (usually excitement); impaired cognition and incoordination.

  >21.7 mmol/l; vestibular and cerebellar signs, autonomic dysfunction with hypotension and hypothermia, stupor and eventually coma as the plasma level rises.

  >108.5 mmol/l; usually results in death from respiratory depression.

  In addition, heavy alcohol consumption over short periods of time may result in episodes of amnesia which cannot be accounted for by either a global depression of consciousness or coincident disorders, such as epileptic seizures.

- Alcohol withdrawal state

  Nausea, vomiting, perceptual difficulties, tremor, visual hallucinations, fits, delirium tremens (DTs). This latter condition is a severe confusional state that is usually seen within the first 4 days of stopping drinking alcohol, and usually lasts for 1–3 days. It consists of profound agitation with insomnia, visual hallucinations and delusions, tremor and autonomic hyperactivity. There may be associated hypophosphataemia.

- Nutritional deficiencies of the nervous system secondary to alcoholism

  Wernicke's acute encephalopathy with (or without) ophthalmoplegia and ataxia precedes a chronic Korsakoff's syndrome which is characterized by a profound anterograde and retrograde memory deficit which may (or, more often, may not) be associated with confabulation.

  Pellagra.

  Peripheral neuropathy: a painful axonal sensorimotor polyneuropathy.

  Optic neuropathy (so-called "tobacco–alcohol amblyopia"): often occurs in association with heavy smoking. It presents with a painless bilateral visual loss that develops over weeks.

- Conditions of uncertain pathogenesis associated with excessive alcohol consumption

  Cerebellar degeneration: M > F, usually in association with peripheral neuropathy. It predominantly involves the rostral vermis, developing over weeks to years, and typically presents with walking difficulties secondary to truncal ataxia. Nystagmus, dysarthria and intention tremor are uncommon. There may be some recovery on stopping the alcohol.

  Marchiafava–Bignami syndrome: characterized by stupor, coma, fits, dementia, and emotional lability. Pathologically there is demyelination, predominantly of the corpus callosum. Said to affect predominantly drinkers of Italian Chianti, M > F.

A

Central pontine myelinolysis (CPM): often associated with rapid electrolyte changes associated with alcoholic liver disease. It typically presents with a rapidly progressive flaccid quadraparesis with brainstem signs and bulbar failure. It can also afford areas outside the brainstem, so-called extrapontine myelinolysis.

Alcoholic myopathy and cardiomyopathy.

Alcoholic dementia (the differential diagnosis of cognitive decline in alcoholic patients includes traumatic subdural haematomas, which must be excluded, since potentially reversible).

Cerebral atrophy.

- Fetal alcohol syndrome (FAS; *q.v.*)

Occurs in ~6% of alcoholic females. There is aberrant fetal neuronal and glial migration with cerebellar dysplasia. Affected babies are microcephalic and have pre- and post-natal growth retardation, facial dysmorphology, neurological deficits, and other systemic abnormalities.

- Neurological disorders associated with alcoholic liver disease

Hepatic encephalopathy.

Chronic hepatocerebral degeneration, or "non-Wilsonian hepatocerebral degeneration".

- Neurological disorders responsive to alcohol

Essential tremor.

Alcohol-responsive dystonia (or myoclonic dystonia sensitive to alcohol): autosomal dominant, starts early in life with combination of dystonia and myoclonic jerks; alcohol in small amounts affects dystonia to some extent but has a dramatic effect on the myoclonic jerks.

Investigations and diagnosis See individual entries

Treatment and prognosis Specific treatment depends on the particular syndrome, but general recommendations include:

Stop alcohol consumption in the context of an alcohol detoxification programme.

Treat with high-dose thiamine, initially intravenously then orally.

Replace any other vitamin deficiencies, normalize any electrolyte abnormalities (e.g. hyponatraemia, hypophosphataemia) slowly.

Check for any other treatable conditions (e.g. subdural haematoma).

References Adams RD, Victor M, Ropper AH. *Principles of Neurology* (6th edition). New York: McGraw-Hill, 1997: 1166–1185.

Charness ME, Simon RP, Greenberg DA. Ethanol and the nervous system. *New England Journal of Medicine* 1989; **321**: 442–454.

Messing RO, Greenberg DA. Alcohol and the nervous system. In: Aminoff MJ (ed.). *Neurology and General Medicine. The Neurological Aspects of Medical Disorders* (2nd edition). New York: Churchill Livingstone, 1995: 615–629.

Other relevant entries Amnesia, Amnesic syndrome; Ataxia; Central pontine myelinolysis; Cerebellar disease: an overview; Dementia: an overview; Drug-induced encephalopathies; Drug-induced myopathies; Epilepsy: an overview;

Fetal alcohol syndrome; Liver disease and the nervous system; Marchiafava–Bignami syndrome; Myopathy: an overview; Neuropathies: an overview; Pellagra; Wernicke–Korsakoff's syndrome.

■ Alexander's disease

Pathophysiology This rare disorder, classified as a leukodystrophy, was first described in 1949 by Alexander in a child with megalencephaly, progressive neurological deterioration and pathological findings of diffuse Rosenthal fibre formation. The condition has very rarely been described in adults. It is progressive and incurable, and the underlying metabolic defect is not known. Recently, dominant mutations in the gene encoding glial fibrillary acidic protein (GFAP) on chromosome 17 have been associated with the condition. The pathological focus is in the white matter, with demyelination and morphological abnormalities in astrocytes. The pathological hallmark is the diffuse accumulation of Rosenthal fibres. These represent a gliotic reaction in which astrocytes appear to have been converted into hyalinized eosinophilic bodies. Whilst not unique to Alexander's disease, Rosenthal fibres are characteristic of it, especially in the subependymal, subpial, and perivascular regions, more so in frontal white matter areas than occipitally. The later the onset of disease the less severe the demyelination.

Clinical features: history and examination

- Infantile group: from birth to early childhood
    - Psychomotor retardation with failure to thrive
    - Epileptic fits
    - Quadriparesis
    - Megalencephaly: progressive head enlargement is a major (but not consistent) feature.
- Juvenile group: age 7–14 years
    - Progressive bulbar/pseudobulbar symptoms
    - Spasticity
    - Epileptic fits and cognitive decline are less common.
- Adult group: age 20–60
    - Similar to juvenile group
    - Occasionally present with a course resembling multiple sclerosis
    - Occasionally asymptomatic.

Investigations and diagnosis *Bloods*: all normal

Imaging: CT and MRI show extensive white matter demyelination; large head in infants, may also have evidence of hydrocephalus.

CSF: usually normal; non-specific protein elevation.

Neurophysiology: EEG may show some epileptiform features; other tests are normal.

Brain biopsy: diagnosis ultimately rests on pathological appearances.

Neurogenetics: mutations in the gene encoding GFAP.

Differential diagnosis Other leukodystrophies, especially Canavan's disease.

Enlarged head:

Hydrocephalus (in juvenile cases)
Canavan's disease
Glutaric aciduria type I
Gangliosidoses
Metachromatic leukodystrophy
L-2-hydroxyglutaric acidaemia.

Treatment and prognosis No specific treatment. Symptomatic measures for epilepsy, spasticity. The younger the onset the worse the prognosis.

Survival:

infantile group ~2.5 years
juvenile group ~8 years.

References Borrett D, Becker LE. Alexander's disease. A disease of astrocytes. *Brain* 1985; **108**: 367–385.

Brenner M, Johnson AB, Boespflug-Tanguy O *et al.* Mutations in GFAP, encoding glial fibrillary acidic protein, are associated with Alexander disease. *Nature Genetics* 2001; **27**: 117–120.

Other relevant entries Adrenoleukodystrophy; Canavan's disease; Hydrocephalus; Krabbe's disease, Krabbe's leukodystrophy; Leukodystrophies: an overview; Metachromatic leukodystrophy; Multiple sclerosis; Pelizaeus–Merzbacher disease.

■ Alexia

Alexia, or dyslexia, is an impairment of reading ability. The term alexia may be reserved for acquired disorders, and dyslexia for developmental problems (particularly in lay parlance), or dyslexia may be used for both and qualified as developmental or acquired.

Alexia may be associated with more widespread problems with language (aphasia, agraphia), with other neurological signs (hemianopia), or occur in relative isolation. Various forms of acquired alexia are described, most often associated with lesions in the region of the angular gyrus and splenium.

Acquired alexias may be divided into:
• Peripheral alexias: deficit is in processing the visual aspects of the stimulus. Examples include:

Alexia without agraphia/pure alexia/letter-by-letter reading: lesion is in left occipital cortex and input to this region (splenio-occipital syndrome).

Neglect alexia: parietal lobe lesions (especially right).

Attentional alexia: preserved reading of single words but impaired reading in the context of other words or letters.

- Central alexias: impairment is in functions which mediate access to meaning. Examples include:

  Deep dyslexia: semantic errors.

  Phonological alexia: a selective deficit of the procedure mediating translation of print-to-sound.

  Surface dyslexia: inability to read words with "irregular" or exceptional print-to-sound correspondences.

Alexia without agraphia is one of the commonest of the alexias. First described by Déjerine in 1892, patients cannot read their own written work. Speech output, comprehension and repetition are normal but they may have some naming difficulties, especially for colours. The reading defect may be so severe that even single letters may not be recognized, but as recovery occurs patients tend to spell the word out before being able to recognize it. There may be an associated right visual field defect with deficiencies of short-term memory, and if the lesion is more extensive there may be alexia with agraphia or even Gerstmann syndrome (acalculia, finger agnosia and right–left disorientation) due to damage to the left angular gyrus.

Developmental dyslexia (previously known as congenital word blindness), first described by Hinshelwood in 1896, is a childhood inability to read and spell correctly, despite normal intelligence and the ability to see and recognize letters. In some cases there are additional cognitive deficits involving verbal and visual memory or difficulties using numbers. Up to 10% of schoolchildren have a degree of dyslexia, usually mild, and this often runs in families and may be associated with left-handedness. The anatomical substrate for this condition is not known, but there is some evidence that there may be abnormalities in the M visual pathway and the normal asymmetry of the planum temporale is lost and that this area is of comparable size in both hemispheres.

References Coslett HB. Acquired dyslexia. In: Heilman KM, Valenstein E (eds). *Clinical Neuropsychology* (4th edition). Oxford: OUP, 2003: 108–125.

McCarthy RA, Warrington EK. *Cognitive Neuropsychology. A Clinical Introduction.* San Diego: Academic, 1990: 214–240.

Leff AA. *Advances in Clinical Neuroscience and Rehabilitation* 2004; **4**(3): 21–22.

Other relevant entries Acalculia; Agraphia; Agnosia; Aphasia; Disconnection syndromes; Gerstmann syndrome.

■ Algodystrophy – see Complex regional pain syndromes

■ Allgrove's syndrome
Triple A syndrome (AAAS) • 4A syndrome

A rare, probably autosomal-recessive condition, characterized by the 4As: alachrima, achalasia, autonomic neuropathy (with reduced heart rate variability, orthostatic hypotension, and impaired response to deep breathing), and adrenocortical insufficiency. The latter may be delayed, hence the condition may be known as 3A or triple A syndrome (AAAS). Other neurological features may also occur including spasticity, ataxia, learning difficulty, neuropathy (axonal, motor), and velopharyngeal incompetence. The complete syndrome is characteristic but may be confused with hereditary motor neuropathy, juvenile amyotrophic lateral sclerosis (ALS), spinal muscular atrophy, and Worster–Drought syndrome.

Mutations in the AAAS gene on chromosome 12q13 have recently been demonstrated. The gene product ALADIN (for *a*lachrima–achalasia–*ad*renal *in*sufficiency *n*eurologic disorders) has a structure, which suggests it may be involved in peroxisomal function. If so, Allgrove syndrome may be related to Refsum's disease and X-linked adrenoleukodystrophy.

References Allgrove J, Clayden GS, Grant DB *et al.* Familial glucocorticoid deficiency with achalasia of the cardia and deficient tear production. *Lancet* 1978; **1**: 1284–1286.

Tullio-Peret A, Salomon R, Hadj-Rabia S *et al.* Mutation of a novel WD-repeat protein gene in Allgrove (Triple A) syndrome. *Nature Genetics* 2000; **26**: 332–335.

Other relevant entry Peroxisomal disorders: an overview.

▓ Alpers disease

Alpers–Huttenlocher syndrome • Diffuse cerebral degeneration in infancy • Progressive cerebral/infantile poliodystrophy • Progressive neuronal degeneration of childhood with liver disease

Pathophysiology This rare autosomal-recessive condition, first described in 1931, usually presents in early childhood with psychomotor retardation, intractable seizures originating in posterior cortical areas, and progressive liver failure. It has rarely been described in young adults. It is progressive, incurable, and leads to death within months to a few years. The cause and pathophysiology of the disease is largely unknown, although various inborn errors of metabolism may be responsible, particularly pyruvate dehydrogenase deficiency and mitochondrial electron transport chain defects. In the brain there is diffuse, non-specific, destruction of cortical neurones, especially in the striate cortex. The marked atrophy of cerebral convolutions with relative preservation of the white matter leads to an appearance described as "walnut brain". There is usually some cortical and adjacent subcortical gliosis. The liver changes are characterized by bile duct proliferation, fatty change, fibrosis, and cirrhosis.

Clinical features: history and examination Alpers disease usually presents between the ages of 2–5 years.

- Psychomotor retardation is the usual presenting feature, with a loss of smiling and disinterest in the surroundings. This is associated with growth retardation, increasing microcephaly and hypotonia.
- Intractable epileptic seizures then develop. These are usually focal initially, but progress to generalized seizures, myoclonic or tonic–clonic, which are difficult to control; epilepsia partialis continua may occur. Seizures may be triggered by systemic illness and may be accompanied by an encephalopathy.

- Liver failure tends to occur late in the course of the illness. The liver undergoes fatty degeneration and cirrhosis.
- Blindness and optic atrophy may occur.
- Diffuse myoclonic jerks occur from early infancy, followed by incoordination of movement (ataxia) and progressive spasticity.
- Episodic tachypnoea.

Investigations and diagnosis *Bloods*: lactic acidosis is common, and may become severe during intercurrent infections; abnormal liver function tests occur late in the disease, but ammonia is usually raised early on.

Imaging: MRI may demonstrate progressive cortical atrophy posteriorly +/− non-specific white matter changes suggestive of patchy gliosis.

CSF: may show raised protein (non-specific), which may relate to the epileptic seizures.

Neurophysiology: EEG: very abnormal, often with occipital epileptic changes.

Visual evoked potentials (VEPs): markedly abnormal in an asymmetric fashion; ultimately lost.

Differential diagnosis

Leigh's disease (seizures, cortical blindness more evident in Alpers disease).

Mitochondrial encephalomyopathy.

Reye's syndrome.

Encephalitis.

Hepatic encephalopathy (for whatever reason).

Metabolic encephalopathies (e.g. hypoglycaemia, hypoxia).

Treatment and prognosis No specific treatment. Symptomatic treatment of seizures with anticonvulsants, although sodium valproate should be avoided, as children with this condition are thought to be susceptible to hepatoxicity induced by this drug. The disease is universally fatal with death within 1–2 years of onset.

References Harding BN, Egger J, Portmann B, Erdohazi M. Progressive neuronal degeneration of childhood with liver disease. A pathological study. *Brain* 1986; **109**: 181–206.

Harding BN, Alsanjari N, Smith SJM *et al.* Progressive neuronal degeneration of childhood with liver disease (Alpers' disease) presenting in young adults. *Journal of Neurology, Neurosurgery and Psychiatry* 1995; **58**: 320–325.

Other relevant entries Encephalitis: an overview; Encephalopathies: an overview; Epilepsy: an overview; Leigh's disease, Leigh's syndrome; Liver disease and the nervous system; Mitochondrial disease: an overview; Reye's syndrome.

■ Alport's syndrome

Pathophysiology A rare X-linked condition characterized by nephritis, haematuria, progressive renal failure, and nerve deafness; ocular abnormalities may also occur. Mutations in one of the collagen genes have been identified.

Clinical features: History and examination
- Haematuria: usual presenting symptom, often related to upper respiratory tract infection.
- Sensorineural hearing loss.
- Ocular defects: cataract, lenticonus, lens dislocation.

Investigations and diagnosis
Diagnosis by clinical picture.

Renal biopsy: irregular thickening of glomerular basement membrane.

Audiometry: high-frequency deafness in most (but not all) cases.

Differential diagnosis Unlikely to be confused with other inherited causes of nerve deafness.

Treatment and prognosis Tends to progress to renal failure, requiring dialysis. Renal transplantation may be complicated by immune response against, and loss of, the allograft.

> **Reference** Barker DF, Hostikka SL, Zhou J *et al.* Identification of mutations in the COL4A5 collagen gene in Alport syndrome. *Science* 1990; **248**: 1224–1227.

> **Other relevant entries** Hearing loss: differential diagnosis; Renal disease and the nervous system.

■ Alström syndrome
Alström–Hallgren syndrome

Pathophysiology An hereditary autosomal recessive syndrome with pigmentary retinopathy and hearing loss.

Clinical features: history and examination
- Obesity, hypogonadism, diabetes mellitus.
- Pigmentary retinal degeneration (cone-rod dystrophy).
- Sensorineural hearing loss.
- Sometimes mental retardation.
- Family history of similar problems.

Investigations and diagnosis *Bloods*: raised glucose, low gonadotrophins.

Neurophysiology: ERG is typically abnormal.

Audiometry.

Differential diagnosis Other inherited syndromes of retinitis pigmentosa (e.g. Laurence–Moon–Biedl syndrome).

Other inherited syndromes of hearing loss (e.g. Usher's syndrome, Refsum's disease, Small's disease, Rosenberg–Chutorian syndrome, Richards–Rundle syndrome).

Prader–Willi syndrome has similar morphological changes but no eye problems.

Treatment and prognosis No specific treatment.

> **Reference** Alström CH. The Lindenov–Hallgren, Alström–Hallgren and Weiss syndromes. In: Vinken PJ, Bruyn GW (eds). *Handbook of Clinical Neurology: Volume 13 Neuroretinal Degenerations.* Amsterdam: North-Holland, 1972: 451–467.

> **Other relevant entries** Bardet–Biedl syndrome; Diabetes mellitus and the nervous system; Hearing loss: differential diagnosis; Laurence–Moon syndrome;

Prader–Willi syndrome; Refsum's disease; Retinitis pigmentosa; Richards–Rundle syndrome; Rosenberg–Chutorian syndrome; Small's disease; Tunbridge–Paley syndrome; Usher's syndrome.

■ Altitude illness

Acute mountain sickness • Chronic mountain sickness • Monge disease

Pathophysiology High-altitude environments (i.e. >5300 ft) are characterized by a lower atmospheric partial pressure of oxygen and hence the risk of hypoxia in humans. All travellers to high altitude will experience varying degrees of acute mountain sickness (AMS), but only in a small percentage does this become life threatening with acute pulmonary and/or cerebral oedema. This most often occurs with rapid ascent to over 12 000 ft in unacclimatized individuals. The symptoms of AMS are headache, insomnia, anorexia, nausea, and dizziness; the more serious manifestations are vomiting, dyspnoea, muscle weakness, oliguria, peripheral oedema, and retinal haemorrhage. Prevention of AMS requires adequate acclimatization, increased fluid intake and a high-carbohydrate, low-fat, low-salt diet. Cerebral oedema may first manifest with slight mental impairments or change in behaviour, accompanied by headache, nausea, vomiting, hallucinations, sometimes with seizures, and ataxia, which may progress to coma and death. In established cases treatment is with supplemental oxygen, descent to lower altitude and rest; dexamethasone is indicated in cases of cerebral oedema. Chronic exposure to high altitude may cause mild cognitive deficits, but of more significance are the neurological manifestations from the secondary polycythaemia induced by hypoxia (the so-called Monge disease).

Clinical features: history and examination

- *AMS*
  - Headache, insomnia, anorexia, nausea and dizziness; a syndrome of burning feet and burning hands is also described.
  - More serious manifestations: vomiting, dyspnoea, muscle weakness, oliguria, peripheral oedema, and retinal haemorrhage; the latter may progress to visual failure. In addition the patient may develop ataxia, abnormal behaviour, drowsiness, and hallucinations, which may progress to coma and death from severe pulmonary and cerebral oedema.
  - Prolonged exposure to high altitude has been reported to cause some mild impairment of neurobehavioral function, especially memory.
- *Chronic mountain sickness (Monge disease)*
  - Pulmonary hypertension, cor pulmonale and secondary polycythaemia, and the systemic effects of long-term habitation at high altitudes.
  - Neurological features may occur, such as mental slowness, fatigue, nocturnal headache, and sometimes papilloedema.

Investigations and diagnosis *Bloods*: may be polycythaemia; hypoxia on arterial blood gases.

Others: imaging, CSF, electrophysiology neither possible nor relevant.

Treatment and prognosis

Prevention:

Slow ascent with acclimization at around 6000–8000 ft
Avoid alcohol
Increase fluid intake
Conditioning exercise before departure, especially if over 35 years old
High-carbohydrate, low-fat, low-salt diet
Carbonic anhydrase inhibitors (acetazolamide or faster acting methazolamide), dex-
amethasone, and nifedipine have been shown to have a prophylactic role in AMS.

Treatment:

Oxygen
Descent to lower altitude
Rest
Dexamethasone in cases of cerebral oedema.

References Barry PW, Pollard AJ. Altitude illness. *British Medical Journal* 2003; **326**:
915–919.

Basnyat B, Murdoch DR. High-altitude illness. *Lancet* 2003; **361**: 1967–1974.

Hornbein TF, Townes BD, Schoene RB, Sutton JR, Houston CS. The cost to the central nervous system of climbing to extremely high altitude. *New England Journal
of Medicine* 1989; **321**: 1714–1719.

Klocke DL, Decker WW, Stepanek J. Altitude-related illnesses. *Mayo Clinic
Proceedings* 1998; **73**: 988–992.

▨ Aluminium toxicity – see Dialysis syndromes; Heavy metal poisoning

▨ Alzheimer's disease

Dementia of the Alzheimer type

Pathophysiology Alzheimer's disease (AD) is a common neurodegenerative disease,
first described by Alzheimer in 1906. It characteristically affects the elderly population and usually presents with episodic memory difficulties. Sporadic and familial
cases are reported, the latter tending to occur earlier. As the disease progresses there
is increasing difficulty with memory, language, and orientation, leading to global
impairment of cognitive faculties within 5–10 years from symptom onset. Death is
usually from secondary causes such as bronchopneumonia.

The pathological accompaniments of intellectual decline are:

- Neurofibrillary tangles composed ultrastructurally of paired helical filaments,
composed largely of the microtubule-associated protein τ.

- Plaques composed largely of amyloid protein, with various morphologies.
- Dystrophic neurites containing paired helical filaments: surrounding some plaques, and in the cortical neuropil (neuropil threads, cortical neuritic dystrophy).
- Synaptic and neuronal loss.

Abnormal cellular processing and subsequent aggregation of certain proteins may be the key pathophysiological process.

The amyloid (cascade) hypothesis remains the most favoured explanation of disease pathogenesis, largely because many of the genetic mutations identified as deterministic for AD (in the genes encoding amyloid precursor protein (APP), presenilin-1, and presenilin-2) lead to increased cellular production of the long variant (42–43 amino acids) of amyloid β-peptide (Aβ42) from its precursor molecule, APP. However, extracellular amyloid brain burden is not sufficient to cause disease; disruption of intraneuronal cytoskeletal integrity leading to formation of neurofibrillary tangles and dystrophic neurites, with synapse loss and neuronal death, is also required for the development of dementia. Apolipoprotein E (ApoE) genotype is a risk factor for the development of AD, the $\varepsilon4/\varepsilon4$ genotype carrying the greatest risk, although this is neither necessary nor sufficient for the development of AD.

The location of the primary pathological event in AD remains uncertain, although neurofibrillary pathology follows a predictable pattern of spread from transentorhinal cortex to neocortex. Gross atrophy of the cerebral cortex with extensive gliosis and neuronal cell loss, associated with atrophy of the cholinergic forebrain nuclei including the basal nucleus of Meynert, and cholinergic insufficiency is the end result.

Clinical features: history and examination

- Cognitive deficits: impairment of episodic memory is the commonest presenting symptom, with preservation of working memory/sustained attention. It is advisable to obtain a history from other family members or carers, to help ascertain the nature, extent and duration of the problems. The patient often makes light of difficulties or attempts to explain them away. (Isolated amnesia insufficient to fulfil diagnostic criteria for AD may be labelled as mild cognitive impairment (MCI), a condition which a high rate of progression to AD.)

  Thereafter cognitive deficits progress to involve other domains, for example:

  Language difficulties, including word finding and comprehension problems
  Visuospatial dysfunction
  Dysexecutive syndrome.

  Impaired activities of daily living (ADL): initially operational (shopping, cooking, finances), but latterly basic (dressing, toileting, feeding).
- Behavioural features: depression may be common in the early stages, and it is sometimes difficult to differentiate cognitive deficits due to depression and dementia. Agitation, wandering, psychosis may also occur. These are the features which most often lead to breakdown of care at home and necessitate institutionalization.
- Neurological features: there are no specific signs. Some patients develop extrapyramidal signs, but these are usually mild. Myoclonus and seizures may occur, with

increasing frequency as the disease progresses and probably more common in familial than sporadic disease.

Clinical variants of AD which have been described include:

- Posterior cortical atrophy (PCA): patients present with a relatively isolated and progressive visual agnosia but with preservation of memory.
- Lewy body variant (LBV) of AD: this name has been applied to those patients with dementia with Lewy bodies (DLB) with additional pathology sufficient to meet standard pathological criteria for AD; this condition may be distinguished from "diffuse Lewy body disease" (DLBD) which lacks concomitant AD pathology.
- A frontal variant of AD.

Various forms of Familial AD (FAD) have been identified, and in certain cases deterministic genetic mutations identified:

- Mutations in the APP gene on chromosome 21: rare families (*ca.* 25 worldwide) in which dominant mutations show complete penetrance by the age of 60, with most cases presenting from 30 to 60 years of age. [One of the amyloid angiopathies, hereditary cerebral haemorrhage with angiopathy, Dutch type (HCHWAD), also results from mutation within the APP gene.]
- Mutations in the presenilin-1 (PS-1) gene on chromosome 14, and in the presenilin-2 gene on chromosome 1: PS-1 mutations are the commonest identified cause of FAD, over 100 different mutations are identified. Mutations usually result in disease with the same age of onset within, but not necessarily between, families; there are occasional cases of incomplete penetrance. These observations suggest a role for other genetic or epigenetic factors (but not ApoE). PS-1 FAD generally presents earlier and runs a more rapid course than sporadic cases of AD. In addition, myoclonus and seizures are more prominent than in sporadic AD.
- In trisomy 21 (Down's syndrome), AD neuropathology usually develops before the age of 40 due to a gene dosage effect of APP.
- Polymorphisms in the gene encoding ApoE on chromosome 19 influence the risk of developing both sporadic and some FAD (e.g. APP mutation families) in a dose-dependent manner; possession of two ApoE ε4 alleles increases risk by about eight-fold; however, this is neither necessary nor sufficient for the development of AD. In contrast the ε2 allele may offer some protection against developing AD.

Other families have been described which do not map to any of the above loci.

Investigations and diagnosis In the absence of definitive treatment for AD, it is important to exclude potentially treatable causes of dementia.

Bloods: usually all normal; should assay thyroid function, calcium, vitamin B_{12}, syphilis serology.

Neuropsychology: extremely helpful in defining the nature and extent of cognitive deficits. Earliest changes are typically in episodic memory, although some patients present with visuospatial problems. Difficulties in language and executive function also emerge with time. Often a global pattern of cognitive impairment is evident by the time of the patient's presentation. Islands of preserved ability may remain (e.g. reading, but without comprehension).

Imaging:

Structural: CT and MRI may show cortical atrophy, but this may overlap with that seen in normal ageing. Longitudinal study of volumetric indices (e.g. hippocampal volume) may be helpful in showing progressive atrophy.

Functional: SPECT and PET changes may demonstrate hypometabolism in the parietotemporal regions. Magnetic resonance spectroscopy may show reductions in neuronal markers (N-acetyl-aspartate).

CSF: usually normal.

Neurophysiology: EEG: non-specific changes only (slowing of background α-rhythm); may be helpful in distinction from frontotemporal dementia where EEG remains normal.

Pathological change remains the "gold standard" for diagnosis, but this is seldom present ante mortem.

Neurogenetics: for early onset AD with a family history suggestive of autosomal-dominant transmission (usually same age at onset, perhaps preserved naming skills), searching for mutations in APP, PS-1, and PS-2 may be worthwhile. Testing for ApoE genotype has little to contribute to diagnosis.

Differential diagnosis

Depression.

Delirium.

The differential diagnosis of dementia *per se* is broad; mixed pathology (AD + vascular change) is also common.

Treatment and prognosis Cholinesterase inhibitors, whose aim is to potentiate the central cholinergic network, are licensed for the symptomatic treatment of mild to moderate AD; perhaps ⅓ to ½ of patients benefit objectively (mini-mental state examination (MMSE), ADL, neuropsychiatric function).

Memantine, an antagonist at NMDA receptors, may also have a therapeutic effect.

Behavioural features may require pharmacotherapy, available agents including quetiapine for agitation.

Disease-modifying drugs are not available, but research into agents influencing amyloidogenesis are ongoing, for example immunomodulatory therapy with amyloid peptides ("vaccine") and secretase inhibitors.

Currently of greater importance in management is support of both the patient and carer(s) at home. Institutionalization may be necessary, often because of behavioural features or incontinence; early intervention may avoid the need for institutionalization.

The disease is progressive and the median survival time from diagnosis to death is around 7–10 years.

References McKhann G, Drachman D, Folstein M *et al.* Clinical diagnosis of Alzheimer's disease. Report of the NINCDS–ADRDA work group under the auspices of the Department of Health and Human Service Task forces on Alzheimer's disease. *Neurology* 1984; **34**: 939–944.

National Institute on Aging and Reagan Institute Working Group on Diagnostic Criteria for the Neuropathological Assessment of Alzheimer Disease. Consensus recommendations for the post-mortem diagnosis of Alzheimer's disease. *Neurobiology of Aging* 1997; **18**(**suppl** 4): S1–S2.

Other relevant entries Amyloid and the nervous system: an overview; Cerebrovascular disease: arterial; Delirium; Dementia: an overview; Dementia with Lewy bodies; Down's syndrome; Frontotemporal dementia; Mild cognitive impairment; Parkinsonian syndromes, parkinsonism; Pick's disease; Vascular dementia.

■ AMAN – see Gangliosides and neurological disorders; Guillain–Barré syndrome

■ Amaurosis fugax – see Transient ischaemic attack

■ Aminoacidopathies: an overview

Pathophysiology Aminoacidopathies are rare, autosomal-recessive, inborn errors of metabolism, in which amino acid synthesis or transport is affected. These disorders do not impair growth, maturation or development *in utero*, but may present in the early months of life with neurological features, which may be episodic or chronically progressive, such as encephalopathy.

Examples of some of the commoner aminoacidopathies with neurological features are given here:

- Phenylketonuria (PKU): phenylalanine hydroxlase deficiency.
  Developmental delay, +/− vomiting from around 2 months; permanent deficits thereafter if untreated. Musty odour.
- Tyrosinaemia: Type I (hepatorenal tyrosinaemia): fumaryl-acetoacetate hydrolase deficiency.
  Neonatal liver failure; cabbage-like odour. Chronic form with hepatic disease and Fanconi syndrome. Episodic porphyric complications.
- Tyrosinaemia: Type II: tyrosine aminotransferase deficiency.
  Corneal, plantar, palmar erosions. Variable neurological involvement with mental retardation and motor delay.
- Homocystinuria: cystathionine β-synthase deficiency.
  Marfanoid habitus, cerebral thromboembolic disease, +/− psychiatric and extrapyramidal features with mental retardation.
- Hartnup's disease: neutral amino acid (e.g. tryptophan) transport defect in kidney and gut.
  Photosensitive dermatitis, personality change, affective disorders and ataxia.

- Maple syrup urine disease (MSUD): disorders of catabolism of branched-chain amino acids.

  Wide range in severity of defects and of clinical presentation: neonatal encephalopathy, later-onset fulminant encephalopathy with mental retardation; episodic encephalopathy in early childhood; ataxia, mental retardation, failure to thrive common; maple syrup odour.

- Non-ketotic hyperglycinaemia (glycine encephalopathy): defect in glycine cleavage system.

  Severe neonatal encephalopathy, myoclonus and apnoea leading to death. Less severe enzyme deficits present with mental retardation, spasticity, and myoclonic fits.

- Histidinaemia: histidase deficiency.

  Association with seizures, mental retardation, attention deficits, tremor, ataxia, and other neurological deficits may be fortuitous rather than causal; many "normals" may be shown to have histidinaemia.

- Lysine intolerance: defect in dibasic amino acid transport mechanism in kidney and gut.

  Feeding difficulties with growth failure, osteoporosis, bone marrow depression and hepatomegaly. Developmental delay with episodic encephalopathy. Mental retardation, psychoses, seizures.

- Cystinosis: intralysosomal accumulation of the amino acid cystine in kidney, cornea, thyroid, and brain.

Clinical features: history and examination See individual entries for further details.

Investigations and diagnosis As a general rule, diagnosis is usually straightforward due to the accumulation of metabolites proximal to the enzyme defect, which being water soluble may be detected in plasma and urine.

Differential diagnosis/treatment and prognosis See individual entries.

References Evans OB, Parker CC, Haas RH, Naidu S, Moser HW, Bock H-GO. Inborn errors of metabolism of the nervous system. In: Bradley WG, Daroff RB, Fenichel GM, Marsden CD (eds). *Neurology in Clinical Practice* (3rd edition). Boston: Butterworth-Heinemann, 2000: 1595–1664.

Gascon GG, Ozand PT. Aminoacidopathies and organic acidopathies, mitochondrial enzyme defects, and other metabolic errors. In: Goetz CG (ed.). *Textbook of Clinical Neurology* (2nd edition). Philadelphia: Saunders, 2003: 629–664.

Menkes JH. Disorders of amino acid metabolism. In: Rowland LP (ed.). *Merritt's Textbook of Neurology* (9th edition). Baltimore: Williams & Wilkins, 1995: 538–546.

Other relevant entries Canavan's disease; Cystinosis; Hartnup's disease; Homocystinuria; Lowe syndrome; Maple syrup urine disease; Non-ketotic hyperglycinaemia; Phenylketonuria; Tyrosinaemia.

Aminolaevulinic acid dehydratase deficiency – see Plumboporphyria

Amnesia, amnesic syndrome

Amnesia is an inability to store or recall explicit (declarative) memories despite preserved attention and general awareness. This deficit of episodic or autobiographical memory may be contrasted with other aspects of memory, such as semantic memory and implicit or procedural memory, which may be preserved. Amnesia may be described as anterograde if there is a failure to learn new information, and retrograde if old memories cannot be accessed.

The amnesic syndrome reflects damage or dysfunction of medial temporal lobe structures, such as the hippocampus, thought to be important in the laying down and recall of episodic memories.

Causes of amnesia may be transient/temporary or persistent:

Transient global amnesia (TGA)
Transient epileptic amnesia (TEA)
Closed head injury
Drugs
Sequel of herpes simplex encephalitis
Alzheimer's disease (may show isolated amnesia in early disease); mild cognitive impairment
Limbic (paraneoplastic) encephalitis
Hypoxic brain injury
Temporal lobectomy (bilateral; or unilateral with previous contralateral injury, usually birth asphyxia)
Bilateral posterior cerebral artery occlusion
Korsakoff's syndrome
Bilateral thalamic infarction
Acute hypoglycaemia in diabetes mellitus (intensive insulin regime for rigorous control)
Third ventricle tumour, colloid cyst
Psychogenic amnesia.

References Hodges JR, Greene JDW. Disorders of memory. In: Kennard C (ed.). *Recent Advances in Clinical Neurology 8*. Edinburgh: Churchill Livingstone, 1995: 151–169.

Bauer RM, Grande L, Valenstein E. Amnesic disorders. In: Heilman KM, Valenstein E (eds) *Clinical Neuropsychology* (4th edition). Oxford: OUP, 2003: 495–573.

Other relevant entries Alzheimer's disease; Colloid cyst; Herpes simplex encephalitis; Mild cognitive impairment (MCI); Memory; Transient epileptic amnesia; Transient global amnesia; Wernicke–Korsakoff's syndrome.

■ Amoebic infection

Amoebae (*Entamoeba histolytica*) may rarely invade the brain (amoebiasis) producing abscesses, especially in the frontal lobes or basal ganglia. A combination of surgery and antibiotics (metronidazole) may be required, but mortality is very high.

Free-living amoebae of the species *Naegleria* or *Acanthamoeba* may cause acute or granulomatous meningoencephalitis. Amoebic trophozoites may be identified in CSF or in skin nodules. Purulent CSF (raised white cell count, mostly polymorphs, raised protein, low glucose, often haemorrhagic) with negative Gram stain may stimulate a search for amoebae. Treatment is with intravenous and intrathecal amphotericin or miconazole. Though rare, the mortality of these conditions is very high.

Other relevant entries *Acanthamoeba*; Infection and the nervous system: an overview.

■ AMSAN – see Guillain–Barré syndrome

■ Amyloid and the nervous system: an overview

Pathophysiology Amyloid is the name given to predominantly extracellular fibrillar material composed primarily of protein, in the form of insoluble β-pleated sheets, the origin of which varies with the type of amyloidosis and disease state. Amyloid deposits are best visualized using the dye Congo red: using light microscopy amyloid deposits appear pink or red in colour, but under polarized light the Congo red-stained amyloid demonstrates an apple-green birefringence. Antibodies against the specific protein component of amyloid (e.g. amyloid β-peptide) allows its visualization by immunohistochemistry.

Amyloid may be deposited in a number of different organs in a number of different diseases, some of which include, or are exclusive to, the nervous system.

Amyloidosis may be classified as follows:
• Systemic amyloidosis

Primary amyloidosis: amyloid (AL: amyloid light chain) is derived from immunoglobulin light chains associated with aberrant expansion of B-cell clones (e.g. multiple myeloma).

Secondary amyloidosis: amyloid (AA: amyloid fibril protein) is derived from serum amyloid-associated protein (SAA), normally secondary to chronic inflammatory conditions (e.g. bronchiectasis, rheumatoid arthritis).

Heredofamilial amyloidosis:

Neuropathic type.

Non-neuropathic type (e.g. familial Mediterranean fever).
• Localized amyloidosis

Senile cardiac amyloidosis

Amyloid in medullary thyroid carcinoma

? Alzheimer's disease (AD)

? Amyloid angiopathies.

Systemic amyloidosis affects only the peripheral nervous system (PNS) with the development of peripheral and autonomic neuropathy. In the central nervous system (CNS), extracellular amyloid deposition occurs in AD in the form of senile plaques, and in blood vessels as amyloid angiopathy. Whilst the latter is of uncertain pathogenic significance, deposition of amyloid in the cerebral vasculature occurs in a number of other conditions associated with intracerebral haemorrhage, the sporadic and hereditary cerebral amyloid angiopathies (CAA).

Clinical features: history and examination

- PNS

    Hereditary/familial forms

        Familial amyloid polyneuropathies (FAPs; *q.v.*).

        Familial amyloidosis with carpal tunnel syndrome: first described by in 1955, affected members of these families characteristically have amyloid deposition in the connective tissues around the carpal tunnel, compressing the median nerve. Occasionally other upper limb nerves are involved.

    Non-familial forms

        Primary systemic amyloidosis: may be clinically indistinguishable from FAPs but with presentation at a later age; however, in contrast with FAPs, there is nearly always involvement of other organ systems before the neuropathy develops, in particular the gut, bone marrow, heart, and kidney.

        (Secondary amyloidosis: nervous system is not involved.)

- CNS

    CAA; *q.v.*

        Sporadic.

        Hereditary: HCHWA-D, HCHWA-I.

    AD.

        Familial British dementia (FBD; Worster-Drought syndrome); Familial Danish dementia (FDD).

Investigations and diagnosis/differential diagnosis/treatment and prognosis See individual entries.

References Castano EM, Frangione B. Non-Alzheimer's disease amyloidosis of the nervous system. *Current Opinion in Neurology* 1995; **8**: 279–285.

Gambetti P, Russo C. Human brain amyloidoses. *Nephrology Dialysis Transplantation* 1998; **13 (suppl 7)**: 33–40.

Reilly MM, Staunton H. Peripheral nerve amyloidosis. *Brain Pathology* 1996; **6**: 163–177.

Reilly MM, Thomas PK. Amyloid neuropathy. In: Mathias CJ, Bannister R (eds). *Autonomic Failure. A Textbook of Clinical Disorders of the Autonomic Nervous System* (4th edition). Oxford: OUP, 1999: 410–418.

Revesz T, Holton JL, Lashley T *et al*. Sporadic and familial cerebral amyloid angiopathies. *Brain Pathology* 2002; **12**: 343–357.

Other relevant entries Alzheimer's disease; Ankylosing spondylitis and the nervous system; Cerebral amyloid angiopathy; Cerebrovascular disease: arterial; Dementia: an overview; Familial amyloid polyneuropathies; Familial Danish dementia; Gelsolin amyloidosis; Neuropathies: an overview; Worster–Drought syndrome (2).

▨ Amyotrophic lateral sclerosis – see Motor neurone disease

▨ Anaesthesia dolorosa – see Trigeminal neuralgia

▨ Analgesia-induced headache – see Medication overuse headache

▨ Analphalipoproteinaemia – see Tangier disease

▨ Anarthria – see Dysarthria

▨ Andermann's syndrome (1)

An inherited, probably autosomal-recessive, syndrome characterized by complete agenesis of the corpus callosum, mental retardation, sensorimotor neuronopathy with flaccid quadriplegia and dysmorphic features, reported in several French-Canadian kindreds from Quebec.

Reference Andermann E. Sensorimotor neuronopathy with agenesis of the corpus callosum. In: Vinken PJ, Bruyn GW (eds). *Handbook of Clinical Neurology: Volume 42 Neurogenetic Directory Part I*. Amsterdam: North-Holland, 1981: 100–103.

Other relevant entry Agenesis of the corpus callosum.

▨ Andermann's syndrome (2)
Action-myoclonus–renal failure syndrome

Pathophysiology Andermann's syndrome is characterized by tremor, action myoclonus, cerebellar signs, epilepsy, and renal failure, with onset in teenage or early twenties, reported in several French-Canadian kindreds in Quebec and presumed to be an autosomal-recessive disorder. The neurological features do not seem to be related to renal failure *per se* in this condition, which is thought to result from an inherited metabolic defect.

Clinical features: history and examination
- Tremor of fingers, hands: onset age 17–18 years.
- Proteinuria: onset age 17–18.
- Action myoclonus: onset age 19–23; most disabling symptom.
- Renal failure: onset age 20–22.
- Cerebellar signs, ataxia, dysarthria: onset age 21–23; not severe.
- Epilepsy (infrequent generalized seizures): onset age 21–23.
- +/− mild axonal degenerative neuropathy.
- No extrapyramidal, pyramidal signs.
- Intelligence probably normal.

Investigations and diagnosis *Imaging*: MRI shows non-specific cerebral, cerebellar atrophy.

Neurophysiology: EEG: spike wave complexes, slowing, photoparoxysmal discharges.

Brain pathology: pigment granules in astrocytes.

Other: renal biopsy shows a non-specific nephritis.

Differential diagnosis Other causes of hereditary myoclonus, epilepsy, cerebellar syndrome (e.g. sialidosis type I, neuronal ceroid lipofuscinosis (Kuf's disease), Hallervorden–Spatz disease).

Treatment and prognosis Symptomatic treatment of myoclonus, epilepsy; renal dialysis +/− transplantation (no recurrence in transplanted organ).

> **Reference** Andermann E, Andermann F, Carpenter S *et al*. Action myoclonus–renal failure syndrome: a previously unrecognized neurological disorder unmasked by advances in nephrology. *Advances in Neurology* 1986; **43**: 87–103.

> **Other relevant entries** Myoclonus; Neuronal ceroid lipofuscinosis; Renal disease and the nervous system; Sialidosis.

■ Andersen disease – see Glycogen-storage disorders: an overview; Polyglucosan body disease

■ Andersen's syndrome

This is a rare disorder consists of the following triad:
- Periodic paralysis (hyperkalaemic or hypokalaemic).
- Malignant ventricular arrhythmia; this may postdate the periodic paralysis by many years; there may be a prolonged QT interval on ECG.
- Craniofacial dysmorphism: may be subtle.

Mutations in the voltage-independent skeletal muscle potassium channel gene (KCNJ2) have been found in this condition, hence it is a channelopathy.

> **References** Davies NP, Weber A, Mueller R, Hilton-Jones D, Chinnery PF, Hanna MG. Periodic paralysis, malignant ventricular arrhythmia and dysmorphism (Andersen's syndrome): a skeletal muscle potassium channel disorder. *Journal of Neurology, Neurosurgery and Psychiatry* 2002; **73**: 221 (abstract 39).

Tawil R, Ptacek LJ, Pavlakis SG *et al*. Andersen's syndrome: potassium sensitive periodic paralysis, ventricular ectopy, and dysmorphic features. *Annals of Neurology* 1994; **35**: 326–330.
Other relevant entries Channelopathies: an overview; Periodic paralysis; Prolonged QT syndromes.

▇ Anderson–Fabry disease – see Fabry's disease

▇ Andrade disease – see Familial amyloid polyneuropathies

▇ Anencephaly

Anencephaly, or aprosencephaly, is a developmental disorder characterized by a failure of the forebrain, cranium and meninges to close in the midline, due to failure of the anterior neuropore to close at around 24 days gestation. Prenatal diagnosis is possible on the basis of raised serum and amniotic fluid α-fetoprotein and ultrasound imaging. Such infants die shortly after birth.

▇ Aneurysm

Pathophysiology Intracranial aneuryms may be classified in various ways:
- Morphology: helpful in defining different natural history.
     Saccular
     Fusiform
     Dissecting.
- Size
     <3 mm, 3–6 mm, 7–10 mm, 11–25 mm, >25 mm (giant).
- Location
     Anterior, posterior circulation, specific vessels, especially at arterial branch points.

In addition, there are a number of rare disorders and hereditary disorders which may be associated with aneurysms:

Arteriovenous malformations
Dural arteriovenous fistulae, spinal arteriovenous malformations
Cardiac myxoma (tumour metastasis)
Sickle-cell disease
Superficial siderosis of the nervous system
Head trauma
Mycotic aneurysms, most often with infective endocarditis
Cocaine abuse
Coarctation of the aorta.

Hereditary:

Ehlers–Danlos syndrome type IV
Pseudoxanthoma elasticum
Infantile fibromuscular dysplasia
Neurofibromatosis
α_1-antitrypsin deficiency
Osler–Weber–Rendu syndrome (hereditary haemorrhagic telangiectasia)
Autosomal-dominant polycystic kidney disease.

Clinical features: history and examination

- Most cerebral aneurysms are asymptomatic, and do not rupture.
- Symptomatic features other than subarachnoid haemorrhage (SAH), if present, depend on aneurysm location and may be acute: ischaemia, headache, seizure, cranial neuropathy; or chronic due to mass effect: headache, visual loss, pyramidal tract dysfunction, facial pain.

Investigations and diagnosis Many aneurysms are discovered incidentally, when cranial imaging is undertaken for some other purpose. If aneurysms are being specifically sought, then some form of angiography is required; catheter angiography has been the gold standard, although it carries a definite morbidity; other options include MRA and digital subtraction angiography (DSA).

Treatment and prognosis Many questions remain: who should be screened for aneurysm (probably family members when two or more first degree relatives have had a SAH, but not in relatives of patients with sporadic SAH); and when and whether to operate on asymptomatic aneurysms (small aneurysms, <10 mm diameter, have a very low rupture rate, and hence the risks of surgery probably outweigh any potential benefits).

> **References** International Study of Unruptured Intracranial Aneurysms Investigators. Unruptured intracranial aneurysms: natural history, clinical outcome, and risks of surgical and endovascular treatment. *Lancet* 2003; **362**: 103–110.
>
> Raps EC, Rogers JD, Galetta SL *et al.* The clinical spectrum of unruptured intracranial aneurysms. *Archives of Neurology* 1993; **50**: 265–268.
>
> **Other relevant entries** Carotid artery disease; Cavernous sinus disease; Cranial nerve disease: III: Oculomotor nerve; Fibromuscular dysplasia; Intracerebral haemorrhage; Subarachnoid haemorrhage; Thunderclap headache.

■ Angelman syndrome
"Happy puppet syndrome"

Pathophysiology A neurogenetic disorder linked to chromosome 15, and of great biological interest since it demonstrates the phenomenon of imprinting (in this instance maternal linked, i.e. the microdeletion is almost always of maternal inheritance, whereas Prader–Willi syndrome is paternal linked).

Most cases are sporadic but a few familial cases are reported. The 15q11–q13 deletion may lead to reduced amounts of the β_3-subunit of the $GABA_A$/benzodiazepine receptor.

Clinical features: history and examination

- Developmental delay; microcephaly, virtually absent speech, feeding difficulties.
- Happy demeanour (constant), unprovoked laughter (may not be prominent).
- Movement disorder: ambulation age 5–6 years, distinctive gait with jerky ataxia and lower extremity hypertonia (the "happy puppet").
- Seizure disorder: tonic, atonic > tonic–clonic.
- Moderate dysmorphism: prognathism.

Investigations and diagnosis *Neurogenetic testing*: for 15q11–q13 deletion.

EEG: often suggestive of diagnosis: runs of slow 3-Hz waves, especially posteriorly, often notched +/− spikes.

Imaging: CT/MRI: normal.

Differential diagnosis Behavioural features are fairly characteristic; may be mistaken for Rett's syndrome in girls, or ataxic cerebral palsy.

Treatment and prognosis No specific treatment; symptomatic therapy for seizures (ethosuximide, topiramate). Although long-term survival is reported, prognosis is generally poor.

References Angelman H. "Puppet" children: a report on three cases. *Developmental Medicine and Child Neurology* 1965; **7**: 681–688.

Cassidy SB, Schwartz S. Prader–Willi and Angelman syndromes. *Medicine* 1998; **77**: 140–151.

Khan NL, Wood NW. Prader–Willi and Angelman syndromes: update on genetic mechanisms and diagnostic complexities. *Current Opinion in Neurology* 1999; **12**: 149–154.

Other relevant entries Cerebral palsy, cerebral palsy syndromes; Prader–Willi syndrome; Rett's syndrome.

■ Angioendotheliomatosis

Intravascular lymphomatosis • Malignant angioendotheliomatosis • Neoplastic angioendotheliomatosis (NAE)

Pathophysiology Angioendotheliomatosis is an unusual condition in which there is a malignant intravascular proliferation of endothelial cells or lymphocytes. It is more accurately defined as an angiotropic intravascular large-cell lymphoma of B-cell type. It may affect vessels in almost all organs but most usually involves the skin and central nervous system. A number of neurological presentations are recognized of which the commonest is with multifocal ischaemic events, due to vascular occlusion by neoplastic cells within small blood vessels, with subsequent disseminated neurological signs and symptoms (simultaneous events in different vascular territories is typical), or dementia. There are often associated systemic features such as fever, raised ESR, and skin lesions, but the diagnosis can only be made by brain and/or meningeal biopsy. Angioendotheliomatosis responds poorly to chemotherapy.

Clinical features: history and examination

- Systemic abnormalities include fever.
- Skin lesions resembling thrombophlebitis or vasculitis.
- Neurological deficits:

    Progressive multifocal infarcts, may lead to dementia.

    Paraparesis, pain, and incontinence.

    Subacute encephalopathy.

    Cranial and/or peripheral neuropathy.

Investigations and diagnosis *Bloods*: often show raised ESR.

Imaging: MRI/CT of brain may show multifocal infarcts of different ages as well as striking meningeal enhancement.

CSF: may show raised protein.

Neurophysiology: often non-contributory, but may show peripheral neuropathy.

Brain/meningeal biopsy: required for diagnosis.

Differential diagnosis

Isolated angiitis of the central nervous system.

Behçet's disease.

Subacute viral encephalitis.

Gliomatosis cerebri.

CNS lymphoma.

Treatment and prognosis The condition is usually fatal, possibly because it is diagnosed late. If detected early, treatment with chemotherapy and radiotherapy may be tried. Steroids may give a temporary benefit. Overall prognosis is poor.

References Fredericks RK, Walker FO, Elster A, Challa V. Angiotropic intravascular large-cell lymphoma (malignant angioendotheliomatosis): report of a case and review of the literature. *Surgical Neurology* 1991; **35**: 218–223.

Heafield MT, Carey M, Williams AC, Cullen M. Neoplastic angioendotheliomatosis: a treatable "vascular dementia" occurring in an immunosuppressed transplant recipient. *Clinical Neuropathology* 1993; **12**: 102–106.

Lachance DH, Louis DN. Case records of the Massachusetts General Hospital (Case 31 – 1995). *New England Journal of Medicine* 1995; **333**: 992–999.

Other relevant entries Behçet's disease; Isolated angiitis of the central nervous sytem; Lymphoma; Vascular dementia.

■ Angiostrongyliasis

Infection with the rat lungworm *Angiostrongylus cantonensis*, following ingestion of snails, slugs, or undercooked prawns, may cause an eosinophilic meningitis or meningoencephalitis; cranial nerve palsies, seizures, and coma may also be features. The absence of focal features on structural brain imaging helps to distinguish this condition from neurocysticercosis and gnathostomiasis. CSF pressure is elevated and the white cell count is raised with a high percentage of eosinophils. Larvae may be found in the CSF or seen in the eye on ophthalmoscopy or slit-lamp examination. Due to possible toxicity of larvicidal agents, supportive treatment only may be appropriate in patients who are improving since the disease is often self-limiting.

■ Angular gyrus syndrome – see Aphasia; Gerstmann syndrome

■ Anismus – see Focal dystonias

■ Ankylosing hyperostosis – see Diffuse idiopathic skeletal hyperostosis

■ Ankylosing spondylitis and the nervous system
Marie–Strümpel disease • Von Bechterew's disease

Pathophysiology Ankylosing spondylitis (AS) is a chronic spondyloarthropathy caused by an autoimmune-mediated process directed against a cartilage proteoglycan. It is strongly associated with the HLA antigen B27. It affects particularly Europeans, men more than women (prevalence 1–3 : 1000), with onset in the second and third decades of life. Characteristically the sacroiliac joints and lumbosacral spine are affected initially, with symptoms of early morning pain and stiffness. Extra-articular manifestations include uveitis, aortic regurgitation, pulmonary fibrosis and amyloidosis, as well as neurological features. These latter include a cauda equina syndrome (CES), radiculopathy, myelopathy, and spinal stenosis. Spinal fracture may also lead to neurological complications. Treatment is designed to reduce inflammation; in some cases surgery may be necessary.

Clinical features: history and examination

- Systemic features: chronic back pain which is often insidious in onset, worse in the morning and made better by exercise (*cf.* osteoarthritis). Pain often radiates into the groin and thighs and with time is associated with a limitation of movement.
- Non-articular, non-neurological manifestations: include Reiter's syndrome, psoriasis, inflammatory diseases of the bowel, uveitis, pulmonary fibrosis, aortic regurgitation, and amyloidosis.
- Neurological features:

    CES: clinical picture is as for other CESs but sensory and sphincter abnormalities tend to be more common than motor weakness. CES is rare, yet the commonest neurological complication of AS.

    Radiculopathy involving the lumbosacral roots.

Myelopathy is rare in this condition and is usually due to a secondary complication, such as meningeal fibrosis, atlanto-axial dislocation (more commonly seen with rheumatoid arthritis), spinal fracture $+/-$ an epidural haematoma $+/-$ cord concussion (especially in the cervical region, in response to minor trauma, as there is marked osteoporosis in this condition).

Spinal lumbar stenosis.

Investigations and diagnosis *Bloods*: often reveal a non-specific inflammatory response with raised ESR, raised acute phase proteins and mild normochromic normocytic anaemia. Rheumatoid factor and other auto-antibodies are negative but 90% of patients are HLA B27 positive.

Imaging:

Spinal radiographs demonstrate bony bridging of the vertebral bodies to produce the so-called "bamboo spine".

Plain radiographs of the sacroiliac joints reveal sacroiliitis which evolves to obliteration of the joint.

MRI of the spine, and/or myelography, often reveals dorsal arachnoid diverticulae. In addition there may be evidence of radicular involvement, meningeal thickening, enlargement of the thecal sac, and dilatation of the lumbosacral nerve root sleeves. There is usually little or no meningeal enhancement with gadolinium.

CSF: may show a raised protein.

Neurophysiology: may reveal a radiculopathy.

Differential diagnosis The lack of spinal movement may also occur in acute painful conditions such as intervertebral disc prolapse. The loss of lordosis may occur in rigid spine syndrome, extrapyramidal disorders, especially progressive supranuclear palsy; and stiff man/person syndrome may lead to lower back symptoms.

Treatment and prognosis AS has no specific treatment. Joint pain and stiffness may be treated symptomatically with non-steroidal anti-inflammatory medications (e.g. indomethacin) and physiotherapy.

Surgical intervention may be required in some patients with either the CES or a myelopathy. In cases of symptomatic atlanto-axial dislocation surgical intervention is mandatory. Steroids are without benefit in CES.

References Ahn NU, Ahn UM, Nallamshetty L *et al*. Cauda equina syndrome in ankylosing spondylitis (the CES–AS syndrome): meta-analysis of outcome after medical and surgical treatments. *Journal of Spinal Disorders* 2001; **14**: 427–433.

Matthews WB. The neurological complications of ankylosing spondylitis. *Journal of the Neurological Sciences* 1968; **6**: 561–573.

Other relevant entries Cauda equina syndrome and conus medullaris disease; Lumbar cord and root disease; Radiculopathies: an overview; Rigid spine syndrome; Spinal stenosis.

Anorexia nervosa – see Eating disorders

Anosmia – see Cranial nerve disease: I: Olfactory nerve

Anterior choroidal artery infarction

Occlusion of the anterior choroidal artery, most usually a branch of the internal carotid artery before its terminal bifurcation into the anterior and middle cerebral arteries, produces inconsistent deficits, including:
- Contralateral hemiparesis and hemisensory deficit (proprioception often spared).
- +/− impaired language, visuospatial function.
- +/− visual field defect, typically homonymous horizontal sectoranopia (lateral geniculate nucleus involvement).

In situ thrombosis of the artery seems commoner than embolism from proximal sources.

Other relevant entry Cerebrovascular disease: arterial.

Anterior inferior cerebellar artery syndrome – see Cerebellar disease: an overview; Lateral medullary syndrome

Anterior interosseous syndrome
Kiloh–Nevin syndrome

The anterior interosseous nerve is a purely motor branch of the median nerve arising distal to pronator teres and lying anterior to the interosseous membrane. It innervates the flexor digitorum profundus I and II, flexor pollicis longus, and pronator quadratus muscles. Selective palsy of the anterior interosseous nerve is rare but produces a characteristic clinical picture of subacute weakness in the hand, with or without pain. Weakness of the terminal phalanx of the index finger causes the "pinch sign", inability to form a small circle by pinching the thumb and index finger together, and the "straight thumb sign" is evident when making a fist. There is no sensory involvement. Diagnosis may be confirmed by electrophysiological studies showing abnormalities confined to the three muscles innervated by the anterior interosseous nerve. Local trauma or compression by a fibrous band between the two heads of pronator teres is the commonest cause.

Reference Goulding PJ, Schady W. Favourable outcome in non-traumatic anterior interosseous nerve lesions. *Journal of Neurology* 1993; **240**: 83–86.

Other relevant entry Neuropathies: an overview.

▓ Anterior ischaemic optic neuropathy – see Ischaemic optic neuropathy

▓ Anterior opercular syndrome – see Foix–Chavany–Marie syndrome

▓ Anterior spinal artery syndrome
Beck syndrome

Pathophysiology The normal blood supply of the spinal cord is from paired posterior spinal arteries supplying the posterior third of the cord, and from a single anterior spinal artery formed by branches from both vertebral arteries, "reinforced" at thoracic levels by segmental arteries such as the artery of Adamkiewicz (arteria radicularis magna). Thus the anterior two-thirds of the cord is relatively vulnerable to ischaemia and infarction, particularly at middle to lower thoracic levels. Many cases of anterior spinal artery syndrome (ASAS) remain idiopathic, although recognized causes include aortic surgery (for resection of thoracic or thoracolumbar aortic aneurysms), occlusion (e.g. systemic atherosclerosis, embolus), systemic hypotension; and, less commonly, inflammatory vessel disease, arachnoiditis, vasculopathies or thrombophilic syndromes. The symptoms and signs in cases related to surgery may be masked by epidural analgesia.

Fibrocartilaginous embolism of the spinal cord is a rare cause of ASAS, in which fibrocartilaginous emboli are found in the vascular bed; there may be a preceding history of minor trauma or Valsalva manoeuvre.

Clinical features: history and examination

- Paraparesis, paraplegia: initially flaccid with reflex loss, evolving to spasticity, hyperreflexia and extensor plantar responses.
- Sensory level with impaired spinothalamic modalities (pain, temperature) below the level, preserved dorsal column modalities (e.g. proprioception).
- Sphincters: bladder and bowel paralysis usual.

Investigations and diagnosis The clinical picture is often diagnostic.

Imaging: spinal cord MRI may show ischaemic lesions and exclude other structural causes of myelopathy.

Treatment and prognosis No specific treatment, other than in embolic cases where anticoagulation or antiplatelet agents may be used. Risk factors for vascular disease merit treatment in their own right.

Recovery is extremely variable, dependent probably on extent and duration of impaired cord perfusion: one series reported <20% of survivors fully ambulatory, with >20% in-hospital mortality; worse prognosis with increasing patient age.

Neurorehabilitation to maximize potential is indicated.

Reference De la Barrera S, Barca-Buyo A, Montoto-Marqués A *et al*. Spinal cord infarction: prognosis and recovery in a series of 36 patients. *Spinal Cord* 2001; **39**: 520–525.

Other relevant entries Arachnoiditis; Spinal cord vascular diseases.

■ Anthrax

Pathophysiology Anthrax is a zoonotic infection with the sporulating Gram-positive bacillus *Bacillus anthracis*, usually a disease of herbivores, acquired from contact with spores in the soil. Exposure to infected animals is one cause of human disease. The possible use of this bacterium as an agent of bioterrorism, since it is relatively easy to weaponize, has lead to increased awareness of its possible effects.

Clinical features: history and examination Main forms of disease are respiratory, cutaneous, and gastrointestinal.

- Inhalational anthrax rapidly progresses to septicaemia, shock, and respiratory failure with a high mortality despite intensive care.
- Cutaneous anthrax is less likely to produce septicaemia and is common in some parts of the tropics.

A pyogenic meningitis occurs in <5% of cases, the clinical features of which are identical to other causes of pyogenic meningitis. A primary site of infection such as a pustule or pulmonary syndrome should be evident in anthrax meningitis.

Investigations and diagnosis

Imaging:

CXR may show widened mediastinum, hilar lymphadenopathy.

CT/MRI brain may show subarachnoid haemorrhage.

CSF: inflammatory CSF, may also be haemorrhagic; Gram-positive rods on Gram stain.

Differential diagnosis Other causes of bacterial meningitis; once Gram-positive rods are seen in CSF, differential diagnosis includes *Listeria*.

Treatment and prognosis Antibiotic regime, initially intravenous, for example ciprofloxacin, doxycycline, imipenem. Role of dexamethasone unclear. Oropharyngeal oedema may necessitate intubation. High mortality despite appropriate treatment. Cutaneous anthrax may respond to penicillin alone.

> **References** Beeching NJ, Dance DAB, Miller ARO, Spencer RC. Biological warfare and bioterrorism. *British Medical Journal* 2002; **324**: 336–339.
>
> Meselson M, Guillemin J, Hugh-Jones M *et al.* The Sverdlovsk anthrax outbreak of 1979. *Science* 1994; **266**: 1202–1207.
>
> **Other relevant entry** Meningitis: an overview.

■ Anti-Hu syndrome – see Paraneoplastic syndromes

■ Antiphospholipid (antibody) syndrome
Hughes syndrome

Pathophysiology Antiphospholipid antibodies syndrome (APS) may be:
- Primary: not associated with an underlying connective tissue disease.
- Secondary: to systemic lupus erythematosus or other connective tissue disorder.

The presence of these antibodies is associated with a tendency to venous or arterial thromboses; in an individual patient, either venous or arterial problems seem to predominate.

Clinical features: history and examination

- Vascular:

  Venous: limb-deep venous thrombosis; retinal, renal, hepatic venous thrombosis.

  Arterial: transient ischaemic attack (TIA), ischaemic stroke, retinal artery occlusion (all these may be associated with migraine); myocardial infarction, peripheral vascular disease.

- Neurological features other than stroke: may be associated with transverse myelitis, chorea, acute inflammatory neuropathy.
- Pregnancy failure.
- Livedo reticularis.
- Thrombocytopenia.
- Mitral valve vegetations.
- In catastrophic APS, rapidly progressive microvascular thrombosis leads to multiorgan failure.

Investigations and diagnosis Assay for antiphospholipid antibodies syndrome (APS) or prothrombotic screen to look for lupus anticoagulant.

Differential diagnosis Other causes of venous or arterial vascular disease.

Treatment and prognosis General: Modification of cardiovascular risk factors.

Specific: anti-thrombotic therapy: warfarin or, in pregnancy, aspirin + heparin. Reasonable evidence that high target INR (3–4) is more effective in secondary prevention than lower.

Immunotherapy has been suggested but no randomized trials have yet been undertaken. In catastrophic APS, plasma exchange is recommended.

References Greaves M. Antiphospholipid antibodies and thrombosis. *Lancet* 1999; **353**: 1348–1353.

Keswani SC, Chauhan N. Antiphospholipid syndrome. *Journal of the Royal Society of Medicine* 2002; **94**: 336–342.

Khamashta MA (ed.). *Hughes Syndrome. Antiphospholipid Syndrome*. London: Springer, 2000.

Scolding N (ed.). *Immunological and Inflammatory Disorders of the Central Nervous System*. Oxford: Butterworth-Heinemann, 1999: 147–180.

Other relevant entries Cerebrovascular disease: arterial; Cerebrovascular disease: venous; Migraine; Sneddon's syndrome; Systemic lupus erythematosus and the nervous system.

■ Anton–Babinski syndrome

Anton–Babinski syndrome refers to unilateral asomatognosia, the inability to recognize a paralysed (usually left) limb as one's own, with left hemiparesis. In addition there may be anosognosia (denial or unawareness of neurological deficits, left sensory extinction), left homonymous hemianopia, and left visual neglect. This usually follows a destructive lesion (commonly infarction) of the right (non-dominant) superior parietal lobule but is also recorded with non-convulsive status epilepticus.

> **Reference** Thomas P, Giraud K, Alchaar H, Chatel M. Ictal asomatognosia with hemiparesis. *Neurology* 1998; **51**: 280–282.

■ Anton's syndrome
Visual anosognosia

Anton's syndrome is cortical blindness accompanied by denial of the visual defect (visual anosognosia), with or without confabulation. The syndrome most usually results from bilateral posterior cerebral artery territory lesions causing occipital or occipitoparietal infarctions but has occasionally been described with anterior visual pathway lesions associated with frontal lobe lesions. It may also occur in the context of dementing disorders or delirium.

> **References** McDaniel KD, McDaniel LD. Anton's syndrome in a patient with post-traumatic optic neuropathy and bifrontal contusions. *Archives of Neurology* 1991; **48**: 101–105.
>
> Gassel M, Williams D. Visual function in patients with homonymous hemianopia. III. The completion phenomenon: insight and attitude to the defect: and visual function efficiency. *Brain* 1963; **86**: 229–260.
>
> **Other relevant entry** Agnosia.

■ Apallic syndrome – see Vegetative states

■ Apert's syndrome
Acrocephalosyndactyly types I and II

This is one of the syndromes in which craniostenoses (i.e. premature developmental closure of the cranial sutures) result in dysmorphology. In type I ("typical"), there is a clover-shaped skull (turribrachycephaly) with protuberant widely spaced eyes, underdeveloped maxillae with relative prognathism, mental retardation, along with complete syndactyly (mitten hands, sock feet). Other complications may occur (deafness, convulsions, visual loss secondary to papilloedema). In type II ("atypical"), syndactyly is less extensive, probably reflecting a phenotypic variant of type I. The syndrome has been linked to chromosome 10q.

> **Other relevant entries** Acrocephalosyndactyly; Craniostenosis.

■ Aphasia
Dysphasia

Pathophysiology Aphasia is an acquired disorder of language, both verbal and non-verbal (e.g. sign language). Aphasia must be distinguished from dysarthria, a difficulty of articulation. Two major cortical areas in the perisylvian region of the dominant (usually left) hemisphere are primarily responsible for language function:

a sensory or receptive area in the left parietotemporal cortex, centred on Wernicke's area (Brodmann area 22); and

a motor or expressive area in the left frontal cortex, centred on Broca's area (Brodmann area 44).

The above two are connected by the arcuate fasciculus. Lesions at different sites in this network produce different subtypes of aphasia which may be clinically delineated. Subcortical lesions may also on occasion produce an aphasia syndrome. The commonest causes of aphasia are acute cerebrovascular disease, head injury, cerebral tumours, and neurodegenerative disease (e.g. Alzheimer's disease, frontotemporal dementia).

Aphasia subtypes may be classified as follows:

- Broca's aphasia ("motor aphasia", "expressive aphasia")
  Non-fluent; preserved comprehension; impaired repetition, naming, reading, and writing; left frontal cortical lesion; if due to middle cerebral artery territory infarct there may be accompanying right hemiparesis, hemisensory loss, apraxia.
- Wernicke's aphasia ("sensory aphasia", "receptive aphasia")
  Fluent with paraphasic errors; impaired comprehension and as a consequence impaired repetition, naming, reading, and writing; left temporal cortex lesion; +/− right homonymous hemianopia.
- Global aphasia
  Combination of Broca and Wernicke-type picture, may result in mute state; may be seen in acute stage of left middle cerebral artery territory infarct, from which an aphasia more in keeping with either Broca or Wernicke type may emerge with recovery.
- Conduction aphasia
  Fluent with literal paraphasias; comprehension preserved, but marked difficulty with repetition; naming, reading, writing may be impaired; ascribed to lesion involving the arcuate fasciculus; +/− apraxia, right hemiparesis, sensory loss, or homonymous hemianopia.
- Anomic aphasia
  Fluent with circumlocutions; marked difficulty with naming; comprehension, repetition preserved.
- Transcortical motor aphasia
  Akin to Broca aphasia (non-fluent), but with marked preservation of repetition.
- Transcortical sensory aphasia
  Akin to Wernicke's aphasia (fluent), but with marked preservation of repetition.
- Pure word deafness
  Normal spontaneous speech, but impaired comprehension for spoken word and repetition, normal naming, and reading, impaired writing to dictation,

spontaneous writing normal; associated with bilateral lesions of middle part of superior temporal gyri.

- Pure word blindness (alexia without agraphia)
   Impaired naming, especially for colours, impaired reading; left medial temporo-occipital lobe lesion; may be associated with right homonymous hemianopia, memory difficulties.
- Pure alexia and agraphia
   Impaired naming, reading, and writing; lesion in left inferior parietal lobule/angular gyrus, +/− right homonymous hemianopia.
- Syndrome of the angular gyrus
   Impaired naming, reading, and writing; left angular gyrus and adjacent white matter lesion, +/− Gerstmann syndrome.
- Gerstmann syndrome
   Impaired writing, right–left disorientation, acalculia, finger agnosia; left parietal lesion.

Clinical features: history and examination In the assessment of aphasia, it is important to know the handedness of the patient, their native language, their previous level of literacy, and their level of consciousness, as all of these factors may influence the assessment of a language deficit.

Aspects of language function which should be examined include:

- Spontaneous output: fluent or non-fluent? Are there paraphrasic errors: literal or phonemic = malformed or inappropriate words (e.g. "grass" → "greel") or even neologisms ("grass" → "grumps"); semantic or verbal = right word but wrong context (e.g. "camel" → "giraffe").
- Comprehension: for single words and then simple (one step) and more complex (two step, three step) commands.
- Repetition: of single words, more complex phrases.
- Naming: ability to name objects with increasing degrees of difficulty (e.g. from high-frequency items such as "watch" to low frequency items such as "stethoscope").
- Reading: looking for evidence of alexia, including pronunciation of irregular words and comprehension of what is being read.
- Writing: looking for evidence of agraphia, both spontaneous writing and to dictation, including the spelling of irregular words.

Examination for other neurological deficits (e.g. right hemiparesis, hemisensory loss, right-sided neglect and right homonymous hemianopia).

Investigations and diagnosis *Bloods*: usually non-contributory.

Imaging: CT/MRI may help in defining the site of the lesion and its possible aetiology.

CSF: usually non-contributory.

Neurophysiology: can sometimes be of value in patients with pure word deafness, since they often complain that they are deaf, yet BSAEP are normal.

Neuropsychology: testing may be difficult to administer and interpret in patients with profound disorders of language. However it may be helpful in defining whether there are deficits other than those within the language system.

Differential diagnosis The cause of the aphasic syndrome is often obvious. The major aetiological causes are:

Vascular events, involving the left middle cerebral or left internal carotid artery; aphasia may evolve from a global to a more focal nature with recovery.

Brain trauma: often associated with a good recovery.

Brain tumours.

Neurodegenerative diseases: Alzheimer's disease, frontotemporal dementia/Pick's disease, primary progressive aphasia, semantic dementia.

Treatment and prognosis Treatment and prognosis is to a great extent dependent on the pathological cause, the symptoms and their individual severity.

Treatment has to be individualized, and is a collaborative effort involving speech therapists, neurologists, and neuropsychologists.

In general, head injury patients do better than those suffering aphasias associated with progressive neurodegenerative and neoplastic conditions.

Aphasias associated with significant impairments of auditory comprehension or speaking ability do less well when compared to patients with "partial" aphasic syndromes.

References Basso A. *Aphasia and Its Therapy*. Oxford: OUP, 2003.

Benson DF, Ardila A. *Aphasia: A Clinical Perspective*. New York: OUP, 1996.

Caplan D. Aphasic syndromes. In: Heilman KM, Valenstein E (eds). *Clinical Neuropsychology* (4th edition). Oxford: OUP, 2003: 14–34.

Damasio AR. Aphasia. *New England Journal of Medicine* 1992; **326**: 531–539.

Spreen O, Risser AH. *Assessment of Aphasia*. Oxford: OUP, 2003.

Other relevant entries Agraphia; Alexia; Alzheimer's disease; Anarthria; Aphonia; Cerebrovascular disease: arterial; Dysarthria; Gerstmann syndrome; Pick's disease; Primary progressive aphasia.

◼ Aphonia
Dysphonia

Pathophysiology Aphonia, or dysphonia, is defined as an inability or difficulty in speaking due to mechanical difficulties in generating sufficient flow of air past the vocal cords to produce sound. Speech may sound croaky, rasping, whispering, or not be produced at all, despite effort (i.e. this is not mutism). It may thus be characterized as a form of dysarthria, due to disorder of respiratory muscles and/or laryngeal function, affecting the pitch, volume, or quality of the voice; shaping of words is normal, and those with dysphonia are easily understood. The ability to comprehend and express language is unaffected (i.e. there is no aphasia); the patient knows what they want to stay and how to say it (i.e. no apraxia).

It is often due to non-organic disease when there are no associated signs or symptoms, although spasmodic dysphonia needs to be excluded in such circumstances.

Causes of aphonia or dysphonia include:

- Laryngeal disease: laryngitis, laryngeal polyps, laryngeal carcinoma.
- Bulbar lesions: may involve not only laryngeal innervation (recurrent laryngeal nerve) but other respiratory muscles and the pattern of respiration, for example extrapyramidal disorders (especially multiple system atrophy), stroke, multiple sclerosis, tumours, syringobulbia. A distinction between dysphonia and dysarthria may be made in these cases, as it is very unusual for bulbar lesions to produce a pure dysphonic syndrome.
- Peripheral nerve/neuromuscular pathology +/− associated respiratory difficulties: poliomyelitis, Guillain–Barré syndrome, myasthenia gravis. In addition, the recurrent laryngeal nerve may be damaged locally in the neck (e.g. after thyroid surgery) or chest (e.g. carcinoma of the left bronchus).
- Spasmodic dysphonia (q.v.).
- Glottic spasm: as occurs in tetany and tetanus, producing stridulous phonation.
- Hysterical: the vocal cords are usually seen to lie equidistant from the midline, in a position corresponding to quiet respiration. They do not come fully together with speech but do with coughing. The voice is weak and whispering. Symptoms are often episodic, with the recurrent attacks of dysphonia often occurring following a minor upper respiratory tract infection. Care is needed in making this diagnosis: spasmodic dysphonia patients were often considered "hysterical" before the delineation of this condition.

Investigations and diagnosis Assessments by ENT specialist (including indirect laryngoscopy), speech therapist.

Imaging: of the brainstem; chest or larynx as needed.

Treatment and prognosis Of cause, where known. Laryngitis is self-limiting; other laryngeal pathology may require surgery. For neurological conditions, see appropriate entries.

> **Other relevant entries** Aphasia; Cranial nerve disease: X: Vagus nerve; Dysarthria; Dystonia: an overview; Guillain–Barré syndrome; Multiple system atrophy; Myasthenia gravis; Poliomyelitis.

■ Apraxia

Pathophysiology Apraxia, or dyspraxia, a term introduced by Liepmann in 1900, is an inability to execute skilled or learned movements in the absence of any significant motor, sensory, coordination, or attentional deficit. Different forms of apraxia are defined: in ideomotor and ideational apraxia the patient is unable to perform gestures, despite adequate comprehension and normal (or near normal) motor and sensory functions. In such cases the lesion is usually found in the contralateral posterior parietal cortex ("posterior apraxia"), although an "anterior apraxia" has also been described with frontal lobe lesions, affecting the supplementary motor area, which leads to difficulties with tasks requiring bimanual coordination and sequencing. The diagnosis of apraxia may be overlooked in some instances unless specific tests of praxis are undertaken.

Apraxia has also been used to label other difficulties, such as "dressing apraxia" and "constructional apraxia", although these are now conceptualized as disorders of visuospatial function.

Dyspraxia is often used to label clumsy children, and is presumably a developmental problem.

Pathological causes of apraxia include:

Cerebrovascular accidents

Tumour

Neurodegeneration: corticobasal degeneration, focal parietal atrophy with other pathology (e.g. Alzheimer's disease).

Clinical features: history and examination

- Ideomotor apraxia: an inability to carry out a motor command despite near normal power, coordination and sensation. The patient is typically unable to copy gestures, and may have difficulties performing actions to command, for example show me how you use a pair of scissors, but these actions are facilitated by provision of the object (*cf.* ideational apraxia). Ideomotor apraxia is usually associated with damage to the dominant inferior posterior parietal cortex. However, it can also be seen with left hemispheric lesions involving the medial frontal lobe (with involvement of supplementary motor area) and/or basal ganglia.
- Ideational apraxia: an inability to perform a given action, as in ideomotor apraxia, but not facilitated by the provision of the object. Functionally, in terms of daily activities, ideational apraxia is usually of greater importance than ideomotor apraxia.
- Buccofacial apraxia, orofacial dyspraxia: the patient cannot perform learned, skilled movements of the mouth, lips, cheeks, tongue, and throat, such as blowing out a match, whistling, kissing, licking the lips, despite normal motor, sensory, and coordination function. They may be able to perform normally when given the real object. Buccofacial apraxia may be seen with and without ideomotor apraxia and is associated with damage to the frontal operculum.
- Gait apraxia: this name has been given to an inability to walk in the absence of any significant motor, sensory, or coordination deficits. The patient may be able to imitate walking whilst lying on the bed (e.g. pretend cycling), but once standing is unable to move; if ambulation is achieved, there is often a wide-based gait with small steps and a rocking motion, often requiring assistance. It is thought to relate to bihemispheric damage to the medial frontal lobes, and some authors prefer the term frontal gait disorder. It may be seen in normal pressure hydrocephalus, and in some patients with corticobasal degeneration.
- Oculomotor apraxia: this is an inability to move eyes either volitionally or to command, despite normal spontaneous and reflex eye movements. To compensate,

patients characteristically turn or thrust their head in the direction in which they wish to look, and on fixating the target the eyes return to the primary position ready for the next head movement. There is relative preservation of vertical eye movements. Oculomotor apraxia is usually seen in children where it may be due to congenital ocular motor apraxia or Cogan's syndrome; additional subtle neurological deficits may also be present (clumsiness, gait abnormalities). Oculomotor apraxia is also seen in ataxia–telangiectasia, Pelizaeus–Merzbacher disease, and Cockayne's syndrome. It may be difficult to distinguish oculomotor apraxia from the supranuclear gaze palsies seen in Gaucher's disease and Niemann–Pick disease type C. The exact site of the lesion producing oculomotor apraxia is not known.

- Apraxia of eyelid opening: an inability to open the eyes voluntarily, but they will nevertheless close reflexively, in response to tactile stimuli to the cornea or the area of innervation of the supraorbital branch of the trigeminal nerve (brow or bridge of the nose). Some authors deny that this is a true apraxia, and prefer to use the term "levator inhibition" to describe these phenomena. Although apraxia of eyelid opening may occur in isolation, it is commonly seen in parkinsonian syndromes, although the exact site of the lesion is not known.

Investigations and diagnosis *Neuropsychology*: the assessment of apraxia is best undertaken by an experienced neuropsychologist, but some bedside testing may be undertaken, for example:

> Show me how you would to use a hammer/a screwdriver/a pair of scissors/ toothbrush.
> Show me how to wave/salute.
> Here is a hammer/screwdriver/pair of scissors: show me how to use them.
> Copy these hand gestures (a variety of meaningful and meaningless hand postures are demonstrated that the patient has to copy).
> Show me how you blow out a match/whistle/blow a kiss.
> Here is a lit match: blow it out.

Additional investigations for a pathological cause hinge on the history and examination. Brain imaging (CT/MRI) is often required in the search for vascular, neoplastic, or degenerative pathology.

Treatment and prognosis Of cause where established, if possible. Apraxias may lead to significant functional impairment, not amenable to specific treatment. Neurorehabilitation techniques may be helpful.

References Freund HJ. The apraxias. In: Kennard C (ed.). *Recent Advances in Clinical Neurology 8*. Edinburgh: Churchill Livingstone, 1995: 29–49.

Heilman KM, Gonzalez Rothi LJ. Apraxia. In: Heilman KM, Valenstein E (eds). *Clinical Neuropsychology* (4th edition). Oxford: OUP, 2003: 215–235.

Robertson IH. The rehabilitation of visuospatial, visuoperceptual, and apraxic disorders. In: Greenwood RJ, Barnes MP, McMillan TM, Ward CD (eds). *Handbook of Neurological Rehabilitation* (2nd edition). Hove: Psychology Press, 2003: 403–415.

Other relevant entries Agraphia; Aphasia; Blepharospasm; Cogan's syndrome (1); Corticobasal degeneration; Gait disorders.

▪ Aprosencephaly – see Anencephaly

▪ Aqueduct stenosis – see Hydrocephalus

▪ Arachnoid cyst

Pathophysiology Arachnoid cysts are cystic areas bounded by arachnoid membranes; they may occur above or below the tentorium but the commonest site is in the middle cranial fossa. They are congenital (developmental) in origin, secondary to arachnoid maldevelopment, with trapping of arachnoid membrane, often with a one-way valve which communicates with the ventricular CSF system.

Arachnoid cysts are often noted as incidental findings on CT or MRI scanning, but rarely cause symptoms themselves. They can occasionally be symptomatic when they enlarge sufficiently to compress neighbouring structures, and they are associated with a slightly increased risk of subdural haematoma.

Clinical features: history and examination

- Usually asymptomatic, incidental findings on structural brain imaging.
- Headache: may occur with a large cyst in the posterior fossa.
- Subdural haematoma.
- Local compressive symptoms, especially when they originate in the posterior fossa.
- In children they may cause macrocrania.
- Occasionally arachnoid cysts may be found in the suprasellar region where they present in childhood with bobbing and nodding of the head, the so-called "bobble head doll syndrome".
- Occasionally arachnoid cysts have been implicated in cognitive decline.

Investigations and diagnosis *Bloods*: normal.

Imaging: cranial CT/MRI reveals the cyst, most commonly at the anterior pole of the temporal lobe.

CSF: not indicated.

Neurophysiology: non-contributory.

Differential diagnosis If local compression occurs, the differential diagnosis is that of a space-occupying lesion.

Treatment and prognosis They are usually found by chance with imaging; patient reassurance as to their non-malignant, non-progressive nature may be required. If there are focal neurological effects then surgical intervention may be required.

References Shaw C-M, Alvord EC. "Congenital arachnoid" cysts and their differential diagnosis. In: Vinken PJ, Bruyn GW (eds). *Handbook of Clinical Neurology. Volume 31 Congenital Malformations of the Brain and Skull, Part II*. Amsterdam: North-Holland Publishing, 1976: 75–135.

Eustace S, Toland J, Stack J. CT and MRI of arachnoid cyst with complicating intra-cystic and subdural haemorrhage. *Journal of Computer Assisted Tomography* 1992; **16**: 995–997.

Other relevant entries Bobble head doll syndrome; Cysts: an overview; Tumours: an overview.

■ Arachnoiditis

Chronic adhesive arachnoiditis • Idiopathic progressive ascending adhesive arachnoiditis • Meningitis circumscripta spinalis

Pathophysiology Arachnoiditis literally means inflammation of the arachnoid, but in clinical practice the term is used to refer to meningeal scarring (fibrosis) as a consequence of injury or inflammation. There may be subsequent obliteration of the subarachnoid space, adhesions between the cord and dura, and occasionally the development of calcification and ossification (arachnoiditis ossificans). These changes may lead to cord compression. Clumping and adhesion of spinal roots (+/− arachnoid cyst development) may cause further compression. Blood vessel involvement may lead to ischaemia with myelomalacia and cavitations in the cord, which may coalesce to form syringomyelia.

The initiating injury may take various forms, including a prolapsed disc, spinal surgery, or the presence of foreign material in the subarachnoid space such as blood, infection, intrathecal drugs, and radiological contrast dyes used in myelography (particularly Myodil). The advent of improved contrast dyes, MR spinal imaging, better surgical techniques and treatment of spinal infection has meant that arachnoiditis has become much less common. It typically affects men in the fifth and sixth decades of life and presents with lumbosacral radiculopathies. Diagnosis and treatment of this condition is difficult.

Clinical features: history and examination

- Usually occurs between the ages of 40–60 years; M > F. There is often a long latent period between insult and symptom onset, up to 25 years. Many cases are asymptomatic.
- Spinal root involvement: low back pain that worsens with exercise, with lumbosacral radiculopathy that is usually recurrent and bilateral, often causing a cauda equina syndrome.
- Spinal cord compression and ischaemia: this is now relatively rare, but patients used to present with thoracic cord involvement and paraparesis/paraplegia.
- Presentation with syringomyelia may still occur. An anterior spinal artery infarction syndrome secondary to fibrosis and vessel involvement may occur.
- Idiopathic progressive ascending adhesive arachnoiditis: a rare condition that usually leads to death after 5–10 years. It presents with a painful progressive cauda equina syndrome, which then progresses to involve the conus and spinal cord in an ascending fashion. Clinically there is a painful ascending severe paraplegia with sensory loss, muscle wasting and weakness with upper motor neurone features, and autonomic dysfunction.

Investigations and diagnosis *Bloods*: usually normal.

Imaging: ideally MRI (not myelography). This may demonstrate adherent roots +/− thickening of the meninges with little or no enhancement following gadolinium.

CSF: may reveal a mildly elevated protein and occasional pleocytosis.

Neurophysiology: may reveal radiculopathy.

Differential diagnosis

Tumour.

Malignant meningitis.

Arachnoiditis may contribute to the neurological complications in ankylosing spondylitis.

Treatment and prognosis The treatment of arachnoiditis is difficult and controversial. Optimum treament is probably conservative with analgesics; carbamazepine, tricyclic antidepressants, and TENS; anti-inflammatory agents are usually not helpful. Surgical intervention is usually ineffective. Patients often have significant morbidity, although rarely die from their condition unless there is significant cord involvement.

> **References** Caplan LR, Noronha AB, Amico LL. Syringomyelia and arachnoiditis. *Journal of Neurology, Neurosurgery and Psychiatry* 1990; **53**: 106–113.
>
> Jellinek E. Myodil arachnoiditis: iatrogenic and forensic illness. *Practical Neurology* 2002; **2**: 237–239.
>
> **Other relevant entries** Ankylosing spondylitis and the nervous system; Anterior spinal artery syndrome; Cauda equina syndrome and conus medullaris disease; Failed back syndrome; Lumbar cord and root disease; Syringomyelia and syringobulbia.

■ Arbovirus disease

Arboviruses are RNA viruses which are probably the commonest cause of encephalitis worldwide, different types occurring in different geographical areas. The name derives from the fact that they are arthropod-borne: many cycle through mosquitoes. Examples include:

- Flaviviruses
  - Dengue
  - St Louis encephalitis virus
  - Japanese encephalitis virus
  - Murray Valley encephalitis virus (Australian X disease)
  - Tick-borne encephalitis virus
  - Louping ill
  - West Nile virus.
- Bunyaviruses
  - Rift Valley Fever virus
- Alphaviruses
  - Eastern equine encephalitis virus
  - Western equine encephalitis virus.

> **Other relevant entries** Dengue; Encephalitis: an overview.

■ Arginase deficiency; Argininosuccinic acid lyase deficiency; Argininosuccinic acid synthetase deficiency; Argininosuccinic aciduria – see Urea cycle enzyme defects

■ Argyll Robertson pupil

The Argyll Robertson pupil (ARP) is small and irregular, with a variable degree of atrophy of the iris, and fails to react to a light stimulus but does constrict to accommodation albeit slowly (i.e. there is light-near dissociation). ARPs also fail to dilate fully in response to mydriatic drugs. Usually both pupils are involved although often asymmetrically. A distinction is sometimes made with "pseudo-ARPs" in which light-near dissociation is seen but there is no miosis or pupillary irregularity.

ARPs are classically seen in late neurosyphilis, but have also been described in a variety of other conditions, including sarcoidosis, diabetes mellitus, syringobulbia, and multiple sclerosis. The localization of the lesion responsible for ARP is uncertain, but the region of the rostral midbrain, proximal to the oculomotor nuclei, is sometimes implicated.

Reference Miller NR. *Walsh and Hoyt's Clinical Neuro-ophthalmology* (4th edition). Baltimore: Williams & Wilkins, 1985: 483–487.

Other relevant entries Cranial nerve disease: II: Optic nerve; Syphilis.

■ Argyrophilic grain disease
Braak disease

This disorder is characterized morphologically on the basis of abundant neuropathological grains, consisting of abnormally phosphorylated τ-protein, mainly in the CA1 subfield of the cornu ammonis, entorhinal and transentorhinal cortices, amygdala, and hypothalamic lateral tuberal nucleus. Neurofibrillary tangles are also present in entorhinal and limbic areas, but are less prominent than in symptomatic Alzheimer's disease (AD). Oligodendroglial τ-filamentous inclusions (coiled bodies) are also seen. Clinically, argyrophilic grain disease (AGD) is a dementing disorder but with more prominent behavioural features and less prominent memory problems than in AD. Hence some authors consider it distinct from AD.

References Braak H, Braak E. Argyrophilic grain disease: frequency of occurrence in different age categories and neuropathological diagnostic criteria. *Journal of Neural Transmission* 1998; **105**: 801–819.

Tolnay M, Monsch AU, Probst A. Argyrophilic grain disease. A frequent dementing disorder in aged patients. *Advances in Experimental Medicine and Biology* 2001; **487**: 39–58.

Other relevant entry Alzheimer's disease.

■ Arhinencephaly

Arhinencephaly is a developmental anomaly characterized by absence of the olfactory bulbs, tracts, and tubercles. This may occur in isolation, as in Kallmann's syndrome (X-linked or autosomal-dominant hypogonadotrophic hypogonadism) or as part of a more extensive developmental malformation such as holoprosencephaly or septo-optic dysplasia.

Reference Kobori JA, Herrick MK, Urich H. Arhinencephaly. *Brain* 1987; **110**: 237–260.

Other relevant entries Holoprosencephaly; Kallmann's syndrome; Septo-optic dysplasia.

▓ Armadillo syndrome – see Isaacs syndrome; Neuromyotonia

▓ Arnold–Chiari malformations – see Chiari malformations

▓ Arnold's neuralgia – see Occipital neuralgia

▓ ARSACS – see Cerebellar disease: an overview; Charlevoix–Saguenay syndrome

▓ Arsenic toxicity – see Heavy metal poisoning

▓ Arteriovenous malformations of the brain

Pathophysiology Arteriovenous malformations (AVMs) of the central nervous system (CNS) are formed from the abnormal development of blood vessels. Their classification is based on morphology and the location of the nidus or fistula. The key feature is arteriovenous shunting of blood, a *sine qua non* which excludes other intracranial vascular malformations such as cavernomas. Since most published series are small, retrospective, hospital based, and lack adequate radiological investigation, conclusions about the frequency, clinical presentation, and prognosis of AVMs are subject to many biases. However, the incidence of AVMs is probably around 1/100 000 per year in an unselected population, with a point prevalence of around 18/100 000 in adults. AVMs vary in size, from a few millimetres to several centimetres, and location. The commonest presenting features are haemorrhage and epilepsy. A number of treatment modalities are suggested (embolization, surgical resection, stereotactic radiotherapy) but none have been subjected to randomized-controlled trials.

On morphological grounds, AVMs may be distinguished as:

cortical;
deep (basal ganglia, thalamus, central white matter, brainstem);
choroid plexus.

Non-traumatic AVMs are probably present from birth but usually present after 10 and before 50 years of age. Sexes are equally affected. AVMs may be associated with saccular cerebral aneurysms, especially in elderly patients with a large AVM.

Clinical features: history and examination

- The majority of AVMs (two-thirds) present with haemorrhage, half with primary intracerebral haemorrhage (PICH) (>subarachnoid haemorrhage (SAH) >intraventricular haemorrhage). AVMs may account for 1–2% of all strokes, and perhaps 4% in young adults; 9% of SAHs; and about 4% of all PICH, but possibly one-third of PICH in young adults.
- The second commonest presentation is with seizures (20%); AVMs are not a common cause of first presentations with unprovoked seizures (1%).
- Perhaps 15% of AVMs are asymptomatic at the time of detection (brain imaging for some other reason, for example to "reassure" someone about the benign nature of their tension-type headache).
- Progressive neurological deficit can occur with large or strategically placed AVMs (e.g. myelopathy with spinal AVM).
- Rarely, hydrocephalus can develop if the vein of Galen is involved with the AVM. However a more common cause for hydrocephalus is basal meningeal fibrosis secondary to SAH.
- Headache, particularly persistently unilateral migraine, was thought to be a common presentation; in fact, only 0.3% of patients with headache without focal neurological signs harbour an AVM; for migraineurs the figure is 0.07%.
- A bruit may be heard in cases of AVM, over the carotid arteries or eyeballs, especially in young patients after exercise.
- Retinal and cutaneous vascular malformations may be found in patients with AVMs of the CNS and they may be in communication with the centrally placed vascular abnormality.

Investigations and diagnosis *Bloods*: usually all normal.

Imaging: CT with contrast will visualize most AVMs but MRI is more reliable. Although MRA can demonstrate some of the anatomy of AVMs, catheter angiography still remains the investigation of choice to define the origin and extent of arterial supply, and the venous drainage, of AVMs.

CSF: may confirm SAH.

Differential diagnosis Other causes of:

intracranial haemorrhage,
focal seizures,
progressive myelopathy.

Treatment and prognosis Studies of the natural history of AVMs suggest an annual risk of first-ever haemorrhage of about 2%, but the recurrence rate is possibly as high as 18% in the first year. The annual risk of developing *de novo* seizures is around 1%, with good prospects for control with anti-epileptic medications. The long-term crude annual fatality rate is approximately 1–1.5%; 50–70% of deaths are due to haemorrhage. Owing to these risks, palliative treatment would seem to be desirable, and a number of treatment modalities have evolved. The three main options are surgical excision, stereotactic radiotherapy and endovascular embolization. However, there are no randomized-controlled trials of any of these in isolation, let alone in comparison. Some large AVMs located in critical sites (e.g. motor cortex) are not amenable to any treatment.

Surgical excision	Stereotactic radiotherapy	Embolization
Procedure		
Open surgical procedure in which the feeding and draining vessels are ligated and the whole AVM removed.	Radiotherapy is delivered stereotactically to the AVM by either a gamma knife or particle beam irradiation. This induces necrosis and fibrosis with obliteration of the AVM.	Under screening, intra-arterial catheters are placed in the major feeding vessels of the AVM, and embolization achieved by the introduction of "coils" or rapidly setting "glues".
Risks		
2–5% mortality rate 5–25% morbidity rate		
Indications		
Superficial location (and this includes cavernomas). Sometimes this option is followed after partial embolization when the AVM is large.	AVMs < 2.5 cm in diameter usually; larger AVMs can be reduced in size by this therapy but not totally obliterated. Elderly or sick patients too unwell for neurosurgery. AVMs located in critical CNS sites.	AVMs with a few, well-defined, arterial feeding vessels.
Outcome		
The vast majority are completely excised.	Angiographic obliteration occurs in 70–88% of cases. If re-treatment of the patient is felt necessary, a period of 3 years must have elapsed from the first treatment.	

References Al-Shahi R, Warlow CP. A systematic review of the frequency and prognosis of arteriovenous malformations of the brain in adults. *Brain* 2001; **124**: 1900–1926.

Mohr JP. Arteriovenous malformations. In: Hennerici M, Meairs S (eds). *Cerebrovascular Ultrasound: Theory, Practice and Future Developments.* Cambridge: CUP, 2001: 280–296.

Other relevant entries Aneurysm; Cavernoma, cavernous haemagioma; Cerebrovascular disease: arterial; Epilepsy: an overview; Intracerebral haemorrhage; Intracranial vascular malformations: an overview; Migraine; Spinal cord vascular diseases; Subarachnoid haemorrhage; Von Hippel–Lindau disease.

▦ Arteritis – see Vasculitis

▦ Arthrogryposis multiplex congenita

Pathophysiology A syndrome of infants with multiple non-progressive joint contractures, of variable aetiology but often associated with limitations of fetal movement. Although in the majority of cases the cause is unknown, identified causes include genetic factors, intrauterine factors limiting fetal movement, and maternal myasthenia gravis.

Clinical features
- Multiple non-progressive joint contractures (arthrogryposis).
- +/− Polyhydramnios.
- Small palate, jaws.
- Lung hypoplasia.
- Neonatal or prenatal death.

Investigations and diagnosis Diagnosis usually evident. Occasionally occurs in infants of mothers without myasthenia but in whom anti-AChR antibodies are found.

Differential diagnosis Arthrogryposis may occur in neuromuscular disorders such as Emery–Dreifuss syndrome, but not evident at birth.

Treatment and prognosis May cause neonatal or prenatal death.

Reference Vincent A, Newland C, Brueton L *et al*. Arthrogryposis multiplex congenita with maternal autoantibodies specific for a fetal antigen. *Lancet* 1995; **346**: 24–25.

Other relevant entry Myasthenia gravis.

▦ Arylsulphatase A deficiency – see Metachromatic leukodystrophy

▦ Arylsulphatase B deficiency – see Maroteaux–Lamy disease

▦ ASAN – see Gangliosides and neurological disorders; Guillain–Barré syndrome

▦ Ascariasis – see Helminthic diseases

▦ Aseptic meningitis: differential diagnosis

Aseptic meningitis may be defined as a syndrome of clinical meningism with an inflammatory CSF (leukocytosis) but with no organism identified (e.g. by Gram stain,

Ziehl–Nielsen stain, culture, polymerase chain reaction). The differential diagnosis is broad:

Partially treated bacterial meningitis
Viral meningitis or meningoencephalitis
Tuberculous meningitis
Fungal meningitis
Other bacterial/protozoal infections: brucellosis, leptospirosis, malaria
Parameningeal infection: epidural/subdural abscess/empyema
Chemical meningitis: blood (subarachnoid haemorrhage), drugs, myelographic agents
Endocarditis
Malignant meningitis: carcinoma, lymphoma, leukaemia
Venous sinus thrombosis
Autoimmune disorders: vasculitis, Behçet's disease
Sarcoidosis
Mollaret's (recurrent) meningitis: dermoid, epidermoid
Chronic (benign) lymphocytic meningitis.

Reference Hopkins AP, Harvey PKP. Chronic benign lymphocytic meningitis. *Journal of the Neurological Sciences* 1973; **18**: 443–453.

Other relevant entries Meningitis: an overview; Tuberculosis and the nervous system.

■ Aspartoacylase deficiency – see Canavan's disease

■ Aspartylglycosaminuria

A rare lysosomal-storage disease, recessively inherited, with the clinical features including:

psychomotor regression;
delayed speech;
behavioural disturbance;
progressive dementia;
corticospinal tract signs;
retinal abnormalities, cataracts;
coarse facies, thick lips and skin.

Blood may show vacuolated lymphocytes.

Other relevant entry Lysosomal-storage disorders: an overview.

■ Asperger's syndrome

In 1944 Asperger described a group of children with a mild autistic syndrome, often developing around 3 years of age. The diagnostic criteria for this condition suggested by the American Psychiatric Association (DSM 299.80) include:

- Impaired social interaction: impaired use of non-verbal behaviours (eye-to-eye gaze, facial expression, body posture); failure to develop peer relationships; lack of spontaneous seeking to share enjoyment; lack of social or emotional reciprocity.
- Restricted repetitive and stereotyped patterns of behaviour; inflexible adherence to routines, rituals; mannerisms.
- Disturbance causes clinically significant impairment of social, occupational or other important area of functioning.
- No significant delay in language or cognitive development; patients may develop idiosyncratic and highly intellectual interests ("little professor").
- No evidence of pervasive developmental disorder or schizophrenia.

Some authors suggest that this diagnosis is unlikely or impossible as all patients qualify for the alternative diagnosis of autism since a communication impairment is present.

The condition probably has a genetic basis, but this remains obscure. All investigations are usually normal and the treatment is generally behavioural in nature.

References David RB, David CH, Riley LS. Asperger's and related disorders. *Practical Neurology* 2003; **3**: 150–159.

Volkmar FR, Klin A, Schultz RT, Rubin E, Bronen R. Asperger's disorder. *American Journal of Psychiatry* 2000; **157**: 262–267.

Other relevant entries Autism, autistic disorder; Psychiatric disorders and neurological disease.

◼ Aspergillosis

This fungal infection (*Aspergillus fumigatus*) may present as a chronic sinusitis with skull base osteomyelitis, with involvement of cranial nerves adjacent to infected bone. Brain abscess and granuloma are recorded, but not meningitis, although meningomyelitis, through invasion of the spinal epidural space via intervertebral foramina, may occur. Stroke-like syndromes from vasculitis or disseminated infection may occur: immunocompromised individuals, for example following organ transplantation, are particularly vulnerable.

Diagnosis is by culture of the organism, or identification on biopsy specimens; there are no reliable serodiagnostic markers. CSF may show pleocytosis, elevated protein, but normal glucose. Treatment is with amphotericin $+/-$ 5-flucytosine.

Reference Marr KA, Patterson T, Denning D. Aspergillosis. Pathogenesis, clinical manifestations and therapy. *Infectious Disease Clinics of North America* 2002; **16**: 875–894.

◼ Astrocytoma

Astrocytomas are tumours of neuroectodermal origin, most cells containing glial fibrillary acidic protein (GFAP), which fall within the rubric of glioma. Histologically several types are described (fibrillary, pilocytic, protoplasmic, gemistocytic, pleo-morphic xanthoastrocytomas) but the histological features do not correlate well with prognosis.

Other relevant entries Glioma; Tumours: an overview.

Ataxia

Ataxia is a lack of coordination (rate, range, timing, direction, force) of voluntary motor acts, impairing their smooth performance. This may arise from deficits in various neuroanatomical systems, and so needs to be qualified accordingly (if possible), as:

- Cerebellar ataxia: defective timing of contraction of agonist and antagonist muscles (asynergia, dyssynergia) resulting in jerky, staggering, inaccurate move-ments with disturbed rate, rhythm and force (decomposition of movement), such as intention tremor, dysmetria (past pointing), dysdiadochokinesia, ataxic dysarthria, excessive rebound phenomenon, macrographia, head tremor (tituba-tion), gait ataxia, and abnormal eye movements (nystagmus, square-wave jerks, saccadic intrusions). There may be concurrent limb hypotonia. Cerebellar hemi-sphere lesions cause ipsilateral limb ataxia (hemiataxia) whereas midline cerebel-lar lesions involving the vermis produce selective truncal and gait ataxia.

- Sensory ataxia: due to impaired proprioception, with pseudo-athetosis, and markedly exacerbated by removal of visual cues (e.g. in Romberg's sign). Causes include disease of spinal cord dorsal (posterior) columns (hence "spinal ataxia"; e.g. syphilis), sensory neuropathies, and neuronopathies affecting the dorsal root ganglia.

- Optic ataxia: misreaching (dysmetria) for visually presented targets due to a parieto-occipital lesion (e.g. as in Balint's syndrome).

- "Frontal ataxia" is similar to cerebellar ataxia, but results from damage to the con-tralateral frontal cortex or frontopontine fibres which run in the corticopontocere-bellar tract, synapsing in the pons before passing through the middle cerebellar peduncle to the contralateral cerebellar hemisphere.

Reference Klockgether T (ed.). *Handbook of Ataxia Disorders.* New York: Marcel Dekker, 2000.

Larner AJ. *A Dictionary of Neurological Signs: Clinical Neurosemiology.* Dordrecht: Kluwer, 2001: 29–30.

Other relevant entries Balint syndrome; Cerebellar disease: an overview; Paraneoplastic syndrome; Syphilis.

Ataxia telangiectasia
Louis–Bar disease • Louis–Bar syndrome

Pathophysiology Ataxia telangiectasia (AT) is a rare autosomal-recessive condition in which there is defective DNA repair as a consequence of mutations in the ATM gene on chromosome 11, which results in a progressive ataxia with loss of cerebellar

Purkinje cells (possibly due to a failure to protect cells from oxidative stress). ATM is a protein kinase with critical signalling roles in the cellular response to ionizing radiation. Immunological deficiency leads to a susceptibility to pyogenic infection and tumour development. AT may be regarded as a chromosome instability syndrome (along with Fanconi's anaemia, Bloom syndrome, Nijmegen breakage syndrome and AT-like disorder). Patients usually present before the age of 10 years with a progressive motor disorder and a characteristic oculomotor apraxia. At a later stage they develop telangiectasia.

Clinical features: history and examination

- Initial development is usually normal, problems becoming apparent when the child learns to walk.
- Ataxia of gait: typically develops between the ages of 12–18 months; by age 10 years patients are usually unable to walk. The initial presentation may be complicated by athetosis with occasional myoclonic jerks. Progressive dystonia of the fingers may emerge with development.
- Oculomotor apraxia: an impairment of voluntary ocular motility, such that to move the eyes an abrupt head thrust may be required. Disordered smooth pursuit and limitation of upgaze may also occur.
- Dysarthria and drooling due to the cerebellar and extrapyramidal involvement.
- A peripheral polyneuropathy with distal muscular atrophy may be seen in adult patients, as may involvement of spinal cord dorsal columns with loss of proprioception.
- Recurrent infections, especially sinopulmonary, are a major feature. Children tend to be small and underweight. Bronchopulmonary infections may progress to bronchiectasis and atrophy of the secondary lymphoid organs.
- Cutaneous features: telangiectasia develops after the ataxia (3–6 years), and are seen on the conjunctiva and skin (ears, exposed parts of the neck, nose, and cheek in a butterfly pattern, flexor creases of forearm). Hypertrichosis and infrequent grey hairs are also a feature.
- 10–15% of patients develop malignancy in early adulthood, usually T-cell tumours. Many other tumour types have also been reported in AT.
- Significant neuropsychological impairments are unusual; mild mental retardation may occur.

Investigations and diagnosis

Bloods: standard blood tests are normal, but there is usually a raised α-fetoprotein (90%), and hypogammaglobulinaemia (80%); selective deficiency of the IgG2 subclass is characteristic.

Imaging: CT/MRI: cerebellar atrophy with relative sparing of cerebral cortex.

CSF: normal.

Neurophysiology: EMG/NCS: may show a peripheral polyneuropathy.

Neurogenetics: numerous mutations have been identified in the gene *ATM* at chromosome 11q22.23.

Other: cultured fibroblasts have increased radiosensitivity due to faulty repair of DNA.

Pathology: striking loss of cerebellar Purkinje cells, degenerative changes in dentate and inferior olivary nucleus; loss of myelinated fibres in the dorsal columns, spinocerebellar tracts and peripheral nerves; degenerative changes in the dorsal roots, with cell loss in the sympathetic ganglia and some anterior horn cell loss.

Differential diagnosis Young onset cerebellar syndromes. The differential diagnosis for the eye movement disorder includes:

Cogan's congenital oculomotor apraxia
Niemann–Pick type C
Gaucher's disease.

Treatment and prognosis There is no specific treatment. Infections should be treated; postural drainage for bronchiectasis. The disease is relentlessly progressive; survival into adulthood is rare. The usual cause of death is intercurrent bronchopulmonary infection or neoplasia, usually during the second decade of life. Routine surveillance for leukaemia/lymphoma is recommended.

Reference Spacey SD, Gatti RA, Bebb G. The molecular basis and clinical management of ataxia telangiectasia. *Canadian Journal of Neurological Science* 2000; **27**: 184–191.

Other relevant entries Apraxia; Cerebellar disease: an overview; Chorea; Cockayne's syndrome; Cogan's syndrome (1); Dystonia: an overview; Gaucher's disease; Myoclonus, Niemann–Pick disease; Xeroderma pigmentosa and related conditions.

■ Ataxia with oculomotor apraxia – see Cerebellar disease: an overview; Early-onset ataxia with ocular motor apraxia with hypoalbuminaemia

■ Ataxia with vitamin E deficiency

*A*taxia with isolated *v*itamin *E d*eficiency (AVED) is a rare autosomal-recessive disorder with deficiency of vitamin E but without evidence of fat malabsorption and with normal lipoproteins (*cf.* abetalipoproteinaemia). Clinically the features are of progressive cerebellar ataxia, proprioceptive sensory loss (axonal peripheral neuropathy), tendon areflexia, extensor plantar responses, dysarthria, scoliosis, pes cavus, with or without a cardiomyopathy. The features are thus identical to Friedreich's ataxia, emphasizing the importance of measuring vitamin E levels in any progressive ataxia. The mutant gene for AVED has been mapped to chromosome 8q and encodes α-tocopherol, a transfer protein which incorporates tocopherol into very low-density lipoproteins. The condition may be treated with vitamin E supplements, but clinical efficacy is uncertain.

Acquired vitamin E deficiency, for example associated with prolonged fat malabsorption, may be associated with similar neurological features (cerebellar ataxia, spinal cord syndrome, peripheral neuropathy).

Reference Ouahchi K, Arita M, Kayden H *et al*. Ataxia with isolated vitamin E deficiency is caused by mutations in the alpha-tocopherol transfer protein. *Nature Genetics* 1995; **9**: 141–145.

Other relevant entries Abetalipoproteinaemia; Cerebellar disease: an overview; Friedreich's ataxia; Vitamin deficiencies and the nervous system.

▨ Ataxic hemiparesis – see Lacunar syndromes

▨ Athetosis

Athetosis is an involuntary movement disorder in which there are slow twisting writhing movements of the limbs, especially apparent distally. It often coexists with the more flowing, dance-like movements of chorea and is most commonly seen in choreoathetoid cerebral palsy. It may be regarded as a form of dystonia.

Other relevant entries Cerebral palsy, cerebral palsy syndromes; Chorea; Dystonia: an overview.

▨ Atlantoaxial dislocation, subluxation

Dislocation or subluxation of the atlantoaxial articulation often results from failure of the stabilizing function of the odontoid peg of C2. This may occur in:

Cervical trauma
Congenital malformation
Rheumatoid arthritis
Down's syndrome
Ankylosing spondylitis
Foramen magnum lesions
Grisel syndrome
Morquio's disease.

The resulting cord compression results in myelopathy or medullary compression, sometimes resulting in sudden death.

Other relevant entries Cervical cord and root disease; Diastematomyelia.

▨ Atypical facial pain
Idiopathic facial pain

Atypical facial pain is the name given to a syndrome of poorly localized unilateral or bilateral facial pain, often over the cheek or nose, lasting weeks or years, provoked by stress or fatigue, largely unresponsive to typical analgesics, without abnormal neurological signs and for which no structural cause is found. Anxiety, depression and other bodily pains are associated factors. Diagnostic criteria are lacking (some consider it a diagnosis of exclusion) which makes epidemiological surveys difficult, but it is generally agreed to be much commoner in women, occurring usually in the fourth to sixth decades. Treatment is with a tricyclic antidepresant such as amitriptyline or nortriptyline, which may need to be continued for up to 2 years.

Other relevant entry Facial pain: differential diagnosis.

■ "Atypical pneumonias" and the nervous system

The term "atypical pnemonia" has been used to describe pneumonia which, in contrast to typical pneumonia, is characterized by relatively gradual onset, dry cough, shortness of breath, and prominent extrapulmonary symptoms including headache, encephalopathy, myalgia, fatigue, nausea, vomiting, and diarrhoea. Agents considered to be causes of atypical pneumonia include:

Mycoplasma pneumoniae
Chlamydia psittaci (psittacosis)
Coxiella burnetti (Q fever)
Legionella pneumophila (Legionnaires' disease)
Francisella tularensis (tularaemia)
Histoplasma capsulatum
Coccidiodes immitis

as well as others, such as Influenza A virus. These agents may account for up to one-third of pneumonias, for which reason it has been suggested that the term "atypical" be dropped.

These conditions may be accompanied by neurological features.

Other relevant entries Legionnaires' disease; Mycoplasma; Psittacosis; Q fever.

■ Austin disease
Juvenile sulphatidosis ● Multiple sulphatase deficiency

This very rare autosomal-recessive condition, occurring mostly in children, results from multiple sulphatase deficiency, the clinical features being:
- Metachromatic leukodystrophy (arylsulphatase A deficiency).
- Dysostosis multiplex, hepatosplenomegaly (deficiency of mucopolysaccharide sulphatases).
- Ichthyosis (steroid sulphatase deficiency).
This condition may be classified with the mucopolysaccharidoses.

Other relevant entries Leukodystrophies: an overview; Metachromatic leukodystrophy; Mucopolysaccharidoses.

■ Autism, autistic disorder

Kanner syndrome

Pathophysiology The essential features of autism are:

- markedly abnormal or impaired development of social interaction and communication (both verbal and non-verbal skills);
- a restricted repertoire of activities and interests;
- onset before 3 years of age.

In most cases there is associated mental retardation which may range from mild to profound. The condition is much commoner in males. The pathogenesis is not understood; whether this is primarily a neuropsychiatric disorder is debated.

Clinical features: history and examination

- DSM-IV diagnostic criteria require:
  - Qualitative impairment in social interaction.
  - Qualitative impairments in communication.
  - Restricted repetitive and stereotyped patterns of behaviour, interests, and activities.
- Stereotyped body movements (clapping, rocking, swaying), and abnormalities of posture may occur.
- Although the development of cognitive skills is abnormal, abilities are uneven (verbal skills typically weaker than non-verbal), and some may be excellent or even prodigious (e.g. calendar calculation; savant syndrome); long-term memory may be excellent (e.g. train timetables) but the information repeated irrespective of its relevance to social context.
- Behavioural features: impulsivity, aggression, temper tantrums, catastrophic reactions to minor changes in expected routine, eating disorders.

Investigations and diagnosis Although brain imaging studies and EEG may be abnormal, changes are non-specific. Diagnosis therefore rests on history and examination. Other investigations may be undertaken to exclude other diagnoses, such as Rett's syndrome.

Differential diagnosis Asperger's syndrome: no mental retardation.

Rett's syndrome (females only).

Pervasive developmental disorder.

Schizophrenia with childhood onset.

Autism may be observed in association with another neurological condition (e.g. fragile X syndrome, tuberous sclerosis).

Treatment and prognosis No specific treatment is currently known.

> **Reference** Filipek PA, Accardo PJ, Asinwal S *et al*. Practice parameter: screening and diagnosis of autism. Report of the Quality Standards Subcommittee of the American Academy of Neurology and the Child Neurology Society. *Neurology* 2000; **55**: 465–479.
>
> Rapin I. Autism. *New England Journal of Medicine* 1997; **337**: 97–104.
>
> Wing L. The autistic spectrum. *Lancet* 1997; **350**: 1761–1766.
>
> **Other relevant entries** Asperger's syndrome; Rett's syndrome; Savant syndrome.

■ Autonomic failure

Pathophysiology The autonomic nervous system (ANS) is composed of two major components: the sympathetic and parasympathetic nervous systems. They have a common origin from the hypothalamus and are involved with the homeostatic mechanisms maintaining cardiovascular stability as well as providing the neural input to visceral structures. There is a close functional relationship with the endocrine system that is similarly largely controlled from the hypothalamus.

Disorders of the ANS may be due either to central or peripheral damage, disease, or interference from pharmacological agents.

Organizational physiology of sympathetic and parasympathetic nervous systems

Organ	Parasympathetic system		Sympathetic system	
	Origin of input	Action on organ	Origin of input	Action on organ
Eye	III cranial nerve (via ciliary ganglion)	Pupillary constriction Accommodation	T1–T2	Pupillary dilatation Minimal retraction of eyelid through innervation of tarsal muscle
Salivary glands	VII and IX cranial nerves (salivatory nuclei via sphenopalatine, otic and sub-mandibular ganglia)	Stimulation of salivary secretion and vasodilatation Tear formation	T1–T2	Reduce salivary secretions
Heart	X cranial nerve (dorsal vagal nucleus)	Reduces rate and force of cardiac contraction	T1–T6	Increases the rate and force of cardiac contraction
Bronchial tree	X cranial nerve (dorsal vagal nucleus)	Broncho-constriction and stimulation of bronchial secretions	T3–T5	Broncho-dilatation and inhibition of bronchial secretions
Stomach/ small intestine/ large intestine	X cranial nerve (dorsal vagal nucleus)	Increase in peri-staltic rate and tone of smooth muscle Relaxes sphincters Stimulates secretions	T5–T12	Inhibit peristalsis Contraction of sphincters Inhibits secretions

(Continued)

Organ	Parasympathetic system		Sympathetic system	
	Origin of input	Action on organ	Origin of input	Action on organ
Bladder and sexual function	Sacral parasympathetic nerves (S2–S4, this also innervates part of the large intestine)	Contraction of bladder detrusor muscle Erection	T12–L3	Contract muscles in trigone of bladder Ejaculation
Adrenal gland	–	–	T8–T11	Stimulation of catecholamine release (the adrenal medulla is the post-ganglionic process)
Skin/ peripheral blood vessels	–	–	T1–T3	Vasoconstriction in skin and vaso-dilatation in muscles Contraction of smooth muscle in hair follicle causes piloerection Stimulates secretion of sweat from sweat glands (but the sympathetic fibres at this site release ACh not NA)

- Causes of autonomic failure include:
    - Central causes:
        - Primary autonomic failure (PAF)
        - Multiple system atrophy (MSA)
        - Idiopathic Parkinson's disease (PD)
        - Structural lesions involving the hypothalamus and brainstem in the region of the fourth ventricle, spinal cord lesions.
    - Peripheral causes:
        - Diabetes mellitus
        - Amyloidosis
        - Alcohol

Guillain–Barré syndrome

Connective tissue disorders (especially Sjögren's syndrome)

Lambert–Eaton myasthenic syndrome (LEMS)

Porphyria

Fabry's disease

Tangier disease

Vitamin B_{12}-deficiency states (rare)

Hereditary sensory and autonomic neuropathies (HSAN)

Infections: botulism, syphilis, HIV, Chagas' disease

Paraneoplastic syndrome (usually in association with ANNA 1 antibodies)

Renal failure.

Dopamine–β-hydroxylase deficiency.

Drug effects:

Anti-hypertensive agents that block the sympathetic network (e.g. α-adrenoceptor, ganglion blockers).

Antidepressant drugs: tricyclic antidepressants, monoamine oxidase inhibitors.

Major tranquilizers: phenothiazines, barbiturates (possibly central action).

Clinical features: history and examination

- Postural hypotension/orthostatic hypotension/orthostatism: may present as syncope or presyncope, often precipitated by standing, exertion, or meals.
- Sexual impotence in males.
- Urinary symptoms: frequency and nocturia.
- Bowel symptoms: either nocturnal diarrhoea or constipation. In the latter case the patient may present with gastroparesis, recurrent vomiting, or intestinal pseudo-obstruction.
- Heat intolerance: associated with loss of sweating.
- Poor tolerance of bright lights, easily dazzled with difficulty accommodating.

Investigations and diagnosis

- Bedside testing

  Pupillary responses to light.

  Postural blood pressure readings: a drop of >30/15 mmHg is significant if the patient is not fluid depleted.

  Heart rate response to standing: should consist of an increase in rate between 10 and 30 beats per minute.

  Sweat test using quinizarin powder: should be positive when body temperature is raised by 1°C using space and electric blankets.

  Valsalva manoeuvre with ECG monitoring: should demonstrate an increase in heart rate and there should be variation in heart rate with respiration.

- Laboratory testing

Baroreflex sensitivity with changes in posture using a tilt table: on tilting, the normal response is a rise in blood pressure and a drop in heart rate. The test is normally done at 45° and 90° tilts.

Cardiovascular response to liquid meal: in normal individuals there is no significant change in heart rate or blood pressure, but in cases of autonomic failure blood pressure often drops after the meal due to failed compensation for increased splanchnic bed blood flow.

Bladder function: cystometrography.

Gastrointestinal motility: may be measured most simply using a barium meal.

Pupillary testing: record responses at 15 minute intervals for up to 1 hour after instillation of the eyedrops.

	Normal response	Peripheral sympathetic lesion	Central sympathetic lesion	Parasympathetic lesion
Rest	–	Small pupil	Small pupil	Large pupil
4% cocaine (prevents catecholamine uptake)	Dilatation (Mydriasis)	Remains small	Slight dilatation	No effect, remains dilated
0.1% adrenaline (acts on supersensitive adrenergic receptors)	No effect	Dilates	Small effect with dilatation	No effect
1% Hydroxyamphetamine (stimulates catecholamine release)	Dilates	No response	Dilates	No effect
2.5% Metacholine/ 0.125% Pilocarpine (acts on muscarinic receptors)	Constricts	? further constriction	? further constriction	Constriction (Miosis)

Treatment and prognosis Autonomic failure is difficult to treat effectively, but a number of symptomatic measures often help, at least initially.

It is imperative to stop any medication that may be contributing to the symptomatology; for example levodopa in MSA may exacerbate the autonomic failure without producing any significant anti-parkinsonian action.

- Postural hypotension

    Head-up bed tilt of about 15° at night: resets the renin–angiotensin system.

    Non-steroidal anti-inflammatory drugs (e.g. indomethacin): causes some fluid retention.

    Desmopressin spray: causes fluid retention and also helps with nocturnal urinary frequency, a common symptom in autonomic failure.

    Fludrocortisone: causes fluid retention.

    Ephedrine: causes vasoconstriction and some increase in cardiac output.

Midodrine.

"Marmite".

- Impotence

    Papaveretum injections into corpora cavernosa.

    Sildenafil (Viagra).

- Urinary frequency/retention

    Oxybutynin, desmopressin spray for urinary frequency.

    Intermittent self-catheterization if urinary retention or large residual urinary
        volumes.

- Bowel immotility

    Cisapride and/or maxolon can increase gastrointestinal motility.

Overall prognosis is dependent on the cause. In PAF and MSA autonomic failure
tends to worsen and often leads to death.

If the cause of autonomic failure is transient [drugs, structural lesions, Guillain–Barré
syndrome (GBS) and some of the infective and metabolic causes] prognosis is better.

References Low PA (ed.). *Clinical Autonomic Disorders. Evaluation and
    Management* (2nd edition). Philadelphia: Lippincott Raven, 1997.

Mathias CJ, Bannister R (eds). *Autonomic Failure. A Textbook of Clinical Disorders
    of the Autonomic Nervous System* (4th edition). Oxford: OUP, 1999.

Mathias CJ, Kimber JR. Treatment of postural hypotension. *Journal of Neurology,
    Neurosurgery and Psychiatry* 1998; **65**: 285–289.

Other relevant entries Alcohol and the nervous system: an overview; Amyloid and
    the nervous system: an overview; Botulism; Cranial nerve disease: II: Optic
    nerve; Cranial nerve disease: III: Oculomotor nerve; Cranial nerve disease: VII:
    Facial nerve; Cranial nerve disease: IX: Glossopharyngeal nerve; Cranial nerve
    disease: X: Vagus nerve; Diabetes mellitus and the nervous system; Dopamine–β-
    hydroxylase deficiency; Fabry's disease; Guillain–Barré syndrome; Infection and
    the nervous system: an overview; Lambert–Eaton myasthenic syndrome;
    Multiple system atrophy; Neuropathies: an overview; Pandysautonomia;
    Paraneoplastic syndromes; Parkinsonian syndromes, parkinsonism; Parkinson's
    disease; Porphyria; Spinal cord trauma; Syphilis; Tangier disease; Tumours: an
    overview; Urinary system; Vasculitis; Vitamin B_{12} deficiency.

■ Autonomic neuropathies – see Autonomic failure; Neuropathies: an overview

■ Autosomal-dominant cerebellar ataxia

Phenotypic classification of autosomal-dominant cerebellar ataxias (ADCA) was proposed by Harding, as follows:

- ADCA type I

    ataxia with ophthalmoplegia, optic atrophy, dementia, or extrapyramidal
        features, including Machado–Joseph disease.

- ADCA type II
  - ataxia with pigmentary maculopathy, with or without ophthalmoplegia or extrapyramidal features.
- ADCA type III
  - "pure" ataxia.

(ADCA type IV, cerebellar ataxia with myoclonus and deafness, probably represents mitochondrial disease, possibly including May–White syndrome, and so is probably obsolete.)

To these categories should be added:

- ADCA with sensory neuropathy (Biemond's ataxia; SCA4): sensory symptoms affect the face and limbs in this rapidly progressive condition (unlike ADCA I–III).
- Dentatorubropallidoluysian atrophy (DRPLA).
- Episodic or periodic ataxias with autosomal-dominant inheritance.

Harding's phenotypic classification has been superseded to some extent by genotypic classification of the spinocerebellar ataxias (SCAs) based on the discovery of gene loci and specific genes responsible for the various syndromes: around 20 loci have now been described. Locus heterogeneity or phenotypic convergence has been demonstrated, since ADCA type I may be a result of mutations in SCA1, 2, 3, and 4, and ADCA type III may be associated with SCA5, 6, and 11. These are all trinucleotide repeat expansions, as is the causative mutation of DRPLA. The episodic ataxias have been found to result from mutations in ion-channel genes.

Reference Harding AE. *The Hereditary Ataxias and Related Disorders.* Edinburgh: Churchill Livingstone, 1984.

Other relevant entries Cerebellar disease: an overview; Channelopathies: an overview; Dentatorubropallidoluysian atrophy; Episodic ataxias; Spinocerebellar ataxia; Trinucleotide repeat diseases.

■ Autosomal-dominant nocturnal frontal lobe epilepsy

Pathophysiology A rare epilepsy syndrome due to a mutation in ligand-gated nicotinic acetylcholine-receptor channels (i.e. a channelopathy).

Clinical features: history and examination

- Nocturnal seizures, occurring in clusters, onset in childhood with persistence to adult life; seizures characterized by vocalization, thrashing, stiffening, sometimes with preserved consciousness.
- Normal clinical examination.
- Positive family history (although penetrance incomplete).

Investigations and diagnosis *EEG*: may show bifrontal epileptiform discharges.
Imaging: normal.
Neurogenetics: mutations have been identified in either of two neuronal nicotinic acetylcholine-receptor subunits, α_4 and β_2.

Differential diagnosis Parasomnia; dyskinesia.

Treatment and prognosis Carbamazepine monotherapy is often effective.

References Scheffer IE, Bhatia KP, Lopes-Cendes I *et al*. Autosomal dominant frontal epilepsy misdiagnosed as sleep disorder. *Lancet* 1994; **343**: 515–517.

Seinlein OK, Mulley JC, Propping P *et al*. A missense mutation in the neuronal nicotinic acetylcholine receptor alpha 4 subunit is associated with autosomal dominant nocturnal frontal lobe epilepsy. *Nature Genetics* 1995; **11**: 201–203.

Other relevant entries Channelopathies: an overview; Epilepsy: an overview; Parasomnias.

■ AVED – see Ataxia with vitamin E deficiency

■ Avellis' syndrome
Palatopharyngeal paralysis of Avellis

Avellis syndrome is paralysis of the soft palate and vocal cord with contralateral hemihypoaesthesia for pain and temperature, with or without a Horner's syndrome, due to a lesion (infarct or tumour) of the tegmentum of the medulla involving the X cranial nerve (nucleus ambiguus), the spinothalamic tract, and sometimes descending pupillary sympathetic fibres. Laryngeal function is spared because only the more cephalad portion of the nucleus ambiguus is damaged.

Reference Takizawa S, Shinohara Y. Magnetic resonance imaging in Avellis' syndrome. *Journal of Neurology, Neurosurgery and Psychiatry* 1996; **61**: 17.

Other relevant entries Brainstem vascular syndromes; Cranial nerve disease: X: Vagus nerve; Horner's syndrome; Jugular foramen syndrome.

■ Azorean disease – see Cerebellar disease: an overview; Machado–Joseph disease; Spinocerebellar ataxia

Bb

■ Babesiosis – see Malaria

■ Babinski–Froehlich syndrome – see Froehlich's syndrome

■ Babinski–Nageotte syndrome
Hemibulbar syndrome • Medullary tegmental paralysis

A rare syndrome, first described in 1902, resulting from an ischaemic lesion of the medulla, producing contralateral hemiplegia and sensory loss in the limbs and trunk, with ipsilateral hemiataxia and facial sensory loss, along with dysarthria, dysphonia, and dysphagia. Some authorities therefore regard it as a rare variant of lateral medullary syndrome with additional contralateral hemiparesis ("Wallenberg plus").

Some writers have equated Babinski–Nageotte syndrome with the hemimedullary syndrome (lateral + medial medullary syndrome), but the original account did not include mention of hypoglossal nucleus involvement, as would be expected in a medial medullary syndrome. The suggested eponym for the hemimedullary syndrome is Reinhold's syndrome.

References De Freitas GR, Moll J, Araujo AQC. The Babinski–Nageotte syndrome. *Neurology* 2001; **56**: 1604.

Krasnianski M, Neudecker S, Schluter A, Zierz S. Babinski–Nageotte syndrome and hemimedullary (Reinhold's) syndrome are clinically and morphologically distinct conditions. *Journal of Neurology* 2003; **250**: 938–942.

Other relevant entries Brainstem vascular syndromes; Céstan–Chenais syndrome; Lateral medullary syndrome; Medial medullary (infarction) syndrome; Opalski's syndrome.

◼ Balint syndrome

The Balint syndrome, first described by a Hungarian neurologist, consists of a triad of signs:

- Inability to look into and scan the peripheral visual field, despite a full range of eye movements, sometimes called "psychic paralysis of fixation of gaze" or sticky fixation.
- A failure to grasp or touch an object under visual guidance, sometimes labelled optic ataxia. The patient may appear blind, locating objects by touch.
- Visual inattention or disorientation affecting the peripheral visual fields, whilst attention to other sensory modalities is unaffected.

The inability to direct oculomotor function appropriately to explore visual space is associated with bilateral damage to the parieto-occipital areas. This may result from functional disconnection between higher order visual cortical regions and the frontal eye fields, with sparing of the primary visual cortex, hence a disconnection syndrome. Brain imaging, either structural (CT, MRI) or functional (SPECT, PET), may demonstrate this bilateral damage, which is usually of vascular origin, for example due to watershed or borderzone ischaemia. Balint syndrome has also been reported in progressive multifocal leukoencephalopathy, Marchiafava–Bignami disease, X-linked adrenoleukodystrophy and some neurodegenerative conditions. Prognosis depends on cause.

References Husein M, Stein J. Rezso Balint and his most celebrated case. *Archives of Neurology* 1988; **45**: 89–93.

Rizzo M. "Balint's syndrome" and associated visuospatial disorders. In: Kennard C
(ed.). *Visual Perceptual Defects*. London: Ballière-Tindall, 1993: 415–437.

Other relevant entries Apraxia; Ataxia; Disconnection syndromes.

■ Balkan disease – see Neuronal ceroid lipofuscinosis

■ Balò's concentric sclerosis
Encephalitis periaxialis concentrica

This is a rare form of demyelinating disease characterized by concentric alternating
bands of myelin destruction and preservation within the cerebral hemispheres.
Originally a pathological diagnosis, this appearance has also been documented *ante
mortem* using MRI, lesions showing hypointense centre and intermediate rings (which
enhance with gadolinium), and hyperintense inner and outer rings. The nosological
position of this disorder with respect to multiple sclerosis (MS) and acute disseminated
encephalomyelitis (ADEM) has been debated, but the concurrence of such lesions with
lesions otherwise typical of MS suggests that it is simply a variant of the latter.

References Balò J. Encephalitis periaxialis concentrica. *Archives of Neurology and
Psychiatry* 1928; **19**: 242–264.

Kastrup O, Stude P, Limmroth V. Balo's concentric sclerosis. Evolution of active
demyelination demonstrated by serial contrast-enhanced MRI. *Journal of
Neurology* 2002; **249**: 811–815.

Other relevant entry Multiple sclerosis.

■ Baltic myoclonus – see Progressive myoclonic epilepsy; Unverricht–Lundborg disease

■ Band heterotopia – see Heterotopia

■ Bannwarth's syndrome – see Borreliosis

■ "Barber's chair syndrome"

An alternative name for Lhermitte's phenomenon.

■ Bardet–Biedl syndrome

This describes a recessively inherited syndrome of mental retardation, obesity,
hypogonadism, syndactyly, and retinitis pigmentosa. It may overlap with
Laurence–Moon syndrome (hence Laurence–Moon–Bardet–Biedl syndrome),
although there is no spastic paraparesis.

Other relevant entries Laurence–Moon syndrome; Retinitis pigmentosa.

■ Barnard–Scholz syndrome – see Kjellin's syndrome

■ Barth syndrome
Barth's X-linked cardiomyopathy and neutropenia syndrome

An X-linked cardiac and skeletal mitochondrial myopathy, presenting with dilated cardiomyopathy, proximal muscle weakness, short stature, and increased susceptibility to infection in boys. Cyclic neutropenia and 3-methylglutaconic aciduria are also features. The responsible gene, G4.5, expresses up to 10 different proteins, called tafazzins, by alternative splicing. The pathogenesis is uncertain, but altered mitochondrial phospholipid composition has been suggested, an idea supported by the observation of deficiency of tetralinoleoyl–cardiolipin in various tissues.

Reference Bione S, D'Adano P, Maestrini E *et al.* A novel X-linked gene, G4.5, is responsible for Barth syndrome. *Nature Genetics* 1996; **12**: 385–389.

Other relevant entry Mitochondrial disease: an overview.

■ Bartonellosis

Bartonella (*Rochalimaea*) *henselae* is the major cause of cat scratch disease, a febrile illness with lymphadenopathy most often occurring in children after a cat scratch (earlier studies had suggested that *Afipia felis* was the cause). It also causes bacillary angiomatosis, a multisystem disorder characterized by proliferation of small blood vessels, seen primarily in patients with acquired immunodeficiency syndrome. Neurological manifestations have been reported in both, including:
- Encephalopathy/encephalitis
- Myelitis
- Radiculitis
- Cerebellar ataxia
- Compressive neuropathy
- Neuroretinitis, optic neuritis, papillitis.

The organism may be identified by culture, PCR, and serology. Various antibiotics (ciprofloxacin, gentamicin, erythromycin, cotrimoxazole) have been reported of benefit in cat scratch disease, but not bacillary angiomatosis.

In South America, *Bartonella bacilliformis* causes a febrile illness variously known as Oroya fever, verruga peruana, and Carrion's disease, the organism transmitted by the bite of sandflies. Invasion of the central nervous system (CNS) may cause meningoencephalitis, myelitis, or venous thrombosis. The differential diagnosis includes malaria. First line treatment is with chloramphenicol, although penicillin, tetracycline, and cotrimoxazole may be used.

Reference Marra CM. Neurologic complications of *Bartonella henselae* infection. *Current Opinion in Neurology* 1995; **8**: 164–169.

Other relevant entry HIV/AIDS and the nervous system.

■ Basal cell Naevus syndrome – see Naevoid basal cell carcinoma syndrome

■ Basal ganglia calcification

Pathophysiology Deposition of calcium within the basal ganglia has been increasingly noted since the advent of CT brain scanning. It may occur in a wide variety of diseases, as well as in neurologically normal individuals, hence its clinical significance is unclear: it may reflect a response to injury or disease rather than being directly responsible for the neurological abnormalities *per se*. Calcification of other central nervous system (CNS) structures, including cortex (especially the occipital lobe), white matter, and cerebellum, may also be present.

Calcification occurs in the walls of capillaries, arteries, small veins, and perivascular spaces, and may be associated with neuronal degeneration and gliosis.

The most commonly recognized associations include:

> hypoparathyroidism, pseudo-hypoparathyroidism;
> mitochondrial cytopathy [e.g. *m*itochondrial *e*ncephalomyopathy, *l*actic *a*cidosis, and *s*troke-like episodes (MELAS)];
> idiopathic familial syndrome (Fahr's syndrome);
> sporadic ("physiological", no disorder of calcium metabolism).

Basal ganglia calcification has also been reported in:

> Birth anoxia
> Cockayne's syndrome
> Carbon monoxide poisoning
> Lead poisoning
> Tuberous sclerosis
> AIDS
> Radiation therapy
> Methotrexate therapy
> Down's syndrome
> Aicardi–Goutières syndrome.

Clinical features: history and examination

- Features of altered calcium metabolism: hypocalcaemia with hypoparathyroidism and pseudo-hypoparathyroidism; skeletal abnormalities in pseudo-hypoparathyroidism.
- Movement disorder: parkinsonism, choreoathetosis.
- Dementia (learning difficulties in children).
- May be asymptomatic.
- Other conditions that have been associated with basal ganglia calcification include epileptic fits, hemiparesis, neuropsychiatric disorders, myoclonus, and dystonia. In children, it may be associated with an encephalopathy +/− microcephaly, dwarfism, and retinal degeneration.

Investigations and diagnosis *Bloods*: calcium, phosphate, and parathormone level. Dependent on clinical context, analysis for lactate and mitochondrial genome abnormalities may be appropriate.

Imaging: calcification is best seen on CT; MR may be required to diagnose associated neurological conditions.

CSF: lactate may be required if mitochondrial disease is suspected.

Others: if a symptomatic cause of calcification is suspected, endocrinological, renal, and gastrointestinal investigations may be required.

Treatment and prognosis

Dependent on the cause.

Correct any underlying metabolic abnormality (e.g. calcium status).

Symptomatic treatment (e.g. levodopa for parkinsonism).

References Fénelon G, Gray F, Paillard F *et al*. A prospective study of patients with CT detected pallidal calcifications. *Journal of Neurology, Neurosurgery and Psychiatry* 1993; **56**: 622–625.

Kobari M, Nogawa S, Sugimoto Y, Fukuuchi Yl. Familial idiopathic brain calcification with autosomal dominant inheritance. *Neurology* 1997; **48**: 645–649.

Koller WC, Cochran JW, Klawans HL. Calcification of the basal ganglia: computerized tomography and clinical correlation. *Neurology* 1979; **29**: 328–333.

Other relevant entries Aicardi–Goutières syndrome; Chorea; Dementia: an overview; Dystonia: an overview; Endocrinology and the nervous system; Gastrointestinal disease and the nervous system; Leigh's disease, Leigh's syndrome; MELAS; Mitochondrial disease: an overview; Parkinsonian syndromes, parkinsonism; Vasculitis.

■ Basedow's paraplegia

A paraplegia-like weakness occurring in the context of severe hyperthyroidism, with flaccid weakness, absent reflexes, minimal or no sensory disturbance, and without sphincter disturbance, was described in the nineteenth century by various authors including Charcot. It is possible that this reflected coincident postinfective polyneuropathy or Guillain–Barré syndrome (GBS). However, cases of acute asymmetric mixed axonal and demyelinating sensorimotor neuropathy in the context of acute hyperthyroidism, with mitochondrial and cytoskeletal tissue changes compatible with thyrotoxicosis in the absence of GBS-type changes, have been reported.

Reference Pandit L, Shankar SK, Gayathri N, Pandit A. Acute thyrotoxic neuropathy – Basedow's paraplegia revisited. *Journal of the Neurological Sciences* 1998; **155**: 211–214.

Other relevant entries Neuropathies: an overview; Thyroid disease and the nervous system.

■ Basilar (artery) migraine – see Migraine

■ Bassen–Kornzweig disease – see Abetalipoproteinaemia

■ Batten's disease – see Neuronal ceroid lipofuscinosis

■ Battle sign

Bruising (haematoma) over the mastoid area may be seen within 24–72 hours of compound fractures of the middle cranial fossa.

■ Becker Disease – see Myotonia and myotonic syndromes; myotonia congenita

■ Becker muscular dystrophy

This condition is allelic with Duchenne muscular dystrophy (*q.v.*), hence a dystrophinopathy, with the same distribution of muscle wasting and weakness, but more benign: onset is around 12 years, and death not until the fourth or fifth decade, sometimes later. There may be associated mental impairment.

Other relevant entries Duchenne muscular dystrophy; Dystrophinopathy; Muscular dystrophies: an overview.

■ Beevor's sign

This refers to the upward movement of the umbilicus when a supine patient attempts to flex the head onto the chest against the resistance of the examiner's hand, when there is weakness of the lower abdominal muscles due to a lesion at or below T10 level. Reported causes include thoracic cord tumours, syringomyelia, and facioscapulohumeral dystrophy.

Reference Tashiro K. Charles Edward Beevor (1854–1908) and Beevor's sign. In: Rose FC (ed.). *A Short History of Neurology: The British Contribution 1660–1910.* Oxford: Butterworth-Heinemann, 1999: 222–225.

■ Behçet's disease

Pathophysiology Behçet's disease is a chronic, multisystem, inflammatory disorder, named after the Turkish dermatologist Hulusi Behçet who formally described the condition in 1937 (although it was possibly described in the fifth century BC in the Hippocratic corpus). It is found throughout the world, but is more common in Japan and Mediterranean countries. Women are more commonly affected (F : M = 2–5 : 1), with presentation around 20–40 years of age. The disease can present in diverse ways (to dermatologists, chest physicians, ophthalmologists, neurologists), although the cardinal features are mucocutaneous ulceration, uveitis, skin lesions, and thrombotic events. It is best diagnosed using an internationally agreed set of criteria. Management often requires long-term immunosuppressive therapy.

Clinical features: history and examination

- Recurrent oral aphthous ulceration (at least three times in a 12-month period).
- Recurrent genital aphthous ulceration.
- Ophthalmic lesions: anterior or posterior uveitis; retinal vasculitis; cells in vitreous humour in asymptomatic individuals.
- Skin lesions: erythema nodosum; pseudofolliculitis; papulopustular lesions; acneiform nodules.
- Joint involvement: recurrent seronegative arthritis, often involves individual large joints, is subacute, self-limiting and non-deforming.
- Intestinal involvement: ulcerative haemorrhagic lesions of stomach, intestine and anus that may be indistinguishable from ulcerative colitis.
- Vascular complications: include thrombophlebitis, deep venous thrombosis, sagittal sinus thrombosis, hepatic vein occlusion, and rarely arterial occlusions.
- Neurological features

    Parenchymal (80%): brainstem $+/-$ spinal cord, hemisphere, isolated pyramidal; present with pyramidal signs, hemiparesis, behavioural change, sphincter disturbance; peripheral nerve involvement rare (polyneuropathy, mononeuropathy multiplex); aseptic meningitis may occur.

    Secondary/non-parenchymal (20%): raised intracranial pressure due to cerebral venous sinus thrombosis

An International Study Group has suggested diagnostic criteria for Behçet's disease:

    recurrent oral ulceration (*sine qua non*) in combination with two or more of the following:
    recurrent genital ulceration,
    eye lesions,
    skin lesions or a positive pathergy test.

However, Behçet's disease can occasionally present with isolated neurological features; the diagnosis may then rely on biopsy.

Investigations and diagnosis *Bloods*: usually non-specific. There is often an inflammatory response with raised ESR and CRP with raised α-gammaglobulin and leukocytosis. Consider HLA testing.

Imaging: MRI may reveal scattered white matter lesions that often involve the brainstem, $+/-$ basal ganglia. Whilst the cerebral lesions may be clinically silent, brainstem lesions are often extensive and symptomatic. MRA may reveal a thrombosed sagittal sinus.

CSF: may be normal. However there may be raised intracranial pressure in the context of dural sinus thrombosis. With parenchymal central nervous system (CNS) disease, hypercellular CSF (neutrophils, lymphocytes) is found in 60%, occasionally with positive oligoclonal bands.

Ophthalmological assessment using a slit lamp may be helpful in defining ocular involvement.

Dermatological and gastroenterological assessments as appropriate.

Brain biopsy: if diagnosis suspected and not established by any other means.

Differential diagnosis

Neurological disorders
- Multiple sclerosis
- Cerebral vasculitis
- Sarcoidosis
- Vogt–Koyanagi–Harada syndrome.

Systemic disorders
- Reiter's disease
- Stevens–Johnson syndrome
- Systemic lupus erythematosus
- Crohn's disease/Ulcerative colitis
- Ankylosing spondylitis
- Sweet's syndrome.

Treatment and prognosis

Disease course varies
- Relapsing–remitting (40%)
- Secondary progressive (30%)
- Primary progressive (10%)
- Silent neurological involvement (20%).

Local therapy
- Oral ulcers can be treated with topical tetracycline or interferon-α
- Genital ulcers can be treated with topical steroids
- Uveitis can be treated with mydriatics and topical steroids

Systemic therapy for parenchymal disease

Various immunosuppressive treatments have been tried, either singly or in combination. None have been submitted to a randomized-controlled trial:
- Corticosteroids (1 mg/kg/day initially then maintenance dose of 5–10 mg/day)
- Azathioprine 2.5 mg/kg/day
- Chlorambucil 6–8 mg/day
- Cyclophosphamide 2–3 mg/kg/day
- Cyclosporine 5–10 mg/kg/day for 3 months
- Colchicine 1 mg/day for 2–24 months.

Other therapies that have been tried include plasma exchange, thalidomide, and dapsone

Thrombotic events: warfarin may be indicated.

Non-steroidal anti-inflammatory drugs may be used for arthritis.

The prognosis is highly variable. It is worse with parenchymal neurological involvement, raised CSF cell count or protein, brainstem + involvement, primary or secondary progressive course, and relapse during tapering of steroid therapy.

References Akman-Demir G, Serdaroglu P, Tasçi B and the Neuro-Behçet Study Group. Clinical patterns of neurological involvement in Behçet's disease: evaluation of 200 patients. *Brain* 1999; **122**: 2171–2181.

International Study Group for Behçet's disease. Criteria for the diagnosis of Behçet's disease. *Lancet* 1990; **335**: 1078–1080.

Kidd D, Steuer A, Denman AM, Rudge P. Neurological complications in Behçet's syndrome. *Brain* 1999; **122**: 2183–2194.

Other relevant entries Aseptic meningitis: differential diagnosis; Gastrointestinal disease and the nervous system; Immunosupressive therapy and diseases of the nervous system; Isolated angiitis of the central nervous system; Multiple sclerosis; Sarcoidosis; Sweet's syndrome; Vasculitis; Vogt–Koyanagi–Harada syndrome.

■ Behr's syndrome
Behr complicated optic atrophy • Optic atrophy–ataxia syndrome

This autosomal-recessive syndrome comprises:
- Optic atrophy
- Spinocerebellar degeneration: spasticity and cerebellar ataxia
- +/− learning disability
- +/− peripheral neuropathy (sensory axonal)
- +/− deafness.

Onset is in infancy and the condition is slowly progressive.

Behr's syndrome may be classifed as an early-onset ataxia with optic atrophy, and may need to be differentiated from Friedreich's ataxia, leukodystrophies, mitochondrial disease, neuronal ceroid lipofuscinosis, and Wolfram syndrome. Alternatively it may be classified with the hereditary spastic parapareses.

3-methylglutaconic aciduria may be noted in Behr's syndrome, suggesting that it may result from enzyme deficiency or mitochondrial disorder.

Other relevant entries
Cerebellar disease: an overview; Hereditary spastic paraparesis; Optic atrophy.

■ Bell's mania – see Catatonia

■ Bell's Palsy

Pathophysiology Bell's palsy is the commonest cause of a lower motor neurone seventh (facial) cranial nerve palsy. The eponym is reserved for idiopathic facial nerve palsy (there are many recognized symptomatic causes for facial palsy), which is speculated to have a viral aetiology. Men and woman are affected equally. The majority of patients require no investigation and make a full and complete recovery.

A minority (15%) fail to make a full recovery, and in some cases the regenerating nerve forms aberrant connections with symptomatic consequences, for example crocodile tears. The evidence supporting a role for steroids in the management of this condition remains weak, but nonetheless they are usually given.

Clinical features: history and examination

- Onset is usually with pain in or behind the ear on the side that becomes affected. This is followed by a lower motor neurone seventh nerve palsy of varying severity.
- Symptoms of numbness of the face on the ipsilateral side are almost invariable, possibly due to altered sensory return caused by subcutaneous muscle flaccidity; there is usually no objective evidence of sensory loss.
- Unilateral facial weakness evolves over hours, reaching a maximum within 2–3 days of symptom onset.
- Ipsilateral impairment of taste (ageusia, hypogeusia) and hyperacusis, may be features, and have localizing value. Lesions within the facial canal distal to the meatal segment cause both hyperacusis and ageusia; lesions in the facial canal between the nerve to stapedius and the chorda tympani cause ageusia but no hyperacusis; lesions distal to the chorda tympani cause neither ageusia nor hyperacusis (i.e. facial motor paralysis only).
- Idiopathic facial nerve palsy can be recurrent but this is rare (and has a distinct differential diagnosis), as does a bilateral onset of facial weakness.

Investigations and diagnosis   Generally no investigations are required.

Bloods, imaging, CSF: normal.

Neurophysiology: relative inexcitability of the facial nerve: if <10% of the normal side within 14 days of onset, suggests recovery will be incomplete.

Differential diagnosis   Other causes of lower motor neurone facial nerve palsy include:

> geniculate herpes zoster (Ramsay Hunt syndrome);
> diabetes mellitus;
> Lyme disease (borreliosis, Bannwarth's disease);
> sarcoidosis;
> leukaemic infiltration, lymphoma;
> HIV seroconversion;
> neoplastic compression (e.g. cerebellopontine angle tumour, rare);
> entrapment: Paget's disease, hyperostosis cranialis interna;
> facial nerve neuroma;
> idiopathic intracranial hypertension (false-localizing sign).

Recurrent lower motor neurone facial nerve palsy should prompt consideration of

> diabetes mellitus;
> lyme disease;
> sarcoidosis;
> leukaemia, lymphoma;
> Melkersson–Rosenthal syndrome.

Facial weakness may also result from disease of muscle (e.g. facioscapulohumeral dystrophy, myotonic dystrophy, mitochondrial disorders) and of the neuromuscular junction (myasthenia gravis). Upper motor neurone lesions may cause facial weakness, distinguished clinically by sparing of frontalis, which may be unilateral (e.g. hemisphere infarct $+/-$ hemiparesis, lacunar infarct, space-occupying lesions: intrinsic tumour, metastasis, abscess) or bilateral (motor neurone disease, diffuse cerebrovascular disease, pontine infarct).

Treatment and prognosis Steroids (prednisolone) are often prescribed if the patient is seen within 48 hours of onset. The evidence supporting their efficacy in hastening improvement is not strong, but it is thought that they probably are effective in improving facial functional outcome. Evidence in favour of using aciclovir or facial nerve decompressive surgery is insufficient to recommend these at present.

If eye closure is incomplete, eye protection with artificial tears may be required, and antibiotics for any exposure conjunctivitis. Tarsorrhapy may be required if recovery is insufficient to achieve eye closure.

Spontaneous recovery occurs over 3 weeks to 2 months in the majority of patients. Poorer prognosis is associated with older patient age (over 40 years) and if no recovery is seen within 4 weeks of onset.

Aberrant nerve regeneration may occur, leading to:

Autonomic synkineses: involuntary tearing of the eye on the affected side with eating (crocodile tears, Bogorad's syndrome); gustatory sweating (Frey's syndrome);

Synkinesis of the facial musculature with chewing: jaw opening leads to eye closure (jaw winking) on the involved side (Marin–Amat syndrome).

Reference Grogan PM, Gronseth GS. Practice parameter: steroids, acyclovir, and surgery for Bell's palsy (an evidence-based review). Report of the Quality Standards Subcommittee of the American Academy of Neurology. *Neurology* 2001; **56**: 830–836.

Other relevant entries Borreliosis; Cranial nerve disease: VII: Facial nerve; Diabetes mellitus and the nervous system; Frey's syndrome; HIV/AIDS and the nervous system; Marin–Amat syndrome; Melkersson–Rosenthal syndrome; Ramsay Hunt syndrome (2); Sarcoidosis; Varicella zoster virus and the nervous system.

■ Belly Dancer's Dyskinesia

A focal involuntary movement disorder characterized by undulating rhythmical movement of the anterior abdominal wall causing circular rotatory umbilical motion. Most cases follow a laparotomy; there is disagreement amongst the authorities as to whether or not cases may be related to neuroleptic use. Pain may also be present. The movements have no associated neurological lesion in the spinal cord, and are usually refractory to treatment.

Reference Iliceto G, Thompson PD, Day BL *et al*. Diaphragmatic flutter, the moving umbilicus syndrome and "belly dancers' dyskinesia". *Movement Disorders* 1990; **5**: 15–22.

■ Benedikt's syndrome

This brainstem vascular syndrome affecting the midbrain is characterized by an ipsilateral oculomotor nerve palsy and contralateral involuntary movements, such as tremor, chorea, or athetosis (due to involvement of the red nucleus), with or without a contralateral hemiparesis (due to involvement of the corticospinal tract). It may thus be differentiated from Claude's syndrome, Nothnagel's syndrome, and Weber's syndrome.

An almost identical syndrome, but with additional contralateral sensory disturbances, has been described as Chiray–Foix–Nicolesco syndrome.

Reference Liu GT, Crenner CW, Logigian EL *et al.* Midbrain syndromes of Benedikt, Claude and Nothnagel: setting the record straight. *Neurology* 1992; **42**: 1820–1822.

Other relevant entries Brainstem vascular syndromes; Cerebrovascular disease: arterial; Claude's syndrome; Cranial nerve disease: III: Oculomotor nerve; Nothnagel's syndrome; Weber's syndrome.

■ Benign epilepsy syndromes

A number of epilepsy syndromes of childhood have an extremely good prognosis, with spontaneous seizure cessation with increasing age, and hence may be described as benign. These include:

Absence seizures ("petit mal")
Rolandic epilepsy (benign epilepsy with centrotemporal spikes)
Panayiotopoulos syndrome (benign occipital epilepsy)
Gastaut's occipital epilepsy
Benign partial epilepsies:
    with affective symptoms
    with extreme somatosensory evoked potentials
    with frontal spikes
Benign infantile seizures: familial, non-familial (Watanabe–Vigevano syndrome)
Benign myoclonic epilepsy of infancy
Benign familial myoclonus
Benign neonatal seizures: familial, non-familial
Benign neonatal convulsions ("5th day fits").

The syndrome of benign familial neonatal convulsions is an autosomal-dominant condition, shown to be a channelopathy, affecting voltage-gated potassium channels, M-type subunit (mutations in genes KCNQ2 and KCNQ3).

Non-epileptic movement disorders may need to be differentiated from some of these syndromes, for example benign neonatal sleep myoclonus and benign non-epileptic myoclonus of infancy ("shuddering attacks").

Reference Panayiotopoulos CP. *A Clinical Guide to Epileptic Syndromes and their Treatment: Based on the New ILAE Diagnostic Scheme*. Chipping Norton: Bladon, 2002: 89–113.

Other relevant entries Absence epilepsy; Channelopathies: an overview; Epilepsy: an overview; Gastaut's occipital epilepsy; Panayiotopoulos syndrome; Rolandic epilepsy; Watanabe–Vigevano syndrome.

■ Benign essential tremor – see Essential tremor

■ Benign fasciculation with cramps syndrome – see Denny–Brown, Foley syndrome

■ Benign hereditary chorea

This autosomal-dominant condition with childhood onset is characterized by chorea which is non-progressive or only slowly progressive; the first symptom may be delayed walking. There is no dementia, PET brain scans are normal and there is no overt pathological change (*cf.* Huntington's disease). There is genetic heterogeneity: some families have mutations in the TITF-1 gene on chromosome 14.

Reference Kleiner-Fisman G, Rogaeva E, Halliday W *et al*. Benign hereditary chorea: clinical, genetic and pathological findings. *Annals of Neurology* 2003; **54**: 244–247.

Other relevant entries Chorea; Huntington's disease.

■ Benign intracranial hypertension

The term idiopathic intracranial hypertension (IIH) is now generally preferred to benign intracranial hypertension (BIH) for this syndrome, since occasionally its follows an aggressive course, despite treatment, resulting in significant visual impairment or even blindness, and hence cannot be described as "benign".

Other relevant entry Idiopathic intracranial hypertension.

■ Benign paroxysmal positional vertigo

Pathophysiology Benign paroxysmal positional vertigo (BPPV) is a common disorder resulting from damage to the peripheral vestibular apparatus. It is often idiopathic in origin but in a significant number of cases it is associated with a preceding history of head trauma or vestibular neur(on)itis, presumably of viral origin. The condition is characterized by paroxysmal positional vertigo and nystagmus, which is normally induced by certain movements of the head such as lying down or rolling over in bed at night. In all cases there is a disruption of flow of endolymph in the semicircular canals, most usually the posterior but occasionally the horizontal. There are two theories of pathogenesis: *cupulolithiasis* suggests that detached otoconia (calcium carbonate crystals) from the utricle become adherent to the cupula of the posterior semicircular canal, rendering it a gravity-sensitive organ; whereas *canalithiasis* refers to debris, including possibly degenerating otoconia, which becomes free floating in the endolymph and disturbs the endolymph when the head is moved, stimulating the ampulla. The latter is the more compelling explanation for the clinical phenomenology. Moreover, it is readily treatable by manipulation to reposition the debris.

Clinical features: history and examination

- Paroxysms of vertigo with nausea and gait ataxia, and occasionally vomiting; induced by turning the head into certain positions, especially lying down and rolling over in bed or bending forward. The attacks last for a few minutes at most.
- There may be a secondary anxiety disorder.
- Attacks may be induced on clinical examination using the Dix–Hallpike (or Nylen–Barany) manoeuvre. Prior to performing this, the patient should be warned that an attack may be induced, and if these are severe prophylactic prochlorperazine may be given. The patient must be told to keep their eyes open during the manoeuvre despite the vertigo.
  - The patient sits on the side of the examination couch.
  - Examiner turns the patient's head through 45° to right or left, then tips the patient back in this position so that the head lies 30° below the horizontal (i.e. hanging over the end of the couch).
  - The eyes are observed in this position for at least 30 seconds. In a positive test, torsional nystagmus with the upper pole of the eye beating towards the ground will be observed.
  - It must be remembered that there will be a delay before the nystagmus emerges; it rapidly fatigues.
  - The test is done in both directions (i.e. right and left head turning).

Investigations and diagnosis *The positional manoeuvre* (Dix–Hallpike and Nylen–Barany) is diagnostic when positive.

Bloods, imaging, CSF and other tests are only necessary when there is doubt about the diagnosis, and/or a central cause for vertigo is considered possible.

Differential diagnosis

Vestibular neur(on)itis.

Labyrinthine concussion.

Ménière's disease, vestibular-only form.

Posterior fossa (cerebellum, brainstem) disease: vascular, demyelinating, neoplastic.

Vertebrobasilar insufficiency (the labyrinthine artery arises from the vertebrobasilar system).

Treatment and prognosis The condition is often self-limiting, with the majority of attacks passing off within 10 weeks. However, there is a tendency to recurrence.

The mainstay of therapy is manipulation to reposition the displaced otolith crystals or otoconia, of which the most successful is the Epley manoeuvre:

- The patient may need prophylactic prochlorperazine since the procedure begins with a Dix–Hallpike manoeuvre.

- The patient's head is tipped to the side that is affected, provoking vertigo and nystagmus.
- The head is then turned through 90° whilst the body remains in the supine position.
- The head and body are then rotated so that the head is facing down; this may provoke further brief vertigo.
- The patient is then brought into the seated position, still with the head turned toward the shoulder.
- The patient's head is then recentred and the head tipped forward (chin down) by about 20°.

The patient should keep their head in the upright position as much as possible in the first 48 hours after the procedure.

About 80% of patients gain improvement after the first session, and this figure rises to 98% after a second session a week later.

Habituating exercises, such as the Brandt–Daroff exercises, may be undertaken if the patient cannot tolerate the Epley manoeuvre.

Drug treatment is usually ineffective, and surgical elimination of posterior semicircular canal function is rarely needed.

References Epley JM. The canalith repositioning procedure: for treatment of benign paroxysmal positional vertigo. *Otolaryngology Head & Neck Surgery* 1992; **107**: 399–404.

Furman JM, Cass SP. Benign paroxysmal positional vertigo. *New England Journal of Medicine* 1999; **341**: 1590–1596.

Lempert T, Gresty MA, Bronstein AM. Benign positional vertigo: recognition and treatment. *British Medical Journal* 1995; **311**: 489–491.

Other relevant entries Chiari malformations; Cerebellar disease: an overview; Cerebrovascular disease: arterial; Cranial nerve disease: VIII: Vestibulocochlear nerve; Ménière's disease; Multiple sclerosis; Vertigo; Vestibular schwannoma.

■ Bent spine syndrome – see Camptocormia

■ Beriberi
Thiamine deficiency • Vitamin B$_1$ deficiency

Pathophysiology Beriberi is a condition that affects the heart and peripheral nervous system, and is due to thiamine or vitamin B$_1$ deficiency. When the disease predominantly affects the heart, the patient presents with congestive cardiac failure (or "wet beriberi"), whereas when the disease involves the peripheral nerves the patient presents with a painful peripheral neuropathy (or "dry beriberi"). In its pure form it is relatively rare, but thiamine deficiency is not uncommonly found to be an aetiological agent in the neuropathies associated with malnutrition and chronic alcoholism. Pathologically there is axonal degeneration with secondary demyelination involving the largest and most distal myelinated fibres; degeneration may extend to the anterior and posterior roots, anterior horn cells, dorsal root ganglia, and dorsal columns. In the early stages of the disease, the neuropathy may be curable with vitamin supplementation.

Clinical features: history and examination

- Insidious onset, usually over weeks, of pain (ache, cramp-like, burning), paraesthesia and weakness, more apparent distally and especially in the legs where it may be associated with skin changes (glossy, atrophic, hairless).
- On examination, there is usually a symmetrical distal sensorimotor loss, especially in the lower limbs, with hyperaesthesia and allodynia, which may be so severe as to prevent walking. Tendon jerks are usually lost early. Sensory loss is very variable in terms of which modalities are lost and which spared. There is often hyperhidrosis of the hands and feet. Lower cranial and recurrent laryngeal nerve involvement is very rare.
- In addition to the neurological features there may be evidence of malnutrition, alcoholism, and congestive cardiac failure.

Investigations and diagnosis *Bloods*: FBC (may show anaemia), liver function tests, vitamin B_{12}, folate, pyruvate (often raised in thiamine deficiency), and RBC transketolase (reduced).

Imaging:

CXR may reveal features of congestive cardiac failure.

CT/MRI brain is usually normal, unless there is concurrent disease associated with the thiamine deficiency (e.g. Wernicke–Korsakoff's syndrome).

CSF: usually normal, occasionally slightly raised protein.

Neurophysiology: EMG/NCS: evidence of an axonal neuropathy, with denervation on needle EMG.

Others: may require a full cardiac assessment.

Differential diagnosis Other painful neuropathies: include those associated with alcohol, diabetes mellitus, Fabry's disease, AIDS, cryoglobulinaemia, borreliosis (Lyme disease), paraneoplastic syndromes, vasculitis, heavy metal poisoning.

Treatment and prognosis The mainstay of treatment is thiamine replacement, at a dose of 50–100 mg/day, as soon as the diagnosis is considered.

In the short-term aspirin, non-steroidal anti-inflammatory medications and tricyclic antidepressants may be needed to control the pain.

Physiotherapy is required, especially as atrophy and weakness may develop due to disuse secondary to the pain.

Congestive cardiac failure may require specific treatment.

The majority of patients start to improve in days, but in the more severe cases, especially with cardiac involvement, improvement may take months and is incomplete.

Reference Windebank AJ. Polyneuropathy due to nutritional deficiency and alcoholism. In: Dyck PJ, Thomas PK, Griffin JW, Low PA, Podulso JF (eds). *Peripheral Neuropathy* (3rd edition). Philadelphia: WB Saunders, 1995: 1310–1321.

Other relevant entries Alcohol and the nervous system: an overview; Neuropathies: an overview; Vitamin B_{12} deficiency; Vitamin deficiencies and the nervous system; Wernicke–Korsakoff's syndrome.

■ Berman's mucolipidosis
Mucolipidosis type IV (ML type IV)

This mucolipidosis is characterized by severe mental retardation and visual impairment beginning in the first year of life; children display hypotonia, may not walk, never develop language, and have visual impairment with corneal clouding, but have no dysmorphic features, organomegaly, bony changes or seizures. Achlorhydria with raised gastrin concentrations is invariable. Unlike other mucolipidoses, most cases are of Ashkenazi Jewish origin. The biochemical defect is in mucolipin 1, linked to mutations in the MCOLN1 gene on chromosome 19p13.3. This protein is thought to be involved in endocytosis.

Other relevant entry Mucolipidoses.

■ Bernard–Horner syndrome – see Horner's syndrome

■ Bernhardt–Roth syndrome – see Meralgia paraesthetica

■ Besnier–Boeck–Schaumann syndrome – see Sarcoidosis

■ Bethlem myopathy
Early-onset limb-girdle myopathy with contractures

A rare autosomal-dominant muscle disease, with onset from infancy to adolescence, with proximal lower limb weakness, and slow progression; most patients remain ambulant. Contractures of interphalangeal joints, elbows, and ankles are common. There is no facial or cardiac involvement (*cf.* Emery–Dreifuss muscular dystrophy). Creatine kinase may be normal or slightly elevated, EMG is myopathic, and muscle biopsy is non-specific. Mutations in the gene encoding collagen VI, an extracellular matrix protein, have been detected.

Reference Jobsis GJ, Keizers H, Vreijling JP *et al*. Type VI collagen mutations in Bethlem myopathy, an autosomal dominant myopathy with contractures. *Nature Genetics* 1996; **14**: 113–115.

Other relevant entries Emery–Dreifuss muscular dystrophy; Limb-girdle muscular dystrophy; Myopathy: an overview.

■ Bickerstaff's brainstem encephalitis

Pathophysiology A syndrome of acute ophthalmoplegia and cerebellar ataxia, clinically very similar to Miller Fisher syndrome. It is preceded by infection and is probably due to autoimmune attack on brainstem structures; anti-GQ1b ganglioside auto-antibodies, as found in Miller Fisher syndrome, are found in some, but not all, cases. At its most severe ventilatory support may be required, but overall prognosis for recovery is extremely good.

Clinical features: history and examination

- Prodrome: general malaise +/− myalgia
- Evolution of brainstem signs (downwards):
    drowsiness, but easily rousable (not always present); mild headache, occasional vomiting;
    acute ophthalmoplegia (downgaze spared), +/− diplopia, ptosis, fixed dilated pupils;
    motor trigeminal involvement;
    lower motor neurone VII involvement;
    cerebellar ataxia (especially trunk);
    bulbar weakness;
    limb power normal; reflexes brisk to absent; plantars may be extensor;
- Maximum disability within 5–30 days.
- Great improvement thereafter, may be complicated by parkinsonism for 2 weeks, but eventual total recovery.
- Clustering of cases has been noted.

Investigations and diagnosis *Bloods*: serological screening; recognized antecedent infections include Herpes simplex virus, Epstein–Barr virus, cytomegalovirus, shingles (varicella zoster), *Campylobacter jejuni* enteritis; +/− Anti-GQ1b auto-antibodies.

Imaging: MRI/CT: may show brainstem lesions, anywhere from midbrain to medulla.

CSF: may show pleocytosis, raised protein; may be normal.

Differential diagnosis

Miller Fisher syndrome.

Brainstem inflammatory disease: multiple sclerosis, Behçet's disease.

Unusual presentation of herpes simplex encephalitis.

Treatment and prognosis Relapses not recorded. If the patient can be appropriately supported through the acute phase, total recovery occurs. Uncontrolled studies suggest plasma exchange and IVIg may be of benefit.

References Bickerstaff ER. Brain stem encephalitis (Bickerstaff encephalitis). In: Vinken PJ, Bruyn GW (eds). *Handbook of Clinical Neurology: Volume 34 Infections of the Nervous System Part II*. Amsterdam: North-Holland, 1978: 605–609.

Chataway SJS, Larner AJ, Kapoor R. Anti-GQ1b antibody status, magnetic resonance imaging, and the nosology of Bickerstaff's brainstem encephalitis. *European Journal of Neurology* 2001; **8**: 355–357.

Other relevant entries Botulism; Encephalitis: an overview; Encephalitis lethargica; Gangliosides and neurological disorders; Guillain–Barré syndrome; Herpes simplex encephalitis; Miller Fisher syndrome.

■ Bielschowsky–Jansky type – see Neuronal ceroid lipofuscinosis

■ Biemond's ataxia – see Autosomal-dominant cerebellar ataxia; Spinocerebellar ataxia

■ BIH – see Idiopathic intracranial hypertension

■ Bilateral nodular periventricular heterotopia
Familial periventricular heterotopia

An X-linked-dominant disorder with contiguous symmetrical nodular heterotopia lining the lateral ventricles, and manifesting in affected females with epilepsy. Cognitive levels may range from mild retardation to normal. The condition is prenatally lethal in hemizygous males. BNPH is associated with mutations (missense or distal truncations, the former causing milder consequences) in the *filamin 1* (*FLN1*) gene.

> **Reference** Moro F, Carrozzo R, Veggiotti P *et al*. Familial periventricular heterotopia: missense and distal truncating mutations of the *FLN1* gene. *Neurology* 2002; **58**: 916–921.
>
> **Other relevant entry** Epilepsy: an overview.

■ Bilharziasis – see Schistosomiasis

■ Bing–Horton syndrome
Erythroprosopalgia

A syndrome of episodic attacks of facial pain, especially at night, with ipsilateral facial reddening, tearing, and nasal discharge, sometimes with concurrent Horner's syndrome. It is thought to reflect an irritative lesion in the region of the greater petrosal nerve.

> **Other relevant entry** Facial pain: differential diagnosis.

■ Bing–Neel syndrome

This describes slowing of the retinal and cerebral circulation in blood hyperviscosity states, which may cause episodic visual disturbances, confusion, strokes and sometimes coma. It is most commonly seen in Waldenstrom's macroglobulinaemia.

■ Binswanger's disease
Binswanger's encephalopathy • Subcortical arteriosclerotic encephalopathy (SAE)

Pathophysiology Binswanger in 1894 described a vascular disorder consisting of a subcortical obliteration of small arteries and arterioles, often in association with systemic hypertension, leading to pathological periventricular demyelination and clinical dementia. The condition was judged relatively rare until the advent of neuroimaging, when radiological evidence of white matter disease lead to increased use of this diagnostic category. However, such white matter changes, now sometimes labelled leukoaraiosis, are relatively common in the elderly both without and with dementia (which may be of Alzheimer type or vascular in origin). The term Binswanger's disease is probably best reserved for pathological changes, modern reports of which are relatively few, and suggest hypertensive small artery disease as the pathological substrate. Diagnostic criteria have been suggested.

Clinical features: history and examination The classic history is of stepwise deterioration, with episodes of acute deterioration from lacunar syndromes, and periods of stability and occasionally even improvement. However, a considerable proportion of patients present with steadily progressive neurological deficits. The clinical picture is of:

Abnormal gait: wide based, shuffling; due to a combination of pyramidal and, particularly, extrapyramidal dysfunction.
Urinary incontinence.
Mood changes including apathy, inertia, abulia.
Pseudobulbar palsy.
Dementia: typically frontal subcortical pattern of deficits.
+/− Focal cerebrovascular deficits.
+/− Epileptic seizures.
Immobility.

Investigations and diagnosis *Bloods*: usually normal apart from possibly renal impairment secondary to hypertension; exclude hyperlipidaemia, thrombophilia.
Imaging: CT/MRI show an ischaemic periventricular leukoencephalopathy often with sparing of subcortical U-fibres; patchy periventricular white matter changes (leukoaraiosis) with lacunar infarcts in the basal ganglia +/− brain atrophy, ventricular dilatation. Carotid angiography shows no significant extra- or intracranial abnormality.
CSF: usually normal.
Neuropsychology: subcortical frontal executive dysfunction is prominent.
Others: investigation for other hypertensive end-organ damage (e.g. echocardiogram, renal ultrasound).

Differential diagnosis Other causes of leukoaraiosis:

Hypertensive small vessel disease (lacunar infarcts):
Multi-infarct dementia
Vascular syndromes including CADASIL and cerebral amyloid angiopathy
Vasculitis
Normal pressure hydrocephalus
Inflammatory CNS disease including sarcoidosis, Behçet's disease, and multiple sclerosis.

Treatment and prognosis Reduce the risk of further vascular events: control blood pressure, hypercholesterolaemia; low dose aspirin. The disease usually progresses, regardless of blood pressure control, with mean survival between 5 and 10 years.

References Bennett DA, Wilson RS, Gilley DW, Fox JH. Clinical diagnosis of Binswanger's disease. *Journal of Neurology, Neurosurgery and Psychiatry* 1990; **53**: 961–965.

Caplan LR, Binswanger's disease revisited. *Neurology* 1995; **45**: 626–633.

Fisher CM. Binswanger's encephalopathy: a review. *Journal of Neurology* 1989; **236**: 65–79.

Other relevant entries Amyloid and the nervous system: an overview; Behçet's disease; CADASIL; Cerebrovascular disease: arterial; Dementia: an overview; Multiple sclerosis; Sarcoidosis; Vascular dementia.

▥ Biopterin deficiency

A syndrome of developmental delay, generalized hypotonia, myoclonic and tonic–clonic seizures, and swallowing difficulty, with increased serum concentrations of phenylalanine but normal phenylalanine hydroxylase levels (*cf.* phenylketonuria). Lack of tetrahydrobiopterin, a cofactor of phenylalanine hydroxylase, is the cause, and hence treatment is with tetrahydrobiopterin and a low phenylalanine diet. Early recognition is essential to prevent irreversible brain injury.

Other relevant entry Phenylketonuria.

▥ Biotin-responsive encephalopathy

Biotin is a cofactor for several carboxylase enzymes which incorporate carbon dioxide into intermediary metabolites. Holocarboxylase synthetase is the enzyme which activates the inactive carboxylase apoenzymes by attaching biotin; deficiency of this enzyme therefore affects all the enzymes requiring biotin cofactor (multiple carboxylase deficiency). Biotinidase is required to free biotin for reuse.

Hence both holocarboxylase deficiency and biotindase deficiency may result in biotin deficiency (as may dietary deficiency or a failure of absorption). Clinical features include:

- Holocarboxylase deficiency
    usually presents in infants aged 3 to 6 months;
    failure to thrive;
    apnoea, hypotonia;
    metabolic (lactic) acidosis;
    dermatological changes: rash resembling seborrhoeic dermatitis, alopecia;
    seizures +/− myoclonus, ataxia (progressive myoclonic epilepsy);
    T and B lymphocyte dysfunction.
- Biotinidase deficiency
    usually later onset and less severe, although considerable clinical overlap.
    Central deafness usual. Candidal dermatitis.

Diagnosis is by urinary organic acid analysis, and blood enzyme assay. Treatment is with biotin (20 mg/day) and is dramatic.

Reference Wolff B, Grier RE, Lukvoy JRS *et al.* Biotinidase deficiency: a novel vitamin recycling defect. *Journal of Inherited and Metabolic Disease* 1985; **8(suppl 1)**: 53–58.

Other relevant entries Inherited metabolic diseases and the nervous system; Progressive myoclonic epilepsy.

■ Biotinidase deficiency– see Biotin-responsive encephalopathy

■ Bismuth toxicity – see Heavy metal poisoning

■ Black widow spider bite

The venom of the black widow spider effectively releases all acetylcholine in presynaptic nerve terminals at neuromuscular junctions and autonomic ganglia. The clinical picture is therefore of muscle cramps and spasms, and painful rigidity of trunk and leg muscles, followed by weakness and autonomic instability. Death may occur within the first 48 hours, but if the patient survives this with appropriate supportive therapy a full recovery occurs.

■ Blackouts – see Epilepsy: an overview; Syncope

■ Blastomycosis

A fungal infection causing a self-limiting respiratory illness, but which may occasionally cause chronic non-specific meningitis or intracranial abscess, more often in immunocompromised individuals. The organism, *Blastomyces dermatitidis*, is seldom identified from the CSF; culture from extraneural sites may be possible. Treatment is with intravenous amphotericin, followed by itraconazole.

Other relevant entry Meningitis: an overview.

■ Blepharospasm

Pathophysiology Blepharospasm is a form of focal dystonia characterized by the involuntary closure of the eyelids as a result of contraction of orbicularis oculi. It may occur in isolation ("benign essential blepharospasm"), or as part of a more complex cranial dystonia (e.g. Meige's syndrome), or in association with another neurological disorder such as Parkinson's disease. Other examples of "secondary blepharospasm" include drug therapy (neuroleptics, levodopa) and lesions of brainstem, and more rarely cerebellum and striatum. Women are affected more often than men; age of onset is usually over 40 years of age. Blepharospasm may be effectively treated with botulinum toxin injections.

Clinical features: history and examination

- Blepharospasm is usually bilateral in origin and begins as an increase in frequency of blinking that leads to clonic and then forced tonic closure of the eyelids. All three states are encompassed by the term blepharospasm. Most patients reach the latter stage within 3 years of the disease onset. Eyelid closure may be so prolonged as to cause functional blindness. There may be an associated grittiness in the eyes.
- Like other forms of dystonia, blepharospasm may be relieved by sensory tricks (*geste antagoniste*) such as talking, yawning, singing, humming, or touching the eyelid. This feature is helpful in diagnosis. Blepharospasm may be aggravated by reading, watching television, exposure to wind, or bright light.
- Blepharospasm may be associated with dystonia of other cranial muscles, including face, jaw, tongue, or neck, and is then termed Meige's syndrome or blepharospasm–oromandibular dystonia.

Investigations and diagnosis Investigations are usually normal, unless blepharospasm is occurring secondary to a basal ganglia lesion or disease.

Differential diagnosis Apraxia of eyelid opening: failure to activate levator palpebrae superioris, rather than involuntary contraction of orbicularis oculi; hence sometimes known as "levator inhibition".

Hemifacial spasm.

Facial myokymia.

Myotonia.

Disease of the eyelid and associated ocular structures, including keratitis, conjunctivitis, uveitis

Photophobia, for example in meningitis, migraine.

Frequent blinking has been reported as a presenting feature of myasthenia gravis.

Treatment and prognosis Botulinum toxin injected into orbicularis oculi at three sites around the eye, to weaken dystonic muscle, is now the treatment of choice. Injections need to be repeated every 3 months or so.

Oral drugs are generally ineffective in the treatment of this condition, but anticholinergics, baclofen, clonazepam, tetrabenazine, carbamazepine, and tricyclic antidepressants have all been tried.

Surgical myectomy may be considered in drug-resistant cases, along with the possibility of chemical myectomy with local injection of doxorubicin.

Reference Hallett M, Daroff RB. Blepharospasm: report of a workshop. *Neurology* 1996; **46**: 1213–1218.

Other relevant entries Apraxia; Botulinum toxin therapy; Dystonia: an overview; Meige's syndrome.

■ Blindsight

Blindsight describes a rare phenomenon in which patients with bilateral occipital lobe damage affecting the primary visual cortex are nonetheless able to discriminate certain visual events within their "blind" fields, but are not aware of their ability to do so.

Reference Weiskrantz L. *Blindsight. A Case Study and Implications.* Oxford: Clarendon, 1986.

■ Bloch–Sulzberger syndrome – see Incontinentia pigmenti (Achromians)

■ Blue rubber Bleb Naevus syndrome

A rare viscero-cutaneous haemangiomatosis, in which bluish rubbery naevi occur on the skin and also in the lungs, liver, skeletal muscle, and, rarely, the central nervous system (CNS). Neurological presentations include focal seizures and cerebellar syndrome. MRI shows high signal intensity lesions on T_2-weighted scans. Haemorrhage and calcification may also be observed. Surgical ablation is possible but conservative management is often adequate. The differential diagnosis encompasses hereditary haemorrhagic telangiectasia.

References Fernandes C, Silva A, Coelho A, Campos M, Pontes F. Blue rubber bleb naevus: case report and literature review. *European Journal of Gastroenterology and Hepatology* 1999; **11**: 455–457.

Wills AJ, Marsden CD (eds). *Fifty Neurological Cases from the National Hospital.* London: Martin Dunitz, 1999: 133–135 [Case 41].

Other relevant entry Phakomatosis.

■ Bobble head doll syndrome

Structural lesions around the third ventricle, such as a tumour, cyst, or aqueduct stenosis, with slowly progressive hydrocephalus, may cause stereotyped head nodding at 2–3 Hz in children. This condition enters the differential diagnosis of spasmus nutans.

Reference Benton JW, Nellhaus G, Huttenlocher PR *et al.* The bobble-head doll syndrome: report of a unique truncal tremor associated with third ventricular cyst and hydrocephalus in children. *Neurology* 1966; **16**: 725–729.

Other relevant entries Arachnoid cyst; Hydrocephalus.

■ Body dysmorphic disorder – see Obsessive–compulsive disorder; Somatoform disorders

■ Bogorad's syndrome – see Bell's Palsy

■ Bonnet syndrome – see Charles Bonnet syndrome

■ Bornholm disease – see Myositis

■ Borreliosis

Bannwarth's syndrome • Garin–Bujadoux meningopolyneuritis •
Lyme disease • Neuroborreliosis

Pathophysiology Infection with the spirochaete *Borrelia burgdorferi*, transmitted by
the bite of infected *Ixodes* ticks, is the cause of borreliosis, a condition endemic in
various areas (coastal north-eastern USA, New Forest UK, Germany). Sequelae of
infection may be dermatological, cardiological, and neurological; the latter may
include aseptic meningitis +/− multiple radicular or peripheral nerve lesions
(Garin–Bujadoux meningopolyneuritis), myelitis, cranial neuropathy (especially
facial nerve) +/− meningoradiculitis of the cauda equina (Bannwarth's syndrome).

Clinical features: history and examination

- *Stage I*: early local infection: rash (erythema migrans chronicum); diagnostic, but
  often missed, occurs 3–30 days after tick bite.
- *Stage II*: early disseminated Lyme disease: cardiac conduction abnormalities,
  polyarthropathy (large joints > distal), myalgia, fatigue, fever, meningitis,
  cranial +/− peripheral neuropathy, radiculitis, transverse myelitis.
- *Stage III*: late Lyme disease: progressive encephalopathy, +/− sensorimotor
  polyradiculoneuropathy.

Investigations and diagnosis *Bloods*: serology for antibodies to *B. burgdorferi*; if positive indicates exposure (may be positive in asymptomatic individuals in endemic
areas).

Neurophysiology: EMG/NCS: neuropathy, radiculopathy.

CSF: lymphocytic pleocytosis, elevated protein, normal glucose.

Differential diagnosis *Facial palsy*: Bell's palsy, other causes of facial weakness.
Differential diagnosis of radiculopathy, meningitis, encephalopathy.

Treatment and prognosis *Antibiotics*: oral doxycycline may be adequate for facial
nerve palsy, whereas intravenous antibiotics (e.g. ceftriaxone, penicillin G) are
required for other neurological complications.

With appropriate treatment, improvement of neurological features should be
expected in days to weeks, although encephalopathy may not improve. An inverse
correlation between time to diagnosis and treatment, and degree of clinical improvement has been noted.

Vaccine does exist for patients deemed at risk (e.g. travel to endemic areas).

References Finkel MF. Lyme disease and its neurologic complications. *Archives of
Neurology* 1988; **45**: 99–104.

Report of the Quality Standards Subcommittee of the American Academy of
Neurology. Practice parameter: diagnosis of patients with nervous system Lyme
borreliosis (Lyme disease) – summary statement. *Neurology* 1996; **46**: 881–882.

Steere AC. Lyme disease. *New England Journal of Medicine* 1989; **321**: 586–596.

Other relevant entries Aseptic meningitis: differential diagnosis; Bell's palsy; Encephalopathies: an overview; Meningitis: an overview; Radiculopathies: an overview.

■ Botulinum toxin therapy

The therapeutic use of botulinum toxin by local injection has revolutionized the treatment of dystonia. Selective injection into dystonic muscles may weaken them sufficiently to ameliorate abnormal involuntary movements. The use of botulinum toxin has also been extensively explored as a therapeutic agent in spasticity, particularly focal spasticity.

Once established on an appropriate dose, botulinum toxin injections need to be repeated around every 3 months. Some patients develop antibodies to the toxin, and in such cases therapy often loses its efficacy. The mechanism of action is detailed in the entry on botulism.

Conditions currently treated with botulinum toxin injections include:
- Ocular disorders
    Strabismus.
- Dystonias
    Blepharospasm
    Spasmodic torticollis
    Oromandibular dystonia
    Spasmodic dysphonia
    Writer's cramp
    Other task-specific dystonias.
- Dyskinesias
    Hemifacial spasm
    Tremor.
- Spasticity, for example in multiple sclerosis, cerebral palsy syndromes.

Many other potential applications have been considered, including tinnitus, chronic tension-type headache, migraine, Parkinson's disease, palatal myoclonus, drooling, hyperhidrosis.

Side-effects include excessive weakness if too large a dose is used; dysphagia may follow even distant injections, for example for spasmodic torticollis.

References Anonymous. New uses for botulinum toxin. *Expert Opinion on Therapeutic Patents* 2002; **12**: 593–596.

Jankovic J. Use of botulinum toxin in neurology. In: Kennard C (ed.). *Recent Advances in Clinical Neurology 8*. Edinburgh: Churchill Livingstone, 1995: 89–110.

Jost WH (ed.). Evidence-based medicine (EBM) in botulinum toxin treatment. *Journal of Neurology* 2001; **248(suppl 1)**.

Moore P, Naumann M (eds). *Handbook of Botulinum Toxin Treatment* (2nd edition). Oxford: Blackwell Scientific, 2003.

Other relevant entries Blepharospasm; Botulism; Dystonia: an overview; Hemifacial spasm; Rigid spine syndrome; Spasmodic dysphonia; Spasmodic torticollis; Writer's cramp.

■ Botulism

Pathophysiology Botulism is an extremely rare condition resulting from infection with the Gram-positive anaerobic bacillus *Clostridium botulinum* that produces a polypeptide exotoxin which exerts neurological effects. Botulinum toxin (Btx) blocks synaptic transmission at the neuromuscular junction (and indeed has been used as a therapeutic agent for dystonic movement disorders and spasticity). Specifically, holotoxin comprises heavy (H) and light (L) chains joined by a disulphide bond; a sequence at the carboxyl end of the heavy (H_C) chain binds with high affinity to a specific presynaptic neuronal surface receptor at cholinergic synapses, allowing toxin to cross the plasma membrane via receptor-mediated endocytosis. From the endosome, toxin enters cell cytoplasm via a pH-dependent conformational change mediated by the amino end of the heavy chain (H_N). Reduction of the disulphide bond releases the L chain, the toxic moiety, an endopeptidase which selectively cleaves proteins essential for the recognition and docking of neurotransmitter-containing vesicles with the plasma membrane [e.g. synapto-brevin or vesicle-associated membrane protein (VAMP), syntaxin, SNAP-25]. This prevents the quantal release of acetylcholine (ACh), and hence clinical features (autonomic dysfunction, muscle paralysis) appear 12–36 hours after toxin ingestion.

Bacterial contamination of foodstuffs is the commonest cause of botulism, but it may also occur in wounds, and as an infantile infection. The clinical presentation is with autonomic failure and muscle paralysis. Treatment is supportive; recovery may be prolonged and incomplete.

Clinical features: history and examination Three variants are recognized:
- Infantile botulism: infants between 2 weeks and 11 months of age are susceptible to intestinal colonization by *C. botulinum*, leading to flaccid paralysis, cranial nerve signs, and autonomic signs.
- Foodborne botulism: causes an afebrile descending paralysis with autonomic and cranial nerve signs.
- Wound botulism: conditions predisposing to this are similar to those encountered in tetanus.

In infantile and foodborne botulism, first symptoms after toxin ingestion (12–36 hours) are anorexia, nausea, vomiting, and diarrhoea (gastroenteritis); not a feature of wound botulism.

Parasympathetic features generally precede muscle weakness: blurred vision and diplopia with an ophthalmoplegia, ptosis and large unreactive pupils, and concurrent bulbar failure.

Descending flaccid paralysis, and signs of autonomic failure (bradycardia, postural hypotension, dry mouth) then occur.

Sensory and cognitive functions are normal.

In foodborne botulism, there may be a history of other people with similar symptoms, or of home canning or bottling of foods (spores can survive for long periods of time and germinate in anaerobic conditions of increased alkalinity with a rise in temperature).

Drug abuse is a risk factor for the development of wound botulism.

Investigations and diagnosis *Bloods*: usually normal; may be able to assay for the toxin in blood.

Imaging: usually normal.

CSF: usually normal.

Neurophysiology: key investigation, showing decreased amplitude of the evoked compound muscle action potentials and, characteristically, an incremental response on rapid repetitive nerve stimulation but a decrement with slow repetitive nerve stimulation. Nerve conduction studies reveal normal conduction velocities (i.e. no neuropathy).

Differential diagnosis

Myasthenia gravis.

Miller Fisher variant of Guillain–Barré syndrome.

Bickerstaff's brainstem encephalitis.

Diphtheria.

Poliomyelitis.

Brainstem vascular lesions.

Treatment and prognosis Treatment is supportive, with respiratory monitoring and, if necessary, ventilation in the intensive care unit. Prolonged parenteral feeding may be required due to autonomic involvement of the gut.

Antibiotic treatment may be given but aminoglycosides should be avoided since they can potentiate neuromuscular blockade.

In the early stages, trivalent equine antitoxin is recommended (after intradermal hypersensitivity testing).

The recovery phase may be prolonged, up to years, and is often incomplete. Botulism is a notifiable disease.

> **Reference** Critchley EMR, Mitchell JD. Human botulism. *British Journal of Hospital Medicine* 1990; **43**: 290–292.
>
> **Other relevant entries** Bickerstaff's brainstem encephalitis; Botulinum toxin therapy; Brainstem vascular syndromes; Diphtheria: Miller Fisher syndrome; Myasthenia gravis; Neuromuscular junction diseases: an overview; Poliomyelitis.

■ Boucher–Neuhauser syndrome

A syndrome comprising:

- spinocerebellar ataxia,
- hypogonadotropic hypogonadism,
- choroidal dystrophy.

Reference Limber ER, Bresnick EH, Lebovitz RM *et al.* Spinocerebellar ataxia, hypogonadotropic hypogonadism and choroidal dystrophy (Boucher–Neuhauser syndrome). *American Journal of Medical Genetics* 1989; **33**: 409–414.

■ Bourneville disease – see Tuberous sclerosis

■ Bovine spongiform encephalopathy – see Prion disease: an overview; Variant Creutzfeldt–Jakob disease

■ Braak disease – see Argyrophilic Grain disease

■ Brachial plexopathies

Pathophysiology The brachial plexus is a collection of nerves, taking their origin from the C5 to T1 anterior and posterior nerve roots, which is located in the region from the lateral aspect of the neck to the axilla, just superior to the apex of the lung. The brachial plexus gives rise to all the nerves of the upper limb. It may be selectively involved in disease processes, and is subject to traumatic injury (e.g. motorbike injuries). Recovery is dependent on the aetiology and extent of the insult.

Recognized causes of brachial plexopathy include:
- Trauma
    Upper plexus: C5–C6 roots and upper trunk (Erb–Duchenne paralysis; *q.v.*)
    Lower plexus: C8–T1 roots and lower trunk (Klumpke paralysis; *q.v.*)
- Inflammatory
    acute brachial neuropathy/plexitis, brachial neuritis, neuralgic amyotrophy
    (*q.v.*), Parsonage–Turner syndrome (synonymous terms).
- Neoplastic
    Upper plexus:
        Primary: neurofibroma, schwannoma, neurogenic sarcoma/fibrosarcoma (rare)
        Secondary: metastatic disease from lung, breast.
    Lower plexus:
        Primary: Pancoast tumour (lung apex)
        Secondary: metastatic disease from lung, breast.
- Postirradiation
- Inherited: hereditary liability to pressure palsies (HNLPP), hereditary neuralgic amyotrophy
- Structural: thoracic outlet syndrome (*q.v.*)
- Drug abuse: heroin.

Clinical features: history and examination Upper limb sensory and/or motor dysfunction (depressed or absent tendon reflexes) in the territory of more than one cervical root or peripheral nerve (i.e. not explicable as single root or nerve lesion).

- Pain may be a feature (striking in neuralgic amyotrophy, tumour infiltration) or may be absent (postirradiation).
- Historical features may suggest aetiology:

  Trauma, for example motorbike accidents, obstetric trauma, gunshot wounds, carrying heavy rucksack, electrical injury.

  Previous tumour, radiation.

  Drug abuse.

  Individual or family history of previous entrapment neuropathies (HNLPP).

A particularly difficult situation occurs when women previously treated for breast cancer, including radiation therapy of axillary nodes, present with a brachial plexopathy, the differential lying between neoplastic infiltration and postirradiation change. Clues to correct diagnosis include:

Pain: typically absent in postirradiation change; may be major clinical symptom in neoplastic infiltration.

Lower plexus more likely to be involved in postirradiation change (upper plexus relatively protected by other anatomical structures).

Neurophysiology: myokymia typical of postirradiation change.

Investigations and diagnosis *Bloods*: usually normal.

Imaging: MRI scanning of the cervical cord and plexus for focal lesions, swelling. Apical views on a chest X-ray, $+/-$ high resolution CT scan through chest, lung apices and plexus.

Neurophysiology:

EMG/NCS: usually critical in distinguishing plexus lesions from cervical radiculopathies if this cannot be done clinically. A reduced sensory action potential implies the lesion is postganglionic and therefore not a radiculopathy. The distribution and size of reduction of SAPs and CMAPs helps localize the site of the lesion within the plexus, as does the pattern of denervation on EMG sampling. In particular, denervation in the cervical paraspinal muscles implies a root lesion, since the plexus does not innervate these muscles. Myokymia is seen in postradiation plexopathy and not in neoplastic plexopathies.

SSEPs: from the upper limb can help localize site of lesion, in terms of plexus versus cervical roots.

CSF: usually normal; may be non-specific elevation of protein.

Other: Axon reflex test: scratching the skin with 1% histamine or intradermal injection will normally induce a wheal and vasodilatory response. If there is a postganglionic lesion this reaction is lost. This test may be used for localization of the level of the lesion by applying it to different dermatomes.

Differential diagnosis

Cervical radiculopathies:

Multiple mononeuropathies.

Motor neurone disease.

Neurogenic thoracic outlet syndrome.

Focal upper limb chronic inflammatory demyelinating polyneuropathy.

Rotator cuff injuries.

Acute poliomyelitis.

Treatment and prognosis Of cause, where identified. Inflammatory lesions may be treated with steroids. Traumatic injury may sometimes be amenable to microsurgical repair.

> **References** Harris W. *The Morphology of the Brachial Plexus*. Oxford: OUP, 1939.
>
> Russell JW, Windebank AJ. Brachial and lumbar neuropathies. In: McLeod JG (ed.). *Inflammatory Neuropathies*. London: Baillière Tindall, 1994: 173–191.

Other relevant entries Cervical cord and root disease; Chemotherapy and radiotherapy-induced neurological disorders; Chronic inflammatory demyelinating neuropathy; Entrapment neuropathies; Erb's palsy, Erb–Duchenne palsy; Hereditary neuropathy with liability to pressure palsies; Klumpke's paralysis; Lumbosacral plexopathies; Motor neurone disease; Multifocal motor neuropathy; Neuralgic amyotrophy; Neuropathies: an overview; Pancoast syndrome; Poliomyelitis; Rucksack paralysis; Thoracic outlet syndromes.

■ Bradbury–Eggleston syndrome – see Autonomic failure; Pure autonomic failure

■ "Brain attack" – see Cerebrovascular disease: arterial

■ Brain death, brainstem death

Pathophysiology Brain death is the permanent cessation of all brain function, both cerebral cortex and brainstem. Brainstem death is the permanent cessation of all brainstem function. Patients are unconscious, apnoeic, and have lost all brainstem reflexes. These are clinical diagnoses. Because individuals suffering brain or brainstem death are potential donors of organs for transplantation, the necessity to establish such diagnoses definitively has become increasingly important. This remains an area of some ethical dispute.

The diagnosis of brainstem death should not normally be considered until at least 6 hours has elapsed from the onset of coma or 24 hours if coma was secondary to anoxia and/or a cardiac arrest. The diagnosis requires a number of criteria to be fulfilled by two independent medical doctors, one of whom is a neurologist. It is normally convenient for one to do the testing and the other to witness. Respiratory disconnection is usually supervised by an anaesthetist and witnessed by the assessors.

The cause of the irreversible brain damage needs to be established, and the reasons why it is irremediable. The time of onset of coma needs to be known.

Clinical features: history and examination Criteria vary in different countries

- Preconditions
  1. Could primary hypothermia, drugs, metabolic–endocrine abnormalities be contributing significantly to the apnoeic coma? (Where appropriate check plasma and urine for drugs, as well as plasma pH, glucose, sodium, and calcium.)
  2. Have any neuromuscular blocking drugs been administered during the preceding 12 hours?
  3. Is the rectal temperature over 35°C? If not, warm the patient up and reassess.

Only if all the preconditions have been met can the examination be undertaken.

- Examination

  All questions must be answered in the negative for the diagnosis to be made.
  1. Doll's eye (oculocephalic) movements: is there any contraversive conjugate deviation of the eyes when the head is gently and fully rotated to either side (i.e. doll's eye movements intact)?
  2. Do the pupils react to light?
  3. Is there any response to corneal stimulation on either side?
  4. Do the eyes deviate when either ear is irrigated with 50 ml of ice cold water for 30 seconds (i.e. oculovestibular reflexes intact)? Check the tympanic membranes are intact first.
  5. Is there a gag reflex?
  6. Is there a cough reflex following bronchial stimulation by a suction catheter?
  7. Is there any motor response within the cranial nerve distribution to a painful stimulus?
  8. Is there any spontaneous ventilation?

If not then preoxygenate the patient for 10 minutes with 100% oxygen and record arterial blood gases (ABG). The $PaCO_2$ must exceed 5.3 kPa before disconnection from the ventilator. Disconnect the patient from the ventilator and give oxygen at 6 l/min via a suction catheter in the trachea and wait 10 minutes before repeating the ABG: the $PaCO_2$ must exceed 6.65 kPa at the end of the disconnection period. Is there any spontaneous respiratory movement?

Investigations and diagnosis As mentioned this is a clinical diagnosis.

It has been suggested that investigations such as the EEG, transcranial Doppler ultrasonography, or brain PET scanning might be helpful in establishing the diagnosis, but these have not been incorporated in accepted diagnostic criteria in the UK.

Differential diagnosis Possibly reversible brain dysfunction, as a consequence of drug/toxin ingestion or hypothermia, must be considered.

Treatment and prognosis The diagnosis implies that there is no hope of recovery.

References O'Brien MD. Criteria for diagnosing brainstem death. *British Medical Journal* 1990; **301**: 108–109.

Pallis C, Harley DH. *ABC of Brainstem Death*, 2nd edition. London: BMJ, 1996.

The Quality Standards Subcommittee of the American Academy of Neurology. Practice parameters for determining brain death in adults (summary statement). *Neurology* 1995; **45**: 1012–1014.

■ Brainstem encephalitis – see Bickerstaff's brainstem encephalitis; Encephalitis: an overview

■ Brainstem vascular syndromes

Numerous eponymous brainstem vascular disorders are described, characterized on the basis of the particular combination of neurological signs, encompassing cranial nerve palsies, cerebellar signs, and long tract signs. These include:

- Midbrain

  Weber's syndrome: ipsilateral oculomotor nerve palsy and contralateral hemiplegia.

  Benedikt's syndrome: ipsilateral oculomotor nerve palsy and contralateral involuntary movements (tremor, chorea, athetosis, due to red nucleus involvement), +/− contralateral hemiparesis.

  Claude's syndrome: ipsilateral oculomotor nerve palsy and contralateral cerebellar ataxia including asynergy, and dysdiadochokinesis.

  Nothnagel's syndrome: ipsilateral oculomotor nerve palsy and contralateral cerebellar ataxia +/− trochlear nerve palsy, +/− sensory loss, +/− nystagmus.

- Pons

  Millard–Gubler syndrome: ipsilateral VI and VII nerve palsies with contralateral hemiplegia

  Raymond syndrome: ipsilateral VI nerve palsy with contralateral hemiplegia.

  Locked-in syndrome (de-efferented state): with bilateral ventral lesions.

  Foville syndrome: ipsilateral gaze paresis (looking away from the lesion), ipsilateral lower motor neurone VII nerve palsy with contralateral hemiplegia.

  Raymond–Céstan syndrome: ipsilateral cerebellar ataxia, contralateral hypoaesthesia (all modalities), +/− contralateral hemiparesis.

  Marie–Foix syndrome: ipsilateral cerebellar ataxia, contralateral hemiparesis, +/− contralateral hypoaesthesia (pain and temperature).

- Medulla

  Medial medullary syndrome (Déjerine's anterior bulbar syndrome): ipsilateral tongue (XII) paresis, contralateral hemiplegia, contralateral hypoaesthesia (position and vibration sensation).

  Céstan syndrome (medial medullary tegmentum): ipsilateral vocal cord and palatal paralysis, ipsilateral Horner's syndrome, ipsilateral ataxia, contralateral hemiplegia, contralateral hemianaesthesia for proprioception, discriminative touch.

  Lateral medullary syndrome (Wallenberg's syndrome): ipsilateral facial hypoaesthesia (pain and temperature), contralateral body hypoaesthesia (pain and temperature), ipsilateral Horner's syndrome, palatal, pharyngeal and vocal cord paralysis, ipsilateral cerebellar signs.

Avellis syndrome: soft palate and vocal cord paralysis with contralateral hemi-anaesthesia.

Babinski–Nageotte syndrome: contralateral hemiplegia and sensory loss, ipsilateral hemiataxia and facial sensory loss, dysarthria, dysphonia, and dysphagia but no tongue (XII) involvement.

Reinhold's syndrome, hemimedullary syndrome = lateral + medial medullary syndrome.

Opalski's (submedullary) syndrome: lateral medullary (Wallenberg) syndrome with ipsilateral hemiplegia.

The clinical features, investigations, and treatment are further described in individual entries.

Some take the view that splitting brainstem vascular syndromes into eponymous syndromes implies differences that are not helpful in management, since the latter depends on aetiology; treatment is irrespective of the precise clinical picture.

References Gan R, Noronha A. The medullary vascular syndromes revisited. *Journal of Neurology* 1995; **242**: 195–202.

Thomas DJ. Basilar thrombosis. In: Welch KMA, Caplan LR, Reis DJ *et al.* (eds). *Primer on Cerebrovascular Diseases*. San Diego: Academic, 1997: 771–773.

Other relevant entries Cerebrovascular disease: arterial; Top of the basilar syndrome.

■ Branched-chain ketoaciduria – see Maple syrup urine disease

■ Branching enzyme deficiency – see Glycogen-storage disorders: an overview

■ Bresolin's disease – see Glycogen-storage disorders: an overview; Phosphoglycerate kinase deficiency

■ Briquet syndrome
Somatization disorder

This polysymptomatic disorder beginning in earlier life is commoner in women, who present recurrently with a variety of somatic complaints that defy medical explanation; it may be defined as a "conversion disorder" or an "hysterical illness". Symptoms may include:

- Neurological (or pseudoneurological): amnesia, dysphagia, aphonia, deafness, double vision, blurred vision, blindness, loss of consciousness/fainting, seizure, or convulsion, difficulty walking, paralysis, muscle weakness, urinary retention, difficulty urinating.

- Gastrointestinal: nausea, vomiting, bloating, pain, diarrhoea, food intolerance.
- Cardiopulmonary: dyspnoea, palpitations, chest pain, dizziness.
- Pain: back, joints, extremities, during urination; headache.
- Sexual/reproductive: dyspareunia, sexual indifference, impotence, menstrual pain, menstrual irregularity.

Management is avoidance of invasive procedures or investigations, and of addictive medications.

Other relevant entry Somatoform disorders.

■ Brissaud syndrome, Brissaud–Sicard syndrome

A brainstem syndrome comprising facial hemispasm with contralateral hemiparesis due to a pontine lesion, caudo-ventrally.

■ Broca's aphasia – see Aphasia

■ Brody's disease

A rare disease of childhood characterized by poor relaxation of muscles, initially in the limbs, then in face and trunk. Mild muscle atrophy and weakness may develop. Despite the clinical resemblance to myotonia, EMG shows no myotonic discharges, hence this is a pseudomyotonia syndrome. It is thought to result from abnormalities of the sarcoplasmic reticulum Ca^{2+} ATPase, and some cases with recessive inheritance have mutations in the gene encoding SERCA1, the fast-twitch skeletal muscle sarcoplasmic reticulum Ca^{2+} ATPase.

Reference Odermatt A, Taschner PE, Scherer SW *et al*. Mutations in the gene encoding SERCA1, the fast-twitch skeletal muscle sarcoplasmic reticulum Ca^{2+} ATPase, are associated with Brody disease. *Nature Genetics* 1996; **14**: 191–194.

Other relevant entry Myotonia and myotonic syndromes.

■ Brown's syndrome
Superior oblique tendon sheath syndrome

Brown's syndrome is restriction of active and passive elevation of the eye in adduction (i.e. compromised superior oblique muscle action) resulting in intermittent vertical diplopia. There may be an associated pulling sensation or clicking noise in the orbit; there may be focal pain at the corner of the orbit. This is due to a restriction of free movement through the trochlea pulley mechanism. The condition may be congenital or acquired, recognized causes including trauma and inflammation (e.g. collagen vascular diseases, such as SLE and Sjögren's syndrome). The previous name of "superior oblique tendon sheath syndrome" is not justified, surgery to the sheath seldom produces clinical benefit. Spontaneous resolution may occur; treatment of the underlying cause (e.g. inflammation) may be required. Superior oblique tenotomy with or without ipsilateral inferior oblique recession may be appropriate in congenital cases.

Reference Wilson ME, Eustis HS, Parks MM. Brown's syndrome. *Survey of Ophthalmology* 1989; **34**: 153–172.

Other relevant entry Cranial nerve disease: IV: Trochlear nerve.

■ Brown–Séquard syndrome

Pathophysiology Anatomical or functional hemisection of the spinal cord produces a reproducible pattern of clinical deficits which is of localizing value, as first described by Brown–Séquard. Spinal cord lesions causing this syndrome may be either extramedullary or intramedullary, with the former said to be more common.

Clinical features: history and examination

- Ipsilateral spastic weakness (involvement of corticospinal tract);
- Segmental lower motor neurone signs at the level of the lesion (roots, anterior horn cells);
- Ipsilateral proprioceptive loss (dorsal columns) with contralateral pain and temperature loss (crossed spinothalamic tract) = dissociated sensory loss.

Investigations and diagnosis *Imaging*: MRI for focal cord lesion (extramedullary or intramedullary).

Differential diagnosis

Multiple sclerosis.

Spinal cord tumour (intrinsic or extrinsic).

Prolapsed cervical intervertebral disc.

Trauma.

Myelitis.

Radiation-induced myelopathy.

Treatment and prognosis Dependent on cause.

Reference Tattersall R, Turner B. Brown–Séquard and his syndrome. *Lancet* 2000; **356**: 61–63.

Other relevant entries Myelopathy: an overview; Spinal cord disease: an overview; Spinal cord trauma.

■ Brown–Vialetto–Van Laere Syndrome
Pontobulbar palsy with deafness

A rare, fatal brainstem degeneration occurring in childhood, with early and prominent sensorineural hearing deficit. Involvement of all muscles supplied by cranial nerves below the fifth occurs (bulbar spinal muscular atrophy). Spinal motor neurones and the pyramidal tract may also be affected. The condition is probably recessive.

Reference Francis DA, Ponsford JR, Wiles CM, Thomas PK, Duchen LW. Brown–Vialetto–van Laere syndrome. *Neuropathology and Applied Neurobiology* 1993; **19**: 91–94.

Other relevant entries Hearing loss: differential diagnosis; Motor neurone diseases: an overview; Spinal muscular atrophy.

■ Brownell–Oppenheimer variant – see Creutzfeldt–Jakob disease

■ Brucellosis
Neurobrucellosis

Pathophysiology *Brucella melitensis*, a Gram-negative coccobacillus, is the commonest of the *Brucella* species to cause human disease. *B. abortus*, *B. suis*, and *B. canis* (naturally found in goats/sheep/camels; cattle; pig, and dog, respectively) may also cause human disease. Acquisition is often through consumption of contaminated (unpasteurized) milk or its products, or contact with infected animals. Spread is from gastrointestinal tract to bloodstream, organs particularly affected being bone, spleen, lungs, as well as brain. Chronic relapsing illness, often involving the nervous system, is typical. Brucellosis is diagnosed by serological testing, and when treated early has a good prognosis.

Clinical features: history and examination

Protean!

Acute:

meningoencephalitis.

Chronic:

lymphocytic meningitis;

demyelination, for example retrobulbar neuritis;

radiculopathy, especially lumbar;

cranial nerve mononeuritis, particularly VIII;

cerebral arteritis, subarachnoid haemorrhage;

spinal cord compression by granuloma;

extrapyramidal syndrome.

Investigations and diagnosis *Culture* of organism from blood, CSF, lymph node, or bone marrow.

Serology: Rose-Bengal/agglutination tests may be positive in endemic areas without active disease; ELISA is more sensitive and specific.

Imaging: CT/MRI may show periventricular change; spinal MRI may identify extradural compressive granulomatous disease.

CSF: raised protein, lymphocytic pleocytosis, low glucose in 20%. May have oligoclonal bands. Elevated adenine deaminase (ADA) is non-specific. PCR for *Brucella* may be helpful.

Neurophysiology:

EEG: in meningoencephalitis shows slowing and sometimes epileptiform features; may be helpful to differentiate other causes of encephalopathy.

EMG: in cases of radiculopathy.

Others: plain radiology, bone scan: for sacroiliitis, lumbar spine involvement. ECG, Echocardiogram: for endocarditis.

Differential diagnosis Broad neurological differential diagnosis:

Tuberculosis
Neurosyphilis
Neuroborreliosis
Neurosarcoidosis
Neuro-Behçet's
CNS lymphoma
CNS vasculitis
Extradural spinal cord compression
Multiple sclerosis.

Treatment and prognosis Rifampicin (600–900 mg/day) and doxycycline (100–200 mg/day) with co-trimoxazole or (if no deafness) streptomycin (0.5–1 g/day intramuscularly). In chronic disease this cocktail should be given for 3–6 months (recheck CSF to look for resolution).

Recovery is the norm for acute episodes. In chronic disease, the outlook is good for cord compression if recognized and treated early, but less good for radiculopathy and meningoencephalitis.

References Madkour MM (ed.). *Brucellosis*. London: Butterworth, 1989.

Shakir RA. Brucellosis. In: Shakir RA, Newman PK, Poser CM (eds). *Tropical Neurology*. London: Saunders, 1996: 167–181.

Other relevant entry Endocarditis and the nervous system.

■ Bruck–DeLange syndrome

This syndrome consists of:

- congenital muscle hypertrophy,
- mental retardation,
- extrapyramidal movement disorder (athetosis).

The Bruck–DeLange syndrome enters the differential diagnosis of myotonia congenita because of the muscle hypertrophy.

Other relevant entry Myotonia congenita.

■ Brueghel's syndrome

This is the name given to a dystonia of the motor trigeminal nerve causing gaping or involuntary opening of the mouth, so named after Brueghel's painting *De Gaper* of

1558, thought to illustrate a typical case. Additional features may include paroxysmal hyperpnoea and upbeating nystagmus. Brueghel's syndrome should be distinguished from other syndromes of cranial dystonia featuring blepharospasm and oromandibular dystonia, better termed Meige's syndrome.

(NB some texts give "Breughel's" syndrome.)

> **Reference** Gilbert GJ. Brueghel syndrome: its distinction from Meige syndrome. *Neurology* 1996; **46**: 1767–1769.
>
> **Other relevant entries** Dystonia: an overview; Meige's syndrome.

■ Brun–Garland syndrome

This describes the asymmetric proximal neuropathy of the lower limb seen in diabetes mellitus, alternatively known as lumbosacral radiculoplexopathy or diabetic amyotrophy.

> **Other relevant entry** Diabetes mellitus and the nervous system.

■ Brushfield spots

Brushfield spots are small grey–white specks of depigmentation that can be seen in the irides of some (90%) patients with Down's syndrome; they may also occur in normal individuals.

> **Other relevant entry** Down's syndrome.

■ Bruxism

Bruxism is grinding of the teeth, which is very common, especially at night (hence a parasomnia). Severe forms, sufficient to mandate wearing tooth or gum shields, are less common, and seen particularly in patients with mental retardation and/or orobuccal dyskinesias. The neuroanatomical substrate for this disorder is not known.

> **Other relevant entry** Parasomnias.

■ Buccolingual syndrome

This is a form of tardive dyskinesia that involves involuntary movements of the facial muscles and protrusion of the tongue.

> **Other relevant entry** Drug-induced movement disorders.

■ Buerger's disease – see Von Winiwarter–Buerger's disease

■ Bulbar Palsy – see Dysarthria

■ Bulimia – see Eating disorders; Kleine–Levin syndrome

■ Bull's eye retinopathy

Retinopathy may occur as an ocular side-effect of anti-malarial drug therapy (chloroquine, hydroxychloroquine); these drugs may also be used in the management of rheumatoid arthritis, SLE, and sarcoidosis. Retinopathy is rare, usually mild and non-progressive, dose related and commoner with chloroquine. An intermediate stage of this pigmentary degeneration is characterized by reduced visual acuity and central foveolar hyperpigmentation surrounded by depigmentation encircled by hyperpigmentation ("bull's eye"). Maculopathy may progress even if the drug is stopped at this stage, hence the importance of screening (visual acuity, fundoscopy) in any patient receiving long-term anti-malarials (these drugs also commonly cause corneal deposits which are innocuous).

High-dose phenothiazine therapy may produce a similar picture.

■ Burning feet burning hands syndrome – see Altitude illness

Cc

■ CADASIL

Cerebral autosomal-dominant arteriopathy with subcortical infarcts and leukoencephalopathy • Chronic familial vascular encephalopathy • Hereditary multi-infarct dementia

Pathophysiology Cerebral *a*utosomal-*d*ominant *a*rteriopathy with *s*ubcortical *i*nfarcts and *l*eukoencephalopathy (CADASIL) is a genetic vasculopathy resulting from mutations within the gene encoding the notch 3 protein. The mechanisms by which mutations lead to disease are not currently understood. An autosomal-recessive variant (CARASIL) has also been described.

Clinical features: history and examination
- Ischaemic stroke, often recurrent, subcortical (lacunar syndromes).
- Migraine with aura: often adult onset.
- Psychiatric disturbance.
- Dementia of "subcortical" type (late).
- Pseudobulbar palsy (late).
- Acute encephalopathy: "CADASIL coma"; self-limiting, may be recurrent.
- There is marked variability in disease course and phenotype.

Investigations and diagnosis *Imaging*: MRI of brain shows confluent high signal in periventricular and deep white matter, plus focal areas of lacunar infarction and basal ganglia lesions. Anterior temporal pole and external capsule high signal may point to diagnosis.

Skin biopsy: granular osmophilic material, an abnormal protein deposit, may be seen adjacent to the basement membrane of smooth muscle cells of arterioles in the dermis; this is highly specific but sensitivity may be only around 50%.

Neurogenetics: *Notch 3* mutations, especially in exons 3, 4, 11, 19.

Brain biopsy: largely superseded by neurogenetic testing and skin biopsy.

Differential diagnosis Other causes of vascular dementia, although risk factors for stroke are often absent in CADASIL.

Treatment and prognosis No specific treatment currently known. Aspirin or other antiplatelet agents may be used; the place of warfarin remains uncertain. Acetazolamide has been reported of benefit for migraine.

References Bousser M-G, Tournier-Lasserve E. Cerebral autosomal dominant arteriopathy with subcortical infarcts and leukoencephalopathy: from stroke to vessel wall physiology. *Journal of Neurology, Neurosurgery and Psychiatry* 2001; **70**: 285–287.

Lammie GA, Rakshi J, Rossor MN, Harding AE, Scaravilli F. Cerebral autosomal dominant arteriopathy with subcortical infarcts and leukoencephalopathy (CADASIL) – confirmation by cerebral biopsy in 2 cases. *Clinical Neuropathology* 1995; **14**: 201–206.

Martin R, Markus H. CADASIL: a genetic form of subcortical vascular dementia. *Dementia Reviews* 2001; **4**(1): 1–6.

Schon F, Martin RJ, Prevett M, Clough C, Enevoldson TP, Markus HS. "CADASIL coma": an underdiagnosed acute encephalopathy. *Journal of Neurology, Neurosurgery and Psychiatry* 2003; **74**: 249–252.

Yanagawa S, Ito N, Arima K, Ikeda S. Cerebral autosomal recessive arteriopathy with subcortical infarcts and leukoencephalopathy. *Neurology* 2002; **58**: 817–820.

Other relevant entries Cerebrovascular disease: arterial; Lacunar syndromes; Migraine; Vascular dementia.

■ Caisson disease

Decompression sickness

Caisson disease or decompression sickness results from too rapid an ascent from a deep underwater dive, leading to the production of nitrogen bubbles within the circulation ("the bends"). These primarily affect the spinal vessels (especially posteriorly), characteristically in the upper thoracic region, producing myelopathic symptoms. Occasionally cerebral involvement is seen. Treatment is immediate hyperbaric oxygen therapy.

References Dick AP, Massey EW. Neurological presentations of decompression sickness and air embolism in sport divers. *Neurology* 1985; **35**: 667–671.

Hallenbeck JM, Bove AA, Elliott DH. Mechanisms underlying spinal cord damage in decompression sickness. *Neurology* 1975; **25**: 308–316.

Other relevant entries Myelopathy: an overview; Spinal cord vascular diseases.

■ Camptocormia

Bent spine syndrome • Souques disease

Camptocormia was first described as a "war neurosis", a psychiatric phenomenon occurring in men facing armed conflict. Subsequently it has been realized that reducible lumbar kyphosis may also result from neurological disorders, including muscle disease (paravertebral myopathy, nemaline myopathy), Parkinson's disease, dystonia, and, possibly, as a paraneoplastic phenomenon. Cases with associated lenticular (putaminal) lesions have also been described. Camptocormia may be related in some instances to dropped head syndrome.

References Djaldetti R, Mosberg-Galili R, Sroka H, Merims D, Melamed E. Camptocormia (bent spine) in patients with Parkinson's disease: characterisation and possible pathogenesis of an unusual phenomenon. *Movement Disorders* 1999; **14**: 443–447.

Umapathi T, Chaudhry V, Cornblath D *et al*. Head drop and camptocormia. *Journal of Neurology, Neurosurgery and Psychiatry* 2002; **72**: 1–7.

Other relevant entries Dropped head syndrome; Myopathy: an overview.

■ Camptodactyly

Isolated crooked little fingers • Streblomicrodactyly

Pathophysiology Camptodactyly is angulation at the proximal interphalangeal joint of the little finger. This may occur as part of a dysmorphic syndrome, or in isolation, the latter either as a sporadic or a familial condition. Inheritance in the latter is probably autosomal dominant with variable penetrance. It is seen incidentally in neurological outpatients more frequently than ulnar neuropathy with which it may be confused.

Clinical features: history and examination Camptodactyly ("bent finger") is a non-traumatic, painless, flexion deformity at the proximal interphalangeal joint of the little finger. Other fingers, and occasionally toes (especially the second), may also be affected. There are no sensory or motor signs. A non-inflammatory arthropathy may coexist with the flexion deformity.

Differential diagnosis

Trauma to little finger.

Ulnar neuropathy causing claw hand (*main en griffe*).

Dupuytren's contracture.

Scleroderma.

Focal dystonia or neuromyotonia.

Diabetic cheiroarthropathy.

Treatment and prognosis Various surgical approaches have been suggested, but there are no trial data. There is little functional compromise as a result of this deformity, which is non-progressive.

Reference Larner AJ. Camptodactyly in a neurology outpatient clinic. *International Journal of Clinical Practice* 2001; **55**: 592–595.

Other relevant entry Ulnar neuropathy.

■ Canavan's disease

Aspartoacylase deficiency • Canavan–van Bogaert–Bertrand disease • Canavan's diffuse sclerosis • Spongy degeneration of cerebral white matter

Pathophysiology Canavan's disease is a rare autosomal-recessive leukodystrophy, occurring mainly in Ashkenazi Jewish families, first described clinically by Canavan in 1931 and pathologically by van Bogaert and Bertrand in 1949. It presents as a progressive encephalopathy in the first months of life, with developmental regression, progressive macrocephaly, blindness with optic atrophy, and hypotonia, progressing to spasticity and seizures. There is no effective treatment and death occurs within 1–5 years. It is caused by a deficiency of the enzyme aspartoacylase, due to mutations in the encoding gene on the short arm of chromosome 17 (17p13), resulting in accumulation of N-acetyl-aspartic acid (NAA) and spongiform degeneration of the brain. Accumulation of N-acetyl-aspartate may also be detected in CSF, plasma, urine, and amniotic fluid.

Clinical features: history and examination Presentation is classically around 2–3 months of age with:

- Mental retardation: an absence or regression of neurological development, failure to thrive.
- Blindness with optic atrophy (between 6 and 18 months) $+/-$ deafness, $+/-$ bulbar symptoms.
- Hypotonia initially, overtaken by increasing spasticity with tonic extensor spasms.
- Progressive enlargement of the head (megalencephaly) to >3 standard deviations above the mean.
- Focal or tonic–clonic seizures are not uncommon.
- Dysautonomia: paroxysmal sweating, hyperthermia, vomiting.

Neonatal and juvenile forms are also described.

Investigations and diagnosis *Bloods*: raised plasma N-acetyl-aspartate.

Urine: raised N-acetyl-aspartate.

Imaging: CT/MRI shows extensive white matter demyelination, with high signal throughout the white matter on T_2-weighted images; MR spectroscopy shows marked elevation of NAA peak, diagnostic for this condition.

CSF: usually normal although on occasions a slightly high protein has been reported; raised N-acetyl-aspartate.

Neurophysiology:

EMG/NCS usually normal;
EEG shows variable non-specific abnormalities.

Others: cultured skin fibrobalsts have reduced aspartoacylase activity; raised N-acetyl-aspartate may be found in amniotic fluid.

Neurogenetics: a single mutation (E285A) in the aspartoacylase gene accounts for 80–85% of mutant alleles.

Pathology: spongy change in cerebral cortex, subcortical white matter and cerebellar cortex; demyelination; enlarged abnormal astrocytic nuclei; increased brain weight.

Differential diagnosis

Alexander's disease (generally later onset, slower course).

Hydrocephalus.

GM2 gangliosidosis: Tay–Sachs disease.

Treatment and prognosis No effective treatment is available. The disease is progressive and death occurs after 1–5 years.

> **Reference** Gordon N. Canavan disease: a review of recent developments. *European Journal of Paediatric Neurology* 2001; **5**: 65–69.

> **Other relevant entries** Alexander's disease; Gangliosidoses: an overview; Hydrocephalus; Leukodystrophies: an overview.

Candidiasis

Moniliasis

Systemic infection with the fungus *Candida* may occur in the context of immunosuppression (including diabetes mellitus), burns, and total parenteral nutrition, affecting the brain as microabscesses, non-caseating granulomata, meningitis, meningoencephalitis, and ependymitis. CSF shows pleocytosis but the organism is rarely identified by culture; extraneural sites (blood, urine, skin) are usually more helpful. Systemic infection carries a grave prognosis, even with intravenous amphotericin treatment.

> **Other relevant entry** Immunosuppressive therapy and diseases of the nervous system.

CANOMAD

CANOMAD is a rare neuropathy, the name is an acronym denoting the key features, viz.:

chronic *a*taxic *n*europathy,
*o*phthalmoplegia,
Ig*M* paraprotein,
cold *a*gglutinins,
*d*isialosyl antibodies.

Clinically there is a chronic neuropathy causing sensory ataxia and areflexia, but with preserved motor function in the limbs. Ocular and bulbar weakness may be fixed or relapsing–remitting. EMG/NCS and nerve biopsy reveal both axonal and demyelinating features. The anti-disialosyl antibodies react with an epitope common to the gangliosides GD1b, GD3, GT1b, and GQ1b. The differential diagnosis includes Miller Fisher syndrome. A partial response to IVIg may be observed.

Reference Willison HJ, O'Leary CP, Veitch J *et al.* The clinical and laboratory features of chronic sensory ataxic neuropathy with anti-disialosyl IgM antibodies. *Brain* 2001; **124**: 1968–1977.

Other relevant entries Gangliosides and neurological disorders; Neuropathies: an overview; Paraproteinaemic neuropathies.

■ Capgras' syndrome

This is one of the classical delusional syndromes of psychiatry, in which patients recognize a close family relative, or other loved object, but believe them to be have been replaced by an exact alien or "double" (illusion of doubles). Initially described in patients with psychiatric disorders, it may also occur in traumatic, metabolic, and neurodegenerative disorders (*e.g.* Alzheimer's disease, dementia with Lewy bodies). Neurologists have encompassed this phenomenon under the term reduplicative paramnesia.

Some believe this syndrome to be the "mirror image" of prosopagnosia, in which faces are not recognized but emotional significance is. Capgras' syndrome may be envisaged as a Geschwindian disconnection syndrome, in which the visual recognition system is disconnected from the limbic system, hence faces can be recognized but no emotional significance ascribed to them.

Reference Ramachandran VS, Blakeslee S. *Phantoms in the Brain. Human Nature and the Architecture of the Mind*. London: Fourth Estate, 1998: 158–173.

Other relevant entries Cotard's syndrome; Disconnection syndromes.

■ Capsular warning syndrome

A syndrome characterized by a cluster of transient ischaemic attacks (TIAs), typically causing weakness of the whole of one side of the body without cognitive or language deficit (hence a pure motor lacunar TIA), followed within hours to days usually by a lacunar infarct of the internal capsule. The syndrome is presumed to reflect intermittent and then complete closure of a single lenticulostriate or other perforating artery. As in other lacunar infarcts, proximal arterial or cardiac cause is unlikely.

Reference Donnan GA, O'Malley HM, Quang L, Hurley S, Bladin PF. The capsular warning syndrome: pathogenesis and clinical features. *Neurology* 1993; **43**: 957–962.

Other relevant entries Cerebrovascular disease: arterial; Lacunar syndromes; Transient ischaemic attack.

■ CARASIL – see CADASIL

■ Carbamoylphosphate synthase I deficiency – see Urea cycle enzyme defects

■ Carbon monoxide poisoning

Acute carbon monoxide (CO) poisoning causes depression of central nervous system (CNS) function which may be fatal. Various symptoms may occur, including headache, dizziness, weakness, nausea, impaired concentration, shortness of breath, and visual changes; loss of consciousness is unusual. The diagnosis may be established by measuring carboxyhaemoglobin level in venous blood. Treatment is by removal of the patient from the CO source, and administration of normobaric or hyperbaric oxygen until the carboxyhaemoglobin level returns to normal.

Some patients with CO poisoning develop a delayed encephalopathy with motor and/or cognitive deficits, a few days to weeks after recovering from the acute poisoning, or without history of acute poisoning. Motor features are usually extrapyramidal and dystonic, including a progressive akinetic-mute syndrome or a delayed parkinsonian syndrome, although pyramidal signs may be seen. There may be additional personality changes (sometimes psychosis), and cognitive deficits such as impaired executive function, slowed mental processing and impaired visuospatial function; deficits may be very focal (e.g. visual agnosia). MRI may show white matter changes in periventricular or centrum semiovale, although these are less common in unselected patients than cognitive sequelae; MR changes may also be seen in caudate nucleus, globus pallidus, cerebellum, or hippocampus.

Patients typically improve with time, but may be left with permanent neurological and/or neuropsychological sequelae.

References Ernst A, Zibrak JD. Carbon monoxide poisoning. *New England Journal of Medicine* 1998; **339**: 1603–1608.

Lee MS, Marsden CD. Neurological sequelae following carbon monoxide poisoning: clinical course and outcome according to the clinical types and brain computed tomography scan findings. *Movement Disorders* 1994; **9**: 550–558.

Parkinson RB, Hopkins RO, Cleavinger HB *et al*. White matter hyperintensities and neuropsychological outcome following carbon monoxide poisoning. *Neurology* 2002; **58**: 1525–1532.

■ Carcinoid syndrome

Tumours secreting serotonin metabolites, detectable as 5-hydroxyindole acetic acid (5-HIAA) in the urine, may be associated with neurological features, for example:

headache ("erythrocyanotic");
proximal myopathy with atrophy of type 2 muscle fibres.

Other relevant entries Erythrocyanotic headache; Myopathy: an overview; Pellagra.

■ Carcinomatous meningitis – see Meningeal carcinomatosis

■ Cardiofacial syndrome
Asymmetrical crying facies

This is a congenital condition in which there is facial asymmetry during crying but not at rest: smiling and sucking are normal and there is no drooling. Weakness may be confined to the depressor anguli oris and depressor labii inferioris muscles. There may be associated congenital heart defects and other abnormalities but usually this is a benign condition.

■ Carney complex

This is a familial multiple neoplasia and lentiginosis syndrome, featuring skin and cardiac myxomas, and testicular, adrenal and pituitary tumours, which has been linked to chromosome 2.

> **Reference** Stratakis CA, Carney JP, Lin JP *et al.* Carney complex, a familial multiple neoplasia and lentiginosis syndrome: analysis of 11 kindreds and linkage to the short arm of chromosome 2. *Journal of Clinical Investigation* 1996; **97**: 699–705.
>
> **Other relevant entries** Endocrinology and the nervous system; Pituitary disease and apoplexy.

■ Carnitine deficiency

Pathophysiology Mitochondrial fatty acid β-oxidation depends on the availability of carnitine, which is synthesized endogenously (from lysine and methionine in liver and kidney; stored in muscle) and is usually plentifully available in the diet (especially in meat). The carnitine cycle transports metabolites across mitochondrial membranes.

Carnitine deficiency may be:
- Primary: due to deficiency of the transporter enzymes which maintain intracellular carnitine levels (no primary disorder of carnitine biosynthesis has yet been identified); or
- Secondary: due to decreased biosynthesis (chronic liver or renal disease, extreme prematurity), inadequate intake (protein calorie malnutrition, total parenteral nutrition, intestinal malabsorption), or increased losses (uraemia, renal tubular loss; organic acidopathies such as propionic acidaemia and methylmalonic acidaemia; urea cycle enzyme defects treated with sodium benzoate).

Carnitine deficiency may be:
- Systemic: causing encephalopathy.
- Limited to muscle; causing myopathy, cardiomyopathy.

Since carnitine deficiency often responds dramatically to oral carnitine supplements, it is an important diagnosis to consider.

Clinical features: history and examination Two major forms are defined:

- *Type I lipid-storage myopathy*: myopathic carnitine deficiency
  Progressive skeletal myopathy and cardiomyopathy, usually with onset after the first year of life.
- *Type II lipid-storage myopathy*: systemic carnitine deficiency
  Recurrent episodes of acute encephalopathy in the first few months of life, with lactic acidosis, hyperammonaemia, hypoketotic hypoglycaemia, and hepatic injury (elevated liver-related enzymes, normal bilirubin).

Investigations and diagnosis *Bloods*: carnitine deficiency may be diagnosed by measuring the level of carnitine in serum:

Type I (muscle) carnitine deficiency: normal serum carnitine but low muscle carnitine concentration.

Type II (systemic) carnitine defiency: very low levels of serum carnitine ($<$5–10 μmol/l).

Secondary carnitine deficiency: moderately decreased serum carnitine concentrations.

Type I and II carnitine deficiency: ratio of esterified : free carnitine markedly increased.

Encephalopathy: hypoglycaemia, lactic acidosis, hyperammoniaemia, and abnormal liver function tests. Total serum carnitine concentration (= free carnitine + acylcarnitine esters) between attacks normally $>$30 μmol/l, with a ratio of esterified : free carnitine of $<$0.4.

Urine: organic acid analysis in any child presenting with cardiomyopathy.

Differential diagnosis Systemic: Reye's syndrome.

Treatment and prognosis Whether primary or secondary, carnitine deficiency often responds to dietary carnitine supplements (L-carnitine 100–200 or 60 mg/kg/day intravenously).

> **Reference** Kerner J, Hoppel C. Genetic disorders of carnitine metabolism and their nutritional management. *Annual Review of Nutrition* 1998; **18**: 179–206.

> **Other relevant entries** Carnitine palmit(o)yltransferase deficiency; Fatty acid oxidation defects; Organic acidaemia; Reye's syndrome; Urea cycle enzyme defects.

■ Carnitine palmit(o)yltransferase deficiency
DiMauro syndrome

Pathophysiology Carnitine palmit(o)yltransferase (CPT) is an enzyme involved in the transport of fatty acid across the mitochondrial membrane: from outside to inside (CPT I) and unhooking carnitine once the complex is inside (CPT II). Two types of deficiency are recognized, both are defects of acylcarnitine synthesis–translocation. CPT II deficiency is the more commonly encountered.

Clinical features: history and examination

- *Type I (CPT I)*: presents in neonatal period with hepatomegaly and severe hepato-cellular dysfunction (hypoglycaemia), encephalopathy, hyperammonaemia, metabolic acidosis, and hypotonia.
- *Type II (CPT II)*: may present in neonatal period as for CPT I; also presents in young adults with a history of episodic muscle stiffness, pain, tenderness, and weakness, induced by exercise, cold, fasting, or intercurrent infection. Accompanying myoglobinuria may precipitate acute renal failure. No "second wind phenomenon" (*cf.* McArdle's disease). A chronic myopathy is also described.

Investigations and diagnosis

- *Type I (CPT I)*: plasma carnitine concentration often elevated, acylcarnitines unremarkable; CPT I deficiency demonstrated in fibroblasts or white cells.
- *Type II (CPT II)*:

  Bloods: plasma carnitine concentration elevated; creatine kinase elevated during attacks; raised triglycerides.

  Muscle biopsy: lipid accumulation (not all cases).

  CPT II deficiency demonstrated in fibroblasts or white cells.

  Neurogenetics: mutations in CPT II gene have been identified.

Differential diagnosis *Type I*: carnitine deficiency.

Type II (CPT II): glutaric aciduria type II (GAII); McArdle's disease (myophosphorylase deficiency).

Treatment and prognosis *Neonatal*: protective therapy: avoid fasting, frequent feeding to avoid mobilizing fatty acids; dietary supplementation with medium-chain triglycerides.

Adult CPT II: avoid strenuous exercise, avoid muscle pain, or exercise when fasted. In cases of rhabdomyolysis, forced alkaline diuresis may be helpful.

References DiMauro S, Melis-DiMauro PM. Muscle carnitine palmityltransferase deficiency and myoglobinuria. *Science* 1973; **182**: 929–931.

Hug G, Bove KE, Soukup S. Lethal neonatal multiorgan deficiency of carnitine palmitoyltransferase II. *New England Journal of Medicine* 1991; **325**: 1862–1864.

Other relevant entries Fatty acid oxidation disorders; Glutaric aciduria; McArdle's disease; Rhabdomyolysis.

■ Carotid artery disease

Pathophysiology The carotid artery is vulnerable to occlusive (stenotic) atheromatous disease, particularly at the bifurcation of the common carotid artery and in the proximal internal carotid artery, which may lead to embolic cerebrovascular disease. The extent of narrowing and the presence or absence of symptomatic consequences are the most important determinants of treatment. Carotid artery dissection, usually following trauma, is also a cause of embolic disease. Aneurysmal disease and fistula formation are less common diseases of the carotid arteries.

Clincal features: history and examination

- Stenosis, asymptomatic: mild narrowing common in the elderly, hypertension, hypercholesterolaemia; a bruit may be present due to turbulent flow but is not an indication for investigation/treatment *per se*.
- Stenosis, symptomatic: may be associated with TIAs (ocular, hemispheric), from emboli breaking off ulcerated surface of atheromatous plaque, or, less commonly, haemodynamic (e.g. limb shaking attacks); total occlusion in childhood may lead to collateral vessel formation at the base of the brain with resultant risk of cerebral haemorrhage (Moyamoya). Cognitive disorder as a consequence of occlusive disease is also possible.
- Dissection: unilateral facial pain, often periorbital, +/− Horner's syndrome +/− hemispheric infarct with "stuttering" onset +/− lower cranial nerve palsies. May be history of trauma to neck; other associations of carotid dissection include fibromuscular dysplasia, Ehlers–Danlos syndrome (type IV), Marfan's syndrome, pseudoxanthoma elasticum.
- Aneurysm: trauma, surgery, irradiation, fibromuscular dysplasia may lead to internal carotid artery aneurysm formation, which may be a source of brain embolism; intracranial aneurysms more likely to rupture and bleed (subarachnoid haemorrhage).
- Fistula: in neck, may follow trauma, especially penetrating (e.g. gunshot and stabbing); in cavernous sinus [see Carotid–cavernous fistula (CCF)].

Investigations and diagnosis *Imaging of carotid artery*: options are Doppler ultrasound, MRA, and catheter angiography. First two adequate for detecting degree of stenosis.

  Bloods: cholesterol, glucose

  Specific investigations for possible underlying vasculopathy (fibromuscular dysplasia, Ehlers–Danlos syndrome).

Differential diagnosis *Stenosis, symptomatic*: consider emboli from other sources (e.g. cardiac, aortic arch). See also differential diagnosis of transient ischaemic attack.
Dissection: Raeder's paratrigeminal syndrome, although many of these may be dissections which are "missed" by imaging.

Treatment and prognosis *Stenosis, asymptomatic*: mainstay of management has been no specific treatment, but control of modifiable risk factors (hypertension, hypercholesterolaemia, smoking); recently the results from the Asymptomatic Carotid Artery Study suggest that early surgery is associated with a reduced risk of subsequent stroke and death, provided cardiovascular status is sufficiently good (major cause of post-operative deaths).

  Stenosis, symptomatic: if stenosis <70%, antiplatelet agents recommended (aspirin, dipyridamole, clopidogrel, ticlopidine); if TIAs continue despite these, formal anticoagulation with warfarin may be considered. Stenosis >70% probably merits carotid endarterectomy, but decision must also take into account cardiovascular status (the commonest cause of morbidity and mortality). Control of risk factors.

  Dissection: anticoagulation with warfarin usually recommended (notwithstanding the current absence of randomized-controlled trials) if patient seen soon after dissection. If delayed dissection, recommend anti-platelet therapy.

Aneurysm: if a source of embolism, may require medical/surgical intervention.

References Bakker FC, Klijn CJM, Jennekens-Schinkel A, Kappelle LJ. Cognitive disorder in patients with occlusive disease of the carotid artery: a systematic review of the literature. *Journal of Neurology* 2000; **247**: 669–676.

Kappelle LJ. Symptomatic carotid artery stenosis. *Journal of Neurology* 2002; **249**: 254–259.

Schievink WI. Spontaneous dissection of the carotid and vertebral arteries. *New England Journal of Medicine* 2001; **344**: 898–906.

Other relevant entries Aneurysm; Carotid–cavernous fistula; Carotidynia; Cerebrovascular disease: arterial; Ehlers–Danlos syndrome; Fibromuscular dysplasia; Horner's syndrome; Limb shaking; Marfan's syndrome; Moyamoya; Pseudoxanthoma elasticum; Raeder's paratrigeminal syndrome; Transient ischaemic attack; Vertebral artery dissection.

■ Carotid–cavernous fistula

Pathophysiology These common dural arteriovenous fistulas link the internal carotid artery with a portion of the cavernous sinus; they may occur spontaneously or following trauma, or in association with connective tissue disorders such as Ehlers–Danlos syndrome.

Clinical features: history and examination
- Injected sclera, chemosis, proptosis (may be pulsatile).
- Ophthalmoplegia, diplopia.
- Pain.
- Ocular bruit.
- $+/-$ visual loss.

Investigations and diagnosis Brain imaging may show a mass in the cavernous sinus. The shunt may be visualized by transcranial Doppler ultrasonography, but to define the anatomy precisely, and as a possible prelude to treatment, catheter angiography is required.

Differential diagnosis Other causes of painful ophthalmoplegia.

Treatment and prognosis Embolization via a catheter may be possible, dependent on the precise anatomy.

Occlusion by intermittent pressure on the carotid artery is also an option.

Carotid–cavernous fistulae rarely cause subarachnoid haemorrhage when they occur spontaneously; those due to trauma are more likely to cause intracerebral bleeding. A significant number of carotid–cavernous fistulae thrombose spontaneously. All treatments are designed to prevent progression and haemorrhage, and will do nothing for the physical appearance of the proptosed eye.

Reference Barrow DL, Spector RH, Braun IF *et al.* Classification and treatment of spontaneous carotid–cavernous sinus fistulas. *Journal of Neurosurgery* 1985; **62**: 248–256.

Other relevant entries Carotid artery disease; Cavernous sinus disease; Ehlers–Danlos syndrome; Ophthalmoplegia.

■ Carotidynia

Carotidynia describes idiopathic neck, and sometimes face, pain with tenderness over the ipsilateral carotid bifurcation. Whether this represents a distinct nosological entity has been debated, but reports of abnormal enhancing tissue around the symptomatic carotid bifurcation on MRI have suggested that it is a distinct condition. Pain may be aggravated by swallowing and head movement. Pain over the carotid artery may also occur with carotid dissection, giant cell arteritis, cluster headache, or tumours in the region of the carotid bifurcation.

References Biousse V, Bousser M-G. The myth of carotidynia. *Neurology* 1994; **44**: 993–995.

Burton BS, Syms MJ, Petermann GW, Burgess LP. MR imaging of patients with carotidynia. *American Journal of Neuroradiology* 2000; **21**: 766–769.

Other relevant entries Carotid artery disease; Cluster headache; Facial pain: differential diagnosis.

■ Carpal tunnel syndrome

Pathophysiology Compression of the median nerve in the carpal tunnel by the transverse carpal ligament (flexor retinaculum) is probably the commonest entrapment neuropathy, commoner in women, often between the ages of 40–60 years. Although a number of clinical tests have been described for carpal tunnel syndrome (CTS), electrophysiological testing is still the gold standard for diagnosis.

Recognized associations include:

rheumatoid arthritis
acromegaly
hypothyroidism
uraemia, dialysis
amyloidosis.

Most instances occur in otherwise healthy people.

Clinical features: history and examination

- Pain: in the hand, classically involving the thumb, index, middle and radial half of ring finger, but on occasion reported to involve all digits; may extend to the whole hand and, in some cases, also up the forearm, occasionally even to the shoulder. Often causes nocturnal waking, when patients may shake or "flick" their hands ("to get the circulation going again") or get up and walk about to relieve symptoms.
- Sensory disturbance: hypoaesthesia generally confined to median nerve distribution in the hand, but anomalous findings may be made.
- Motor wasting and/or weakness affecting the median innervated muscles of the thenar eminence may occur.

- Often bilateral.
- A number of clinical tests have been described which aim to provoke the typical symptoms of tingling (Tinel's "sign of formication") in the cutaneous distribution of the damaged nerve ("peripheral reference"). These include:

   Tinel's sign: tapping over transverse carpal ligament, for example with a tendon hammer (sensitivity 60–67%; specificity 59–77%).

   Phalen's sign: prolonged forced wrist flexion.

   Carpal tunnel compression test: application of moderate pressure over the transverse carpal ligament (sensitivity 52.5%; specificity 61.8%).

   Pressure provocative test: pressure cuff + direct median nerve pressure (sensitivity 54.5%; specificity 68.4%).

   "Flick test": clinical history of relieving symptoms by flicking or shaking hands (occurs with same frequency in cases with and without EMG confirmation).

Investigations and diagnosis *Bloods*: thyroid function tests, rheumatoid factor, may be assayed if clinical features suggest relevant underlying diagnosis.

Neurophysiology: EMG/NCS: the gold standard for the diagnosis of carpal tunnel syndrome remains electrophysiological testing: decreased amplitude and prolonged median motor and sensory latencies; EMG shows denervation abnormalities in advanced cases. In some cases may be part of a more generalized neuropathy.

Differential diagnosis

Sensory polyneuropathy.

Radiculopathy.

Hyperventilation.

Treatment and prognosis Splinting of wrist, analgesia; surgical decompression. A recent randomized-controlled trial has suggested that surgery is the more efficacious. Short-term (2–4 weeks) low-dose oral steroids are also effective.

References Chang MH, Ger LP, Hsieh PF, Huang SY. A randomised clinical trial of oral steroids in the treatment of carpal tunnel syndrome: a long term follow up. *Journal of Neurology, Neurosurgery and Psychiatry* 2002; **73**: 710–714.

Gerritsen AAM, de Vet HCW, Scholten RJPM, Bertelsmann FW, de Krom MCTFM, Bouter LM. Splinting vs surgery in the treatment of carpal tunnel syndrome. A randomized controlled trial. *Journal of American Medical Association* 2002; **288**: 1245–1251.

Heller L, Ring H, Costeff H, Solzi P. Evaluation of Tinel's and Phalen's signs in the diagnosis of the carpal tunnel syndrome. *European Neurology* 1986; **25**: 40–42.

Kanaan N, Sawaya RA. Carpal tunnel syndrome: modern diagnosis and management techniques. *British Journal of General Practice* 2001; **51**: 311–314.

Kaul MP, Pagel KJ, Wheatley MJ, Dryden JD. Carpal compression test and pressure provocative test in veterans with median-distribution paresthesias. *Muscle and Nerve* 2001; **24**: 107–111.

McNamara B. Clinical anatomy of the median nerve. *Advances in Clinical Neuroscience and Rehabilitation* 2003; **2(6)**: 19–20.

Rosenbaum RB, Ochoa JL. *Carpal Tunnel Syndrome and Other Disorders of the Median Nerve* (2nd edition). Boston: Butterworth-Heinemann, 2002.

Other relevant entries Entrapment neuropathies: an overview; Familial amyloid polyneuropathies; Renal disease and the nervous system; Rheumatoid arthritis; Thyroid disease and the nervous system.

■ Carpenter syndrome
Acrocephalopolysyndactyly

This is an autosomal-recessive condition in which there is premature closure of all cranial sutures with a number of facial and skeletal abnormalities, such as flattened nasal bridge, epicanthal folds, micrognathia, and polysyndactyly. In addition there may be subnormal intelligence, cardiac abnormalities, and hypogenitalism in males.

Other relevant entry Craniostenosis.

■ Carrion's disease – see Bartonellosis

■ Castleman disease – see POEMS syndrome

■ Cat scratch disease – see Bartonellosis

■ Cataplexy

Pathophysiology Cataplexy is the sudden loss of axial and lower limb muscle tone, often provoked by excitement or emotion and usually resulting in the patient falling to the ground. There is no loss of consciousness in cataplectic attacks, which may occur several times a day. Status cataplecticus rarely occurs, after withdrawal of medications. Occasionally the face, jaw, and neck muscles are involved, leading to neck sagging or jaw opening, but the oculomotor and respiratory muscles are never affected. During attacks, there is muscle atonia as seen in rapid eye movement (REM) sleep but without other REM features and with a wakeful EEG; hence there is muscular hypotonia and transient areflexia.

Cataplexy is most commonly associated with the features making up the narcoleptic tetrad (narcolepsy, sleep paralysis, hypnagogic hallucinations), usually developing after the narcoleptic sleep attacks have become apparent. Cataplexy may rarely be secondary, associated with structural lesions of the hypothalamus and brainstem (e.g. postencephalitic parkinsonism), and may occur in other conditions such as Niemann–Pick's disease type C, Norrie disease.

Investigations and diagnosis Diagnosis is generally clinical; other investigations only required if secondary causes are suspected.

Differential diagnosis

Epilepsy.

Syncope; cardiac arrhythmias.

Vestibular disorders.

Drop attacks.

Hyperekplexia.

Periodic paralyses.

Treatment and prognosis

Tricyclic antidepressants (e.g. protriptyline, imipramine, clomipramine).

Selective serotonin reuptake inhibitors (e.g. fluoxetine).

Amphetamines (as for narcolepsy).

> **Other relevant entries** Drop attacks; Hyperekplexia; Narcolepsy, narcoleptic syndrome.

■ Cataracts

Cataracts occur in a number of neurological diseases; their presence may be helpful in reaching a diagnosis in the appropriate clinical setting:

Alport's syndrome

Cerebrotendinous xanthomatosis

Cockayne's syndrome

Congenital rubella syndrome

Conradi–Hünerman syndrome

Dystrophia myotonica (may be the sole feature)

Fabry's disease

Flynn–Aird syndrome

Galactosaemia

Lowe syndrome

Marinesco–Sjögren syndrome

Peroxisomal disorders

Proximal myotonic myopathy

Rothmund–Thomson syndrome

Usher's syndrome

Wilson's disease (sunflower)

Zellweger syndrome.

> **Other relevant entry** See individual entries.

■ Catatonia

Pathophysiology Catatonia is a neurobehavioural disorder characterized by unresponsiveness, muteness, marked decrease in motor activity often punctuated by outbursts of agitated excitement, refusal to eat and drink, limb rigidity, maintenance of abnormal body postures (catalepsy) with waxy flexibitlity (*flexibilitas cerea*), negativism, echophenomena and stereotypies. Urinary incontinence or retention may occur. Following recovery, patients may be able to recall events which occurred during the catatonic state.

Although initially described in the context of psychiatric disease, it is now well recognized that catatonia may occur in the context of structural or metabolic neurological conditions:

- Psychiatric disorders
  Manic–depressive illness
  Schizophrenia.
- Neurological disorders
  Cerebrovascular disease (posterior circulation)
  Tumours (especially around third ventricle, corpus callosum)
  Head trauma
  Encephalitis
  Syphilis
  Extrapyramidal disorders
  Epilepsy.
- Systemic illnesses
  Endocrine: hyperthyroidism, Addison's disease, Cushing's disease, diabetic ketoacidosis
  Metabolic: uraemia, hypercalcaemia, hepatic encephalopathy
  Others: Systemic lupus erythematosus (SLE).

Various subtypes of catatonia are enumerated by some authorities, including:

Retarded catatonia (Kahlbaum's syndrome)

Excited catatonia (manic delirium, Bell's mania)

Malignant catatonia, lethal catatonia: also encompasses the neuroleptic malignant syndrome (NMS) and the serotonin syndrome

Periodic catatonia.

Differential diagnosis

Abulia.

Locked-in syndrome.

Parkinsonian off state.

Depression.

Treatment Correct any underlying abnormality where possible.

Symptomatic treatment with lorazepam is the treatment of choice; ECT has been tried. Anti-psychotic agents are best avoided.

References Fink M, Taylor MA. *Catatonia: A Clinician's Guide to Diagnosis and Treatment.* Cambridge: CUP, 2003.

Moore DP. *Textbook of Clinical Neuropsychiatry.* London: Arnold, 2001: 112–116.

Muqit MMK, Rakshi JS, Shakir RA, Larner AJ. Catatonia or abulia? A difficult differential diagnosis. *Movement Disorders* 2001; **16**: 360–362.

Rosebush PI, Mazurek MF. Catatonia: reawakening to a forgotten disorder. *Movement Disorders* 1999; **14**: 395–397.

Other relevant entries Neuroleptic malignant syndrome; Schizophrenia; Serotonin syndrome.

■ Cauda equina syndrome and conus medullaris disease

Pathophysiology The conus medullaris is the most distal part of the spinal cord (adjacent to the vertebral body of L1 in normal adults) and the cauda equina ("the horse's tail") is the sheaf of nerve roots which lies below it, the roots running distally to the intervertebral foramina of the lower lumbar, sacral and coccygeal vertebrae. Local pathology may involve both structures or, less likely, affect them individually. Although this anatomical distinction may be attempted on clinical grounds, it is often difficult and of little practical value.

Recognized causes of cauda equina and conus medullaris syndromes include:

Central disc herniation
Tumour: primary (e.g. ependymoma, meningioma, schwannoma); metastasis.
Haematoma.
Abscess.
Lumbosacral fractures.
Inflammation (e.g. cauda equina syndrome in sarcoidosis; rare).
Ankylosing spondylitis (cauda equina syndrome in association with dorsal arach-
   noid diverticula: rare).

Clinical features: history and examination

- Pain: lumbar region, thighs, buttocks, perineum, legs (may be symmetric or asym-metric); may be worse in recumbent position and increased by Valsalva manoeuvre.
- Sphincter disturbance: bladder symptoms (impaired initiation of micturition, loss of bladder sensation) said to occur earlier in conus lesions; constipation.
- Impotence: impaired erection, ejaculation.
- Wasting: glutei, posterior thigh, anterolateral leg and foot muscles; more evident in cauda equina lesions.
- Fasciculations: if conus involved.
- Weakness of legs: flaccid paralysis in cauda equina syndrome; hip flexor weakness said to be relatively specific for conus lesion.
- Reflex loss or diminution, especially ankle jerk.
- Sensory loss: so-called saddle anaesthesia (sacral dermatomes), dorsal aspect of thigh; more asymmetric in cauda equina syndromes. Sensory deficits may extend to trunk in conus lesion, and position sense may be affected (*cf.* cauda equina syndrome).

Hence, disease confined to the conus medullaris is said to produce early sphincter involvement, late pain, and symmetrical sensory involvement, whereas pure cauda equina lesions produce early pain, late sphincter involvement, and asym-metric sensory deficits.

Investigations and diagnosis *Imaging*: MRI is the modality of choice (e.g. for disc dis-ease, tumours and inflammation).

Neurophysiology: EMG/NCS: electrophysiological studies may help determine whether roots are affected.

CSF: may show non-specific raised protein.

Differential diagnosis Polyneuropathy, multiple radiculopathy, lumbar spinal stenosis.

Treatment and prognosis Dependent on cause; discs, tumours, haematomas, abscesses may be surgically resected or aspirated; inflammatory disease may require steroids; the cauda equina syndrome of ankylosing spondylitis may be stabilized by lumboperitoneal shunting. Recovery is said to be more likely with lesions of the conus than the cauda equina.

> **Reference** Swash M, Katifi HA. The conus medullaris and cauda equina syndromes. *Journal of Neurology, Neurosurgery and Psychiatry* 1996; **61**: 216–217.

> **Other relevant entries** Ankylosing spondylitis and the nervous system; Arachnoiditis; Lumbar cord and root disease; Radiculopathies: an overview; Sarcoidosis; Spinal stenosis; Tumours: an overview.

■ Caudal vermis syndrome – see Cerebellar disease: an overview

■ Causalgia – see Complex regional pain syndromes

■ Cavernoma, cavernous haemagioma

Cavernomas, or cavernous haemagiomas, are thin-walled vascular spaces, lacking a shunt [hence not arteriovenous malformations (AVMs)]. More often supratentorial than infratentorial, they may be single or multiple ("cavernomatosis"), sporadic or familial (mapped to chromosome 7q11–q22, mutations in Krit1 gene). Although readily identified by MRI, cerebral angiography is usually negative because of the absence of AV shunting. They may present as space-occupying lesions, with seizures, or with haemorrhage; sometimes with relapsing–remitting symptoms which may be confused with multiple sclerosis, especially if located in the brainstem. Many are asymptomatic and found by chance when the brain is imaged for other reasons.

> **References** Cader MZ, Winer JB. Cavernous haemangioma mimicking multiple sclerosis. *British Medical Journal* 1999; **318**: 1604–1605.

> Moran NF, Fish DR, Kitchen N, Shorvon S, Kendall BE, Stevens JM. Supratentorial cavernous haemangiomas and epilepsy: a review of the literature and case series. *Journal of Neurology, Neurosurgery and Psychiatry* 1999; **66**: 561–568.

> **Other relevant entries** Arteriovenous malformations of the brain; Intracranial vascular malformations: an overview.

■ Cavernous sinus disease

Cavernous sinus syndrome

Pathophysiology The cavernous sinus lies behind the eye and lateral to the pituitary gland. It contains the internal carotid artery, the nerves that innervate the extraocular muscles and the first two divisions of the trigeminal nerve. A number of disease processes may affect the cavernous sinus and present with a progressive ophthalmo-plegia with or without involvement of the first and second divisions of the trigeminal nerve. A cavernous sinus syndrome may result from:

Granulomatous inflammatory conditions: sarcoidosis; Wegener's; idiopathic inflammation (so-called Tolosa–Hunt syndrome).
Aneurysms of the carotid artery.
Thrombophlebitis and thrombosis: cavernous sinus thrombosis may be a conse-quence of sepsis, associated with infections of the orbit, paranasal sinuses and teeth, usually resulting in bilateral signs and symptoms.
Carotid–cavernous fistula (CCF; *q.v.*).
Metastatic disease: especially from the nasopharynx.
Meningioma, glioma.
Mucormycosis (especially in context of diabetes mellitus).

The advent of MRI has greatly improved the visualization of the cavernous sinus and diagnosis of conditions involving it.

Clincal features: history and examination

- Diplopia: due to the involvement of third, fourth, or sixth cranial nerves; isolated palsies or any combination of nerves can be involved. The sixth cranial nerve lies adjacent to the carotid artery in the cavernous sinus and so an aneurysm may present with an isolated sixth nerve palsy.
- Sensory loss: with a depressed corneal reflex. If the lesion is far back in the cavernous sinus then the second division of the trigeminal nerve can be involved; a lesion in the posterior part of the cavernous sinus may present with a sixth nerve palsy and a Horner's syndrome, as a branch of the sympathetic chain briefly links up with the abducens nerve in the posterior part of the cavernous sinus (Parkinson's syndrome).
- Proptosis: may occur in any of the conditions involving the cavernous sinus. In the case of carotid–cavernous fistula, the exophthalmos is often pulsatile and associ-ated with an ocular bruit.
- Pain: located retro-orbitally is common, especially with metastatic and granuloma-tous conditions involving the cavernous sinus.
- Reduced visual acuity: may occur on occasion, due to compression of the optic nerve at the apex of the cavernous sinus, or in the case of carotid–cavernous fistula due to ischaemia.
- Chemosis and injected conjunctival vessels: may be found in cases of carotid–cavernous fistula.

In the case of a cavernous sinus thrombosis the signs are bilateral and often develop acutely in the context of local infection in the orbit, paranasal sinuses or teeth. The patient is usually systemically unwell with prominant retro-orbital pain with chemosis, proptosis, orbital congestion with a variable ophthalmoplegia and sensory loss over the forehead. There is often ocular oedema or optic nerve compression which can lead to blindness, which may also occur secondary to occlusion of the ophthalmic artery.

Investigations and diagnosis *Bloods*: including FBC, ESR, CRP, serum ACE, ANCA.

Imaging: may include:

CXR (? sarcoid; Wegener's; neoplasm).
Brain MRI$+/-$ gadolinium.
CT to ascertain if any bone erosion.
MRA or angiogram to localize any aneurysm/fistula.

CSF: usually normal.

Others: may need to consider further investigations for sarcoidosis and Wegener's; ENT opinion for exclusion of a nasopharyngeal carcinoma.

Differential diagnosis

Orbital disease:

Thyroid eye disease.
Orbital pseudotumour.
Metastatic orbital disease.
Primary tumours of the eye (e.g. melanoma).
Sarcoidosis within the orbit.

A similar clinical picture may occur with lesions at the orbital apex or the superior orbital fissure; the term Foix–Jefferson syndrome has been used to describe a combination of third, fourth, fifth and sixth cranial nerve palsies with exophthalmos and eyelid oedema associated with tumour, aneurysm, or thrombosis of the cavernous sinus.

Treatment and prognosis Dependent on cause.

Granulomatous disease normally responds dramatically to steroids (e.g. prednisolone initially at a dose of 80 mg/day). Long-term follow-up is recommended and some patients may require long-term treatment with steroids.

Tumours, whether primary or secondary, are usually inoperable. The treatment of choice is therefore chemo- or radiotherapy.

Aneurysms of the carotid artery in the cavernous sinus do not cause subarachnoid haemorrhage. If they are saccular they can be embolized, if fusiform then the only option is occlusion of the ipsilateral carotid artery. Often the treatement of choice is to do nothing.

Reference DiNubile MJ. Septic thrombosis of the cavernous sinus. *Archives of Neurology* 1988; **45**: 567–572.

Other relevant entries Aneurysm; Cluster headache; Cranial nerve disease: II: Optic nerve; Cranial nerve disease: III: Oculomotor nerve; Cranial nerve disease: IV: Trochlear nerve; Cranial nerve disease: V: Trigeminal nerve; Cranial nerve disease: VI: Abducens nerve; Facial pain: differential diagnosis; Headache: an overview; Parkinson's syndrome; Sarcoidosis; Tolosa–Hunt syndrome; Tumours: an overview.

■ Cayman disease
Cayman cerebellar ataxia

An autosomal-recessive cerebellar ataxia, confined to one area of Grand Cayman in the Cayman Islands, described in 1978. It is characterized by psychomotor retardation, non-progressive ataxia, nystagmus, intention tremor, and hypotonia, without retinal changes or optokinetic nystagmus. Linkage to chromosome 19p13.3 has been established.

Reference Nystuen A, Benke PJ, Merren J, Stone EM, Sheffield VC. A cerebellar ataxia locus identified by DNA pooling to search for linkage disequilibrium in an isolated population from the Cayman Islands. *Human Molecular Genetics* 1996; **5**: 525–531.

Other relevant entry Cerebellar disease: an overview.

■ Central and peripheral demyelinating disease
Chronic demyelinating neuropathy with multifocal CNS demyelination

A rare syndrome comprising the features of both multiple sclerosis and chronic inflammatory demyelinating polyradiculopathy; the latter tends to dominate the clinical picture.

Reference Thomas PK, Walker RWH, Rudge P *et al*. Chronic demyelinating peripheral neuropathy associated with multifocal central nervous system demyelination. *Brain* 1987; **110**: 53–76.

Other relevant entry Demyelinating diseases of the nervous system: an overview.

■ Central cord syndrome – see Cervical cord and root disease

■ Central core disease

This rare autosomal-dominant myopathy was the first congenital myopathy to be described. Infants present in the neonatal period with hypotonia, areflexia, delayed motor milestones, proximal limb, and facial weakness. Associated features include pes cavus, short stature, kyphoscoliosis, and dislocation of the hips. The condition is usually non-progressive. Adult presentation with muscle cramps or limb girdle weakness may occur, or the condition may remain asymptomatic. Susceptibility to anaesthesia-related malignant hyperthermia occurs in one-third of patients.

Creatine kinase is usually normal but may be mildly elevated. Neurophysiology shows non-specific myopathic change.

Muscle histology reveals densely packed and disorganized myofibrils ("cores") in the centre of most type 1 muscle fibres, seen as central pallor with stains for mitochondrial enzymes.

Central core disease may be associated with mutations in the gene (*RYR1*) on chromosome 19q13.1 encoding the ryanodine receptor of the sarcoplasmic membrane, hence this is a channelopathy. The malignant hyperthermia phenotype is also associated with mutations in this gene.

There is no specific treatment.

References Quane KA, Healy JM, Keating KE *et al*. Mutations in the ryanodine receptor gene in central core disease and malignant hyperthermia. *Nature Genetics* 1993; **5**: 51–55.

Zhang Y, Chen HS, Khanna VK *et al.* A mutation in the human ryanodine receptor gene associated with central core disease. *Nature Genetics* 1993; **5**: 46–50.
Other relevant entries Channelopathies: an overview; Congenital muscle and neuromuscular disorders: an overview; Malignant hyperthermia.

■ Central pontine myelinolysis
Extrapontine myelinolysis

Pathophysiology This disorder is characterized by the destruction, usually symmetrical, of myelin sheaths in the basal pons, sometimes extending beyond (hence "pontine myelinolysis" may be a misnomer). Reported cases are most often, but not exclusively, associated with hyponatraemia and its rapid correction with intravenous fluids. Other recognized associations include chronic alcoholism and undernutrition, dehydration associated with vomiting (e.g. pregnancy) and diarrhoea, diuretic therapy, postoperative overhydration, compulsive water drinking (dipsomania), organ (especially liver) transplantation, and following severe burns. A feature common to many of these situations is change in plasma osmolality, leading to the notion that CPM may represent an "osmotic demyelination syndrome". Why the neurones of the pons should be particularly susceptible to such changes has not been clearly explained.

Clinical features: history and examination Broad! May affect pyramidal, extrapyramidal, and cerebellar pathways and lower cranial nerves:

behavioural changes;
eye movement disorders;
bulbar/pseudobulbar palsy;
quadriplegia, locked-in syndrome;
seizures;
coma;
delayed onset movement disorders;
some cases are asymptomatic being discovered only at autopsy.

Investigations and diagnosis *Bloods*: monitor sodium, + / − osmolality.

Imaging: MRI is best suited to demonstrate signal changes in the pons and elsewhere in the brainstem, cerebellum, basal ganglia; these signal changes represent demyelination.

Neurophysiology: BSAEP: may demonstrate prolonged latencies consistent with pontine lesions.

Pathology: demyelination, often symmetrical in pons.

Differential diagnosis

Inflammatory demyelination unlikely to be confused with CPM from the context. Brainstem infarction (basilar artery occlusion).

Treatment and prognosis Prevention is the best treatment; hence judicious (slow) correction of hyponatraemia is advisable, although the precise rate remains debatable (*ca.* 12 mmol/l/day). For those with malnutrition and/or alcoholism, vitamin supplemetation (e.g. thiamine) is appropriate. Once the damage is done, only symptomatic treatment is available.

References Adams RD, Victor M, Mancall EL. Central pontine myelinolysis: a hitherto undescribed disease occurring in alcoholic and malnourished patients. *Archives of Neurology and Psychiatry* 1959; **81**: 154–172.

Lampl C, Yazdi K. Central pontine myelinolysis. *European Neurology* 2002; **47**: 3–10.

Sterns RH, Riggs JE, Schochet SS. Osmotic demyelination syndrome following correction of hyponatraemia. *New England Journal of Medicine* 1986; **314**: 1535–1542.

Other relevant entry Alcohol and the nervous system: an overview.

■ Central sleep apnoea – see Sleep apnoea syndromes

■ Centronuclear myopathies
Myotubular myopathies

This is a group of congenital myopathies. The most common is an X-linked disorder presenting in boys at birth with hypotonia, ventilatory insufficiency, and feeding difficulties. There is an elongated expressionless face, tent-shaped mouth, high-arched palate (as in nemaline myopathy) and kyphoscoliosis and pes cavus may be present. Autosomal-dominant and -recessive forms have a later onset, in childhood or early adulthood, with facial weakness, ophthalmoplegia, ptosis, and proximal limb weakness. Seizures may be a feature.

Creatine kinase may be normal or slightly elevated. Neurophysiology shows a non-specific myopathy.

All variants show the histological feature of centrally placed internal nuclei in small muscle fibres, in addition to the normal peripherally located nuclei. Multiple internal nuclei may also be seen in myotonic dystrophy.

Linkage to mutations in the *MTM1* gene which encodes myotubularin, a non-receptor protein tyrosine phosphatase, has been demonstrated.

There is no specific treatment. Respiratory support may be appropriate for ventilatory insufficiency.

Other relevant entries Congenital muscle and neuromuscular disorders: an overview; Dystrophia myotonica; Nemaline myopathy; Respiratory failure.

■ Ceramidase deficiency – see Farber's lipogranulomatosis

■ Cerebellar disease: an overview

Pathophysiology The cerebellum, located in the posterior fossa behind the brainstem and below the tentorial membrane, is part of the motor system. Its organization may best be thought of in terms of three systems:

- vestibulo- or archeocerebellum: involved in balance and eye movement control;

- spino- or paleocerebellum: primarily involved with the control of axial movement and posture;
- ponto- or neocerebellum: coordinates limb movements.

A number of clinical cerebellar syndromes are recognized, related to cerebellar anatomy:

- Rostral vermis syndrome (anterior lobe): wide-based stance and gait; little limb ataxia, hypotonia, nystagmus, dysarthria (e.g. alcoholic cerebellar degeneration).
- Caudal vermis syndrome (flocculonodular and posterior lobe): axial disequilibrium, staggering gait, no limb ataxia, sometimes nystagmus (e.g. medulloblastoma in children).
- Cerebellar hemispheric syndrome: ipsilateral limb ataxia, dysarthria.
- Pancerebellar syndrome: combination of all the above, with bilateral signs in trunk, limbs, and axial musculature.

Recognized causes of cerebellar syndromes are many, including:

- Inherited: of the hereditary degenerative disorders, recessive conditions tend to present early (before age 20 years) whereas late onset (after age 20 years) is more suggestive of an autosomal-dominant disorder:

    Autosomal dominant

    Clinically classified as ADCA types I, II, and III; now increasingly reclassified on the basis of underlying genetic mutations as spinocerebellar ataxias (SCA)

    Episodic ataxias: channelopathies involving potassium (type 1) and calcium (type 2) channels

    Huntington's disease (HD)

    Dentatorubral–pallidoluysian atrophy (DRPLA)

    Inherited prion diseases, especially Gerstmann–Sträussler–Scheinker (GSS) disease.

    Autosomal recessive

    Friedreich's ataxia (FA)

    Ataxia with isolated vitamin E deficiency (AVED)

    Ataxia telangestasia (AT)

    Ataxia with oculomotor apraxia (AOA)/Early-onset ataxia with hypoalbuminaemia/early-onset ataxia with ocular motor apraxia with hypoalbuminaemia (EAOH)

    Charlevoix–Saguenay syndrome (autosomal-recessive spastic ataxia of Charlevoix–Saguenay, ARSACS)

    Refsum's disease.

- Other inherited metabolic disorders associated with progressive ataxia.

    Abetalipoproteinaemia (Bassen–Kornzweig disease)

    Adrenoleukodystrophy (X-ALD)

    Behr's syndrome

    Cerebrotendinous xanthomatosis (CTX)

Cockayne's syndrome

GM2 gangliosidosis: adult onset (partial hexosaminidase A deficiency)

Gillespie's syndrome

Hartnup's disease

Joubert syndrome

Marinesco–Sjögren syndrome

Mitochondrial disorders

Neuronal ceroid lipofuscinoses (NCL)

Niemann–Pick disease (NPD) type B ("non-neuropathic")

Paine syndrome

Pontocerebellar hypoplasia

Sialidosis

Sjögren–Larsson syndrome

Unverricht–Lundborg disease

Urea cycle enzyme defects (UCED)

Wilson's disease

Xeroderma pigmentosa (XP).

Pathogenetic mechanisms are starting to be defined, including impaired defence from oxidative stress (e.g. FA, AVED, abetalipoproteinaemia), impaired DNA repair (e.g. AT, Cockayne's syndrome, XP), and impaired metabolic homeostasis.

- Acquired

  Vascular

  Cerebellar infarction: 40% posterior inferior cerebellar artery (PICA) territory; 5% anterior inferior cerebellar artery (AICA) territory; 35% superior cerebellar artery (SCA) territory; and 20% watershed infarcts

  Cerebellar haemorrhage: patient may present with an acute cerebellar syndrome +/− hydrocephalus secondary to brainstem compression and/or tonsillar herniation. There may also be brainstem signs. Urgent imaging is required; with tonsillar herniation, urgent neurosurgical intervention may be necessary in the form of posterior fossa decompression or shunt.

  Infective

  Viral infection: for example EBV, varicella, congenital rubella syndrome.

  Bacterial: direct spread from middle ear disease or mastoiditis, with possible abscess formation, in which case the patient is usually unwell and toxic with severe headache.

  Parasitic: cysticercosis.

  Prion disease: CJD (sporadic, iatrogenic), Gerstmann–Sträussler–Schenker disease, kuru.

  Inflammatory

  Multiple sclerosis: often with other signs of disseminated CNS lesions.

  Other CNS inflammatory conditions: sarcoidosis, Behçet's disease, vasculitis.

Miller Fisher variant of Guillain–Barré syndrome.

Bickerstaff's brainstem encephalitis.

Metabolic/endocrine

Gluten ataxia (with or without gluten-sensitive enteropathy = coeliac disease).

Vitamin E deficiency (isolated deficiency, acquired with gastrointestinal disease).

Wernicke–Korsakoff's syndrome.

Hypothyroidism (rare).

Neoplasia

Primary CNS tumour: including hamangioblastoma, medulloblastoma, glioma, ependymoma, vestibular schwannoma, meningioma.

Secondary metastatic tumours: lung, breast, kidney, thyroid, gastrointestinal, melanoma.

Paraneoplastic cerebellar degeneration: especially with breast and gynaecological tumours.

Drug/toxin induced

Alcohol: acute (reversible), chronic (truncal ataxia+/− peripheral neuropathy).

Anticonvulsants (phenytoin, carbamazepine).

Chemotherapy (e.g. 5-fluorouracil, cytosine arabinoside).

Toluene (glue sniffing).

Thallium poisoning (rare).

Degenerative

Multiple system atrophy (MSA): MSA-C.

Idiopathic late-onset cerebellar ataxia (ILOCA).

Clinical features: history and examination

- Ataxia: if the vermal structures are involved there is truncal ataxia with little or no limb, speech or eye involvement. The patient walks with a wide-based, staggering gait. With severe vermal/paravermal damage, there may be an inability to stand or sit. If lateral cerebellar structures are involved there is ipsilateral limb ataxia, manifest as inaccurate reaching for targets. (NB Ataxia *per se* may result from disorders in sensory and optic, as well as cerebellar, pathways.)

- Decomposition of movement (asynergia): a loss of smooth fluid movement in the performance of skilled tasks, leading to clumsiness or jerkiness.

- Dysmetria or pastpointing: errors may be made in reaching for targets. Tremor may become more evident as the target is approached (intention tremor).

- Dysdiadochokinesis: clumsiness in performing rapid alternating movements, for example supination/pronation of the forearm.

- Dysarthria: speech may be slurred and broken up, often referred to as scanning dysarthria. This is associated with damage in the region of the paravermal zone of the rostral cerebellum. In some cases of severe acute bilateral cerebellar damage, particularly in children, there maybe muteness that can last for months (cerebellar mutism).

- Nystagmus; eye movment abnormalities: various eye movement abnormalities have been described with cerebellar disease, many of which are also seen with brainstem lesions. These include gaze-evoked nystagmus (nystagmus directed towards the side of the lesion, *cf.* vestibular nystagmus), ocular dysmetria and opsoclonus.
- Hypotonia: reduced muscular tone in ipsilateral limbs, +/− reduced tendon jerks, may be seen with acute cerebellar lesions. The hypotonia is more evident in arm than leg, and proximal more than distal. It may result from reduced cerebellar outflow to the muscle spindle. (Hypertonia is often seen in cerebellar lesions due to involvement of adjacent brainstem and the descending motor pathways.)

Investigations and diagnosis See individual entries for further details.

Investigation scheme for an ataxic individual will be tailored to the specific situation but may involve:

Imaging: CT/MRI for atrophy, structural lesion, inflammatory change.

CSF: especially if inflammatory cause suspected, for example for oligoclonal bands.

Bloods/neurogenetics: as appropriate. Testing for SCA6 should be considered in late-onset ataxia even without a family history.

Differential diagnosis/Treatment and prognosis See individual entries for further details.

References Brazis PW, Masdeu JC, Biller J. *Localization in Clinical Neurology* (4th edition). Philadelphia: Lippincott Williams & Wilkins, 2001: 371–386.

Duus P. *Topical Diagnosis in Neurology: Anatomy, Physiology, Signs, Symptoms* (3rd edition). Stuttgart: Thieme, 1998: 164–179.

Manto MU, Pandolfo M (eds). *The Cerebellum and Its Disorders.* Cambridge: CUP, 2002.

Wood NW, Harding AE. Cerebellar and spinocerebellar disorders. In: Bradley WG, Daroff RB, Fenichel GM, Marsden CD (eds). *Neurology in Clinical Practice* (3rd edition). Boston: Butterworth-Heinemann, 2000: 1931–1951.

Other relevant entries Ataxia; Autosomal-dominant cerebellar ataxia; Chemotherapy and radiotherapy-induced neurological disorders; Dementia: an overview; Dysarthria; Episodic ataxias; Idiopathic late-onset cerebellar ataxia; Mitochondrial disease: an overview; Nystagmus: an overview; Paraneoplastic syndromes; Spinocerebellar ataxia; Tremor: an overview.

■ Cerebellopontine angle syndrome

Extra-axial mass lesions at the cerebellopontine angle, abutting the internal auditory meatus, produce a typical constellation of neurological signs ipsilaterally:

depression of the corneal reflex (V; early);
lower motor neurone facial (VII) weakness;

sensorineural hearing loss (VIII);
hemiataxia.

The commonest cause of this syndrome is a vestibular schwannoma (acoustic neuroma) but it may also occur with a meningioma, dermoids, epidermoids (cholesteatoma), and chordoma.

Reference Baloh RW, Konrad HR, Dirks D *et al.* Cerebellar-pontine angle tumors. *Archives of Neurology* 1976; **33**: 507–512.

Other relevant entries Cholesteatoma; Chordoma; Meningioma; Vestibular schwannoma.

▇ Cerebral abscess – see Abscess: an overview

▇ Cerebral amyloid angiopathy
Congophilic angiopathy • Dyshoric angiopathy

Pathophysiology Cerebral amyloid angiopathy (CAA) is used to refer to conditions characterized by the deposition of amyloid within cerebral blood vessels, and may be regarded as an organ-specific form of amyloidosis. In many cases, the protein is predominantly amyloid β-peptide, but other proteins may also be responsible for CAA, such as cystatin c in the Icelandic form of hereditary cerebral haemorrhage with amyloidosis (HCHWA-I).

CAA may be observed in:

Alzheimer's disease.
Down's syndrome.
Dementia pugilistica.
Post-irradiation.
Normal elderly.
HCHWA – Dutch type (HCHWA-D).
HCHWA – Icelandic type (HCHWA-I).

Clinical features: history and examination
- May be asymptomatic.
- Recurrent lobar haemorrhages: headache, nausea, vomiting, focal neurological deficit +/– impaired consciousness.
- Dementia.
- Transient neurological symptoms: transient ischaemic events, focal seizures, myoclonus +/– positive family history.

Investigations and diagnosis Definitive diagnosis relies on the examination of brain tissue, but this is seldom available: brain biopsies may be taken at the time of evacuation of cerebral haemorrhages if this is clinically indicated.

Neurogenetics: for HCHWA-D (APP gene); HCHWA-I (cystatin c).

Imaging: MRI reveals new and old haemorrhages predominantly involving the subcortical white matter.

Differential diagnosis Primary intracerebral haemorrhage, for example from hypertension, excessive anticoagulation (INR > 3.0), blood dyscrasias.

Head trauma.

Vascular malformations.

Vasculitis.

CNS tumour, metastases.

Treatment and prognosis No specific treatment. Surgical evacuation of lobar haemorrhages may be indicated on occasion.

In HCHWA-D, there is a 50% mortality rate at presentation with a cerebral haemorrhage; gradual development of dementia syndrome occurs with repeated haemorrhage, and cognitive decline has been noted in some patients even in the absence of haemorrhage.

References Coria F, Rubio I. Cerebral amyloid angiopathies. *Neuropathology and Applied Neurobiology* 1996; **22**: 216–227.

Revesz T, Ghiso J, Lashley T *et al.* Cerebral amyloid angiopathies: a pathologic, biochemical and genetic view. *Journal of Neuropathology and Experimental Neurology* 2003; **62**: 885–898.

Vinters HV. Cerebral amyloid angiopathy: a critical review. *Stroke* 1987; **18**: 311–324.

Other relevant entries Alzheimer's disease; Amyloid and the nervous system: an overview; Intracerebral haemorrhage.

■ Cerebral autosomal-dominant arteriopathy with subcortical infarcts and leukoencephalopathy – see CADASIL

■ Cerebral palsy, cerebral palsy syndromes

Pathophysiology Cerebral palsy (CP) denotes a variety of persisting and evolving disorders of movement and motor function caused by non-progressive brain lesions. CP is a common (1–2 per 1000 births) cause of persisting neurological disability. In the majority of cases, the cause is unknown, with <15% of cases following perinatal complications. Although relatively underinvestigated in the past, thorough evaluation is now recommended; many cases labelled as CP may have another disorder. A trial of levodopa to try to identify cases of dopa-responsive dystonia is recommended by some authorities.

Clinical features: history and examination CP may be classified according to:

Topography: tetraplegic, hemiplegic, diplegic (Little's disease).

Clinical features: spastic, dystonic, dyskinetic, hypotonic, ataxic.

However, these labels should not be used as a substitute for thorough investigation of potential underlying causes.

Investigations and diagnosis No specific investigation is diagnostic, but some may be helpful, for example MRI of the brain may show a vascular insult in hemiplegic CP.

Investigations may be used principally to establish alternate diagnosis (see below), for example MRI brain, blood/urine analysis for amino acids, urine organic acid analysis, white blood cell enzymes.

Differential diagnosis CP needs to be differentiated from developmental coordination disorder (clumsy child, "developmental dyspraxia") and global developmental delay. Other conditions need to be considered in specific situations:

- in the absence of a history of perinatal insult;
- a positive family history of "CP";
- developmental regression;
- presence of oculomotor abnormalities, ataxia, muscle atrophy, sensory loss, involuntary movements;

Conditions which may be confused with CP may be listed according to the clinical features:

- With apparent or real muscle weakness
  Duchenne/Becker muscular dystrophy
  Infantile neuroaxonal dystrophy
  Mitochondrial cytopathy.
- With predominant diplegia/tetrapelgia
  Adrenoleukodystrophy/adrenomyeloneuropathy (X-ALD/AMN)
  Arginase deficiency
  Metachromatic leukodystrophy (MLD)
  Hereditary spastic paraparesis (HSP)
  Holocarboxylase synthetase deficiency.
- With significant dystonia/involuntary movements
  Dopa-responsive dystonia (DRD)
  Glutaric aciduria type I
  Pyruvate dehydrogenase complex deficiency
  Lesch–Nyhan disease
  Rett's syndrome
  Juvenile neuronal ceroid lipofuscinosis
  Pelizaeus–Merzbacher disease (PMD)
  3-methylglutaconic aciduria
  3-methylcrotonyl CoA carboxylase deficiency.
- With significant ataxia
  Ataxia telangiectasia (AT)
  Angelman syndrome
  Chronic/adult GM1 gangliosidosis
  Mitochondrial cytopathy (especially NARP, 8993 mutation)
  Niemann–Pick disease type C
  Pontocerebellar atrophy/hypoplasia
  Posterior fossa tumour
  X-linked spinocerebellar ataxia.

- With significant bulbar/oromotor dysfunction

  Worster-Drought syndrome (perisylvian, opercular, Foix–Chavany–Marie syndrome).

Treatment and prognosis Treatment is of the underlying cause if identified. The most important treatable cause is DRD which responds to small doses of levodopa.

Symptomatic treatment of spasticity. Physiotherapy. Orthopaedic interventions generally unhelpful.

References Gupta R, Appleton RE. Cerebral palsy: not always what it seems. *Archives of Disease in Childhood* 2001; **85**: 356–360.

Lin J-P. The cerebral palsies: a physiological approach. *Journal of Neurology, Neurosurgery and Psychiatry* 2003; **74(suppl I)**: i23–i29.

Miller G, Clark GD (eds). *The Cerebral Palsies: Causes, Consequences and Management*. Boston: Butterworth-Heinemann, 1998.

Other relevant entries Dopa-responsive dystonia; Little's disease.

■ Cerebral salt wasting syndrome

Natriuresis with consequent hyponatraemia is a recognized complication of sub-arachnoid haemorrhage, space-occupying lesions (or following neurosurgery for these conditions), and, occasionally, meningitis or encephalitis. Clinically it may be mistaken for the syndrome of inappropriate antidiuretic hormone secretion (SIADH), since hyponatraemia is common to both.

Variable	CSW	SIADH
Serum sodium	↓	↓
Weight	↓	↑
Central venous pressure (CVP)	↓	↑ or N
Orthostatic hypotension	+	−
Serum osmolality	↑ or N	↓
Serum uric acid	N	↓
Plasma urea	N or ↑	↓ or N
Packed cell volume (PCV)	↑	↓ or N
Urine sodium	↑↑	↑
Urine volume	↑↑	↓ or N

N = normal; + = present; − = absent; ↑ = increased; ↓ = decreased.

The distinction is important since the management is different. In CSW, hypona-traemia results from natriuresis resulting in renal sodium and water loss with reduced intravascular volume, whereas in SIADH renal conservation of water results in dilutional hyponatraemia. Hence the appropriate management of CSW is intravenous saline (under central venous pressure guidance) with intravenous hydrocortisone or fludrocortisone, the mineralocorticoid effects of which reduce renal sodium loss.

Reference Harrigan MR. Cerebral salt wasting syndrome: a review. *Neurosurgery* 1996; **38**: 152–160.

Other relevant entry Syndrome of inappropriate diuretic hormone secretion.

■ Cerebral venous thrombosis – see Cerebrovascular disease: venous

■ Cerebrohepatorenal syndrome – see Zellweger syndrome

■ Cerebrosidoses – see Gaucher's disease

■ Cerebrotendinous xanthomatosis
Cholestanolosis

Pathophysiology Cerebrotendinous xanthomatosis (CTX) is a rare autosomal-recessive lipid-storage disorder in which there is impaired bile acid synthesis due to various mutations in the gene encoding the mitochondrial enzyme 27-sterol hydroxylase (CYP27) on the distal portion of chromosome 2p: no genotype/phenotype correlations have been identified. The enzyme deficiency causes an absence of chenodeoxycholic acid in the bile with consequent elevated cholestanol in the plasma and other tissues (e.g. neurones, tendons and lungs). The condition may present in late childhood with bilateral cataracts and diarrhoea, followed by an ataxic syndrome, spasticity, dementia, peripheral neuropathy, and tendon xanthomata. It is a progressive disorder; early treatment with chenodeoxycholic acid can be effective.

Clinical features: history and examination
- Juvenile bilateral cataracts (97%).
- Diarrhoea (50%).
- Tendon xanthomata, especially Achilles tendon (visible or palpable; 41%).
- Pyramidal signs: spasticity (81%).
- Cerebellar ataxia (56%).
- Dementia, around age 20 years (66%).
- Peripheral neuropathy (31%).
- Osteoporosis secondary to abnormal vitamin D metabolism.
- Premature atherosclerosis.

Investigations and diagnosis *Bloods*: raised serum cholestanol; low to normal cholesterol.
Urine: elevated bile alcohols
Imaging: CT/MRI shows global cerebral atrophy and parenchymal demyelination.
CSF: usually normal.
Neurophysiology:

EMG/NCS: peripheral neuropathy
Evoked potentials: delayed central conduction
EEG: diffuse slowing.

Neurogenetics: mutations in 27-sterol hydroxylase gene.

Treatment and prognosis Treatment with chenodeoxycholic acid (750 mg/day) can be effective if early diagnosis is made.

> **References** Verrips A, Hoefsloot LH, Steenbergen GCH *et al*. Clinical and molecular genetic characteristics of patients with cerebrotendinous xanthomatosis. *Brain* 2000; **123**: 908–919.
>
> Verrips A, van Engelen BGM, Wevers RA *et al*. Presence of diarrhea and absence of tendon xanthomas in patients with cerebrotendinous xanthomatosis. *Archives of Neurology* 2000; **57**: 520–524.

> **Other relevant entries** Abetalipoproteinaemia; Leukodystrophies: an overview; Vitamin deficiencies and the nervous system.

■ Cerebrovascular disease: arterial

Pathophysiology Arterial cerebrovascular disease is one of the commonest causes of morbidity and mortality in the adult population. The diagnosis is suggested on the basis of a clinical history of sudden onset, focal neurological deficit, without alternative explanation (although the differential diagnosis is broad); moreover, cerebrovascular disease may sometimes have a subacute or stuttering onset. Most usually "stroke" reflects atheromatous and/or thrombotic disease of cerebral vasculature, less often embolism (including arterial dissection) or haemodynamic compromise. A wide variety of vasculopathies, both inflammatory (vasculitides) and non-inflammatory may also result in cerebrovascular disease.

Once the diagnosis of acute cerebrovascular disease is made, a number of other considerations, relevant to pathophysiology and management, need to be addressed:

- Thromboembolic or haemorrhagic: The majority of strokes (85%) are ischaemic in origin, due to thromboembolic disease, with some due to arterial dissection, other vasculopathies, vasculitides, and migraine. A smaller percentage (*ca.* 10%) results from haemorrhage, the remainder being accounted for by subarachnoid haemorrhage. These various possibilities cannot be reliably differentiated on clinical grounds alone; imaging is required.
- Cardioembolic or vascular: For ischaemic strokes of embolic origin, either from heart or major vessels, anticoagulation may be indicated. A search for an embolic source may sometimes be necessary.
- Anterior or posterior circulation: Events in carotid artery territory may be distinguished from those in vertebrobasilar artery territory, the latter affecting brainstem, cerebellum, and occipital lobes. In up to 20% of people, a single anterior cerebral artery supplies both anterior territories, which may lead to bilateral signs following an infarct.

Clinical features: history and examination A number of clinical syndromes have been defined on the basis of the primary site of the vascular lesion and the resulting neurological signs:

- Total anterior circulation infarct/syndrome (TACI/TACS)

For example, due to carotid occlusion: hemiparesis, hemianopia, $+/-$ cortical dysfunction (aphasia, agnosia, apraxia, visuospatial dysfunction); generally has a poor prognosis.

- Partial anterior circulation infarct/syndrome (PACI/PACS)

    Two out of three of hemiparesis, hemianopia, and cortical dysfunction; better prognosis than TACI.

- Posterior circulation infarct/syndrome (POCI/POCS)

    Brainstem strokes and/or occipital infarction with homonymous hemianopia with macular sparing, for example top of the basilar syndrome. Variable prognosis. There are many eponymous brainstem stroke syndromes (some of which are interpreted differently by different authors) including:

    Midbrain:

        Benedikt's syndrome
        Claude's syndrome
        Nothnagel's syndrome
        Weber's syndrome.

    Pons:

        Foville syndrome
        Locked-in syndrome
        Marie–Foix syndrome
        Millard–Gubler syndrome
        Raymond syndrome
        Raymond–Céstan syndrome.

    Medulla:

        Avellis syndrome
        Babinski–Nageotte syndrome
        Céstan syndrome
        Lateral medullary syndrome (Wallenberg's syndrome)
        Medial medullary syndrome (Déjerine's anterior bulbar syndrome)
        Opalski's syndrome.

    (for further details see entry on Brainstem vascular syndromes).

- Lacunar syndromes (LACS; *q.v.*)

    Thrombosis of perforating cerebral arteries supplying the basal ganglia, pons, and internal capsule. Miller Fisher defined a number of lacunar syndromes including:

        Pure motor hemiparesis
        Dysarthria–clumsy hand syndrome
        Pure sensory stroke
        Ataxic hemiparesis (especially crural paresis).

    Multiple subcortical infarcts can lead to a syndrome of gait and cognitive disturbance sometimes referred to as Binswanger's disease or encephalopathy (*q.v.*).

    Lacunar syndromes are generally not associated with a proximal embolic cause.

- Transient ischaemic attacks (TIAs; *q.v.*)

    Focal neurological deficits of <24 hours duration (usually <30 minutes), with complete recovery, affecting either the eye (ocular TIA, amaurosis fugax), one hemisphere, or both homolateral eye and hemisphere (high risk situation). Reversible neurological deficits of >24 hours duration may be labelled minor stroke or reversible ischaemic neurological deficit (RIND). For patients seen within 24 hours of onset of focal neurological deficit, one cannot know whether the diagnosis is stroke or TIA, and hence the name "brain attack" has been suggested, emphasizing the need for prompt assessment and, possibly, treatment.
- Borderzone/watershed infarcts.
- Intracerebral haemorrhage (ICH, *q.v.*).

Investigations and diagnosis *Bloods*: glucose (hyperglycaemia associated with worse prognosis); ESR, FBC, clotting, electrolytes; auto-antibodies if vasculitis suspected; VDRL; lactate/pyruvate if mitochondrial disorder suspected; thrombophilia screen sometimes indicated.

ECG: looking particularly for atrial fibrillation.

Imaging:

    CXR: enlarged heart, unfolded aorta.

    Brain CT/MRI may confirm vascular cause for neurological events, and is the only reliable way to differentiate haemorrhage from infarction; also helps to localize pathology. MRI/MRA may assist in the diagnosis of dissection.

Echocardiogram: (transthoracic and/or transoesophageal): if it is appropriate to search for cardiac embolic source.

Carotid doppler ultrasonography: to search for carotid stenosis if anterior circulation infarct, transient ischaemic attack (some centres, depending upon local expertise, prefer MRA or formal angiography).

Differential diagnosis

Decompensation of previous stroke.

Venous cerebrovascular disease.

Migraine (especially hemiplegic migraine).

Seizure.

Traumatic brain injury.

Subdural haematoma.

Cerebral abscess.

Tumour (especially meningioma).

Demyelination.

Mitochondrial encephalomyopathies.

Treatment and prognosis *Acute*: nursing in a dedicated stroke unit, rather than a general medical ward, is associated with a better outcome. This may be related to improved access to medical, nursing, and ancillary care (physiotherapy, speech therapy, occupational therapy).

    Aspirin reduces mortality and stroke recurrence following thromboembolic stroke but is contraindicated in haemorrhagic stroke (it causes a small increase in haemorrhagic events in ischaemic stroke). Thrombolysis may have a role in certain situations if given early (probably within 3–6 hours of stroke onset) but carries a risk of intracranial bleeding.

For patients in atrial fibrillation, anticoagulation is the treatment of choice, probably beginning 2 weeks after stroke to avoid risk of haemorrhagic transformation of an ischaemic stroke.

For patients with symptomatic carotid stenosis >70–80% surgery (endarterectomy) is advised; <70% antiplatelet agents (aspirin, aspirin + dipyridamole, clopidogrel, ticlopidine).

Control of risk factors (secondary prevention) is important:

hypertension (probably should not be reduced acutely, because of loss or impairment of cerebral autoregulation associated with acute stroke);
atrial fibrillation (anticoagulation);
smoking cessation;
optimal control of diabetes;
control of cholesterol levels.

Neuropsychiatric sequelae of stroke are well recognized, particularly depression, which mandate specific treatment in their own right.

References Adams Jr HP, Bendixen BH, Kappelle LJ *et al*. Classification of subtype of acute ischemic stroke: definitions for use in a multicenter clinical trial. *Stroke* 1993; **24**: 35–41.

Bamford J, Sandercock P, Dennis M, Burn J, Warlow C. Classification and natural history of clinically identifiable subtypes of cerebral infarction. *Lancet* 1991; **337**: 1521–1526.

Bogousslavsky J, Caplan L (eds). *Stroke Syndromes* (2nd edition). Cambridge: CUP, 2002.

Bogousslavsky J, Caplan L (eds). *Uncommon Causes of Stroke*. Cambridge: CUP, 2002.

Gubitz G, Sandercock P. Acute ischaemic stroke. *British Medical Journal* 2000; **320**: 692–696.

Lees KR, Bath PMW, Naylor AR. Secondary prevention of transient ischaemic attack and stroke. *British Medical Journal* 2000; **320**: 991–994.

Robinson RG. *The Clinical Neuropsychiatry of Stroke: Cognitive, Behavioral and Emotional Disorders following Vascular Brain Injury*. Cambridge: CUP, 1998.

Warlow CP, Dennis MS, Van Gijn J, Hankey GJ, Sandercock PAG, Bamford JM, Wardlaw JM. *Stroke. A practical Guide to Management* (2nd edition). Oxford: Blackwell Science, 2001.

Welch KMA, Caplan LR, Reis DJ *et al*. (eds) *Primer on Cerebrovascular Diseases*. San Diego: Academic, 1997.

Other relevant entries Arteriovenous malformations of the brain; Binswanger's disease; Brainstem vascular syndromes; Carotid artery disease; Cerebrovascular disease: venous; Fibromuscular dysplasia; Horner's syndrome; Intracerebral haemorrhage; Intracranial vascular malformations: an overview; Lacunar syndromes; Lateral medullary syndrome; Locked-in syndrome; Mitochondrial disease: an overview; Sneddon's syndrome; Subarachnoid haemorrhage; Subdural haematoma; Top of the basilar syndrome; Transient ischaemic attack; Tuberculosis and the nervous system; Vasculitis; Weber's syndrome.

■ Cerebrovascular disease: venous

Cerebral venous thrombosis (CVT) • Cortical venous thrombosis (CVT) • Sagittal sinus thrombosis (SST) • Sinus thrombosis • Venous sinus thrombosis (VST)

Pathophysiology Thrombosis of the venous sinuses (sagittal, lateral) or cortical veins may have an acute or subacute onset and produce a variety of clinical features. Although many cases are idiopathic, recognized risk factors, some of which are amenable to modification, include use of the oral contraceptive pill, other drugs (tetracyclines), localized intracranial infection (e.g. middle ear, $+/-$ cholesteatoma, leading to lateral sinus thrombosis), thrombophilia, malignancy, vasculopathic inflammatory disease [systemic lupus erythematosus (SLE), Behçet's, polyarteritis nodosa], the puerperium, and possibly sarcoidosis.

Clinical features: history and examination Very variable.
- Headache: non-specific, sometimes "thunderclap" $+/-$ papilloedema (especially sagittal sinus thrombosis).
- Seizures.
- Focal signs: motor, sensory, visual deficits (often bilateral), aphasia (especially with cortical venous thrombosis causing infarction).

Investigations and diagnosis *Imaging*: infarction not confined to a single arterial territory is suggestive, $+/-$ oedema, haemorrhage (may even be subarachnoid blood). Delta sign may be evident on contrast-enhanced CT in sagittal sinus thrombosis, but not reliably so. MRI with attention to the veins (MRV) may confirm absence of flow voids; catheter angiography with attention to the venous phase may be required on occasion.

Other investigations attempt to define cause, especially studies of the clotting system (anti-thrombin III, protein C, protein S).

CSF: may show increased pressure, protein, pleocytosis.

Differential diagnosis

Broad:

Headache: from acute onset severe (e.g. subarachnoid haemorrhage) to chronic mild (tension-type headache)

Seizures: encephalitis, meningitis

Focal signs: arterial stroke, haemorrhage; cerebral abscess; subdural haematoma

CSF: aseptic, lymphocytic meningitis, idiopathic intacranial hypertension (IIH).

Treatment and prognosis Anticoagulation with heparin/warfarin, even in the presence of cerebral haemorrhage, is the treatment of choice, although robust evidence (systematic reviews, randomized-controlled trials) is not available. It should probably be maintained for 3–12 months. Thrombolysis is unproven.

Symptomatic treatment of seizures; prophylactic anticonvulsants are sometimes recommended, with withdrawal at 6–12 months if the patient remains seizure free.

Symptomatic treatment of raised intracranial pressure (deteriorating consciousness, visual failure).

If established, the underlying cause may mandate specific treatment.

The mortality of the acute condition is up to 30%. Although some patients make a full recovery, neurological sequelae may occur.

References De Bruijn SFTM, Stam J, for the Cerebral Venous Sinus Thrombosis Group. Randomized, placebo-controlled trial of anticoagulant treatment with low-molecular-weight heparin for cerebral sinus thrombosis. *Stroke* 1999; **30**: 484–488.

Bousser M-G, Ross Russell RW. *Cerebral Venous Thrombosis*. London: Saunders, 1997.

Other relevant entries Behçet's disease; Cerebrovascular disease: arterial; Cholesteatoma; Polyarteritis nodosa; Systemic lupus erythematosus and the nervous system.

■ Cervical cord and root disease
Cervical myelopathy, • Cervical radiculopathy

Pathophysiology The cervical spine consists of seven vertebrae, C1–C7, and the cervical spinal cord provides eight sets of cervical nerves, each arising above the corresponding numbered vertebra with the exception of C8 which emerges between the C7 and T1 vertebrae. The cervical nerves provide motor innervation for the muscles in the upper limb, the shoulder and upper chest and back, and sensory innervation of the upper limb, shoulder, neck, and back of the head. Damage to the nerve roots (cervical radiculopathy) causes wasting and weakness in the upper limb often with pain and sensory loss, and is most commonly due to degenerative cervical spine disease: hypertrophic facet joint osteophytes, degenerative ligaments, and bulging/herniation of intervertebral discs. In such cases there is often narrowing of the cervical canal which may lead to compression of the spinal cord (cervical myelopathy) causing spastic paraparesis, triparesis, or quadriparesis, depending on the level of the compression. A similar clinical picture may be produced by other pathologies, including inflammation, tumours, trauma, and anterior horn cell disease. The advent of MRI has greatly improved the ability to visualize adequately this part of the neuraxis and hence diagnostic precision.

Causes of cervical myelopathy +/− radiculopathy include:

Extradural:
　Degenerative disease of cervical spine (cervical spondylotic myelopathy)
　Vertebral collapse (e.g. secondary to metastatic disease, tuberculosis)
　Traumatic vertebral fracture/dislocation

Craniocervical junction anomalies: platybasia, basilar invagination, odontoid peg abnormalities, ankylosing spondylitis, Paget's disease, rheumatoid arthritis.

Intradural, extramedullary:

Meningioma

Neurofibroma

Epidural abscess.

Intramedullary:

Tumour: glioma, ependymoma, haemangioblastoma

Vascular lesions: anterior spinal artery occlusion, spinal AVMs, Caisson disease

Syringomyelia: may be associated craniovertebral anomaly, spinal tumour

Inflammation: MS, Devic's syndrome, acute disseminated encephalomyelitis, sarcoidosis, systemic lupus erythematosus (SLE), vasculitis; parainfectious (e.g. mycoplasma)

Subacute combined degeneration of the cord (vitamin B_{12} deficiency)

HIV/AIDS vacuolar myelopathy

Post-radiation myelopathy

Spinal cord abscess (rare)

Lightning or electrical injuries (rare).

Clinical features: history and examination

Myelopathy:

- History

    Pain may or may not be a feature

    Complaint of limb weakness; legs giving way, dragging, tripping especially after walking for some time

    May be sphincter involvement, especially if intramedullary lesion.

- Examination

    Upper motor neurone signs: spasticity, pyramidal pattern of weakness (flexors > extensors), hyperreflexia, Babinski sign

    Minor sensory signs: when present involve joint position sense and vibration perception (i.e. dorsal column); occasionally a Brown–Séquard syndrome.

    May have radicular signs in one or both upper limbs.

Radiculopathy:

- History

    Dermatomal pain

    Paroxysmal pain, increased by coughing, sneezing, straining at stool.

- Examination

    Paresis appropriate to root

    Reflex loss appropriate to root.

Specific roots:

C1: motor only; minor weakness of head flexion, extension

C2: posterior scalp sensory change, $+/-$ minor weakness of head flexion, extension

C3: sensory disturbance lower occiput, angle of jaw, upper neck; "red ear syndrome" (*q.v.*); weakness of scalene and levator scapulae muscles, $+/-$ diaphragm

C4: sensory signs on lower neck; weakness of scalene, levator scapulae and rhomboid muscles, $+/-$ diaphragm

C5: neck, shoulder, upper anterior arm pain; weakness of levator scapulae, rhomboid, serratus anterior, supraspinatus, infraspinatus, deltoid, biceps, brachioradialis muscles, $+/-$ (rarely) diaphragm; biceps and supinator reflexes may be depressed

C6: pain in lateral arm, dorsal forearm, first and second digits; weakness of serratus anterior, biceps, pronator teres, flexor carpi radialis, brachioradialis, extensor carpi radialis longus and brevis muscles; biceps and supinator reflexes may be depressed; inverted reflex may be seen if concurrent cord compression at C5–C6

C7: pain in dorsal forearm; sensory change in third and fourth digits; weakness of serratus anterior, pectoralis major, latissimus dorsi, biceps, pronator teres, flexor carpi radialis, triceps, extensor carpi radialis longus and brevis muscles, extensor digitorum; triceps reflex may be depressed

C8: pain in medial arm and forearm; sensory signs on medial forearm and hand, and fifth digit; weakness of flexor digitorum superficialis, flexor pollicis longus, flexor digitorum profundus, pronator quadratus, small hand muscles; finger flexor reflex may be depressed; $+/-$ ipsilateral Horner's syndrome.

(T1: sensory signs on medial arm; weakness of small hand muscles; finger flexor reflex may be depressed; $+/-$ ipsilateral Horner's syndrome).

In terms of frequency, roots most commonly involved are C7 >>>C6≥C8>C5.

Specific levels:

C3–C4 central cord syndrome:

"Numb and clumsy hands" syndrome

Often follows hyperextension neck injury, in elderly patients; ischaemia, syringomyelia

No obvious wasting but increased tone and hyperreflexia in upper limbs

Loss of joint position sense and light touch in upper limbs

Numbness in fingertips and palms, $+/-$ pain in shoulder girdle

Loss of vibration perception in lower limbs.

Investigations and diagnosis *Bloods*: may include FBC, ESR, vitamin B_{12}, auto-antibody profile, serum ACE.

Imaging: MRI is imaging technique of choice for cervical spine; occasionally a myelogram is required if a dural AVM is suspected but not seen with MRI.

CSF: to exclude an inflammatory or malignant process.

Neurophysiology:

EMG/NCS

to exclude peripheral neuropathy or widespread anterior horn cell disease;

to define level of radiculopathy, the sites of greatest denervation are:

C5 radiculopathy: spinati, deltoid, biceps, brachioradialis

C6 radiculopathy: 50% are similar to C5 radiculopathy with additional involvement of pronator teres; the other 50% are identical to the findings in a C7 radiculopathy

C7 radiculopathy: pronator teres, flexor carpi radialis, triceps

C8 radiculopathy: first dorsal interosseous, abductor digiti minimi, abductor pollicis brevis, flexor pollicis longus.

Others: occasionally evoked potentials and central motor conduction times are useful in diagnosing demyelinating CNS disease and upper motor neurone involvement.

Differential diagnosis Other causes of arm pain, weakness, sensory disturbance, for example brachial plexopathy (such as neuralgic amyotrophy).

Treatment and prognosis Dependent on the cause of the cervical cord syndrome. In the case of spondylotic cervical radiculomyelopathy, conservative management is normally the first line of treatment (collar, physical therapy). However, surgery may become necessary when there is a progressive impairment of function with no remission. Best results are expected with only a single level of compression diagnosed clinically with appropriate radiological correlate. Multiple compressive lesions may be approached surgically, but pose greater problems. The aim of surgery is to prevent progression rather than reverse the neurological deficits. However in a significant number of cases there is some neurological improvement postoperatively. The surgical approach may be either posterior, with laminectomy and foraminotomy, or anterior (Cloward's procedure) with laminectomy and osteophyte-posterior ligament removal. The latter approach gives a better decompression and has a complication rate of between 2% and 8%.

Comparative studies suggest that discectomy, collar, or physical therapy, all give similar outcomes at 12-month follow-up.

References Braakman R. Management of cervical spondylotic myelopathy and radiculopathy. *Journal of Neurology, Neurosurgery and Psychiatry* 1994; **57**: 257–263.

Laing RD. Management of cervical spondylotic radiculopathy and myelopathy. In: Scolding NJ (ed.). *Contemporary Treatments in Neurology*. Oxford: Butterworth-Heinemann, 2001: 114–128.

Levin KH, Maggiano HJ, Wilbourn AJ. Cervical radiculopathies: comparison of surgical and EMG localization of single root lesions. *Neurology* 1996; **46**: 1022–1025.

Nakajima M, Hirayama K. Midcervical central cord syndrome: numb and clumsy hands due to midline cervical disc protrusion at the C3–4 intervertebral level. *Journal of Neurology, Neurosurgery and Psychiatry* 1995; **58**: 607–613.

Yoss RE, Corbin KB, MacCarty CS, Love JG. Significance of symptoms and signs in localization of involved root in cervical disc protrusion. *Neurology* 1957; **7**: 673–683.

Other relevant entries Acute disseminated encephalomyelitis; Ankylosing spondylitis and the nervous system; Atlantoaxial dislocation, subluxation; Brown–Séquard syndrome; Chiari malformations; Chemotherapy- and radiotherapy-induced neurological disorders; Devic's disease, Devic's syndrome; Foramen magnum lesions, Foramen magnum syndrome; Horner's syndrome; Intervertebral disc prolapse; Klippel–Feil anomaly; Lumbar cord and root disease; Motor neurone disease; Multiple sclerosis; Myelitis: an overview; Myelopathy: an overview; Ossification of the posterior longitudinal ligament; Paraparesis: acute management and differential diagnosis; Radiculopathies: an overview; Red ear syndrome; Rheumatoid arthritis; Sarcoidosis; Spinal cord trauma; Spinal cord vascular diseases; Spinal muscular atrophy; Syringomyelia and syringobulbia; Thoracic outlet syndromes; Tumours: an overview; Vasculitis; Vitamin B_{12} deficiency.

■ Cervical dystonia – see Dystonia: an overview; Spasmodic torticollis

■ Cervical rib syndrome – see Thoracic outlet syndromes

■ Cervical spondylosis

Osteoarthritic change and spondylosis in the cervical spine is ubiquitous with increasing age; cervical dystonia may exacerbate such change. The role of cervical spondylosis *per se* in causing neck ache, brachialgia, or headache is doubtful. Compressive cervical radiculopathy and myelopathy may occur as a consequence of cervical spondylosis.

Other relevant entries Cervical cord and root disease; Intervertebral disc prolapse.

■ Cervical spondylotic myelopathy – see Cervical cord and root disease; Myelopathy: an overview

■ Céstan syndrome
Céstan–Chenais syndrome

Infarction of the medial part of the medullary tegmentum as a result of vertebral artery occlusion causes a syndrome of unilateral palatal and vocal cord paralysis, Horner's syndrome, contralateral hemiplegia, and contralateral hemianaesthesia for proprioception and discriminative touch (medial lemniscus involvement) with sparing of pain and temperature (spinothalamic) sensation. This syndrome may be characterized as equivalent to Wallenberg's lateral medullary syndrome without the ipsilateral ataxia, but with additional contralateral hemiparesis. Some authorities therefore regard it as a rare variant of lateral medullary syndrome ("Wallenberg plus").

Céstan's name is also coupled with that of Raymond describing a syndrome of rostral–tegmental pontine pathology (*q.v.*).

Other relevant entries Babinski–Nageotte syndrome; Brainstem vascular syndromes; Lateral medullary syndrome; Raymond syndrome, Raymond–Céstan syndrome.

■ Cestode infection – see Helminthic diseases

■ Chagas' disease – see Gastrointestinal disease and the nervous system; Trypanosomiasis

■ Channelopathies: an overview

Channelopathy is the generic name applied to a wide variety of neurological diseases caused by dysfunction of ion channels in excitable membranes. Many of these are due to inherited mutations of genes encoding ion channels in muscle, neurones, and glia. Acquired channelopathies, of autoimmune and transcriptional pathogenesis, may also occur.

The channelopathies may be classified as:
- Muscle channelopathies
  Voltage-gated channels

Sodium channels:	Hyperkalaemic periodic paralysis
	Hypokalaemic periodic paralysis (rare)
	Paramyotonia congenita
	Potassium-aggravated myotonia (PAM)
Potassium channels:	Hypokalaemic periodic paralysis
	Andersen's syndrome
Calcium channels:	Hypokalaemic periodic paralysis (common)
	Malignant hyperthermia
	Central core disease
Chloride channels:	Myotonia congenita (Becker, Thomsen types)

  Ligand-gated channels
  Nicotinic acetylcholine

receptors:	Congenital myasthenic syndromes

- Neuronal channelopathies:
  Voltage-gated channels

Sodium channels:	Generalized epilepsy with febrile seizures plus (GEFS+)
	Severe myoclonic epilepsy of infancy
Potassium channels:	Episodic ataxia type 1
	Benign familial neonatal convulsions
Calcium channels:	Familial hemiplegic migraine (FHM)

	Spinocerebellar ataxia type 6 (SCA6)
	Episodic ataxia type 2
Ligand-gated channels	
Nicotinic acetylcholine receptors:	Autosomal-dominant nocturnal frontal lobe epilepsy (ADNFLE)
Glycine receptors:	Familial hyperekplexia
GABA receptors:	Generalized epilepsy with febrile seizures plus

• Glial channelopathies

| Gap junction proteins: | Charcot–Marie–Tooth disease CMT-X or CMT-1X |

Some of the inherited prolonged QT syndromes are also channelopathies.

Clinical features: history and examination/Investigations and diagnosis/Differential diagnosis/Treatment and prognosis See individual entries.

> **References** Kleopka KA, Barchi RL. Genetic disorders of neuromuscular ion channels. *Muscle and Nerve* 2002; **26**: 299–325.
>
> Kullmann DM, Hanna MG. Neurological disorders caused by inherited ion-channel mutations. *Lancet Neurology* 2002; **1**: 157–166.
>
> Rose MR, Griggs RC (eds). *Channelopathies of the Nervous System*. Boston: Butterworth-Heinemann, 2001.

Other relevant entries Andersen's syndrome; Autosomal-dominant nocturnal frontal lobe epilepsy; Central core disease; Charcot–Marie–Tooth disease; Ciguatera; Congenital myasthenic syndromes; Dystrophia myotonica; Epilepsy: an overview; Episodic ataxias; Febrile convulsions; Hyperekplexia; Malignant hyperthermia; Migraine; Myotonia and myotonic disorders; Paramyotonia; Periodic paralysis; Prolonged QT syndromes.

◾ Charcot–Bouchard aneurysms

These are small dissecting aneurysms (microaneurysms) arising from the small perforating arteries of the brain, possibly as a consequence of vessel wall weakening from lipohyalinosis and often in the context of hypertension. They may be implicated in hypertensive brain haemorrhage affecting the basal ganglia, thalamus, pons, and subcortical white matter.

Other relevant entry Intracerebral haemorrhage.

◾ Charcot–Marie–Tooth disease

Pathophysiology Charcot and Marie, and independently, Tooth, in 1886 described hereditary peripheral neuropathy with a peroneal muscular atrophy phenotype: distal weakness and atrophy, distal sensory loss, areflexia, and foot deformity (pes cavus). The heterogeneity of this group of conditions soon became apparent, falling within the rubric of "hereditary motor and sensory neuropathy" (HMSN) in the classification of hereditary neuropathies proposed by Dyck and Lambert in 1968. The observation that nerve conduction velocities might be low or normal, implying demyelinating and axonal variants respectively, led to the division into HMSN I (or CMT-I) and HMSN II (or CMT-II). The definition of the genetic basis of some of these inherited neuropathies has forced a revision of classification.

Currently the following varieties fall within the rubric of Charcot–Marie–Tooth disease:

- CMT-1: Autosomal-dominant, hypertrophic demyelinating neuropathy

    CMT-1A: duplications or point mutations in peripheral myelin protein 22 (PMP22) gene

    CMT-1B: mutations in myelin protein zero (MPZ or P_0) gene: includes Roussy–Lévy syndrome

    CMT-1C: linked to chromosome 16p13.1–p12.3; gene unknown

    CMT-1D: mutations in early growth response element 2 (EGR2) gene.

- CMT-2: Autosomal-dominant, axonal neuropathy

    CMT-2A: mutations in kinesin motor protein 1B (KIF-1Bβ) gene

    CMT-2B: linked to chromosome 3q13–q22

    CMT-2D: linked to chromosome 7p14

    CMT-2E: mutations in neurofilament light chain (NEFL) gene

    CMT-2F: linked to chromosome 7q11–21

    CMT-2 phenotype with mutations in myelin protein zero (MPZ or P_0) gene: allelic with CMT-1B.

- CMT-4: this nomenclature has been used to described autosomal-recessive types of CMT-1, (hypertrophic demyelinating neuropathy) and, confusingly, autosomal-recessive forms of CMT-2 (as CMT-4C, also known as AR-CMT)

    CMT-4A: mutations in ganglioside-induced differentiation-associated protein 1 (GDAP1) gene

    CMT-4B1: mutations in myotubularin-related protein 2 (MTMR2) gene

    CMT-4B2: linked to chromosome 11p15

    CMT-4C: linked to chromosome 5q23–q33

    CMT-4C1 = AR-CMT-2A: mutations in lamin A/C nuclear envelope protein (LMNA); mutations in this gene also reported in Emery–Dreifuss muscular dystrophy, limb-girdle muscular dystrophy

    CMT-4C2: linked to chromosome 8q21.3

    CMT-4C3: linked to chromosome 19q13.3

    CMT-4C4: mutations in ganglioside-induced differentiation-associated protein 1 (GDAP1) gene, hence allelic with CMT-4A

    CMT-4D: mutations in N-myc-downstream regulated gene 1 (NDRG1)

    CMT-4E: mutations in early growth response element 2 (EGR2) gene, hence allelic with CMT-1D

    CMT-4F: mutations in periaxin (PRX) gene.

- CMT-X: X-linked, intermediate motor conduction velocities

    CMT-X or CMT-1X: mutations in gap junction protein β-1 (GJB1) gene, also
       known as Connexin 32

    CMT-2X: linked to chromosome Xq24–q26

    CMT-3X: linked to chromosome Xp22.2

    CMT-4X: linked to chromosome Xq26.q28.

- Dominant intermediate CMT (DI-CMT): conduction velocities intermediate
  between those of CMT-1 and CMT-2

    DI-CMT-A: linked to chromosome 10q24.1–q25.1

    DI-CMT-B: linked to chromosome 19p12–p13.2

    HMSN-P (=proximal): linked to chromosome 3p14.1–q13.

Of these, the most common are CMT-1A, CMT-1B, and CMT-1X.

Clinical features: history and examination In addition to distal sensory and motor findings (see Hereditary motor and sensory neuropathy [(HMSN)] there may in addition be other features such as deafness (CMT-4D, CMT-2 with MPZ or P_0 mutations, CMT-2X), mental retardation (CMT-2X, CMT-3X).

Investigations and diagnosis *Neurophysiology*: EMG/NCS: motor conduction velocities allow assignment to CMT-1, CMT-2, or DI-CMT groups. Genetic tests are available for some of these neuropathies.

Differential diagnosis Other demyelinating or axonal neuropathy, but the clinical phenotype with positive family history is unlikely to lead to confusion, with possible exception of CMT-1B and Friedreich's ataxia.

Treatment and prognosis

No specific therapy.

Variable prognosis according to subclassification.

References Kuhlenbäumer G, Young P, Hünermund G, Ringelstein B, Stögbauer F. Clinical features and molecular genetics of hereditary peripheral neuropathies. *Journal of Neurology* 2002; **249**: 1629–1650.

Reilly MM, Hanna MG. Genetic neuromuscular disease. *Journal of Neurology, Neurosurgery and Psychiatry* 2002; **73(suppl II)**: ii12–ii21.

Other relevant entries Channelopathies: an overview; Emery–Dreifuss muscular dystrophy; Hereditary motor and sensory neuropathy; Limb-girdle muscular dystrophy; Neuropathies: an overview; Roussy–Lévy syndrome.

■ Charcot's disease – see Motor neurone disease

■ Charcot's triad

This refers to the combination of nystagmus, dysarthria ("scanning speech") and intention tremor, most commonly seen in multiple sclerosis, usually in its advanced stages.

Other relevant entry Multiple sclerosis.

■ Charles Bonnet syndrome

Bonnet syndrome

Charles Bonnet, an eighteenth century Swiss physician, reported on visual hallucinations occurring in blind or partially sighted people; a similar phenomenon may occur in visual field defects. Deafferentation may thus be crucial to the origin of the hallucinations, which are often vivid and bizarre. They often disappear when the eyes are shut, implying that some of the hallucinatory properties are driven by peripheral visual stimuli. The phenomenology may also overlap with that of palinopsia in which multiple copies of an object are seen after it moves. The pathophysiology of Charles Bonnet syndrome is still not fully understood, but the syndrome is common.

References Manford M, Andermann F. Complex visual hallucinations. Clinical and neurobiological insights. *Brain* 1998; **121**: 1819–1840.

Teunisse RJ, Cruysberg JRM, Verbeek A *et al*. The Charles Bonnet syndrome: a large prospective study in the Netherlands. *British Journal of Psychiatry* 1995; **166**: 234–257.

Ffytche D. Visual hallucination and illusion disorders: a clinical guide. *Advances in Clinical Neuroscience and Rehabilitation* 2004; **4**(2): 16–18.

Other relevant entry Palinopsia.

■ Charlevoix–Saguenay syndrome

An autosomal-recessive disorder of childhood, initially reported from Quebec, Canada, characterized by a slowly progressive pyramidal syndrome, dysarthria, ataxia, abnormal eye movements (vertical pursuit), sphincter involvement, mitral incompetence and motor neuropathy, linked to chromosome 13q11–q12. It may be classified as a "complicated" hereditary spastic paraparesis or as an early-onset autosomal-recessive cerebellar ataxia with retained reflexes (autosomal-recessive spastic ataxia of Charlevoix–Saguenay, ARSACS).

Reference Mrissa N, Belal S, Ben-Hamida M *et al*. Linkage to chromosome 13q11–q12 of an autosomal recessive cerebellar ataxia in a Tunisian family. *Neurology* 2000; **54**: 1408–1414.

Other relevant entries Cerebellar disease: an overview; Hereditary spastic paraparesis; Troyer syndrome.

■ Charlin's syndrome

Ciliary neuralgia

This syndrome comprises bouts of severe pain in the corner of one eye and ipsilateral nasal root, associated with lacrimation and rhinorrhoea. It is thought to result from irritation of the ciliary ganglion. The conjunction of ipsilateral pain and autonomic features suggest that this may be a variant of cluster headache.

Other relevant entry Cluster headache.

■ Chédiak–Higashi syndrome

Pathophysiology Chédiak–Higashi syndrome, first described in the early 1950s independently by Chédiak and Higashi and given the eponym in 1955 by Soto, is a rare autosomal-recessive condition characterized by partial oculocutaneous albinism due to a defect in tyrosine metabolism, with neurological abnormalities (nystagmus, cerebellar syndrome, pyramidal signs, papilloedema, peripheral neuropathy), and frequent pyogenic infections due to a defect in phagocyte function. It is progressive and incurable with death usually before 10 years of age from infection or lymphoreticular malignancy.

Clinical features: history and examination

- Systemic:
    Partial oculocutaneous albinism (may not be present)
    Recurrent pyogenic infections (may not occur)
    Lymphadenopathy
    Hepatosplenomegaly.
- Neurological:
    Gait ataxia and nystagmus
    Mental retardation
    Raised intracranial pressure with papilloedema
    Sensorimotor peripheral neuropathy.

Investigations and diagnosis *Bloods*: FBC may show neutropenia, anaemia. Blood film may show abnormal cytoplasmic inclusions in neutrophils which are pathognomonic of this condition.

CSF: may show a raised opening pressure $+/-$ raised white cell count and protein.

Neurophysiology: EMG/NCS: may demonstrate sensorimotor neuropathy.

Differential diagnosis

Cerebral palsy.

Xeroderma pigmentosa.

Treatment and prognosis

Treatment is largely symptomatic (e.g. antibiotics for recurrent infections).

Bone marrow transplantation may be helpful.

The condition is progressive and the patients die of either overwhelming sepsis or develop a lymphoreticular malignancy.

> **Reference** Blume RS, Wolff SM. The Chédiak–Higashi syndrome: studies in four patients and a review of the literature. *Medicine (Baltimore)* 1972; **51**: 247–280.

> **Other relevant entries** Albinism; Cerebellar disease: an overview; Neuropathies: an overview; Xerodermal pigmentosa and related conditions.

■ Cheiralgia paraesthetica
Handcuff neuropathy

Cheiralgia paraesthetica describes paraesthesia and pain in the distribution of the superficial dorsal sensory branch of the radial nerve (radial side of the thumb, dorsoradial side of hand). Ulnar flexion of the hyperpronated forearm may exacerbate the pain. It is a sensory mononeuropathy of the superficial ramus of the radial nerve which may result from pressure trauma to the nerve from handcuffs or tight wristbands and is usually self-limiting. It has also been recorded with diabetes mellitus.

> **Reference** Massey EW, Pleet AB. Handcuffs and cheiralgia paresthetica. *Neurology* 1978; **28**: 1312–1313.

> **Other relevant entries** Diabetes mellitus and the nervous system; Entrapment neuropathies: an overview; Neuropathies: an overview; Radial neuropathy.

■ Cheiro-oral syndrome
Restricted acral sensory syndrome

An abnormal sensory syndrome involving the perioral region, sometimes bilaterally, and the ipsilateral palm, sometimes only certain digits ("pseudoradicular"), +/− ipsilateral foot. Most commonly this reflects thalamic pathology (VPN), usually stroke, but may also occur with lesions of the corona radiata and sensory cortex (the latter especially if isolated pseudoradicular syndrome).

> **Reference** Kim JS. Restricted acral sensory syndrome following minor stroke: further observations with special reference to differential severity of symptoms among individual digits. *Stroke* 1994; **25**: 2497–2502.

> **Other relevant entry** Thalamic syndromes.

■ Chemodactoma – see Glomus jugulare tumour

■ Chemotherapy- and radiotherapy-induced neurological disorders

Pathophysiology Drug and radiation therapies, most often given to inhibit or destroy neoplastic cells, are non-specific in their effects and may adversely affect normal neuronal function in brain, spinal cord and peripheral nervous system, transiently or permanently. Neurotoxicity is more likely with high-dose therapy, combined therapies, and intrathecal drug administration.

Some of the commoner adverse effects are listed here, along with the drugs most often culpable.

Clinical features: history and examination
• Chemotherapy

Encephalopathy: acute, subacute, chronic, with focal signs, seizures, cognitive deficit, coma: methotrexate, cytosine arabinoside, 5-fluorouracil, intra-arterial nitrosoureas, ifosfamide, L-asparaginase; radiotherapy

Chemical meningitis: intrathecal drugs (e.g. methotrexate, cytosine arabinoside)

Cerebellar syndrome: cytosine arabinoside, 5-fluorouracil

Peripheral neuropathy: vinca alkaloids, taxanes, cis-platinum, procarbazine, etoposide

Ototoxicity: cis-platinum

Ocular toxicity: intra-arterial nitrosoureas, tamoxifen

Syndrome of inappropriate ADH secretion: vincristine, cis-platinum.

- Radiotherapy

    Cerebral injury: acute encephalopathy, early delayed encephalopathy, late encephalopathy (focal cerebral necrosis, diffuse cerebral injury: leuko-encephalopathy)

    Cerebrovascular disease: occlusive disease

    Optic neuropathy, other cranial neuropathies (especially XII, X, XI)

    Myelopathy: transient, delayed progressive

    Brachial plexopathy: usually delayed progressive; lumbosacral plexopathy

    Intracranial tumours: meningioma, glioma, sarcoma; long latency.

Investigations and diagnosis Usually the clinical picture is clearly related to drug use, but investigations to exclude other diagnostic possibilities, especially opportunistic infection, may be appropriate. Radiotherapy effects may occur after some delay (months to years) and must be differentiated from tumour recurrence or metastatic disease. Depending on the clinical presentation, imaging, EMG/NCS, and CSF analysis may be appropriate, but these seldom produce diagnostic information. One possible exception is the finding of myokymic discharges in the EMG in radiation-induced brachial plexopathy, not found in brachial plexopathy due to metastatic disease (lung, breast).

Differential diagnosis Metastatic disease, opportunistic infection, metabolic derangement, other drug toxicities.

Treatment and prognosis Therapeutic options are often limited. Drug withdrawal may be appropriate if acute toxicity occurs. Some toxicities reverse spontaneously, others do not. Corticosteroids (e.g. dexamethasone) may reduce both the risk and the effects of radiation-induced acute encephalopathy.

References Dropcho EJ. Neurologic complications of radiation therapy. In: Biller J (ed.). *Iatrogenic Neurology*. Boston: Butterworth-Heinemann, 1998: 461–483.

Keime-Guibert F, Napolitano M, Delattre JY. Neurological complications of radio-therapy and chemotherapy. *Journal of Neurology* 1998; **245**: 695–708.

Paleologos NA. Complications of chemotherapy. In: Biller J (ed.). *Iatrogenic Neurology*. Boston: Butterworth-Heinemann, 1998: 439–459.

Quasthoff S, Hartung HP. Chemotherapy-induced peripheral neuropathy. *Journal of Neurology* 2002; **249**: 9–17.

Other relevant entries Brachial plexopathies; Encephalopathy: an overview; Immunosuppressive therapy and diseases of the nervous system; Neuropathies: an overview; Syndrome of inappropriate ADH secretion; Tumours: an overview.

■ Cherry red spot-myoclonus syndrome – see Sialidosis

■ Chiari malformations
Arnold–Chiari malformations

Pathophysiology Chiari in the 1890s described a number of congenital anomalies at the base of the brain, which have become known as Chiari (or Arnold–Chiari) malformations. They are characterized by descent of the cerebellar tonsils and parts of the brainstem into the cervical canal, often with associated hydrocephalus. Two types of Chiari malformation are recognized: type I without, and type II with, an associated myelomeningocoele and other signs of dysraphism. Diagnosis has become easier with the advent of magnetic resonance imaging. Management by surgery is controversial and complex.

Several hypotheses have been advanced to explain the mechanism whereby hindbrain anomalies cause associated hydrocephalus and syringomyelia and syringobulbia, with the hope that this will inform surgical approaches. The issues are not entirely resolved. Descent of the brainstem and cerebellum into the cervical canal occludes the foramen magnum; in addition there may be narrowing of the cerebral aqueduct, and obstruction to the outflow of CSF from the foramina of Luschka and Magendie. A piston-type mechanism may then lead to hydrocephalus and syrinx formation. There may be associated developmental abnormalities such as cervical myelomeningocoele, polymicrogyria, and a low termination of the spinal cord.

Clinical features: history and examination

- Type I Chiari malformation: not associated with meningocoele or other signs of dysraphism
    - Symptoms and signs usually develop in adolescence or adult life
    - Symptom onset may be sudden, especially after neck manipulation (especially extension)
    - A significant number of patients have an abnormally short ("bull") neck
    - Raised intracranial pressure
    - Progressive cerebellar ataxia
    - Syringomyelia
    - Lower cranial nerve palsies+/− long tract signs and sensory loss due to spinal cord compression+/− cerebellar ataxia
    - Downbeat nystagmus
    - Cough/hindbrain headache
- Type II Chiari malformation: associated with meningocoele
    - Symptoms usually develop early in life, in the neonatal period
    - Progressive hydrocephalus
    - Progressive lower cranial nerve abnormalities (VI to XII)
    - Signs as for type I anomaly

Investigations and diagnosis *Imaging*: MRI is the diagnostic investigation.
CSF: may show raised protein and pressure.

Differential diagnosis

Type I

    Multiple sclerosis

    High cervical tumour

    Skull base tumour with foramen magnum involvement.

Type II

    Other causes of hydrocephalus

    Spina bifida

    Brainstem/cerebellar tumour.

Treatment and prognosis The optimal management of Chiari malformations remains uncertain. If the clinical picture is stable, then conservative management may be most appropriate. If the signs and disability are progressing surgical intervention may be indicated, for example upper cervical laminectomy and foramen magnum decompression. Associated syringomyelia may merit treatment in its own right.

References Anson JA, Benzel EC, Awad IA (eds). *Syringomyelia and the Chiari Malformations*. Park Ridge, Illinois: American Association of Neurological Surgeons, 1997.

Arnett B. Arnold–Chiari malformation. *Archives of Neurology* 2003; **60**: 898–900.

Hadley DM. The Chiari malformations. *Journal of Neurology, Neurosurgery and Psychiatry* 2002; **72(suppl II)**: ii38–ii40.

Pillay PK, Awad IA, Little JR, Hahn JF. Symptomatic Chiari malformation in adults: a new classification based on magnetic resonance imaging with clinical and prognostic significance. *Neurosurgery* 1991; **28**: 639–645.

Saez RJ, Onofrio BM, Yanagihara T. Experience with Arnold–Chiari malformation, 1960–1970. *Journal of Neurosurgery* 1976; **45**: 416–422.

Other relevant entries Cervical cord and root disease; Cough headache; Hydrocephalus; Multiple sclerosis; Nystagmus: an overview; Syringomyelia and syringobulbia; Tumours: an overview.

■ Chiggers – see Rickettsial diseases

■ Childhood ataxia with central nervous system hypomyelination – see Vanishing white matter disease

■ Chinese paralytic syndrome – see Guillain–Barré syndrome

■ Chiray–Foix–Nicolesco syndrome – see Benedikt's syndrome

■ Chlamydia – see Psittacosis

■ Chloroma
Balfour disease

This name has been applied to a solid mass of acute or chronic myelogenous leukaemic cells, with a greenish tinge, affecting brain (e.g. cerebellopontine angle), dura or orbit. The syndrome is uncommon, and of doubtful nosological value.

Other relevant entry Lymphoma.

■ Cholestanolosis – see Cerebrotendinous xanthomatosis

■ Cholesteatoma

Cholesteatoma (epidermoid) of the ear is a skin cyst within the middle ear space that behaves like a localized tumour. It may be congenital or acquired; the fact that the incidence of cholesteatoma has not fallen since the introduction of antibiotic therapy for middle ear infection suggests that most are congenital (like epidermoids elsewhere). Cholesteatoma predisposes to repeated acute middle ear infections and mastoid infections (and is usually found in the presence of chronic otitis media), and also erodes bone in the vestibular labyrinth which may lead to a perilymphatic fistula (causing vertigo, sensorineural deafness) and facial nerve palsy. Central extension may cause meningitis, venous sinus thrombosis, or dural abscess.

On clinical grounds alone, it may not be possible to differentiate chronic otitis media from cholesteatoma; this requires debridement of the external ear and otological examination.

Cholesteatoma may invade the cerebellopontine angle from the middle ear, mimicking a vestibular schwannoma or other cerebellopontine angle pathology. Clinical signs reported with cholesteatomas also include Gradenigo's syndrome and spontaneous periodic hypothermia. Glomus jugulare tumours also enter the differential diagnosis.

Surgical approach to cholesteatoma necessitates tumour excision and exteriorizing the skin cyst.

Other relevant entries Cerebellopontine angle syndrome; Cerebrovascular disease: venous; Epidermoid; Gradenigo's syndrome; Vestibular schwannoma.

■ Cholesterol embolization syndrome

In patients with widespread atheroma, cholesterol emboli may enter the circulation spontaneously or, more commonly, as a consequence of instrumentation, and possibly anticoagulant or thrombolytic therapy. Cholesterol emboli occlude the microcirculation causing a syndrome of malaise, fever, renal failure, abdominal pain, skin petechiae, confusion, and even peripheral gangrene. Blood tests show anaemia, thrombocytopenia, leukocytosis, eosinophilia, and raised ESR. The differential diagnosis includes infective endocarditis and systemic vasculitis.

> **Reference** Fine MJ, Kapoor W, Falanga V. Cholesterol crystal embolisation: a review of 221 cases in the English literature. *Angiology* 1987; **38**: 769–784.

> **Other relevant entries** Cerebrovascular disease: arterial; Endocarditis and the nervous system; Vasculitis.

■ Cholesterol ester-storage disease – see Wolman's disease

■ Chordoma

Pathophysiology Chordomas are rare tumours that originate from the remnant of the notochord. They are found most commonly either at the level of the clivus, sellar or parasellar region, or sacrococcygeal region. Tumours are locally invasive, have a tendency to recurrence, and potential to metastasize.

They present most often in the 30–50-year-age group.

Clinical features: history and examination
- Cerebral lesions: diplopia +/− other cranial nerve palsy; headache.
- Sacrococcygeal lesions: conus +/− cauda equina syndrome; lower back pain.

Investigations and diagnosis *Imaging*: MRI shows a circumscribed, extrinsic lesion, often heterogeneous signal intensity.

Biopsy: required for definitive diagnosis, the characteristic microscopic feature is the presence of physaliphorous cells.

Differential diagnosis Other mass lesions: meningioma, neurofibroma, and carcinoma of the local tissue.

Consider also Wegener's granulomatosis.

Treatment and prognosis *Surgery*: clival lesions may be difficult to access. Although full removal may be possible, there is a tendency to recurrence.

Chordomas are largely refractory to both radio- and chemotherapy, although some centres report improved survival with surgery + radiotherapy; proton beam therapy may be helpful.

5-year survival is around 60%.

> **Reference** Watkins L, Khudados ES, Kaleoglu M *et al*. Skull base chordomas: a review of 38 cases, 1958–1988. *British Journal of Neurosurgery* 1993; **7**: 241–248.

> **Other relevant entries** Cranial polyneuropathy; Tumours: an overview.

■ Chorea

Pathophysiology Chorea is an involuntary hyperkinetic movement disorder characterized by a series of unpredictable, brief, jerky movements that randomly affect different parts of the body; the name derives from the Greek word meaning "dance-like".

It is important to differentiate the movements of chorea from myoclonus or tics, not only in order to arrive at the correct diagnosis, but also because some diseases associated with chorea have major implications for the whole family (e.g. Huntington's disease). Chorea may be seen in large number of conditions, only some of which are treatable.

Although the exact pathogenesis of chorea is not known, one model suggests that, whatever the primary site of pathology, there is a reduction in output from the basal ganglia to the thalamus leading to a disinhibition in the relay nuclei of this structure, in turn leading to increased cortical excitability which is then translated through the descending motor pathways, resulting in chorea.

Recognized causes of chorea include:

- Inherited disorders

    Autosomal dominant:

        Huntington's disease

        Spinocerebellar ataxias: including SCA, Machado–Joseph disease, DRPLA

        Benign hereditary chorea (BHC).

    Autosomal recessive:

        Aminoacidopathies

        Ataxia telangectasia (AT)

        Basal ganglia calcification

        Hallervorden–Spatz disease

        Lesch–Nyhan syndrome

        Lysosomal disorders

        Neuroacanthocytosis

        Porphyria

        Tuberous sclerosis

        Urea cycle disorders

        Wilson's disease.

    Others:

        Leigh's syndrome

        Mitochondrial disease.

- Drug induced

    Neuroleptics

    Propofol

    Anticonvulsants.

    Anti-parkinsonian medication

    Oral contraceptive

    Amphetamines and tricyclic antidepressants (rare).

- Toxic/metabolic

    Alcohol

    Anoxia

    Carbon monoxide poisoning

    Cocaine

Heavy metal poisoning

Hyperthyroidism

Hypoparathyroidism

Pregnancy

Hyper- or hyponatraemia, magnesaemia, calcaemia

Hyper- or hypoglycaemia

Acquired hepatocerebral degeneration

Nutritional.

- Infection

  Sydenham's chorea/PANDAS

  Brainstem encephalitis, encephalitis lethargica

  Prion disease: Creutzfeldt–Jakob disease, vCJD

- Immunological

  Systemic lupus erythematosus

  Henoch–Schonlein purpura

  Sarcoidosis

  Multiple sclerosis

  Behçet's disease (rare)

  Vasculitis

  Hashimoto's encephalopathy.

- Vascular

  Infarction (including Binswanger's encephalopathy)

  Haemorrhage

  Arteriovenous malformation

  Polycythaemia

  Migraine

  Cerebral palsy.

- Tumours

  Primary and secondary (rare).

- Others

  Trauma

  Physiological chorea of infancy

  Senile chorea

  Paroxysmal choreoathetosis

  Post-pump (cardiac bypass) chorea

  Psychogenic.

Of these, probably the most important in terms of frequency are Huntington's disease, drug-induced, Sydenham's chorea/PANDAS, and senile chorea.

Clinical features: history and examination Patients appear fidgety; there is a complaint (often voiced by relatives rather than the patient) of clumsiness and incoordination rather than abnormal movement.

Chorea may evolve to the point of interfering with activities of daily living, such as feeding and walking.

On examination, patients usually demonstrate a range of choreiform movements which can be made worse by standing and walking. Respiratory muscles may be involved resulting in grunting, sniffing, and respiratory gulps. There may be other abnormal movements associated, including athetosis, dystonia, parkinsonism, tics, myoclonus, and tremor.

Cognitive impairment may coexist, or may be the presenting feature in some choreiform disorders.

Investigations and diagnosis Dependent on clinical context, some or all of the following may be required:

Bloods: FBC, ESR, haematocrit, thyroid function tests and thyroid antibodies, calcium, phosphate and parathyroid hormone level, electrolytes including magnesium, liver-related blood tests, auto-antibodies, plasma amino acids, ammonia, lactate, glucose, copper, and caeruloplasmin; vitamin B_{12}, red cell folate, α-fetoprotein (if AT suspected), white cell enzymes (lysosomal-storage diseases), fresh blood film (3 times; for acanthocytes); uric acid (Lesch–Nyhan syndrome), heavy metal screen, vitamin B_6 levels, RBC transketolase. Lipoprotein electrophoresis.

Urine: porphobilinogen, organic acids.

Imaging: CT for calcification, hamartomas; $+/-$ MRI: basal ganglia lucencies in mitochondrial disease, "eye of the tiger" in Hallervorden–Spatz.

CSF: looking for evidence of inflammation, infection, oligoclonal bands.

Neurogenetics: for Huntington's disease, spinocerebellar ataxias (triplet repeat; appropriate genetic counselling before testing); mitochondrial mutations.

Others: slit-lamp examination (Wilson's disease); muscle biopsy (mitochondrial disease).

Differential diagnosis Other involuntary hyperkinetic movement disorders to be considered include:

- Tardive dyskinesia: usually stereotypic movements involving the orolingual region.
- Myoclonus: usually very brief, shock-like involuntary movements, either due to active muscle contraction or to inhibition of ongoing muscle activity.
- Tics: usually abrupt transient stereotyped coordinated movements which are often irregular in periodicity and which may be voluntarily suppressed.
- Dystonia: sustained muscle contraction, leading to the adoption of abnormal postures, which may have a jerky component to it.
- Epilepsia partialis continua: usually a rhythmic contraction of muscles in a localized area, not under voluntary command and which is stereotypic in nature.

Treatment and prognosis Some causes may be amenable to specific treatment (e.g. metabolic conditions, drug induced), but many are not, hence requiring symptomatic treatment. The options include:

anti-dopaminergic drugs (neuroleptics, sulpiride);
dopamine depleting agents (tetrabenazine).

Prognosis is determined by cause.

References Barker R. Chorea: diagnosis and management. *Advances in Clinical Neuroscience and Rehabilitation* 2003; **3(4)**: 19–20.

Shoulson I. On chorea. *Clinical Neuropharmacology* 1986; **9(suppl 2)**: S85–S99.
Other relevant entries Benign hereditary chorea; Drug-induced movement disorders; Huntington's disease; Spinocerebellar ataxia.

■ Choreoacanthocytosis – see Neuroacanthocytosis

■ Choriocarcinoma

A germ-cell tumour characterized by differentiation into trophoblastic tissue, highly vascular and prone to haemorrhage. It may occur as a metastasis in the pineal region, cauda equina, spinal canal, often after a molar pregnancy or abortion, presenting with seizures, haemorrhages, or gradually progressive deficits. It is associated with increased CSF levels of β-human chorionic gonadotrophin. The management may involve chemotherapy, radiotherapy, and surgery.

Other relevant entries Germ-cell tumours; Pineal tumours.

■ Choroid plexus papilloma

A rare tumour, which may cause headache with hydrocephalus and raised intracranial pressure due to excessive CSF secretion, or may remain asymptomatic.

Other relevant entry Hydrocephalus.

■ Chronic daily headache – see Headache: an overview

■ Chronic demyelinating neuropathy with multifocal CNS demyelination – see Central and peripheral demyelinating disease

■ Chronic inflammatory demyelinating polyneuropathy

Pathophysiology Chronic inflammatory demyelinating polyneuropathy, or polyradiculoneuropathy, (CIDP) is an acquired peripheral sensorimotor neuropathy of presumed immunological pathogenesis. Although its presentation and course is heterogeneous, CIDP may be clinically distinguished from Guillain–Barré syndrome (GBS) by its progressive worsening over a period of at least 8 weeks. The key features are electrophysiological (and pathological) evidence of demyelination and elevated CSF protein concentration. CIDP is often responsive to immunosuppressive therapy.

Clinical features: history and examination

- Variable course: relapsing–remitting, progressive, subacute monophasic. Unlike GBS the neurological deficits are still developing 8 weeks after disease onset and often continue to evolve over months or years.

- Symmetrical demyelinating sensorimotor polyradiculoneuropathy: involves distal and proximal musculature, although the distal weakness is usually more prominent. The degree of weakness is usually much greater than muscle atrophy, and deep tendon reflexes are depressed or absent. About 65% of cases have sensory loss, paraesthesiae, or pain in the limbs, with occasional involvement of the trunk. Pure sensory variants have been described.
- The nerves may be thickened and palpable; rarely cord compression from hypertrophied nerve roots has been described.
- Occasionally patients have cranial nerve or autonomic involvement; presentation with subacute progressive sensory ataxia may occur.
- Focal forms of the disease are described, for example with involvement of only one limb; ophthalmoplegic migraine may be a focal variant of demyelinating neuropathy.
- In some patients there is evidence of concurrent central demyelination.

Investigations and diagnosis *Bloods*: serum electrophoresis and quantitation of immunoglobulins should be performed to exclude paraproteinaemic neuropathy; raised anti-ganglioside antibodies (anti-GM1) may be found, although this is more typical of multifocal motor neuropathy (MMN) with conduction block.

Imaging: periventricular white matter lesions on brain MRI, similar to those seen in multiple sclerosis, are sometimes seen, and may cause clinical manifestations. Thickened nerve roots on spinal MRI may be seen, which may narrow the spinal canal and cause cord compression if very large.

CSF: protein is raised to between 0.9–2.5 g/l. There are usually no cells, normal glucose ratio, and no oligoclonal bands. However patients with central demyelination may have oligoclonal bands.

Neurophysiology: EMG/NCS: electrophysiological criteria for a diagnosis of CIDP include:
- reduced motor conduction velocities, >75% of lower limit of normal (i.e. demyelinating neuropathy);
- prolonged distal motor latencies, >140% of normal;
- conduction block and/or temporal dispersion of compound muscle action potential;
- increased F wave latency, >120% of normal.

Although CIDP is usually clinically symmetrical, there are often electrophysiological differences between limbs, which, like conduction block, are not seen in the hereditary demyelinating neuropathies.

Nerve biopsy: shows features of multifocal demyelination, principally proximal, and remyelination with onion bulb formation+/− a mononuclear cell (macrophage and lymphocyte) infiltration.

Differential diagnosis Guillain–Barré syndrome: it is extremely rare to have recurrent GBS with complete recovery between attacks. Furthermore GBS does not progress after 6 weeks by definition, although the patient may still be severely debilitated at this and later stages.

Hereditary motor and sensory neuropathy (HMSN) type I: a symmetrical neuropathy with a long history; pes cavus frequent.

Paraproteinaemic polyneuropathy.

Paraneoplastic polyneuropathies, including the POEMS syndrome.

Metabolic neuropathies.

Polyradiculoneuropathy associated with HIV and Lyme disease.

Vasculitic neuropathy, including non-systemic vasculitic neuropathy.

Treatment and prognosis In mild cases there may be no need of treatment. In those disabled by their condition or continuing to progress, the mainstay of treatment is immunosuppression.

Steroids+/− steroid sparing agent: most patients with CIDP respond to 8 weeks of steroid therapy, starting with high doses (*cf.* MMN, often does not respond and may actually get worse).

Plasma exchange (PEx).

Intravenous immunoglobulin (IVIg: 0.4 g/kg/day for 5 days; or 1 g/kg/day for 2 days). Both IVIg and PEx are equally effective in CIDP.

A typical treatment programme would be courses of IVIg every 4–6 weeks for 3–6 months, to see whether there is any response (this may include an assessment of muscle strength using myometry). Steroid therapy would be introduced midway through the IVIg regime, in order to try to sustain the response with IVIg that often only lasts from 6 to 10 weeks. If this fails, then repeated IVIg with the introduction of cyclophosphamide may be considered.

The majority of patients with CIDP respond to therapy and remain ambulant and employed. Only a minority fail to respond and become wheelchair bound.

References Choudhary PP, Hughes RAC. Long-term treatment of chronic inflammatory demyelinating polyradiculoneuropathy with plasma exchange or intravenous immunoglobulin. *Quarterly Journal of Medicine* 1995; **88**: 493–502.

Hughes RAC, Bensa S, Willison H *et al.* Randomized controlled trial of intravenous immunoglobulin versus oral prednisolone in chronic inflammatory demyelinating polyneuropathy. *Annals of Neurology* 2001; **50**: 195–201.

Mendell JR. Chronic inflammatory demyelinating polyradiculoneuropathy. *Annual Review of Medicine* 1993; **44**: 211–219.

Report from an Ad Hoc Subcommittee of the American Academy of Neurology AIDS Task Force. Research criteria for diagnosis of chronic inflammatory demyelinating polyneuropathy (CIDP). *Neurology* 1991; **41**: 617–618.

Said G. Chronic inflammatory demyelinative polyneuropathy. *Journal of Neurology* 2002; **249**: 245–253.

Other relevant entries Central and peripheral demyelinating disease; Cryoglobulinaemia, Cryoglobulinaemic neuropathy; Demyelinating diseases of the nervous system: an overview; Gangliosides and the nervous system; Guillain–Barré syndrome; HIV/AIDS and the nervous system; Immunosuppressive therapy and diseases of the nervous system; Leukodystrophies: an overview; Motor neurone disease; Multifocal motor neuropathy; Multiple sclerosis; Neuropathies: an

overview; Ophthalmoplegic migraine; Paraneoplastic syndromes; Paraproteinaemic neuropathies; POEMS syndrome; Proximal weakness; Vasculitis.

■ Chronic paroxysmal hemicrania
Episodic hemicrania ● Sjaastad syndrome

This rare headache syndrome is similar in nature to cluster headache, in terms of the type of headache experienced, and indeed may be envisaged as a variant of cluster headache. It occurs predominantly in middle-aged women. Stereotyped attacks, occurring 5–20 times a day, last up to minutes, pain being intense and strictly unilateral. CPH almost invariably responds to indomethacin (75–150 mg/day).

Reference Sjaastad O, Dale I. A new (?) headache entity "chronic paroxysmal hemicrania". *Acta Neurologica Scandinavica* 1976; **54**: 140–159.

Other relevant entries Cluster headache; Headache: an overview; SUNCT syndrome.

■ Chronic progressive external ophthalmoplegia

Pathophysiology Chronic progressive external ophthalmoplegia (CPEO) is a mitochondrial disorder. Sporadic and familial cases are recognized; the latter may be autosomal dominant or recessive. The phenotype may result from a number of mutations, including multiple deletions of mitochondrial DNA (mtDNA), single base pair mutations of mtDNA (e.g. bp 3243, 4977), mitochondrial tRNA mutations, and defects in nuclear genes encoding mitochondrial proteins.

In CPEO, the mutated mtDNA is confined to muscle, unlike the situation in Pearson's syndrome and Kearns–Sayre syndrome (KSS) wherein mutated mtDNA is found in a wide variety of tissues.

Clinical features: history and examination CPEO is perhaps more loosely defined than KSS, consisting clinically of:

slowly progressive paresis of eye musculature;
bilateral ptosis;
+/− cardiac conduction defects;
+/− proximal muscle weakness, fatigue (especially in later stages);
+/− pigmentary retinopathy.

Onset is usually in the third or fourth decade, but may be as late as the fifth or sixth decade. Hence it shares many features in common with the definition of KSS but with later onset.

Investigations and diagnosis *Muscle biopsy*: COX-negative fibres, ragged red fibres on Gomori trichrome stain.

Neurogenetics: muscle mtDNA deletions or point mutations may be found.
Ophthalmology consultation for fundus photography, ERG.

Differential diagnosis
Other mitochondrial disorders.
Ocular myasthenia.

Thyroid ophthalmopathy.

Ocular abnormalities may be similar to those of progressive supranuclear palsy, but additional features should rule this out.

Multisystem involvement: Systemic lupus erythematosus (SLE), Lyme, Whipple's disease.

Local orbital disease

Treatment and prognosis No specific treatment, although coenzyme Q10 and carnitine may be used. Supportive treatment as appropriate (e.g. treatment of diabetes mellitus, cardiac pacemaker).

> **Reference** Bindoff L, Brown G, Poulton J. Mitochondrial myopathies. In: Emery AEH (ed.). *Diagnostic Criteria for Neuromuscular Disorders* (2nd edition). London: Royal Society of Medicine Press, 1997: 85–90.

> **Other relevant entries** Kearns–Sayre syndrome; Mitochondrial disease: an overview; Ophthalmoplegia.

■ Chronic relapsing inflammatory optic neuropathy – see CRION

■ Churg–Strauss syndrome

A systemic vasculitic illness with many features in common with polyarteritis, with excess circulating and tissue eosinophils. The clinical features include:

Pulmonary: asthma, allergic rhinitis.

Cutaneous: erythema multiforme, leukocytoclastic vasculitis.

Neurological: acute painful mononeuritis multiplex most common, but distal symmetric polyneuropathy, radiculopathy, ischaemic optic neuropathy/visual loss, and bilateral trigeminal neuropathy have also been recorded; cerebrovascular disease rare.

Steroids usually lead to improvement or stabilization of disease.

> **Reference** Sehgal M, Swanson JW, DeRemee RA, Colby TV. Neurologic manifestations of Churg–Strauss syndrome. *Mayo Clinic Proceedings* 1995; **70**: 337–341.

> **Other relevant entries** Hypereosinophilic syndrome; Mononeuritis multiplex, Mononeuropathy multiplex; Polyarteritis nodosa; Renal disease and the nervous system; Vasculitis.

■ CIDP – see Chronic inflammatory demyelinating polyneuropathy

■ Ciguatera

This is a form of marine food poisoning, common in the tropics, follows consumption of reef fish (barracuda, grouper, red snapper) which are transvectors for dinoflagellates which produce the toxins ciguatoxin, maitotoxin, and scaritoxin.

These act by activating sodium and calcium ion channels in excitable membranes. Initial gastrointestinal features are followed within hours of eating reef fish by paraesthesiae (limbs, oral cavity, trunk, genitalia), headache, myalgia, and occasionally ataxia and limb weakness. Cardiovascular effects may also occur. Neurophysiology shows slowing of sensory and motor nerve conduction velocities. Supportive care is indicated, with eventual recovery. Mannitol has been found helpful although the mechanism is unclear. Chronic pain may be a sequela.

Reference Pearn J. Neurology of ciguatera. *Journal of Neurology, Neurosurgery and Psychiatry* 2001; **70**: 4–8.

Other relevant entry Channelopathies: an overview.

■ Ciliary neuralgia – see Charlin's syndrome

■ CIPA – see Hereditary sensory and autonomic neuropathy

■ Citrullinaemia – see Pyruvate carboxylase deficiency; Urea cycle enzyme defects

■ CJD – see Creutzfeldt–Jakob disease; Prion disease: an overview

■ Claude's syndrome

This brainstem vascular syndrome affecting the midbrain is characterized by an ipsilateral oculomotor nerve palsy and contralateral cerebellar ataxia, asynergia, and dysdiadochokinesis, due to a lesion in the region of the brachium conjunctivum. It may be differentiated on clinical grounds from other midbrain syndromes (Benedikt's syndrome, Nothnagel's syndrome, and Weber's syndrome).

Reference Liu GT, Crenner CW, Logigian EL *et al*. Midbrain syndromes of Benedikt, Claude and Nothnagel: setting the record straight. *Neurology* 1992; **42**: 1820–1822.

Other relevant entries Benedikt's syndrome; Brainstem vascular syndromes; Cerebrovascular disease: arterial; Nothnagel's syndrome; Weber's syndrome.

■ Claude–Bernard syndrome

This describes intermittent focal sympathetic overactivity with pupillary dilatation in association with lid retraction, facial hyperhidrosis and headache.

■ Clinically isolated syndromes

Focal demyelination in the central nervous system may be the first manifestation of an illness which subsequently recurs, leading to a diagnosis of multiple sclerosis

(MS). Prior to the advent of neuroimaging, this required a second clinical episode, separated spatially and temporally from the first. With neuroimaging, particularly MRI, evidence may be found for clinically silent but spatially distinct disease at the time of clinical presentation of an isolated syndrome. These individuals certainly have a higher probability of converting to MS. Tentative evidence that intervention with MS "disease-modifying" drugs reduces the conversion rate has been presented, although the treatment is not currently licensed for this indication in the UK.

Clinically isolated syndromes may be classified as:

Optic neuritis (*q.v.*)
Spinal cord syndromes: Transverse myelitis (partial more likely to be MS than complete)
Brainstem syndrome
Acute disseminated encephalomyelitis (ADEM) and variants.

References Jacobs LD, Beck RW, Simon JH *et al*. Intramuscular interferon β-1a therapy initiated during a first demyelinating event in multiple sclerosis. CHAMPS Study Group. *New England Journal of Medicine* 2000; **343**: 898–904.

O'Riordan JI, Thompson AJ, Kingsley DPE *et al*. The prognostic value of brain MRI in clinically isolated syndromes of the CNS. A 10-year follow-up. *Brain* 1998; **121**: 495–503.

Other relevant entries Acute disseminated encephalomyelitis; Multiple sclerosis; Optic neuritis; Transverse myelitis, transverse myelopathy.

▪ Clostridia infection – see Botulism; Tetanus

▪ Clumsy hand–dysarthria syndrome – see Lacunar syndromes

▪ Cluster breathing

Damage at the pontomedullary junction may result in a breathing pattern characterized by a cluster of breaths following one another in an irregular sequence (*cf.* ataxic breathing). This sign may be of localizing value in comatose patients.

Other relevant entry Coma.

▪ Cluster headache
Erythroprosopalgia • Harris's syndrome • Horton's headache, Horton's neuralgia • Migrainous neuralgia

Pathophysiology Cluster headache (CH) is an episodic stereotypic headache of extreme severity, occurring more often in men than women (3.5–7 : 1). Headache is strictly unilateral and associated with cranial autonomic features. Onset is most commonly in the third or fourth decade of life although it may begin at any age. Circannual and circadian periodicity of the headaches is typical. CH typically responds to a number of drugs, hence correct diagnosis is important.

Clinical features: history and examination

- Cluster attack

    Orbital/temporal pain of abrupt onset and cessation, strictly unilateral, of extreme severity, lasting minutes to hours, usually 45–90 minutes. Frequency of attacks ranges from 8 per day to 1 every 2nd day; attacks may occur at identical times each day. During an attack, cranial autonomic features are present: lacrimation, nasal congestion, rhinorrhoea, forehead/facial sweating, miosis and ptosis (partial Horner's syndrome), eyelid oedema, conjunctival injection. These features are transient, with the possible exception of the partial Horner's syndrome. Occasionally there may be migrainous phenomena such as nausea, vomiting, photophobia, and phonophonia. Sufferers are often restless and irritable during an attack, preferring to move about (*cf.* migraine); the pain may be so severe that they will bang their head against a wall for relief.

    Recognized precipitants: alcohol (usually within an hour; *cf.* migraine, several hours), nitroglycerine, exercise, elevated environmental temperature.

    There is usually no family history (*cf.* migraine). CH may be associated with a higher incidence of peptic ulceration.

- Cluster bout

    Episodic cluster headache (80–90%): recurrent bouts lasting .1 week and separated by remissions of .2 weeks.

    Chronic cluster headache (10–20%): no remissions within 1 year, or remissions <2 weeks.

Investigations and diagnosis History, and examination during the attack, is diagnostic.

Bloods: usually normal.

Imaging: structural imaging is normal. PET may show focal hypothalamic activity.

CSF: not necessary.

Differential diagnosis

Migraine.

Chronic paroxysmal hemicrania/episodic hemicrania; Charlin's syndrome (ciliary neuralgia): these may be variants of CH.

Hypnic headache.

*S*hort-lasting *U*nilateral *N*euralgiform headache with *C*onjunctival injection and *T*earing (SUNCT) syndrome.

Trigeminal neuralgia.

Carotid dissection; Raeder's paratrigeminal syndrome.

Granulomatous disease of the cavernous sinus ("Tolosa–Hunt syndrome").

Glaucoma.

Giant cell arteritis.

Sinusitis.

Dental disease.

Treatment and prognosis

- Acute treatment

    Avoid triggers (alcohol, vasodilator drugs)

    Sumatriptan 6 mg subcutaneously (bd if necessary); no evidence to support oral treatment

    Oxygen 100% at flow rate 7–12 l/min

    Intranasal lignocaine 20–60 mg: adjunct, rarely adequate alone

    Ergotamine tartrate oral/rectal (1–2 mg): onset generally too slow.

- Prophylactic treatment

    Short term (episodic CH):

    Verapamil = drug of choice; 240–960 mg daily with baseline ECG and monitoring for PR interval prolongation

    Prednisolone: short intensive courses, 2–3 weeks in tapering doses, for example 60 mg/day for 5 days, taper dose by 10 mg every 3 days (often associated with relapse)

    Methysergide: 4–10 mg/day (~60% improve); monitor for retroperitoneal fibrosis (drug scheduled to be withdrawn)

    Ergotamine: oral or rectal, 1–2 mg.

    Long term (prolonged episodic CH, chronic CH):

    Verapamil = drug of choice; 240–960 mg daily with baseline ECG and monitoring for PR interval prolongation

    Lithium: 300 mg bd, titrated (following British National Formulary) to serum lithium concentration in upper part of therapeutic range; monitoring blood tests for renal and thyroid function required

    Methysegide: require drug holiday every 6 months.

    Other treatments used, but currently lacking compelling clinical evidence:

    Greater occipital nerve injection

    Thermocoagulation of the gasserian ganglion or section of sensory root of trigeminal nerve

    Pizotifen

    Valproate

    Topiramate

    Gabapentin.

Reference Bahra A, May A, Goadsby PJ. Cluster headache: a prospective clinical study in 230 patients with diagnostic implications. _Neurology_ 2002; **58**: 354–361.

Other relevant entries Cavernous sinus disease; Charlin's syndrome; Chronic paroxysmal hemicrania; Facial pain: an overview; Headache: an overview; Hypnic headache; Migraine; SUNCT syndrome; Trigeminal neuralgia; Vasculitis.

■ Coarctation of the aorta

Neurological complications of this condition, which may be congenital or acquired (e.g. following childhood irradiation, or in Takayasu's disease), are variable, and include:

- Ruptured intracerebral aneurysm/subarachnoid haemorrhage: may be related or coincidental.
- Headache (secondary to proximal hypertension?): may be related or coincidental.
- Spinal cord ischaemia/infarction (possibly as a consequence of a steal phenomenon): may result in neurogenic intermittent claudication.
- Spinal cord compression: from enlarged collateral vessels; may also cause spinal subarachnoid haemorrhage.
- Episodic loss of consciousness: syncope? seizures?.
- Left recurrent laryngeal nerve palsy: compression by aneurysmal dilatation proximal to coarctation.

  Reference Goodin DS. Neurological sequelae of aortic disease and surgery. In: Aminoff MS (ed.). *Neurology and General Medicine. The Neurological Aspects of Medical Disorders*. New York: Churchill Livingstone, 1989: 23–48.

  Other relevant entries Spinal cord vascular diseases; Subarachnoid haemorrhage.

■ Coats' disease
Unilateral retinal telangiectasis

This condition is characterized by abnormal retinal vascular development causing intraretinal and subretinal lipid accumulation and exudative retinal detachment. As a rule the condition is isolated, unilateral, and confined to males. Cases associated with facioscapulohumeral (FSH) dystrophy and with facial port-wine stain have been reported. Somatic mutation of the NDP gene, which underlies Norrie disease, has been reported in one case.

  Other relevant entry Norrie disease.

■ Cobb syndrome
Cutaneomeningospinal angiomatosis

In this sporadic neurocutaneous syndrome, a dural angioma is associated with a cutaneous angioma in the corresponding dermatome. The former may behave as an extradural mass lesion, compressing the spinal cord or roots.

  Other relevant entry Klippel–Trénaunay–Weber syndrome.

■ Cocaine

Neurological consequences of cocaine use include stroke (a significant cause in young adults), seizures, encephalopathy, acute headache, and unusual transient neurological effects. Psychiatric effects ranging from mania and delusions to depression (following drug withdrawal) are also recognized. Rare cases of true (histologically proven) vasculitis are reported, prompting speculation on the value of steroid treatment for some of these conditions.

The potent vasoconstrictor (sympathomimetic) action of cocaine may account for some of these features, as may its action in blocking sodium channels. The use of "crack" cocaine, the free base, produces high blood levels almost instantaneously after smoking and increases the likelihood of toxicity. The only treatment is abstinence.

Reference Rowbotham MC, Lowenstein DH. Neurologic consequences of cocaine use. *Annual Review of Medicine* 1990; **41**: 417–422.

Other relevant entry Drug-induced encephalopathies.

■ Coccidioidomycosis

This is a fungal infection, due to the soil fungus *Coccidioides immitis*, common in the south-western United States, that presents with an influenza-like illness with pulmonary infiltrates and is usually self-limiting. Occasionally disease becomes disseminated, and meningitis may be a feature, with papilloedema and sixth nerve palsy, and CSF findings similar to tuberculous meningitis. The organism is hard to culture from CSF but may be identified in lung, lymph node, and skin lesions. The differential diagnosis also encompasses other fungal causes of meningitis (histoplasmosis, blastomycosis) and actinomycosis. Treatment is with intravenous amphotericin, often required for months, and CSF drainage if hydrocephalus occurs, despite which the condition may be fatal.

Other relevant entry Tuberculosis and the nervous system.

■ Coccydynia

Coccydynia, or coccygodynia, is pain in the region of the coccyx. It may result from damage to the bony structures, as well as diseases involving local structures, of both inflammatory and neoplastic origin, but often does not yield a symptomatic diagnosis.

■ Cockayne's syndrome

This is a rare autosomal-recessive condition caused by defective repair of transcriptionally active DNA, leading to peripheral and central demyelination.

It generally presents in late infancy with the following clinical features:

Stunting of growth
Photosensitivity of the skin
Microcephaly
Retinitis pigmentosa ("salt and pepper" retinopathy)

Cataracts

Blindness, deafness, and nystagmus

Delayed psychomotor and speech development

Ataxia

Areflexic, weak and wasted limbs (demyelinating neuropathy)

Dysmorphic face with progeric features.

Investigations show normal blood tests and CSF analysis is normal. On EMG/NCS there is slowing of nerve conduction; brain stem auditory evoked potentials are abnormal. CT may show basal ganglia calcification. Pathologically there is severe cerebellar atrophy with a leukodystrophy and demyelinating peripheral neuropathy.

Genetically the condition is heterogeneous; it may be associated with mutations also known to cause xeroderma pigmentosum.

Clinically some cases may be confused with Pelizaeus–Merzbacher disease.

Death occurs by the third decade.

Reference Ozdirim E, Topcu M, Ozon A *et al*. Cockayne syndrome: review of 25 cases. *Pediatric Neurology* 1996; **15**: 312–316.

Other relevant entries Ataxia telangiectasia; Basal ganglia calcification; Pelizaeus–Merzbacher disease; Xeroderma pigmentosa and related conditions.

■ Coeliac disease (gluten-sensitive enteropathy)

Coeliac disease may rarely (<10% of cases) be associated with a variety of neurological complications, including:

Epilepsy

Migraine

Cerebellar syndrome

Spinocerebellar ataxia

Peripheral neuropathy: predominantly sensory axonopathy; may be demyelinating, mixed

Myelopathy

Myoclonus

Intracerebral calcification, especially occipital

Encephalopathy: ? cerebral vasculitis

Dementia

Disseminated enteropathic T-cell lymphomatosis, presenting with cranial nerve palsies, radiculopathies

Secondary nutritional deficiencies from malabsorption.

Although vitamin deficiencies (e.g. vitamin B_{12}) have been implicated in the neuropathic features, as a consequence of malabsorption, repletion seldom leads to clinical improvement.

The diagnosis of coeliac disease is based on the clinical picture of malabsorption, with anti-gliadin, anti-endomysial, and anti-reticulin antibodies, and the finding of subtotal villous atrophy on a duodenal biopsy. Response to a gluten-free diet is typical.

Some patients with cerebellar ataxia have only anti-gliadin antibodies without intestinal changes, so-called gluten ataxia. It has also been suggested that some cases labelled as "idiopathic late-onset cerebellar ataxia" in fact have gluten ataxia, with or without underlying enteropathy, that is, this may be understood as an isolated, immune-mediated, disease of brain rather than a subclinical affection of the gut.

References Cooke WT, Smith WT. Neurological disorders associated with adult coeliac disease. *Brain* 1966; **89**: 683–722.

Hadjivassiliou M, Grunewald RA, Chattopadhyay AK *et al*. Clinical, radiological, neurophysiological, and neuropathological characteristics of gluten ataxia. *Lancet* 1998; **352**: 1582–1585.

Pengiran Tengah DSNA, Wills AJ, Holmes GKT. Neurological complications of coeliac disease. *Postgraduate Medical Journal* 2002; **78**: 393–398.

Other relevant entries Gastrointestinal disease and the nervous system; Idiopathic late-onset cerebellar ataxia.

■ Coenurosis

Infection with the larval form of the dog tapeworm *Taenia multiceps* or *Taenia serialis*, a cestode helminth, may produce space-occupying cysts within the central nervous system (CNS), causing headaches, raised intracranial pressure, and focal signs. The grape-like cysts may be visualized by brain imaging, most often in the posterior fossa, and removed surgically. The differential diagnosis includes echinococcosis.

Other relevant entries Cysts: an overview; Echinococcosis; Helminthic disease.

■ Cogan's lid-twitch sign

This is a twitch of the upper eyelid seen a moment after the eyes are moved from downgaze to the primary position. It is said to be a characteristic finding in myasthenia gravis.

Other relevant entry Myasthenia gravis.

■ Cogan syndrome (1)

Congenital oculomotor apraxia • Oculomotor apraxia of Cogan

This is a congenital condition in which there is an isolated apraxia of ocular movements, primarily in the horizontal direction (hence, a congenital lack of lateral gaze). To overcome this, patients use a thrusting movement of the head in the desired direction of gaze, often overshooting so that the eyes can fixate by slowly drifting back. Reflex eye movements (e.g. optokinetic nystagmus) can be elicited normally. A similar apraxia of eye movement is seen in ataxia telangectasia.

Other relevant entries Apraxia; Ataxia telangectasia.

■ Cogan syndrome (2)
Non-syphilitic interstitial keratitis

This is an autoimmune disorder characterized by episodic vertigo, tinnitus, hearing loss, and interstitial keratitis.

References Cogan DG. Syndrome of non-syphilitic interstitial keratitis and vestibuloauditory symptoms. *Archives of Ophthalmology* 1945; **33**: 144–149.

Lunardi C, Bason C, Leandri M *et al*. Autoantibodies to inner ear and endothelial antigens in Cogan's syndrome. *Lancet* 2002; **360**: 915–921.

■ Coital cephalalgia, coital headache

Lance described two types of headache which may occur during sexual intercourse:

- Headache which develops during the build up to intercourse and relates to increased tension in the neck musculature.
- Headache which occurs at orgasm and is similar clinically to the headache of sub-arachnoid haemorrhage (SAH). It is probably vascular in origin, associated with tachycardia and hypertension of orgasm. Idiopathic thunderclap headache has also been described in this context.

Both types of headache are benign with an excellent prognosis. It is often, however, necessary to perform investigations to exclude SAH in orgasm-associated headache: with acute presentation, CT brain scan to look for subarachnoid blood; if negative, LP for xanthochromia; proceeding to angiography if SAH identified. With delayed presentation, MRA is often performed.

Reassurance is usually the only treatment required, as the headaches are benign. With recurrent type 2 headache, a course of indomethacin propanolol or ergotamine may be helpful.

Reference Lance JW. Headaches related to sexual activity. *Journal of Neurology, Neurosurgery and Psychiatry* 1976; **39**: 1226–1230.

Other relevant entries Headache: an overview; Migraine; Subarachnoid haemorrhage; Thunderclap headache.

■ Collagen vascular disorders and the nervous system: an overview

There is no universally agreed classification for conditions which may be labelled as collagen vascular disorders, connective tissue disorders, and vasculitides, but conditions recognized to fall within these groupings include:

- Connective tissue disease
    Rheumatoid arthritis
    Systemic lupus erythematosus (SLE)
    Systemic sclerosis (scleroderma)

Dermatomyositis

Polymyositis

Ankylosing spondylitis

Sjögren's syndrome

Mixed connective tissue disease (MCTD).

- Vasculitides

Polyarteritis nodosa (PAN)

Churg–Strauss syndrome

Wegener's granulomatosis

Temporal arteritis

Takayasu's arteritis

Isolated angiitis of the nervous system.

The potential effects of these conditions upon the nervous system, both central and peripheral, are protean, including encephalopathy, stroke-like episodes, relapsing–remitting syndromes, radiculopathy, neuropathy, and myopathy.

References Scolding N. Neurological complications of rheumatological and connective tissue disorders. In: Scolding N (ed.). *Immunological and Inflammatory Disorders of the Central Nervous System*. Oxford: Butterworth-Heinemann, 1999: 147–180.

Shannon KM, Goetz CG. Connective tissue diseases and the nervous system. In: Aminoff MJ (ed.). *Neurology and General medicine. The Neurological Aspects of Medical Disorders* (2nd edition). New York: Churchill Livingstone, 1995: 447–471.
Other relevant entries See individual entries.

■ Collet–Sicard syndrome

Collet–Sicard syndrome consists of a unilateral deficit of the lower four cranial nerves (IX to XII), causing palatal and pharyngeal anaesthesia, palatal and vocal cord paresis, weakness of sternocleidomastoid, trapezius, and the tongue. This is usually due to trauma or tumour at the skull base (retroparotid lesion), but has also been reported with cerebral vein thrombosis. Additional involvement of the cervical sympathetic chain is known as Villaret's syndrome.

Lannois–Jouty syndrome and Mackenzie syndrome share similar clinical features.

Other relevant entries Cranial nerve disease: XII: hypoglossal nerve; Cranial polyneuropathy; Jugular foramen syndrome; Vernet's syndrome; Villaret's syndrome.

■ Collier's sign

Collier's sign, first described in 1927, is pathological upper eyelid retraction causing a staring appearance ("posterior fossa stare") which occurs with upper dorsal midbrain lesions, such as Parinaud's syndrome.

Other relevant entry Parinaud's syndrome.

■ Colloid cyst
Neuroepithelial cyst

Colloid cysts are thought to arise from ependymal cells in the vestigial paraphysis in the anterior portion of the third ventricle, where they may block the third ventricle and cause obstructive hydrocephalus. Presentation from late childhood onwards is with either an intermittent obstructive syndrome ("ball valve" arrangement) causing severe bifrontal–biooccipital headache, unsteady gait, incontinence, visual impairment, and drop attacks without loss of consciousness, or with a normal pressure hydrocephalus. Behavioural changes may also be noted. Some instances are now found incidentally when undergoing brain imaging for other reasons. The differential diagnosis encompasses glioma, choroid plexus papilloma, craniopharyngioma, pineal and pituitary tumours. Surgical resection may be undertaken, although symptoms may be more easily controlled with shunting or stereotactic decompression of the cyst. Damage to the fornix, either from the cyst or as a consequence of surgery may result in persistent amnesia.

Reference Hodges JR, Carpenter K. Anterograde amnesia with fornix damage following removal of a third ventricle colloid cyst. *Journal of Neurology, Neurosurgery and Psychiatry* 1991; **54**: 633–638.

Other relevant entries Amnesia, Amnesic syndrome; Cysts: an overview; Drop attacks; Normal pressure hydrocephalus.

■ Colpocephaly

Colpocephaly is a developmental disorder of the nervous system in which there is dilatation of the occipital horns of the lateral ventricles, but not the frontal or temporal horns, due to loss of surrounding white matter. This may be a neuronal migration disorder, or follow infarction and cystic degeneration of the posterior cerebral hemispheres. There may be concurrent agenesis of the corpus callosum. Patients typically have severe mental retardation, spastic diplegia, epilepsy, and visual loss.

Other relevant entries Agenesis of the corpus callosum; Cerebral palsy, cerebral palsy syndromes; Holoprosencephaly; Lissencephaly; Septo-optic dysplasia.

■ Coma

Pathophysiology Coma is a state of unresponsiveness, with eyes closed, from which a patient cannot be roused by verbal or mechanical stimuli. It represents a greater degree of impairment of consciousness than stupor or obtundation, all three forming part of a continuum, rather than discrete stages, between being fully alert and being comatose. The causes of coma include:

drugs and toxins;
metabolic causes: hypoglycaemia, hepatic failure;
infections;

epilepsy: non-convulsive status epilepticus;

cerebrovascular insults: haemorrhage, infarction.

Clinical features: history and examination Although coma may be graded by means of a lumped "score", such as the Glasgow Coma Scale (*q.v.*), description of the individual aspects of neurological function in unconscious patients, such as eye movements, limb movements, vocalization, and response to stimuli, may be preferable since this conveys more information.

Signs should be documented serially to assess any progression of coma. Changes in eye movements and response to central noxious stimuli indicate change in depth of coma: roving eye movements are lost before oculocephalic responses followed by caloric responses; pupillary reflexes are last to go. The switch from flexor to extensor posturing (decorticate versus decerebrate rigidity) also indicates increasing depth of coma.

Investigations and diagnosis *Bloods*: electrolytes, glucose, arterial blood gases; drug screen.

Imaging: CT, MRI for intracranial lesion (infarct, haemorrhage).

CSF: if meningitis or encephalitis possible.

Neurophysiology: EEG: if non-convulsive status epilepticus a possibility.

Differential diagnosis

Abulia.

Akinetic mutism.

Catatonia.

Locked-in syndrome.

Treatment and prognosis General supportive treatment of respiration, circulation; specific treatments dependent on cause. Some drug-induced comas may be promptly reversible (e.g. benzodiazepines with flumazenil, opiates with naloxone).

References Plum F, Posner JB. *The diagnosis of Stupor and Coma* (3rd edition). Philadelphia: Davis, 1980.

Young GB, Ropper AH, Bolton CF (eds). *Coma and Impaired Consciousness: a Clinical Perspective*. New York: McGraw-Hill, 1998.

Other relevant entries Catatonia; Concussion; Decerebrate rigidity, Decorticate rigidity; Encephalopathies: an overview, Glasgow Coma Scale.

■ Coma vigil – see Vegetative states

■ Common peroneal nerve palsy – see Peroneal neuropathy

■ Common variable immunodeficiency

Common variable immunodeficiency (CVID) is one of the commonest syndromes of primary antibody deficiency, characterized by profound hypogammaglobulinaemia. Various neurological complications may occur, including: pneumococcal meningitis, acute and chronic meningoencephalitis due to enteroviral infection, and subacute combined degeneration of the spinal cord due to vitamin B_{12} deficiency secondary to chronic gastritis or pernicious anaemia.

Reference Hermaszewski RA, Webster ADB. Primary hypogammaglobulinaemia: a survey of clinical manifestations and complications. *Quarterly Journal of Medicine* 1983; **86**: 31–42.

Other relevant entries Meningitis: an overview; Vitamin B_{12} deficiency.

■ Communicating hydrocephalus – see Hydrocephalus

■ Compartment syndromes

Swelling of muscles, for example following ischaemia or trauma, within a semirigid fibro-osseous compartment may compromise capillary blood flow, leading to a vicious circle of further ischaemic damage and swelling. Such compartment syndromes are particularly described for the anterior tibial muscles and the volar muscles of the forearm. Sensory and motor features following compression of peripheral nerves within the compartment may occur. Excessive muscle damage results in rhabdomyolysis, myoglobinuria, and possibly renal failure. Eventual fibrosis of damaged muscle may lead to contracture (Volkman's ischaemic contracture).

Acute treatment is subcutaneous fasciotomy to relieve pressure.

Other relevant entries Pretibial syndrome; Rhabdomyolysis.

■ Complex regional pain syndromes

Algodystrophy • Causalgia • Causalgia–dystonia syndrome • Reflex sympathetic dystrophy (RSD)

Pathophysiology Complex regional pain syndrome is the term now used to describe ill-understood chronic pain disorders, first described by S Weir Mitchell in 1864 as a consequence of traumatic peripheral nerve injury (causalgia, complex regional pain syndrome type 2), although there may be no definable nerve injury (complex regional pain syndrome type 1). There is some evidence for maintained sympathetic nerve activity in the early (but not the late) stages of the disease.

Clinical features: history and examination

- Pain: greater than expected for the degree of tissue damage; chronic burning pain, often initially dermatomal but gradually spreading to be regional; hyperalgesia, allodynia, hyperpathia, leading to sleep disturbance and secondary depression.
- Autonomic dysfunction: sudomotor, vasomotor change.
- Oedema: limb swelling (? neurogenic inflammation).
- +/− Dystrophy/Atrophy: nails, hair, skin (livedo reticularis, mottling), bone [cystic and subchondral erosion, diffuse osteoporosis (Sudeck's atrophy, Sudeck–Leriche syndrome)].
- Movement disorder: inability to initiate movement, weakness, tremor, muscle spasms, dystonia.

Investigations and diagnosis Clinical diagnosis; no specific tests. EMG/NCS may be used to define underlying nerve injury.

Differential diagnosis If movement disorder is prominent, other causes of dystonia may need to be excluded.

Treatment and prognosis The natural history varies from stability to progression. Regional sympathetic blockade, along with physical therapy, may alleviate motor manifestations in early stages only; efficacy questionable in later stages. Drugs for neuropathic pain and spinal cord stimulation may improve pain; intrathecal baclofen helps (may abolish) dystonia.

References Dotson RM. Causalgia – reflex sympathetic dystrophy – sympathetically maintained pain: myth and reality. *Muscle and Nerve* 1993; **16**: 1049–1055.

Ficat CCJ (ed.). *Reflex Sympathetic Dystrophy*. London: Baillière Tindall, 1996.

Paice E. Reflex sympathetic dystrophy. *British Medical Journal* 1995; **310**: 1645–1648.

Scadding JW. Neuropathic pain. *Advances in Clinical Neuroscience and Rehabilitation* 2003; **2**(3): 8–14.

Schott GD. Mechanisms of causalgia and related clinical conditions. The role of the central and of the sympathetic nervous systems. *Brain* 1986; **109**: 717–738.

Schwartzman RJ. New treatments for reflex sympathetic dystrophy. *New England Journal of Medicine* 2000; **343**: 654–656.

Other relevant entries Dystonia: an overview; Shoulder–hand syndrome.

Concussion

Pathophysiology Cerebral concussion is defined as an immediate and transient impairment of consciousness following head injury; there need not be loss of consciousness although this usually occurs briefly. There is usually amnesia for the events surrounding the injury (retrograde and anterograde). Modern classification of head injury has tended to abandon the term concussion in favour of descriptions of the extent (diffuse versus focal) and severity of head injury (as measured, e.g. by the Glasgow Coma Scale); there are also scales for measuring the severity of post-traumatic amnesia.

Clinical features: history and examination Because of the impaired consciousness with or without amnesia, the patient may not be able to give a history; a witness account may be helpful.

Depending on how soon the patient is seen, there may not be any signs; if seen acutely, the amnesia may be demonstrated.

Investigations and diagnosis Patients generally need to be observed for 24 hours.

Imaging may be indicated to exclude more severe cerebral injury (e.g. extradural haematoma, subarachnoid haemorrhage).

Differential diagnosis Other causes of amnesia: transient global amnesia, transient epileptic amnesia, psychogenic amnesia.

Treatment and prognosis The outlook is generally good with no lasting sequelae. A post-concussion syndrome of headaches, dizziness, difficulty concentrating, irritability, loss of confidence, anxiety and depression is common. This syndrome is of variable severity and is not related to the severity of the original injury; psychological factors, perhaps related to legal claims ("accident neurosis", "compensation neurosis") may contribute in some circumstances. Epidemiological studies suggest that head injuries severe enough to produce concussion are a risk factor for the later development of Alzheimer's disease.

Reference McCrory PR, Berkovic SF. Concussion. *Neurology* 2001; **57**: 2283–2289.

Quality Standards Committee of the American Academy of Neurology. The management of concussions in sports. *Neurology* 1997; **48**: 581–585.

Other relevant entries Coma; Glasgow Coma Scale; Memory.

■ Conduction aphasia – see Aphasia; Disconnection syndromes

■ Confusion

Confusion, understood as the inability to think with one's customary clarity and coherence, is a feature of delirium, but also of other situations (encephalopathies, attentional disorders). Moreover, as there is a lack of correlation of meaning when this term is used by different health professionals, it has become unhelpful.

Reference Simpson CJ. Doctors' and nurses' use of the word confusion. *British Journal of Psychiatry* 1984; **145**: 441–443.

Other relevant entry Delirium.

■ Congenital insensitivity to pain
Congenital indifference to pain

Congenital insensitivity to pain and anhydrosis (CIPA) is now classified with the hereditary sensory and autonomic neuropathies (HSAN), as types IV and V, associated with mutations in a gene encoding a receptor for nerve growth factor (NGF). Other syndromes which in the past were labelled as congenital insensitivity or indifference to pain, or pain asymbolia, with clinical features of acroparaesthesia and Charcot joints, probably also represent varieties of hereditary sensory and autonomic neuropathy.

Reference Larner AJ, Moss J, Rossi ML, Anderson M. Congenital insensitivity to pain: a 20 year follow up. *Journal of Neurology, Neurosurgery and Psychiatry* 1994; **57**: 973–974.

Other relevant entries Hereditary sensory and autonomic neuropathy; Osuntokun's syndrome.

■ Congenital muscle and neuromuscular disorders: an overview

Many neuromuscular disorders are inherited and hence might be labelled "congenital", viz.:

- muscular dystrophies,
- spinal muscular atrophies,

- hereditary neuropathies,
- myotonic disorders,
- various myopathies.

However, the label "congenital" has been used specifically for:

- congenital muscular dystrophies (CMD) (*q.v.*);
- congenital myasthenic syndromes (CMS) (*q.v.*);
- congenital myopathies:
    central core disease,
    nemaline myopathy,
    centronuclear (myotubular) myopathy,
    minicore–multicore disease,
    desmin-related myopathy,
    myofibrillar myopathy.

References Rakowicz W. Congenital myopathies and muscular dystrophies. *Advances in Clinical Neuroscience and Rehabilitation* 2003; **2(6)**: 11–13.

Taratuto AL. Congenital myopathies and related disorders. *Current Opinion in Neurology* 2002; **15**: 553–561.

Other relevant entries See individual entries.

■ Congenital muscular dystrophies

This heterogeneous group of autosomal-recessive disorders presents with hypotonia and weakness at birth or in the first few months of life, with or without mental retardation. Some are static, some progress, with or without respiratory muscle involvement. A number of phenotypes are defined within this group, including:

"Pure" congenital muscular dystrophy
Fukuyama-type congenital muscular dystrophy
Muscle–eye–brain (MEB) disease
Rigid spine syndrome
Walker–Warburg syndrome (WWS).

Neurogenetic studies have defined a number of loci and proteins aberrant in these disorders:

Gene locus	Protein defect
6q	Laminin α_2 (merosin)
12q	Laminin receptor (α_7-integrin)
9q	Fukutin (Fukuyama dystrophy)
1p	Selenoprotein (rigid spine syndrome)
1p	Glycosyltransferase (muscle–eye–brain disease)

Clinical features: history and examination
- Muscle weakness presenting at birth or within the first few months of life.

- $+/-$ hypotonia, arthrogryposis.
- Mental retardation and epilepsy are prominent in Fukuyama dystrophy.
- Cardiac function is normal.

Investigations and diagnosis *Bloods*: creatine kinase may be elevated, consistently in Fukuyama type.

Neurophysiology: EMG/NCS: no specific abnormality.

Muscle biopsy: dystrophic changes.

Others: Imaging, EEG: may be abnormal in some types; white matter change in merosin deficiency.

Differential diagnosis Other childhood myopathies, dystrophia myotonica.

Treatment and prognosis No specific treatment available. Few walk; contractures may be prominent. Feeding and respiratory problems are the usual cause of death.

Reference Dubowitz V. Congenital muscular dystrophies. In: Emery AEH (ed.). *Diagnostic Criteria for Neuromuscular Disorders* (2nd edition). London: Royal Society of Medicine Press, 1997: 23–26.

Other relevant entries Arthrogryposis multiplex congenita; Dystrophia myotonica; Muscular dystrophies: an overview; Myasthenia gravis; Myopathy: an overview; Muscle–eye–brain disease; Neuropathies: an overview; Rigid spine syndrome; Spinal muscular atrophy; Walker–Warburg syndrome.

■ Congenital myasthenic syndromes

Pathophysiology The congenital myasthenic syndromes are classified according to the pattern of inheritance and the site of the defect:

- Type I: Autosomal recessive:

    CMS type 1a: familial infantile myasthenia syndrome

    CMS type 1b: limb girdle myasthenic syndrome

    CMS type 1c: acetylcholinesterase-deficiency syndrome

    CMS type 1d: acetylcholine-receptor-deficiency syndrome.

- Type II: Autosomal dominant:

    CMS type 2a: slow channel syndrome.

- Type III: No family history:

    CMS type 3: all other patients younger than 12 years of age with AChR antibody negative fatiguable weakness and neurophysiological evidence of neuromuscular transmission defect and lacking features of any of the other categories.

Transient neonatal myasthenia and arthrogryposis multiplex congenita in the off-spring of mothers with myasthenia gravis, although presenting at birth, are not included under the rubric of congenital myasthenic syndromes because of the association with anti-AChR antibodies of maternal origin which cross the placenta.

Mutations in ligand-gated nicotinic acetylcholine-receptor channels (subunits α_1, β_1, δ, and ε) have been identified in some of these syndromes, hence they may be classified with the channelopathies.

Investigations and diagnosis *Bloods*: antibodies to AChR are not present and indeed are counted as exclusion criteria for these diagnoses.

Neurophysiology: EMG/NCS: key investigation, showing decremental response with repetitive stimulation and jitter/block on single fibre studies, indicative of neuromuscular transmission defect.

Muscle biopsy: tubular aggregates in type 1b; morphological evidence of AChE deficiency in type 1c; reduced AChR in type 1d.

Differential diagnosis Other forms of neonatal/infantile weakness.

Other defects of neuromuscular transmission.

Treatment and prognosis No specific treatment available; unlike autoimmune myasthenia, CMS do not respond to plasma exchange and immunosuppressive therapy.

> **References** Engel AG, Ohno K, Sine SM. Congenital myasthenic syndromes: recent advances. *Archives of Neurology* 1999; **56**: 163–167.
>
> Middleton LT. Congenital myasthenic syndromes. In: Emery AEH (ed.). *Diagnostic Criteria for Neuromuscular Disorders* (2nd edition). London: Royal Society of Medicine Press, 1997: 91–97.

> **Other relevant entries** Arthrogryposis multiplex congenita; Channelopathies: an overview; Myasthenia gravis; Neuromuscular junction diseases: an overview.

Congenital nystagmus

Congenital nystagmus is a pendular nystagmus with the following characteristics:

Usually noted at birth or in early infancy; sometimes may only become apparent in adult life

Irregular waveforms

Conjugate

Almost always horizontal

Accentuated by fixation, attention, anxiety

Decreased by convergence, active eyelid closure

Often a null point or region

No complaint of oscillopsia

It may appear with blindness of childhood onset.

Acquired pendular nystagmus may be a result of neurological disease which may be present in childhood, such as Pelizaeus–Merzbacher disease, mitochondrial disease, multiple sclerosis, Whipple's disease.

> **Other relevant entry** Nystagmus: an overview.

Congenital rubella syndrome – see Rubella

Congophilic angiopathy – see Cerebral amyloid angiopathy

■ Connective tissue disorders – see Collagen vascular disorders and the nervous system: an overview; Vasculitis

■ Conradi–Hünerman syndrome
Chondrodysplasia punctata ● Chondrodystrophia calcificans congenita

An autosomal-dominant or -recessive disorder of craniocephalic skeletal anomalies, including facial dysmorphism (flat nose, prominent forehead, hypertelorism), cataracts, short neck, kyphoscoliosis, limb shortening (epiphyseal calcification), dry atrophic skin, and alopecia. Mental retardation is sometimes present.

■ Conus medullaris syndrome – see Cauda equina syndrome and conus medullaris disease

■ Conversion disorder, Conversion hysteria – see Somatoform disorders

■ Coproporphyria – see Porphyria

■ Cori–Forbes disease – see Glycogen-storage disorders: an overview

■ Cortical dementia, cortical syndrome – see Dementia: an overview

■ Corticobasal degeneration
Cortical-basal ganglionic degeneration

Pathophysiology Corticobasal degeneration (CBD) is a rare late-onset neurodegenerative disorder of unknown aetiology that is characterized by a movement disorder, an asymmetric akinetic-rigid syndrome with marked dyspraxia, involuntary movements and alien limb/hand behaviour, in combination with a cognitive disorder (cortical dementia). Early descriptions emphasized the movement disorder, but subsequently the prominence of the cognitive disorder has been increasingly recognized.

Pathologically, the condition is distinct, characterized by nerve cell loss and gliosis in the cortex, underlying white matter, thalamus, lentiform nucleus, subthalamic nucleus, red nucleus, midbrain tegmentum, substantia nigra, and locus ceruleus. Many residual nerve cells are swollen and chromatolysed with eccentric nuclei (achromasia). Neuronal inclusions resembling the globose neurofibrillary tangles of progressive supranuclear palsy may be present in the substantia nigra.

There is currently no effective pharmacotherapy.

Clinical features: history and examination

- Movement disorder: "classical" clinical picture is of a chronic progressive asymmetric rigidity with apraxia [Progressive *a*symmetrical *r*igidity and *a*praxia (PARA) syndrome]:
    1/2 apraxic limb sometimes displaying an alien limb syndrome;
    +/− cortical sensory dysfunction;
    +/− dystonia;
    +/− myoclonus: action induced, stimulus sensitive;
    +/− less common features include supranuclear gaze palsy, dysarthria, ataxia, chorea, blepharospasm, corticospinal tract signs.
- Cognitive disorder: deficits of sustained attention and verbal fluency + deficits of praxis, finger tapping and motor programming.

    Cases presenting with features of frontotemporal dementia (FTD) without motor disorder have been reported, as have patients with parieto-occipital (Balint-like) cortical dysfunction, and a combination of dementia, parkinsonism, and motor neurone disease.
- Neuropsychiatric/behavioural disorders may also occur.

Investigations and diagnosis *Bloods*: normal

Imaging: structural imaging (CT/MRI) may show asymmetric frontoparietal atrophy; functional imaging (SPECT, PET) may show reduced tracer uptake in striatum and medial frontal cortex.

CSF: may show non-specific elevation of protein.

Electrophysiology: no diagnostic features in EEG, EMG/NCS, SSEP, although non-specific abnormalities may occur.

Neuropsychology: may show cortical deficits, especially of frontal type, with deficits of praxis.

Differential diagnosis Neurodegenerative conditions with parkinsonian features: idiopathic Parkinson's disease (usually begins asymmetrically but then spreads contralaterally); progressive supranuclear palsy; multiple system atrophy; Creutzfeldt–Jakob disease (CJD).

A number of cortical dementias may also enter the differential: AD, FTD.

Phenocopies with non-CBD pathology are well described, including AD, FTD of Pick type, and occasional cases of motor neurone disease (MND)–dementia, CJD, or non-specific histology. Hence it is suggested that all clinically diagnosed cases be labelled "CBD syndrome" until histology is available to permit definitive classification. Occasionally a vascular phenocopy of the condition can occur.

Treatment and prognosis The syndrome is essentially unresponsive to levodopa, although a therapeutic trial is often given.

Clonazepam may be useful for action tremor/myoclonus.

Severe rigidity with immobility is common within 3–5 years of disease onset.

Death usually occurs within 7–10 years of onset.

References Dickson DW, Bergeron C, Chin SS *et al*. Office of Rare Diseases neuropathologic criteria for corticobasal degeneration. *Journal of Neuropathology and Experimental Neurology* 2002; **61**: 935–946.

Doran M, du Plessis DG, Enevoldson TP, Fletcher NA, Ghadiali E, Larner AJ. Pathological heterogeneity of clinically diagnosed corticobasal degeneration. *Journal of the Neurological Sciences* 2003; **216**: 127–134.

Lang AE, Riley DE, Bergeron C. Cortical-basal ganglionic degeneration. In: Calne DB (ed.). *Neurodegenerative diseases*. Philadelphia: WB Saunders, 1994: 877–894.

Other relevant entries Alzheimer's disease; Apraxia; Frontotemporal dementia; Myoclonus; PARA syndrome; Parkinsonian syndromes, parkinsonism; Parkinson's disease; Pick's disease; Progressive supranuclear palsy.

■ Costen syndrome

This is a syndrome of craniofacial pain ascribed to temporomandibular joint dysfunction. There is often local tenderness over the joint with limited jaw opening, pain in the muscles of mastication made worse by jaw movements such as chewing, and noises in the joint during mastication. Malocclusion of the teeth or missing molars may predispose to this condition, as may rheumatoid arthritis. Treatment usually involves a dental surgical approach.

Other relevant entries Bruxism; Facial pain: differential diagnosis; Rheumatoid arthritis.

■ Cotard's syndrome

A delusional syndrome, first described in the 1890s, characterized by the patient's denial of their own existence, or of part of their body. The patient may assert that they are dead, and able to smell rotten flesh or feel worms crawling over their skin. Although this may occur in the context of psychiatric disease, especially depression and schizophrenia, it may also occur in association with organic brain abnormalities, specifically lesions of the non-dominant temporoparietal cortex, or migraine.

Some envisage Cotard's syndrome as a more pervasive form of Capgras' syndrome, originating similarly as a consequence of Geschwindain disconnection between the limbic system and all sensory areas, leading to a loss of emotional contact with the world. Antidepressant treatment and/or ECT may sometimes be helpful in Cotard's syndrome of psychiatric origin.

References Cotard J. *Etudes sur les maladies cerebrales et mentales*. Paris: Bailliere, 1891.

Pearn J, Gardner-Thorpe C. Jules Cotard (1840–1889): his life and the unique syndrome which bears his name. *Neurology* 2002; **58**: 1400–1403.

Other relevant entries Capgras' syndrome; Disconnection syndromes.

■ Cough headache

Cough headache may occur as an isolated benign condition, in which a sudden severe headache, usually occipital or suboccipital in location, develops on coughing or other activities, such as sneezing, laughing, or lifting heavy objects, which involve a Valsalva manoeuvre. Headache lasts seconds to minutes, occasionally hours, and is described as bursting or explosive. It is not associated with persistently raised intracranial pressure and treatment is rarely required; analgesic preparations such as indomethacin or anti-migraine therapies may be tried. However, structural causes must be sought for cough headache, particularly lesions of the foramen magnum (e.g. Chiari malformations) or posterior fossa [e.g. tumour, arteriovenous malformations (AVM)].

Reference Pascual J, Iglesias F, Oterino A *et al*. Cough, exertional, and sexual headaches: an analysis of 72 benign and symptomatic cases. *Neurology* 1996; **46**: 1520–1524.

Other relevant entry Chiari malformations.

Cough syncope – see Syncope

Cowden's disease
Multiple hamartoma syndrome

This rare autosomal-dominant phakomatosis usually presents to dermatologists with multiple focal papules, palmar and plantar keratoses, and oral papillomas. Associations include thyroid adenoma, gastrointestinal polyposis, ovarian cysts, benign fibrocystic breast disease, and (possibly) meningioma.

Reference Lyons CJ, Wilson CB, Horton JC. Association between meningioma and Cowden's disease. *Neurology* 1993; **43**: 1436–1437.

Other relevant entries Meningioma; Phakomatosis.

Coxiella – see Q Fever; Rickettsial diseases

CPEO – see Chronic progressive external ophthalmoplegia

Crack – see Cocaine

Cramp fasciculation syndrome – see Denny–Brown, Foley syndrome

Cramps

Pathophysiology Cramps are defined as involuntary contractions of a number of muscle units which results in a hardening of the muscle with pain due to a local lactic acidosis. Cramps are not uncommon in normal individuals but in a minority of cases they are associated with an underlying neurological or metabolic disorder. Cramps need to be distinguished from spasticity, neuromyotonia, and myokymia. Recognized associations of cramp include:

- Normal individuals
    Especially during periods of dehydration with salt loss; pregnancy
    Benign cramp syndrome, there is a family history of cramps.
- Metabolic causes
    Hypothyroidism
    Haemodialysis
    Hypocalcaemia; hyperventilation (with secondary hypocalcaemia).
- Neurological causes
    Chronic peripheral neuropathy
    Metabolic myopathies (e.g. myophosphorylase deficiency, carnitine palmit(o)yltransferase II (CPT II) deficiency, lactate dehydrogenase (LDH) deficiency, with exercise intolerance and myoglobinuria)
    Muscular dystrophies (especially Becker, Duchenne)
    Motor neurone disease
    Stiff man syndrome.

Investigations and diagnosis *Bloods*: FBC, serum electrolytes, calcium, thyroid function tests and creatine kinase levels. Blood tests pertinent to the investigation of peripheral neuropathy, multifocal motor neuropathy with conduction block (anti-GM1 antibodies) and stiff man syndrome (anti-GAD antibodies) may need to be sent, dependent on clinical features.

Neurophysiology: EMG/NCS to exclude primary muscle disease, peripheral neuropathy, motor neurone disease. EMG changes during a cramp are critical in defining its significance.

Differential diagnosis

Benign cramp syndrome.

Myokymia.

Neuromyotonia (Isaacs syndrome).

Stiff people.

Treatment and prognosis Avoid precipitants; treat any underlying metabolic abnormality.

Symptomatic treatment of cramps includes: quinine sulphate; carbamazepine; phenytoin, procainamide; benadryl (no randomized-controlled trials).

Prognosis depends on the cause.

Reference Layzer RB. The origin of muscle fasciculations and cramps. *Muscle and Nerve* 1994; **17**: 1243–1249.

Other relevant entries Denny–Brown, Foley syndrome; Endocrinology and the nervous system; Lactate dehydrogenase deficiency; Motor neurone disease; Muscular dystrophies: an overview; Neuromyotonia; Neuropathies: an overview; Painful legs and moving toes; Renal disease and the nervous system; Stiff people: an overview.

■ Cranial nerve disease: I: Olfactory nerve

Anosmia, the principal symptom of olfactory nerve pathology, is unusual in neurological practice. Sometimes patients will present with a complaint of loss of taste.

The commonest causes of anosmia are:

- Trauma: head injury may cause shearing of olfactory nerve fibres as they pass through the cribriform plate, for example in anterior cranial fossa fracture.
- Tumour: olfactory bulb and tract meningioma (may cause Foster–Kennedy syndrome, *q.v.*), nasopharyngeal carcinoma, neuroblastoma (esthesioneuroblastoma).
- Congenital: for example in X-linked hypogonadotrophic hypogonadism (Kallmann's syndrome, *q.v.*).

Olfactory dysfunction is also reported in neurodegenerative diseases (e.g. Alzheimer's disease, Parkinson's disease); and in multiple sclerosis with plaques in inferior frontal and temporal regions.

> **Reference** Brazis PW, Masdeu JC, Biller J. *Localization in Clinical Neurology* (4th edition). Philadelphia: Lippincott Williams & Wilkins, 2001: 127–132.
>
> **Other relevant entries** Esthesioneuroblastoma; Foster–Kennedy syndrome; Kallmann's syndrome.

■ Cranial nerve disease: II: Optic nerve

Pathophysiology Optic nerve disease may present with impairment of vision, sometimes with a complaint of a veil covering the eye which cannot be wiped away (particularly if acute).

Causes of optic neuropathy include:

Inflammatory disease: multiple sclerosis (MS), acute demyelinating encephalomyelitis (ADEM), sarcoidosis, chronic relapsing inflammatory optic neuropathy (CRION), Wegener's granulomatosis

Structural: Tumour: glioma, meningioma (neurofibromatosis), lymphoma
    Mucocele: sphenoidal, ethmoidal

Ischaemia: giant cell arteritis, cavernous sinus thrombosis, pituitary apoplexy, atherosclerotic disease

Infection: AIDS, Lyme, syphilis

Nutritional: tobacco–alcohol amblyopia; vitamin B_{12} deficiency; "epidemic" optic neuropathy (e.g. Jamaica, Cuba, Tanzania)

Metabolic: thyroid ophthalmopathy

Hereditary: autosomal-dominant optic atrophy, autosomal-recessive optic atrophy, Leber's hereditary optic neuropathy (LHON), Wolfram syndrome

Degenerative: secondary to prolonged raised intracranial pressure ("secondary optic atrophy", e.g. idiopathic intracranial hypertension)

Drugs: methanol, ethambutol, chloramphenicol

Radiation.

Unilateral or bilateral symptoms may be more suggestive of particular pathologies, for example MS, tumour more likely to be unilateral.

Clinical features: history and examination Complaint of visual impairment.

- Check visual acuity, without and with pinhole (latter corrects refractive problems): Snellen chart, reading type.
- Check colour vision: Ishihara pseudo-isochromatic plates (colour vision may be impaired in absence of abnormalities of acuity, e.g. following optic neuritis).
- Check visual fields: look for presence of field cut, scotoma, enlargement of blind spot; some patterns of field loss more suggestive of pathology elsewhere than optic nerve.
- Fundoscopy: may be normal; may see papilloedema, disc swelling; other features such as pigmentary retinal degeneration (retinitis pigmentosa).
- Pupillary responses: relative afferent pupillary defect may be seen with unilateral optic neuropathy (e.g. demyelination).
- Look for clues to other possible causes: dietary history (e.g. alcohol, veganism), drug history, family history of early visual loss.

Investigations and diagnosis Automated field testing may be required (Humphrey, Goldman).

Neurophysiology

VER may be delayed with optic nerve demyelination.
ERG may be reduced or absent with primary retinal pathology.

Other investigations as appropriate to suspected neurological cause, for example MR brain + gadolinium (MS), MR optic nerve (tumour, sarcoidosis); mitochondrial DNA (LHON).

Differential diagnosis Primary diseases of retina (retinopathy), macular dystrophies (maculopathy), eye (glaucoma) with loss of ganglion cells may present with visual impairment, visual field defects (scotoma).

Chiasmal disease may present with visual field defects (typically heteronymous hemianopias): pituitary adenoma, craniopharyngioma.

Optic radiation, visual cortical lesions may present with visual field defects (typically homonymous hemianopias).

Cavernous sinus and orbital apex lesions will be attended by additional cranial nerve involvement.

Treatment and prognosis Dependent on cause. See individual entries.

References Acheson J. Optic nerve and chiasmal disease. *Journal of Neurology* 2000; **247**: 587–596.

Kanski JJ, Thomas DJ. *The Eye in Systemic Disease* (2nd edition). London: Butterworth-Heinemann, 1990.

Other relevant entries Acute demyelinating encephalomyelitis; Alcohol and the nervous system: an overview; CRION; Glaucoma; Idiopathic intracranial hypertension; Ischaemic optic neuropathy (ION); Multiple sclerosis; Neurofibromatosis; Optic atrophy; Optic neuritis; Retinitis pigmentosa; Sarcoidosis; Strachan's syndrome.

Cranial nerve disease: III: Oculomotor nerve

Pathophysiology The oculomotor (third) nerve supplies levator palpebrae superioris (LPS); medial, inferior and superior rectus (MR, IR, SR) muscles and the inferior oblique (IO) muscle; as well as supplying the parasympathetic innervation to the pupil. Hence in a complete third nerve palsy one would expect ptosis, ophthalmoplegia with sparing of trochlear (superior oblique) and abducens (lateral rectus) nerve function, and mydriasis. Partial third nerve palsies also occur, in which case diagnosis may be less easy. However, an understanding of third nerve anatomy and its relationship to other cranial nerves facilitates localization.

Oculomotor nerve lesions may be:

* Intramedullary (brainstem)

    Nuclear: very rare; SR subnucleus lesion causes bilateral denervation; + expect other signs: pupils (Edinger–Westphal nucleus), medial longitudinal fasciculus involvement.

    Fascicular (within substance of midbrain): all muscles or specific muscles + expect other signs: contralateral ataxia (Claude's syndrome), hemiparesis (Weber's syndrome).

* Extramedullary

    Subarachnoid space: peripherally located pupillomotor fibres often spared by ischaemic lesions, not by space-occupying lesions (e.g. aneurysm).

    Cavernous sinus: oculomotor nerve runs over trochlear nerve; other ocular motor nerves +/− trigeminal often affected.

    Superior orbital fissure: superior division/ramus to SR, LPS; inferior to MR, IR, IO; proptosis with space-occupying lesions; may get selective (=divisional) palsy.

    Orbit: Paresis of isolated muscle almost always from orbital lesion or muscle disease.

    Pathologies responsible for third nerve palsy include:

* Microangiopathy: hypertension, diabetes.
* Structural lesions: midbrain (stroke, tumour; rarely demyelination); posterior communicating artery aneurysm; cavernous sinus pathology; orbital lesions.

Clinical features: history and examination Ptosis may be obvious or subtle; need to differentiate from "pseudoptosis" (redundant skin fold, especially in older patients).

Pupillary responses: pupil may be involved (mydriasis) or spared in third nerve palsy; latter is said to be more common with "surgical" causes of palsy, such as posterior communicating artery aneurysm, but the distinction is not absolute.

Eye movements: weakness of superior, medial, and inferior rectus, combined with inferior oblique; if all involved, then eye may look downwards and outwards (unopposed action of lateral rectus (VI) and superior oblique (IV) muscles, although the latter has its greatest effect on the adducted eye); if partial third nerve palsy, weakness may be confined, for example to superior rectus in a divisional palsy, or individual muscles with orbital pathology.

Other features may suggest location of pathology, for example contralateral hemiparesis suggests midbrain pathology, other ocular motor nerves + trigeminal nerve suggests cavernous sinus.

Measure blood pressure.

Investigations and diagnosis *Imaging*: MR indicated for structural lesion; some would argue that imaging is not necessary in a complete third nerve palsy in the presence of diabetes mellitus.

Additional investigations as appropriate, for example bloods for diabetes, CSF if malignancy suspected.

Differential diagnosis Myasthenia gravis may sometimes produce ptosis and weakness of eye movements, but usually bilateral.

Thyroid ophthalmopathy should also be considered.

Treatment and prognosis Dependent on cause; microangioapthic third nerve palsies related to diabetes or hypertension often recover gradually with no specific treatment. Posterior communicating artery aneurysm may require surgical intervention (clipping).

References Brazis PW. Subject review: Localization of lesions of the oculomotor nerve: recent concepts. *Mayo Clinic Proceedings* 1991; **66**: 1029–1035.

Coles A. The third cranial nerve. *Advances in Clinical Neuroscience and Rehabilitation* 2001; **1(1)**: 20–21.

Larner AJ. Proximal superior division oculomotor nerve palsy from metastatic subarachnoid infiltration *Journal of Neurology* 2002; **249**: 343–344.

Other relevant entries Aneurysm; Cavernous sinus disease; Claude's syndrome; Diabetes mellitus and the nervous system; Hypertension and the nervous system; Internuclear ophthalmoplegia; Ophthalmoplegia; Ophthalmoplegic migraine; Weber's syndrome.

■ Cranial nerve disease: IV: Trochlear nerve

Palsies of the fourth cranial nerve cause diplopia on looking downwards and inwards (e.g. when going downstairs) due to weakness of the superior oblique muscle (contralateral with nuclear lesions, ipsilateral with lesions in the subarachnoid space or beyond). Clinically there is hypertropia, exacerbated by tilting the head towards the paralysed side (Bielschowsky's test); head tilt away from the paralysed side may be evident, to compensate for the diplopia.

Isolated trochlear nerve palsies may be congenital or acquired, the latter most often due to trauma. Other recognized causes include ischaemia, superior cerebellar artery aneurysm, primary trochlear nerve neoplasm; rarely a pituitary lesion, diffuse meningeal process, or idiopathic intracranial hypertension. Lesions of the cavernous sinus may cause a fourth nerve palsy in conjunction with involvement of other ocular motor nerves (III, VI) and the ophthalmic branch of the trigeminal (V) nerve. Nuclear lesions may result fom ischaemia, tumour, or demyelination and are usually accompanied with other signs referable to the midbrain (e.g. Nothnagel's syndrome).

Myasthenia gravis may on occasion cause isolated superior oblique muscle weakness, as may thyroid ophthalmopathy. Restriction of the superior oblique tendon may result in vertical diplopia (Brown's syndrome).

Superior oblique myokymia (*q.v.*) may be a consequence of trochlear nerve palsy.

Reference Brazis PW. Palsies of the trochlear nerve: diagnosis and localization: recent concepts. *Mayo Clinic Proceedings* 1993; **68**: 501–509.

Other relevant entries Brown's syndrome; Cavernous sinus disease; Nothnagel's syndrome; Superior oblique myokymia.

■ Cranial nerve disease: V: Trigeminal nerve

Pathophysiology The trigeminal nerve is the motor nerve to muscles of mastication (masseter, temporalis, lateral pterygoids), the sensory nerve to the face through ophthalmic, maxillary, and mandibular divisions (V_1, V_2, V_3, respectively), and is involved in the afferent limb of the corneal and jaw reflexes.

Fifth nerve involvement may result from:

- Nuclear lesions: for example hemimasticatory spasm, or trismus; lateral medullary syndrome; herpes zoster ophthalmicus represents recrudescence of varicella infection in the trigeminal sensory ganglion.
- Peripheral lesions: for example cerebellopontine angle lesions may cause depression of the corneal reflex; cavernous sinus/superior orbital fissure pathology; Gradenigo's syndrome; trigeminal sensory neuropathy (*q.v.*) may be related to inflammatory disease, skull base tumour, or be a false-localizing sign of raised intracranial pressure; trigeminal neuralgia (*q.v.*, Fothergill's disease) is believed to result from neurovascular compression at the root entry zone. Metastatic disease may cause a numb cheek or numb chin syndrome.

Clinical features: history and examination

- Sensory impairment in any of the divisions of the trigeminal nerve (remember V_1 extends to vertex; angle of jaw spared by trigeminal innervation: may be helpful in defining sensory complaints as non-dermatomal).
- Weakness of jaw opening, masticatory muscles may occur, but wasting likely to be evident before weakness.
- Impaired corneal reflex, jaw jerk.

Investigations and diagnosis *Bloods*: trigeminal sensory neuropathy should prompt investigation for underlying inflammatory disease such as Sjögren's syndrome (autoantibodies).

Imaging: dependent on additional neurological signs, imaging may be focused upon the cerebellopontine angle, cavernous sinus.

CSF: for malignant cells may be undertaken if numb cheek/chin syndrome.

Neurophysiology: blink and jaw reflexes may be recorded for latency.

Differential diagnosis Facial pain has a broad differential, but objective facial sensory loss indicates trigeminal nerve involvement.

Treatment and prognosis Dependent on cause.

Reference Brazis PW, Masdeu JC, Biller J. *Localization in Clinical Neurology* (4th edition). Philadelphia: Lippincott Williams & Wilkins, 2001: 271–287.

Other relevant entries Cavernous sinus disease; Cerebellopontine angle syndrome; Facial pain: differential diagnosis; Gradenigo's syndrome; Neurovascular compression syndromes; Numb cheek syndrome, numb chin syndrome; Trigeminal neuralgia; Trigeminal sensory neuropathy; Vestibular schwannoma.

Cranial nerve disease: VI: Abducens nerve

Palsies of the VI cranial nerve cause diplopia on looking laterally due to weakness of the lateral rectus muscle. There may be a head turn away from the paralysed side to compensate for diplopia.

In isolation, VI nerve palsy is most often due to ischaemia (microangiopathy), in the context of hypertension or diabetes mellitus. Intracranial hypertension, for example of the idiopathic variety, may cause bilateral VI nerve palsy as a false-localizing sign. Pathology in the pontine region may cause VI nerve palsies in combination with facial diplegia (Möbius syndrome), with ipsilateral facial paresis and either contralateral dysmetria (Foville syndrome), or with contralateral hemiplegia (Millard–Gubler syndrome). Lesions at the petrous apex may cause VI nerve palsy with deafness and retro-orbital pain (Gradenigo's syndrome), and cavernous sinus disease may produce a combination of cranial nerve palsies involving III, IV, Va, VI, and Horner's syndrome. Combined VI and XII nerve palsies (Godtfredsen's syndrome) suggest malignant infiltration, as in nasopharyngeal carcinoma.

Impaired lateral gaze may be seen with internuclear ophthalmoplegia and the one-and-a-half syndrome. Isolated lateral rectus weakness, mimicking an abducens nerve palsy, may also occur in myasthenia gravis.

Other relevant entries Cavernous sinus disease; Foville syndrome; Godtfredsen's syndrome; Gradenigo's syndrome; Internuclear ophthalmoplegia; Idiopathic intracranial hypertension; Millard–Gubler syndrome; Möbius syndrome; One-and-a-half syndrome.

Cranial nerve disease: VII: Facial nerve

Pathophysiology The facial nerve is motor to facial muscles (including orbicularis oculi, buccinator, orbicularis oris) and to stapedius in the middle ear. It conveys taste sensation from the anterior two-thirds of the tongue via the chorda tympani, and cutaneous sensation from the skin of the external auditory meatus, lateral pinna, and mastoid. Concurrence of loss of taste sensation and hyperacusis may permit more accurate localization of pathology (facial canal syndrome), whereas after the nerve leaves the temporal bone lesions cause only weakness of the mimetic muscles (stylomastoid foramen syndrome). The facial nerve is involved in the efferent limb of the blink reflexes.

Isolated facial nerve palsy is common, and usually idiopathic (Bell's palsy), but many other disease processes may present with facial nerve involvement.

Clinical features: history and examination

- History of facial weakness: drooping, pulling; difficulty closing eyes (may lead to conjunctivitis), dysarthria, escape of liquid from corner of mouth.
- There may be complaints of facial sensory involvement in Bell's palsy, but no sensory signs.
- On examination, lagophthalmos, loss or smoothing of nasolabial fold, absence of frontalis action (lower motor neurone), weak eye closure (may expose Bell's phenomenon), weak blowing out of cheeks, inability to whistle, may be found; emotional movement may be preserved with upper motor neurone lesions.
- +/− loss of taste anterior two-thirds of the tongue, hyperacusis (nerve to stapedius).

Investigations and diagnosis Bell's palsy *per se* probably requires no specific investigation.

If other features are suggestive, or there is a history of a prior visit to an endemic region, Borrelia serology may be appropriate (esp. if there is bilateral VII nerve palsy). May also pursue diagnosis of sarcoidosis.

Bilateral and/or recurrent facial nerve palsy mandates further investigation for diabetes, lymphoma/leukaemia, sarcoidosis and borreliosis.

Upper motor neurone lesions require brain imaging.

Neurophysiology: analysis of blink reflexes may indicate facial nerve involvement.

Differential diagnosis Upper motor neurone facial weakness (e.g. due to cerebrovascular event, tumour) may be differentiated from lower motor neurone weakness by the sparing of frontalis with the former; however, in a recovering Bell's palsy, frontalis function may recover first, thus producing a picture akin to upper motor neurone weakness.

Facial weakness may also occur in myasthenia gravis (especially eye closure, often with frontalis overactivity) and Guillain–Barré syndrome; myopathy may involve facial musculature, as in facioscapulohumeral (FSH) muscular dystrophy or myotonic dystrophy.

Treatment and prognosis Dependent on cause.

> **Reference** Brazis PW, Masdeu JC, Biller J. *Localization in Clinical Neurology* (4th edition). Philadelphia: Lippincott Williams & Wilkins, 2001: 289–307.
>
> **Other relevant entries** Bell's palsy; Blepharospasm; Hemifacial spasm.

■ Cranial nerve disease: VIII: Vestibulocochlear nerve

Pathophysiology The eighth cranial nerve consists of two parts, subserving hearing (cochlea) and vestibular function (utricle, saccule, semicircular canals). These may be affected separately or jointly by pathological processes, which declare themselves as hearing impairment or vestibular dysfunction (vertigo). For pathological causes of vestibular dysfunction and hearing loss, see individual entries.

Clinical features: history and examination

- *Vestibular*: dysfunction typically manifests as vertigo (*q.v.*); neuro-otological examination may include search for spontaneous nystagmus, testing of vestibulo-ocular reflex, positional testing.
- *Hearing*: impairment may be obvious from conversation, or by field testing (whispering a number or word some distance from the ear, with the contralateral ear muffled); conductive hearing loss may be distinguished from sensorineural hearing loss by means of the tuning fork tests of Rinne (compares air conduction with bone conduction) and Weber (lateralization of bone conduction).
- The presence of other neurological signs may give clues as to aetiology, for example of central vertigo, or of specific cause for hearing loss (e.g. ipsilateral cerebellar ataxia and depressed corneal reflex with cerebellopontine angle tumour).

Investigations and diagnosis *Vestibular*: caloric testing, rotational testing and videooculography without visual fixation (Frenzel goggles, infrared sensors in darkened environment).

Hearing: audiometry may be required.

Other tests as appropriate to suspected cause.

Differential diagnosis *Vestibular*: vertigo of peripheral origin may be differentiated from central vertigo by its lack of neurological company (long tract signs, cerebellar dysfunction) and its tendency to habituate.

Hearing: central hearing loss is uncommon, due to the bilateral representations of the pathways, but may sometimes occur, often with other neurological signs.

Treatment and prognosis Dependent on cause.

Reference Brazis PW, Masdeu JC, Biller J. *Localization in Clinical Neurology* (4th edition). Philadelphia: Lippincott Williams & Wilkins, 2001: 309–327.

Other relevant entries Cerebellopontine angle syndrome; Hearing loss: differential diagnosis; Vertigo; Vestibular disorders: an overview.

■ Cranial nerve disease: IX: Glossopharyngeal nerve

Isolated glossopharyngeal nerve palsy is rare, most usually there is concurrent involvement of neighbouring cranial nerves, especially the vagus. The glossopharyngeal nerve is the motor supply to stylopharyngeus muscle, which is difficult to test, and the sensory nerve supplying the posterior tongue (including taste), tonsils, soft palate, nasopharynx and, via the tympanic branch (Jacobson's nerve) the tympanic membrane, Eustachian tube and mastoid region. It is the afferent (sensory) component of the reflex arc underpinning the gag reflex.

Glossopharyngeal nerve palsy may occur with intramedullary lesions involving the nucleus, such as vascular disease, malignancy, demyelination, or syringobulbia; or as part of a jugular foramen syndrome or with lesions of the retropharyngeal or retroparotid space.

Reference Brazis PW, Masdeu JC, Biller J. *Localization in Clinical Neurology* (4th edition). Philadelphia: Lippincott Williams & Wilkins, 2001: 329–336.

Other relevant entries Collet–Sicard syndrome; Cranial nerve disease: X: Vagus nerve; Glossopharyngeal neuralgia; Jugular foramen syndrome.

Cranial nerve disease: X: Vagus nerve

Pathophysiology The vagus nerve is motor to the soft palate, pharynx, and larynx, and is the efferent (motor) arc of the gag reflex. Its sensory distribution is limited to the pinna and overlaps with other nerves so is not amenable to specific examination. The vagus also carries autonomic fibres to the lungs, heart, and abdominal viscera.

Clinical features: history and examination

- Impaired phonation (dysphonia), swallowing (dysphagia). Unilateral vagal palsy evident as flattening of palatal arch, failure of elevation with attempted phonation; impaired gag reflex.
- Often concurrent glossopharyngeal nerve involvement, +/− other lower cranial nerves involved at jugular foramen or retropharyngeal or retroparotid space (syndromes of Vernet, Schmidt, Jackson, Collet–Sicard, *q.v.*). Nuclear lesions may be vascular (lateral medullary syndrome, Avellis' syndrome), neoplastic, structural (syringobulbia), degenerative (motor neurone disease) or inflammatory.

Investigations and diagnosis Dependent on clinical picture, imaging of jugular foramen or retropharyngeal space may be indicated.

Differential diagnosis Dysphagia may result from disease of the neuromuscular junction (myasthenia gravis) or muscles *per se* (e.g. oculopharyngeal muscular dystrophy). Likewise dysphonia, which may also relate to disease of vocal cords (tumour, nodule) or dystonia (spasmodic dysphonia) or weakness (multiple system atrophy).

Treatment and prognosis Dependent on cause.

> **Reference** Brazis PW, Masdeu JC, Biller J. *Localization in Clinical Neurology* (4th edition). Philadelphia: Lippincott Williams & Wilkins, 2001: 329–336.

> **Other relevant entries** Aphonia; Avellis' syndrome; Cranial nerve disease: IX: Glossopharyngeal nerve; Dysphagia; Jugular foramen syndrome.

Cranial nerve disease: XI: Accessory nerve

Isolated lesions of this purely motor nerve, innervating the sternocleidomastoid and trapezius muscles, are rare. Involvement of sternocleidomastoid causes weakness of head turning to the opposite side and of head flexion, although wasting of the muscle may be evident on palpation before clinical weakness appears. Weakness of trapezius causes the shoulder on the affected side to be lower, the scapula is displaced downwards and laterally and there is slight winging.

Accessory nerve lesions most commonly occur at the foramen magnum or at the jugular foramen, often involving neighbouring cranial nerves IX, X, and XII, for example syndromes of Collet–Sicard, Villaret, Schmidt, Jackson, Tapia, and Garcin (see individual entries for further details).

> **Reference** Brazis PW, Masdeu JC, Biller J. *Localization in Clinical Neurology* (4th edition). Philadelphia: Lippincott Williams & Wilkins, 2001: 337–343.

■ Cranial nerve disease: XII: Hypoglossal nerve

Isolated lesions of the hypoglossal nerve, the motor nerve of the tongue, resulting in wasting and weakness of the tongue, are unusual. Often they are bilateral, resulting most commonly from:

malignant tumours (metastases, chordoma, nasopharyngeal carcinoma, lymphoma);
trauma to the neck (e.g. gunshot wounds).

Other recognized causes include:

stroke
Guillain–Barré syndrome
infection
neck surgery
Chiari malformation
multiple sclerosis.

Due to its close spatial relationship to cranial nerves IX, X, and XI at the skull base, the hypoglossal nerve may be involved with these in various eponymous syndromes (e.g. Collet–Sicard, Villaret, Jackson, Tapia and Garcin).

Combined VI and XII nerve palsies (Godtfredsen's syndrome) suggest malignant infiltration as in nasopharyngeal carcinoma.

Central lesions involving the hypoglossal nuclei in the medulla oblongata may result in tongue paresis, atrophy, and fasciculation, for example motor neurone disease, poliomyelitis. The central ramifications of the nerve may be involved by intramedullary tumour, demyelination, syringobulbia, and vascular disease (medial medullary syndrome or Déjerine's anterior bulbar syndrome).

A spastic tongue may be evident with upper motor neurone lesions involving corticobulbar fibres, for example of the internal capsule, corona radiata, or basal pons.

References Brazis PW, Masdeu JC, Biller J. *Localization in Clinical Neurology* (4th edition). Philadelphia: Lippincott Williams & Wilkins, 2001: 345–351.

Keane JR. Twelfth-nerve palsy. Analysis of 100 cases. *Archives of Neurology* 1996; **53**: 561–566.

Other relevant entries Cranial polyneuropathy; Galloping tongue syndrome; Garcin syndrome; Godtfredsen's syndrome; Medial medullary (infarction) syndrome.

■ Cranial polyneuropathy

Pathophysiology Multiple cranial nerve palsies may accompany intrinsic brainstem disease, in which case long tract signs are also usually evident. The differential diagnosis of multiple cranial nerve palsies without evidence of intrinsic brainstem disease is broad, including:

Infective: Chronic meningitides:
spirochaetal (syphilis)
fungal (cryptococcus, aspergillosis)

mycobacterial (tuberculosis)

mycoplasma

viral (EBV, VZV).

Granulomatous/vasculitis:

sarcoidosis

Wegener's granulomatosis

polyarteritis nodosa (rare)

giant cell arteritis (rare).

Metabolic:

diabetes mellitus (usually mononeuropathy).

Structural: Neoplasia:

Primary: chordoma, meningioma of sphenoid ridge, glomus jugulare tumour

Secondary: metastasis, carcinomatous/lymphomatous meningitis.

Aneurysm/dissection (rare).

Oligosymptomatic Guillain–Barré syndrome.

Idiopathic cranial polyneuropathy (*q.v*).

Investigations and diagnosis *Bloods*: ESR; serology for possible infective agents.

Imaging: CT/MRI may demonstrate structural lesions; enhancement of the meninges may suggest inflammatory or malignant infiltration.

CSF: in addition to cell count, protein, and glucose, other studies may be needed, including indian ink staining, cryptococcal antigen, cytology; may need to repeat CSF if initial study is inconclusive.

Tissue: meningeal biopsy may be contemplated if other investigations provide no specific diagnosis.

Treatment and prognosis See individual entries.

Reference Beal MF. Multiple cranial nerve palsies – a diagnostic challenge. *New England Journal of Medicine* 1990; **322**: 461–463.

Other relevant entries Garcin syndrome; Idiopathic cranial polyneuropathy; Jugular foramen syndrome.

■ Craniopharyngioma

Pathophysiology Craniopharyngiomas are tumours of the pituitary region which are thought to arise from the remnant of the embryological pouch of Rathke. Most occur in childhood; they are less common than tumours of the pituitary gland.

Clinical features: history and examination Craniopharyngiomas present with local compressive features, viz.:

- Visual symptoms: bitemporal hemianopia: often progressing from inferior to superior (*cf.* pituitary tumours, superior to inferior)
- Hypothalamic dysfunction: growth failure, diabetes insipidus, Froehlich's syndrome.
- Raised intracranial pressure, headache.

Investigations and diagnosis *Bloods*: for hypothalamic dysfunction, especially evidence of diabetes insipidus.

Imaging: MRI: tumour often gives increased signal on T_1-weighted scans due to cholesterol content.

Differential diagnosis Other pituitary mass lesions.

Treatment and prognosis There is a debate as to whether surgery should attempt total resection or partial resection followed by radiotherapy. If the capsule is densely adherent to surrounding structures partial removal is preferred. There is a tendency to recurrence; some advocate periodic postoperative MRI.

> **Reference** Hoffman HJ. Craniopharyngiomas. *Canadian Journal of Neurological Sciences* 1985; **12**: 348–352.

> **Other relevant entries** Froehlich's syndrome; Pituitary disease and apoplexy; Tumours: an overview.

■ Craniostenosis
Craniosynostosis

Craniostenosis or craniosynostosis is a premature closure of cranial sutures, resulting in an abnormally shaped skull. The frequency of this condition is estimated at 1 : 1000 births. This is often associated with other developmental abnormalities, including varying degrees of mental retardation. Raised intracranial pressure may also be a feature.

Craniostenosis is a feature of a number of conditions:

Acrocephalosyndactyly:
Types I and II: Apert's syndrome
Type III: Saethre–Chotzen syndrome
Type IV: Pfeiffer syndrome
Acrocephalopolysyndactyly: Carpenter syndrome

Craniostenosis may also be found, but not consistently, in:

Crouzon syndrome
Conradi–Hünerman syndrome
Baller–Gerold syndrome
Autley–Bixler syndrome.

> **Reference** Hayward R, Jones B, Dunaway D, Evans R (eds). *The Clinical Management of Craniosynostosis*. Cambridge: Mac Keith Press, 2003.

■ Cree leukoencephalopathy – see Vanishing white matter disease

■ CREST syndrome – see Systemic sclerosis

■ Cretinism – see Endocrinology and the nervous system

■ Creutzfeldt–Jakob disease

Pathophysiology Creutzfeldt–Jakob disease (CJD) is the prototypical human prion disease, occurring in sporadic, familial, and iatrogenic forms. The inherited (familial) form results from mutations within the prion protein (PrP) gene (*PRNP*). All forms of CJD are associated with accumulation of abnormal isoforms of the cellular prion protein, PrP^{Sc} or PrP^{Res}, within the brain. Variant Creutzfeldt–Jakob disease (vCJD) has been recently described, probably resulting from the agent which caused the epidemic of bovine spongiform encephalopathy (BSE) in British cattle in the 1980s, hence sometimes known as "human BSE".

Clinical features: history and examination

- Sporadic cases may present subacutely; inherited and iatrogenic variants may have a more insidious onset.
- Clinical features are heterogeneous and include:
    Dementia: subcortical and cortical features
    Cortical blindness (Heidenhain or visual variant)
    Cerebellar syndrome: Brownell–Oppenheimer (ataxic) variant
    Myoclonus
    Encephalopathy (Nevin–Jones syndrome); "epileptic" presentation (mimicking complex partial status epilepticus)
    Extrapyramidal syndrome; akinetic mutism
    Pyramidal signs
    Psychiatric disturbance (commoner in vCJD, although may occur in CJD)
    Sensory symptoms and signs (especially vCJD: hyperpathia)
    Amyotrophy (muscle wasting).

If the diagnosis is suspected, a family history of similarly affected relatives should be sought, along with enquiries about exposure to recognized iatrogenic factors: corneal transplantation, dura mater grafts, intracranial electrodes, human pituitary-derived hormones (growth hormone, gonadotrophins).

Investigations and diagnosis *Bloods*: all normal.

Imaging: on CT/MRI brain atrophy may be evident; MR high signal change may be seen in the putamen and caudate head in sporadic CJD, and in posterior thalamus in vCJD (pulvinar sign). Functional imaging (SPECT, PET) may show multiple patchy perfusion abnormalities.

CSF: moderately elevated protein may be seen in sporadic CJD; protein markers of neuronal injury (Neurone-Specific Enolase, 14-3-3) and glial activation (S100β) may be elevated but this finding is non-specific.

EEG: periodic complexes at a frequency of 1–2 per second in a markedly abnormal background are the classical changes in CJD, although they may not develop until late in the disease (hence repeated EEGs may be needed); atypical changes (focal changes, periodic lateralized epileptiform discharges) sometimes reminiscent of complex partial status epilepticus may also be seen. EEG is typically normal in vCJD.

Neuropsychology: common features include epsiodic unresponsiveness, interference effects, verbal, and motor perseverations, reflecting subcortical disease; $+/-$ cortical features such as cortical blindness, auditory agnosia, language deficits.

Brain biopsy: (with precautions for dealing with the instruments) spongiform vacuolation affecting any part of the cerebral grey matter (cases without spongiform change have also been described); astrocytic proliferation, gliosis; neuronal loss, synaptic degeneration; PrP-immunopositive amyloid plaques.

Tonsil biopsy: may be helpful in diagnosis of vCJD if PrP-immunopositive staining is present.

Neurogenetics: screening PrP gene for mutations (missense deletions, insertions) in inherited cases; in sporadic CJD gene analysis is normal.

Differential diagnosis

Hashimoto's encephalopathy.

Complex partial status epilepticus.

Cerebrovascular disease with vasculitis.

Lithium intoxication.

Dementia with Lewy bodies.

Alzheimer's disease (rare).

Treatment and prognosis No specific treatment currently known. Disease is uniformly fatal, often within weeks to months in sporadic CJD, although some inherited forms may survive for many years. Survival in vCJD may be more than a year.

References Collie DA, Sellar RJ, Zeidler M, Colchester ACF, Knight R, Will RG. MRI of Creutzfeldt–Jakob disease: imaging features and recommended MRI protocol. *Clinical Radiology* 2001; **56**: 726–739.

Collinge J, Palmer MS (eds). *Prion Diseases*. Oxford: OUP, 1997.

Snowden JA, Mann DMA, Neary D. Distinct neuropsychological characteristics in Creutzfeldt–Jakob disease. *Journal of Neurology, Neurosurgery and Psychiatry* 2002; **73**: 686–694.

Zerr I, Pocchiari M, Collins S *et al.* Analysis of EEG and CSF 14-3-3 proteins as aids to the diagnosis of Creutzfeldt–Jakob disease. *Neurology* 2000; **55**: 811–815.

Other relevant entries Dementia: an overview; Prion disease: an overview; Variant Creutzfeldt–Jakob disease.

■ Cri–du–chat syndrome

A chromosomal dysgenetic syndrome (deletion of 5q) in which the cry of the affected child sounds like that of a kitten mewing. In addition there is severe mental retardation, hypotonia, and facial dysmorphism (hypertelorism, epicanthal folds, antimongoloid slant of palpebral fissures, moon face, brachycephaly, micrognathia).

■ Criggler–Najjar syndrome

Lack or deficiency of the enzyme glucuronosyl transferase may result in neonatal hyperbilirubinaemia which in turn may cause kernicterus.

Other relevant entry Kernicterus.

CRION

Chronic relapsing inflammatory optic neuropathy (CRION) describes a rare syndrome of subacute, painful visual loss, often bilaterally sequential, in which the degree of visual loss is usually more severe than in other causes of demyelinating optic neuropathy. The condition is exquisitely corticosteroid responsive, but quickly relapses once steroids are weaned, often requiring long-term immunosuppression. VERs show prolonged latency but preserved amplitude, and ERG shows reduced amplitude of the N95 peak, indicating that this is a purely optic nerve disease. CSF is normal. Superficially CRION resembles the granulomatous optic neuropathy of sarcoidosis, but with prolonged follow-up patients do not develop signs of widespread disease.

Reference Kidd D, Burton B, Plant GT, Hughes EM. Chronic relapsing inflammatory optic neuropathy (CRION). *Brain* 2003; **126**: 276–284.

Other relevant entries Cranial nerve disease: II: Optic nerve; Optic neuritis; Sarcoidosis.

Critical illness myopathy

Three principal patterns of muscle involvement are recognized in patients requiring intensive care:

- Non-necrotizing "cachectic" myopathy
- Myopathy with selective loss of myosin filaments ("thick filament myopathy")
- Acute necrotizing myopathy of intensive care.

The latter two entities may be triggered by use of steroids and neuromuscular blocking agents, but otherwise pathogenesis is obscure, presumed related to mediators of inflammation and multiple organ failure.

Reference Hund E. Neurological complications of sepsis: critical illness polyneuropathy and myopathy. *Journal of Neurology* 2001; **248**: 929–934.

Other relevant entries Critical illness polyneuropathy; Myopathy: an overview.

Critical illness polyneuropathy

Patients who have protracted stays on intensive care units may develop an acute or subacute symmetrical axonal polyneuropathy, especially if their course is complicated by sepsis and multiple organ failure. The motor nerves seem particularly affected, whereas cranial nerves and autonomic functions are spared. Unlike the situation in Guillain–Barré syndrome, which enters the differential diagnosis, CSF is normal. Slow recovery over a period of months may occur. Pathogenesis is not understood, but contributing factors may include drug toxicity, nutritional deficiency, and hyperpyrexia.

References Hund E. Neurological complications of sepsis: critical illness polyneuropathy and myopathy. *Journal of Neurology* 2001; **248**: 929–934.

Wilmshurst PT, Treacher DF, Lantos PL, Wiles CM. Critical illness polyneuropathy following severe hyperpyrexia. *Quarterly Journal of Medicine* 1995; **88**: 351–355.

Zochodne DW, Bolton CF, Wells GA *et al.* Polyneuropathy associated with critical illness: a complication of sepsis and multiple organ failure. *Brain* 1987; **110**: 819–842.

Other relevant entries Critical illness myopathy; Neuropathies: an overview.

■ Crocodile tears – see Bell's palsy

■ Crouzon's syndrome
Craniofacial dysostosis

This is an autosomal-dominant condition in which there are varying degrees of craniosynostosis. Typically, however, patients have hypoplasia of many of the midline facial structures, with shallow orbit and proptosis, in association with mild mental retardation.

Other relevant entry Craniostenosis.

■ Crow–Fukase syndrome – see POEMS syndrome

■ Cryoglobulinaemia, Cryoglobulinaemic neuropathy

Cryoglobulins are proteins that precipitate in the cold and dissolve when heated. They can occur in isolation or in association with either lymphoproliferative disorders or chronic viral hepatitis (both hepatitis B and C). Cryoglobulinaemia may be asymptomatic, as in mixed essential cryoglobulinaemia, or symptomatic. The clinical features of cryoglobulinaemia include purpura, polyarthralgia, Raynaud's phenomenon, skin vasculitis, and glomerulonephritis. The commonest neurological feature is a vasculitic peripheral neuropathy. Central nervous system complications are rare, although a relapsing encephalopathy with abdominal pain, presumed ischaemic, has been reported.

Management involves avoidance of cold conditions, and treatment of the underlying condition, which in the majority of cases is a lymphoproliferative disorder.

Reference Ince PG, Duffey P, Cochrane HR, Lowe J, Shaw PJ. Relapsing ischemic encephaloenteropathy and cryoglobulinemia. *Neurology* 2000; **55**: 1579–1581.

Other relevant entries Neuropathies: an overview; Paraproteinaemic neuropathy; Raynaud's disease, Raynaud's phenomenon, Raynaud's syndrome.

■ Cryptococcosis
Torulosis

Pathophysiology *Cryptococcus neoformans* is a saprophytic fungus. Central nervous system (CNS) infections with this organism were formerly rare, but are now commonly seen in the context of AIDS, where it is the third most common CNS infection (and most common fungal infection) after HIV encephalopathy and toxoplasma encephalitis. It occurs most commonly in those with CD4 cell count <200 per microlitre. Organ transplant recipients are also susceptible to this infection.

Clinical features: history and examination

- Cryptococcal meningitis: fever, headache, stiff neck, photophobia, although symptoms may be minimal or absent.
- Cryptococcoma (toruloma): mass lesion of brain parenchyma; may cause raised intracranial pressure, cranial nerve palsy, hemiparesis, seizures.
- Spinal lesions: rare.

Investigations and diagnosis *Bloods*: main diagnostic test is cryptococcal antigen testing which has high sensitivity and specificity; HIV status; CD4 count.

Imaging:

CT: low-density cyst-like lesions in basal ganglia, mesencephalon;
MRI: T_1 low intensity, T_2 high signal intensity, lesions +/− meningeal enhancement; enhancement of mass lesions uncommon.

CSF: elevated opening pressure; protein, cell count, and glucose may be normal or only marginally abnormal; Indian ink stain for hyphal threads is necessary, fungal culture; detection of cryptococcal antigen.

Differential diagnosis Toxoplasma encephalitis.
Lymphoma.

Treatment and prognosis Anti-fungal agents such as amphotericin or fluconazole may be used intravenously for 2–3 weeks or until symptoms resolve. Relapses occur and hence maintenance oral fluconazole may be given.

> **Reference** Chuck SL, Sande MA. Infections with *Cryptococcus neoformans* in the acquired immunodeficiency syndrome. *New England Journal of Medicine* 1989; **321**: 580–584.

> **Other relevant entries** HIV/AIDS and the nervous system; Immunosuppressive therapy and diseases of the nervous system.

■ Cubital tunnel syndrome

Pathophysiology This refers to entrapment of the ulnar nerve within the fibroosseous canal formed by the medial ligament of the elbow joint and the aponeurosis of flexor carpi ulnaris. Compression at this point may occur with ("tardy ulnar palsy") or without a prior history of elbow trauma.

Clinical features: history and examination

- Sensory: paraesthesia, pain in ulnar division of fingers, hand and wrist.
- Motor: weakness of interossei, abductor digiti minimi, adductor pollicis, flexor pollicis brevis; atrophy, claw hand; flexor carpi ulnaris remains strong; median/radial innervated muscles unaffected (but beware "all ulnar hand").

Investigations and diagnosis *Neurophysiology*: EMG/NCS: reduced ulnar SNAP and CMAP, +/− conduction block in motor fibres at the level of the elbow; fibrillation potentials in ulnar-innervated hand muscles.

Treatment and prognosis Surgical decompression may be considered; splinting.

Other relevant entries Entrapment neuropathies: an overview; Ulnar neuropathy.

◼ Cushing reflex, Cushing response

This is the triad of hypertension, bradycardia, and slow irregular breathing associated with either stimulation of regions in the paramedian caudal medulla or elevation of intracranial pressure, for example with posterior fossa masses or subarachnoid haemorrhage.

◼ Cushing's disease, Cushing's syndrome – see Drug-induced myopathies; Endocrinology and the nervous system; Pituitary disease and apopolexy

◼ Cyanide poisoning

Cyanide poisoning may occur acutely as a deliberate act, or chronically through exposure at work. Acute cases may be rapidly fatal since cyanide disrupts cellular mechanisms for carrying and utilizing oxygen with resultant tissue hypoxia. Survivors may manifest parkinsonism, dementia, and dystonia. In more chronic cases patients may develop seizures, delirium, and visual failure.

◼ Cyclists' palsy – see Ramsay Hunt syndrome (3); Ulnar neuropathy

◼ Cystathionine β-synthase deficiency – see Homocystinuria

◼ Cysticercosis

Pathophysiology Infection with the larval stage (cysticercus) of the helminth cestode *Taenia solium*, the pork tapeworm, usually results from eating undercooked pork, and may lead to diverse neurological syndromes when cysticerci reach the central nervous system (CNS); muscle, eye, and subcutaneous tissues may also be involved. In some tropical countries it is the commonest cause of epilepsy.

Clinical features: history and examination

Focal or generalized epilepsy.

Focal neurological deficits, for example episodic ataxia (nausea, projectile vomiting, fever, malaise).

Raised intracranial pressure.

Cognitive decline.

Meningitis (acute, chronic)

Myelopathy, spinal epidural abscess.

Fulminant encephalitis (rare).

Focal or generalized muscle enlargement: examine subcutaneous tissues for calcified cysts.

Investigations and diagnosis *Bloods*: eosinophilia (not often helpful); ELISA (high false-positive rate).

Stool: ova (not often helpful).

Imaging: CT for granuloma, calcified cysts; MRI for cysts; may see lesions at different stages of development.

CSF: mononuclear or lymphocytic pleocytosis; raised pressure.

Brain biopsy: may be required for definitive diagnosis.

Differential diagnosis

Broad!

Echinococcosis
Cryptococcosis
Paragonimiasis
Cystic astrocytoma
Epidermoid.

Intermittent ataxias of genetic aetiology.

Other symptomatic causes of epilepsy.

Treatment and prognosis *Active disease*: anti-helminthic therapy with albendazole or praziquantel, with steroid (dexamethasone) cover.

Inactive disease: symptomatic treatment, for example anti-epileptic drugs.

Shunting for hydrocephalus.

References Pal DK, Carpio A, Sander JWAS. Neurocysticercosis and epilepsy in developing countries. *Journal of Neurology, Neurosurgery and Psychiatry* 2000; **69**: 137–143.

Wadia NH. Neurocysticercosis. In: RA Shakir, PK Newman, CM Poser (eds). *Tropical Neurology*. London: Saunders, 1996: 247–273.

Other relevant entries Cerebellar disease: an overview; Cryptococcosis; Echinococcosis; Helminthic disease.

■ Cystinosis

Pathophysiology A genetic metabolic disorder in which there is intralysosomal accumulation of the amino acid cystine in kidney, cornea, thyroid, and brain; hence, a lysosomal-storage disease.

Clinical features: history and examination

- Proximal tubulopathy: De Toni–Debre–Fanconi syndrome, characterized by hyperphosphaturia, hyperaminoaciduria, and glucosuria; polyuria and proteinuria may lead to rickets.
- Ocular damage: corneal cystine crystals, retinopathy.

- Neuropsychological deficits.
- Distal vacuolar myopathy also described.

Investigations and diagnosis *Bloods*: renal impairment, hypoalbuminaemia.

Urine: polyuria; hyperphosphaturia, hyperaminoaciduria, glucosuria.

Neuropsychology: impaired spatial processing; perceptual processing largely intact.

Neurogenetics: mutations in the CTNS gene which encodes cystinosin, a lysosomal cystine transporter.

Differential diagnosis De Toni–Debre–Fanconi syndrome may also occur in mitochondrial disorders such as Kearns–Sayre syndrome.

Treatment and prognosis Cysteamine reduces intracellular cystine levels, and should be commenced as soon as diagnosis is made, since it delays disease progression, although its use is associated with limiting side-effects.

Renal transplantation: corrects renal tubular dysfunction, and consequences thereof, but not the underlying metabolic defect, and hence disease may recur in the transplanted organ.

Reference Charnas LR, Luciano CA, Dalakas M *et al*. Distal vacuolar myopathy in nephropathic cystinosis. *Annals of Neurology* 1994; **35**: 181–188.

Other relevant entries Aminoacidopathies: an overview; Kearns–Sayre syndrome.

■ Cytomegalovirus and the nervous system

Infection with cytomegalovirus (CMV), a member of the herpesvirus family, may be associated with various neurological syndromes:

Intrauterine infection:

Stillbirth, prematurity; granulomatous encephalitis

Seizures, focal signs, mental retardation in survivors

Periventricular calcification seen on skull radiographs, brain CT

Meningitis, myelitis, deafness and vertigo.

Adult infection (rare):

Infectious mononucleosis-like illness

Encephalitis

Meningitis

Guillain–Barré syndrome.

CMV has also been implicated in some cases of Reye's syndrome, and Rasmussen's syndrome.

Opportunistic CMV infection in HIV/AIDS may cause retinitis, encephalitis, mononeuritis multiplex, cauda equina syndrome.

Complement fixation tests, neutralization tests, and polymerase chain reaction tests are available for diagnosis, as well as culture from urine, saliva, or liver biopsy specimens.

Ganciclovir may be beneficial for some CMV infections.

Other relevant entries Epstein–Barr virus (EBV) and the nervous system; HIV/AIDS and the nervous system; Rasmussen's encephalitis, Rasmussen's syndrome; Reye's syndrome; Varicella zoster virus and the nervous system.

■ Cysts: an overview

Pathophysiology The term cyst is used of a number of fluid-filled lesions which may affect the nervous system.

- Developmental malformations representing trapped embryonic remnants. Lesions with an epithelial lining (mucus secreting columnar epithelium that may vary from low cuboidal to pseudostratified) may be called:

    Neuroenteric cyst: in the spinal cord, posterior fossa; presumably of enteric origin
    Neuroepithelial cyst: in the hemispheres; of ependymal origin
    Colloid cyst: in the third ventricle
    Rathke cleft cyst: in the sella; stomodeal origin
    Dermoid, epidermoid cysts: misplaced ectoderm (may also be acquired)
    Tarlov cyst: sacral nerve root.

- Cystic space bounded by arachnoid membranes: arachnoid cyst.
- Cysts associated with parasitic infection:

    Cysticercosis, coenurosis, echinococcosis, paragonimiasis, trichinosis.

- Cystic swellings associated with tumours (e.g. glioma, haemangioblastoma).

Investigations and diagnosis *Imaging*: CT usually shows cysts as low attenuation lesions; contrast enhancement may be absent or confined to the rim. There may be compression of adjacent structures.

Pathology: developmental cysts immunostain positive for cytokeratin or epithelial membrane antigen (EMA) but not for glial fibrillary acidic protein (GFAP).

Differential diagnosis They may be present as space-occupying lesions, requiring differentiation from tumour, haematoma, and abscess.

Treatment and prognosis Surgical decompression or removal may be required if there are compressive symptoms. Parasitic cysts require appropriate chemotherapy; there may be difficulties with surgical approach (e.g. echinococcosis).

Other relevant entries Abscess: an overview; Arachnoid cyst; Colloid cyst; Coenurosis; Cysticercosis; Dermoid; Echinococcosis; Epidermoid; Glioma; Haematoma: an overview; Paragonimiasis; Trichinosis; Tumours: an overview.

Dd

■ "Dancing eyes, Dancing feet" – see Myoclonus; Opsoclonus; Paraneoplastic syndromes

■ Dandy's syndrome

Dandy's syndrome is the combination of oscillopsia and gait ataxia caused by bilateral loss of vestibular function. In Dandy's original cases, this was due to vestibular nerve section for Ménière's disease, but nowadays it may result from use of ototoxic drugs.

Reference Dandy WE. Ménière's disease: its diagnosis and methods of treatment. *Archives of Surgery* 1928; **16**: 1127.
Other relevant entries Ménière's disease; Oscillopsia.

Dandy–Walker syndrome

The Dandy–Walker syndrome is a developmental abnormality characterized by a failure of development of the midline portion of the cerebellum which results in cyst-like enlargement of the fourth ventricle, with bulging of the occipital bone posteriorly and upward displacement of the tentorium and torcula. There may be associated agenesis of the corpus callosum, dilatation of the central aqueduct and third and lateral ventricles, and aplasia of the cerebellar vermis.

Danon disease

Danon disease is a rare X-linked disorder characterized by cardiomyopathy, vacuolar myopathy, and variable mental retardation. The myopathy is proximal and often mild in comparison with the cardiomyopathy. Creatine kinase may be elevated (*ca*. 1000 U/l), muscle biopsy shows a vacuolar myopathy and there may be deposition of membrane attack complex on vacuolated fibres. Clinically the condition may appear similar to Pompe disease, but α-glucosidase levels are normal.

Danon disease has been shown to be due to mutations in the gene encoding the lysosomal-associated membrane protein LAMP-2. Affected males die in the second to third decade; carrier females may manifest a cardiomyopathy and die in the third to fifth decade.

References Davies NP, Beesley C, Elliott PM *et al*. Intronic and missense mutations within the LAMP-2 gene in Danon disease (X-linked vacuolar cardiomyopathy and myopathy). *Journal of Neurology, Neurosurgery and Psychiatry* 2002; **72**: 139 (abstract).

Nishino I, Fu J, Tanji K *et al*. Primary LAMP-2 deficiency causes X-linked vacuolar cardiomyopathy and myopathy (Danon disease). *Nature* 2000; **406**: 906–910.
Other relevant entries Myopathy: an overview; X-linked myopathy with excessive autophagy.

Davidoff–Dyke–Masson syndrome – see Cerebral palsy, cerebral palsy syndromes

Dawidenkow syndrome
Kaeser syndrome • Scapuloperoneal syndrome

A rare neurogenic scapuloperoneal syndrome, with amyotrophy and associated distal sensory loss, nerve hypertrophy, and pes cavus. It resembles myogenic scapuloperoneal syndromes, for example in facioscapulohumeral dystrophy,

Emery–Dreifuss syndrome, and phosphofructokinase deficiency, but is thought to be related to the hereditary motor and sensory neuropathies.

Reference Serratrice G, Pélissier JF, Pouget J. Trois cas d'amyotrophie scapulopéronière neurogène (syndrome de Dawidenkow): situation nosologique par rapport à la maladie de Charcot–Marie–Tooth. *Revue Neurologique* 1984; **140**: 738–740.

Other relevant entries Neuropathies: an overview; Scapuloperoneal syndrome.

■ De-afferentation syndrome

De-afferentation, for example after brachial root avulsion in a motorcycle accident, may result in a syndrome of spontaneous painful dysaesthesia without allodynia or hyperalgesia, known as de-afferentation syndrome. Management of the painful useless limb is difficult; amputation does not result in pain relief. If pharmacotherapy fails, surgical options include dorsal root entry zone section.

■ Decerebrate rigidity, Decorticate rigidity

- Decerebrate rigidity, or extensor posturing, describes the position of a comatose patient with extension and pronation of the upper limbs, extension of the legs, and plantar flexion of the feet. Painful stimuli may induce opisthotonos, hyperextension and hyperpronation of the upper limbs. Decerebrate rigidity occurs with upper brainstem dysfunction (e.g. following anoxia/ischaemia, drugs, trauma) and is thought to represent a loss of inhibitory brainstem input to the spinal cord producing an exaggeration of the normal standing posture.
- Decorticate rigidity, or flexor posturing, describes comatose patients with adduction of the shoulders and arms, and flexion of the elbows and wrists. The responsible lesion is higher than that in decerebrate rigidity, often being diffuse cerebral hemisphere or diencephalic disease; despite the name, it may occur with upper brainstem lesions.

Decerebrate rigidity indicates a deeper level of coma than decorticate rigidity; the transition from the latter to the former is associated with a worsening of prognosis.

Other relevant entry Coma.

■ Decompression sickness – see Caisson disease

■ De-efferented state – see Locked-in syndrome

■ Degos disease – see Kohlmeier–Degos disease

■ Déjerine anterior bulbar syndrome – see Medial medullary (infarction) syndrome

■ Déjerine–Klumpke palsy – see Klumpke's paralysis

■ Déjerine–Mouzon syndrome
Pseudothalamic syndrome

Déjerine–Mouzon syndrome, first described in 1914–1915, is a parietal lobe syndrome in which there is severe impairment of all primary sensory modalities (touch, pain, temperature, vibration, and joint position sense) contralateral to the lesion. It is usually due to a vascular event involving the parietal branch of the middle cerebral artery. It often improves with time. It is easily confused with the sensory loss seen with a thalamic lesion affecting the sensory relay nuclei (the Déjerine–Roussy syndrome) and hence is sometimes known as the pseudothalamic syndrome.

■ Déjerine–Roussy syndrome

Déjerine–Roussy syndrome describes contralateral sensory loss due to a lesion (typically vascular, occasionally neoplastic) in the ventroposterolateral (VPL) and posteromedial (VPM) nuclei of the thalamus. The sensory loss is most frequently for joint position sense, pain, and temperature. There may be associated transient hemiparesis $+/-$ homonymous hemianopia, with on occasions taste distortion, athetosis of the hand, and depression. With partial recovery the patient may be left with spontaneous pain or discomfort in the region of the sensory loss, so-called thalamic pain, which has an unpleasant, diffuse, and lingering quality, often resistant to standard analgesia.

Delayed onset of involuntary movements following stroke in the posterolateral thalamus was also reported by Déjerine and Roussy. This may take the form of dystonia, athetosis, and chorea, associated with position sensory loss (hence appropriately designated "pseudochoreoathetosis"); or tremor and myoclonus, associated with cerebellar ataxia.

Reference Kim JS. Delayed onset mixed involuntary movements after thalamic stroke. Clinical, radiological and pathophysiological findings. *Brain* 2001 **124**: 299–309.

Other relevant entries Déjerine–Mouzon syndrome; Thalamic syndromes.

■ Déjerine–Sottas syndrome
Hereditary motor and sensory neuropathy type III (HMSN III)

Although not a distinct genetic entity, this term describes a severe peripheral neuropathy with early age at onset, reduced motor nerve conduction velocities, absent sensory nerve action potentials (usually) and pronounced demyelination in nerve biopsy specimens. These patients probably fall into the rubric of Charcot–Marie–Tooth (CMT) 1 or 4 (respectively, CMT-1 and CMT-4) since dominant and/or recessive mutations have been identified in the genes encoding PMP22, MPZ (P_0), EGR2 and PRX, known to be associated with these types of CMT disease.

Other relevant entries Charcot–Marie–Tooth disease; Hereditary motor and sensory neuropathy; Neuropathies: an overview.

■ DeLange syndrome

DeLange syndrome is a developmental disorder characterized by intrauterine growth retardation resulting in severe mental retardation along with a combination of some of the following abnormalities: short stature, microbrachycephaly; generalized hirsutism (including bushy eyebrows that may cross the midline = synophrys), small nose and anteverted nostrils, long upper lip, micromelia, and skeletal abnormalities (flexion of the elbows, webbing of the second/third toes, clinodactyly of fifth fingers, and transverse palmar crease). There may be a low-pitched weak growling cry. No chromosomal abnormalities have yet been identified in DeLange syndrome.

■ Delirium

Acute brain syndrome • Acute confusional state

Pathophysiology Delirium (from the Latin meaning "out of furrow") is an organic neurobehaviourial disorder characterized by the acute onset of a fluctuating level of attention; there is disorganized thinking and global cognitive or behaviourial abnormalities, with or without an altered level of consciousness (ranging from drowsiness to hypervigilance). It is a common occurrence in hospital in-patients, especially in the elderly and in the ITU setting. It is more likely to occur in individuals with pre-existing cerebral pathology or cognitive impairment, and therefore overlaps with dementia. No consistent pathological abnormalities are seen at post-mortem.

The pathogenesis is usually multifactorial, although no cause is identified in 5–20% of cases:

- Metabolic and endocrine abnormalities: hypoglycaemia, diabetes mellitus, renal failure, hyponatraemia, liver failure, anaemia, hypercalcaemia, thyroid disease, disseminated intravascular coagulopathy, thrombotic thrombocytopenic purpura (TTP), hyperviscosity states.
- Infection

    Systemic: urinary tract infection, septicaemia, pneumonia (especially the atypical pneumonias) particularly in the elderly; malaria.

    Central nervous system (CNS): meningitis, encephalitis; occasionally AIDS.
- Vascular: cerebrovascular accidents in the elderly, especially right middle cerebral artery and left posterior cerebral artery territory events; hypertensive encephalopathy.
- Epileptic: either post-ictally or in some cases of non-convulsive status epilepticus.
- Drug induced

    Drug/solvent abuse in the younger patient.

    Sedatives, hypnotics, antidepressants, anticholinergics, anti-parkinsonian, and steroid therapy, especially in the elderly.

- Drug withdrawal: for example, alcohol (Wernicke's encephalopathy) with delirium tremens; barbiturates, benzodiazepines, amphetamine and cocaine.
- Significant head injury.
- Brain tumours.
- Others: fractured bones $+/-$ fat emboli; paraneoplastic (limbic) encephalitis; systemic lupus erythematosus; some auto-immune channelopathies; porphyria; vitamin B_{12} deficiency; heavy metal poisoning.

Recognized risk factors for the development of delirium include:

older age groups,
pre-existing cerebral pathology or cognitive impairment,
previous history of delirium,
history of substance abuse or dependency,
use of psychotropic and analgesic medication,
medical procedures,
active infective processes,
AIDS,
serious burns,
numerous co-morbid conditions.

Overall, delirium occurs in 10–35% of all patients in a general hospital.

Clinical features: history and examination
- Acute onset with fluctuating course, developing over hours or days; often with periods of normality, but typically worse at night.
- Attentional deficits: the patient is distractable, shows disorganized thinking, may have rambling incoherent speech with a degree of perseveration. This is associated with disorientation (in time > place > person) and memory disturbances.
- There are often perceptual disturbances with misidentifications (illusions) more common than hallucinations (usually visual).
- Altered level of consciousness may occur, varying from hypoactivity and mutism to hyperactivity and general motor overactivity (e.g. in cases of alcohol withdrawal).
- In addition there is often disruption of the normal sleep–wake cycle.
- Mood disturbances are common, often with marked lability.
- Collateral history from the family, friends (e.g. cognitive state prior to admission); drug history.

Investigations and diagnosis
Bloods:

First line investigations in all patients: FBC, ESR, blood film, U&Es, glucose, liver function tests, calcium and phosphate, blood cultures, and arterial blood gases.

Additional investigations if no cause identified with first line investigations: clotting, fibrin degradation products (FDPs), blood viscosity, ammonia, thyroid function tests, and serology (infection; syphilis; HIV disease; auto-antibodies including anti-neuronal and K^+ channel antibodies).

Urinalysis: infection, porphyria screen, drug screen, fat.

Imaging: CXR; CT/MRI head, $+/-$ search for fractured bones/neoplasia.

Neurophysiology: EEG may typically show slowing, the degree of which correlates well with the clinical status of the patient. Occasionally faster activity is seen (e.g. in delirium tremens), or ictal activity.

CSF: cell count, protein, glucose, oligoclonal bands, Gram stain, culture (infection, inflammation), fat.

Differential diagnosis *Dementia*: chronic confusional state; but may underlie episodes of delirium.

Psychiatric disorders: for example, schizophrenia, depression, mania, attention deficit disorder, autism, dissociative disorders, Ganser's syndrome.

Aphasic syndromes (especially Wernicke-type aphasia).

Treatment and prognosis Find reversible causes and correct them; particularly, give thiamine and/or glucose if any possibility of alcoholism or hypoglycaemia.

Reduce conflicting and changing sensory stimuli: patient should ideally be nursed in a simple, uncluttered, unchanging immediate environment and remain in the same bed whilst on the ward, with adequate lighting and limited noise. Contact should be restricted to few nurses and doctors; all instructions should be clear and simple; ensure glasses, hearing aids, dentures are all in place. Relatives and friends may visit regularly and encourage patient with questions on orientation and objects from home.

Do not interrupt sleep.

Avoid drug therapy; if needed (especially in the hyperactive patient) may use haloperidol ($\sim$1.5–20 mg/day orally) or lorazepam (initially 0.5–1 mg od).

The outlook is generally good but depends on precipitant and underlying condition of patient. Overall the diagnosis of delirium carries with it an increased mortality rate, especially if it is not recognized and treated.

References Andrefsky JC, Frank JI. Approach to the patient with acute confusional state (delirium/encephalopathy). In: Biller J (ed.). *Practical Neurology* (2nd edition). Philadelphia: Lippincott Williams & Wilkins, 2002: 3–18.

Brown TM, Boyle MF. Delirium. *British Medical Journal* 2002; **325**: 644–647.

Caracini A, Grassi L. *Delirium: Acute Confusional States in Palliative Medicine*. Oxford: OUP, 2003.

Lindesay J, Rockwood K, Macdonald A (eds). *Delirium in Old Age*. Oxford: OUP, 2002.

Meagher DS, O'Hanlon D, O'Mahoney E, Casey PR. The use of environmental strategies and psychotropic medication in the management of delirium. *British Journal of Psychiatry* 1996; **168**: 512–515.

Other relevant entries Alcohol and the nervous system: an overview; Aphasia; Atypical pneumonias and the nervous system; Cerebrovascular disease: arterial; Dementia: an overview; Drug-induced encephalopathies; Encephalitis: an overview; Encephalopathies: an overview; Endocrinology and the nervous system; Epilepsy: an overview; Fat embolism syndrome; HIV/AIDS and the nervous system; Lead and the nervous system; Meningitis: an overview; Paraneoplastic syndromes; Porphyria; Psychiatric disorders and neurological disease; Systemic lupus erythematosus and the nervous system; Vitamin B_{12} deficiency.

■ Delirium tremens – see Alcohol and the nervous system: an overview; Delirium

■ Dementia: an overview
Chronic brain syndrome

Pathophysiology Dementia is variously defined as a progressive loss of cognitive function, usually but not invariably with memory impairment, without a deficit of arousal or attention (*cf.* delirium), which interferes with social or occupational function. Dementia occurs in many conditions, most often (over 90% of cases) due to neurodegeneration, as in Alzheimer's disease (AD) and frontotemporal dementia (FTD), or due to cerebrovascular disease, for example due to multiple infarcts. The prevalence of dementia increases exponentially with age: 1% of people aged 60 years old are affected, up to 50% by the age of 85 years. Although rare, treatable causes of dementing illness must be sought.

Dementia may be classified according to the pattern of neuropsychological deficits, which correlate with areas of involvement within the central nervous system (CNS), and by histopathology (although this is seldom available *ante mortem*). A distinction is sometimes made on neuropsychological grounds between cortical and subcortical dementia syndromes. Cortical dementias are characterized by amnesia, aphasia, apraxia, agnosia, in isolation or combination: examples include AD and FTD. Subcortical dementias are associated with slowing of cognitive speed with a frontal pattern of cognitive deficits (ranging from apathy to disinhibition, with or without extrapyramidal signs such as akinesia); examples include progressive supranuclear palsy (PSP) and Huntington's disease (HD). However, the division between cortical and subcortical dementias is not absolute and this terminology is not universally used.

The clinical picture does not always reliably predict the neuropathological substrate. Imaging techniques and electrophysiological studies may sometimes assist in the diagnosis of dementing disorders.

Dementia may be classified according to aetiology:
* Neurodegeneration
  Relatively pure dementia syndrome
    AD, or dementia of the Alzheimer type (DAT): accounts for ~70% of all dementia cases
    FTD/Pick's disease: accounts for ~1–5% of all cases of dementia
  "Dementia plus" syndromes
    + motor neurone involvement

FTD with motor neurone disease (FTD/MND)
  + basal ganglia involvement
  Parkinson's disease with dementia (PD-D)
  Dementia with Lewy bodies (DLB)
  HD
  Progressive supranuclear palsy (PSP)
  Corticobasal degeneration (CBD)
  + cerebellar involvement
  Some autosomal-dominant cerebellar ataxias (ADCA type I)
- Cerebrovascular diseases
  Multiple infarcts
  Strategic infarcts (e.g. bilateral paramedian thalamic infarction)
  Binswanger's disease/encephalopathy
  Recurrent haemorrhages (e.g. cerebral amyloid angiopathy)
  Subdural haematomas
  Cerebral autosomal-dominant arteriopathy with subcortical infarcts and
    leukoencephalopathy (CADASIL)
- Metabolic disorders
  Wilson's disease
  Leukodystrophies
  Aminoacidopathies
  Lipid-storage disorders
  Mitochondrial disease
  Obstructive sleep apnoea syndrome (OSAS)
- Endocrine and nutritional disorders
  Thiamine deficiency
  Hypothyroidism; Hashimoto's encephalopathy
  Cushing's disease
  Vitamin B_{12} deficiency
- Inflammatory CNS disease
  Multiple sclerosis
  Sarcoidosis
  Behçet's disease
  Cerebral vasculitis or vasculopathy (e.g. SLE, Sjögren's syndrome)
- Neoplasia
  Brain tumours
  Paraneoplastic syndromes (limbic encephalitis)
- Structural disorders
  Normal pressure hydrocephalus (NPH)
  Chronic subdural haematomas
  Strategically placed tumours
- Infection
  Neurosyphilis

HIV, and complications thereof: cryptococcus, progressive multifocal leukoencephalopathy (PML)

Whipple's disease

Coeliac disease

Prion disease

- Drug induced

    Alcoholism, $+/-$ thiamine deficiency

    Drug-induced cognitive impairment

Clinical features: history and examination

- History of memory difficulties, behavioural change, functional capacities (instru-
mental and basic activities of daily living), psychiatric symptoms (hallucinations,
delusions).
- Drug history, dietary history.
- Family history of cognitive disorder.
- History taking should include independent (collateral) history from spouse or
carer, where possible.

Investigations and diagnosis *Neuropsychology or psychometry*: simple bedside
screening tests [e.g. mini-mental state examination (MMSE), Addenbrooke's
Cognitive Examination (ACE)]; more detailed assessments including IQ (e.g. NART),
memory, language, perception, frontal lobe or executive function.

Bloods:

First line investigations in all patients: FBC, ESR, U&Es, glucose, liver function
tests, calcium and phosphate, vitamin B_{12}, thyroid function tests, VDRL–TPHA.

Additional investigations in certain circumstances: blood film; auto-antibodies,
red blood cell transketolase, full vasculitic screen, copper and caeruloplasmin, white
cell enzymes, urinary amino acids and organic acids, HIV test, *Borrelia* serology,
anti-neuronal antibodies, thyroid antibodies, voltage gated K^+ channel antibodies.

Imaging:

Structural: CT/MRI to exclude structural causes (NPH, subdural haematoma,
tumour, lymphoma) which may potentially be reversible; for global or focal atrophy
(AD, FTD); vascular disease (may be incidental).

Functional: SPECT scan may reveal perfusion deficits of possible diagnostic value
(e.g. temporoparietal in AD, frontal in FTD).

CSF: to exclude infective or inflammatory causes.

Neurogenetics: familial AD [amyloid precursor protein (APP), presenilin], FTD (τ),
subcortical dementias (HD), and some ADCA.

Neurophysiology: not often helpful, except in cases of suspected prion disease
(periodic EEG changes in sporadic Creutzfeldt–Jakob disease) or seizure
disorders; EEG remains normal in FTD whereas slowing is usually seen in AD.

Brain biopsy: reserved for cases in which there is a high suspicion of potentially
reversible cause, such as inflammatory conditions.

Other tests, according to suspected cause: carotid artery ultrasonography, echocardiography (multi-infarct disease), duodenal biopsy (Whipple's disease or coeliac disease).

Differential diagnosis

Delirium.

Psychiatric illness, especially depression and anxiety states.

Drug-induced cognitive impairment.

Poorly controlled epilepsy, non-convulsive status.

Purely subjective memory impairment, "worried well".

Treatment and prognosis Reversible causes of dementia are rare. Treatment is most often palliative. Prognosis in terms of survival depends on the underlying cause.

References Cummings JL, Benson DF. *Dementia: A Clinical Approach* (2nd edition). Boston: Butterworth-Heinemann, 1992.

Doran M. Diagnosis of presenile dementia. *British Journal of Hospital Medicine* 1997; **58**: 105–110.

Geldmacher DS, Whitehouse PJ. Evaluation of dementia. *New England Journal of Medicine* 1996; **335**: 330–336.

Growdon JH, Rossor MN (eds). *The Dementias*. Boston: Butterworth-Heinemann, 1998.

Hodges JR (ed.). *Early-Onset Dementia. A Multidisciplinary Approach*. Oxford: OUP, 2001.

O'Brien J, Ames D, Burns A (eds). *Dementia* (2nd edition). London: Arnold, 2000.

Other relevant entries Alzheimer's disease; Cerebellar disease: an overview; Cerebrovascular disease: arterial; Collagen vascular diseases and the nervous system; Corticobasal degeneration; Dementia with Lewy bodies; Endocrinology and the nervous system; Epilepsy: an overview; Frontotemporal dementia; Gastrointestinal diseases and the nervous system; HIV/AIDS and the nervous system; Huntington's disease; Infection and the nervous system: an overview; Leukodystrophies: an overview; Mild cognitive impairment; Motor neurone disease; Multiple sclerosis; Normal pressure hydrocephalus; Paraneoplastic syndromes; Parkinsonian syndromes, parkinsonism; Parkinson's disease; Pick's disease; Prion disease: an overview; Progressive subcortical gliosis; Progressive supranuclear palsy; Sarcoidosis; Syphilis; Vascular dementia; Vitamin B_{12} deficiency; Whipple's disease; Wilson's disease.

■ Dementia of Alzheimer's type – see Alzheimer's disease; Dementia: an overview

■ Dementia with Lewy bodies

Cortical Lewy body disease • Diffuse Lewy body disease • Lewy body dementia • Senile dementia of the Lewy body type

Pathophysiology A neurodegenerative disorder causing a syndrome of dementia and parkinsonism, claimed by some to be second in frequency only to Alzheimer's disease (AD) as a cause of dementia.

Clinical features: history and examination

- Cognitive disorder: usually the presenting feature; cortical dementia similar to AD but with more severe and early impairment of visuospatial function and visual memory. Also, cognitive performance tends to fluctuate from day to day, thought to represent an "unstable platform of attention".
- Visual hallucinations: very common; usually non-threatening; often children or animals, often the patient retains insight that these are not really there; the report of figures emerging from the television into the room may be given.
- Marked neuroleptic sensitivity: causes clinical deterioration (both cognitively and extrapyramidally) and may hasten death [not exclusive to dementia with Lewy bodies (DLB), but much commoner than in other dementia syndromes].
- Falls, syncopal episodes: autonomic failure, due to Lewy body pathology in autonomic ganglia, is the presumed cause, and autonomic failure may precede the emergence of DLB.
- Parkinsonism: usually mild, and follows cognitive disorder; rarely asymmetrical, tremor not prominent (*cf.* idiopathic Parkinson's disease).
- Myoclonus may be observed.
- Possible additional features include:
  REM sleep behaviour disorder,
  depression.

A very similar neuropsychological and neuropsychiatric picture may emerge in individuals with established idiopathic Parkinson's disease, and it seems likely that the pathological substrate of this Parkinson's disease with dementia (PD-D) is identical to that in DLB, but with differing regional predominance at clinical onset. A convenient distinction is that patients with DLB have marked cognitive problems within a year of being diagnosed with their Parkinsonism.

Investigations and diagnosis *Bloods*: unremarkable.

Imaging: CT/MRI may show medial temporal lobe atrophy as in AD, or more generalized atrophic change. Functional imaging (SPECT/PET) may show the temporoparietal deficits said to be typical of AD but with additional occipital changes, perhaps reflecting the visuospatial dysfunction in DLB.

Neurophysiology: EEG may show non-specific abnormalities such as diffuse slowing; very occasionally a periodic EEG, similar to that seen in sporadic Creutzfeldt–Jakob disease, may be seen, which may lead to diagnostic confusion.

CSF: usually normal.

Neuropsychology: visuospatial deficits may be prominent, as may attentional deficits (leading to fluctuating performance), more so than memory deficits; in light of this, it has been claimed that a score derived from the mini-mental state examination (MMSE) [attention − 5/3(memory) + 5(visuospatial)] reliably differentiates DLB from AD, but this has not been corroborated.

Other: sleep studies may be indicated if there is a clinical history suggesting concurrent sleep disorder (e.g. REM sleep behaviour disorder).

Pathology: Lewy bodies, positive for ubiquitin and α-synuclein, are evident throughout the cerebral cortex as well as in the brainstem; neuritic changes (Lewy neurites) are also seen, primarily in the hippocampus. Concurrent Alzheimer pathology may be seen.

Differential diagnosis Other cognitive disorders: AD, vascular dementia (fluctuations), prion disease (myoclonus; periodic EEG).

Other parkinsonian syndromes: progressive supranuclear palsy (PSP) has a different clinical and cognitive profile.

The relationship of DLB to the dementia syndrome which may emerge in some patients with established idiopathic Parkinson's disease is uncertain, but there is pathological and therapeutic evidence to suggest that they are similar, merely the pathology is preponderant in a different location (substantia nigra, cortex) at clinical onset of disease. A marked cholinergic deficit, even greater than that in AD, is noted in DLB.

Treatment and prognosis Anti-parkinsonian medication may help parkinsonian features but exacerbate hallucinations.

Cholinesterase inhibition with rivastigmine has been shown in a randomized double-blind controlled trial to improve attentional deficits and reduce hallucinations.

Symptomatic treatment may be given for concurrent sleep disorder (e.g. clonazepam for REM sleep beheviour disorder).

Avoid neuroleptics in any patient in whom this diagnosis is suspected.

Untreated, the pace of the illness is said to be quicker than AD, with survival of 5–8 years.

References Briel RC, McKeith IG, Barker WA *et al*. EEG findings in dementia with Lewy bodies and Alzheimer's disease. *Journal of Neurology, Neurosurgery and Psychiatry* 1999; **66**: 401–403.

Downes JJ, Priestley NM, Doran M, Ferran J, Ghadiali E, Cooper P. Intellectual, mnemonic and frontal functions in dementia with Lewy bodies: a comparison with early and advanced Parkinson's disease. *Behavioral Neurology* 1998; **11**: 173–183.

McKeith I, Del Ser T, Spano P *et al*. Efficacy of rivastigmine in dementia with Lewy bodies: a randomised, double-blind, placebo-controlled international study. *Lancet* 2000; **356**: 2031–2036.

McKeith IG, Galasko D, Kosaka K *et al*. Consensus guidelines for the clinical and pathologic diagnosis of dementia with Lewy bodies (DLB): report of the consortium on DLB international workshop. *Neurology* 1996; **47**: 1113–1124.

McKeith IG, Perry EK, Perry RH. For the consortium on Dementia with Lewy Bodies. Report of the second dementia with Lewy body international workshop. *Neurology* 1999; **53**: 902–905.

Other relevant entries Alzheimer's disease; Dementia: an overview; Lewy body disease: an overview; Parkinsonian syndromes, parkinsonism; Parkinson's disease; Prion disease: an overview; REM sleep behaviour disorder.

■ Dementia paralytica – see Syphilis

■ Dementia pugilistica

Pugilistic encephalopathy • "Punch drunk syndrome"

Originally described in boxers (hence "punch drunk syndrome"), this is a syndrome of cognitive impairment following repeated head trauma; it may also occur in steeple-chase jockeys after repeated falls. In addition to cognitive impairment, there may be dysarthria and a parkinsonian syndrome dominated by akinesia and variably responsive to levodopa. Brain imaging may show ventricular dilatation and a cavum septum pellucidum. Pathologically the condition is reminiscent of Alzheimer's disease, with neurofibrillary tangles, deposition of amyloid β-peptide and diffuse neuronal loss.

Other relevant entries Alzheimer's disease; Dementia: an overview; Parkinsonian syndromes, parkinsonism.

■ De Morsier's syndrome – see Septo-optic dysplasia

■ Demyelinating diseases of the nervous system: an overview

The demyelinating disorders of the nervous system are dealt with in individual entries, but the differential diagnosis is broad, encompassing:
- Central demyelinating disorders, for example
    Multiple sclerosis, and its variants.
    Acute disseminated encephalomyelitis (ADEM) and its variants.
    Devic's disease/syndrome, neuromyelitis optica.
    Leukodystrophies.
    Bickerstaff's brainstem encephalitis (BBE).
    Marchiafava–Bignami syndrome.
- Peripheral demyelinating disorders, for example
    Chronic inflammatory demyelinating poly(radiculo)neuropathy (CIDP).
    Guillain–Barré syndrome (GBS) and its variants.
    Leukodystrophies.
    Inherited demyelinating peripheral neuropathies.
Combined central and peripheral demyelinating disease may occur, usually with the central or peripheral component predominating.

Myelin damage may be the principal neuropathological finding in other disorders such as central pontine myelinolysis and subacute combined degeneration of the spinal cord secondary to vitamin B_{12} deficiency.

Other relevant entries See individual entries; Neuropathies: an overview.

◼ Dengue

Dengue is the most common arthropod-borne viral disease of humans, caused by a flavivirus of the togaviridae family which is transmitted by the mosquito *Aedes aegypti*. It occurs predominantly in the tropics and subtropics, especially Asia but also Africa, Australia and the Americas.

There is a 3–7-day incubation period before the development of a fever with a relative bradycardia, arthralgia, myalgia, and a macular rash that blanches on pressure. This may progress to a more severe form of the disease, dengue haemorrhagic fever, especially in children, in which the patient develops vomiting, collapse, and spontaneous haemorrhages. This is thought to be a vascular leak syndrome.

Neurological complications are uncommon (1% of dengue admissions in one series), and include:

Encephalopathy/encephalitis: seizures, coma, stiff neck, and paresis.
Cranial and peripheral neuropathies: VII, IX–X, ulnar, sciatic.
Guillain–Barré (GBS)-like syndrome.
Reye's syndrome.

There may be a mild CSF leukocytosis. Diagnosis is by serology or PCR.

Treatment is supportive and symptomatic. The prognosis for pure dengue fever is very good, but the more fulminant forms of the disease have 50% mortality in the untreated state.

Reference Solomon T, Dung NM, Vaughn DW *et al.* Neurological manifestations of dengue infection. *Lancet* 2000; **355**: 1053–1059.

◼ Denny–Brown, Foley syndrome
Benign fasciculation with cramps syndrome • Cramp fasciculation syndrome

This is the suggested eponym for the syndrome of benign fasciculations with cramps, in honour of two of the earliest characterizations of the condition. There is no associated wasting or weakness, distinguishing it from progressive anterior horn cell disease. Electrophysiologically there is continuous motor unit activity which differs only quantitatively, rather than qualitatively, from that seen in neuromyotonia. If troublesome, cramps may be treated with phenytoin, quinine or chlorpromazine. The condition may lead to muscle hypertrophy.

Other relevant entries Cramps; Motor neurone disease; Neuromyotonia.

◼ Dentatorubral–pallidoluysian atrophy
Dentatorubropallidoluysian atrophy • "Haw River" syndrome

Pathophysiology Dentatorubral–pallidoluysian atrophy (DRPLA) was first described by Smith *et al.* in the 1950s, although it was only in the early 1980s that it was recognized to be inherited. DRPLA is an autosomal-dominant condition in which there is an exonic CAG trinucleotide repeat expansion on chromosome 12p13.31 (normal = 3–36 repeats, expansion = 49–88 in DRPLA), encoding polyglutamine. The mechanism by which the genetic abnormality produces the degenerative pathological changes is currently not known.

Occasional sporadic forms have been described. It is most commonly reported in Japanese families but not exclusively. The phenotype is variable, consisting of ataxia with an extrapyramidal disorder (dystonia, parkinsonism or choreoathetosis), myoclonus, seizures, and dementia. It can present at any age and is incurable.

Clinical features: history and examination Can present at any age (mean age of onset ~32 years old) with:

cerebellar ataxia;

extrapyramidal disorder: dystonia, parkinsonism or choreoathetosis;

myoclonus which may be associated with seizures;

psychiatric manifestations;

dementia;

positive family history.

Type	Type 1	Type 2
Age of onset (years)	Adult >20	Juvenile <20
Triplet repeat number	~50–60	>60
Disease severity	Mild–moderate	Moderate–severe
Ataxia	+++	++
Choreoathetosis	++	+
Cognitive deficit	++/+++ (dementia)	+++ (mental retardation)
Myoclonus	+	++/+++
Epilepsy	+	+++

+: mild; ++: moderate; +++: severe.

Hence there is a correlation between longer triplet expansion, usually inherited from an affected father, and with both early onset and the progressive myoclonic epilepsy phenotype.

Investigations and diagnosis *Bloods*: normal, aside from genetic test for the expanded triplet repeat which is diagnostic.

Imaging: MRI shows atrophy of basal ganglia, midbrain and cerebellum.

CSF: usually normal.

Neurophysiology: EEG can show spike and wave abnormalities especially in those patients with epilepsy.

Pathology: neuronal loss with atrophy and gliosis of dentate nucleus in cerebellum and red nucleus in midbrain (dentatorubral system); pallidum (especially GP$_e$) and subthalamic nucleus (pallidoluysian system).

Differential diagnosis Huntington's disease (especially in older patients). Other autosomal-dominant cerebellar ataxias.

In the absence of a family history other conditions to consider include:

neuronal ceroid lipofuscinosis (in younger patients);
Lafora body disease (in younger patients);
mitochondrial disease.

(i.e. conditions causing progressive myoclonic epilepsy).

Prion disease.
Whipple's disease.

Treatment and prognosis Symptomatic treatment only (e.g. for seizures, myoclonus).

References Ikeuchi T, Koide R, Tanaka H *et al*. Dentatorubral–pallidoluysian atrophy: clinical features are closely related to unstable expansions of trinucleotide (CAG) repeat. *Annals of Neurology* 1995; **37**: 769–775.

Komure O, Sano A, Nishino N *et al*. DNA analysis in hereditary dentatorubral–pallidoluysian atrophy: correlation between CAG repeat length and phenotypic variation and the molecular basis of anticipation. *Neurology* 1995; **45**: 143–149.

Tsuji S. Dentatorubral–pallidoluysian atrophy (DRPLA). *Journal of Neural Transmission Supplement* 2000; **58**: 167–180.

Other relevant entries Cerebellar disease: an overview; Chorea; Dementia: an overview; Dystonia: an overview; Epilepsy: an overview; Huntington's disease; Parkinsonian syndromes, parkinsonism; Prion disease: an overview; Progressive myoclonic epilepsy; Trinucleotide repeat diseases; Whipple's disease.

▪ Dermatomyositis

Pathophysiology Dermatomyositis is an inflammatory disorder of skeletal muscle and dermis, the former of B-cell origin. The condition involves complement-mediated microvascular injury by antibodies within blood vessels of the dermis and muscle. Classically the patient presents with proximal muscle weakness; in addition, a purple discolouration of the skin around the eyes, extensor surfaces of the arms and fingers may be evident. Dermatomyositis typically requires aggressive immunotherapy. In older patients there may be an associated underlying malignancy.

Dermatomyositides may be classified as follows:
- Childhood dermatomyositis with vasculitis.
- Adult dermatomyositis.
- Adult dermatomyositis associated with connective tissue disorders, especially systemic sclerosis (scleroderma), rheumatoid arthritis, Sjögren's syndrome, and mixed connective tissue disease: overlap syndrome (e.g. sclerodermatomyositis).
- Adult dermatomyositis with underlying malignancy, typically breast, lung, ovary, stomach (i.e. a paraneoplastic syndrome).

Clinical features: history and examination Children > Adults, F > M.

- Skin involvement often precedes or accompanies muscle weakness, and may take the form of:

  Purple discolouration over the upper eyelids with oedema (heliotrope rash).

  Flat red rash on face and upper trunk.

  Erythema on knuckles with a raised violaceous scaly eruption (Gottron's sign) which can spread to involve elbows, knees, malleoli, neck (V-sign), back and shoulders (shawl sign).

  Rash can be made worse by sunlight.

  In the nailbed there are looped and dilated capillaries in association with either small haemorrhages or thrombosed vessels.

  In time the skin may become fragile and shiny with pigmentary changes. In children there can be marked soft tissue calcification.

- Muscle involvement may begin with myalgia before progressing to frank weakness:

  Typically symmetrical, proximal muscle involvement of subacute onset (6–12 weeks), progressing with time to proximal muscle weakness, firstly of the lower limbs (e.g. difficulty getting out chairs, climbing stairs).

  Respiratory, neck, bulbar and facial muscles may be involved in severe cases.

  Muscle wasting gradually develops; muscles may be swollen and tender with acute disease (inflammation), or firm and indurated with chronic disease (fibrosis and fatty infiltration).

- Occasionally the disease can present in a florid fashion with development of acute renal failure secondary to myoglobinuria, in which case the muscles are often swollen and tender.

- Systemic involvement may occur: fever, malaise, fatigue, weight loss, arthralgia, Raynaud's phenomenon (especially with underlying connective tissue disorder).

- Extraocular muscles, sphincter function, and sensation are typically spared, and the reflexes are present unless muscles are severely atrophied.

Investigations and diagnosis *Bloods*: may reveal leukocytosis, raised ESR, positive ANA; none are diagnostic. Creatine kinase is elevated in over 95% of cases; if this is markedly raised there may be secondary renal failure. Serology for auto-antibodies may reveal an underlying connective tissue disorder. A similar myopathy may occur with HIV and HTLV-1 in appropriate geographical areas, hence it is sensible to check for these.

Neurophysiology: EMG shows myopathic changes, but these may be patchy requiring sampling of more than one site; fibrillation potentials, excessive insertional activity and spontaneous discharges may also be seen. Indolent disease with fibrotic muscle may not show characteristic changes.

Muscle biopsy: the definitive test, showing perifascicular atrophy with other fibres undergoing degeneration and necrosis so that they lose the staining characteristics with many enzyme reactions (so-called ghost fibres). There is also an intense inflammatory infiltrate centred on the blood vessels with endothelial hyperplasia, fibrin thrombi, intracapillary tubular inclusions and obliteration of capillaries.

Imaging: not usually helpful, although MRI of muscle does show some abnormalities.

CSF: not necessary.

Others: search for an underlying malignancy should be undertaken in patients (especially men) presenting after the age of 50 years; this may include CXR, pelvic ultrasound, CT chest and abdomen, barium swallow, GI endoscopy, as appropriate. Check ECG to exclude cardiomyopathy; respiratory function (spirometry) to exclude respiratory muscle involvement.

Differential diagnosis

Polymyositis (+ / − overlap syndrome).

Sporadic inclusion body myositis (IBM).

Drug-induced myopathies (e.g. amiodarone, statins).

Muscular dystrophies (especially limb girdle dystrophies).

Treatment and prognosis High-dose prednisolone in the first instance: 100 mg/day, or 2 mg/kg/day in children, reducing to 60 mg/day (or 1 mg/kg/day in children) over the next 2 months. Thereafter the dose should be reduced by about 5–10 mg a month according to disease activity; this may be measured according to clinical symptoms, quantitative myometry, and creatine kinase level.

If symptoms recur or are not controlled then options include the introduction of:

azathioprine 1.5–2 mg/kg/day (monitor FBC, LFT weekly in first instance);
methotrexate (15–25 mg/week orally);
intravenous immunoglobulin (0.4 g/kg/day for 5 days; repeated every 6–8 weeks);
cyclosporin, cyclophosphamide and plasma exchange have all been tried with only marginal benefit.

Supportive treatment may also be neceesary (e.g. respiratory support, nasogastric feeding).

Physiotherapy is essential to avoid disuse atrophy and development of contractures. Persistent subcutaneous calcifications are difficult to treat.

References Byrne E, Dennett X. Idiopathic inflammatory myopathies: clinical aspects. *Baillière's Clinical Neurology* 1993; **2(3)**: 499–526.

Dalakas MC. Polymyositis, dermatomyositis, and inclusion body myositis. *New England Journal of Medicine* 1991; **325**: 1487–1498.

Dalakas MC, Sivakumar K. The immunopathologic and inflammatory differences between dermatomyositis, polymyositis and sporadic inclusion body myositis. *Current Opinion in Neurology* 1996; **9**: 235–239.

Other relevant entries Collagen vascular diseases and the nervous system; Drug-induced myopathies; Immunosuppressive therapy and diseases of the nervous system; Inclusion body myositis; Muscular dystrophies: an overview; Myopathy: an overview; Paraneoplastic syndromes; Polymyositis; Proximal weakness; Systemic sclerosis.

■ Dermoid

Dermoids are benign cystic tumours, similar to epidermoids, the exception being that they contain skin appendages and hair follicles as well as the keratin found in epidermoids. They tend to be more common in children, presenting as midline lesions anywhere from the cerebellum to the lower cord; presenting symptoms depend on location. Like epidermoids they may rupture into the CSF causing chemical (aseptic) meningitis.

Dermoids occur in Goldenhar syndrome, along with lipomas of the corpus callosum.

Other relevant entries Aseptic meningitis; Cysts: an overview; Epidermoid; Goldenhar syndrome, Goldenhar–Gorlin syndrome.

■ De Sanctis–Cacchione syndrome – see Xeroderma pigmentosum and related conditions

■ Desmin myopathy, desminopathy

Desmin is a structural protein of muscle. Although diffuse and focal non-specific increases in desmin may be seen in biopsies from a variety of muscle diseases, the term desminopathy is largely reserved for an autosomal-dominant distal myopathy of middle adulthood associated with frequent cardiac involvement. Leg weakness leading to gait disturbance is followed over 5–10 years by weakness of all extremities, bulbar, facial and respiratory muscle weakness, and cardiac problems (arrhythmia, conduction block, congestive failure). EMG shows prominent spontaneous activity, short duration motor unit potentials, and polyphasia. Muscle biopsy shows central nuclei, and subsarcolemmal material in both type I and type II fibres which stains positive with antibodies to desmin and ubiquitin. Electron microscopy shows aggregates of granular and filamentous material arising from the Z-bands.

There is no specific treatment. Supportive treatment may include anti-arrhythmic drugs or cardiac pacing for heart block.

References Goebel HH. Desmin-related neuromuscular disorders. *Muscle and Nerve* 1995; **18**: 1306–1320.

Horowitz SH, Schmalbruch H. Autosomal dominant distal myopathy with desmin storage: a clinicopathologic and electrophysiologic study of a large kinship. *Muscle and Nerve* 1994; **17**: 151–160.

Other relevant entry Distal muscular dystrophy, distal myopathy.

■ Detoni–Debre–Fanconi syndrome – see Cystinosis; Kearns–Sayre syndrome

■ Devic's disease, Devic's syndrome
Neuromyelitis optica (NMO)

Pathophysiology In 1894 Eugene Devic described a distinct syndrome characterized by acute or subacute onset of optic neuropathy with visual impairment in one or both eyes, associated with a severe transverse myelitis. This syndrome may be seen in a number of conditions including multiple sclerosis (MS), acute demyelinating encephalomyelitis (ADEM), connective tissue disorders (e.g. systemic lupus erythematosus, SLE) and tuberculosis, but it is often an isolated condition with distinctive MRI appearances (neuromyelitis optica), the precise relationship of which to MS remains a subject of debate. The idiopathic syndrome may occur more frequently in Japan. Whilst it is thought to have an immunological basis, IgG oligoclonal bands are frequently not found in the CSF (*cf.* MS) and the patient responds poorly to immunotherapy with steroids and so is typically left with severe disability.

Hence, Devic's syndrome encompasses three entities:

- Conventional MS with greatest burden of disease falling on optic nerves/spinal cord: brain MRI may be typical of MS, CSF oligoclonal bands positive.
- Inflammatory/infective optico-spinal disease of other origins (e.g. lupus, sarcoid).
- Devic's disease: pure optico-spinal inflammatory demyelination; brain MRI normal, CSF oligoclonal bands negative.

Clinical features: history and examination

- Acute severe transverse myelitis, causing paraparesis or quadriparesis +/− sphincter involvement.
- Acute unilateral or bilateral optic neuropathy, often with poor recovery (typically blind or counting fingers only).
- Typically a mono- or multiphasic illness with little in the way of relapsing–remitting symptoms.
- There is no clinical evidence for involvement of other cranial nerves or other parts of the nervous system.

Investigations and diagnosis
Bloods: usually normal, although some patients may have raised markers of inflammation and/or positive serology to indicate an underlying infection or connective tissue disorder.

Imaging:

CXR to exclude pulmonary TB.

Spinal MRI reveals a diffuse abnormality of the cord (typically cervical and thoracic) with a long high signal lesion associated with oedema.

Brain MRI is normal in about 50% of cases; in the other 50% there are non-specific scattered and clinically silent white matter lesions (some suggested criteria demand an entirely normal brain MRI).

CSF: usually normal with only about 20% of cases having a raised white cell count and evidence of intrathecal IgG production (i.e. oligoclonal bands).

Neurophysiology: not usually necessary, but SSEPs and visual evoked potentials (VEPs) are abnormal.

Pathology: shows demyelination, gliosis, and sometimes necrosis and cavitation of the spinal cord and optic nerve.

Differential diagnosis
MS

ADEM

Sarcoidosis

Vasculitis
Leber's hereditary optic neuropathy
Vitamin B_{12} deficiency
Strachan's syndrome.

Treatment and prognosis The syndrome responds poorly to steroid therapy, including intravenous methylprednisolone. Other immunosuppressive drugs are of unproven efficacy, although there is some emerging evidence that plasma exchange may be effective in some patients. The patients are usually left with permanent and severe deficits.

References Devic E. Myelite subaigue compliquee de nevrite optique. *Bulletin of Medicine* 1894; **8**: 1033–1034.

Mandler RN, Davis LE, Jeffery DR, Kornfeld M. Devic's neuromyelitis optica: a clinicopathological study of 8 patients. *Annals of Neurology* 1993; **34**: 162–168.

O'Riordan JI, Gallagher HL, Thompson AJ *et al*. Clinical, CSF, and MRI findings in Devic's neuromyelitis optica. *Journal of Neurology, Neurosurgery and Psychiatry* 1996; **60**: 382–387.

Weinshenker BG. Neuromyelitis optica: what it is and what it might be. *Lancet* 2003; **361**: 889–890.

Wingerchuk DM, Hogancamp WF, O'Brien PC, Weinshenker BG. The clinical course of neuromyelitis optica (Devic's syndrome). *Neurology* 1999; **53**: 1107–1114.

Other relevant entries Acute disseminated encephalomyelitis; Collagen vascular diseases and the nervous system, Cranial nerve disease: II: Optic nerve; Leber's hereditary optic neuropathy; Mitochondrial disease: an overview; Multiple sclerosis; Sarcoidosis; Vasculitis; Vitamin B_{12} deficiency.

■ *De Vivo* disease – see Glucose transporter-deficiency syndrome

■ Diabetes insipidus

Diabetes insipidus (DI) is a syndrome of polyuria and polydipsia resulting from failure of antidiuretic hormone (ADH, vasopressin) production or secretion from the hypothalamo-posterior pituitary axis (central DI) or of renal response to secreted ADH (nephrogenic DI). There is an inability to concentrate the urine (failure to increase urine osmolality to >750 mosmol/l after a water deprivation test), which in the case of central DI may be corrected by exogenous DDAVP; plasma osmolality is high with hypernatraemia.

Most instances of central DI are idiopathic, but various disease processes affecting the hypothalamus and/or posterior pituitary gland may cause DI, including:

Trauma, local surgery.
Local tumours (e.g. craniopharyngioma, pineal tumours).
Inflammatory or granulomatous disease (e.g. sarcoidosis).
Vascular lesions.

Various other syndromes: Froehlich, Wolfram, Friedreich's ataxia, anorexia nervosa, Langerhans cell histiocytosis (LCH).

Reference Baylis PH. Investigation of suspected hypothalamic diabetes insipidus. *Clinical Endocrinology* 1995; **43**: 507–510.

Other relevant entries Craniopharyngioma; Endocrinology and the nervous system; Froehlich's syndrome; Langerhans cell histiocytosis; Pineal tumours; Pituitary disease and apoplexy; Sarcoidosis; Syndrome of inappropriate ADH secretion; Vernant's syndrome; Wolfram syndrome.

■ Diabetes mellitus and the nervous system

Pathophysiology Diabetes mellitus results from a failure either of adequate insulin production from the endocrine pancreas or of end-organ responsiveness to insulin (insulin resistance), with resultant hyperglycaemia, polyuria and polydipsia. Diabetes mellitus may affect both the PNS and CNS. In the PNS hyperglycaemia causes capillary damage with nerve ischaemia, glycosylation of structural nerve proteins, depletion of myoinositol and accumulation of sorbitol and fructose, leading to reduced axonal transport and axonal loss. In the CNS the main consequences of diabetes occur as a result of the aetiological role of hyperglycaemia in atherosclerosis.

Clinical features: history and examination *PNS complications*: 7–80% of patients with diabetes mellitus develop neuropathies but only about a fifth are symptomatic. Neuropathies include:

• Symmetrical polyneuropathies

Distal sensory or sensorimotor polyneuropathy is the most common type of diabetic neuropathy. It is predominantly sensory, producing a glove and stocking sensory loss with some distal weakness and wasting. Two major types of this form of neuropathy exist: one in which large fibres are predominantly involved produces a non-painful loss of joint position sense and vibration perception. The other type affects the small fibres and is often painful, with allodynia, loss of pinprick and temperature sensation and a degree of autonomic involvement. These neuropathies can progress to ulceration and destruction of soft tissue and joints (neuropathic or Charcot's joints); the picture may resemble tabes dorsalis (pseudotabes).

An acute painful neuropathy is occasionally seen after treatment initiation with insulin, so-called insulin-induced neuropathy. This may persist for a number of weeks or months and is thought to represent active axonal degeneration/regeneration.

Diabetic neuropathic cachexia is a condition in which there is an acutely painful diabetic polyneuropathy associated with a sudden and severe weight loss, typically in the context of a depressive illness. It is more common in men, especially when the control of diabetes is poor. Recovery occurs with better control of the blood glucose and weight gain.

- Focal and multifocal neuropathies

  Lumbosacral radiculoplexopathy (diabetic amyotrophy; Brun–Garland syndrome) typically presents in the older non-insulin-dependent diabetic, when it may be the first presentation of their condition. The patient presents with a painful asymmetric weakness and wasting of proximal leg muscles, typically the quadriceps femoris and hip flexors, with loss of the knee jerk. The onset is either abrupt or stepwise and is often seen in conjunction with a distal symmetrical polyneuropathy (so additional loss of ankle jerks). The sensory deficits are mild and recovery is slow (up to 2 years) and incomplete. It is thought to be due to infarction of the proximal nerve roots as they emerge from the spinal canal or in the plexus itself.

  Limb mononeuropathy is usually due to nerve entrapment or infarction. Typically when the nerve infarcts the patient presents with pain and a focal nerve deficit, whereas in entrapment neuropathies the sensorimotor loss occurs more insidiously and without pain. On occasion patients may present with a mononeuritis multiplex.

  Truncal neuropathy/radiculopathy is typically seen in older NIDDM patients and often occurs with the lumbosacral radiculoplexopathy. It presents with a sudden onset of root pain and dysaesthesia in the T4–T12 dermatomes, which spontaneously resolves over several months, but may leave a degree of abdominal wall weakness.

  Cranial neuropathy may occur, involving especially the third, sixth and fourth cranial nerves. Occasionally other cranial nerves can be involved, for example seventh.

- Autonomic neuropathy

  This usually correlates with the severity of the somatic neuropathy and results in orthostatic hypotension, fixed heart rate, delayed gastric emptying and constipation with faecal incontinence, and urinary retention with impotence. The symptoms develop insidiously and this may result in blunted responses to hypoglycaemia. Occasionally sudomotor abnormalities produce distal anhidrosis which may be associated with a compensatory hyperhidrosis including "gustatory sweating", profuse facial sweating following food intake.

CNS complications:

- Cerebrovascular accidents secondary to accelerated atherosclerosis; hypertension secondary to diabetic renal disease may also contribute, as well as embolic phenomena if there has been a history of myocardial infarction.
- Encephalopathy secondary to hyperosmolar states (hyperosmolar non-ketotic syndrome, HONKS) which may be complicated by hemichorea, sagittal sinus thrombosis and rarely focal fits.
- Hypoglycaemic seizures and coma, secondary to excessive treatment.
- Retinopathy.
- There is an association between diabetes and stiff man syndrome; it may also be a feature of Friedreich's ataxia, mitochondrial diseases, myotonic dystrophy, Wolfram syndrome.

- Fungal infection (mucormycosis) may occur in the context of diabetic acidosis.
- A focal amnesic syndrome, sometimes with hippocampal changes on MR brain scanning, may occur with intensive glycaemic control leading to profound hypoglycaemia.

Investigations and diagnosis *Bloods*: to confirm diabetes: fasting glucose >8 mmol/l, random (non-fasting) glucose >11 mmol/l. If results are equivocal, an oral glucose tolerance test may be performed. Glycaemic control may be assessed by measurement of glycosylated haemoglobin (HbA_{1c}).

Neurophysiology: EMG/NCS: typically reveals a mixed axonal-demyelinating polyneuropathy with more sensory than motor involvement and with a predilection for the lower limbs. EMG shows denervation, which is particularly useful in the diagnosis of the lumbosacral radiculoplexopathy.

Nerve biopsy: confirms axonal-demyelinating polyneuropathy, with some inflammatory infiltrate of uncertain significance.

Imaging: CT/MRI may reveal multiple cerebral infarcts.

CSF: may reveal raised protein.

Treatment and prognosis

Optimal control of hyperglycaemia.

Symptomatic treatment of painful neuropathies with either tricyclic antidepressants (amitriptyline) or carbamazepine, gabapentin.

Symptomatic treatment of autonomic neuropathies.

Many patients improve when the above therapies are followed.

There is limited evidence that some cases of diabetic amyotrophy have a diabetes-related vasculitic origin and that immunotherapies, such as intravenous immunoglobulin (IVIg), may have a therapeutic role.

References Said G. Diabetic neuropathy: an update. *Journal of Neurology* 1996; **243**: 431–440.

Thomas PK, Tomlinson DR. Diabetic and hypoglycemic neuropathies. In: Dyck PJ, Thomas PK, Griffin JW, Low PA, Podulso JF (eds). *Peripheral Neuropathy* (3rd edition). Philadelphia: WB Saunders, 1995: 1219–1250.

Other relevant entries Amnesia, amnesic syndrome; Autonomic failure; Bell's palsy; Cerebrovascular disease: arterial; Cerebrovascular disease: venous; Cranial nerve disease: III: Oculomotor nerve; Cranial nerve disease: VI: Abducens nerve; Entrapment neuropathies; Mononeuritis multiplex, Mononeuropathy multiplex; Mucormycosis.

■ Dialysis syndromes

There are a number of conditions associated with dialysis for renal failure:

- Dialysis disequilibrium syndrome: this presents acutely either during or immediately after dialysis with features of cerebral irritation (headache, irritability, disorientation, agitation, somnolence and generalized tonic–clonic seizures), and muscle cramps, tremor, nausea, and vomiting; exophthalmos may occur. It is probably due to cerebral oedema, as the urea concentration within the brain remains much higher than that in the blood during rapid dialysis. Characteristically the EEG shows slowing and there is raised opening pressure on lumbar puncture.

- Dialysis dementia syndrome: now very rare, this syndrome used to be seen in chronic dialysis patients and is thought to be related to aluminium in the dialysate; the reduction of aluminium in the dialysate fluids has greatly reduced the incidence of this condition. Clinically, patients develop hesitant speech and even speech arrest, which progresses to cognitive decline with delusions, hallucinations, fits, myoclonus, asterixis, and gait abnormalities. The EEG shows slowing with multifocal bursts of more profound slowing and spikes. Patients typically die within 6–12 months. There is evidence that aluminium plays a role in the development of Alzheimer's disease-like paired helical filaments in exposed subjects.

- Wernicke's encephalopathy: probably related to nutritional deficiencies (especially protein intake).

- Carpal tunnel syndrome: due to ischaemia/venous congestion or amyloidosis.

Reference Harrington CR, Wischik CM, McArthur FK, Taylor GA, Edwardson JA, Candy JM. Alzheimer's-disease-like changes in tau protein processing: association with aluminium accumulation in brains of renal dialysis patients. *Lancet* 1994; **343**: 993–997.

Other relevant entries Alzheimer's disease; Carpal tunnel syndrome; Dementia: an overview; Renal disease and the nervous system; Wernicke–Korsakoff's syndrome.

■ Diaphragmatic flutter – see Leeuwenhoek's disease

■ Diastematomyelia
Split notochord syndrome

Diastematomyelia is a congenital malformation of the spinal cord such that there is sagittal division of part of the cord into two hemicords, usually in the lower thoracic or lumbar region. Usually there is a bony or cartilaginous spur and dura in the cleft between the two parts of the cord and to which the cords are tethered, and often there are overlying skin abnormalities. It may occur in the context of congenital atlanto-axial dislocation. Although often asymptomatic, neurological dysfunction (lower limbs, sphincters) may develop in adolescence or adulthood, and may be progressive. MR imaging confirms the diagnosis. Surgical attempts to untether the cord may be undertaken.

Other relevant entries Achondroplasia; Atlantoaxial dislocation, subluxation; Tethered cord syndrome.

■ DIDMOAD syndrome – see Wolfram syndrome

■ Diencephalic epilepsy – see Shapiro syndrome; Spontaneous periodic hypothermia

■ Diencephalic syndrome
Russell's syndrome

The diencephalic syndrome, also known as Russell's syndrome, is a rare condition of children, usually below the age of 3 years, in which there is progressive emaciation and failure to thrive despite adequate food intake. In addition there may also be pallor (but no anaemia), motor hyperactivity, euphoria, vomiting, excessive sweating, and optic atrophy with nystagmus. MRI shows an anterior hypothalamic mass lesion, usually a low-grade astrocytoma. There may also be raised plasma levels of growth hormone and CSF levels of β-HCG.

Other relevant entries Eating disorders; Endocrinology and the nervous system; Hypothalamic disease: an overview.

■ Diffuse idiopathic skeletal hyperostosis
Ankylosing hyperostosis • Forestier's disease

Excessive calcification along the lateral and anterior portions of the vertebral bodies without loss of disc height may be asymptomatic, or may cause back pain and limited spinal movement. Myelopathy may rarely develop if calcification is present within the spinal canal. Diffuse idiopathic skeletal hyperostosis (DISH) may predispose to spinal fracture after relatively minor trauma.

Other relevant entries Ankylosing spondylitis and the nervous system; Myelopathy: an overview; Ossification of the posterior longitudinal ligament.

■ Diffuse Lewy body disease – see Dementia with Lewy bodies; Lewy body disease: an overview

■ Diffuse sclerosis – see Canavan's disease; Schilder's disease

■ DiMauro syndrome – see Carnitine palmit(o)yltransferase deficiency

■ Diogenes syndrome

Diogenes of Sinope (*ca.* 412–323 BC), not to be confused with Diogenes of Apollonia (*fl.* fifth century BC) and Diogenes Laertius (*fl.* second century AD), was a cofounder of the Cynic school of philosophy in Athens, and was noted for his austere asceticism and self-sufficiency and his disregard for domestic comforts: he lived in a barrel or tub. Hence, the term Diogenes syndrome was coined to refer to a syndrome characterized by severe self-neglect, domestic squalor, hoarding behaviour, and social withdrawal. Most patients are elderly, single or living alone, of average or above average intelligence, and often with a good income (i.e. the condition is not the result of poverty). A distinction is drawn between primary Diogenes syndrome, when it is unrelated to any mental illness (50–70%), and secondary when it is related to depression, schizophrenia, dementia (particularly of frontotemporal type) or alcoholism. There may be concurrent physical illness, indeed this may prompt admission to hospital. Management is often difficult because of patients' refusal to cooperate, perhaps a reflection of the suspicious, quarrelsome and even aggressive traits associated with the syndrome. Treatment of underlying mental and physical illness, involvement of social worker/health visitor or nurse, and attendance at a day centre to develop a social network may help, but long-term outlook is generally poor ("relapse", death).

Reference Clarke ANG, Manikar GO, Gray I. Diogenes syndrome. A clinical study of gross neglect in old age. *Lancet* 1975; **i**: 366–368.

Other relevant entries Frontotemporal dementia; Psychiatric disorders and neurological disease.

■ Diphtheria

Pathophysiology Diphtheria is an acute infectious disease, now very rare in the developed world since the introduction of widespread vaccination, but still encountered in the underdeveloped world. It is caused by the organism *Corynebacterium diphtheriae*, the effects of which may be local or, more seriously, remote, the latter due to the production of a pathogenic exotoxin. Toxigenic *Corynebacterium diphtheriae* causes neurological illness by inhibiting protein synthesis through ADP ribosylation and inactivation of ribosomal GTPase by toxin subunit A. This produces a gradual onset of bulbar palsy followed by a demyelinating neuropathy, with full recovery over a similar time period.

Clinical features: history and examination

- Initial infection may be asymptomatic, or symptomatic with malaise, irritability, anorexia, headache, arthralgia.
- Primary infection may be faucial, cutaneous, vaginal, or, in neonates, umbilical.

    Primary (faucial) infection: inflamed throat with patchy white exudate and membrane, +/− cervical lymphadenopathy ("bull neck") after incubation period of 2–6 days.

    Secondary toxic features – early local: after 3–6 weeks, bulbar problems: palatal paralysis, lower cranial neuropathies but facial weakness rare (*cf.* Guillain–Barré syndrome).

- Autonomic (myelinated parasympathetic) involvement can produce blurred vision (bilateral ciliary paralysis with loss of accommodation), impaired pupillary reactions, and vagal block, 3–4 weeks into the illness. Cardiomyopathy with congestive cardiac failure, arrhythmias and death may occur without appropriate supportive therapy.

- *Secondary toxic features – late remote*: after around 8 weeks, following haematoge-nous dissemination, a generalized sensorimotor demyelinating peripheral neur-opathy develops with a proximal to distal spread of weakness (*cf.* Guillain–Barré syndrome). There may be additional oculomotor nerve palsy and phrenic nerve palsy. The severity of the neuropathy varies from sensory symptoms to a severe large fibre sensory neuropathy (the so-called diphtheritic pseudotabes) with inability to walk and the need for ventilatory support.
- Rarely infection is localized to the skin (primary cutaneous diphtheria) in which case there is an anaesthetic zone around the skin ulcer +/− muscle weakness in the surrounding muscles. In just under 50% of such cases the patient goes on to develop more generalized disease.
- Central nervous system (CNS) involvement in diphtheria has only rarely been described and in these cases a vascular origin, secondary to the cardiomyopathy, is the most likely explanation.

Investigations and diagnosis *Bloods*: typically unhelpful, apart from pointing towards an infective process. Throat swabs can be taken but special media are required to culture the organism.

Neurophysiology: EMG/NCS are normal in the early stages of the illness, but after 4 weeks a demyelinating peripheral neuropathy with features similar to Guillain–Barré syndrome is found.

Imaging: not usually helpful, although CXR may reveal cardiomegaly in cases of cardiac involvement.

CSF: usually normal except in severe cases when there is an elevated white cell count and protein level. In the case of the delayed neuropathy the protein is typically raised.

Nerve biopsy: shows a demyelinating neuropathy.

Differential diagnosis

Guillain–Barré syndrome/CIDP in the case of the delayed neuropathy.

Botulism.

Brainstem lesion/demyelination.

Basal meningitis (infective/inflammatory/malignant).

Myasthenia gravis.

Polymyositis.

Treatment and prognosis Prevention is the primary aim, with diphtheria toxoid given in childhood as part of the triple vaccination. Booster shots of the toxoid should be given every 10 years.

In the established case, antitoxin should be given as soon as possible within the first 48 hours (although this can produce anaphylactic reactions). Antitoxin reduces the incidence and severity of the neuropathic complications.

Antibiotics should be given (penicillin or erythromycin) even when the effect of the toxin is apparent.

Supportive therapy may be required once neurological features occur, and this may include ventilatory support.

Only very occasionally have patients been described having more than one attack of diphtheria.

References McAuley JH, Fearnley J, Laurence A, Ball JA. Diphtheritic neuropathy. *Journal of Neurology, Neurosurgery and Psychiatry* 1999; **67**: 825–826.

McDonald WI, Kocen RS. Diphtheritic neuropathy. In: Dyck PJ, Thomas PK, Griffin JW, Low PA, Podulso JF (eds). *Peripheral Neuropathy* (3rd edition). Philadelphia: WB Saunders, 1995: 1412–1417.

Other relevant entries Autonomic failure; Guillain–Barré syndrome; Neuropathies: an overview.

Diphyllobothriasis

Infection with the cestode fish tapeworm *Diphyllobothrium latus* from ingestion of undercooked fish can lead to vitamin B_{12} deficiency with the haematological and neurological consequences thereof due to absorption of this vitamin by the parasite.

Other relevant entries Helminthic diseases; Vitamin B_{12} deficiency.

Discitis

Discitis is an inflammatory, usually infective, process affecting the intervertebral discs, with sparing of the vertebral body (although the discovertebral junction may be affected). The process may also spread to the epidural space and paraspinal soft tissues producing neurological features. The clinical picture is one of severe localized back pain, with fever, with or without neurological signs which may be radicular, meningeal, or myelopathic. There may be a history of recent instrumentation of the spine (e.g. epidural anaesthesia) or evidence for underlying immunosuppression. Bloods may show a raised ESR. Imaging with plain radiographs may suggest the diagnosis but MRI is the investigation of choice. Commonly encountered organisms are staphylococci, salmonella, and *Mycobacterium tuberculosis*. Direct biopsy may be required to establish the microbiological diagnosis and decide on appropriate antibiotic therapy. Clinical outcome is usually good.

Reference Hopkinson N, Stevenson J, Benjamin S. A case ascertainment study of septic discitis: clinical, microbiological and radiological features. *Quarterly Journal of Medicine* 2001; **94**: 465–470.

Disconnection syndromes
Disconnexion syndromes

Pathophysiology As the name implies, disconnection syndromes are conditions in which there is an interruption of inter- and intrahemispheral fibre tracts. This concept was originally put forward in the 1890s but was taken up and modernized by Norman Geschwind in the 1960s. The disconnection syndromes essentially fall into either those resulting from interruption of fibres within the corpus callosum or commissures (interhemispheric disconnection syndromes) or of fibres within a hemisphere (intra-hemispheric disconnection syndromes). The former is most graphically seen with "split-brain" patients, whilst the latter syndromes are best described in the domain of language.

Clinical features: history and examination

- Interhemispheric disconnection

  Complete, for example tumour or surgical section of the corpus callosum

  A blindfolded patient can correctly name objects placed in the right hand, but not those in left, and objects in the left hemifield cannot be named or matched to a similar object in the right hemifield.

  Posterior callosal section (at splenium; e.g. left posterior cerebral artery occlusion)

  Cannot read or name colours, as information cannot pass to the left hemispheric language areas.

  Copying of words and writing, both spontaneously and to dictation, is intact as the information passes to the left hemisphere anterior to the site of damage.

- Intrahemispheric disconnection syndromes

  Conduction aphasia

  The patient has fluent but paraphasic speech and writing, with greatly impaired repetition despite relatively normal comprehension of the spoken and written word. This is traditionally explained as due to a lesion in the arcuate fasciculus.

  Ideomotor apraxia in Broca's aphasia

  An apraxia of left hand movements to command. It is due to lesions disconnecting the cortical motor areas anterior to the primary motor cortex.

  Pure word deafness

  Patients are able to hear and identify non-verbal sounds but unable to understand spoken language. It is due to a lesion in the white matter of the left temporal lobe which isolates Wernicke's area from the auditory cortex.

Speculations that unusual delusional syndromes (Capgras', Cotard's) are also disconnection syndromes have also been advanced.

Investigations and diagnosis *Imaging*: may disclose structural cause for disconnection (stroke, tumour).

Treatment and prognosis Of underlying cause.

References Absher JR, Benson DF. Disconnection syndromes: an overview of Geschwind's contributions. *Neurology* 1993; **43**: 862–867.

Geschwind N. Disconnexion syndromes in animals and man. *Brain* 1965; **88**: 237–294; 585–644.

Other relevant entries Aphasia; Apraxia; Balint syndrome; Capgras' syndrome; Cerebrovascular disease: arterial; Cotard's syndrome; Marchiafava–Bignami syndrome; Tumours: an overview.

■ Disinhibition–dementia–parkinsonism–amyotrophy complex

Disinhibition–dementia–parkinsonism–amyotrophy complex (DDPAC) is a form of frontotemporal dementia with parkinsonism linked to chromosome 17 caused by mutations within the τ-gene.

Reference Lendon CL, Lynch T, Norton J *et al.* Hereditary dysphasic disinhibition dementia. *Neurology* 1998; **50**: 1546–1555.

Other relevant entries Dementia: an overview; Tauopathy.

■ Dissection – see Carotid artery disease; Ehlers–Danlos syndrome; Vertebral artery dissection

■ Disseminated sclerosis – see Multiple sclerosis

■ Distal muscular dystrophy, distal myopathy

In distal muscular dystrophy, muscle wasting and weakness are predominantly distal. A number of variants are recognized on the basis of their age of onset, clinical features, and inheritance pattern.

- Late-adult onset (>40 years)
    Type 1: autosomal-dominant, Welander's disease.
    Type 2: autosomal-dominant, Markesbery–Griggs/Udd disease.
- Early-adult onset (<30 years)
    Type 1: autosomal-recessive, Nonaka type.
    Type 2: autosomal-recessive, Miyoshi type (dysferlinopathy).
    Type 3: autosomal-dominant, Laing type.

Other myopathies which may manifest with predominantly distal weakness and which need to be differentiated from distal muscular dystrophies include:

- dystrophia myotonica;
- desmin myopathy;
- facioscapulohumeral (FSH) muscular dystrophy, scapuloperoneal myopathy;
- inclusion body myositis/myopathy (IBM);
- metabolic myopathies: acid-maltase deficiency, debrancher deficiency;
- congenital myopathies: central core, nemaline;
- occasionally myasthenic limb weakness may be predominantly distal.

Neuropathies and neuronopathies may present with isolated distal weakness, for example Charcot–Marie–Tooth, distal spinal muscular atrophy, motor neuropathies (e.g. porphyria).

References Illa I. Distal myopathies. *Journal of Neurology* 2000; **247**: 169–174.

Udd B, Griggs R. Distal myopathies. *Current Opinion in Neurology* 2001; **14**: 561–566.

Other relevant entries Desmin myopathy, Desminopathy; Dysferlinopathy; Miyoshi myopathy; Muscular dystrophies: an overview; Myasthenia gravis; Myopathy: an overview; Nonaka myopathy; Proximal weakness.

▓ DNET – see Dysembryoplastic neuroepithelial tumours

▓ Dolichoectasia

Dolichoectasia describes the presence of dilated, elongated or tortuous intracranial arteries (vertebrobasilar, carotid, or both) with or without thrombus or calcification (there are no specific diagnostic criteria). Dolichoectasia may cause brain infarction by thrombosis, embolism, stenosis, or occlusion of deep penetrating arteries. There may be a combination of focal brainstem findings (e.g. sixth nerve palsy) due to local compression from a dilated vessel, and embolic cerebral hemisphere events. The most common cause is atherosclerosis, but dolichoectasia has been noted in Fabry's disease.

A retrospective study of nearly 400 cases of first cerebral infarction identified dolichoectasia on CT or MRI in 3% of patients, the majority in the vertebrobasilar circulation. These patients were more likely to have a lacunar pattern of infarction, and a better rate of survival but higher rate of recurrence. Anticoagulation with warfarin may have a place in the management of some of these cases, although no controlled trials have been performed.

References Ince B, Petty GW, Brown Jr RD, Chu C-P, Sicks JD, Whisnant JP. Dolichoectasia of the intracranial arteries in patients with first ischemic stroke: a population-based study. *Neurology* 1998; **50**: 1694–1698.

Sacks JG, Lindenberg R. Dolicho-ectatic intracranial arteries. Symptomatology and pathogenesis of arterial elongation and distension. *Johns Hopkins Medical Journal* 1969; **125**: 95–106.

Other relevant entries Cerebrovascular disease: arterial; Fabry's disease.

▓ Domoic acid poisoning
Amnesic shellfish poisoning

An outbreak of poisoning with domoic acid following ingestion of mussels infested with the phytoplankton *Nitzschia pungens* occurred in Prince Edward Island, Canada, in 1987. Domoic acid acts as an excitotoxin, binding to kainate receptors. Patients presented within hours of eating mussels with diarrhoea, vomiting, abdominal cramps, with or without headaches. Other features included delirium, seizures, myoclonus, ataxia, alternating hemiparesis, and complete external opthalmoplegia. EEG showed slowing in the acute stages and PET scanning showed reduced perfusion of the amygdala and hippocampus. Limited autopsy studies show cell loss and astrocytosis in the amygdala and hippocampus. Treatment of the acute illness is supportive and symptomatic, diazepam and phenobarbitone being useful for seizures. Gradual and spontaneous recovery occurs over 3 months but there may be residual anterograde amnesia, temporal lobe epilepsy, motor neuronopathy or sensorimotor axonal neuropathy. The diagnosis can be made using a mouse bioassay for the toxin, although the condition is no longer seen in Canada as shellfish are now screened for the toxin.

> **Reference** Perl TM, Bedard L, Kosatsky T *et al*. An outbreak of toxic encephalopathy caused by eating mussels contaminated with domoic acid. *New England Journal of Medicine* 1990; **322**: 1775–1780.

■ Doose syndrome
Epilepsy with myoclonic-astatic seizures

An idiopathic generalized epilepsy of childhood, in which previously normal children develop myoclonic–astatic seizures which often occur with atonic, myoclonic, and absence seizures; non-convulsive status epilepticus is common. By definition, all tests other than the EEG are normal, hence differentiating Doose syndrome from other syndromes such as Lennox–Gastaut, West, and Dravet, and the progressive myoclonic epilepsies. Drug therapy is determined by the predominant seizure type, sodium valproate is probably most efficacious, with or without lamotrigine.

> **Reference** Panayiotopoulos CP. *A Clinical Guide to Epileptic Syndromes and Their Treatment: Based on the New ILAE Diagnostic Scheme*. Chipping Norton: Bladon, 2002: 124–129.

> **Other relevant entries** Epilepsy: an overview; Progressive myoclonic epilepsy.

■ Dopamine-β-hydroxylase deficiency

A rare inborn error of metabolism, presenting with autonomic dysfunction. Dopamine-β-hydroxylase synthesizes noradrenaline from dopamine; its deficiency leads to virtual absence of circulating noradrenaline and adrenaline. Clinically there is postural hypotension and partial ptosis, but sweating, bladder function, and cognitive function are preserved.

> **Reference** Mathias CJ, Bannister R. Dopamine-β-hydroxylase deficiency – with a note on other genetically determined causes of autonomic failure. In: Mathias CJ, Bannister R (eds). *Autonomic Failure. A Textbook of Clinical Disorders of the Autonomic Nervous System* (4th edition). Oxford: OUP, 1999: 387–401.

> **Other relevant entry** Autonomic failure.

■ Dopa-responsive dystonia
DYT5 ● Hereditary dystonia with marked diurnal fluctuations ● Segawa syndrome

Pathophysiology This rare dystonic condition usually presents before the age of 10 years and is commoner in females (F : M = 2 : 1). It shows autosomal-dominant inheritance with variable penetrance and is linked to chromosome 14q22.1–q22.2.

It has been shown to result from mutations in the gene encoding GTP cyclohydrolase I (GTPCH I) which is responsible for the synthesis of tetrahydrobiopterin, an essential cofactor for a number of enzymes, including tyrosine hydroxylase which is the first enzyme in the synthetic pathway of dopamine. There is therefore a functional dopamine denervation but, unlike the situation in Parkinson's disease, without anatomical loss of the dopaminergic neurones in the nigrostriatal tract. DRD is exquisitely sensitive to small doses of levodopa and, again unlike the situation in PD, response fluctuations generally do not develop over time. For these reasons, it is advocated that all children with dystonia of unknown cause, or "dystonic cerebral palsy", should be given an adequate trial of levodopa.

Clinical features: history and examination

- Dystonic posturing; initially of foot, spreads eventually to all limbs. May be associated with a tremor, postural retrocollis, and hyperreflexia with a striatal toe; pyramidal signs and spasticity may be present in addition to the extrapyramidal features. The patients typically complain of difficulty walking and of falls.
- Cognitive impairment and seizures do not occur.
- In many (but not all cases) the dystonia shows diurnal variation, at its best in the morning and worsening during the day or with exertion; if present, this historical point is highly suggestive of DRD.
- In some family members disease manifests with adult-onset parkinsonism or a tremor.

Investigations and diagnosis *Imaging*: normal brain

CSF: reduced dopamine metabolites and tetrahydrobiopterin; these tests now superseded by neurogenetics.

Neurogenetics: for mutations in GTP cyclohydrolase I gene: deletion, point mutation. Therapeutic response to levodopa.

Differential diagnosis May be misdiagnosed as cerebral palsy of athetoid or spastic diplegic type, or hereditary spastic paraparesis.

Treatment and prognosis There is a dramatic and sustained improvement with low dose levodopa (100–300 mg/day), without the development of response fluctuations or the loss of efficacy.

DRD progresses until the age of 20 years, then stabilizes or improves and may be inapparent after the fourth decade.

Reference Ichinose H, Ohye T, Takahashi E *et al*. Hereditary progressive dystonia with marked diurnal fluctuations caused by mutations in the GTP cyclohydrolase I gene. *Nature Genetics* 1994; **8**: 236–242.

Other relevant entries Cerebral palsy, cerebral palsy syndromes; Dystonia: an overview.

▪ Dorsal midbrain syndrome – see Parinaud's syndrome

▪ Double cortex syndrome – see Heterotopia

■ Down's syndrome
Mongolism ● Trisomy 21

This common chromosomal dysgenesis, due to either a triplication of chromosome 21 or a translocation, is usually easily recognized clinically because of its morphological features.

Round head, palpebral fissures slanting upwards and outwards ("mongoloid slant"), medial epicanthi, low set ears, hypoplastic maxilla, macroglossia, Brushfield spots, palmar simian crease, short stature.

Neurologically there is learning disability which may range from mild to severe. Congenital heart disease is a feature, which may lead to embolic strokes or brain abscesses. Atlanto-axial anomalies may lead to spinal cord compression. There is an increased incidence of hypothyroidism in children with Down's syndrome. With age, all Down's syndrome patients develop the typical neuropathological changes of Alzheimer's disease, presumably due to overexpression of the amyloid precursor protein (APP) gene on chromosome 21 and hence production of amyloid β-peptide, and many will also have progressive cognitive deficits. Seizures may also be a feature.

Reference Berg JM, Karlinsky H, Holland AJ (eds). *Alzheimer Disease, Down Syndrome and Their Relationship*. Oxford: OUP, 1993.

Other relevant entry Alzheimer's disease.

■ Dracunculiasis

Infection with the nematode Guinea worm *Dracunculus medinensis* through ingestion of infected water (Africa, Arabia, Asia) can lead to burning dysaesthesia at the ulcer site where the female worm emerges after migrating through the subcutaneous tissues; compressive mononeuropathy may result. Up to 120 cm in length, these worms can cause periorbital and spinal epidural abscesses, as well as peripheral nerve thickening.

Other relevant entry Helminthic diseases.

■ Dravet syndrome
Severe myoclonic epilepsy in infancy

This rare progressive epileptic encephalopathy, commoner in boys, and usually beginning before the age of 3 years, is characterized by:

early infantile clonic febrile convulsions,
myoclonic jerks,
atypical absences,
complex partial seizures.

After a mild period with seizures occurring only during febrile periods, there is a "seismic" phase of relentless seizures with, if survived, residual mental and neurological abnormalities. Control of seizures with anti-epileptic drugs is not usually possible. No underlying metabolic abnormality has been identified.

Reference Panayiotopoulos CP. *A Clinical Guide to Epileptic Syndromes and Their Treatment: Based on the New ILAE Diagnostic Scheme.* Chipping Norton: Bladon, 2002: 63–66.

Other relevant entry Epilepsy: an overview.

■ Drop attacks

Pathophysiology Drop attacks may be defined as sudden falls with or without a loss of consciousness: the term has also been used to describe sudden falls without warning secondary to either a transient ischaemic attack or intracranial tumour in the third ventricle or posterior fossa. Drop attacks may be due to a loss of muscle tone (atonic attacks) or abnormal muscle contraction (tonic drops), although in clinical practice it is difficult to distinguish these two conditions. A large number of conditions are associated with drop attacks of which the commonest causes are cardiac arrhythmias. However the majority of patients do not yield to a diagnosis after thorough investigation. Such idiopathic drop attacks are commoner in the elderly, and have sometimes been labelled as due to "cerebrovascular insufficiency" although there is no particular evidence to support such a pathogenesis.

Recognized causes of drop attacks include:

- Symptomatic drop attacks (20–30%)

  Syncope

  Cardiac arrhythmias, including Stokes–Adams attacks.

  Postural hypotension and vasovagal attacks: always have preceding symptoms. These episodes may include convulsive syncope where a patient who has fainted exhibits tonic–clonic movements which are not epileptic. This is especially associated with breath-holding attacks in children, prolonged QT syndromes, blood donation, and trigeminal neuralgia.

  Congenital cyanotic heart disease.

  Epilepsy

  Lennox–Gastaut syndrome, infantile spasms, and occasionally juvenile myoclonic epilepsy.

  Complex partial seizures of frontal or temporal lobe origin.

  Myoclonic jerks

  Post-hypoxic action myoclonus and progressive myoclonic epilepsy syndromes.

  Transient ischaemic attacks (TIA)

  Bilateral anterior cerebral artery ischaemia which is usually secondary to carotid artery disease.

  Vertebrobasilar ischaemia which may be precipitated by certain head movements in patients with degenerative cervical spine disease. There may be no warning in such attacks, but often the patient complains of other posterior circulation TIA symptoms.

Peripheral vestibular disorder

Ménière's disease, including Tumarkin's otolithic crisis, where there is sudden falling without vertigo.

Startle reactions

Exaggerated normal physiological startle reaction.

Hyperekplexia.

Stiff man syndrome.

Cataplexy, typically with narcolepsy

Paroxysmal kinesigenic choreoathetosis

Structural lesions of the central nervous system (CNS)

Brainstem and posterior fossa lesions: tumour, arachnoid cyst, Chiari malformation, odontoid process fracture.

Cerebral hemisphere lesions such as frontal lobe tumours.

Hydrocephalus

Normal pressure hydrocephalus.

Obstructive hydrocephalus due to third ventricular colloid cysts or meningioma, fourth ventricular ependymoma and aqueduct stenosis.

Neurodegenerative disorders

Alzheimer's disease, Parkinson's disease, progressive supranuclear palsy, Huntington's disease, multiple system atrophy, corticobasal degeneration.

Neuromuscular

Muscle disease, myasthenia gravis, neuropathy, myelopathy and intermittent spinal ischaemia.

Psychogenic attacks.

Prognosis with symptomatic drop attacks is dictated by the coexistent medical condition, and thus is poorest in patients with cardiac disease.

- Idiopathic drop attacks (60–70%)

Typically these attacks first occur in patients between the ages of 40 and 60 years, and increase with advancing age. Some, but not all, studies find the condition to be commoner in middle-aged females. Patients typically collapse to the ground with no impairment of consciousness and get up immediately with no sequelae. More than 90% of such patients have recurrent attacks (on average 2–12 per year), but the remission rate is not known accurately, figures vary from 25% to 80%, depending on the study.

Patients with idiopathic drop attacks usually suffer only minor injuries and have a favourable prognosis with no increased risk of stroke or death compared to an age- and sex-matched population. However in older patients the drop attacks cause more serious injuries including fractures of the femur.

No symptomatic treatment is available to patients with idiopathic drop attacks.

Investigations and diagnosis *Bloods*: FBC, ESR, U&E, glucose, LFTs, lipids. Additional tests may be requested if a specific symptomatic cause is suspected.

Imaging: CXR, CT/MRI brain. May need to consider magnetic resonance angiography (MRA), catheter angiography, or myelography depending on suspected cause.

CSF: not usually necessary.

Neurophysiology: EEG; may need ambulatory EEG recordings +/- telemetry.

Other investigations: ECG, 24-hour ECG, echocardiography; neuro-otological assessment.

Reference Meissner I, Wiebers DO, Swanson JW, O'Fallon WM. The natural history of drop attacks. *Neurology* 1986; **36**: 1029–1034.

Other relevant entries Autonomic failure; Cataplexy; Cerebrovascular disease: arterial; Epilepsy: an overview; Hydrocephalus; Hyperekplexia; Ménière's disease; Myoclonus; Parkinsonian syndromes, parkinsonism; Progressive myoclonic epilepsy; Progressive supranuclear palsy; Prolonged QT syndromes; Syncope; Tumarkin's otolithic crisis; Tumours: an overview; Vertigo.

▓ Dropped head syndrome

Floppy head syndrome • Suarez–Kelly syndrome

This is a disorder in which there is weakness of neck extension, such that the head may fall forward onto the chest. This may occur in a number of disorders such as myasthenia gravis, motor neurone disease, inflammatory myopathies, facioscapulo-humeral muscular dystrophy, inflammatory neuropathies (GBS, CIDP) and carnitine deficiency. A rare isolated neck extensor myopathy has been described in middle-aged to elderly people, which may on occasion be responsive to corticosteroids. Dropped head syndrome may be related to the "bent spine syndrome" or camptocormia.

References Katz JS, Wolfe GI, Burns DK, Bryan WW, Fleckenstein JL, Barohn RJ. Isolated neck extensor myopathy. A common cause of dropped head syndrome. *Neurology* 1996; 46: 917–921.

Lange DJ, Fetell MR, Lovelace RE, Rowland LP. The floppy head syndrome. *Annals of Neurology* 1986; **20**: 133 (abstract P37).

Other relevant entry Camptocormia.

▓ Drug-induced encephalopathies

Drug overdose is very common and a number of agents when taken in high dose may induce an encephalopathy. Drugs may also cause decompensation in other causes of encephalopathy (e.g. hepatic encephalopathy).

Some of the commoner drug-induced encephalopathies are:

• Ethanol

Blood alcohol levels can be checked acutely if diagnosis is clinically uncertain. Patients need to be monitored for aspiration and hypoglycaemia.

If admitted to hospital, may later develop withdrawal-related symptoms.

- Benzodiazepines (BDZs)

   May cause profound respiratory depression.

   If suspected, flumazenil, a BDZ-receptor antagonist, may be tried; its half-life is shorter than that of most BDZs, so repeated doses may be needed.

- Paracetamol (acetaminophen)

   Impaired consciousness is not a feature early after overdose unless paracetamol is combined with another central nervous system (CNS) depressant, for example dextropropoxyphene (Distalgesic).

   Paracetamol hepatotoxicity leading to hepatocellular necrosis, failure, and encephalopathy is not usually evident until the 3rd to 5th day after overdose; early administration of sulphydryl donors such as cysteamine prevents hepatocellular damage. For late presentation, full supportive care may lead to survival. Liver transplantation may also be considered.

- Salicylates (aspirin)

   Level can be checked.

   Usual symptoms of salicylate poisoning are hyperventilation, tinnitus, deafness, vasodilatation and sweating. CNS depression (delirium, agitation, confusion, coma, convulsions) is more commonly seen in children; in adults it implies a huge overdose and carries a grave prognosis.

- Barbiturates

   Blood levels can be checked.

   May cause profound respiratory depression, hypotension and hypothermia in addition to drowsiness, ataxia, dysarthria, and coma.

   Skin blistering may occur.

- Tricyclic antidepressants (TCADs)

   May cause cardiac arrhythmias, hypotension, dry mouth, hyperreflexia, extensor plantar responses, convulsions, respiratory failure and occasionally dilated pupils and urinary retention (anticholinergic effects).

   The encephalopathy may be complicated by a metabolic acidosis.

- Opiates

   May cause pinpoint pupils and respiratory depression.

   If suspected, naloxone, an opiate-receptor antagonist, may be tried.

- Lithium

   Typically overdose with lithium induces nausea, vomiting and diarrhoea, with later CNS effects: increased muscle tone, myoclonus, which may progress to convulsions, coma, hypotension, and renal failure.

- Recreational drugs/illicit drugs

   Amphetamines

      CNS stimulation: wakefulness, hyperactivity, paranoia, hallucinations and hypertension followed by exhaustion, seizures, hyperthermia, cardiac arrhythmias, and coma.

   "Ecstasy" (MDMA; 3,4-methylenedioxymethamphetamine)

      Hyperpyrexia, seizures, intracerebral haemorrhage.

Cocaine

May cause agitation, dilated pupils, tachycardia, hypertension, hallucinations, hypertonia and hyperreflexia followed by coma, convulsions and metabolic acidosis.

- Organophosphate/carbamate poisoning (insecticides)

Cholinesterase inhibition may cause anxiety, restlessness, dizziness, headache, miosis, nausea, hypersalivation, vomiting, abdominal colic, diarrhoea, bradycardia and sweating; may progress to muscle weakness and fasciculations, flaccid paralysis, seizures, coma and pulmonary oedema +/− hyperglycaemia.

Treatment is supportive with the administration of atropine +/− pralidoxime mesylate.

Reference Proudfoot A. *Diagnosis and Management of Acute Poisoning*. Oxford: Blackwell, 1982.

Other relevant entries Alcohol and the nervous system: an overview; Brainstem vascular syndromes; Cerebrovascular disease: arterial; Cocaine; Coma; Encephalitis: an overview; Encephalopathies: an overview, Epilepsy: an overview; Hepatic encephalopathy.

■ Drug-induced movement disorders

A large number of drugs may induce movement disorders. Many of the drug-induced movement disorders are predictable in terms of known drug pharmacology, typically affecting the dopaminergic network. However in some cases the drugs act peripherally, typically with tremor. In other instances the pathogenetic mechanism is not known. This entry summarizes proven associations and gives details of treatment where necessary.

- Postural tremor

May be induced by agents enhancing physiological tremor via peripheral β_2 adrenoreceptors:

Sympathomimetics
Tricyclic antidepressants
Amphetamines
Lithium
Bronchodilators
Sodium valproate
Levodopa
Hypoglycaemic agents
Caffeine
Corticosteroids
Thyroxine
Alcohol withdrawal
(amiodarone; ciclosporin A: uncommon).

Drug withdrawal ameliorates tremor.

- Acute dystonic reactions

    May be induced by dopaminergic blockers; those with stronger anticholinergic activity are less likely to do so, suggesting that excessive cholinergic activity may be involved in pathogenesis, as well as dopaminergic mechanisms:

    > Metoclopramide
    > Neuroleptics (anti-psychotic drugs)
    > (Anti-malarials: uncommon).

    Typically the patients develop dystonia within hours to days of starting therapy. Typically there is involvement of cranial, nuchal and axial muscles (e.g. oculogyric crisis, opisthotonos, retrocollis, torticollis). It lasts from a few seconds up to 48 hours and may be aborted by giving benztropine (1–2 mg intravenously) or procyclidine (5 mg i.v.) and oral anticholinergics given for 2–3 days to prevent recurrences.

- Akathisia

    May be induced by dopamine antagonists (and also seen in Parkinson's disease):

    > Neuroleptics (anti-psychotic drugs)
    > Metoclopramide
    > Reserpine
    > Tetrabenazine
    > (SSRIs, L-dopa and dopamine agonists: uncommon.)

    Akathisia usually develops within a few days of either starting the drug or increasing the dose of it. Occasionally it can take months to appear (tardive akathisia). Usually subsides on stopping therapy, but occasionally does not. It may respond to anticholinergics, amantadine, β-blockers and opiate-like drugs.

- Parkinsonism

    > Neuroleptics (anti-psychotic drugs)
    > Metoclopramide
    > Catecholamine depletors (reserpine, tetrabenazine)
    > (Selective serotonin reuptake inhibitors (SSRI); α-methyldopa, alcohol withdrawal, toxins including MPTP; manganese, cyanide, carbon monoxide and carbon disulphide)
    > Phenytoin and sodium valproate.

    Parkinsonism typically develops in about 15% of patients on anti-psychotic medication within the first 3 months, with older patients being the most susceptible. Treatment of choice for this condition, in cases where the offending agent cannot be stopped or exchanged to a newer anti-psychotic agent, is amantadine or anticholinergic drugs. The drug-induced parkinsonism normally resolves in a few weeks but has been known to persist for up to 18 months after discontinuation of the therapy before resolving. There is some evidence that those affected are more likely to develop "idiopathic Parkinson's disease" in time.

- Chorea, including tardive dyskinesia and orofacial dyskinesia
  - Anti-psychotic drugs
  - Metoclopramide
  - Levodopa
  - Dopamine agonists including amphetamine
  - Oral contraceptives (oestrogen containing)
  - Phenytoin
  - (Anticholinergic agents; antihistamines: uncommon).

  Tardive dyskinesia develops after the long-term use of dopamine depleting agents, and typically involves the orolingual musculature (buccolingual syndrome, rabbit syndrome), with occasional involvement of the trunk and limbs, usually without distress to the patient. Tardive dyskinetic movements may persist for months to years after discontinuation of the causative therapy. Prevention is the best form of treatment but in established cases benefit may be achieved with clonazepam, baclofen or tetrabenazine.

  The withdrawal–emergent syndrome describes the generalized chorea that occurs soon after the withdrawal of neuroleptic therapy in children with schizophrenia. It typically occurs in 50% of cases within the first month of drug withdrawal, and always resolves spontaneously.
- Dystonia, including tardive dystonia (excluding acute dystonic reactions):
  - Anti-psychotic drugs
  - Metoclopramide
  - Levodopa
  - Dopamine agonists
  - (SSRIs; phenytoin: uncommon).

  This typically presents as a focal or segmental dystonia, especially retrocollis and partial opisthotonos, and typically occurs after brief exposure to neuroleptic therapy. It may persist after drug withdrawal and is refractory to most therapies, although tetrabenazine, anticholinergics and botulinum toxin have all been used with benefit.
- Neuroleptic malignant syndrome (NMS):
  - Anti-psychotic drugs, especially haloperidol, chlorpromazine and flupenthixol decanoate.

  This is a highly unpredictable response to neuroleptic therapy. It typically occurs when the drug is started or the dose increased rapidly but may arise at any time during treatment. Patients develop fluctuating levels of consciousness with extreme rigidity, fever and autonomic instability over a few days. Treatment involves withdrawal of the offending drug, supportive therapy and the administration of bromocriptine and/or dantrolene, or lorazepam/ECT; without specific treatment up to 25% of patients die. An identical syndrome may develop in patients with Parkinson's disease when dopaminergic treatment is suddenly withdrawn. A "non-NMS" has also been proposed following use of agents such as zopiclone.

- Tics

    Levodopa

    Dopamine agonists

    Amantadine

    Anti-psychotic drugs

    Amphetamines

    Carbamazepine.

    Tardive tic syndrome, consisting of both motor and vocal tics, can occasionally be seen with chronic neuroleptic therapy.

- Myoclonus

    Levodopa

    Dopamine agonists

    Anticonvulsants

    Tricyclic antidepressants

    (And other agents causing a toxic encephalopathy).

- Asterixis

    Anticonvulsants

    Hepatotoxins

    Respiratory depressants

    (And other agents causing a toxic encephalopathy).

"Anti-psychotic drugs" includes phenothiazines (e.g. chlorpromazine and thioridazine); butyrophenones (e.g. haloperidol); diphenylbutylpiperidines (e.g. pimozide); thioxanthenes (e.g. flupenthixol); substituted benzamides (e.g. sulpiride) and the newer atypical anti-psychotic drugs such as clozapine, olanzapine, sertindole and risperidone.

References Comella C. Drug-induced movement disorders. In: Sawle G (ed.). *Movement Disorders in Clinical Practice.* Oxford: Isis, 1999: 165–182.

Tanner CM, Klawans HL. Tardive dyskinesia – a historical review. In: Sen AK, Lee T (eds). *Receptors and Ligands in Neurological Disorders.* Cambridge: CUP, 1988: 52–63.

Van Harten PN, Hoek HW, Kahn RS. Acute dystonia induced by drug treatment. *British Medical Journal* 1999; **319**: 623–626.

Wojcieszek J. Drug-induced movement disorders. In: Biller J (ed.). *Iatrogenic Neurology.* Boston: Butterworth-Heinemann, 1998: 215–231.

Other relevant entries Akathisia; Catatonia; Chorea; Dystonia: an overview; Myoclonus; Neuroleptic malignant syndrome; Parkinsonian syndromes, parkinsonism; Parkinson's disease; Tics; Tremor: an overview.

Drug-induced myopathies

There are a number of drug-induced myopathic conditions.

- Corticosteroids

    Long-term use of corticosteroid therapy is associated with Cushing's syndrome, one feature of which is a proximal myopathy involving the arms and legs. The creatine kinase level is rarely raised and the EMG is either normal or mildly myopathic. Typically myopathy develops in patients on high-dose corticosteroid therapy, although there is no direct correlation between the total dose of steroid and the development of myopathy.

In addition an acute myopathy may occur in patients on the intensive care unit associated with high-dose corticosteroid therapy and neuromuscular junction blocking agents (critical illness myopathy). These patients present with an acute, diffuse, flaccid weakness of the proximal muscles with a necrotizing myopathy on EMG and a normal or slightly raised creatine kinase.

- Thyroid replacement therapy

    Thyrotoxicosis may be associated with a chronic proximal myopathy, and this may also occur with overtreatment in patients receiving thyroid replacement therapy. Typically this involves the proximal leg muscles more than the arms, although they can be involved, and there may be a marked degree of atrophy. The creatine kinase and EMG are usually normal, and muscle biopsy may show a degree of atrophy.

- L-tryptophan

    The ingestion of L-tryptophan has been associated with the acute onset of fatigue, fever, eosinophilia with muscle pain, tenderness, weakness and skin induration: the eosinophilia–myalgia syndrome. Many patients developed a florid inflammatory myopathy. As a result of this condition, the use of L-tryptophan has been prohibited in some countries.

- Alcohol (see entry on Alcohol and the nervous system: an overview)

- Others

    Amiodarone can induce a myopathy.

    Chloroquine can induce a painful vacuolar myopathy, with a raised creatine kinase and abnormal inclusion bodies on biopsy (curvilinear bodies).

    Colchicine can induce a subacute proximal myopathy with raised creatine kinase.

    Simvastatin.

Drugs may also interfere with the neuromuscular junction transmission (e.g. penicillamine-induced myasthenia gravis, MG) or exacerbate MG (see entry on MG).

Reference Schultz CE, Kincaid JC. Drug-induced myopathies. In: Biller J (ed.). *Iatrogenic Neurology*. Boston: Butterworth-Heinemann, 1998: 305–317.

Other relevant entries Alcohol and the nervous system: an overview; Critical illness myopathy; Endocrinology and the nervous system: Eosinophilia–myalgia syndrome; Myasthenia gravis; Myopathy: an overview; Thyroid disease and the nervous system.

■ Drug-induced neuropathies

A number of drugs have been associated with the development of neuropathies, in particular those used in cancer chemotherapy. In general drugs produce axonal neuropathies, although occasionally they may cause a neuronopathy or demyelinating polyneuropathy. In most instances removal of the drug eventually leads to improvement or a cessation of progression; initial progression ("coasting") may be seen after drug withdrawal.

- Axonal neuropathies

Sensory

Almitrine: produces a painful distal sensory neuropathy; CSF protein may be raised. Recovery is slow and often incomplete.

Arsenic.

Cis-platinum: induces a large fibre sensory polyneuropathy (with doses of $225–500$ mg/m^2 in total), which improves on cessation of therapy.

$2',3'$-Dideoxycytidine (ddC): induces a painful sensory neuropathy that recovers on cessation of the drug therapy.

Hydralazine: rarely produces a distal, predominantly sensory, polyneuropathy which is unrelated to its ability to induce a lupus-like syndrome. Symptoms improve with stopping the drug or the administration of vitamin B_6.

Metronidazole: can produce a large and small fibre sensory polyneuropathy. It slowly improves on stopping the medication.

Nitrous oxide: can induce a sensory polyneuropathy and myelopathy when there is heavy exposure, due to its ability to interfere with the vitamin B_{12} pathway.

Taxol: can induce a sensory polyneuropathy when given in high doses.

Thallium.

Motor

Dapsone: can induce a predominantly distal motor neuropathy with weakness and wasting $+/-$ optic neuropathy. Slow recovery on discontinuing the drug.

Sensorimotor

Chloramphenicol: can produce a painful sensorimotor polyneuropathy. Complete recovery following drug withdrawal if recognized early on.

Chloroquine: can occasionally induce a sensorimotor axonal polyneuropathy; steady improvement seen after stopping therapy.

Colchicine: can induce a mild distal axonal polyneuropathy that improves on stopping the drug. In addition there may be a compounding myopathy.

Disulfiram: can induce a neuropathy $+/-$ optic neuritis and encephalopathy. It is dose related and improves slowly on stopping the drug.

Gold: occasionally induces a distal axonal polyneuropathy.

Isoniazid: induces an axonal polyneuropathy especially in those individuals who are slow acetylators. It takes a number of months to develop, and can be avoided by the co-administration of vitamin B_6 (pyridoxine).

Nitrofurantoin: can produce a delayed (weeks to months) distal sensorimotor polyneuropathy; pre-existing renal impairment may predispose to this complication.

L-tryptophan: as part of the eosinophilia–myalgia syndrome can cause an axonal sensorimotor polyneuropathy, which is inflammatory in nature but not responsive to steroids.

Vincristine: induces a dose-related sensorimotor polyneuropathy, which begins with limb paraesthesias before evolving into sensory loss, areflexia and weakness. Autonomic involvement can also occur.

- Neuronopathy or ganglionopathy (i.e. loss of the nerve cell bodies)

  Methyl-mercury compounds.

  Pyridoxine: in very high doses can induce a severe sensory polyneuropathy that is probably axonal in nature, rather than a neuronopathy, although the latter has been shown experimentally. Most patients recover on stopping the drug.

  Thalidomide: can cause a dorsal root ganglion degeneration with selective loss of the large myelinated nerve fibres which results in a permanent sensory ataxia.

  Doxorubicin.

- Demyelinating neuropathies.

  Amiodarone: sensorimotor involvement with characteristic lamellar membranous inclusions in Schwann cells, fibroblasts and endothelial cells on nerve biopsy. There may be other side-effects with this drug, including a myopathy.

  Gold: can induce a Guillain–Barré-like syndrome with a demyelinating polyneuropathy and raised CSF protein.

  Perhexiline: when given chronically can induce a painful demyelinating sensorimotor polyneuropathy, with a raised CSF protein. Recovery occurs if the drug is stopped.

  Phenytoin: may cause an asymptomatic polyneuropathy with reduced motor conduction velocities. The severity of the polyneuropathy is proportional to the duration of the treatment and is not related to the folate abnormalities that can develop with phenytoin use.

  Suramin: can cause a severe demyelinating polyneuropathy which may involve the bulbar and respiratory muscles and be associated with a raised CSF protein level.

Reference Laycock MA. Drug-induced peripheral neuropathies. In: Biller J (ed.). *Iatrogenic Neurology*. Boston: Butterworth-Heinemann, 1998: 269–282.

Other relevant entries Autonomic failure; Chemotherapy- and radiotherapy-induced neurological disorders; Chronic inflammatory demyelinating polyneuropathy; Drug-induced myopathies; Guillain–Barré syndrome; Heavy metal poisoning; Neuropathies: an overview; Vitamin B_{12} deficiency.

▓ Drusen

Drusen are hyaline bodies that are typically seen on and around the optic nerve head, and may be mistaken for papilloedema ("pseudopapilloedema"). Drusen are thought to be due to altered axonal flow with axonal degeneration. They occur sporadically or may be inherited in an autosomal-dominant fashion, and are common, occurring in 2% of the population. In children the drusen are buried whilst in adults they are on the surface.

Drusen are usually asymptomatic but can cause visual field defects (typically an inferior nasal visual field loss) or occasionally transient visual obscurations, but not changes in visual acuity; these require investigation for an alternative cause. When there is doubt whether papilloedema or drusen is the cause of a swollen optic nerve head, retinal fluorescein angiography is required.

■ Duane's syndrome
Duane's retraction syndrome

Duane's syndrome is a congenital eye movement abnormality causing strabismus, in which there is paradoxical anomalous lateral rectus innervation by misdirected oculomotor nerve axons destined for the medial rectus (this is a syndrome of anomalous axonal guidance); effectively there is loss of the abducens nerve innervation to the lateral rectus. Clinically there is palpebral fissure narrowing and retraction of the affected eyeball on attempted adduction, with a variable degree of horizontal eye movement limitation: in type I, abduction is defective, in type II adduction is defective, and in type III both abduction and adduction are defective. Up to 10% of cases are familial with autosomal-dominant inheritance. Linkage to chromosome 2q31 has been reported.

Reference Gutowski NJ. Duane's syndrome. *European Journal of Neurology* 2000; **7**: 145–149.

Other relevant entries Cranial nerve disease: III: Oculomotor nerve; Cranial nerve disease: VI: Abducens nerve.

■ Duchenne muscular dystrophy (DMD)
Meryon's disease • Pseudohypertrophic muscular dystrophy

Pathophysiology The commonest of the muscular dystrophies, this X-linked condition was first described in detail by Meryon in the 1850s but his work was neglected. DMD is linked to chromosome Xp21 and results from deficiency of dystrophin, a sarcolemmal protein; it is allelic with Becker muscular dystrophy (BMD).

Clinical features: history and examination
- Affected boys are clinically normal at birth, and develop normally until about 5–7 years when they develop progressive difficulty running and climbing stairs; proximal myopathy is then evident, along with calf enlargement (pseudohypertrophy).
- Gowers manoeuvre may be observed in rising from the floor: "climbing up the legs".
- Boys usually become wheelchair bound around 12 years.
- Scoliosis.
- +/− mild mental impairment (IQ < 70 in 20% of boys).
- Cardiac involvement: cardiac conduction defects, dilated cardiomyopathy.

- Nocturnal hypoventilation in later disease may lead to excessive daytime somnolence.
- 5–10% of female carriers (heterozygotes) have muscle weakness, enlarged calves, +/− dilated cardiomyopathy.

Investigations and diagnosis *Bloods*: creatine kinase is raised from birth, usually in the thousands.

Electrophysiology:

EMG: myopathy.

ECG: prominent R waves in right precordial leads, deep Q waves in left precordial and limb leads.

Echocardiogram: may be required if cardiomyopathy present.

Muscle biopsy: variation in fibre size, fibre necrosis (broken down sarcolemma), macrophage invasion, muscle replaced with fat and connective tissue; deficient dystrophin on immunohistochemistry.

Neurogenetics: mutations in dystrophin gene.

Lung function: measure FVC if excessive daytime somnolence, +/− sleep studies.

Differential diagnosis The clinical picture is so characteristic that it is not likely to be mistaken for other disorders.

Treatment and prognosis

Prognosis is poor, most boys die in their 20s from pneumonia +/− cardiac complications.

Cardiac problems: pacemaker for conduction defects.

Respiratory problems: scoliosis surgery may help to preserve lung function (but avoid succinylcholine as this may cause myoglobinuria); elective tracheostomy and/or nocturnal intermittent positive-pressure ventilation for nocturnal hypoventilation.

Reference Emery AEH, Muntoni F. *Duchenne Muscular Dystrophy* (3rd edition). Oxford: OUP, 2003.

Other relevant entries Becker muscular dystrophy; Dystrophinopathy; Muscular dystrophies: an overview.

■ Dural arteriovenous fistula – see Spinal cord vascular diseases

■ Dwarfism

Dwarfism may be defined as extreme short stature (<135 cm), with, in addition, bodily proportions which are also abnormal. Recognized syndromes of short stature associated with neurological abnormalities include:

Silver–Russell syndrome (*q.v.*)

Pierre Robin syndrome (*q.v.*)

DeLange syndrome (*q.v.*)

Smith–Lemli–Opitz syndrome (*q.v.*)

Rubinstein–Taybi syndrome (*q.v.*)

Nanocephalic dwarfism (Seckel bird-headed dwarfism); severe mental retardation + dysmorphic features

Tryptophanuria with dwarfism: resulting from tryptophan pyrrolase deficiency

Ellis–van Creveld syndrome: chondroectodermal dysplasia.

Congenital growth hormone (GH) deficiency is a cause of dwarfism without neurological features; it may be autosomal recessive, X-linked, or autosomal dominant. Laron dwarfism is an autosomal-recessive condition with characteristic morphology: small facies and mandible, prominent forehead, saddle nose, delayed and discoloured dentition, slow and sparse hair growth, small hands and feet. Unlike GH deficiency, GH levels are elevated in Laron dwarfism but levels of insulin-like growth factor-1, which mediates the effects of GH, are low. At least some cases result from a genetic defect in the GH-receptor gene.

■ Dysarthria

Pathophysiology Dysarthria is a disorder of speech, as opposed to language (*cf.* aphasia), because of impairments in the actions of the speech production apparatus *per se*, due to paralysis, ataxia, tremor or spasticity, in the presence of intact mental function, comprehension, and memory of words. In its most extreme form, anarthria, there is no speech output.

Dysarthria is a symptom, which may be caused by a number of different conditions, all of which ultimately affect the function of pharynx, palate, tongue, lips and larynx, be that at the level of the cortex, lower cranial nerve nuclei or their motor neurones, neuromuscular junction or bulbar muscles themselves. Dysarthrias affect articulation in a highly reliable and consistent manner, the errors reflecting the muscle group involved in the production of specific sounds.

Dysarthria must be distinguished from aphasia, a primary language disorder, and aphonia, a difficulty in sound production.

Recognized neurological causes of anarthria and dysarthria include:

- Muscle disease

  For example, oculopharyngeal muscular dystrophy: nasal speech; weak pharynx/drooling.

- Neuromuscular disorder

  For example, myasthenia gravis: nasal speech; fatiguability (development of hypophonia with prolonged conversation, counting).

- Lower motor neurone disease = bulbar palsy.

  For example, motor neurone disease (rasping monotones, wasted and fasciculating tongue), poliomyelitis, Guillain–Barré syndrome, diphtheria.

- Upper motor neurone disease = pseudobulbar palsy.

  For example, motor neurone disease (spastic tongue), cerebrovascular disease.

- Cortical dysarthria

    Damage to left frontal cortex, usually with associated right hemiparesis; may be additional aphasia.
- Extrapyramidal disease

    For example, hypokinetic disorders: Parkinson's disease: slow, hypophonic, monotonic; multiple system atrophy (may have vocal cord palsy).

    For example, hyperkinetic disorders: Huntington's disease: loud, harsh, variably stressed, and poorly coordinated with breathing; myoclonus of any cause (hiccup speech); dystonia of any cause.
- Ataxic dysarthria

    Disease of or damage to cerebellum: slow, slurred, monotonous, with incoordination of speech with respiration; may therefore be quiet and then explosive; unnatural separation of syllables; slow tongue movements
- Acquired stuttering

    Involuntary repetition of letters or syllables, may be acquired with aphasia; developmental stutter, the commoner cause, most commonly affects the beginnings of words and with plosive sounds, whereas the acquired form may be evident throughout sentences and affect all speech sounds.

Clinical features: history and examination

- *Context may be obvious*: stroke, Parkinson's disease, motor neurone disease.
- Variability may suggest myasthenia gravis or dystonia.
- Examination of speech:

    Listen to conversational speech, noting speed and articulatory difficulties.

    Check strength of lip closure, jaw opening and blowing out cheeks.

    Check movement, speed and strength of tongue.

    Check palatal movement and gag reflex.

    Check pronunciation of individual letters "p", "t", and "k", which tests labial, lingual and guttural (throat and soft palate) components of speech respectively.

Investigations and diagnosis Investigations are governed by the suspected cause. Important exclusions/considerations are:

    Structural lesion: for example thoracic lesion affecting left recurrent laryngeal nerve.

    Myasthenia gravis: consider tensilon test.

    Focal dystonia: consider ENT referral.

    Consider psychogenic causes.

Differential diagnosis

Aphasia: may be difficult to distinguish in cases of cortical dysarthria.
Dysphonia.
Treatment and prognosis Dependent on cause. Help from a speech therapist is frequently required.

Reference Darley FL, Aronson AE, Brown JR. Differential diagnostic patterns of dysarthria. *Journal of Speech and Hearing Research* 1969; **12**: 246–249.
Other relevant entries Aphasia; Aphonia; Cerebellar disease: an overview; Chorea; Diphtheria; Dystonia: an overview; Huntington's disease; Motor neurone disease; Multiple system atrophy; Muscular dystrophies: an overview; Myasthenia gravis; Myoclonus; Parkinsonian syndromes, parkinsonism; Poliomyelitis; Spasmodic dysphonia.

Dysarthria–clumsy hand syndrome – see Lacunar syndromes

Dysautonomia – see Autonomic failure; Pandysautonomia

Dysembryoplastic neuroepithelial tumours (DNET)

Dysembryoplastic neuroepithelial tumours (DNET) are low-grade tumours, possibly even hamartomas, of mixed neuronal/glial cell lineage, although often categorized with neuronal tumours. They occur throughout childhood, most often in the temporal lobe, causing intractable complex partial and secondary generalized seizures. They are multinodular and may be associated with cortical dysplasia. Prognosis after surgical resection is generally good.

Ganglioglioma and other low-grade tumours with a predilection for the temporal lobe causing an intractable seizure disorder enter the differential diagnosis.

Reference Daumas-Duport C. Dysembryoplastic neuroepithelial tumors. *Brain Pathology* 1993; **8**: 283–295.
Other relevant entries Epilepsy: an overview; Ganglioglioma; Tumours: an overview.

Dysexecutive syndrome – see Frontotemporal dementia

Dysferlinopathy

Dysferlinopathy is a generic term for allelic disorders associated with mutations in the gene encoding dysferlin. The clinical phenotype of these conditions is variable, including:

- Limb girdle muscular dystrophy (type 2B).
- Miyoshi myopathy.
- Distal anterior compartment myopathy.

Reference Ueyama H, Kumamoto T, Nagano S *et al.* A new dysferlin gene mutation in two Japanese families with limb-girdle muscular dystrophy 2B and Miyoshi myopathy. *Neuromuscular Disorders* 2001; **11**: 139–145.
Other relevant entries Distal muscular dystrophy, distal myopathy; Limb-girdle muscular dystrophy; Miyoshi myopathy; Myopathy: an overview.

■ Dyslexia – see Alexia

■ Dyspeptic dystonia – see Sandifer's syndrome

■ Dysphagia

Pathophysiology Dysphagia is defined as difficulty in swallowing. This may be due to mechanical obstruction, primary gastroenterological disease or connective tissue disease (e.g. peptic stricture, oesophageal malignancy, dysphagia lusoria, systemic sclerosis) but may also be a consequence of neurological disease.

Dysphagia may be:

- Neurogenic
  - Central nervous system (CNS)
    - Cerebrovascular disease: hemisphere, brainstem stroke.
    - Extrapyramidal disease: Parkinson's disease, progressive supranuclear palsy, Huntington's disease, Wilson's disease, tardive dyskinesia, dystonia.
    - Inflammatory disease: multiple sclerosis.
    - Neoplasia: primary, secondary; cerebral, brainstem (skull base).
    - Other structural disorders of the brainstem: syringobulbia, cerebellar disease.
    - Developmental disorders: cerebral palsy syndromes, Chiari malformations.
  - Neuronopathy
    - Motor neurone disease.
  - Neuropathy
    - Guillain–Barré syndrome.
    - Autonomic neuropathy (diabetes mellitus, amyloidosis, Chagas' disease, autonomic failure).
  - Neuromuscular
    - Myasthenia gravis.
- Myogenic
  - Inflammatory muscle disease: polymyositis, inclusion body myositis.
  - Myotonia: dystrophia myotonica.
  - Muscular dystrophy: oculopharyngeal muscular dystrophy.
  - Symptomatic oesophageal peristalsis ("nutcracker oesophagus").
- Functional
  - "Hysterical", globus hystericus (diagnosis of exclusion).

Clinical features: history and examination

- What sticks (food > drink = mechanical problem, usually).
- Where food sticks: usually of poor-localizing value.
- Nasal regurgitation: especially with bulbar palsy.
- Choking or chest infections.
- Degree of weight loss; cachexia.

- Pain.
- Associated features: change in voice (dysarthria, dysphonia); fatiguability; other neurological symptoms, signs suggestive of underlying neurological illness.

Investigations and diagnosis *Bloods*: usually non-contributory but need to check FBC (for anaemia); iron status, vitamin B_{12}, folate (for deficiencies); acetylcholine-receptor antibodies; auto-antibodies (for autoimmune disorders such as systemic sclerosis and Sjögren's syndrome).

Imaging:

Barium swallow $+/-$ videofluoroscopy to ascertain level of dysphagia, $+/-$ CXR to assess for aspiration; assessment by speech therapist, ENT opinion, may be required.

CT/MRI brain if intracranial or skull base pathology suspected.

CT chest (if myasthenia suspected).

Neurophysiology: EMG/NCS if neuromuscular disorders, anterior horn cell disease, neuropathy suspected.

CSF: only indicated if an infiltrative or inflammatory CNS/PNS disease is suspected.

Others: gastroscopy, oesophageal manometry, biopsy of skin/salivary gland/rectum etc. depending on possible cause of dysphagia; psychiatric opinion may be indicated if diagnosis is globus hystericus.

Differential diagnosis Gastrointestinal causes of dysphagia, for example

Intrinsic
  Oesophageal carcinoma
  Metastatic or extrinsic tumour spread
  Peptic (post-inflammatory) stricture
  Hiatus hernia
Extrinsic
  Thoracic aortic aneurym
  Abnormal origin of right subclavian artery (dysphagia lusoria)
  Posterior mediastinal mass
  Large goitre.
  Retropharyngeal mass

Treatment and prognosis Dependent on cause; see individual entries.

Reference Logemann JA. Approach to the patient with dysphagia. In: Biller J (ed.). *Practical Neurology* (2nd edition). Philadelphia: Lippincott Williams & Wilkins, 2002: 227–235.

Other relevant entries Amyloid and the nervous system: an overview; Autonomic failure; Brainstem vascular syndromes; Cerebellar disease: an overview; Cerebrovascular disease: arterial; Chiari malformations; Collagen vascular disorders and the nervous system: an overview; Dermatomyositis; Diphtheria; Gastrointestinal disease and the nervous system; Guillain–Barré syndrome;

Motor neurone disease; Multiple sclerosis; Multiple system atrophy; Myasthenia gravis; Myopathy: an overview; Neuropathies: an overview; Parkinsonian syndromes, parkinsonism; Parkinson's disease; Polymyositis; Progressive supranuclear palsy; Syringomyelia and syringobulbia; Tumours: an overview.

▦ Dysphasia – see Aphasia

▦ Dyssynergia cerebellaris myoclonica – see Unverricht–Lundborg disease

▦ Dystonia: an overview

Pathophysiology Dystonia is defined as a motor syndrome of sustained involuntary muscle contractions causing twisting and repetitive movements and/or abnormal postures. Dystonic movements may be slow and twisting (athetosis), rapid or rhythmic (dystonic tremor), or apparent only with certain actions (action dystonia). Hence examination of the dystonia and the actions that induce it is important. Pathophysiology remains ill understood; central and peripheral mechanisms may be important, and motor and sensory systems, perhaps to different degrees in different syndromes.

The dystonias may be defined by their anatomical extent, in terms of which body parts are involved:

focal,
segmental (i.e. two or more adjacent body parts),
multifocal (i.e. two or more non-contiguous body parts),
generalized.

The dystonias may also be classified according to their aetiology, hence family history and perinatal history are important.
- Primary or idiopathic dystonia.
    Hereditary
        Generalized dystonia [primary torsion dystonia (PTD), dystonia musculorum deformans, idiopathic torsion dystonia: usually autosomal dominant)]
        X-linked dystonia–parkinsonism syndrome (Lubag disease)
        Alcohol-responsive dystonia, myoclonus–dystonia syndrome (autosomal dominant)
        Dopa-responsive dystonia (DRD) (Segawa syndrome; autosomal dominant)
        Paroxysmal kinesigenic or non-kinesigenic dystonia (? autosomal dominant)
        Dystonia in mitochondrial disease.
    Non-hereditary
        Sporadic generalized dystonia

Sporadic paroxysmal non-kinesigenic dystonia

Focal dystonias

    Cranial dystonia: Meige's syndrome, blepharospasm $+/-$ oromandibular dystonia

    Spasmodic torticollis (cervical dystonia)

    Writer's cramp (graphospasm)

    Other occupational or task-specific dystonias

    Spasmodic dysphonia

    Dystonic dysphagia

    Axial dystonia

    Leg dystonia

    Anismus.

- Symptomatic or secondary dystonia

    Inherited metabolic causes

      Wilson's disease, Menkes' disease

      Gangliosidoses: GM1, GM2

      Metachromatic leukodystrophy

      Lesch–Nyhan disease

      Organic acidurias (e.g. glutaric aciduria type I)

      Homocystinuria

      Hexosaminidase A and B deficiency

      Hartnup's disease

      Rett syndrome

      Triose phosphate isomerase deficiency.

    Non-inherited metabolic causes

      Kernicterus.

    Inherited possible metabolic causes

      Hallervorden–Spatz disease

      Basal ganglia calcification

      Leigh's syndrome

      Bilateral necrosis of basal ganglia ($+/-$ Leber's hereditary optic neuropathy)

      Niemann–Pick disease.

    Inherited non-metabolic causes

      Ataxia telangectasia

      Neuroacanthocytosis

      Neuronal ceroid lipofuscinosis

      Huntington's disease

      Spinocerebellar ataxias (especially Machado–Joseph disease).

    Non-inherited, non-metabolic causes

      Degenerative disorders

        Parkinson's disease and its treatment

        Progressive supranuclear palsy

Multiple system atrophy

Pallidopyramidal degeneration.

Trauma

Head trauma, cervical cord and peripheral nerve injury, often with a delay before the onset of the dystonia. In peripheral nerve damage, focal dystonia may develop in conjunction with reflex sympathetic dystrophy.

Anoxia/ischaemia

Perinatal anoxia causing immediate and delayed (i.e. up to 20 years) dystonia

Cerebrovascular disease

Arteriovenous malformations

Tumours: of the basal ganglia can present with hemidystonia

Toxins: manganese, carbon monoxide, carbon disulphide, methanol, mercury.

Infections, postinfectious disorders: encephalitis, Reye's syndrome, subacute sclerosing panencephalitis (SSPE)

Post-operative: especially after thalamotomy

Multiple sclerosis (often paroxysmal).

Drug induced

Neuroleptics

Dopamine agonists

Dopamine

Anticonvulsants

Selective serotonin reuptake inhibitors

Tetrabenazine

Flecainide

Propranolol

Cimetidine

Psychogenic.

The dystonias may also be classified according to their age of onset:

- Childhood onset (<13 years of age)

    65% generalize

    Leg involvement common

    Cause found 40%.

- Adolescent onset (13–20 years of age)

    35% generalize

    Leg involvement often

    Cause found 30%.

- Adult onset (>20 years of age)

    3% generalize

    Leg involvement very rare

    Cause found 13%.

Increasingly dystonias may now be classified according to their genetic basis; a number of genetic mutations and chromosomal linkages have been defined:

Gene	Locus	Inheritance	Clinical classification	Protein
DYT1	9q34	Autosomal dominant (AD)	PTD	Torsin A
DYT2	Unknown	Autosomal-recessive (AR)	PTD	Unknown
DYT3	Xq13.1	X-linked	X-linked dystonia–parkinsonism, Lubag	Unknown
DYT4	Unknown	AD	"Non-DYT1" PTD	Unknown
DYT5	14q22.1–q22.2	AD	DRD	GTP cyclohydrolase I (GTPCH I)
DYT6	8p21–q22	AD	Adolescent, mixed PTD	Unknown
DYT7	18p11.3	AD	Adult-onset focal PTD	Unknown
DYT8	2q25–q33	AD	Paroxysmal dystonic choreoathetosis (PDC)	Unknown
DYT9	1p13.3–p21	AD	Paroxysmal choreoathetosis with episodic ataxia, spasticity	Unknown
DYT10	16p11.2	AD	Paroxysmal kinesigenic choreoathetosis (PKC)	Unknown
DYT11	7q21–q31	AD	Myoclonus–dystonia	D2 receptor, ε-sarcoglycan
DYT12	19q13	AD	Rapidly progressive dystonia parkinsonism	Unknown
DYT13	1p36.13	AD	Focal or segmental dystonia	Unknown

Investigations and diagnosis A large number of investigations may be appropriate in a patient with a dystonia, particularly if the dystonia is generalized.
Bloods:

  FBC, three (fresh) blood films for acanthocytes
  ESR
  Biochemical screen (U&E; glucose; liver and thyroid function tests)
  Copper/caeruloplasmin
  Lactate/pyruvate ratio
  Syphilis serology
  Creatine kinase

Antinuclear antibodies, rheumatoid factor and immunoglobulins
Uric acid
α-fetoprotein
White cell enzymes
Plasma amino acids
Toxicology screen.

Urine:

Organic acids
amino acids
24-hour protein excretion; creatinine clearance; copper excretion
Mucopolysaccharides/oligosaccharides.

Imaging: MRI brain +/− cervical cord.
CSF: including lactate, oligoclonal bands, +/− lactate/pyruvate ratio.
Neurophysiology: EMG/NCS; EEG; ERG; evoked potentials.
Ophthalmology: Kayser–Fleischer rings, retinal vasculitis.
Neurogenetics: Huntington's disease, spinocerebellar ataxias, DYTI.
Other: Bone marrow aspirate; Skin/muscle biopsy.

Differential diagnosis Some cases labelled as cerebral palsy may in fact have a dystonic syndrome (e.g. dopa-responsive dystonia and glutaric aciduria type I).

Treatment and prognosis Of cause if possible, for example Wilson's disease.

Owing to the exquisite and long-lasting sensitivity of dopa-responsive dystonia to levodopa preparations, it is recommended that all patients with young onset generalized dystonia should receive a trial of levodopa (e.g. two tablets of Sinemet plus or Madopar 125 tds) for 2–3 months.

In other generalized dystonias, treatment is often disappointing and involves polypharmacy. Other agents that can be used in generalized dystonias include:

Anticholinergic agents
Benzhexol 2.5 mg bd increasing by 2.5 mg/day every 1–2 weeks to a maximum dose of 180 mg. Treatment is usually limited by side-effects, although most benefit is seen with very high doses of these agents.
Benzodiazepines
Diazepam, often in high dose.
Others
Baclofen.
Carbamazepine (may be useful for paroxysmal kinesigenic or non-kinesigenic dystonia).
Haloperidol, phenothiazines.
Tetrabenazine.
Pimozide.

In difficult cases the patient often requires high-dose anticholinergic drugs with diazepam, tetrabenazine +/− pimozide.

5% of all idiopathic dystonias have spontaneous improvement or even resolution of movement disorder, typically within the first 5 years of the illness. However subsequent relapses are common. Childhood dystonias tend to stabilize in adulthood. Most adult dystonias are focal in nature and remain so; they respond poorly to drug therapy and are best treated with local injections of botulinum toxin.

Stereotactic surgery for dystonia is the subject of resurgent interest; pallidotomy seems to be more effective than thalamotomy in alleviating dystonia (likewise dyskinesia) especially in DYTI-PTD.

Other treatments such as physiotherapy and supportive psychotherapy are useful but mechanical braces and other surgical appliances are useless.

References Carvalho Aguiar PM de, Ozelius LJ. Classification and genetics of dystonia. *Lancet Neurology* 2002; **1**: 316–325.

Fahn S, Marsden CD. The treatment of dystonia. In: Marsden CD, Fahn S (eds). *Movement Disorders 2*. London: Butterworth, 1987: 359–382.

Fahn S, Marsden CD, Calne DB. Classification and investigation of dystonia. In: Marsden CD, Fahn S (eds). *Movement Disorders 2*. London: Butterworth, 1987: 332–358.

Németh AH. The genetics of primary dystonias and related disorders. *Brain* 2002; **125**: 695–721.

Other relevant entries See individual entries; Basal ganglia calcification; Botulinum toxin therapy; Cerebral palsy, cerebral palsy syndromes; Complex regional pain syndromes; Drug-induced movement disorders; Dysphagia; Focal dystonias; Mohr–Tranebjaerg syndrome; Status dystonicus.

■ Dystonia musculorum deformans – see Primary torsion dystonia

■ Dystrophia myotonica
Myotonic dystrophy type 1 (DM1) • Steinert's disease

Pathophysiology Dystrophia myotonica (DM) is an autosomal-dominant disorder caused by a trinucleotide repeat expansion in the myotonin protein kinase gene, a serine/threonine protein kinase which is expressed in muscle >>> heart and brain, encoded on chromosome 19. It is the most common inherited myopathy seen in adulthood, occurring in 1:8000 live births. As in other trinucleotide repeat disorders, disease severity is proportional to the number of repeats, although the mechanism by which trinucleotide repeats cause disease is still unknown.

At its most severe (>2000 repeats), disease presents in the neonatal period; mild disease with adult onset occurs with 50–80 repeats. The clinical phenotype is variable, features including frontal baldness, cataracts, myopathic facies, weakness (usually distal > proximal), myotonia, a cardiomyopathy, diabetes mellitus and testicular atrophy.

Clinical features: history and examination

- Neonatal disease (very large repeats)
     Extreme hypotonia with facial paralysis
     Feeding difficulties and failure to thrive
     Club feet and mental retardation are common
     Prone to URTI, pneumonia and death.
- Adult disease
  - Muscle
       Myotonia: difficulty in relaxing contracted muscle, manifest as difficulty letting go of objects, especially in cold weather. Myotonia may be induced clinically by voluntary contraction or percussion of muscle. It tends to disappear with advancing disease and loss of muscle.

       Wasting and weakness, typically involves the distal limb muscles, the neck muscles (especially sternocleidomastoid) and facial muscles (especially masseter and temporalis). This produces a "hollowed" face with hooded eyes (ptosis), and a tented or slack mouth which can cause dislocation of the jaw. In advanced cases there is proximal muscle involvement, including the respiratory musculature, as well as involvement of the palate and pharynx causing dysphagia and dysarthria.
  - Somnolence +/− respiratory depression may occur due to respiratory muscle involvement and an abnormal central ventilatory response to carbon dioxide.
  - Smooth muscle involvement may account for dysphagia and aspiration, constipation, symptoms akin to irritable bowel syndrome, faecal soiling; and impaired uterine contraction.
  - Cardiac: cardiomyopathy occurs with advanced disease, causing conduction abnormalities, arrhythmias, heart failure and sudden death.
  - Ophthalmological: cataracts are very common.
  - Endocrine: testicular atrophy with infertility; ovarian dysfunction with infertility; diabetes mellitus; frontal balding.

Investigations and diagnosis Detailed family history; check for cataracts in other family members.

Bloods: creatine kinase is usually normal; check glucose for diabetes mellitus. Arterial blood gases may be useful if respiratory depression is suspected, contributing to somnolence and/or heart failure.

Imaging: CXR for cardiomyopathy. CT/MRI brain not required.

CSF: not required.

Neurophysiology: EMG/NCS shows myopathic changes and myotonic discharges.

Muscle biopsy: (seldom necessary with advent of genetic testing) shows random variability in size of fibres with fibrosis, along with numerous ring fibres in which small bundles of myofibrils are oriented at 90° to majority.

Neurogenetics: trinucleotide CTG repeat in the 3′ untranslated region of myotonin protein kinase (DMPK) gene on chromosome 19q13.3 is definitive: normal = 5–40 repeats; abnormal = 44–3000. Prenatal diagnosis can now be made using genetic test with tissue samples from chorionic villous biopsy.

ECG/24-hour ECG: for conduction abnormalities.

Differential diagnosis

Proximal myotonic myopathy (PROMM) or myotonic dystrophy type 2 (DM2) Other myotonic syndromes.

Treatment and prognosis There is no curative treatment and the condition is progressive.

Supportive treatment involves the use of:

Prostheses: foot and/or wrist splints.

Symptomatic treatment of myotonia: phenytoin; quinine; procainamide or acetazolamide (but need to watch for respiratory depression with phenytoin).

Cardiac and respiratory treatment may involve pacemakers or respiratory support (e.g. CPAP), Symptomatic treatment of diabetes mellitus.

Ophthalmologists may need to do cataract extraction.

Genetic counselling may be required.

Reference Harper PS (ed.). *Myotonic Dystrophy* (3rd edition). Philadelphia: Saunders, 2001.

Other relevant entries Cataracts; Diabetes mellitus and the nervous system; Dysarthria; Dysphagia; Endocrinology and the nervous system; Myopathy: an overview; Myotonia and myotonic syndromes; Proximal myotonic myopathy; Trinucleotide repeat diseases.

■ Dystrophinopathy

The term dystrophinopathy has been used to describe conditions in which the primary genetic disorder is in the gene encoding the sarcolemmal protein dystrophin, viz. Duchenne muscular dystrophy and Becker muscular dystrophy, in which there is immunohistochemical evidence of absence or deficiency, respectively, of dystrophin in muscle biopsies.

Other relevant entries Becker muscular dystrophy; Duchenne muscular dystrophy; Muscular dystrophies: an overview.

Ee

■ Eales' disease

This rare disorder, mostly affecting young males, is a retinal "perivasculitis" which causes recurrent bilateral retinal and vitreous haemorrhage. Stroke and transient ischaemic attack (TIA) have occasionally been reported with associated cerebral and leptomeningeal vasculitis.

Reference Gordon MF, Coyle PK, Golub B. Eales' disease presenting as stroke in the young adult. *Annals of Neurology* 1988; **24**: 264–266.

■ Early-onset ataxia with ocular motor apraxia and hypoalbuminaemia

Ataxia with ocular motor apraxia (AOA)

This autosomal-recessive syndrome is characterized by:

cerebellar ataxia,
peripheral neuropathy,
ocular motor apraxia,
hypoalbuminaemia,
hypercholesterolaemia,
+ / − generalized dystonia.

CT/MRI shows cerebellar atrophy. Sural nerve biopsy shows depletion of large myelinated fibres. Mutations in the gene encoding aprataxin have been discovered; this may be a nuclear protein with a role in DNA repair.

The differential diagnosis includes ataxia telangiectasia (AT) and Friedreich's ataxia (FA).

Reference Shimazaki H, Takiyama Y, Sakoe K *et al.* Early-onset ataxia with ocular motor apraxia and hypoalbuminemia: the aprataxin gene mutations. *Neurology* 2002; **59**: 590–595.

Other relevant entries Ataxia telangiectasia; Cerebellar disease: an overview; Friedreich's ataxia.

■ Eastern equine encephalitis – see Arbovirus disease; Encephalitis: an overview

■ Eating disorders

Anorexia nervosa and bulimia have been considered as psychiatric diseases but in light of the known roles of the hypothalamus in controlling feeding behaviour some consider them hypothalamic diseases. Both occur predominantly in young women. Antidepressant medications may help in both conditions.

• *Anorexia nervosa*: Characterized by extreme emaciation as a result of voluntary starvation, related to a distorted body image with fear of gaining weight. Occasional cases have been described in association with hypothalamic tumours, akin to the diencephalic syndrome of infants; mild diabetes insipidus may occur. There are no characteristic neurological signs, although "hung-up" tendon reflexes have been described.

• *Bulimia*: This eating disorder (literally "ox-eating") is characterized by binge eating followed by induced vomiting and excessive use of laxatives. Hyperphagia akin to that seen in bulimia may occur as one feature of the Kleine–Levin syndrome.

Disorders of eating may also occur in frontotemporal dementia.

Reference Fairburn CG, Harrison PJ. Eating disorders. *Lancet* 2003; **361**: 407–416.

Other relevant entries Diencephalic syndrome; Frontotemporal dementia; Gourmand syndrome; Hypothalamic disease: an overview; Kleine–Levin syndrome.

■ Echinococcosis
Hydatid disease

Infection with the cestode larval tapeworms of the genus Echinococcus (*E. granulosus*, *E. multilocularis* or *E. vogeli*) may cause cystic lesions (hydatid cysts). The disease occurs in areas where dogs (definitive host) and sheep or cattle (intermediate hosts) are common, hence Wales, Australasia, Eastern Europe, Argentina and Chile, Africa, and the Middle East. The ova are found in canine faeces and, on human ingestion, escape from their eggs, enter the portal circulation, and spread to various organs, including on occasion brain and muscle. In these sites, as in other organs, cysts cause symptoms by local compression, for example seizures, compressive myelopathies (spinal epidural abscess; hydatid Pott's disease). Imaging reveals single or multiple cysts, often with scolices evident within them; different cysts may be at different stages of maturity. There may be a peripheral eosinophilia. Serology (ELISA, indirect haemagglutination) may assist with diagnosis but is not reliable. Differential diagnosis includes cysticercosis. Treatment of choice is surgical resection of the cyst(s), taking care to avoid rupture as this can be associated with anaphylaxis or recurrent disease. Treatment with albendazole or mebendazole may shrink cysts, and non-resectable cysts may be treated with albendazole (400 mg bd).

Other relevant entries Coenurosis; Cysticercosis; Cysts: an overview; Helminthic diseases; Pott's disease.

■ Eclampsia

Pathophysiology Eclampsia is the most feared neurological complication of pregnancy, defined as the development of seizures with or without coma on the background of pre-eclampsia, the latter defined as raised blood pressure (>140/90 mmHg), proteinuria, and oedema after 20 weeks of gestation. Hence eclampsia requires the onset of symptoms, specifically seizures. Eclampsia may be subdivided as:

- antepartum (three-fourths of all eclampsia: before 28 weeks = "early");
- intrapartum (no pre-eclampsia prior to labour);
- postpartum (within 7 days of delivery).

Eclampsia may complicate as many as 1 : 2000 deliveries and is a significant cause of maternal deaths during pregnanacy (~10%). The pathophysiology is uncertain; presumably hypertension in some way triggers a vasculopathy with haemorrhages and microinfarcts within cerebral white matter. Seizures are best treated with high doses of parenteral magnesium. Eclampsia may occasionally be seen with hydatiform moles.

Clinical features: history and examination

- Pre-eclampsia: hypertension (>140/90 mmHg), proteinuria, and oedema after 20 weeks of gestation.
- Headache.
- Seizures: usually tonic–clonic.
- Obtundation, stupor, coma.
- Focal neurological signs may develop, including visual scintillations, visual loss, hemiparesis.
- HELLP syndrome: *h*aemolysis, *e*levated *l*iver function tests, *l*ow *p*latelet count.

Investigations and diagnosis *Bloods*: may show pregnancy-induced anaemia; clotting studies may show the development of disseminated intravascular coagulopathy, an alarming finding. Renal function may be abnormal.

Urine: proteinuria.

Imaging: CT/MRI may be normal, but may show white matter (especially occipital) hypodensity/T_2-weighted hyperintensity; occasionally multiple small haemorrhages may be seen.

Neurophysiology: EEG is abnormal in 80% of cases, with slowing +/− spikes.

CSF: not usually necessary.

Differential diagnosis Other causes of seizures during pregnancy: pre-existing epilepsy, cerebral venous thrombosis, cerebrovascular events, space-occupying lesion, infection, metabolic disorder (e.g. hypoglycaemia).

Subarachnoid haemorrhage (SAH).

Pituitary apoplexy.

Posterior leukoencephalopathy syndrome.

Treatment and prognosis

Maternal–fetal monitoring for pre-eclampsia (prevention is the best treatment).

Adequate oxygenation.

Control blood pressure: hydralazine, labetalol, nifedipine if rapid control required.

Control seizures: magnesium sulphate is now the treatment of choice (preferable to phenytoin, benzodiazepines):

4 g intravenously over 5–20 minutes;

then an infusion of 1 g/hour for 24 hours, or 5 g each buttock + single 5 g injection every 4 hours;

if seizures recur, then 2–4 g magnesium over 5 minutes intravenously.

Need continuous monitoring of ECG, blood pressure, and clinical signs; look for evidence of hypermagnesaemia (loss of knee jerks, weakness, nausea, sensation of warmth, flushing, drowsiness, diplopia, and dysarthria), if present treat with calcium gluconate.

Management/prevention of organ failure.

Safe delivery of the fetus.

Eclampsia is a significant cause of maternal perinatal mortality. Prevention cannot therefore be too heavily emphasized.

References Kaplan PW, Repke JT. Eclampsia. *Neurologic Clinics* 1994; **12**: 565–582.

The Eclampsia Trial Collaborative Group. Which anticonvulsant for women with eclampsia? Evidence from the Collaborative Eclampsia Trial. *Lancet* 1995; **345**: 1455–1463.

Thomas SV. Neurological aspects of eclampsia. *Journal of the Neurological Sciences* 1998; **155**: 37–43.

Other relevant entries Cerebrovascular disease: venous; Epilepsy: an overview; Headache: an overview; Hypertension and the nervous system; Posterior leukoencephalopathy syndrome; Pregnancy and the nervous system: an overview; Subarachnoid haemorrhage.

■ Ehlers–Danlos syndrome

This inherited disorder of connective tissue, of which several subtypes are recognized, may be complicated by various neurological features, in addition to the hyperelasticity of skin, hyperextensibility of joints, and easy bruising. Type IV is particularly associated with neurovascular complications. Mutations in the COL3A1 gene on chromosome 2, which codes for the α_1 chain of type III collagen are associated with this variant:

Dissection/rupture of intra- and extracranial arteries (usually spontaneous).
Intra- and extracranial aneurysm formation; subarachnoid haemorrhage (SAH).
Carotid–cavernous fistula (CCF).
Mitral valve prolapse.

Reference North KN, Whiteman DAH, Pepin MG *et al.* Cerebrovascular complications in Ehlers–Danlos syndrome Type IV. *Annals of Neurology* 1995; **38**: 960–964.

Other relevant entries Carotid–cavernous fistula; Cerebrovascular disease: arterial; Occipital horn syndrome; Subarachnoid haemorrhage.

■ Ehrlichiosis

Infection with tick-borne *Ehrlichia*, an intraleukocytic bacterium which resembles the *Rickettsiae*, may cause meningitis, seizures, and encephalopathy.

Reference Fishbein DB, Dawson JE, Robinson LE. Human Ehrlichiosis in the United States, 1985–1990. *Annals of Internal Medicine* 1994; **120**: 736–743.

Other relevant entry Rickettsial disease.

■ Eight-and-a-half syndrome

The eight-and-a-half syndrome is the combination of a facial (VII) nerve palsy with a one-and-a-half syndrome due to a pontine lesion. These patients may develop oculopalatal myoclonus months to years after the onset of the ocular motility problem.

References Eggenberger EJ. Eight-and-a-half syndrome: One-and-a-half syndrome plus cranial nerve VII palsy. *Journal of Neuro-ophthalmology* 1998; **18**: 114–116.

Wolin MJ, Trent RG, Lavin PJM, Cornblath WT. Oculopalatal myoclonus after the one-and-a-half syndrome with facial nerve palsy. *Ophthalmology* 1996; **103**: 177–180.

Other relevant entries Cranial nerve disease: VII: Facial nerve; One-and-a-half syndrome.

▓ Ekbom's syndrome (1) – see Restless legs syndrome

▓ Ekbom's syndrome (2)

Delusional parasitosis

This is a delusional disorder in which patients believe with absolute certainty that insects, maggots, lice, or other vermin infest their skin or other parts of the body. Sometimes other psychiatric features may be present, particularly if the delusions are part of a psychotic illness, such as schizophrenia or depressive psychosis. Females are said to be more commonly affected. Clinical examination may sometimes show evidence of skin picking, scratching, or dermatitis caused by repeated use of antiseptics. The patient may produce skin fragments or other debris as "evidence" of infestation. Treatment should be aimed at the underlying condition if appropriate; if the delusion is isolated, anti-psychotics, such as pimozide, may be tried.

Reference Enoch MD, Ball HN. *Uncommon Psychiatric Syndromes* (4th edition). London: Arnold, 2001: 209–223.

Other relevant entry Psychiatric disorders and neurological disease.

▓ Electrical injuries and the nervous system

Electrical injury to the nervous system can occur through lightning strikes or accidental contact with mains electricity. In many cases it is fatal due to heat damage to the brain or ventricular fibrillation.

The injury sustained with electrical insults is dependent on the course of the current through the body; flow from the head to limbs will damage brain and spinal cord, whilst current between one arm and the other or to the leg will only affect the spinal cord.

Minor electrical injuries produce pain and paresthesiae that quickly resolve.

More serious injuries may induce a number of neurological deficits, some of which are expressed at the time of the injury, others of which are delayed by 1–6 weeks. These include:

• Brain: loss of consciousness, headache, tinnitus, and seizures in the immediate post-injury period with recovery in a few days. Occasionally patients have a delayed vascular event that presents acutely and is thought to be thrombotic in origin. Occasional patients have been described who develop parkinsonism. Recurrent seizures are rare, but an encephalopathy may develop in some patients with electrical injuries traversing the head, often in association with spinal cord and limb signs.

- Spinal cord: clinical manifestation of cord injury is often delayed: a syndrome of segmental wasting (spinal atrophic paralysis) may occur, progression of which may mimic motor neurone disease or a transverse myelopathy.
- Peripheral nervous system: damage may be so severe that repair does not occur, resulting in the development of a chronic pain syndrome.

References Sirdofsky MD, Hawley RJ, Manz H. Progressive motor neurone disease associated with electrical injury. *Muscle and Nerve* 1991; **14**: 977–980.

Winkelman MD. Neurological complications of thermal and electrical burns. In: Aminoff MJ (ed.). *Neurology and General Medicine. The Neurological Aspects of Medical Disorders* (2nd edition). New York: Churchill Livingstone, 1995: 915–929.

■ Elephantiasis – see Filariasis

■ Elephantiasis neuromatosis

This is one of the terms given to the plexiform neuromas which are found on the face, scalp, neck and chest in neurofibromatosis type 1. They are very disfiguring and can undergo sarcomatous change.

Other relevant entry Neurofibromatosis.

■ Elsberg syndrome
Sacral myeloradiculitis

A syndrome of sensorimotor dysfunction affecting sacral dermomyotomes due to polyradiculitis, associated with urinary retention and CSF pleocytosis. It may resemble idiopathic lumbosacral plexopathy.

Reference Komar J, Szalay M, Dalos M. Acute retention of urine due to isolated sacral myeloradiculitis. *Journal of Neurology* 1982; **228**: 215–217.

Other relevant entry Lumbosacral plexopathies.

■ Embryonal carcinoma – see Germ-cell tumours

■ Emery–Dreifuss muscular dystrophy

Pathophysiology This rare muscular dystrophy is characterized by the early development of joint contractures, sometimes even before clinical signs of weakness are apparent. X-linked-recessive and autosomal-dominant/autosomal-recessive (AD/AR) forms are described, resulting from mutations in different genes. Cardiac complications are common and may account for early death, sometimes in young adults without other evidence of muscular disorder; hence screening is important.

The X-linked form is linked to chromosome Xq28, STA gene, and defect of the protein emerin.

AD/AR forms are linked to chromosome 1q21, LMNA gene, and defect of the protein lamin A/C [allelic with one form of limb girdle muscular dystrophy (LGMD)].

Clinical features: history and examination

- Early development of joint contractures: Achilles tendon, elbows, posterior cervical/neck.
- Slowly progressive muscle wasting and weakness: Proximal arms, distal legs (scapulohumeroperoneal pattern), extending to limb girdle muscles.
- Cardiomyopathy: Cardiac conduction defects (e.g. prolonged PR interval, complete heart block) by the age of 30 years. Cardiac manifestations may occur in the absence of muscle disease, and in female carriers of the disease, presenting with sudden death.

Investigations and diagnosis *Bloods*: creatine kinase may be moderately elevated.

Neurophysiology: EMG: myopathic.

ECG: for cardiac conduction abnormalities: sinus bradycardia, prolonged PR interval, complete heart block.

Muscle biopsy: dystrophic, with scattered necrotic and regenerating fibres; variation in fibre diameter, increased number of hypertrophic fibres, splitting fibres, internal nuclei; disorganized intermyofibrillary networks producing a "moth-eaten" appearance.

Neurogenetics: dependent on pattern of inheritance (from the family history), analysis for mutations in the emerin or lamin A/C gene may be undertaken.

Differential diagnosis Unlikely to be confused with any of the other muscular dystrophies because of the prominence of contractures. Bethlem myopathy lacks cardiac involvement.

Rigid spine syndrome.

Scapuloperoneal syndrome (*q.v.*).

AD/AR form is allelic with LGMD type 1B and Dunnigan partial lipodystrophy.

Treatment and prognosis EMD is a progressive, incurable condition. Cardiac involvement is the commonest cause of death through arrhythmia and cardiac failure. Pacemaker insertion may prolong life.

References Emery AEH, Dreifuss FE. Unusual type of benign X-linked muscular dystrophy. *Journal of Neurology, Neurosurgery and Psychiatry* 1966; **29**: 338–342.

Tsuchiya Y, Arahata K. Emery–Dreifuss syndrome. *Current Opinion in Neurology* 1997; **10**: 421–425.

Other relevant entries Bethlem myopathy; Limb-girdle muscular dystrophy; Muscular dystrophies: an overview; Rigid spine syndrome; Scapuloperoneal syndrome.

■ Emotional lability: differential diagnosis

The term "emotional lability" may be used to refer generally to any failure of inhibition of emotion incongruent with prevailing social norms, or more specifically to an easy alternation between tears and laughter, these emotions being appropriate to the stimulus and mood congruent (*cf.* pathological crying and laughter):

- True emotional lability (moria) is usually associated with bilateral corticobulbar damage, and so conditions that predominantly affect the frontal lobe and descending pathways express this sign (orbitofrontal syndrome). It may be seen in cerebrovascular disease, motor neurone disease, Alzheimer's disease, progressive supranuclear palsy, multiple sclerosis, and diffuse hypoxic–ischaemic encephalopathy.

- Placidity and apathy are usually seen with damage of the frontostriatal connections (frontal convexity syndrome). They may be seen in the context of degenerative dementias (e.g. frontotemporal, Alzheimer's), tumours, normal pressure hydrocephalus, as well as degenerative extrapyramidal disorders (e.g. Parkinson's disease) and focal basal ganglia lesions (e.g. vascular events).

- Sudden rage can be part of a personality disorder, but may also (albeit rarely) represent ictal activity originating from the amygdaloid nucleus. It may occasionally be seen in vascular lesions of the temporal lobe or early in an encephalitic illness. Rage reactions may be one feature of the Klüver–Bucy syndrome. Sudden outbursts of laughter may represent gelastic epilepsy, which is associated with hypothalamic lesions.

- Acute panic attacks may occur in severe anxiety states, but may also be manifestations of epilepsy or part of an hallucinatory experience as occurs in schizophrenia and some neurodegenerative conditions, such as dementia with Lewy bodies.

  Reference Heilman KM, Blonder LX, Bowers D, Valenstein E. Emotional disorders associated with neurological diseases. In: Heilman KM, Valenstein E (eds). *Clinical Neuropsychology* (4th edition). Oxford: OUP, 2003: 447–478.

  Other relevant entries Frontal lobe syndrome; Gelastic epilepsy; Klüver–Bucy syndrome.

■ Empty sella syndrome

The empty sella syndrome, or non-tumourous enlargement of the sella, is a radiological diagnosis in which there appears to be no pituitary gland in an expanded pituitary fossa. The presumed pathogenesis is a defect in the dural diaphragm which allows arachnoid to bulge downwards, gradually enlarging the sella, possibly as a consequence of pressure pulsations in the CSF. It is commonly seen in idiopathic intracranial hypertension and is not associated with clinical or biochemical evidence of pituitary insufficiency, as the gland remains functional as a thin ribbon of tissue along the wall of the expanded sella. Downward herniation of the optic chiasm may also occur, producing visual disturbances similar to those seen with a pituitary adenoma.

  Other relevant entries Idiopathic intracranial hypertension; Pituitary disease and apoplexy.

■ Empyema – see Subdural empyema

■ Encephalitis: an overview

Pathophysiology Encephalitis is inflammation of the brain parenchyma. This inflammation is usually due to direct invasion of brain tissue by infectious agents, most usually viral but sometimes protozoan, rickettsial or fungal; there may be concurrent meningitic features (meningoencephalitis). Post-infectious encephalitis, due to allergic or immune reactions, may be clinically indistinguishable. Clinical clues as to the causative agent may be found, but often no specific microbe is identified. Encephalitis is also described with underlying malignancy (paraneoplastic or limbic encephalitis). Infective encephalitides usually present acutely or subacutely, although chronic presentations and sequelae are not infrequent. The term "encephalitis" has sometimes been used for disorders in which brain inflammation is not obviously apparent (e.g. prion disorders).

Encephalitides may be classified in a number of ways:

- Location
    Diffuse (panencephalitis).
    Focal, for example herpes simplex encephalitis (HSE), Rasmussen's encephalitis, paraneoplastic (limbic) encephalitis, transmissible spongiform encephalitis, brainstem encephalitis, encephalitis lethargica.

- Disease incidence
    Epidemic encephalitis
        arboviral: including dengue, Russian spring–summer, Japanese encephalitis, St Louis encephalitis, Eastern equine and Western equine encephalitis (Von Economo's) encephalitis lethargica.
    Sporadic encephalitis
        herpes simplex type 1
        mumps virus
        Epstein–Barr virus (EBV)
        adenovirus (especially type 7 in children)
        other viruses (including hepatitis, rotavirus, CMV).
    Zoonotic encephalitis
        rabies
        others including lymphocytic choriomeningitis.
    Chronic encephalitides
        subacute sclerosing panencephalitis (SSPE)
        progressive measles encephalitis
        progressive rubella encephalitis
        AIDS encephalopathy
        progressive multifocal leukoencephalopathy (PML)
        Rasmussen's encephalitis.

- Specific encephalitides include

  Viral

  Herpes simplex (HSV, *q.v.*)

  Varicella zoster (VZV)

  Cytomegalovirus (CMV)

  Epstein–Barr virus

  Measles

  Mumps

  Arboviruses: Japanese, California, St Louis, Murray Valley, Eastern equine, Western equine, Russian spring–summer

  Human immunodeficiency virus (HIV)

  ? Rasmussen's encephalitis.

  Protozoal

  Malaria (*q.v.*)

  Rabies (*q.v.*).

  Bacterial

  Brucellosis

  Legionnaire's disease

  Mycoplasma pneumoniae

  Listeria monocytogenes

  Lyme disease.

  Fungal

  Nocardia.

  Paraneoplastic: limbic, brainstem.

  Transmissible spongiform encephalitis (prion disease).

  Inflammatory disorders: sarcoid, systemic lupus erythematosus (SLE), antiphospholipid syndrome, anti-voltage gated K^+ channels.

Clinical features: history and examination The presentation can be very dramatic with the patient becoming profoundly unwell and unconscious in a few hours. More typically the patient presents with:

- Prodrome (days): myalgia, fever, malaise, anorexia; rash (may be characteristic for varicella or measles); parotitis suggests mumps.
- Headache, mental change, drowsiness (i.e. encephalopathy), with or without meningitic features.
- Coma.
- Seizures.
- +/− focal signs, for example hemiparesis, aphasia, cerebellar deficits, neuro-psychological deficits (memory).
- +/− raised intracranial pressure.

Inquiries should be made about travel to areas where certain encephalitides are endemic.

Investigations and diagnosis *Bloods*: evidence of systemic infection (raised ESR, CRP; leukocytosis; blood cultures, immunoglobulins, electrophoretic strip); other organ involvement (U&E, LFTs); viral serology; film for malaria if recent travel to endemic areas.

Imaging: CT/MRI to exclude mass lesions, oedema, infarction; may well be normal in the first 2–3 days. Bilateral temporal lobe hyperintensity may be seen in HSE, the commonest encephalitic illness in non-tropical countries.

Neurophysiology: EEG: may show non-specific diffuse slow-wave activity +/− epileptic activity; focal temporal lobe spike and wave activity is suggestive of HSE.

CSF: standard investigations may be normal. Blood may be seen in some cases of severe encephalitis where there is haemorrhagic infarction of the brain. CSF may be under increased pressure; white count may be raised (10 to several thousands/µl), usually lymphocytes, sometimes polymorphs. Protein raised, glucose normal, organisms not seen on Gram stain. Indian ink stain if fungal infection suspected. CSF PCR for common viral causes of encephalitis (HSV, VZV, CMV, EBV).

Brain biopsy: not favoured in some centres; may be a case for it in immunocompromised patients where diagnosis not forthcoming by other means, or if there is a focal lesion on imaging.

Other tests: usually not necessary unless the presentation is atypical. Auto-antibodies (including anti-neuronal, anti-thyroid, anti-ENA, anti-VGKC antibodies) may be sent. Investigations appropriate to rare causes of an encephalitic illness may need to be considered (e.g. prion disease, Whipple's disease, coeliac disease).

Differential diagnosis Other encephalopathies, for example:

Infection
    Meningitis, especially bacterial
    Septicaemia
    Endocarditis
    Intracranial abscess.
Drug abuse.
Central nervous system (CNS) vasculitis.
Epilepsy.
Organ failure, for example liver failure.

Treatment and prognosis Assess patient and decide on level of dependency: may require supportive therapy on ITU.

Aciclovir (antiviral chemotherapy): start as soon as diagnosis is contemplated, especially HSE.

Anti-epileptic medications for seizures.

Treat any secondary infections with antibiotic therapy, or if meningitis cannot be excluded.

Consider steroids if a vasculitis cannot be excluded.

Cerebral oedema: hyperventilation; glycerol; mannitol; dexamethasone.

Symptomatic treatment: oxygenation (ventilation if necessary), hydration, nutrition.

Condition may be fatal; this was commonly the case before the advent of aciclovir. Recovery may be complete or there may be neurological and/or neuropsychological sequelae, especially an amnesic syndrome after HSE.

Reference Anderson M. Encephalitis and other brain infections. In: Donaghy M (ed.). *Brain's Diseases of the Nervous System* (11th edition). Oxford: OUP, 2001: 1117–1180.

Other relevant entries Atypical pneumonias and the nervous system; Bickerstaff's brainstem encephalitis; Borreliosis; Brucellosis; Cytomegalovirus and the nervous system; Encephalitis lethargica; Epstein–Barr virus and the nervous system; Herpes simplex encephalitis; HIV/AIDS and the nervous system; Malaria; Paraneoplastic syndromes; Prion disease: an overview; Rabies; Rasmussen's encephalitis, Rasmussen's syndrome; Rubella; Subacute sclerosing panencephalitis; Syphilis; Vasculitis.

■ Encephalitis lethargica
Post-encephalitic parkinsonism ● Von Economo disease

Encephalitis lethargica is a profound parkinsonian syndrome of unknown cause, but presumed viral, which occurred in epidemic form in the years after the First World War, but is now rare. Clinical features are initially of fever, somnolence, personality changes, and cranial nerve involvement, especially ophthalmoplegia. A prolonged convalescent period is characterized by parkinsonism and oculogyric crises; myoclonus, dystonia, bulimia, obesity, and sleep disturbances are also reported. Imaging findings are non-specific: bilateral substantia nigra changes may be seen. Response to levodopa has been demonstrated, and in refractory cases intravenous methylprednisolone has been reported of benefit. Myoclonus may be treated with clonazepam.

Although presumed to be related to the influenza pandemic following the First World War, archival brain tissue examined for influenza RNA has been negative. This virus may not have been neurotropic and hence not directly responsible. More recently the condition has been thought to be due to anti-basal ganglia antibodies.

References Blunt SB, Lane RJ, Turjanski N, Perkin GD. Clinical features and management of two cases of encephalitis lethargica. *Movement Disorders* 1997; **12**: 354–359.

Dickman MS. Von Economo encephalitis. *Archives of Neurology* 2001; **58**: 1696–1698.

Other relevant entries Bickerstaff's brainstem encephalitis; Encephalitis: an overview; Parkinsonian syndromes, parkinsonism; Rubella; Subacute sclerosing panencephalitis.

■ Encephalocele – see Exencephaly

■ Encephalomyelitis: differential diagnosis

Encephalomyelitis, the simultaneous involvement of the brain and spinal cord by an inflammatory process, has a differential diagnosis which differs from that of encephalitis, including:

> acute disseminated encephalomyelitis (ADEM);
> multiple sclerosis;
> vasculitides;
> paraneoplasia, including progressive encephalomyelitis with
> > rigidity $+/-$ myoclonus (PERM): especially with small-cell carcinoma of bronchus;
> infective causes: viral, Bartonellosis.

Other relevant entries Acute disseminated encephalomyelitis; Bartonellosis; Encephalitis: an overview; Myelitis; Paraneoplastic syndromes.

■ Encephalopathies: an overview

Pathophysiology Encephalopathy describes a state of diffuse or global cerebral dysfunction in which patients are typically confused, delirious or comatose, with abnormal eye movements and asterixis (flapping tremor). Epileptic seizures may occur. Encephalopathies most commonly result from acute (or acute on chronic, or decompensated) metabolic disturbances or toxic insults (including drugs) to the CNS, although the term has also been used in the context of vascular (e.g. Binswanger), epileptic, or neurodegenerative (e.g. Alzheimer's, Creutzfeldt–Jakob) disease.

The differential diagnosis of encephalopathy is broad, but essentially the causes fall into three large groups: metabolic, infective (septic), and drug/toxin induced:

- Metabolic encephalopathies.
    > Hepatic encephalopathy (*q.v.*): liver failure.
    > Wernicke's encephalopathy: thiamine deficiency.
    > Uraemic encephalopathy.
    > Anoxic–ischaemic encephalopathies: may be acute (at the time of the original or ongoing insult), or delayed, emerging after a number of days to weeks [post-anoxic encephalopthy, e.g. carbon monoxide (CO) poisoning].
    > Lactic acidosis: (e.g. mitochondrial disease); typically these patients (usually children) become encephalopathic with an intercurrent illness such as a viral infection.
    > Electrolyte disturbances: (e.g. $\uparrow\downarrow Na^+$, $\uparrow\downarrow Ca^{2+}$, $\uparrow\downarrow Mg^{2+}$); disorders of glucose homeostasis (e.g. hyperosmolar state).

Hypertensive encephalopathy: (e.g. with uncontrolled hypertension).

Endocrine encephalopathies: e.g. Cushing's disease, hyper- and hypothyroidism, Hashimoto's encephalopathy (irrespective of thyroid status)

Mitochondrial disorders, urea cycle enzyme defects.

- Septic encephalopathies

    Marked brain dysfunction in the context of systemic sepsis with or without multiorgan failure, (e.g. infective endocarditis).

- Drug/toxin-induced encephalopathies

    Not uncommon; may be precipitated by a number of agents including:

    alcohol;

    sedatives (e.g. benzodiazepines, opiates);

    antidepressants;

    metals: lead in children; bismuth;

    radiation;

    (see individual entries).

Clinical features: history and examination History of prior illness (hepatic, renal, respiratory); drug/toxin exposure

- Global signs

    Disturbance of consciousness: drowsy to comatose

    Seizures

    Delirium.

- Focal signs

    Hemiplegia, hemisensory signs, ataxia, myoclonus

    Aphasia, apraxia

    Brainstem signs: orofacial automatisms, posturing, asterixis, tremor.

Investigations and diagnosis *Bloods*: consider FBC + film, ESR, clotting including fibrin degradation products (FDPs), urea and electrolytes, glucose, calcium, magnesium, other electrolytes, thyroid function tests, blood cultures, serology, ammonia, lactate, and arterial blood gases.

Imaging: includes CXR, CT/MRI (+MRV) brain +/− echocardiography, abdominal ultrasound.

CSF: including lactate.

Neurophysiology: EEG.

Other: ECG; assays for defects typical of inherited metabolic disease (e.g. organic and amino acids).

Differential diagnosis

Of encephalopathy:

Encephalitis/meningitis

Non-convulsive status epilepticus

Cerebral vasculitis

Cerebral venous sinus thrombosis

Hypothalamic damage.

Of uraemic encephalopathy: encephalopathy secondary to the underlying cause of the renal failure (e.g. hypertension, diabetes mellitus, systemic lupus erythematosus, thrombotic thrombocytopenic purpura), and encephalopathy secondary to the treatment of renal failure (e.g. dialysis syndromes).

Treatment and prognosis Of cause where identified. If in doubt, there is little to be lost and possibly much to be gained by administration of thiamine. Therapeutic trials of naloxone (opiate antagonist) and flumazenil (benzodiazepine antagonist) may also be considered if the clinical picture is compatible. Otherwise, supportive care; symptomatic treatment of seizures.

> **Reference** Kunze K. Metabolic encephalopathies. *Journal of Neurology* 2002; **249**: 1150–1159.

> **Other relevant entries** Carbon monoxide poisoning; Drug-induced encephalopathies; Encephalitis: an overview; Endocarditis and the nervous system; Endocrinology and the nervous system; Hashimoto's encephalopathy; Heavy metal poisoning; Hepatic encephalopathy; Hypertension and the nervous system; Lead and the nervous system; Renal disease and the nervous system; Wernicke–Korsakoff's syndrome.

▮ Encephalotrigeminal angiomatosis – see Phakomatosis; Sturge–Weber syndrome

▮ Endocarditis and the nervous system

Pathophysiology Infective endocarditis is a microbial infection of the endocardial surface of the heart, most commonly on valves (especially if prosthetic or deformed) but also on chordae tendinae or mural endocardium. The characteristic lesions are vegetations formed of platelets, fibrin, microorganisms, and inflammatory cells. Distinction is sometimes made between acute and subacute-chronic endocarditis, dependent on the pace of the disease. Various microorganisms may be involved, including:

- Bacteria
    Streptococci; if *bovis*, investigate for bowel neoplasm
    Staphylococci
    Pseudomonas, other Gram-negative bacilli
    Brucella
    Enterobacteria.
- Fungi: for example *Candida.*
- Rickettsia: for example *Coxiella* (Q fever).

Intravenous drug abuse and prolonged intravenous access (e.g. for parenteral nutrition) may predispose to endocarditis by providing a route for infection to enter the circulation.

Neurological consequences of endocarditis occur in about a third of cases and typically are embolic in nature, with vegetations embolizing to the cerebral circulation causing infarcts or the development of mycotic aneurysms that can rupture. Multiple septic emboli may cause a meningoencephalitis or encephalopathy. Treatment is with antibiotics.

Clinical features: history and examination

- *Cardiac*:

    Fever, variable heart murmurs, cardiac failure.

    Embolic stigmata: nail bed infarcts (*cf.* nail trauma), Roth spots, Janeway lesions, Osler's nodes.

- *Neurological*:

    10–30% of patients with infective endocarditis present with neurological symptoms.

    Focal deficits: secondary to embolic infarcts, due to vessel occlusion by septic embolus. May undergo haemorrhagic transformation. Most occur early in course of disease. Patients with Q fever are thought particularly prone to embolism.

    Intracranial haemorrhage: secondary to rupture of a cerebral mycotic aneurysm; infected emboli lodge at the distal bifurcation points in the cerebral circulation, and typically are multiple. On occasions the vessel may rupture with haemorrhage in the absence of aneurysm formation, due to a septic arteritis.

    Meningoencephalitis or diffuse encephalopathy: due to multiple septic emboli, presenting with confusion, meningism, and headache.

    Seizures.

    Abscess: brain, paraspinal.

Of those patients with infective endocarditis and neurological complications, infection with *Staphylococcus aureus* and history of IV drug abuse are over represented compared to those with endocarditis and no neurological features.

Investigations and diagnosis *Bloods*: FBC (anaemia), ESR (elevated), C-reactive protein (CRP) (elevated), and repeated blood cultures (3–6); INR if anticoagulated.

Imaging:

CXR

Echocardiogram: transthoracic, transoesophageal

CT/MRI +/− MR/catheter angiography when intracranial haemorrhage has occurred.

CSF: often normal, although a slight polymorph leukocytosis with some red cells and normal glucose is not uncommon. Large numbers of red cells may be seen in cases of intracerebral haemorrhage.

Neurophysiology: usually not required.

Others: cardiological and microbiological advice.

Differential diagnosis There is usually little doubt about the diagnosis, but in patients with a high ESR and cerebral events consider:

atrial myxoma;

marantic or non-bacterial endocarditis (e.g. lupus, Libman–Sacks);

vasculitis (including temporal arteritis);

angioendotheliomatosis (intravascular lymphomatosis);

hyperviscosity syndromes (e.g. Waldenström's macroglobulinaemia);

cholesterol embolization syndrome;

paraneoplastic encephalitis.

Treatment and prognosis Untreated the condition is fatal.

Aggressive intravenous antimicrobial therapy appropriate for the infective agent is the mainstay of treatment, which may be required for several weeks, and with which most symptoms improve or resolve, including the neurological abnormalities.

Embolic phenomena do not mandate anticoagulant treatment in patients with native valve endocarditis. In patients already receiving anticoagulation (e.g. for prosthetic valves), this should not be stopped unless there is intracranial haemorrhage, when cessation of treatment for a short period (? 2 days) is thought advisable.

Mycotic aneurysms usually resolve with antibiotic therapy and do not require surgical intervention.

Involvement of cardiologists and cardiothoracic surgeons is necessary, as the patient may require treatment for heart failure +/− valve replacement.

Despite treatment, overall mortality remains 20–25%; mortality is twice as high in group with neurological complications.

References Kanter MC, Hart RG. Neurologic complications of infective endocarditis. *Neurology* 1991; **41**: 1015–1020.

Lerner PI. Neurological manifestations of infective endocarditis. In: Aminoff MJ (ed.). *Neurology and General Medicine. The Neurological Aspects of Medical Disorders* (2nd edition). New York: Churchill Livingstone, 1995: 97–117.

Mylonakis E, Calderwood SB. Infective endocarditis in adults. *New England Journal of Medicine* 2001; **345**: 1318–1330.

Other relevant entries Angioendotheliomatosis; Brucellosis; Cholesterol embolization syndrome; Paraneoplastic syndromes; Q fever; Vasculitis.

▪ Endocrinology and the nervous system

Disorders of the endocrine system can affect the nervous system in a number of different ways. This may be developmental (e.g. in hypothyroidism), or acquired, global (e.g. encephalopathy) or focal (e.g. carpel tunnel syndrome). This entry briefly reviews associations of endocrine disease and neurological dysfunction, with the exception of diabetes mellitus which is discussed separately.

- Thyroid disorders

    Hypothyroidism

        In children:

            Cretinism: manifest as prolonged neonatal jaundice, followed a few weeks later by the development of coarse facial features, thick tongue, protruding abdomen, irritability, and a coarse cry. If untreated it causes permanent mental retardation, with spasticity and cerebellar ataxia. Screening programmes in the UK, USA, and most developed countries, have greatly reduced the incidence.

In adults:

Myopathy, sluggish reflexes, hypothermia, mental slowing, dementia.

Rare (and sometimes debatable) accounts of cerebellar syndrome, peripheral neuropathy, and pyramidal syndrome responding to thyroxine therapy.

Hyperthyroidism

Myopathy

Tremor

Ocular involvement: chemosis, proptosis, and ophthalmoplegia in Graves disease

Cognitive and mental changes, delirium

Seizures

Headache: migraine or tension type

Polyneuropathy (distal sensorimotor)

Chorea

Hashimoto's encephalopathy may occur with hypo-, hyper-, or euthyroidism.

Thyroid disease may be associated with other neurological disorders (e.g. myasthenia gravis, periodic paralyses).

Embolic phenomena secondary to paroxysmal atrial fibrillation.

- Adrenal gland

  Deficiencies in adrenocortical hormones: Addison's disease may present with fatigue, generalized weakness, weight loss, headache, skin hyperpigmentation, and syncopal attacks. Adrenal failure is a feature of X-linked adrenoleukodystrophy (X-ALD).

  Excessive adrenocortical secretion: Cushing's disease may present with hypertension, proximal myopathy, a psychiatric syndrome or with an encephalopathy.

- Pituitary gland

  Anterior

  Growth hormone:

  - Deficiency: in children causes a reduction in growth that responds to replacement therapy. Recombinant growth hormone (GH) is now used; use of GH from cadaveric pituitaries was discontinued after some children developed iatrogenic Creutzfeldt–Jakob disease (CJD).

  - Excess: in children this causes gigantism, in adults acromegaly. In both cases there may be secondary diabetes mellitus, proximal myopathy, and carpal tunnel syndrome.

    In the diencephalic syndrome, GH secretion can be increased or decreased.

Gonadotrophins:
- Deficiency: causes delayed puberty and amenorrhoea in women; delayed puberty, reduced libido and body hair in men.
- Excess: precocious puberty in children, as seen in a number of conditions affecting the hypothalamic–pituitary axis (e.g. hamartomas, germinomas).

Posterior
Antidiuretic hormone:
- Deficiency: causes diabetes insipidus, with polyuria and polydipsia; seen in children and adults when there is damage to the hypothalamus and/or posterior pituitary.
- Excess: syndrome of inappropriate ADH secretion.

- Parathyroid glands
  - Hypoparathyroidism (parathormone deficiency) leads to hypocalcaemia which causes tetany, paraesthesia, muscle cramps, laryngeal spasm and even fits. In adults it may be associated with intracranial calcification involving the basal ganglia and cerebellum, usually incidental but in some cases the patient may manifest a movement disorder (e.g. parkinsonism).
  - Hyperparathyroidism, usually due to a parathyroid adenoma, may on occasion be complicated by proximal and bulbar myopathy, ataxia, ophthalmoplegia, and pyramidal signs.

Reference Schipper HM, Abrams GM. Other endocrinopathies and the nervous system. In: Aminoff MJ (ed.). _Neurology and General Medicine. The Neurological Aspects of Medical Disorders_ (2nd edition). New York: Churchill Livingstone, 1995: 383–400.

Other relevant entries Acromegaly; Adrenoleukodystrophy; Basal ganglia calcification; Creutzfeldt–Jakob disease; Cushing's disease, Cushing's syndrome; Diabetes insipidus; Diabetes mellitus and the nervous system; Diencephalic syndrome; Dwarfism; Fibrous dysplasia; Hashimoto's encephalopathy; Parkinsonian syndromes, parkinsonism; Pituitary disease and apoplexy; Prion disease: an overview; Syndrome of inappropriate ADH secretion; Thyroid disease and the nervous system.

▇ Endolymphatic hydrops – see Ménière's disease

▇ Engel's disease – see Acid-maltase deficiency; Glycogen-storage disorders: an overview

▇ Entrapment neuropathies: an overview

Pathophysiology Entrapment or compression is the commonest cause of mononeuropathy. Various entrapment neuropathies are described, some due to compression within anatomical structures [e.g. carpal tunnel syndrome (CTS)], many more involving extraneous pressure. Concomitant alcohol use greatly increases the risk of nerve entrapment due to external compression, as does any diffuse clinical or subclinical neuropathy. Pressure on nerves during anaesthesia for surgical procedures is a potentially avoidable cause of entrapment. More than one episode of entrapment neuropathy, or a strong family history, should raise suspicion of an underlying hereditary neuropathy with liability to pressure palsies.

Commonly occurring peripheral nerve entrapment syndromes include the following (see individual entries for more information):

- Upper limb:

Median nerve:	Forearm:	Anterior interosseous syndrome
		Pronator teres syndrome
	Wrist:	Carpal tunnel syndrome
Ulnar nerve:	Elbow:	Medial epicondyle (ulnar groove)
		Cubital tunnel syndrome
	Hand:	Canal of Guyon (Ramsay Hunt syndrome)
Radial nerve:	Arm:	Spiral groove of the humerus ("Saturday night palsy")
	Forearm:	Posterior interosseous syndrome
		Superficial sensory branch
Suprascapular nerve:		Suprascapular notch
Dorsal scapular nerve:		Scalene muscle
Lower brachial plexus:		(Neurogenic) thoracic outlet syndrome (TOS)

- Lower limb:

Ilioinguinal:	Abdominal wall
Lateral cutaneous nerve of the thigh:	Meralgia paraesthetica (Bernhardt–Roth syndrome)
Femoral nerve:	Psoas sheath haematoma, abscess
	Inguinal ligament
Obturator nerve:	Obturator canal
Sciatic nerve:	Sciatic notch
	Piriformis syndrome
	Popliteal fossa
Tibial nerve:	Medial malleolus (posterior tibial)
	Tarsal tunnel
Common peroneal nerve:	Fibular head; prolonged squatting (e.g. strawberry pickers)
	Anterior compartment
Plantar interdigital nerves:	Morton's metatarsalgia

- Other possible nerve entrapment syndromes:

Cheiralgia paraesthetica:	Radial side of thumb; distal dorsal digital nerve
Notalgia paraesthetica:	Medial margin of scapula; dorsal branches of roots T2 to T6
Gonyalgia paraesthetica:	Patella; infrapatellar branch of saphenous nerve

Investigations and diagnosis The diagnosis is often possible on clinical grounds alone, but if in doubt NCS showing focal slowing or even conduction block and EMG showing denervation of muscles innervated by the nerve in question may be helpful.

Differential diagnosis Mononeuropathies are unlikely to be confused with peripheral polyneuropathies or radiculopathies but may overlap with inflammatory neuropathy (mononeuritis, mononeuritis multiplex).

Treatment and prognosis Many entrapment neuropathies due to external pressure ("neurapraxia") recover spontaneously. For anatomical entrapment surgical decompression may be possible (e.g. carpal tunnel syndrome). Often symptomatic treatment with local splinting and/or analgesic medications may suffice. Drugs with particular efficacy for neuropathic pain include amitriptyline, carbamazepine, and gabapentin.

> **References** Dawson DM, Hallett M, Wilbourn AJ (eds). *Entrapment Neuropathies* (3rd edition). Philadelphia: Lippincott, Williams & Wilkins, 1999.
>
> Nakano KK. The entrapment neuropathies. *Muscle and Nerve* 1978; **1**: 264–279.
>
> Pecina MM, Krmpotić-Nemanić J, Markiewitz AD. *Tunnel Syndromes*. Boca Raton: CRC Press, 1991.
>
> Staal A, van Gijn J, Spaans F. *Mononeuropathies: Examination, Diagnosis and Treatment*. London: WB Saunders, 1999.
>
> **Other relevant entries** Anterior interosseous syndrome; Carpal tunnel syndrome; Cheiralgia paraesthetica; Cubital tunnel syndrome; Gonyalgia paraesthetica; Hereditary neuropathy with liability to pressure palsies; Median neuropathy; Meralgia paraesthetica; Notalgia paraesthetica; Piriformis syndrome; Posterior interosseous syndrome; Pronator teres syndrome; Radial neuropathy; Ramsay Hunt syndrome (3); Thoracic outlet syndrome; Ulnar neuropathy.

▧ Environmental dependency syndrome

This name has been given to the acting out of behavioural sequences appropriate to the environment without being asked to do so, hence utilization behaviour as a component of frontal lobe pathology.

> **Reference** Lhermitte F. Human anatomy and the frontal lobes. Part II. Patient behaviour in complex and social situations: the "environmental dependency syndrome". *Annals of Neurology* 1986; **19**: 335–343.
>
> **Other relevant entry** Frontal lobe syndrome.

▧ Eosinophilia–Myalgia syndrome

This is a systemic illness characterized by severe generalized myalgia and peripheral blood eosinophilia, an epidemic of which occurred in 1989–1990 due to ingestion of L-tryptophan tablets contaminated with a ditryptophan aminal of acetaldehyde.

Clinically there is subacute onset of fatigue, fever, myalgia, cramps, acroparaesthesiae, and skin induration, in association with a raised eosinophil count ($>1000/mm^3$). Severe axonal neuropathy may be associated with some cases. Creatine kinase may be elevated, along with liver function tests. Pathologically there is evidence for a microangiopathy and an inflammatory reaction in connective tissue structures in the skin, muscle, and peripheral nerve. These features closely resemble those of the toxic oil syndrome described in Spain in 1981 in which ingestion of contaminated rapeseed oil was incriminated.

Eosinophilia–myalgia may respond to corticosteroids, although the axonal neuropathy may not resolve completely, but the mainstay of therapy is removal of the offending drug.

References Medsger TA Jr. Tryptophan-induced eosinophilia–myalgia syndrome. *New England Journal of Medicine* 1990; **322**: 926–928.

Ricoy JR, Cabello A, Rodriguez J, Téllez I. Neuropathological studies on the toxic syndrome related to adulterated rapeseed oil in Spain. *Brain* 1983; **106**: 817–835.

Other relevant entry Drug-induced myopathies.

■ Eosinophilic fasciitis
Shulman's syndrome

This is a rare entity of unknown aetiology, predominantly seen in men between 30 and 60 years of age, in which fever and myalgia, often after exercise, precedes diffuse cutaneous thickening, likened to scleroderma, and limitation of joint movement which may develop into contractures. Proximal muscle weakness may occur. Blood tests reveal raised ESR, eosinophilia (in most cases), and raised gammaglobulins. Subcutaneous tissues are infiltrated with plasma cells, lymphocytes and eosinophils; eosinophilic infiltration of muscle may be seen in those with proximal weakness (hence the condition may overlap with eosinophilic myopathy, *q.v.*), in which there is a predominantly eosinophilic inflammation of the fascia but not the muscle, without evidence for a eosinophilia.

Clinical improvement may occur spontaneously, or may follow use of steroids.

Reference Shulman LE. Diffuse fasciitis with hypergammaglobulinemia and eosinophilia: a new syndrome? *Journal of Rheumatology* 1984; **11**: 569–570.

Other relevant entry Eosinophilic myopathy.

■ Eosinophilic granuloma – see Langerhans cell histiocytosis

■ Eosinophilic myopathy

Muscle weakness with biopsy evidence of inflammation and eosinophilic infiltration may occur in a number of situations, which may represent overlapping conditions or separate nosological entities, viz.:

• Eosinophilic fasciits (*q.v.*).

- Eosinophilic (mono)myositis: painful swelling, often of the calf muscle(s); responds to steroids.
- Eosinophilic polymyositis: predominantly proximal weakness, evolving over weeks, as part of a systemic illness typical of the hypereosinophilic syndrome (HES) (*q.v.*), hence with other manifestations such as involvement of lung, heart, skin, and blood (eosinophilia, anaemia, hypergammaglobulinaemia).

In eosinophilic mono- and polymyositis, there may be raised ESR and creatine kinase, +/− positive rheumatoid factor and antinuclear antibody. EMG usually reveals a myopathic pattern with fibrillation potentials. Steroids may be used, usually with benefit to the muscle symptoms and signs, but overall prognosis depends on involvement of other organs (HES).

Eosinophilia and muscle symptoms +/− signs may also coexist in eosinophilia–myalgia syndrome, drug-induced muscle disorders (phenobarbitone, tranilast, as well as L-tryptophan), parasitic diseases, Lyme disease, and mixed connective tissue disease.

Reference Layzer RB, Shearn MA, Satya-Murti S. Eosinophilic polymyositis. *Annals of Neurology* 1977; **1**: 65–71.

Other relevant entries Eosinophilia–myalgia syndrome; Eosinophilic fasciitis; Hypereosinophilic syndrome.

▓ Ependymoma

Pathophysiology Ependymomas are tumours derived from the ependymal cells which line the surface of the ventricular system of the brain and the central canal of the spinal cord; hence they may be classified as a subtype of glioma. They account for about 5% of all brain tumours. They are typically found in the posterior fossa in childhood, but may occur at any age and involve the spinal cord as commonly as the brain in adults. They present insidiously and generally respond to surgical debulking and radiotherapy. Contact with CSF pathways permits seeding of ventricular surfaces and subarachnoid pathways.

Pathologically ependymomas are often grey–pink exophitic growths, often well demarcated. Microscopically tumour cells form rosettes and pseudorosettes (circular arrangements around blood vessels). Distinction may be drawn between benign, well-differentiated tumours which form papillae, and more malignant, anaplastic lesions with high mitotic activity, which may be termed ependymoblastomas; some classify these with primitive neuroectodermal tumours (PNET). Subependymona has features of both ependymoma and astrocytoma.

Clinical features: history and examination
- Supraspinal tumours: most arise in the fourth ventricle, hence patients present with posterior fossa signs and raised intracranial pressure from obstructive hydrocephalus: headache, nausea, vomiting, ataxia and nystagmus. Cerebral lesions present as space-occupying lesions with seizures.

- Spinal ependymomas: most occur in the lumbosacral region, conus or filum termi-nale. Unlike supraspinal ependymomas these tumours are only found in adults, and men more commonly than women (M : F = 2 : 1). They typically present with a slowly progressive spinal cord syndrome and back pain, with the spinothalamic tract in particular being affected.

Investigations and diagnosis *Bloods*: usually non-contributory.

Imaging: CT/MRI; typically these tumours enhance homogenously with gadolinium contrast.

Differential diagnosis Other tumours:

Medulloblastoma in fourth ventricle
Glioma in cerebral cortex
Astrocytoma in spinal cord.

Treatment and prognosis Treatment is surgical debulking with radiotherapy, except in the case of the benign myxopapillary tumour of the filum terminale where surgery alone can be curative. Chemotherapy with platinum-containing regimens has been shown to induce remission at tumour recurrence.

Prognosis depends on the location of the tumour, the degree of seeding (which occurs in about 5–10% of tumours), the age of the patient (better prognosis in adult patients) and the grade of the tumour.

Reference Lyons MK, Kelly PJ. Posterior fossa ependymomas: report of 30 cases and review of the literature. *Neurosurgery* 1991; **28**: 659–665.

Other relevant entries Glioma; Tumours: an overview.

■ Epidermal naevus syndrome
Jadassohn's naevus phakomatosis • Schimmelpenning's syndrome

This name has been used to describe a number of rare congenital neurocutaneous disorders in which an epidermal naevus or linear sebaceous naevus is associated with various neurological features, including thickening of the skull on the side of the skin lesion, mental retardation, hemiparesis, seizures, cranial nerve palsies (VI, VII, VIII) and intracranial vascular abnormalities (arteriovenous malformations, vessel atresia). Brain tumours have also been reported in association with ENS. The alterna-tive names may be used when neurological features dominate.

Reference Baker RS, Ross PA, Baumann RJ. Neurologic complications of the epidermal nevus syndrome. *Archives of Neurology* 1987; **44**: 227–232.

Other relevant entry Phakomatosis.

■ Epidermoid
Cholesteatoma • Pearly tumour

Epidermoids are benign cystic tumours which develop from misplaced ectodermal tissue. They may be congenital, one of the commonest embryonal intracranial tumours, or acquired. The congenital forms are often found in association with dysraphism, whereas acquired forms occur secondary to invasive procedures (e.g. lumbar puncture) or infection (e.g. cholesteatoma: these may also be congenital).

Epidermoids may be found in a variety of central nervous system (CNS) sites, including cerebellopontine angle, suprasellar region, skull base, brainstem or intraventricular cavity, presenting with symptoms and signs of local pressure effects. They are usually encapsulated and contain keratin producing squamous epithelium +/− partly calcified collagenous walls. Rupture of the cyst into the CSF may produce a syndrome akin to Mollaret's meningitis (recurrent aseptic meningitis).

MRI shows a lesion with low signal on T1 and high signal on T2.

Surgical removal is possible, sometimes complete, although the tendency to envelop neurovascular structures may make this difficult. Recurrences may occur.

Other relevant entries Aseptic meningitis; Cerebellopontine angle syndrome; Cholesteatoma; Cysts: an overview; Dermoid; Mollaret's meningitis; Tumours: an overview.

Epidural abscess – see Abscess: an overview

Epidural haematoma – see Haematoma: an overview

Epilepsia partialis continua – see Rasmussen's encephalitis, Rasmussen's syndrome; Status epilepticus

Epilepsy: an overview

Pathophysiology Epileptic seizures are currently classified, using the International League Against Epilepsy (ILAE) classification, according to seizure phenomenology and EEG findings:

- Partial (focal, local) seizures
    Simple partial seizures, with motor, somatosensory, autonomic, or psychic symptoms.
    Complex partial seizures: simple partial seizure followed by impaired consciousness, or with impairment of consciousness at onset, with or without automatisms.
    Partial seizures evolving to secondarily generalized seizures (tonic–clonic, tonic, or clonic).
- Generalized seizures (convulsive and non-convulsive)
    Absence seizures: typical ("petit mal"), atypical.
    Myoclonic seizures.
    Clonic seizures.
    Tonic seizures.
    Tonic–clonic seizures.

Atonic seizures.

Combinations.

- Unclassified epileptic seizures.

Essentially, all epileptic seizures are thought to reflect abnormal, synchronous, electrical discharges within neuronal circuits.

Clinical features: history and examination A clear history of seizure morphology is the most important factor in reaching a correct diagnosis, but may be difficult or impossible to obtain if there is impairment or loss of consciousness. Collateral (witness) history may (or may not) add useful information. If possible, a video of a seizure should be obtained by family, friends.

Additional neurological signs may suggest an underlying symptomatic cause for epilepsy (e.g. tuberous sclerosis).

Investigations and diagnosis Diagnosis is essentially based on a description of the seizure. Other investigations seek to identify seizure type and aetiology.

Neurophysiology: routine interictal EEG is often normal, it cannot "exclude" or "confirm" epilepsy, unless by chance it coincides with a clinical seizure; sleep-deprived EEG may offer more information. Prolonged recording with telemetry may increase the chance of recording a seizure; if performed in an in-patient setting, this is combined with video recording. Depth electrodes may be helpful in identifying a focus of seizure onset, not evident from surface recording.

Imaging: MRI is increasingly of value, especially in focal seizures, to identify underlying structural lesions, for example indolent temporal lobe tumours (e.g. gangli-oglioma), neuronal migration disorders.

Wada test: if surgery is contemplated, intracarotid phenobarbital is used to anaesthetize one temporal lobe during which neuropsychological functioning may be assessed to determine lateralization of language and memory.

Despite investigation, many seizures remain cryptogenic.

Differential diagnosis

Syncope.

Drop attacks.

Cataplexy.

Pseudoseizures, non-epileptic seizures.

Panic attacks.

Microsleeps.

Movement disorders (e.g. paroxysmal dyskinesias).

Treatment and prognosis Prognosis for many seizures is good, with spontaneous remission and no requirement for long-term medication or follow-up.

Anti-epileptic medications are the mainstay of management. Monotherapy is preferred, since no anti-epileptic drug is without side-effects and the potential for interactions is high. First line medications are carbamazepeine and sodium valproate; although the evidence from randomized-controlled trials is inconclusive, carbamazepine is probably the most effective drug for seizures of partial onset, sodium valproate for seizures of generalized onset. Second line medications include older drugs such as phenytoin and phenobarbitone, and newer add-on therapies such as lamotrigine, gabapentin, topiramate, levetiracetam, oxcarbazepine. Some of these newer drugs have now obtained licences for monotherapy, but whether they are better than the established medications remains to be determined.

Certain seizure types are best treated with particular anti-epileptic drugs, for example juvenile myoclonic epilepsy responds best to sodium valproate.

For the manangement of status epilepticus, see individual entry.

With focal seizures caused by a focal lesion (tumour, neuronal migration defect), surgery is sometimes possible which may reduce or abolish seizures.

Mortality in epilepsy is higher than for a matched seizure-free population.

References Chadwick D. Seizures, epilepsy, and other episodic disorders in adults. In: Donaghy M (ed.). *Brain's Diseases of the Nervous System* (11th edition). Oxford: OUP, 2001: 651–709.

Duncan JS. Imaging and epilepsy. *Brain* 1997; **120**: 339–377.

Duncan JS, Shorvon SD, Fish DR. *Clinical Epilepsy*. New York: Churchill Livingstone, 1995.

Engel J, Pedley TA (eds). *Epilepsy. A Comprehensive Textbook*. Philadelphia: Lippincott-Raven, 1997.

Panayiotopoulos CP. *A Clinical Guide to Epileptic Syndromes and their Treatment: Based on the New ILAE Diagnostic Scheme*. Chipping Norton: Bladon, 2002.

Shorvon SD. *Handbook of Epilepsy Treatment*. Oxford: Blackwell Science, 2001.

Smith D, Chadwick D. The management of epilepsy. *Journal of Neurology, Neurosurgery and Psychiatry* 2001; **70 (suppl II)**: ii15–ii21.

Other relevant entries Absence epilepsy; Benign epilepsy syndromes; Cataplexy; Doose syndrome; Dravet syndrome; Drop attacks; Fetal hydantoin syndrome; Fetal valproate syndrome; Ganglioglioma; Gastaut's occipital epilepsy; Gelastic epilepsy; Jacksonian fit; Jeavons syndrome; Juvenile myoclonic epilepsy; Panayiotopoulos syndrome; Progressive myoclonic epilepsy; Pseudoseizures; Reflex epilepsy; Status epilepticus; Sudden unexplained death in epilepsy; Syncope; Traumatic brain injury.

▓ Epiloia – see Tuberous sclerosis

▓ Episodic ataxias

Pathophysiology The episodic ataxias are syndromes in which incoordination occurs intermittently, either spontaneously or in association with factors such as stress, fatigue, or certain foods. Two types of autosomal-dominant paroxysmal cerebellar ataxia, episodic ataxia types 1 and 2, have been recognized on clinical grounds, and subsequently characterized at the molecular level as channelopathies.

Clinical features: history and examination

- Episodic ataxia type 1 (EA1), episodic ataxia/myokymia syndrome:
    Autosomal-dominant disorder characterized by brief (minutes) attacks of cerebellar ataxia, usually without abnormal eye signs (*cf.* EA2). Attacks may be

provoked by stress, emotion, sudden movement. Myokymia or neuromyotonia may be evident as continuous spontaneous repetitive discharges on EMG, but this is not always evident clinically. Some families have seizures.

- Episodic ataxia type 2 (EA2):

    Autosomal-dominant paroxysmal cerebellar disorder; attacks reponsive to acetazolamide; migraine-like symptoms, interictal nystagmus, cerebellar atrophy. Attacks last hours to days. Progressive cerebellar dysfunction.

	Episodic ataxia type 1	Episodic ataxia type 2
Chromosomal location	12p13	19p13
Gene	KCNA1 (potassium channel)	CACNL1A4 (calcium channel)
Age of onset	Early childhood	Adolescence; late childhood
Provoking factors	Startle, exercise	Stress, exercise, fatigue, but not startle
Duration of attack	Seconds to minutes	Hours to days
Ataxia	+++	+++
Dysarthria	+++	+++
Blurred vision	+++	+
Myokymia	+++	−
Nausea, vomiting	+	+++
Vertigo	+	+++
Nystagmus	+	+++
Headache	−	+++
Fixed signs		
Myokymia	+++	−
Nystagmus	−	+++
Ataxia	−	+++
Response to		
Acetazolamide	Marked	Marked

(Key: −, absent; +, present in 1–25% of cases; +++, present in 75–100% of cases.)

Investigations and diagnosis

Neurogenetics:

EA1 caused by mutations in the potassium channel gene KCNA1 on chromosome12p13.

EA2 caused by mutations in the P/Q-type calcium channel gene (CACNL1A4) on chromosome 19p13; this disorder is allelic with familial hemiplegic migraine and spinocerebellar ataxia (SCA) type 6 (CAG trinucleotide repeat expansions in the carboxyl terminus of the gene are responsible for SCA6), thus demonstrating phenotype divergence. EA2 is associated with premature stop codons and splice-site mutations (*cf.* missense mutations in familial hemiplegic migraine).

Imaging: MRI: cerebellar atrophy in EA2, not EA1.

Neurophysiology: EMG: neuromyotonia in EA1.

Differential diagnosis Other conditions in which intermittent episodes of ataxia have been described include:

basilar migraine;

cysticercosis;

inborn errors of metabolism, especially "small molecule disorders" such as urea cycle enzyme defects (e.g. ornithine transcarbamoylase deficiency), organic acidopathies, variants of maple syrup urine disease, pyruvate dehydrogenase deficiency;

inner ear disease.

Treatment and prognosis EA1: some families respond to carbamazepine, acetazolamide; phenytoin. Some families are drug resistant.

EA2: some families respond to acetazolamide.

References Browne DL, Gancher ST, Nutt JG *et al.* Episodic ataxia/myokymia syndrome is associated with point mutations in the human potassium channel gene, KCNA1. *Nature Genetics* 1994; **8**: 136–140.

Kullmann DM, Rea R, Spauschus A, Jouvenceau A. The inherited episodic ataxias: how well do we understand the disease mechanism? *Neuroscientist* 2001; **7**: 80–88.

Ophoff RA, Terwindt GM, Vergouwe MN *et al.* Familial hemiplegic migraine and episodic ataxia type-2 are caused by mutations in the Ca^{2+} channel gene CACNL1A4. *Cell* 1996; **87**: 543–552.

Other relevant entries Autosomal-dominant cerebellar ataxia; Cerebellar disease: an overview; Channelopathies: an overview; Cysticercosis; Maple syrup urine disease; Migraine; Myokymia; Neuromyotonia; Organic acidopathies; Ornithine transcarbamoylase deficiency; Paroxysmal dyskinesias; Periodic paralysis; Pyruvate dehydrogenase deficiency; Trinucleotide repeat diseases; Urea cycle enzyme defects.

▮ Episodic hemicrania – see Chronic paroxysmal hemicrania

▮ Epley manoeuvre – see Benign paroxysmal positional vertigo

▮ Epstein–Barr virus infection and the nervous system

Epstein–Barr virus (EBV) is a DNA virus which causes infectious mononucleosis (IM), the syndrome of glandular fever, with fever, pharyngitis and lymphadenopathy. Diagnosis is based on blood tests which reveal a lymphocytosis with atypical lymphocytes and a positive monospot test. Serology for EBV can also be performed.

EBV has been associated with the development of a number of neurological conditions, which can occur in the absence of overt IM:

Encephalitis with predominant cerebellar involvement (imaging and CSF analysis is typically normal in such patients).

Myelitis.

Aseptic meningitis.

Guillain–Barré syndrome (GBS).

Lumbosacral plexopathy.

Facial palsy.

Neuropathy: sensory, autonomic: rarely described.

Postviral fatigue syndrome.

There is no specific treatment, other than supportive care. Although recovery is the norm, there may be neurological sequelae after encephalitis.

In immunocompromised individuals, Epstein–Barr virus infection is implicated in the development of primary central nervous system (CNS) lymphoma, as well as Burkitt's lymphoma.

References Cohen JI. Epstein–Barr virus infection. *New England Journal of Medicine* 2000; **343**: 481–492.

Majid A, Galetta SL, Sweeney CJ *et al.* Epstein–Barr virus myeloradiculitis and encephalomyeloradiculitis. *Brain* 2002; **125**: 159–165.

Other relevant entries Aseptic meningitis; Cerebellar disease: an overview; Encephalitis: an overview; Guillain–Barré syndrome; Lymphoma.

◼ Erb–Goldflam disease – see Myasthenia gravis

◼ Erb's palsy, Erb–Duchenne palsy
Superior plexus paralysis

This describes an upper brachial plexus lesion involving fibres from the C5/C6 roots, as a consequence of which the affected arm hangs at the side, internally rotated and extended at the elbow ("waiter's tip" posture). There is sensory loss down the lateral arm to the hand; biceps and supinator jerks may be lost or depressed.

Erb–Duchenne palsy typically occurs in traumatic injuries when there is a sudden and severe increase in the angle between the neck and shoulder, for example during a traumatic delivery or, more commonly, with motorcycle accidents. A similar picture may occur after carrying a heavy rucksack for prolonged periods ("rucksack paralysis", *q.v.*). If severe trauma has occurred then little recovery may be expected but often there is only neurapraxia or a short distance for axon regrowth. Occasionally exploratory surgery and microsurgical nerve repair may be necessary; good recovery may occur, aided with physiotherapy.

Other relevant entries Brachial plexopathies; De-afferentation syndrome; Klumpke's paralysis; Rucksack paralysis.

Erdheim–Chester disease

Erdheim–Chester disease is a rare sporadic non-Langerhans cell histiocytosis (LCH) which may affect multiple organs, including the central nervous system (CNS), which may manifest as a cerebellar syndrome, diabetes insipidus, orbital lesions, extra-axial masses, and, exceptionally, dementia.

Reference Wright RA, Hermann RC, Parisi JE. Neurological manifestations of Erdheim–Chester disease. *Journal of Neurology, Neurosurgery and Psychiatry* 1999; **66**: 72–75.

Other relevant entry Langerhans cell histiocytosis.

Erethism – See Heavy metal poisoning

Ergotism
St Anthony's fire

Poisoning with ergot, derived from the rye fungus *Claviceps purpurea*, is now rare, but in the Middle Ages was commoner from the consumption of infected rye bread, leading to the syndrome known as St Anthony's fire. Nowadays, chronic overdosage of ergot-containing drugs is the most likely cause, especially of ergotamine used in the treatment of migraine.

Ergotism may take one of two forms:

- Gangrenous: severe vasospasm and occlusive infarction of the distal small arteries in the limbs.
- Convulsive/neurogenic: fasciculations, myoclonus, muscle spasms, + / − seizures. An ataxic disorder with areflexia and sensory loss, clinically similar to tabes dorsalis, may follow. Pathologically this is due to loss of the dorsal columns, dorsal root ganglia and peripheral nerves, for reasons that are not clear.

Erythrocyanotic headache

This name has been applied to a severe throbbing generalized headache that may be associated with flushing of the face and hands and numbness of the fingers (erythromelalgia). It may be seen with:

mastocytosis,
carcinoid tumour producing high levels of serotonin,
phaeochromocytoma,
some pancreatic islet cell tumours.

Other relevant entry Headache: an overview.

▮ Erythromelalgia

Erythermalgia • "Inverse Raynaud's phenomenon" • Weir Mitchell syndrome

In this rare condition, first described by Silas Weir Mitchell in 1878, there is burning pain in the toes and forefoot, associated with change in ambient temperature. Specifically, above a certain temperature the feet become bright red and warm and symptoms appear, for which reason socks and stockings are often eschewed. Walking on a cold surface or bathing the feet with cold water may relieve the symptoms. Examination usually shows no neurological deficits, although sometimes there may be an accompanying peripheral neuropathy, and peripheral pulses are normal.

Erythromelalgia is thought to be disorder of the microvasculature. Some authors distinguish three varieties, viz.:

Erythromelalgia with thrombocythaemia (e.g. polycythaemia rubra vera, myelo-fibrosis): improves with aspirin.

Primary erythromelalgia: very rare, refractory to all treatments.

Secondary erythromelalgia: associations include gout, occlusive vascular disease, vasoactive drugs (e.g. calcium channel blockers), systemic lupus erythematosus (SLE), cryoglobulinaemia, diabetes mellitus. In these cases, treatment is aimed at the underlying illness.

This classification has been criticized.

Reference Drenth JPH, Michiels JJ. Three types of erythromelalgia. *British Medical Journal* 1990; **301**: 454–455.

Other relevant entries Raynaud's disease, Raynaud's phenomenon, Raynaud's syndrome.

▮ Essential hypersomnolence – see Idiopathic hypersomnia

▮ Essential myoclonus

This name has been given to a syndrome characterized by myoclonic jerks, usually affecting various body sites (polymyoclonus), usually with childhood onset, generally without any other neurological deficit. The condition is usually sporadic in nature but some cases are familial, with probable autosomal-dominant inheritance with variable penetrance. It is a non-progressive condition, and the myoclonus is thought to have a subcortical origin.

In some cases there may be additional dystonia. In most cases the myoclonus responds dramatically to alcohol ("alcohol-responsive myoclonus"), as can the dystonia in those rare patients who have both conditions. These patients would now be classified as having myoclonus–dystonia syndrome (*q.v.*). The relationship of essential myoclonus to essential tremor is uncertain: families with both conditions have been described.

Many patients accept their movements without complaint, but in those requiring treatment, clonazepam is the drug of choice. Anticholinergic agents and sodium valproate may be tried with some benefit.

Other relevant entries Dystonia: an overview; Myoclonus; Myoclonus–dystonia syndrome; Sarcoglycanopathy.

▧ Essential tremor

Pathophysiology Essential tremor (ET) is one of the commonest movement disorders. Some argue that there must be a family history (autosomal-dominant condition with variable penetrance), with at least three generations affected, for the diagnosis of ET to apply, others are prepared to accept sporadic cases. ET may present at any age, and tends to worsen with age. Although not life threatening, it may nevertheless be very disabling, both physically and psychologically; hence the previous name of "benign essential tremor" has fallen into disuse. Hands, head, and voice are commonly involved, and the tremor often improves following modest alcohol consumption. The pathophysiology is not well understood: PET studies suggest tremor may originate in the cerebellum. The current treatment of choice is with β-blockers.

Clinical features: history and examination

- Upper limb involvement: distal, may be asymmetric. Tremor may be present at rest but worsens with action and posture (e.g. writing, holding cups) but is not an intention tremor. As the patient gets older the frequency of the tremor often decreases but the amplitude increases. Classically the tremor improves with alcohol.
- Head titubation occurs in about 50% of cases, and voice may also be involved. This may precede the upper limb tremor, but more typically follows it.
- Tongue, trunk, and lower limbs are rarely involved.
- There are no other abnormal findings aside from tremor in patients with ET. The presence of mild extrapyramidal features has been described, but this is very unusual and may suggest that the tremor is symptomatic of another disorder. Eye movements are normal.
- Criteria for diagnosis have been suggested.
- Drug history: β-agonist drugs may cause a tremor, as can valproate and a range of other drugs.

Investigations and diagnosis *Bloods*: usually normal; may need to exclude Wilson's disease and other metabolic causes of an extrapyramidal syndrome in young patients. Liver function tests may also require checking if there is a history of heavy alcohol consumption. Thyroid function tests, serum electrophoresis, immuno-globulins to exclude symptomatic causes of tremor.

Imaging: normal; may need to exclude other causes of a tremor (e.g. MS).

CSF: not usually required.

Neurophysiology: not required unless the tremor is thought to be secondary to a demyelinating peripheral neuropathy (e.g. paraprotein-associated demyelinating neuropathy). In some centres where tremor analysis is undertaken, EMG may reveal a tremor frequency of 5–8 Hz (in PD: 4–5 Hz; physiological tremor 8–12 Hz).

Differential diagnosis Parkinson's disease: many patients come to clinic fearing this diagnosis, sometimes in part because other family members are affected, itself a clue to the true diagnosis.

Other extrapyramidal disorders, such as Wilson's disease.

Demyelinating peripheral neuropathies (neuropathic tremor).

Exaggerated physiological tremor (endocrine abnormalities, especially thyroid over-activity; drug induced).

Cerebellar or midbrain tremor (typically seen in MS).

Certain toxins may induce a coarse action tremor (e.g. methyl bromide, bismuth).

Treatment and prognosis Most therapies probably act centrally, including alcohol.

Propanolol: 80–120 mg/day (contraindicated in patients with asthma or peripheral vascular disease); occasionally higher doses are required (240–320 mg).

Primidone starting at very low dose 25 mg/day, increasing slowly to a maximum of 750 mg/day if tolerated (soporific side-effects are problematic).

Clonazepam may help, especially in cases of severe kinetic tremor (i.e. worse with action) or orthostatic tremor.

Nicardipine 30 mg/day.

Topiramate (anecdotal evidence only at present).

Occasionally stereotactic surgery is indicated (refractory cases with severe disability): ventrolateral thalamotomy or the use of thalamic stimulators is the surgical treatment of choice.

Therapy is often unsatisfactory.

References Bain PG, Findley LJ, Thompson PD *et al.* A study of hereditary essential tremor. *Brain* 1994; **117**: 805–824.

Deuschl G, Bain P, Brin M and an Ad Hoc Scientific Committee. Consensus statement of the Movement Disorder Society on tremor. *Movement Disorders* 1998; **13(suppl 3)**: 2–23.

Schrag A, Münchau A, Bhatia KP, Quinn NP, Marsden CD. Essential tremor: an overdiagnosed condition? *Journal of Neurology* 2000; **247**: 955–959.

Other relevant entries Drug-induced movement disorders; Tremor: an overview.

■ Esthesioneuroblastoma
Olfactory neuroblastoma

This is a rare tumour that originates in the olfactory epithelium in the upper nasal cavity, often adjacent to the ethmoid sinus. It presents with anosmia, nasal obstruction and epistaxis, and may occasionally involve the orbit causing proptosis, diplopia, and visual loss.

Reference Morita A, Ebersold MJ, Olsen KD *et al.* Esthesioneuroblastoma: prognosis and management. *Neurosurgery* 1993; **32**: 706–714.

Other relevant entries Cranial nerve disease: I: Olfactory nerve; Tumours: an overview.

Ethylene oxide poisoning

Ethylene oxide is an alkylating agent used in the chemical industry and for the sterilization of medical equipment. Acute poisoning produces an encephalopathy, whilst chronic exposure may produce cognitive impairment with, in addition, a reversible distal symmetrical axonal sensorimotor neuropathy. CSF analysis is normal. Recovery is usually complete once exposure to the agent is stopped.

Ethylmalonic–adipic aciduria – see Glutaric aciduria

Eulenburg's disease – see Paramyotonia

Excessive daytime somnolence – see Sleep disorders: an overview

Exencephaly
Encephalocele

Exencephaly is a midline cranial defect in which there is failure of development of the occipitoparietal bones leading to a posterior encephalocele, containing cerebellar tissue. Less commonly, frontal or anterior encephaloceles may occur. The central nervous system (CNS) tissue within an encephalocele is often abnormal, and may be covered with skin or meninges. CSF leaks are common and the risk of infection high. Visceral developmental abnormalities often coexist.

Affected children typically have severe mental handicap, epilepsy, motor impairment and cortical blindness. Hydrocephalus may develop. In severe cases the child may not survive, but in less severe cases surgical excision of a small encephalocele with closure of the overlying neurocutaneous defect may be undertaken.

"Exploding head syndrome"

The "exploding head syndrome" is characterized by a terrifying sensation of a painless explosion in the head, experienced as a crack, snap or bang, occurring often at sleep onset, but sometimes during sleep. Although frightening, the syndrome is benign, and reassurance may be the only treatment required. Reports of benefit with clomipramine and nifedipine have appeared. The clinical description differs from hypnic headache although both occur at night.

References Green MW. The exploding head syndrome. *Current Pain and Headache Reports* 2001; **5**: 279–280.

Pearce JM. Clinical features of the exploding head syndrome. *Journal of Neurology, Neurosurgery and Psychiatry* 1989; **52**: 907–910.

Other relevant entries Headache: an overview; Hypnic headache.

■ Extradural abscess – see Abscess: an overview

■ Extradural haematoma – see Haematoma: an overview

■ Extrapyramidal syndromes – see Parkinsonian syndromes, Parkinsonism

■ Eyelid myoclonia with absences – see Jeavons syndrome

Ff

■ Fabry's disease

Anderson–Fabry disease ● Angiokeratoma corporis diffusum ● Hereditary dystopic lipidosis

Pathophysiology This rare X-linked disorder, linked to chromosome Xq22.1, is due to α-galactosidase A deficiency, which results in the accumulation of glycosphingolipids, specifically ceramidetrihexoside (also known as globotriaosylceramide or Gb_3), in most visceral tissues and body fluids, especially the lysosomes of the vascular endothelium (hence a lysosomal-storage disorder). It is a multisystem disorder affecting skin, eyes, heart and circulation, kidneys, gastrointestinal tract, respiratory tract, and bone as well as the peripheral, central and autonomic nervous systems. Patients typically present in childhood and adolescence with characteristic skin lesions (angiokeratomas) and intermittent lancinating pains or dysaesthesias in the limbs (acroparaesthesia) which are often precipitated by fever, exercise, or hot weather. Heterozygote females may be asymptomatic or exhibit some symptoms and signs of the disease if they have partial deficiency of α-galactosidase. Diagnosis is by assay of enzyme activity in white cells. The condition is currently incurable but the advent of enzyme replacement therapy may offer new hope to patients.

Clinical features: history and examination Typically affects males in childhood or adolescence, although it does display variable expression in men. Female carriers may be asymptomatic or have limited forms of the disease. Diagnosis may require questioning and examination of female family members who may be carriers with mild symptoms, as well as a dermatological examination for angiokeratomas.

• Neurological

  Peripheral nervous system: a small fibre polyneuropathy is often an early feature of the disease. This presents with distal limb pain and dysaesthesia (acroparaesthesia) often with autonomic involvement, and the lancinating pains are often made worse by exertion, hot weather, or a fever. In children these symptoms may be erroneously labelled as "growing pains".

Central nervous system: cerebrovascular events, typically infarcts, affecting the posterior more than the anterior circulation around the fourth decade. Cognitive decline as a result of vascular events may occur. Dolichoectasia may be present, and occasional patients have been described with focal cranial nerve problems related to the abnormal dolichoectatic intracranial arteries, including optic atrophy, oculomotor paralysis, trigeminal neuralgia, eighth nerve dysfunction, and hypoglossal nerve palsy.

Autonomic nervous system: this is often involved early, usually manifest as diminished sweating, impaired tear and saliva formation and gut hypomotility.

- Non-neurological

Skin: angiokeratoma corpus diffusum universale, dark red telangiectasia, is a skin lesion that is primarily found on the scrotum, buttocks, thighs, and back +/− mucosal involvement.

Kidney: progressive renal failure leads to hypertension, which can accelerate the cardiac and cerebrovascular complications of this disease.

Eye: whorl-like corneal opacifications (cornea verticillata) are characteristic; slit-lamp examination may be required. Anterior cataracts and tortuous retinal vessels (tortuositas vasorum) may also be seen.

Heart: cardiac arrhythmias due to involvement of pacemaker tissue. Later, myocardial ischaemia and infarction, cardiac failure and mitral regurgitation may occur. There is also a relatively high incidence of mitral leaflet prolapse which may play a role in the cerebral ischaemia seen in the younger patients.

Other: a facial appearance akin to acromegaly, lymphoedema of the arms and legs, respiratory compromise from obstructive airways disease (late), and arthritis have all been described. A characteristic deformity of the distal interphalangeal joint of the fingers limiting joint extension is described.

Investigations and diagnosis *Bloods*: the definitive test is assay of the white cell enzymes for α-galactosidase activity. Renal function tests (urea, creatinine, creatinine clearance) may indicate the degree of renal damage.

Imaging:

CXR may reveal cardiomegaly, heart failure.

Skeletal radiography: degenerative changes may be seen in distal interphalangeal joints.

Brain CT/MRI may reveal multiple infarcts (haemorrhages are rare), dolichoectasia.

Angiography may reveal irregular abnormal vessels with both stenoses and dilatation (e.g. renal artery).

Urine: microscopic examination may reveal Maltese cross-shaped crystals.

CSF: not necessary.

Neurophysiology: for neuropathy.

ECG: may reveal old ischaemia/infarcts and hypertension.

Skin biopsy: may show lipid inclusions in vascular epithelial cells.

Differential diagnosis Other causes of painful peripheral neuropathy. Other causes of young stroke.

Similar angiokeratoma may occur in fucosidosis, sialidosis.

Treatment and prognosis Treatment is essentially symptomatic. Painful dysaesthesias related to neuropathy may be helped with gabapentin, carbamazepine, phenytoin, or amitriptyline. Heart rhythm abnormalities may require anti-arrhythmics and/or a pacemaker. Hypertension must be controlled. Renal failure may require dialysis. Renal transplantation is feasible, the transplanted organ is not affected, but its production of normal enzyme is insufficient, although the neuropathy may improve.

Genetic counselling is essential; prenatal screening through chorionic villous biopsies is possible. Most patients die in their 40s.

Recently, enzyme replacement therapy with genetically engineered α-galactosidase A (agalsidase alpha), given as an intravenous infusion, has become available. This is reported to be associated with improved cardiac and renal function and amelioration of neuropathic pain.

References Beck M, Ries M. *Fabry Disease: Clinical Manifestations, Diagnosis and Therapy*. Oxford: TKT Europe, 2001.

Mehta A. New developments in the management of Anderson–Fabry disease. *Quarterly Journal of Medicine* 2002; **95**: 647–653.

Mitsias P, Levine SR. Cerebrovascular complications of Fabry's disease. *Annals of Neurology* 1996; **40**: 8–17.

Morgan SH, Rudge P, Smith SJ *et al.* The neurological complications of Anderson–Fabry disease (α-galactosidase A deficiency) – investigation of symptomatic and presymptomatic patients. *Quarterly Journal of Medicine* 1990; **75**: 491–507.

Other relevant entries Dolichoectasia; Gaucher's disease; Lysosomal-storage disorders: an overview.

Facial canal syndrome – see Cranial nerve disease: VII: Facial nerve

Facial hemiatrophy of Romberg – see Parry–Romberg syndrome

Facial migraine – see Migraine

Facial myokymia

Facial myokymia is a rare form of facial dyskinesia, comprising fine continuous undulating movements of the facial muscles which may be likened to a "bag of worms". This may be associated with facial weakness or contracture. Facial myokymia most often denotes a pontine tegmental lesion involving the postnuclear facial (VII) nerve, and has been postulated to represent a disinhibition of the facial nucleus ("release phenomenon"). Although many pathological substrates are described, the commonest causes are demyelination and tumour.

Spread of myokymia from orbicularis oculi to involve one side of the face may lead to tonic contracture of the involved muscles and reduced voluntary facial movement (spastic paretic facial contracture). This is associated with dorsal pontine lesions in the region of the facial nucleus, particularly tumours.

Facial myokymia may need to be differentiated from hemifacial spasm, which is much commoner. Periocular myokymia is a common and benign condition.

Other relevant entries Hemifacial spasm; Myokymia.

▓ Facial nerve palsy – see Bell's palsy; Cranial nerve disease: VII: Facial nerve

▓ Facial pain: differential diagnosis

Facial pain has a broad differential diagnosis, including the following entities, many of which are discussed in individual entries: history is generally the most important factor in reaching a diagnosis:

Trigeminal neuralgia (TN)
Atypical facial pain
Giant cell arteritis
Post-herpetic neuralgia
Cluster headache (CH)
Costen syndrome
Raeder paratrigeminal syndrome
Carotidynia
Dissection of the carotid artery
Occipital neuralgia (Arnold's neuralgia)
Cavernous sinus pathology
Glossopharyngeal neuralgia
Geniculate neuralgia
Otalgia
Neck–tongue syndrome.

Certain headache syndromes may produce pain which is distributed over the face, in addition to or rather than the head: migraine, CH, tension headache, meningitis, meningeal irritation (e.g. after a subarachnoid haemorrhage), raised intracranial pressure, and temporal arteritis, as well as a variety of non-neurological conditions, such as hypertension, erythrocyanotic headache, and disorders of the upper cervical cord.

Local disease of the teeth, sinuses, nasopharynx, temporomandibular joint (Costen's syndrome), ear (otalgia), and bones may also cause facial pain.

Vascular pathology must also be considered (dissection of carotid artery; carotidynia), including disease within the cavernous sinus.

Investigation and diagnosis *Bloods*: ESR if giant cell arteritis suspected; standard haematological and biochemical screening tests.

Imaging: CT if bony lesion suspected; MRI if meningeal disease, cavernous sinus or brainstem pathology suspected; MRA/angiography if carotid artery dissection suspected.

CSF: only necessary if meningeal disease suspected.

Others: may include ENT, maxillofacial, oral surgical, psychiatric opinion.

Treatment and prognosis/Other relevant entries See individual entries.

■ Facioscapulohumeral muscular dystrophy
Landouzy–Déjerine dystrophy

Pathophysiology Facioscapulohumeral muscular dystrophy (FSH) is an autosomal-dominant muscular dystrophy, with weakness in the areas described by the name, which may be asymmetric and of variable expression within families. It has been linked to a deletion of an integral number of 3.3 kb KpnI repeats (D4Z4) in the sub-teleomeric region of chromosome 4 (4q35) in many, but not all, families; the actual genetic defect awaits clarification. Bigger deletions may be associated with younger onset and more severe forms of the disease.

The condition has very variable expression within families but has 95% penetrance by the age of 20 years. It typically presents with facial weakness and winging of the scapulae, and then spreads to involve other proximal muscles of the upper limb.

Clinical features: history and examination Weakness, often asymmetric, affects:

- Facial muscles: often the first feature of disease, although facial expression is relatively well preserved. The mouth may have a pouting quality: *bouche de tapir*.
- Shoulder muscles: particularly the scapular fixators, so that winging of the scapulae is an early feature. However the deltoid muscle is normally well preserved, whilst biceps and triceps are weak and wasted, giving rise to an appearance of so-called "Popeye arms" or "chicken wings" in the upper limbs.
- Quadriceps and hip flexor muscle involvement is not uncommon; ankle dorsiflexion, wrist extensors may be involved as the disease progresses.

A severe form of FSH exists in infancy in which there is typically no facial movement and severe limb weakness, confining the child to a wheelchair by the age of about 10 years. In addition there may be a severe high tone hearing loss and vascular degeneration of the retina (Coats' disease).

Scapulohumeral and scapuloperoneal muscular dystrophies may, in some instances, represent variants of FSH.

A facial-sparing variant of FSH is described.

Extraocular and pharyngeal muscles are not involved; there is no cardiac involvement; mentation is normal.

Family history may be positive for the disorder, although intrafamilial heterogeneity is recognized.

Investigations and diagnosis *Bloods*: raised creatine kinase to several times above the normal range.

Neurophysiology: EMG shows myopathic change.

Muscle biopsy: general dystrophic features $+/-$ scattered tiny fibres, with an inflammatory infiltrate which may lead to confusion with polymyositis. Changes are sometimes minimal.

Neurogenetics: typical deletion of chromosome 4q35 is very helpful in diagnosis, and may obviate the need for EMG and muscle biopsy.

Imaging, CSF: not usually necessary.

ECG: normal.

Differential diagnosis

Dystrophia myotonica.

Polymyositis.

Nemaline rod myopathy.

Mitochondrial disease.

Congenital muscular dystrophies.

The severe childhood form may be mistaken for Möbius syndrome.

Treatment and prognosis There is no specific treatment. Supportive treatment with physiotherapy and surgical procedures may be helpful, such as stabilization of the scapulae; ankle–foot orthosis; transposition of the posterior tibial tendon to the dorsum of the foot. Immunosuppressive therapy is usually of no value.

In its most severe form the patient may become wheelchair bound in the first decade of life. However the disease often follows a more benign course and overall only 20% of patients with FSH are wheelchair bound by the age of 40 years.

References Padberg GW, Lunt PW, Koch M, Fardeau M. Facioscapulohumeral muscular dystrophy. In: Emery AEH (ed.). *Diagnostic Criteria for Neuromuscular Disorders* (2nd edition). London: Royal Society of Medicine Press, 1997: 9–15.

Tawil R, Figlewicz DA, Griggs RC *et al*. Facioscapulohumeral dystrophy: a distinct regional myopathy with a novel molecular pathogenesis. FSH consortium. *Annals of Neurology* 1998; **43**: 279–282.

Other relevant entries Coats' disease; Dystrophia myotonica; Möbius syndrome; Muscular dystrophies: an overview; Polymyositis.

■ Fahr syndrome – see Basal ganglia calcification

■ Failed back syndrome

Failed back syndrome (FBS) refers to the situation in which surgery for lumbar radiculopathy, claudication, or instability fails to alleviate symptoms, particularly pain, and indeed the patient may have more severe chronic pain than pre-operatively. In some cases the persistent symptoms relate to inadequate surgical technique (wrong level, incomplete removal of lumbar intervertebral disc fragments) in which case reoperation may be appropriate. More commonly, however, symptoms relate to progression of spinal degenerative disease, post-operative arachnoiditis, or inappropriate initial indication for surgery, in which cases further surgery is best avoided. Reimaging (MRI, CT with contrast enhancement) may be helpful in re-evaluation. Psychological factors may also play a role in the persistence of pain. Distant causes for pain such as hip osteoarthritis, abdominal, or gynaecological pathology also need to be excluded. Pain management for FBS using tricyclic antidepressants, non-steroidal anti-inflammatory drugs (NSAIDs) and physical measures, and possibly input from a pain psychologist, may be needed. All such cases require very careful evaluation.

> **Reference** Groff MW. Approach to the patient with failed back syndrome. In: Biller J (ed.). *Practical Neurology* (2nd edition). Philadelphia: Lippincott Williams & Wilkins, 2002: 315–320.

> **Other relevant entries** Arachnoiditis; Lumbar cord and root disease; Sciatica; Spinal stenosis.

▨ Familial amyloid polyneuropathies
Andrade disease

Pathophysiology Familial amyloid polyneuropathy (FAP), a small fibre neuropathy, was first described by Andrade in 1952. Since then other hereditary neuropathies with autosomal-dominant inheritance and characterized pathologically by amyloid deposition in nerves have been described. They may be classified as:

> Type I (Andrade, Portuguese type): deposition of abnormal transthyretin.
> Type II (Indiana/Swiss/Rukavina type): deposition of abnormal transthyretin.
> Type III (Iowa/Van Allen type): deposition of mutant apolipoprotein A-I.
> Type IV (Finnish): deposition of gelsolin.

However, with the definition of the genetic basis of these disorders, the conditions are increasingly defined by mutational analysis.

Clinical features: history and examination The clinical picture is similar (but not identical) in all types:

> Autonomic dysfunction: impotence, postural hypotension, pupillary abnormalities; gastrointestinal abnormalities (constipation, diarrhoea)
> Paraesthesia, neuropathic pain; carpal tunnel syndrome
> Muscle weakness: distal to proximal spread; areflexia
> Bulbar involvement: dysphagia, dysarthria
> No nerve thickening (*cf.* primary systemic amyloidosis).

Variations

> Type II: carpal tunnel syndrome; no renal, sphincter involvement
> Type IV: corneal lattice dystrophy; facial and auditory nerve involvement.

Amyloid deposition may also occur in other organs:

Heart: cardiomyopathy
Vitreous body: opacities
Kidney: nephrotic syndrome
Leptomeninges: subarachnoid haemorrhage.

Investigations and diagnosis *Neurophysiology*: EMG/NCS: shows axonal neuropathy (non-specific).

CSF: protein often raised.

Tissue diagnosis: nerve biopsy, rectal mucosa, skin, abdominal fat pad, may show amyloid deposits; in nerve, unmyelinated and small myelinated fibres may be lost, and amyloid preferentially accumulates around endoneurial vessels.

Neurogenetics: mutations in genes encoding transthyretin (chromosome 18q11.2–q12.1); gelsolin (chromosome 9q34).

ECG/Echocardiography: arrhythmia, cardiomyopathy (enlarged interventricular septum).

Slit lamp: vitreous opacities.

Urine: for protein.

Differential diagnosis Other causes of axonal neuropathy, if autonomic features overlooked.

Treatment and prognosis Liver transplantation is curative, if performed early in the course of disease, that is, no improvement in neuropathy but no further axonal loss.

References Adams D. Hereditary and acquired amyloid neuropathies. *Journal of Neurology* 2001; **248**: 647–657.

Adams D, Didier S, Goulon-Goeau C *et al*. The course and prognostic factors of familial amyloid polyneuropathy after liver transplantation. *Brain* 2000; **123**: 1495–1504.

Reilly MM, King RH. Familial amyloid polyneuropathy. *Brain Pathology* 1993; **3**: 165–176.

Other relevant entries Amyloid and the nervous system: an overview; Carpal tunnel syndrome; Cerebral amyloid angiopathies; Gelsolin amyloidosis.

▓ Familial British dementia – see Worster-Drought syndrome (1)

▓ Familial Danish dementia

This novel form of cerebral amyloidosis is associated with mutations in a gene (BRI2) on chromosome 13, which leads to the production of an extended precursor protein and of an amyloidogenic fragment (A-Dan), similar to the involvement of A-Bri in the pathogenesis of familial British dementia (Worster-Drought syndrome, *q.v*). Pathologically there is cerebral amyloid amyloidosis, parenchymal protein deposits, and neurofibrillary change.

Reference Holton JL, Lashley T, Ghiso J *et al*. Familial Danish dementia: a novel form of cerebral amyloidosis associated with deposition of both amyloid-Dan

and amyloid-β. *Journal of Neuropathology and Experimental Neurology* 2002;
61: 254–267.

Other relevant entries Amyloid and the nervous system: an overview; Cerebral
amyloid angiopathy; Dementia: an overview; Worster-Drought syndrome (1).

■ Familial dysautonomia – see Hereditary sensory and autonomic neuropathy; Riley–Day syndrome

■ Familial hemiplegic migraine – see Episodic ataxias; Migraine

■ Farber's lipogranulomatosis
Farber's syndrome

This is a very rare autosomal-recessive condition caused by deficiency of the lysosomal enzyme ceramidase, leading to accumulation of ceramide in lysosomes and disseminated lipogranulomatosis. The typical presentation is in the first year of life with arthropathy and subcutaneous nodules. The nodules may occur in periarticular skin, larynx (causing a hoarse cry), scalp, or near pressure points. In addition there may be interstitial lung disease, psychomotor retardation, hepatosplenomegaly with lymphadenopathy, macroglossia, cherry-red spot at the macula, conjunctival nodules and cardiac disease. Neurological features resulting from abnormal lipid storage include myoclonus, seizures, dementia, hypotonia, and muscle wasting. Diagnosis is made by assaying the enzyme, and by observation of the typical lysosomal inclusion bodies in the reticuloendothelial system ("banana bodies") and neurones ("zebra bodies"). There is no specific treatment and patients die in the first decade of life.

Other relevant entry Lysosomal-storage disorders: an overview.

■ Fasciitis – see Eosinophilic fasciitis

■ Fat embolism syndrome

The fat embolism syndrome (FES) is a post-traumatic neurological syndrome occurring in 3–4% of patients with long bone fractures, typically 12 hours to 3 days after trauma (although cases up to 11 days have been reported). Diagnosis is based on clinical criteria, the features being respiratory distress, encephalopathy, retinal haemorrhages, and cutaneous petechiae; in addition anaemia, coagulopathy, fever, or urinary fat globules may be found. Some patients may have neurological focal deficits in addition to encephalopathy. MRI may show transient patchy lesions of low intensity on T_1-weighted imaging and high intensity on T_2-weighted imaging in the white matter and subcortical grey matter; these may represent transient perivascular oedema. FES is a self-resolving illness and most patients make a full recovery with supportive therapy at the time of respiratory distress.

Reference Dominguez-Morán JA, Martinez-San Millán J, Plaza JF, Fernández-Ruiz LC, Masjuan J. Fat embolism syndrome: new MRI findings. *Journal of Neurology* 2001; **248**: 529–532.

■ Fatal familial insomnia

This is a rare, inherited autosomal-dominant prion disorder that presents with progressive insomnia and autonomic dysfunction, with motor and cognitive abnormalities developing later in the course of the illness. The sleep disorder is characterized by loss of slow-wave sleep and abnormal rapid eye movement sleep behaviour. Endocrine and vegetative circadian rhythms are lost. The dysautonomia may cause hyperhidrosis, hypertension, hyperthermia, tachycardia, and sphincter disturbances. Similar features have been observed in Morvan's syndrome, mediated by auto-antibodies directed to voltage-gated potassium channels. Motor features of fatal familial insomnia (FFI) include ataxia, myoclonus, pyramidal features, and tremor. The condition occurs in middle age and is progressive, causing coma and death in 1–2 years. There is no specific treatment. Pathologically, thalamic nuclei seem to be predominantly affected (anterior ventral, dorsomedial). Mutations in codons 178 and 200 of the prion protein (PrP) gene have been reported in FFI. One sporadic case (sporadic fatal insomnia) has been reported to date. The condition has also been transmitted to primates by experimental inoculation.

References Lugaresi E, Medori R, Montagna P *et al.* Fatal familial insomnia and dysautonomia with selective degeneration of thalamic nuclei. *New England Journal of Medicine* 1986; **315**: 997–1003.

Medori R, Tritschler HJ, LeBlanc A *et al.* Fatal familial insomnia, a prion disease with a mutation at codon 178 of the prion protein gene. *New England Journal of Medicine* 1992; **326**: 444–449.

Other relevant entries Insomnia; Morvan's syndrome; Prion disease: an overview; Sleep disorders: an overview.

■ Fatal infantile leukodystrophy – see Vanishing white matter disease

■ Fatty acid oxidation disorders

Pathophysiology A number of inborn fatty acid oxidation disorders (FAOD) are recognized, affecting transport and β-oxidation of long-, medium-, and short-chain fatty acids which takes place in the mitochondrial matrix:

- Medium-chain acyl-CoA dehydrogenase (MCAD) deficiency: the commonest of these disorders, presenting in older infants with recurrent episodes of acute encephalopathy with hepatocellular dysfunction, or a Reye-like syndrome; rarely a cause of severe illness in the newborn.

- Systemic carnitine deficiency: Reye-like syndrome with evidence of skeletal myopathy and cardiomyopathy (*cf.* MCAD).
- Long-chain acyl-CoA dehydrogenase (LCAD) deficiency: Reye-like syndrome with evidence of skeletal myopathy and cardiomyopathy (*cf.* MCAD).
- Short-chain acyl-CoA dehydrogenase (SCAD) deficiency: very rare, presenting in the newborn period with non-specific encephalopathy, poor feeding, failure to thrive, hypotonia, seizures, myopathy and cardiomyopathy, with metabolic acidosis.
- Long-chain hydroxyacyl-CoA dehydrogenase (LCHAD) deficiency: as for LCAD but with very prominent cardiomyopathy (*cf.* MCAD).
- Carnitine palmitoyltransferase I (CPT I) deficiency.
- Carnitine palmitoyltransferase II (CPT II) deficiency.
- Carnitine-acylcarnitine translocase deficiency (CACT).

Clinical features: history and examination See individual entries.

- Basically, symptoms are provoked by fasting, exercise or infection; commonly hypoketotic hypoglycaemia; metabolic myopathy may be evident, sometimes complicated by exercise-induced rhabdomyolysis.
- MCAD, LCAD, SCAD have infantile presentation; CPT I and LCHAD have childhood presentation; CPT II may present in infancy or adulthood (classical exercise-induced myoglobinuria).
- FAOD have been associated with sudden infant death syndrome (SIDS), severe liver injury, and complications of pregnancy (e.g. HELLP syndrome). Search for evidence of FAOD is recommended in these situations, and screeening of siblings.

Investigations and diagnosis *Bloods*: hypoglycaemia, hyperammonaemia, hepatocellular dysfunction; plasma acylcarnitines; α-fetoprotein normal (*cf.* tyrosinaemia).

Urine: organic acid abnormalities, but these may be evanescent, for example:

- MCAD: large amounts of dicarboxylic acids: adipic, suberic, sebacic; very low levels of 3-hydroxybutyrate.
- SCAD: large amounts of ethylmalonic acid, glutarate, butyrylglycine, and hexanoylglycine (similar to glutaric aciduria type II).
- LCAD, LCHAD: long-chain dicarboxylic and monocarboxylic acids.

Enzyme analysis in cultured skin fibroblasts is diagnostic test.

Differential diagnosis Aminoacidopathies, for example hepatocellular dysfunction and cardiomyopathy resembles hepatorenal tyrosinaemia (but hypoalbuminaemia and coagulopathy not prominent in FAOD).

Neonatal hepatitis, haemochromatosis.

Hereditary fructose intolerance.

Reye's syndrome.

Treatment and prognosis No specific treatment, but reduction of fatty acid oxidation by ensuring avoidance of fasting. A high-calorie high-carbohydrate diet, and elimination of fat from the diet, is recommended. Riboflavin, polyunsaturated fatty acid supplementation may be recommended.

References Boles RG, Buck EA, Blitzer MG *et al.* Retrospective biochemical screening of fatty acid oxidation disorders in postmortem livers of 418 cases of sudden death in the first year of life. *Journal of Pediatrics* 1998; **132**: 924–933.

Pourfarzam M, Schaefer J, Turnbull DM *et al.* Analysis of fatty acid oxidation intermediates in cultured fibroblasts to detect mitochondrial oxidation disorders. *Clinical Chemistry* 1994; **40**: 2267–2275.

Other relevant entries Carnitine deficiency; Carnitine palmitoyl transferase deficiency; Glutaric aciduria (GA); Hereditary fructose intolerance; Medium-chain acyl-CoA dehydrogenase deficiency; Tyrosinaemia.

Fazio–Londe disease
Progressive bulbar paralysis of childhood

This is a rare inherited (autosomal-dominant) childhood disorder characterized by bulbar failure due to selective loss of the anterior horn cells in the lower cranial nerve nuclei. The disorder is progressive and fatal.

Other relevant entry Spinal muscular atrophy.

Febrile convulsions
Febrile seizures

Pathophysiology Febrile convulsions may be defined as epileptic seizures occurring between the ages of 3 months and 5 years, in association with a temperature of $\geqslant 38°C$, in the absence of central nervous system infection or metabolic disturbance.

Clinical features: history and examination Febrile convulsions may be classified as:

- Simple: primary generalized, usually tonic–clonic seizure, lasting not >15 minutes and not recurring within 24 hours.
- Complex: prolonged, focal, and/or recurrent within 24 hours.

Generalized epilepsy with febrile seizures plus (GEFS+) is an autosomal-dominant syndrome of variable phenotype characterized by multiple febrile seizures and various afebrile generalized seizures (tonic–clonic, absence, myoclonic, atonic). Three forms have been characterized, all linked to mutations in genes encoding voltage- or ligand-gated ion channels, hence channelopathies:

Syndrome	Inheritance	Locus	Gene	Protein
GEFS+1	AD	19q13	SCN1B	β_1 subunit, voltage-gated Na$^+$ channel
GEFS+2	AD	2q23–q31	SCN1A	α-subunit, voltage-gated Na$^+$ channel
GEFS+3	AD	5q31–q33	GABRG2	GABA(A) receptor γ_2-subunit

AD: autosomal dominant

Investigations and diagnosis *CSF*: recommended in infants below 18 months of age to exclude meningitis.

Bloods, EEG, neuroimaging not mandatory in a child with a first simple febrile seizure, although these may be indicated in the context of complex febrile seizure(s).

Differential diagnosis Meningitis, especially in those under 18 months.

Treatment and prognosis During fever: antipyretics; prophylactic anti-epileptic drugs such as diazepam may reduce the risk of febrile seizure. A febrile seizure lasting >2–3 minutes may be treated with diazepam.

Regular phenobarbitone may reduce the risk of further seizures, but this benefit needs to be balanced against the risk of cognitive and behavioural adverse effects.

Febrile seizures are a risk factor for the development of epilepsy later in life, occurring in about 2–7% of children, predictors being complex febrile seizures, neuro-developmental abnormalities, family history of epilepsy, recurrent febrile seizures.

> **Reference** Mikati MA, Rahi AC. Febrile seizures in children. *Practical Neurology* 2003; **3**: 78–85.

> **Other relevant entries** Channelopathies: an overview; Epilepsy: an overview.

■ Fegeler syndrome – see Sturge–Weber syndrome

■ Femoral neuropathy

Pathophysiology Palsy of the femoral nerve, which arises from L2 to L4 roots, most often follows surgical trauma, stretch or traction injuries, or direct compression.

Clinical features: history and examination

- Motor
     weak leg: quadriceps, absent or diminished patellar reflex; adductor muscles should not be affected (innervated by obturator nerve).
- Sensory
     loss over anterior thigh and, if the saphenous branch is involved, medial aspect of leg and foot.

Investigations and diagnosis EMG/NCS: EMG involvement of paraspinal muscles or adductor muscles refutes the diagnosis.

Differential diagnosis

L2–L4 radiculopathy; "diabetic amyotrophy".

Lumbosacral plexopathy.

> **Reference** Staal A, Van Gijn J, Spaans F. *Mononeuropathies: Examination, Diagnosis and Treatment.* London: WB Saunders, 1999: 103–108.

> **Other relevant entries** Diabetes mellitus and the nervous system; Neuropathies: an overview; Saphenous neuropathy.

■ FENIB

Familial encephalopathy with neuroserpin inclusion bodies

An autosomal-dominant disorder characterized clinically by progressive dementia with frontal and frontal subcortical deficits and relative sparing of recall memory, and pathologically by cytoplasmic neuroserpin inclusions (Collins bodies) within the deep cortical layers, substantia nigra, and subcortical nuclei. It is linked to a point mutation in the gene on chromosome 3 encoding neuroserpin, a serine-proteinase inhibitor, the mutant protein undergoing polymerization. Mutations causing greater conformational change (G392E) cause early onset progressive myoclonus epilepsy, whereas lesser degrees of conformational change (S49P) cause dementia in the fifth decade.

References Davis RL, Shrimpton AE, Holohan PD *et al.* Familial dementia caused by polymerization of mutant neuroserpin. *Nature* 1999; **401**: 376–379.

Davis RL, Shrimpton AE, Carrell RW *et al.* Association between conformational mutations in neuroserpin and onset and severity of dementia. *Lancet* 2002; **359**: 2242–2247.

Other relevant entries Dementia: an overview; Progressive myoclonic epilepsy.

Ferguson–Critchley syndrome

This is the combination of a hereditary spastic paraplegia with spinocerebellar ataxia and disorders of gaze + / − emotional lability, bladder instability and extrapyramidal features. It may also be characterized as an autosomal-dominant cerebellar ataxia type I.

Other relevant entries Autosomal-dominant cerebellar ataxia; Hereditary spastic paraparesis.

Fetal alcohol syndrome

Babies born to alcoholic mothers may show a number of characteristic features, labelled fetal alcohol syndrome (FAS), most particularly growth retardation and intellectual deficits. In addition to small size (length >> weight), morphological abnormalities may include short palpebral fissures and epicanthal folds, maxillary hypoplasia, micrognathia, cleft palate, hip dislocation, flexion deformities of the fingers, cardiac abnormalities, anomalous external genitalia, and capillary haemangiomas. These babies may feed poorly and always have a degree of mental retardation. Neonatal seizures may occur. Disordered neurite growth, with reduced number and abnormal geometry of dendritic spines of cortical neurones, is thought to be a consequence of excessive alcohol exposure *in utero*.

Reference Spohr H-L, Willms J, Steinhausen H-C. Prenatal alcohol exposure and long-term developmental consequences. *Lancet* 1993; **341**: 907–910.

Other relevant entries Agenesis of the corpus callosum; Alcohol and the nervous system: an overview.

Fetal hydantoin syndrome
Acrofacial syndrome

All anticonvulsant drugs are potentially teratogenic, but a distinct syndrome of growth retardation, developmental delay, dysmorphism (e.g. broad depressed nasal bridge, hypertelorism), and distal limb abnormalities (e.g. hypoplastic distal phalanges, nails) has been labelled fetal hydantoin syndrome; it may follow use not only of phenytoin but also barbiturates, valproate, and alcohol.

Other relevant entries Alcohol and the nervous system: an overview; Fetal valproate syndrome.

Fetal valproate syndrome

Exposure to valproate in utero has been occasionally associated with a specific syndrome of dysmorphism:

Eyes: epicanthal folds, hypertelorism
Nose: flat nasal bridge, long philtrum
Mouth: microstomia, prominent lower lip
Digits: distal phalangeal hypoplasia, nail hypoplasia.

Associated malformations may include:

Neural tube defects
Congenital heart disease
Cleft lip/palate
Genitourinary malformations
Tracheomalacia
Radial ray defects
Abdominal wall defects
Arachnodactyly/overlapping digits.

In addition, use of valproate as monotherapy or as part of polytherapy during pregnancy may be associated with increased educational needs in the offspring.

References Adab N, Jacoby A, Smith D, Chadwick D. Additional educational needs in children born to mothers with epilepsy. *Journal of Neurology, Neurosurgery and Psychiatry* 2001; **70**: 15–21.

Clayton-Smith J, Donnai D. Fetal valproate syndrome. *Journal of Medical Genetics* 1995; **32**: 724–727.

Other relevant entries Epilepsy: an overview; Fetal hydantoin syndrome.

Fibrocartilaginous embolism of the spinal cord – see Anterior spinal artery syndrome

Fibrodysplasia ossificans progressiva – see Myositis ossificans

Fibromuscular dysplasia

Pathophysiology A rare, non-atheromatous and non-inflammatory, segmental disease of small- and medium-sized arteries, first described in renal arteries but which can affect craniocervical arteries, especially the internal carotid artery; intracranial involvement is rare. It is usually bilateral, much more common in women, and most often manifests after the age of 40 years. It may be associated with transient ischaemic attacks, strokes, arterial dissection, and intracranial aneurysm formation.

Clinical features: history and examination
- May be asymptomatic; probably most cases.
- May cause cerebral ischaemia, possibly embolic (possibly following a dissection).
- Concurrent saccular intracranial aneurysms (in *ca.* 25%) may cause subarachnoid haemorrhage.
- May be concurrent hypertension from renal artery involvement.

Investigations and diagnosis *Imaging*: carotid arteriography: multifocal stenoses ("string of beads" appearance), tubular narrowing, usually bilateral; +/− intracranial aneurysms.

Histology: degeneration of elastic tissue, proliferation of fibroblasts, smooth muscle hyperplasia, +/− atherosclerosis.

Differential diagnosis Other causes of cerebral ischaemia; atheromatous carotid artery disease; carotid dissection.

Treatment and prognosis If asymptomatic, no treatment may be necessary. If symptomatic, endovascular dilatation or excision of the affected segment may be necessary. Anticoagulation sometimes given. No controlled trials of any of these treatments have been performed.

> **Reference** Luscher TF, Lie JT, Stanson AW *et al.* Arterial fibromuscular dysplasia. *Mayo Clinic Proceedings* 1987; **62**: 931–952.

> **Other relevant entries** Aneurysm; Carotid artery disease; Cerebrovascular disease: arterial; Subarachnoid haemorrhage.

▓ Fibromyalgia syndrome
Myofascial pain syndrome

Fibromyalgia syndrome (FMS) is characterized by diffuse muscle aches and pains ("myalgia"), with an emphasis on the shoulder girdle musculature and tender spots in the muscle. There is no associated clinical or investigative abnormality to indicate a disease of joints, bones, connective tissue, muscle, or nervous system. Symptoms of fatigue, sleep disturbance, and headache are common; there may be an underlying depressive illness. Symptomatic treatment may be helpful; the condition may be self-limiting, lasting for a period of weeks to months.

> **Reference** Wolfe F, Smythe HA, Yunus MB *et al.* The American College of Rheumatology 1990 Criteria for the Classification of Fibromyalgia. Report of the Multicenter Criteria Committee. *Arthritis and Rheumatism* 1990; **33**: 160–172.

▓ Fibrous dysplasia

Small areas of bone destruction or massive sclerotic overgrowth involving the skull vault and/or base may occur in isolation, causing headache and cranial nerve involvement (e.g. visual loss, hearing loss), or as part of the McCune–Albright syndrome (in addition, café-au-lait spots, endocrinopathy such as precocious puberty, thyrotoxicosis, primary hyperparathyroidism, hyperprolactinaemia). Malignant transformation to fibrosarcoma may occur. Surgical resection or radiation therapy may be used to relieve symptoms.

Other relevant entries Hyperostosis cranialis interna; McCune–Albright syndrome; Van Buchem's syndrome.

Filariasis

Lymphatic or Bancroftian filariasis results from infection with nematodes (e.g. *Wuchereria bancrofti*) spread by mosquito bite in equatorial Africa and south-east Asia, causing fever and lymphadenitis. Lymphoedema may follow resulting in swelling of limbs (elephantiasis) or genitalia. Nerve compression palsies may occur as a consequence of enlarged or calcified lymph nodes or dilated lymphatic channels, and Guillain–Barré syndrome has been reported in the context of acute filariasis. Diagnosis may be based on clinical features, or use of antibody detection tests, or visualization of adult worms or microfilariae in tissue sections.

Finnish amyloidosis – see Familial amyloid polyneuropathies; Gelsolin amyloidosis

Fisher syndrome – see Miller Fisher syndrome

Flail arm syndrome

Probably a variant of motor neurone disease (MND) in which there is symmetrical wasting and weakness of the arms without, or with only minimal, leg and bulbar involvement. This syndrome may correspond to what was previously called Vulpian–Bernhardt syndrome. It has been suggested that prognosis may be relatively good in this variant as compared to other manifestations of MND.

References Gamez J, Cervera C, Codina A. Flail arm syndrome or Vulpian–Bernhart's [*sic*] form of amyotrophic sclerosis. *Journal of Neurology, Neurosurgery and Psychiatry* 1999; **67**: 258.

Hu MTM, Ellis CM, Al-Chalabi A, Leigh PN, Shaw CE. Flail arm syndrome: a distinctive variant of amyotrophic lateral sclerosis. *Journal of Neurology, Neurosurgery and Psychiatry* 1998; **65**: 950–951.

Other relevant entry Motor neurone disease.

Flier syndrome

A syndrome, first described by Flier and colleagues in 1980, characterized by:
- Painful muscle cramps with elevated (10–20 times) creatine kinase levels; may be treated with phenytoin.
- Enlarged hands and feet ("acral hypertrophy").

- Acanthosis nigricans.
- Insulin resistance.
    Reference Kingston W, Moxley RT, Griggs RC, Freedman Z, Levy R. Flier syndrome: muscle cramps, acanthosis nigricans, acral hypertrophy, and insulin resistance. *Annals of Neurology* 1982; **12**: 79 (abstract B11).

▒ Floppy head syndrome – see Dropped head syndrome

▒ Fluorosis

Excessive ingestion of fluoride may apparently cause osteophyte overgrowth in the vertebral column with resultant spinal nerve and cord compression.
    Reference Singh A, Jolly SS, Bansal BC. Skeletal fluorosis and its neurological complications. *Lancet* 1961; **1**: 197.

▒ Flying saucer syndrome – see Juvenile myoclonic epilepsy

▒ Flynn–Aird syndrome

A rare syndrome of hereditary hearing loss with a progressive sensorimotor polyneuropathy, dental caries, skin atrophy with ulceration, baldness, cystic bone changes, joint stiffness, and ocular defects (cataracts, atypical pigmentary retinopathy; myopia), with onset in the first or second decade.
    Reference Flynn P, Aird RB. A neuroectodermal syndrome of dominant inheritance. *Journal of the Neurological Sciences* 1965; **2**: 161–182.
    Other relevant entry Hearing loss: differential diagnosis.

▒ Focal dystonias

There are a number of dystonias which involve a single body part. Typically these occur in adult life and are idiopathic in origin. A clue to the dystonic origin of these movements, which, particularly in the past, were sometimes labelled as "hysterical", is the observation of transient relief of the movements by the use of sensory tricks (*geste anatgoniste*).
Focal dystonias include (*q.v.*):

Cranial dystonia
    Meige's syndrome
    Blepharospasm +/− oromandibular dystonia (Brueghel syndrome).

Spasmodic torticollis
Writer's cramp (graphospasm)
Other occupational or task-specific dystonias
Spasmodic dysphonia

Dystonic dysphagia
  A rare dystonia of pharyngeal muscles causing dysphagia; dystonic body movements in children may be induced by gastro-oesophageal reflux (Sandifer syndrome).
Axial dystonia
  Spasms of the trunk which interfere with lying, sitting, standing, or walking.
Leg dystonia
  Inversion and plantar flexion of the foot causing the patient to walk on their toes (toe-walking).
Anismus
  A focal dystonia of the external anal sphincter during attempted defaecation, leading to faecal retention and a complaint of constipation.

Focal dystonias respond poorly to drug therapy and the mainstay of treatment is therefore with local injections of botulinum toxin.

Other relevant entries See individual entries; Botulinum toxin therapy; Dystonia: an overview.

■ Foix–Alajouanine syndrome
Subacute necrotizing myelopathy

First described in 1926, this is a slowly or subacutely progressive paraparesis, often asymmetrical, with distal pain and sensory disturbance and with sphincter and sexual disturbances. It results from a vascular malformation leading to impaired venous outflow from the cord causing a necrotic myelopathy.

Reference Mirch DR, Kucharuczyk W, Weller MA *et al*. Subacute necrotizing myelopathy: MR imaging in four pathologically proved cases. *American Journal of Neuroradiology* 1991; **12**: 1077–1083.

Other relevant entry Spinal cord vascular diseases.

■ Foix–Chavany–Marie syndrome
Anterior opercular syndrome

This is an acquired syndrome in which there is bilateral anterior perisylvian damage involving the primary motor cortex and parietal opercula. There is loss of voluntary control of the facial, pharyngeal, lingual, masticatory +/− ocular muscles, whilst retaining normal reflexive and automatic functions of these muscles. Patients can therefore yawn, blink, and laugh spontaneously but cannot close their eyes or open their mouths to command. Cerebrovascular disease is the commonest cause. A similar syndrome may be seen in children following bilateral opercular damage: the perisylvian syndrome is sometimes designated as "developmental Foix–Chavany–Marie syndrome".

Reference Mao C-C, Coull BM, Golper LAC, Rau MT. Anterior operculum syndrome. *Neurology* 1989; **39**: 1169–1172.

Other relevant entries Cerebral palsy, cerebral palsy syndromes; Perisylvian syndrome; Worster-Drought syndrome (2).

◼ Foix–Jefferson syndrome – see Cavernous sinus disease

◼ Foot drop: differential diagnosis

Pathophysiology The patient presenting with foot drop is not uncommon in neurological practice. The differential diagnosis is wide, reflecting the extensive neuroanatomical pathway subserving foot movement, but division of cases into upper motor neurone ("stiff foot drop") and lower motor neurone ("floppy foot drop") facilitates diagnosis and focuses investigation.

The neural pathway controlling foot movement is as follows; pathology anywhere along this pathway may potentially cause foot drop:

- Motor cortex (parasagittal region)
- Descending motor pathways (corticospinal pathway: internal capsule, cerebral peduncles, corticospinal tracts)
- Anterior horn cells of spinal cord (neuronopathy)
- L4–S1 roots contain motor neurone axons (radiculopathy)
- Lumbosacral plexus (plexopathy)
- Sciatic nerve, common peroneal nerve (mononeuropathy)
- Neuromuscular junction
- Muscles (myopathy)
    Tibialis anterior
    Extensor digitorum and hallucis longus
    Extensor digitorum brevis.

Clincal features: history and examination
- Upper motor nerve lesion: "stiff foot drop"
    Appearance: wasting may be minimal unless lesion is chronic
    Tone: spasticity of leg, foot; may be sustained ankle clonus
    Reflexes: hyperreflexia, extensor plantar response
    Gait: circumduction of leg on walking
    Sensory findings: may be absent
    Potential causes
        Cerebral (e.g. parasagittal) lesion: usually unilateral, for example meningioma; stroke
        Spinal cord lesion: usually bilateral (e.g. demyelination)
        Dystonia.
- Lower motor nerve lesion: "floppy foot drop"
    Appearance: wasting of leg, intrinsic foot muscles may be evident
    Tone: hypotonia, flaccidity of foot, leg
    Power: sparing of ankle inversion and foot plantar flexion differentiates common peroneal nerve palsy from L5 radiculopathy
    Reflexes: depressed or absent ankle jerk; plantar response flexor or mute
    Gait: dragging of foot on walking so often high stepping

Sensory findings: may be root, plexus or peripheral nerve pattern of sensory impairment/loss.

Potential causes

Unilateral

Radiculopathy (L5/S1 root)

Plexopathy

Mononeuropathy: sciatic, common peroneal.

Bilateral

Polyneuropathy

Muscular dystrophy: scapuloperoneal type.

- A combination of upper and lower motor signs may be seen, suggesting motor neurone disease (e.g. fasciculations, weakness, but brisk reflexes, upgoing plantar); absent ankle jerks with extensor plantar responses may be seen in Friedreich's ataxia and subacute combined degeneration of the cord due to vitamin B_{12} deficiency.

Investigations and diagnosis *Bloods*: only if malignancy or peripheral neuropathy suspected.

Imaging: requirements vary. For upper motor neurone type, imaging of brain and whole spinal cord may be required, unless other features point to a more specific localization; in lower motor neurone type, MRI of lumbar spine and/or lumbosacral plexus may be appropriate.

CSF: if infiltrative meningitic process is suspected.

EMG/NCS: often diagnostic in floppy foot drop.

Muscle/nerve biopsy: as appropriate.

Differential diagnosis Dorsal column lesions (e.g. tabes dorsalis) or large fibre sensory neuronopathies (ganglionopathies) causing sensory ataxia may be mistaken for foot drop as the patient slams foot to ground because of the proprioceptive loss.

Treatment and prognosis Dependent on cause. See individual entries.

Reference Katirji B. Peroneal neuropathy. *Neurologic Clinics* 1999; **17**: 567–591.

Other relevant entries Dystonia: an overview; Neuropathies: an overview; Lumbar cord and root disease; Lumbosacral plexopathies; Peroneal neuropathy; Sciatic neuropathy.

■ Footballer's migraine

A migraine attack may be precipitated by exercise such as playing football. It has been speculated that this may be a consequence of sudden jarring of the head, as may occur when a heading the ball, but there is no systematic evidence regarding this.

Reference Matthews WB. Footballer's migraine. *British Medical Journal* 1972; **2**: 326–327.

Other relevant entries Headache: an overview; Migraine.

Foramen magnum lesions, foramen magnum syndrome

Pathophysiology The foramen magnum syndrome is characterized by neck stiffness and suboccipital pain which may be associated with sensorimotor abnormalities from the neck downwards and neuro-ophthalmological abnormalities. It may result from extrinsic or intrinsic lesions. Recognition of the syndrome is important as many of the tumours responsible for it are benign and readily excised, without long-term sequelae. However, the syndrome can be difficult to recognize as the signs are often subtle even with large lesions. The advent of MRI has made this syndrome easier to diagnose.

- Extrinsic lesions causing compression at foramen magnum
  - Meningioma
  - Neurofibroma
  - Metastasis
  - Skull base tumour (e.g. teratoma)
  - Tonsillar ectopia in Chiari malformation
  - Cervical spondylosis
  - Atlantoaxial dislocation (e.g. rheumatoid arthritis)
  - Other craniovertebral junction bony abnormalities.
- Intrinsic lesions
  - Glioma
  - Demyelination (e.g. multiple sclerosis)
  - Syrinx (typically with Chiari malformation).

Clinical features: history and examination

- The history is often indolent and non-specific with progression over years.
- Neck-occipital stiffness and pain with radiation to the shoulder or arm, with Lhermitte's phenomenon. Pain is typically made worse by head movement; the patient may hold the head at an angle, or even develop torticollis.
- Weakness of the limbs, which may be upper and/or lower motor neurone (UMN/LMN) in type. The UMN presentation typically begins in the ipsilateral arm and then spreads sequentially to involve the ipsilateral leg before the contralateral leg and then contralateral arm ("around the clock" presentation, eventually producing hemiparesis, triparesis, or quadriparesis). The LMN presentation is with wasting, weakness, and areflexia in the upper limb which may be false localizing, suggesting involvement of segments well below the level of the lesion, possibly as a result of compromise of the anterior spinal artery blood supply to the cervical cord.
- Numbness and clumsiness of the hands and arms, with a sensory loss to all modalities. There may be a dissociated and suspended sensory loss of syringomyelic type, and there may be pseudo-athetosis if posterior columns are affected. Occasionally there may be patches of sensory loss or dysaethesia on the trunk.
- Lower cranial nerve palsies (e.g. IX–XII) are rare, although facial sensory loss may be present. However down beating nystagmus is highly suggestive of a lesion at the

cervico-medullary junction (although this can be an isolated finding in elderly patients without foramen magnum lesion).

- Papilloedema may be seen if there is obstruction to CSF circulation.
- Occasionally patients with foramen magnum tumours have a relapsing–remitting course.

Investigations and diagnosis *Bloods*: not usually helpful; serology for rheumatoid arthritis may be appropriate.

Imaging: MRI is the most appropriate modality.

CSF: only necessary if demyelination suspected.

Neurophysiology: not usually necessary, unless marked lower motor neurone findings in the arms, although these may be false localizing.

Treatment and prognosis This is dependent on cause. Mass lesions require a complicated neurosurgical approach and as such may have a relatively high morbidity. However, benign tumours may be associated with few neurological sequelae.

Reference Symonds CP, Meadows SP. Compression of the spinal cord in the neighbourhood of the foramen magnum. *Brain* 1937; **60**: 52–84.

Other relevant entry Chiari malformations.

Foreign accent syndrome

A rare disorder of speech production such that the speech sounds as though it is foreign, or different from the speakers native intonation. There is no language disorder since comprehension of spoken and written language is preserved; hence it is qualitatively different from Broca's aphasia. This syndrome probably overlaps with other disorders of speech production, labelled as phonetic disintegration, pure anarthria, aphemia, apraxic dysarthria, verbal or speech apraxia, and cortical dysarthria. Case heterogeneity is noted.

References Graff-Radford NR, Cooper WE, Colsher PL, Damasio AR. An unlearned foreign "accent" in a patient with aphasia. *Brain and Language* 1986; **28**: 86–94.

Kurowski KM, Blumstein SE, Alexander M. The foreign accent syndrome: a reconsideration. *Brain and Language* 1996; **54**: 1–25.

Monrad-Krohn GH. Dysprosody or altered "melody" of language. *Brain* 1947; **70**: 405–415.

Other relevant entries Aphasia; Dysarthria.

Forestier's disease – see Diffuse idiopathic skeletal hyperostosis

Foster–Kennedy syndrome

First described in 1911, this clinical syndrome consists of:

- optic atrophy in one eye,
- papilloedema in the other eye,
- anosmia ipsilateral to optic atrophy.

This is classically due to a tumour, typically an olfactory groove meningioma, which compresses the ipsilateral optic nerve to cause atrophy, and raises intracranial pressure to cause contralateral papilloedema. Similar clinical appearances may occur with sequential anterior ischaemic optic neuropathies, sometimes called a pseudo-Foster–Kennedy syndrome.

Other relevant entries Cranial nerve disease: I: Olfactory nerve; Ischaemic optic neuropathy; Meningioma.

■ Fothergill's disease

The eighteenth century English physician John Fothergill (1712–1780) described cases of a "painful affliction of the face" which probably correspond to the current entity of trigeminal neuralgia.

References Fothergill J. On a painful affliction of the face. *Medical Observations and Enquiries* 1773; **5**: 129–142.

Rose FC. Trigeminal neuralgia. *Archives of Neurology* 1999; **56**: 1163–1164.

Other relevant entry Trigeminal neuralgia.

■ Fotopoulos syndrome

A syndrome of uncertain nosology, characterized by the association of chorea and lower motor neurone disease causing neurogenic atrophy. Acanthocytosis, mitochondrial disease, and trinculeotide repeat disorders may account for many, but not all, cases.

Reference Pageot N, Vial C, Remy C, Chazot G, Broussolle E. Progressive chorea and amyotrophy without acanthocytes: a new case of Fotopoulos syndrome? *Journal of Neurology* 2000; **247**: 392–394.

Other relevant entry Neuroacanthocytosis.

■ *Fou rire prodromique*
Laughing madness

Fou rire prodromique, first described by Féré in 1903, is pathological laughter which heralds the development of a brainstem stroke, usually as a consequence of basilar artery occlusion. Pathological crying as a prodrome of brainstem stroke has also been described ("folles larmes prodromiques").

References Gondim F de A, Parks BJ, Cruz-Flores S. "Fou rire prodromique" as the presentation of pontine ischaemia secondary to vertebrobasilar stenosis. *Journal of Neurology, Neurosurgery and Psychiatry* 2001; **71**: 802–804.

Larner AJ. Basilar artery occlusion associated with pathological crying: "folles larmes prodromiques"? *Neurology* 1998; **51**: 916–917.

Other relevant entries Brainstem vascular syndromes; Locked-in syndrome.

■ Foville's syndrome

A dorsolateral pontine vascular syndrome of crossed paralysis, characterized by ipsilateral gaze paresis (looking away from the lesion), ipsilateral lower motor neurone facial (VII) nerve palsy, and contralateral hemiparesis or hemiplegia. This usually results from infarction in the territory of the anterior inferior cerebellar artery.

Reference Silverman IE, Lui GT, Galetta SL. The crossed paralyses. The original brain-stem syndromes of Millard–Gubler, Foville, Weber and Raymond–Céstan. *Archives of Neurology* 1995; **52**: 635–638.

Other relevant entries Brainstem vascular syndromes; Raymond syndrome, Raymond–Céstan syndrome.

■ Fragile X syndrome

This is the most common chromosomal cause of mental retardation. The higher incidence of mental retardation in males and families with exclusively males affected initially suggested a non-specific X-linked inheritance, sometimes known as Martin–Bell syndrome or Renpenning's syndrome. The current name originates from the identification of an unusual fragile site on the X-chromosome, evident during karyotype preparation in folate-free culture medium.

It is characterized by mental retardation (IQ 40–55), attention deficit disorder, and somatic abnormalities such as prognathism, thick nasal bridge, large ears, enlarged testes, and occasional macrocephaly. Female carriers may sometimes be affected but only to a slight degree.

FRAXE is a trinucleotide repeat disorder in which there is an expanded CGG repeat in the 5′ untranslated region of the *FRX-1* gene.

Other relevant entry Trinucleotide repeat diseases.

■ Franceschetti–Zwahlen–Klein syndrome – see Treacher Collins syndrome

■ Fregoli's syndrome

This is a psychiatric delusional disorder in which the patient believes that a familiar person may be identified in other people even though they bear no resemblance; the supposed persecutor can change his or her appearance and appear as other people. This delusion may occur in schizophrenia.

Other relevant entry Schizophrenia.

■ Frey's syndrome
Auriculotemporal syndrome

When parasympathetic fibres to the salivary glands reinnervate sweat glands, which normally have a sympathetic cholinergic supply, for example after recovery from a Bell's palsy, gustatory sweating may occur.

Other relevant entry Bell's palsy.

■ Friedreich's ataxia

Pathophysiology Friedreich's ataxia (FA), described first by Friedreich in 1861, is the most common of the autosomal-recessive ataxias with an incidence of 1–2 per 100 000 population. The disease typically presents before the age of 20 years with a combination of ataxia, axonal polyneuropathy, optic atrophy, dysarthria, pyramidal weakness of the legs, scoliosis, and cardiac abnormalities.

The discovery of the genetic basis of FA to be an intronic trinucleotide repeat (GAA) in the frataxin gene on chromosome 9q13 (normal = 8–22 repeats, affected = 90–1700 repeats) has led to an expansion of the clinical phenotype. Some FA patients are compound heterozygotes, with GAA expansion on one allele and point mutation on the other. Genetic changes cause reduced expression of frataxin protein, localized in the mitochondrial matrix (hence FA may be regarded as a mitochondrial disorder), resulting in production of reactive oxygen species, inactivation of iron–sulphur proteins in various complexes (I, II, III) of the oxidative phosphorylation pathway, and iron accumulation.

FA is currently incurable and 95% of patients are wheelchair bound by 45 years of age.

Clinical features: history and examination

- FA typically presents between the ages of 8–15 years, but since the discovery of the frataxin gene the age range has expanded, with case onset even into the seventh decade being recorded.
- Progressive limb and gait ataxia with dysarthria (slow, jerky speech) and abnormal eye movements (nystagmus in <50%, but fixation instability with square-wave jerks almost always present); symptoms may begin abruptly after a febrile illness.
- Axonal sensory polyneuropathy with absent tendon reflexes (but preserved abdominal reflexes early in the disease), loss of proprioception, and vibration per-ception, with distal wasting and pes cavus +/− equinovarus deformity of the feet.
- Pyramidal weakness of the legs with extensor plantar responses (90% in later stages of the disease).
- Optic atrophy (25%).
- Sensorineural deafness (10%).
- Head titubation is relatively common and there may be irregular ataxic respiration.
- Sphincter abnormalities are not a major feature of this disease.
- Kyphoscoliosis (50%) can precede neurological deficits.
- Heart disease is seen in 65% of cases, including heart failure with arrhythmias late in the disease; in the early stages the main abnormality is on ECG with widespread T-wave inversion and left ventricular hypertrophy.
- Diabetes mellitus (10%), with an additional 10–20% having an impaired glucose tolerance test.
- Diabetes insipidus is also reported.
- Mentation is preserved, although emotional lability is not uncommon.
- Atypical presentations are also reported, with late-onset spastic ataxia, pure sensory ataxia, ophthalmoplegia, myoclonus, or chorea.

Investigations and diagnosis *Bloods*: usually non-contributory; diabetes mellitus and vitamin E deficiency should be excluded.

Imaging: CT and/or MRI of the brain and spinal cord usually reveals a degree of cerebellar and spinal cord atrophy.

CSF: usually normal; not obligatory.

Neurophysiology:

EMG/NCS: axonal polyneuropathy; severe reduction or loss of sensory action potentials without involvement of motor conduction velocities. This pattern is very useful in distinguishing FA from Hereditary motor and sensory neuropathy (HMSN) type I, in which motor nerve conduction velocity is slowed, and autosomal-dominant ataxias such as SCA3 in which sensory neuropathy may not be clinically apparent.

Evoked potentials: VEP are abnormal in most cases, as are limb SEPs.

ECG: widespread T-wave inversion, left ventricular hypertrophy.

Neurogenetics: search for trinucleotide expansion and mutation in the frataxin gene is now the definitive test; genetic counselling.

Others: may include echocardiography, cardiac opinion, respiratory studies, orthopaedic opinion.

Pathology: degeneration with gliosis of dorsal columns, especially in cervical cord, dorsal root ganglia, pyramidal tracts, especially in lower spinal cord, and spinocerebellar tracts with secondary mild atrophy of cerebellum and neuronal loss in the dentate nucleus and inferior olivary nucleus. Optic and peripheral nerves show loss of large myelinated fibres. Nuclei of cranial nerves VIII, X, and XII all show reduced cell counts.

Differential diagnosis HMSN, especially type I.

Ataxia with isolated vitamin E deficiency (AVED).

Other inherited cerebellar syndromes, autosomal recessive or dominant.

Mitochondrial disease.

Abetalipoproteinaemia.

Complicated hereditary spastic paraparesis (HSP).

Wolfram syndrome.

Treatment and prognosis The rate of progression is very variable: death may occur in the 30s but patients can live upto sixth or seventh decade. Mean time to become wheelchair bound is ~15 years, 95% are wheelchair bound by age of 45 years. Mean survival time from onset is ~36 years.

Symptomatic treatment includes management of diabetes and cardiac abnormalities. Surgery may be needed for foot deformities.

There is currently no treatment for the underlying condition but improved understanding of pathogenesis suggests that antioxidants such as idebenone may be helpful. Randomized trials are awaited.

References Dürr A. Friedreich's ataxia: treatment within reach. *Lancet Neurology* 2002; **1**: 370–374.

Dürr A, Cossee M, Agid Y *et al.* Clinical and genetic abnormalities in patients with Friedreich's ataxia. *New England Journal of Medicine* 1996; **335**: 1169–1175.

Other relevant entries Abetalipoproteinaemia; Ataxia with vitamin E deficiency; Cerebellar disease: an overview; Hereditary motor and sensory neuropathy; Hereditary spastic paraparesis; Mitochondrial disease: an overview; Sylvester disease; Trinucleotide repeat diseases.

Froehlich's syndrome

Adiposogenital dystrophy • Babinski–Froehlich syndrome

This is a rare disorder in which there is obesity in association with gonadal under-development, due to a lesion of the hypothalamic–pituitary axis, for example a tumour such as craniopharyngioma. Other symptoms and signs which may occur include visual loss, mood swings, abulia, and diabetes insipidus, all of which indicate pathology in the hypothalamic region. The Prader–Willi syndrome presents a similar clinical picture.

Other relevant entries Craniopharyngioma; Hypothalamic disease: an overview; Prader–Willi syndrome.

Froin's syndrome

Exceptionally high CSF protein concentration, which may be sufficient to cause the CSF to clot, sometimes associated with low CSF opening pressure, may be seen with spinal block, malignancy, Guillain–Barré syndrome, and vestibular schwannomas.

Froment's sign

Froment's manoeuvre

This is the induction or exaggeration of rigidity in a limb by movement of the contra-lateral limb, also known as activated rigidity or synkinesis.

Froment's (prehensile thumb) sign

Signe du journal

In ulnar nerve lesions, when attempting to pinch the thumb and index finger together (for example to grasp a sheet of paper), an involuntary flexion of the distal phalanx of the thumb may be observed. This movement is mediated by flexor pollicis longus, innervated by the median nerve, to compensate for the weakness of the ulnar-innervated adductor pollicis.

Other relevant entry Ulnar neuropathy.

Frontal lobe syndrome

Pathophysiology Damage to the frontal lobes may produce a constellation of symptoms and signs affecting both cognitive and motor function. Characteristically patients with a frontal lobe syndrome have little or no insight into their problems, which causes greater concern to their family and friends. A frontal lobe syndrome may occur as a consequence of various pathologies:

Neurodegenerative process: especially frontotemporal dementia or Pick's disease; motorneuron disease

Structural lesion: tumour (intrinsic, extrinsic), normal pressure hydrocephalus; Vascular event

Head injury

Inflammatory metabolic disease: multiple sclerosis, X-linked adrenoleuko-dystrophy, metachromatic leukodystrophy.

Clinical features: history and examination

- Motor abnormalities may include:

Contralateral hemiplegia: with involvement of the motor cortex.

Unilateral motor neglect, difficulty with sequencing movements and bimanual coordination: involvement of supplementary motor area, frontal convexity.

Akinesia, akinetic mutism: involvement of medial frontal region.

Gait disorder: frontal gait disorder, frontal disequilibrium, isolated gait ignition failure (subsumes gait apraxia, *marche a petit pas*).

Voluntary saccadic eye movements may be abnormal, although assessment may be difficult in the context of other motor deficits and/or behavioural change.

In addition "primitive reflexes" or "frontal release signs" may be elicited, including the pout, palmomental and grasp reflexes, as well as increased tone in the limbs with passive movement (*gegenhalten*). Imitation and utilization behaviour may also be seen. If the dominant (usually left) hemisphere is involved then speech output will be affected, either in the form of a Broca's aphasia or as a reduction in spontaneous speech and verbal fluency. Urinary incontinence may occur with damage to the superior frontal and anterior cingulate gyri and intervening white matter of either hemisphere.

- Cognitive and intellectual changes may include:

Loss of initiative and spontaneity, a lack of concern and freedom from anxiety, with poor attention and a subsequent impairment of anterograde memory: frontal convexity.

Disinhibition, frivolity, with inappropriate comments and behaviour: orbitofrontal cortex.

Primary psychiatric disorder may be inappropriately diagnosed in some patients with a frontal lobe syndrome.

Large prefrontal lesions, including subfrontal meningiomas, may be relatively silent in terms of clinical expression; anosmia may be the only clinical sign, so testing of olfaction is necessary in all patients with a frontal lobe syndrome. Ophthalmological examination is also suggested (Foster–Kennedy syndrome).

Investigations and diagnosis *Bloods*: syphilis serology and screen for vasculitis may be indicated.

Imaging: CT/MRI for frontal lobe pathology: mass lesion, atrophy.

Neuropsychology: looking specifically for frontal lobe dysfunction (e.g. verbal fluency, go–no go tests, Wisconsin card sorting test, Stroop test). Other neuropsychological deficits may point to possible cause of disorder (e.g. language, memory).

CSF: may be required to diagnose inflammatory or infective cause.

Neurophysiology: EEG typically normal in frontotemporal dementia.

Others: may include ophthalmological, psychiatric opinions and tests for rare metabolic conditions.

Treatment and prognosis Dependent on cause.

References Cummings JL, Mega MS. *Neuropsychiatry and behavioral neuroscience.* Oxford: OUP, 2003: 128–145.

Damasio AR, Anderson SW. The frontal lobes. In: Heilman KM, Valenstein E (eds). *Clinical Neuropsychology* (4th edition). Oxford: OUP, 2003: 404–446.

Other relevant entries Adrenoleukodystrophy; Alzheimer's disease; Aphasia; Apraxia; Cerebrovascular disease: arterial; Dementia: an overview; Emotional lability: differential diagnosis; Encephalitis: an overview; Frontotemporal dementia; Gait disorders; Multiple sclerosis; Normal pressure hydrocephalus; Pick's disease; Psychiatric disorders and neurological disease; Subdural haematoma; Tumours: an overview; Vasculitis.

■ Frontotemporal dementia

Frontotemporal lobar degeneration

Pathophysiology Neurodegenerative disorders with circumscribed atrophy of the frontal and/or temporal regions were first described by Pick. These account for perhaps 20% of cases of primary cerebral atrophy occurring in the presenium. A number of subsyndromes are recognized, dependent on the precise anatomical distribution of pathology, although there is a tendency for clinical merging as the disease progresses:

- Frontotemporal dementia (FTD), dementia of frontal type, frontal lobe degeneration, frontal variant of FTD.
- Progressive non-fluent aphasia, primary progressive aphasia (PPA), temporal variant of FTD.
- Semantic dementia (*q.v.*).

Development of motor neurone disease (MND) (MND–dementia) may occur with a frontotemporal dementia.

Not all cases have the typical pathology of "Pick's disease", as originally described by Alzheimer; some have "dementia lacking distinctive pathology", other have pathology typical of MND.

Familial occurrence is commoner than in Alzheimer's disease (AD). Some families have shown mutations in the τ-gene on chromosome 17.

Clinical features: history and examination

- FTD: a neurobehavioural syndrome with change in personality, impaired judgement (dysexecutive syndrome); patient may be apathetic and lack motivation, or be disinhibited, overactive and fatuous.
- Reduced ability to show emotion or empathize with the emotions of others.
- Stereotyped and perseverative behaviours; rituals, clockwatching. Gluttony, food fads, especially a predilection for sweet or sticky foods to the exclusion of other food. Speech economic, concrete. No amnesia or disorientation. Late akinesia, rigidity.
- Progressive non-fluent aphasia: progressive decline in language production with relative absence of other neuropsychological deficits; comprehension relatively preserved.
- Semantic dementia: loss of word meaning leading to fluent but empty speech.
- Fasciculation may suggest an underlying pathological diagnosis of MND–dementia.

Investigations and diagnosis *Neuropsychology*: deficits appropriate to anatomical distribution of pathology: attentional difficulties in FTD, language problems in progressive non-fluent aphasia, semantic difficulties in semantic dementia.

Imaging: CT/MRI: focal frontotemporal atrophy, often asymmetric; SPECT shows focal deficits of perfusion.

EEG: typically normal (*cf.* AD).

CSF: unremarkable.

EMG/NCS: may be undertaken to look for evidence of anterior horn cell disease.

Differential diagnosis Cases of FTD have probably been labelled as mania or manic–depressive psychosis in the past.

Language disorders need to be distinguished from focal presentations of AD. Semantic dementia is sometimes confused with AD.

Treatment and prognosis No specific treatment currently available. Behavioural agitation may be treated empirically with anticonvulsant medication (carbamazepine, valproate) or "atypical" anti-psychotics such as risperidone, olanzapine, or quetiapine.

References Brun A, Englund B, Gustafson L *et al.* Clinical and neuropathological criteria for frontotemporal dementia. *Journal of Neurology, Neurosurgery and Psychiatry* 1994; **57**: 416–418.

Miller BL, Ikonte C, Ponton M *et al.* A study of the Lund–Manchester research criteria for frontotemporal dementia: clinical and single-photon emission CT correlations. *Neurology* 1997; **48**: 937–942.

Neary D, Snowden JS, Gustafson L *et al.* Frontotemporal lobar degeneration: a consensus on clinical diagnostic criteria. *Neurology* 1998; **51**: 1546–1554.

Snowden JS, Neary D, Mann DMA. *Fronto-temporal Lobar Degeneration: Frontotemporal Dementia, Progressive Aphasia, Semantic Dementia.* New York: Churchill Livingstone, 1996.

Other relevant entries Alzheimer's disease; Dementia: an overview; Dementia with Lewy Bodies; Frontal lobe syndrome; Semantic dementia; Tauopathy.

■ Fructose-1,6-diphosphatase deficiency – see Hereditary fructose intolerance

■ Fructose intolerance – see Hereditary fructose intolerance

■ Fucosidosis

Pathophysiology A rare autosomal-recessive inherited metabolic disorder due to a deficiency of lysosomal α-fucosidase. A distinction may be made between:

Type I (infantile): with onset between 3 and 18 months; in which seizures may occur and progression is rapid.

Type II (juvenile): with onset from 1 to 2 years in which ataxia and behavioural problems may feature, progression somewhat slower.

Type III: signs noted in the first few years of life, but adolescence or adulthood reached before severe mental and motor deterioration.

Clinical features: history and examination
- Chronic encephalopathy with developmental delay; psychomotor retardation; progressive quadriplegia.
- Seizures; ataxia.
- "Storage facies": enlarged salivary glands, coarse facial features, gargoylism, excessive sweating.
- Angiokeratoma.
- Recurrent infection.

Investigations and diagnosis *Bloods*: smears may show vacuolated mononuclear cells; white cell enzymes for fucosidase activity.

Imaging: mild dysostosis multiplex (beaking of the vertebral bodies).

Pathology: skin biopsy electron microscopy may reveal intralysosomal laminated structures and axonal spheroids.

Differential diagnosis

Mannosidoses.

Hurler syndrome.

Angiokeratoma are identical to those seen in Fabry's disease.

Treatment and prognosis No specific treatment. Usually fatal within 4–6 years.

Reference Galluzzi P, Rufa A, Balestri P *et al.* MR brain imaging of fucosidosis type I. *American Journal of Neuroradiology* 2001; **22**: 777–780.

Other relevant entries Lysosomal-storage disorders: an overview; Mannosidoses; Mucopolysaccharidoses.

■ Fukuhara syndrome – see MERRF syndrome

■ Fukuyama muscular dystrophy

This autosomal-recessive condition, found almost exclusively in Japan, is a form of congenital muscular dystrophy, in which a child is born with profound hypotonia, muscle wasting, and weakness. Additional features include severe mental retardation, seizures, skull asymmetry, and the development of joint contractures.

The condition is linked to chromosome 9q, with deficiency of the protein fukutin.

Other relevant entries Congenital muscular dystrophies; Muscle–eye–brain disease; Walker–Warburg syndrome.

▤ Fumaryl-acetoacetate hydrolase deficiency – see Tyrosinaemia

▤ Fungal disease and the nervous system – see Infection and the nervous system: an overview

Gg

▤ Gait disorders

Pathophysiology Disorders of gait are relatively common in neurological practice and may have a number of different causes, acting either individually or collectively; gait disorder may be multifactorial. A thorough neurological examination is indicated in any patient with a gait disorder.

Various forms of gait disorder are recognized:

- Myopathic gait

  Waddling; difficulty climbing stairs, rising from chairs; proximal weakness.

- Neuropathic gait

  May be unsteady, cautious; high stepping gait (steppage); distal weakness and sensory loss, foot drop, areflexia. Focal neuropathies may cause gait difficulties (e.g. lateral popliteal or femoral neuropathies).

- Spastic gait

  Most commonly unilateral, with circumduction of leg, + / − ipsilateral arm held in abduction, internally rotated at the shoulder and flexed at the elbow (hemiplegic); + / − other upper motor neurone signs, aphasia. May be bilateral, with scissoring gait, spastic paraparesis + / − impaired bladder function, sensory level.

- Ataxic gait

  Cerebellar: broad-based, staggering + / − nystagmus, dysarthria, limb ataxia; midline cerebellar lesions cause a gait/truncal ataxia with little in the way of limb or eye signs.

  Sensory: broad-based, staggering, Romberg sign positive, often high stepping with slapping down of foot; distal sensory loss + / − weakness.

- Extrapyramidal gait

    Parkinson's disease (PD): stooped posture, slow initiation, shuffling/festinant ambulation, reduced or absent arm swing, freezing +/− hypomimia, tremor, quiet voice.

    Progressive supranuclear palsy: as for PD but axial rigidity with neck extension (retrocollis); early history of falls, especially on turning; +/− supranuclear gaze palsy.

    Dystonia: abnormal leg posture, often with walking: typically inversion and plantar flexion of the foot but may involve hip; toe-walking; minimal neurological signs examining on the couch, except possibly dystonia; differential diagnosis includes dopa-responsive dystonia (DRD), and paroxysmal kinesigenic choreoathetosis (PKC).

    Choreiform: often only hand and head chorea seen, but may affect legs and cause lurching or stumbling gait which is irregular and unpredictable; +/− cognitive abnormalities (Huntington's disease).

    Post-anoxic action myoclonus: bouncing gait, collapsing; bizarre give-way type walking may be labelled "psychiatric".

    Primary orthostatic tremor (POT): "shaky legs syndrome", unsteady on standing still, often better with walking or sitting; minimal signs; leg tremor is not uncommonly seen in essential tremor (ET) but rarely causes a gait disorder.

- Rigid gait

    Stiff man syndrome: stiff but not scissoring; lumbar hyperlordosis, abdominal rigidity, no abnormal limb signs.

- *Marche à petit pas*

    Short, small steps, upright posture; +/− subcortical dementia, pseudobulbar palsy, history of strokes.

- Gait apraxia

    Unable to start walking means gait ignition failure, associated with frontal lobe involvement; normal examination on bed, can pretend to cycle on bed.

- Painful, antalgic gait

    Staggering, limping; no neurological deficits, may be Trendelenburg sign positive.

- Psychogenic gait disorders

    Often bizarre, staggering but always able to compensate, never falling; inconsistent neurological deficits; consider chorea and action myoclonus as possible causes before applying this diagnosis.

- Cautious gait

    Holding on to objects (e.g. furniture), small steps, fear of falling; no abnormal signs.

- Impaired vision/diplopia, vestibular disorders

    May produce cautious gait, ataxic gait.

Gait disorders may be multifactorial, particularly in the elderly (any combination of painful hips, poor vision, mild neuropathy, vestibular dysfunction).

A number of different gait disorders have been described with frontal lobe pathology, including:

subcortical disequilibrium,
frontal disequilibrium,
isolated gait ignition failure,
frontal gait disorder.

Clinical features: history and examination
- Mechanical stability: joint/skeletal integrity.
- Power: neuromuscular integrity.
- Proprioception, vestibular input, and sensory feedback: peripheral input from somatosensory, vestibular, and visual system.
- Coordination and maintenance of posture: cerebellum and ventromedial motor system.
- Corrective motor responses: motor cortices, basal ganglia, cerebellum, and spinal cordmotor apparatus.

Investigations and diagnosis May be apparent clinically (e.g. PD). If not, may require:

Bloods: investigation of arthropathies
Imaging: focal brain/cord lesion; joints
EMG/NCS: neuromuscular integrity
Other: gait analysis.

Differential diagnosis/treatment and prognosis See individual entries.

References Bronstein AM, Brandt T, Woollacott MH (eds). *Clinical Disorders of Balance, Posture and Gait*. London: Arnold, 1996.

Elble RJ. Approach to the patient with gait disturbances and recurrent falls. In: Biller J (ed.). *Practical Neurology* (2nd edition). Philadelphia: Lippincott Williams & Wilkins, 2002: 84–98.

Nutt JG, Marsden CD, Thompson PD. Human walking and higher-level gait disorders, particularly in the elderly. *Neurology* 1993; **43**: 268–279.

Other relevant entries Cerebrovascular disease: arterial; Foot drop: differential diagnosis; Frontal lobe syndrome; Proximal weakness.

■ Galactosaemia

Pathophysiology This is an autosomal-recessive condition in which there is a defect in the galactose-1-phosphate uridyl transferase (GALT or GPUT) enzyme which normally converts galactose-1-phosphate to galactose uridine diphosphogalactose. Various forms have been described according to the degree of metabolic block; partial enzyme deficiencies are more common and present with milder forms of the disease. Typically the condition presents in the neonatal period following milk ingestion, and has the capacity to produce long-term disability, with cognitive decline, speech abnormalities, and ovarian failure. A rare adult-onset form of the disease has been described. Neurological features may result from accumulation of galactitol in the brain.

Clinical features: history and examination In the neonatal period, the disease presents following the ingestion of galactose-containing milk, with vomiting, diarrhoea, failure to thrive, hypotonia, drowsiness; anaemia, hepatosplenomegaly with jaundice and hypoglycaemia soon develop in the untreated state, along with renal tubular defects; punctate cataracts may form. *Escherichia coli* sepsis is common. Cerebral oedema and intracranial hypertension may develop.

A late presenting form of the disease has been described with ataxia, dystonia, apraxia, and a degree of cognitive impairment.

Investigations and diagnosis *Bloods*: raised blood galactose level, hypoglycaemia; significant hyperbilirubinaemia very common, initially unconjugated, later conjugated + raised transaminases, moderate coagulopathy; low enzyme level in peripheral white blood cells, red cells, and hepatocytes.

Urine: non-glucose reducing substances typical of galactosaemia; high galactitol levels; generalized aminoaciduria if renal tubular damage present.

Imaging: CT/MRI demonstrates atrophy of cerebellum, brainstem, and basal ganglia.

Neurophysiology: central motor conduction time (CMCT) and somatosensory evoked potential (SSEP) may show non-specific abnormalities, but EMG/NCS are normal.

In event of acute deterioration, screening for evidence of *E. coli* sepsis is necessary. Infants with *E. coli* sepsis should be investigated for galactosaemia.

Differential diagnosis Other causes of neonatal hypoglycaemia, especially hereditary fructose intolerance (also has non-glucose reducing substances in urine). Other causes of neonatal jaundice.

Treatment and prognosis Surviving untreated children have a degree of psychomotor retardation, visual impairment, and features of cirrhosis and portal hypertension.

Treatment should be aimed at correcting metabolic and/or infective complications.

Galactose should be excluded from the diet (i.e. milk substitutes required).

Patients with partial enzyme deficiencies, and those diagnosed and treated promptly, do best.

However most children experience late-onset problems including hypergonadotrophic hypogonadism (with ovarian failure), tremor, ataxia, and cognitive deficits.

References Schweitzer S, Shin Y, Jakobs C, Brodehl J. Long-term outcome in 134 patients with galactosaemia. *European Journal of Pediatrics* 1993; **152**: 36–43.

Wang ZJ, Berry GT, Dreha SF *et al*. Proton magnetic resonance spectroscopy of brain metabolites in galactosemia. *Annals of Neurology* 2001; **50**: 266–269.

Other relevant entries Hereditary fructose intolerance; Inherited metabolic diseases and the nervous system.

■ Galactosidase deficiency

α-galactosidase is the deficient enzyme in Fabry's disease; located at chromosome Xq21.33–q22.

β-galactosidase is the deficient enzyme in GM1 gangliosidosis and Morquio's disease type B; located at chromosome 3p21.

Other relevant entries Fabry's disease; Gangliosidoses: an overview; Morquio's syndrome.

■ Galactosylceramide lipidosis – see Krabbe's disease

■ Galloping tongue syndrome

Galloping tongue syndrome is an episodic, rhythmic, involuntary movement of the tongue following head and neck trauma. The episodes begin as posterior midline focal tongue contractions at a frequency of 3 Hz and last for around 10 seconds. The movements differ from branchial myoclonus, are innocuous and self-limiting, resolving in 2–4 months. They do not spread and are not associated with any EEG abnormality.

Reference Keane JR. Galloping tongue: post-traumatic, episodic, rhythmic movements. *Neurology* 1984; **34**: 251–252.

■ Gamstorp's disease – see Periodic paralysis

■ Ganglioglioma

Gangliogliomas are benign tumours, occurring typically in childhood and early adulthood, often occurring in the temporal lobe and causing partial epilepsy. They are occasionally found in other lobes of the cerebral hemisphere, cerebellum, and spinal cord. They are composed of both neuronal and glial elements and are well delineated from surrounding tissues; calcification is common. Local surgical excision is often possible.

Reference Zentner J, Wolf HK, Ostertun B *et al*. Gangliogliomas: clinical, radiological and histopathological findings in 51 patients. *Journal of Neurology, Neurosurgery and Psychiatry* 1994; **57**: 1497–1502.

Other relevant entries Epilepsy: an overview; Tumours: an overview.

■ Ganglionopathy – see Neuropathies: an overview; Paraneoplastic syndromes

■ Gangliosides and neurological disorders

Pathophysiology Gangliosides are acidic glycosphingolipids which form a relatively minor component of total myelin lipids (0.3–0.7%). Ganglioside molecules contain sialic acid in association with a variety of neutral sugars, which generate related but distinct antigens. Antibodies to gangliosides have been detected in a number of neurological conditions, especially peripheral neuropathies, in some of which the antibodies may be of pathogenetic significance. Non-specific, low-titre anti-ganglioside antibodies may also be observed in a number of conditions especially GM1 antibodies in motorneuron disease. Some antibodies do not persist and hence for diagnostic purposes may need to be assayed shortly after disease onset (e.g. anti-GQ1b in Miller Fisher syndrome, MFS).

Gangliosidoses (*q.v.*) are disorders characterized by accumulation of gangliosides GM1 or GM2 in the nervous system due to deficiency of enzymes which break down these compounds.

A number of associations between anti-ganglioside antibodies and neurological disorders are recognized:

> GM1 (binding to nodes of Ranvier): multifocal motor neuropathy (MMN) with conduction block; also seen in some cases of Guillain–Barré syndrome, Chinese paralysis syndrome.
>
> GD1a: acute motor axonal neuropathy (AMAN).
>
> GD1b: acute sensory ataxic neuropathy (ASAN).
>
> GQ1b (binding to presynpatic terminals): MFS, some instances of Bickerstaff's brainstem encephalitis, usually at onset of diplopia.
>
> CANOMAD: anti-disialosyl antibodies (GD1b, GQ1b, GT1a, GD2, GD3).

Therapeutic use of gangliosides, predicated on their *in vitro* ability to cause axonal sprouting, has been associated with peripheral neuropathy, presumably due to antigenic cross reaction.

Investigations and diagnosis Anti-ganglioside antibodies are detected by standard enzyme-linked immunosorbent assay and thin layer chromatography techniques. Assays are difficult and considerable inter-laboratory variation exists.

Differential diagnosis/treatment and prognosis See individual entries.

> **References** O'Leary CP, Willison HJ. The role of antiglycolipid antibodies in peripheral neuropathies. *Current Opinion in Neurology* 2000; **13**: 583–588.
>
> Willison HJ. Antiglycolipid antibodies in peripheral neuropathy: fact or fiction? *Journal of Neurology, Neurosurgery and Psychiatry* 1994; **57**: 1303–1307.
>
> Willison HJ, Yuki N. Peripheral neuropathies and anti-glycolipid antibodies. *Brain* 2002; **125**: 2591–2625.

> **Other relevant entries** Bickerstaff's brainstem encephalitis; CANOMAD; Gangliosidoses: an overview; Guillain–Barré syndrome; Miller Fisher syndrome; Multifocal motor neuropathy; Neuropathies: an overview.

▨ Gangliosidoses: an overview

Pathophysiology Gangliosides are made up of ceramide and sialic acid, and are important components of central nervous system (CNS) and peripheral nervous system (PNS) lipid. Accumulation of various gangliosides in the CNS systemically occurs in the inherited gangliosidoses, of which two main types are recognized:

• GM1 gangliosidosis: due to deficiency of lysosomal β-galactosidase.

- GM2 gangliosidosis: due to deficiency of hexosaminidase activity, though more complex, since three genes may be involved (for the α-locus, the β-locus, and for a heat-stable protein cofactor), and two enzymes, hexosaminidase A (α- and β-subunits) and B (only β-subunit).

Clinical features: history and examination

- GM1 gangliosidosis (familial neurovisceral lipidosis); no ethnic tendencies

  Type 1/Infantile: (birth to <3 months old).

  Coarsened facies at birth, enlarged tongue, hepatosplenomegaly, umbilical hernia; pseudo-Hurler's phenotype.

  Neurology

  Micro- or macrocephaly

  No psychomotor development after 3–6 months

  Blind with macular cherry-red spots (50%) and nystagmus; corneal clouding unusual

  Deafness

  Hypotonia then spasticity

  Seizures (late)

  +/− cardiomyopathy.

  Type 2/Late infantile, Juvenile: (6–18 months old)

  No systemic features (i.e. no visceral storage or bone involvement).

  Neurology

  Weakness (progressive)

  Incoordination

  Spasticity

  Mental retardation

  Seizures

  Vision preserved.

  Type 3/Adult: (mid-childhood to adolescence)

  No systemic features.

  Neurology

  Gait disorder with spasticity

  Dystonia and other extrapyramidal features

  Dysarthria and ataxia

  Mental retardation; may progress to dementia

  No visceral or skeletal changes.

- GM1 gangliosidosis may alternatively be classified as two variants:

  Early infancy

  Rapidly progressive neurovisceral-storage disease with dysmorphic facial features, late-onset dysostosis multiplex

  Cherry-red macular spot

  Late-onset variant

  Gait disturbance

  Dysarthria

Psychomotor retardation

Spasticity

Seizures

Little or no evidence of non-neurological disease.

- GM2 gangliosidosis: predilection for Ashkenazi Jews

  Type 1: Infantile (α-locus: total hexosaminidase A deficiency) Tay–Sachs disease (*q.v.*)

  Type 2: Juvenile (α-locus: reduced hexosaminidase A activity)

  Type 3: Adult (α-locus: partial hexosaminidase A deficiency)

  Sandhoff's disease (*q.v.*; β-locus: hexosaminidase A and B deficiency).

Investigations and diagnosis

GM1 gangliosidosis

  Blood: vacuolated lymphocytes; deficiency of β-galactosidase in leukocytes, fibroblasts.

  Urine: oligosaccharides abnormal.

  Imaging:

  plain radiographs: dysostosis multiplex

  CT/MRI: putaminal lesions in adult form.

  Neurophysiology: Visual evoked response (VER) delayed or absent, ERG abnormal with retinal involvement.

  Neurogenetics: mutations in β-galactosidase gene on chromosome 3p21.

GM2 gangliosidosis

  No biochemical marker

  See entries for Sandhoff disease, Tay–Sachs disease.

Differential diagnosis

GM1 gangliosidosis

  Type 1/Infantile

  Mucopolysaccharidoses: Hurler's syndrome: similar dysmorphism but no corneal clouding

  Sialidosis

  Neuronal ceroid lipofuscinosis

  If cardiomyopathy present, consider Pompe's disease.

GM2 gangliosidosis

  See entries for Sandhoff disease, Tay–Sachs disease.

Treatment and prognosis Neither condition has specific treatment.

GM1 gangliosidosis

  Type 1/Infantile: typically die within first 2–3 years of life; respiratory failure associated with infection.

  Type 2/Juvenile: typically die between the ages of 3–7 years old.

  Type 3/Adult: survival is typically prolonged.

GM2 gangliosidosis

  See entries for Sandhoff disease, Tay–Sachs disease.

References Maertens P, Dyken PR. Storage diseases: neuronal ceroid-lipofuscinoses, lipidoses, glycogenoses, and leukodystrophies. In: Goetz CG (ed.). *Textbook of Clinical Neurology* (2nd edition). Philadelphia: Saunders, 2003: 601–628.

Navon R. Molecular and clinical heterogeneity of adult GM2 gangliosidosis. *Developmental Neuroscience* 1991; **13**: 295–298.

Suzuki K. Neuropathology of late onset gangliosidosis. A review. *Developmental Neuroscience* 1991; **13**: 205–210.

Suzuki Y, Sakuraba H, Oshima A *et al.* Clinical and molecular heterogeneity in hereditary β-galactosidase deficiency. *Developmental Neuroscience* 1991; **13**: 299–303.

Other relevant entries Galactosidase deficiency; Hurler's disease; Morquio's syndrome; Mucopolysaccharidoses; Neuronal ceroid lipofuscinosis; Sandhoff disease; Sialidosis; Tay–Sachs disease.

◼ Ganser phenomenon, Ganser syndrome
Vorbereiden

The Ganser phenomenon consists of giving approximate answers to questions, which can at times verge on the absurd: the classic example is, in answer to the question "how many legs does a horse have?", the answer "Three". This may occur in the context of depression, schizophrenia, and sometimes following head injury or in epilepsy. Some patients may be malingering. A Ganser syndrome is also described, comprising hallucinations, cognitive disorientation, and conversion disorder, but does not appear in DSM-IV-TR.

References Carney MW. Ganser syndrome and its management. *British Journal of Psychiatry* 1987; **151**: 697–700.

Enoch MD, Ball HN. *Uncommon Psychiatric Syndromes* (4th edition). London: Arnold, 2001: 74–94.

Other relevant entries Malingering; Psychiatric disorders and neurological disease.

◼ Garcin syndrome
Hemibasal syndrome

This refers to unilateral palsy of all cranial nerves, often occurring successively. It is most commonly seen with skull base tumours (chordoma, chondrosarcoma of the clivus), rhinopharyngeal tumours (nasopharyngeal carcinoma) or metastases, and basal meningitides.

Reference Hanse MCJ, Nijssen PCG. Unilateral palsy of all cranial nerves (Garcin syndrome) in a patient with rhinocerebral mucormycosis. *Journal of Neurology* 2003; **250**: 506–507.

Other relevant entry Cranial polyneuropathy.

Gardner's syndrome

A dominantly inherited familial polyposis coli syndrome, associated with multiple osteomas, sometimes of the skull, skin, and soft tissue tumours. Brain tumours may sometimes occur.

Reference Foulkes WG. A tale of four syndromes: familial adenomatous polyposis, Gardner syndrome, attenuated APC and Turcot syndrome. *Quarterly Journal of Medicine* 1995; **88**: 853–863.

Other relevant entry Turcot syndrome.

Garin–Bujadoux meningopolyneuritis – see Borreliosis

Gasperini's syndrome

A brainstem syndrome comprising ipsilateral palsy of the fifth, sixth, seventh, and eighth cranial nerves, with contralateral sensory disturbance, with additional nystagmus, due to a lesion of the posterior tegmentum of the pons.

Other relevant entries Brainstem vascular syndromes; Cranial polyneuropathy.

Gasserian ganglion syndrome

This rare syndrome occurs with metastatic infiltration of the Gasserian (or semilunar) ganglion, the origin of the sensory portion of the trigeminal nerve. Patients therefore present with pain and sensory disturbance in the second and third divisions of the trigeminal nerve. There may be additional weakness of the pterygoids and masseter muscle, and occasionally the sixth cranial nerve is involved.

Gastaut–Geschwind syndrome – see Geschwind syndrome

Gastaut's occipital epilepsy

Gastaut-type childhood occipital epilepsy

A rare childhood epilepsy syndrome manifesting mainly with elementary visual hallucinations, blindness, or both, seizures being frequent and brief (seconds). The visual hallucinations consist of small multi-coloured circular patterns often in the periphery of a visual field. Consciousness is not impaired. There may rarely be progression to extra-occipital manifestations. Post-ictal headache may occur, causing potential confusion with migraine, although the visual symptoms are much briefer. Investigations are normal with the exception of the EEG which shows paroxysms of occipital spikes. Prognosis is good, most patients respond to carbamazepine.

Reference Panayiotopoulos CP. *A Clinical Guide to Epileptic Syndromes and their Treatment: Based on the New ILAE Diagnostic Scheme.* Chipping Norton: Bladon, 2002: 103–105.
Other relevant entries Epilepsy: an overview; Panayiotopoulos syndrome.

■ Gastrointestinal disease and the nervous system

Pathophysiology Neurological and gastroenterological problems may be interrelated in a number of ways. Neurological disorders may cause abnormalities of gut motility; gastro-enterological disorders may cause malabsorption with secondary neurological effects.

Clinical features: history and examination

- Disorders of gut motility

     Achalasia: primary, secondary (Chagas' disease)

     Dysphagia (*q.v.*)

      Neurogenic: stroke (hemisphere, brainstem); extrapyramidal disorders (Parkinson's disease, progressive supranuclear palsy, Huntington's disease, Wilson's disease), multiple sclerosis, Guillain–Barré syndrome (GBS), motor neurone disease, myasthenia gravis.

       Myogenic: inflammatory muscle disease (polymyositis, inclusion body myositis), myotonic dystrophy, oculopharyngeal muscular dystrophy.

     Constipation/diarrhoea (with autonomic neuropathy) e.g. diabetes mellitus, and Parkinson's disease/MSA.

- Malabsorption

     Vitamin B_1 deficiency: beriberi, Wernicke–Korsakoff's syndrome; pellagra

     Vitamin B_{12} deficiency: peripheral neuropathy, myelopathy (subacute combined degeneration of the cord), optic neuropathy, disorder of affect or cognition (rarely dementia)

     Vitamin D deficiency: myopathy

     Vitamin E deficiency: spinocerebellar syndrome with peripheral neuropathy

     Coeliac disease (gluten-sensitive enteropathy): epilepsy (usually partial, occipital), cerebellar syndrome, peripheral neuropathy, myelopathy, myoclonus, dementia.

- Inflammatory bowel disease: thromboembolic complications including cerebral venous thrombosis; peripheral neuropathy (? related to nutritional deficiency).

- Whipple's disease: dementia, ophthalmoplegia (supranuclear), myoclonus, hypo-thalamic features (hypersomnia, polydipsia, hyperphagia).

Investigations and diagnosis Videofluoroscopy may help to characterize the location of the swallowing difficulty (oral, pharyngeal, both) and whether there is aspiration. Dependent on clinical context, assays of vitamin B_{12}, vitamin D, vitamin E may be appropriate.

Differential diagnosis Dysphagia: gastroenterological causes: peptic stricture, tumour. Constipation/Diarrhoea: gastroenterological causes: tumour, diverticular disease, irritable bowel syndrome, inflammatory bowel disease or endocrine cause (e.g. thyroid disease, caranoid syndrome etc.).

Treatment and prognosis Treatment of the underlying cause where possible. Speech therapy advice on appropriate feeding methods and diet; in extreme cases percutaneous endoscopic gastrostomy (PEG) or jejunostomy (PEJ) may be required to ensure adequate nutrition.

References Camilleri M. Disturbances of gastrointestinal motility and the nervous system. In: Aminoff MJ (ed.). *Neurology and General Medicine. The Neurological Aspects of Medical Disorders* (2nd edition). New York: Churchill Livingstone, 1995: 267–284.

Mancall EL. Nutritional disorders of the nervous system. In: Aminoff MJ (ed.). *Neurology and General Medicine. The Neurological Aspects of Medical Disorders* (2nd edition). New York: Churchill Livingstone, 1995: 285–301.

Perkin GD, Murray-Lyon I. Neurology and the gastrointestinal system. *Journal of Neurology, Neurosurgery and Psychiatry* 1998; **65**: 291–300.

Other relevant entries Abetalipoproteinaemia; Alcohol and the nervous system: an overview; Beriberi; Coeliac disease (gluten-sensitive enteropathy); Dementia: an overview; Diabetes mellitus and the nervous system; Dysphagia; Dystrophia myotonica; Guillain–Barré syndrome; Huntington's disease; Inclusion body myositis; Motor neurone disease; Multiple sclerosis: Myasthenia gravis; Myoclonus; Oculopharyngeal muscular dystrophy; Parkinson's disease; Pellagra; Polymyositis; Progressive supranuclear palsy; Sandifer's syndrome; Vitamin B$_{12}$ deficiency; Vitamin deficiencies and the nervous system; Wernicke–Korsakoff's syndrome; Whipple's disease; Wilson's disease.

■ Gaucher's disease

Glucosylceramide lipidosis

Pathophysiology This is a rare autosomal-recessive lysosomal-storage condition, in which there is a deficiency of lysosomal β-glucosidase (or glucocerebrosidase) which leads to the accumulation of glucocerebrosides in cells of the reticuloendothelial system. Three forms of the disease are recognized, of which the commonest form, type I, is non-neuronopathic. Type II is a severe form of neuronopathic disease with onset in the first months of life and death usually by 2 years of age. Type III is the late-onset adult form of the condition that has a subacute onset with supranuclear gaze palsies, intellectual decline, and spasticity with hepatosplenomegaly.

Gaucher's disease is linked to genetic mutations in the glucocerebrosidase gene on chromosome 1q21. Rare cases are associated with deficiency of saposin C, a heat-stable cofactor required for the normal catalytic activity of glucocerebrosidase, due to mutations in the prosaposin gene on chromosome 10q21 (allelic to some forms of metachromatic leukodystrophy, MLD).

Clinical features: history and examination
- Type I: non-neuronopathic (commonest)
    Visceromegaly
    Bone changes
    Thrombocytopenia: marked bruising, anaemia.

- Type II: acute infantile neuronopathic

  Typically presents in first months of life

  Neurological features:

      Developmental arrest

      Hypertonia (spasticity)

      Neck retraction, opithotonos

      Strabismus, visual impairment; normal fundi; supranuclear gaze palsy

      Feeding diffiulties, unable to swallow: laryngeal stridor, trismus, and
  dysphagia

      Microcephaly

      Seizures are rare.

  Systemic features

      Hepatosplenomegaly: huge

      Skin and scleral pigmentation

      $+/-$ lymphadenopathy

      No bone changes (*cf.* type I).

- Type III: subacute non-neuronopathic

  Typically presents in early to middle childhood, either with neurological features, or with aggressive visceral disease reminiscent of type I which may cause death from hepatic failure before significant neurological problems develop.

  Neurological features

      Seizures, myoclonus

      Slowly progressive ataxia

      Dysarthria

      Cognitive decline

      Oculomotor disorder (supranuclear gaze palsy).

  Systemic features

      Hepatosplenomegaly: almost always.

Investigations and diagnosis *Bloods*: raised acid phosphatase; pancytopenia if bone marrow significantly involved; deficiency of β-glucosidase (glucocerebrosidase) may be demonstrated in leukocytes or fibroblasts and is diagnostic.

Imaging: widened ends of long bones on plain radiography due to infiltration and expansion by glucocerebroside-containing storage cells ("Erlenmeyer flask" in femur).

CSF: not usually required, although Gaucher cells (swollen by intracytoplasmic accumulation of cerebrosides giving a foamy appearance) may be found in the CSF.

Others: characteristic Gaucher cells may be seen in bone marrow aspirates and liver biopsies.

Neurogenetics: L444P mutation in glucocerebrosidase gene in most patients with types II and III. Mutations in prosaposin gene may be sought if glucocerebrosidase gene is normal.

Differential diagnosis Type I may be clinically indistinguishable from Niemann–Pick type B.

Type III may be clinically similar to MLD but the presence of hepatosplenomegaly assists in differentiating them. It also enters the differential diagnosis of progressive myoclonic epilepsies.

Treatment and prognosis Intravenous enzyme replacement therapy may be effective for treating the systemic features in types I and III, for example to reduce hepatosplenomegaly; however, it delays but does not prevent the neurological complications of type II; outcome uncertain in type III.

Treatment of hypersplenism by splenectomy may be required.

Type II: typically die by the age of 2 years.

Type III: death second to fourth decade.

Reference Cox TM. Gaucher's disease – an exemplary monogenic disorder. *Quarterly Journal of Medicine* 2001; **94**: 399–402.

Other relevant entries Lysosomal-storage disorders: an overview; Metachromatic leukodystrophy; Niemann–Pick disease; Progressive myoclonic epilepsy.

▨ Gegenhalten

Gegenhalten, or paratonia, describes a variable resistance to passive limb movement, such that the more the arm is moved by the clinician the greater the resistance to movement; exhortations to the patient to relax meet with conspicuous failure. This sign is characteristically seen in frontal lobe syndromes (especially when the mesial frontal lobe is involved).

Other relevant entry Frontal lobe syndrome.

▨ Gelastic epilepsy

These are partial epileptic seizures characterized by involuntary laughter. They may be symptomatic, particularly of hypothalamic hamartoma (along with precocious puberty and mental retardation), and of tuberous sclerosis, but may also be cryptogenic in some cases, in which case the prognosis for seizure control with anti-epileptic medications is better.

Reference Striano S, Mea R, Bilo L *et al*. Gelastic epilepsy: symptomatic and cryptogenic cases. *Epilepsia* 1999; **40**: 294–302.

Other relevant entries Emotional lability: differential diagnosis; Epilepsy: an overview.

▨ Gélineau's syndrome – see Narcolepsy, narcoleptic syndrome

▨ Gelsolin amyloidosis
Familial amyloidosis, Finnish type (FAF)

This hereditary systemic amyloidosis, first described in Finland, results from mutation in the gene encoding gelsolin, an actin-binding protein, on chromosome 9, G654A, or G654T ("Danish type"), resulting in the Asp187Asn substitution.

The clinical features are characterisitic, viz.

corneal lattice dystrophy;
polyneuropathy: mild, sensory, principally proximal nerve involvement, with preferential large fibre loss;
cranial neuropathy, especially facial weakness, +/- atrophic bulbar palsy;
+/- gait ataxia;
+/- cognitive impairment;
+/- skin changes: baggy and atrophic.
Pathologically there is meningeal amyloid angiopathy.

Reference Kiuru S. Gelsolin-related familial amyloidosis, Finnish type (FAF), and its variants found worldwide. *Amyloid* 1998; **5**: 55–66.

Other relevant entries Amyloid and the nervous system: an overview; Familial amyloid polyneuropathies .

■ General paresis of the insane – see Syphilis

■ Generalized epilepsy with febrile seizures plus – see Channelopathies: an overview; Febrile convulsions

■ Geniculate herpes zoster – see Herpes zoster and postherpetic neuralgia; Ramsay Hunt syndrome (2)

■ Geniculate neuralgia

This refers to pain of unknown cause in the region of the ear which is not paroxysmal but continuous. There are no associated neurological signs. It is very rare and more commonly occurs in women. Carbamazepine may be of benefit.

Other relevant entry Facial pain: differential diagnosis.

■ Geniospasm

Geniospasm is a focal movement disorder involving tremor of the chin and lower lip, sometimes precipitated by stress, concentration, or emotion. The condition begins in early childhood, and sometimes occurs in families with an autosomal-dominant pattern of inheritance.

Reference Jarman PR, Wood NW, Davis MT *et al.* Hereditary geniospasm: linkage to chromosome 9q13–q21 and evidence for genetic heterogeneity. *American Journal of Human Genetics* 1997; **61**: 928–933.

■ Genitofemoral neuropathy

Lesions of the genitofemoral nerve, arising from the L1 and L2 spinal roots, cause pain and paraesthesiae in the groin and upper medial thigh ("spermatic neuralgia").

Owing to its proximity, the ilioinguinal nerve is also often affected. The cremasteric reflex may be absent. Surgery is probably the commonest cause of neuropathy.

Other relevant entries Ilioinguinal neuropathy; Neuropathies: an overview.

■ Gerhardt syndrome

Bilateral vagus (X) nerve palsies, due to brainstem or skull base pathology, causing bilateral adductor laryngeal paralysis with severe dysphonia and dyspnoea.

Other relevant entry Cranial nerve disease: X: Vagus nerve.

■ Germ-cell tumours

The group of germ-cell tumours encompasses:
- Germinoma
- Teratoma
- Embryonal carcinoma
- Yolk sac tumour
- Choriocarcinoma

Although they may occur at many intracranial locations, the pineal gland is the commonest.

There may be elevations of serum and CSF α-fetoprotein, human chorionic gonadotrophin (HCG), and placental alkaline phosphatase, which may facilitate diagnosis, since MRI findings are usually non-specific. If bloods and imaging prove unhelpful, biopsy should be undertaken to establish tumour type.

Reference Glenn OA, Barkovich AJ. Intracranial germ cell tumors: a comprehensive review of proposed embryologic derivation. *Pediatric Neurosurgery* 1996; **24**: 242–251.

Other relevant entries Parinaud's syndrome; Pineal tumours.

■ Germinoma

Germinoma is a germ-cell tumour, accounting for <1% of primary intracranial tumours, with a predilection for the pineal gland and suprasellar region, rarely the basal ganglia and thalami, and very uncommonly the posterior fossa, with symptoms and signs appropriate to specific location. This is a tumour occurring most commonly in childhood. There may be elevations of serum and CSF α-fetoprotein, human chorionic gonadotrophin, and placental alkaline phosphatase. MRI usually shows a solid lesion, sometimes surrounded by calcium, but there may be cystic areas, with homogenous or heterogeneous enhancement. Biopsy is the key to management, especially for pineal lesions since a variety of tumours may occur in this location. Good remission rates with no detectable disease have been achieved with chemotherapy and local, limited, radiotherapy.

Other relevant entries Germ-cell tumours; Pineal tumours.

Gerstmann syndrome
Angular gyrus syndrome

Gerstmann syndrome refers to the constellation of signs:
- right–left disorientation,
- finger agnosia,
- acalculia,
- agraphia (central type).

It occurs with lesions, most usually of vascular origin, in the region of the dominant (usually left) posterior parietal cortex (angular and supramarginal gyri), and thus may be associated with a visual field defect. All the signs do dissociate, so partial syndromes do occur.

References Benton AL. Gerstmann's syndrome. *Archives of Neurology* 1992; **49**: 445–447.

Mayer E, Martory M-D, Pegna AJ *et al*. A pure case of Gerstmann's syndrome with a subangular lesion. *Brain* 1999; **122**: 1107–1120.

Other relevant entries Acalculia; Agraphia; Agnosia.

Gerstmann–Sträussler–Scheinker disease

This is a rare inherited form of prion disease, first described in 1928, that presents with a slowly evolving cerebellar syndrome followed by dementia, long tract signs, and an extrapyramidal disorder; myoclonus and psychiatric features may occur, visual and sensory signs are rare. Pathologically it is characterized by multicentric amyloid plaques. Few patients survive for >5 years after onset of illness.

GSS is associated with mutations in the PrP gene which encodes the prion protein.

Reference Kovacs GG, Trabattoni G, Hainfellner JA, Ironside JW, Knight RSG, Budka H. Mutations of the prion protein gene: phenotypic spectrum. *Journal of Neurology* 2002; **249**:1567–1582.

Other relevant entries Cerebellar disease: an overview; Prion disease: an overview.

Geschwind syndrome
Gastaut–Geschwind syndrome

This syndrome consists of:
- hypergraphia,
- hyperreligiosity,
- hyposexuality.

It may occur as part of an interictal psychosis in patients with complex partial seizures of temporal lobe origin, particularly with a non-dominant focus.

Reference Trimble MR. The Gastaut–Geschwind syndrome. In: Trimble MR, Bolwig TG (eds). *The Temporal Lobes and the Limbic System*. Petersfield: Wrightson Biomedical, 1992: 137–147.

Giant axonal neuropathy

This is a rare, autosomal-recessive, condition, traditionally classified with the hereditary peripheral neuropathies, although both peripheral nervous system (PNS) and central nervous system (CNS) are affected. It manifests in childhood with:

- psychomotor retardation,
- progressive axonal peripheral neuropathy,
- ataxia,
- dysarthria,
- nystagmus,
- dementia,
- dull blonde curly hair.

In sporadic cases, skeletal and cardiac muscle involvement has been reported.

Nerve biopsy shows pathognomonic large focal axonal swellings that contain neurofilamentous masses, which reflect a defect of the cellular intermediate filaments. The condition is linked to chromosome 16q24 and mutations in the gene encoding gigaxonin have been identified. Prognosis is poor, most patients become wheelchair bound and die before age 30 years.

References Berg BO, Rosenberg SH, Asbury AK. Giant axonal neuropathy. *Pediatrics* 1972; **49**: 894–899.

Bomont P, Cavalier L, Blondeau F *et al*. The gene encoding gigaxonin, a new member of the cytoskeletal BTB/kelch repeat family, is mutated in giant axonal neuropathy. *Nature Genetics* 2000; **26**: 370–374.

Other relevant entry Neuropathies: an overview.

Giant cell arteritis

Cranial arteritis • Extracranial arteritis • Granulomatous arteritis • Horton's syndrome • Polymyalgia arteritica • Temporal arteritis

Pathophysiology An inflammatory arteritis, most commonly affecting the ophthalmic and superficial branches of the external carotid artery, which usually occurs in people over 50 years of age. It most commonly presents with headache and local tenderness of the temporal artery and is often associated with the features of polymyalgia rheumatica (PMR). Almost invariably there is a markedly raised ESR, but temporal artery biopsy is required for definitive diagnosis. However, treatment should be initiated early, often before the diagnosis is established with certainty, since occlusion of branches of the ophthalmic artery may result in irreversible blindness. Other arteries may be involved. Treatment is with steroids.

Clinical features: history and examination

- Headache, with local tenderness over the temporal (and less often occipital) arteries, often noted as scalp tenderness on combing the hair. The temporal artery is typically thickened with reduced pulsation and painful to touch.
- Jaw claudication with eating is relatively rare but almost pathognomonic for this condition. Tongue claudication is very rare.
- Painful proximal muscles and joints with stiffness may be a feature, especially first thing in the morning (PMR).
- Lassitude, fatigue, preceding weight loss may occur.
- Amaurosis fugax is an ominous sign as it often heralds impending visual failure.
- Sudden non-painful visual loss is rarely the presenting symptom of this disease, representing an arteritic acute ischaemic optic neuropathy.
- Other, rare, associations that occur in <10% of patients include:
    peripheral neuropathy,
    extraocular muscle involvement,
    limb (typically arm) claudication,
    TIA/stroke (more common is posterior vascular territories),
    confusional state,
    acute myelopathy.

Incidence is 5–15 per 100 000 in population over the age of 50 years; F : M = 3 : 1, Caucasians affected more often than Asians, Afro-Caribbeans.

Investigations and diagnosis *Bloods*: raised ESR, sometimes in excess of 100 mm/hour; very rarely the ESR may be normal in biopsy-proven giant cell arteritis (GCA). Anaemia, leukocytosis, and thrombocytosis may occur.

Imaging: usually normal; not mandatory.

CSF: not usually indicated.

Neurophyisology: not required.

Temporal artery biopsy: the diagnostic test, so should be performed as soon as possible, although inflammation persists for several days after the initiation of steroid therapy. A long segment of artery should be taken, given the patchy nature of the inflammation (skip lesions). Inflammation of the vessel wall, with lymphocytes, neutrophils, and giant cells, is seen, with intimal proliferation causing vessel stenosis and occlusion.

Differential diagnosis

Metastatic malignant disease or myeloma.

Viral illnesses.

Systemic vasculitis.

Treatment and prognosis If the diagnosis is suspected, treatment with steroids should be started immediately because of the potential risk to vision; biopsy should be arranged as soon as possible thereafter.

Typically doses are prednisolone 80 mg/day for a week, thereafter 60 mg/day for a month or until ESR falls. The steroids should then be slowly tapered by 5–10 mg/day per month, depending on symptoms and the ESR.

If the ESR does not fall within a week, the diagnosis needs re-evaluating if the biopsy was non-contributory.

In cases with visual loss, some clinicians start with intravenous methylprednisolone (1 g/day for 3 days) before commencing high-dose oral steroids.

As the population suffering from this disease is elderly, prophylaxis for gastrointestinal ulceration and osteoporosis may be required.

Once appropriate therapy is commenced the outlook is good, especially from a visual point of view, assuming the steroids are not reduced too dramatically. However, neuropathies and large artery involvement can still occur several months after initiation of the steroid therapy.

Reference Caselli RJ, Hunder GG, Whisnant JP. Neurologic disease in biopsy-proven giant-cell (temporal) arteritis. *Neurology* 1988; **38**: 352–359.

Other relevant entries Ischaemic optic neuropathy; Polymyalgia rheumatica.

Gigantism

Gigantism, the development of excessively high stature, is most often due to a pituitary tumour (micro- or macroadenoma) secreting excess amounts of growth hormone (GH) in childhood or adolescence, before the fusion of the bony epiphyses (after fusion, the syndrome is acromegaly). A purely hypothalamic form of gigantism (or acromegaly) has been postulated, for example in association with hypothalamic gangliocytomas which secrete growth hormone releasing hormone (GHRH).

Partial forms of gigantism may also occur, for example:

cerebral gigantism (Sotos syndrome, *q.v.*);
partial gigantism (e.g. of digits in Proteus syndrome).

Other relevant entries Pituitary disease and apoplexy; Sotos syndrome.

Gilles de la Tourette syndrome – see Tourette syndrome

Gillespie's syndrome

This is a congenital inherited cerebellar ataxia in which there is also mental retardation and aniridia. The inheritance pattern is uncertain.

Reference Gillespie FD. Aniridia, cerebellar ataxia and oligophrenia in siblings. *Archives of Ophthalmology* 1965; **73**: 338–341.

Other relevant entries Cerebellar disease: an overview; Marinesco–Sjögren syndrome.

Glasgow Coma Scale

The Glasgow Coma Scale (GCS) was devised in the 1970s by Jennett and colleagues in Glasgow as a quick, convenient, reproducible, and accurate way of assessing the unconscious patient. It is now used widely throughout the world. Three responses are observed and scored: eye opening; verbal response, and motor response, with the best response being recorded. A score of between 3 and 15 may be achieved (3 worst, 15 best):

Best eye response (E)	
Spontaneously	4
To verbal command	3
To pain	2
No eye opening	1
Best verbal response (V)	
Oriented and converses	5
Confused but converses	4
Incomprehensible words	3
Incomprehensible sounds	2
No verbal response	1
Best motor response (M)	
Obeys commands	6
Localizes to pain	5 (ensure localization, not simply flexing)
Withdrawal from pain	4
Flexion to pain	3
Extension to pain	2
No motor response	1

It is best to break the figure down into its components (e.g. E3V3M5) rather than quote the global score (e.g. GCS = 11), since the latter may result from various combinations. This said, a Coma score of 13 or higher correlates with mild brain injury, 9–12 is moderate injury, 8 or less is a severe injury. The use of GCS to describe patients following other neurological disorders, such as stroke, is not validated.

Reference Teasdale G, Jennett B. Assessment of coma and impaired consciousness: a practical scale. *Lancet* 1974; **2**: 81–84.

Other relevant entries Coma; Concussion; Subarachnoid haemorrhage; Traumatic brain injury.

▮ Glaucoma

Raised intraocular pressure, or ocular hypertension, may be the cause of glaucoma, an excavation of the optic disc with subsequent visual loss, a common cause of blindness. Typically the raised pressure in the anterior chamber is due to reduced outflow of aqueous humour for reasons that are not clear.

Varieties of glaucoma include:

• Open-angle glaucoma (90% of cases): drainage channels appear open; clinical picture is of insidious visual loss with an arcuate field loss and enlarged blind spot.

- Angle-closure glaucoma (5%): narrow, blocked angle between lateral cornea and pupil; may present with a painful red eye (may be mistaken for systemic illness) with orbital headache and acute visual loss; in addition, clinical signs include corneal clouding (from oedema), ocular injection, and a mid-dilated and unreactive pupil.
- Secondary glaucoma: following another ocular event, such as: anterior uveitis; haemorrhage into the anterior chamber (hyphaema); rubeosis iridis following ocular ischaemia (as in diabetes mellitus, carotid artery occlusion). Glaucoma is the main ophthalmological problem encountered in Sturge–Weber syndrome.

Normal tension glaucoma, in which intraocular pressure appears normal, is also described; it is possible that the pressure is elevated in a cyclical manner, missed by a single reading.

In long-standing glaucoma, fundoscopy shows an excavated and atrophic optic disc.

Early diagnosis and appropriate treatment is the mainstay of management; as there may be a genetic factor, relatives of patients with confirmed glaucoma may be screened, or entitled to free eye tests. Treatment consists of reducing intraocular pressure with eye drops: timolol, a β-blocker, is the traditional first line treatment; an alternative is latanoprost, structurally related to prostaglandin $F_2\alpha$, more expensive but with fewer side-effects than timolol. Combinations may be indicated if a single drug does not control intraocular pressure. Surgery may be required, especially in angle-closure glaucoma.

Prolonged ophthalmological follow-up is necessary to monitor intraocular pressure and visual fields.

Reference Dayan M, Turner B, McGhee C. Acute angle closure glaucoma masquerading as systemic illness. *British Medical Journal* 1996; **313**: 413–415.

Other relevant entries Sturge–Weber syndrome; Visual loss: differential diagnosis.

■ Glioblastoma multiforme – see Glioma

■ Glioma

Pathophysiology Gliomas are tumours consisting of abnormal proliferation of glial cells. Within this rubric may be included astrocytomas, oligodendrogliomas, and ependymomas (*q.v.*). Deletions from chromosomes 13, 17, and 22 are found in many gliomas, with tumour suppressor genes being located on chromosomes 13 and 22, and p53 on chromosome 17. Neurofibromatosis (NF) is associated with the development of gliomas (optic chiasm).

Gliomas *per se* may occur with a spectrum of malignancy, ranging from the aggressive (high-grade) glioblastoma multiforme, through anaplastic lesions to more benign (low-grade) tumours. The clinical features depend on their location within the central nervous system (CNS) and the type of tumour. The more aggressive malignancies present with features of raised intracranial pressure and typically arise in the cerebral hemispheres. More indolent tumours may present with seizures and progressive focal neurological deficits. Brainstem tumours tend to be relatively slow growing with a presentation of focal deficits, similar to that seen in the spinal cord. Generally biopsy or excision is necessary to make the diagnosis. Treatment is usually palliative in all but for the most benign tumours, and consists of radiotherapy +/− chemotherapy. Prognosis is dependent on the grade of the glioma, and remains dismal for the high-grade tumours. Gliomas (astrocytomas) may be graded as:

Grade 1
  25–30% of all intracranial gliomas
Grade 2
  Occur in cerebral hemispheres in adults
  Occur more often in the posterior fossa and spinal cord in children;
  Gliomas of the brainstem, optic nerves, and chiasm occur almost always in
    people under the age of 21 years
  Grow very slowly
  Typically present with seizures when growing in the cerebral hemisphere, or
    slowly evolving focal syndrome in other sites (brainstem or spinal cord).
Grade 3: Anaplastic astrocytoma
  Usually presents in fifth decade of life.
Grade 4: Glioblastoma multiforme
  55% of all gliomas
  Typically involves the cerebral hemisphere, may be multicentric
  Usually presents in sixth decade of life.

Clinical features: history and examination

- Raised intracranial pressure: classically with a headache which is worse at night or first thing in the morning, related to change in posture; +/− nausea and vomiting, especially with posterior fossa tumours. In these cases the headache is often occipital in location whilst supratentorial tumours produce more of a frontal headache.
- Papilloedema is usually present; visual obscurations are an ominous sign, suggesting compromised retinal perfusion pressure.
- Seizures: especially with slow-growing tumours; focal onset, secondary generalization.
- Focal neurological deficits.
- Changes in cognitive function may be the presenting feature.
- Dizziness and non-specific symptoms of light-headedness are not uncommon.
- Occasionally presentation is acute, as a stroke following a bleed into the tumour.
- False-localizing signs: most commonly sixth nerve palsies, although others may occur, for example VII nerve palsy; hemiparesis ipsilateral to the side of the lesion when the cerebral peduncle is compressed contralaterally by the herniating cerebral hemisphere (Kernohan's notch syndrome, *q.v.*).
- In the frontal and temporal lobes gliomas may grow to considerable size without producing any significant neurological deficits ("silent areas").

Investigations and diagnosis *Imaging*: MRI is imaging modality of choice to define tumour anatomy; enhancement with contrast is usually absent or limited, although ring enhancement may be seen especially in high-grade tumours; cystic elements may be seen (e.g. low-grade cerebellar glioma).

Imaging of other structures (e.g. lung and kidney) may be undertaken to exclude a primary tumour if metastasis rather than primary brain tumour is suspected, or if NF is suspected.

Bloods: are usually non-contributory, unless there is a concern about metastatic disease or infective causes. Routine haematological and biochemical screen is sufficient in most cases, but in context of HIV, the management is different.

CSF: LP usually contraindicated, especially if evidence of raised intracranial pressure.

Brain biopsy +/− excision: mandatory to make a diagnosis.

Differential diagnosis Other CNS mass lesions include:

tumour: meningioma, metastatic disease, medulloblastoma;
abscess;
cyst, for example infection (cystercosis);
granulomatous or vascultic disease (e.g. sarcoidosis);
infarct with luxury perfusion;
demyelinating disease occasionally presents as a mass lesion.

Treatment and prognosis Dependent on tumour grade and location.
Brainstem and spinal cord tumours are typically low grade and progress over years. Cerebellar astrocytomas in children are often cystic and may be completely resected by surgery.

Early symptomatic improvement may be obtained using dexamethasone (4 mg tds) to reduce local cerebral oedema, which alleviates many of the symptoms of raised intarcranial pressure as well as some of the focal deficits.

Higher-grade gliomas are usually treated with radiotherapy. Chemotherapy and immunotherapy may be tried, particularly at relapse, but in general the results are disappointing. Survival:

Grade 1 with radiotherapy at 5 years: 58%.
Grade 2 with radiotherapy at 5 years: 25%.
Grade 3: 18 month postoperative survival: 62%.
Grade 4: 18 month postoperative survival: 15%; mean survival time with radiotherapy is 42 weeks.

Survival rates are generally better in children.

Reference Galanis E, Buckner JC. Diffuse cerebral gliomas in adults. In: Noseworthy JH (ed.). *Neurological Therapeutics: Principles and Practice.* London: Dunitz, 2003: 737–753.

Other relevant entries Ependymoma; Kernohan's syndrome; Li–Fraumeni syndrome; Neurofibromatosis; Oligodendroglioma; Tumours: an overview.

■ Gliomatosis cerebri

A rare condition in which the whole cerebral hemisphere is diffusely infiltrated by a tumour with no discrete tumour mass being evident.

Other relevant entry Glioma.

■ Globoid cell leukodystrophy – see Krabbe's disease, Krabbe's leukodystrophy; Leukodystrophies: an overview

■ Glomus jugulare tumour
Chemodactoma • Paraganglioma

Pathophysiology Tumours of the glomus jugulare, derived from the glomus body in the jugular bulb, just below the floor of the middle ear, are rare. The tumour is derived from non-chromaffin paraganglioma cells in the adventitia of the jugular bulb. The tumour is slow growing, over 10–20 years, and may invade locally into the middle ear, cranial nerves, brainstem, and temporal lobe, presenting with slowly evolving lower cranial nerve palsies in association with a vascular polyp in the ear and a mass in the neck. Treatment is radical surgery and radiotherapy.

Clinical features: history and examination
- Conductive deafness, otalgia +/− pulsatile tinnitus with a vascular polyp in the external auditory meatus.
- Local cranial nerve palsies: facial nerve, hypoglossal, glossopharyngeal, and vagus with dysphagia and dysarthria.
- Mass in the neck anterior to the mastoid eminence, with a bruit.
- Occasionally brainstem and temporal lobe involvement, with raised intracranial pressure from partial occlusion of the jugular vein.

Investigations and diagnosis *Bloods*: usually normal.

Imaging: CT/MRI shows a mass originating from the jugular foramen with erosion of the skull base (CT is often imaging modality of choice initially); angiography to define tumour blood supply may be desirable pre-operatively.

CSF: shows raised protein, but usually not indicated.

As these lesions are highly vascular, biopsy is contraindicated. Caution should be exercised when considering biopsy of any mass lesion in the ear.

Differential diagnosis
Metastatic disease.
Tumours originating from bone.
Meningioma.
Inflammatory disease, such as cholesteatoma, Wegener's granulomatosis.

Treatment and prognosis Radical mastoidectomy followed by radiotherapy may affect cure.

> **Reference** Spector GJ, Druck NS, Gado M. Neurologic manifestations of glomus tumors in the head and neck. *Archives of Neurology* 1976; **33**: 270–274.

> **Other relevant entries** Cranial polyneuropathy; Hearing loss: differential diagnosis; Tumours: an overview.

■ Glossodynia
Burning mouth syndrome • Glossopyrosis

Glossodynia is a sensation of burning pain of the tongue and oral mucosa of unknown aetiology. There is no associated erythema, tongue weakness, or alterations in taste.

It is commoner in women, and in the middle-aged and elderly. Vitamin B_{12} deficiency has been cited as a causative factor in some cases, others may be psychogenic.

▧ Glossopharyngeal nerve palsy – see Cranial nerve disease: IX: Glossopharyngeal nerve

▧ Glossopharyngeal neuralgia
Reichert syndrome

This is a condition in which there is severe, unilateral, paroxysmal pain in the throat, radiating to the neck, nasopharynx, and pinna. Pain is usually triggered by swallowing, talking, and coughing and may cause coughing paroxysms, excessive salivation, and occasionally symptomatic bradycardia with syncope (deglutition syncope, swallow syncope). It most often develops in people over the age of 40 years, for reasons that are not clear. Occasionally it is seen with local malignancies in the skull base and oropharynx, as well as after tonsillar infections. Multiple sclerosis is an exceedingly rare cause of glossopharyngeal neuralgia.

Treatment is as for trigeminal neuralgia, with which glossopharyngeal neuralgia shares many features, using drugs such as carbamazepine, phenytoin, gabapentin; or surgery (microvascular nerve decompression or section). A pacemaker may be required to prevent syncopal episodes.

Reference Jacobson RR, Ross Russell RW. Glossopharyngeal neuralgia with cardiac arrhythmia: a rare but treatable form of syncope. *British Medical Journal* 1979; **1**: 379–380.

Other relevant entries Facial pain: differential diagnosis; Syncope; Trigeminal neuralgia.

▧ Glucocerebrosidase deficiency – see Gaucher's disease

▧ Glucose transporter-deficiency syndrome
De Vivo disease

Glucose transporter (GLUT1)-deficiency syndrome is a primary deficiency of glucose transport into the brain, characterized clinically by:

  seizures, resistant to anti-epileptic drug therapy,
  acquired microcephaly,
  developmental delay (intellectual and motor retardation),
  ataxia.

Investigations show persistent hypoglycorrhachia (CSF : blood glucose <0.33). Neuroimaging and EEG are normal.

Mutations in the GLUT1 (SLC2A1) gene on chromosome 1p are deterministic. Treatment is with ketogenic diet for seizure control. With early diagnosis and adequate seizure control, prognosis is good.

References De Vivo DC, Trifiletti RR, Jacobson RI *et al*. Defective glucose transport across the blood–brain barrier as a cause of persistent hypoglycorrhachia, seizures and developmental delay. *New England Journal of Medicine* 1991; **325**: 703–709.

Wang D, Kranz-Eble P, De Vivo DC. Mutational analysis of GLUT1 (SLC2A1) in Glut-1 deficiency syndrome. *Human Mutation* 2000; **16**: 224–231.

■ Glucuronidase deficiency – see Mucopolysaccharidoses; Sly disease

■ Glue sniffing – see Solvent exposure

■ Glutaric aciduria

Pathophysiology Glutaric aciduria (GA) may be primary, due to disorders of glutaric acid metabolism (GA types I and II), or, more commonly, secondary, for example to mitochondrial electron transport chain defects.

Clinical features: history and examination

- Type I: glutaric aciduria type I (GAI), mitochondrial glutaryl-CoA dehydrogenase (GCDH) deficiency

    Acute onset in infancy of episodic encephalopathy with vomiting and ketoacidosis, often after an infectious episode:

    hypotonia;

    seizures;

    movement disorder: choreoathetosis, dystonia, posturing (arching or opisthotonos, grimacing, tongue thrusting, fisting);

    recovery from episodes is incomplete with extrapyramidal features persisting.

    A Reye-like syndrome may also occur without neurological signs.

- Type II: glutaric aciduria type II (GAII), multiple acyl-CoA dehydrogenase deficiency

    Hetereogeneous presentation:

    Neonatal disease, severe

        With dysmorphism (face, abdominal wall, hypospadias), hypotonia, hepatomegaly, hypoketotic hypoglycaemia, metabolic acidosis, hyperammonaemia, +/− cardiomyopathy.

        Odour of sweaty feet.

        Without dysmorphism, but other metabolic features present.

    Later onset, mild

        Acute metabolic acidosis, failure to thrive, hypoglycaemia, hyperammonaemia.

Investigations and diagnosis

- Type I

  Bloods: metabolic acidosis, ketosis, hypoglycaemia, hyperammonaemia, hepato-cellular dysfunction; plasma carnitine levels reduced, excess glutarylcarnitine.

  Urine: usually contains large amounts of glutaric acid, +3-hydroxyglutarate and glutaconic acid; raised glutarylcarnitine.

  Imaging: early cortical atrophy; attenuation of white matter, basal ganglia (especially caudate, putamen).

  CSF: mild increase in protein.

  Neurogenetics: mutations in GCDH gene on chromosome 19p13.2.

- Type II

  Bloods: metabolic acidosis, ketosis, hypoglycaemia, hyperammonaemia, hepato-cellular dysfunction; elevations of several amino acids in plasma, especially proline and hydroxyproline.

  Urine: very large amounts of glutarate, ethylmalonate, dicarboxylic acids; mild GAII is also known as ethylmalonic–adipic aciduria in consequence of the predominant urinary findings.

  Imaging: MRI brain shows disorganized cerebral cortex, reflecting a neuronal migration disorder; ultrasound shows cystic disease of the kidneys in severe disease.

Differential diagnosis Other causes of neonatal encephalopathy, metabolic acidosis. GAI may be mistaken for meningitis or encephalitis because of acute deterioration in context of infective episode with raised CSF protein (also been observed after immunizations). Some cases labelled as "cerebral palsy" may in fact be GAI.

GAII may be difficult to distinguish from severe neonatal carnitine palmitoyltransferase II (CPT II) deficiency.

Treatment and prognosis

GAI:

> Dietary restriction of tryptophan and lysine recommended in GAI, +
>> L-carnitine, riboflavin, baclofen.
>
> Symptomatic treatment of metabolic derangements.
>
> Prognosis poor for late diagnosis.

Other relevant entries Dystonia: an overview; Organic acidopathies.

■ Gluten ataxia, gluten-sensitive enteropathy – see Coeliac disease (Gluten-sensitive enteropathy)

■ Glycine encephalopathy – see Aminoacidopathies: an overview; Non-ketotic hyperglycinaemia

■ Glycogen-storage disorders: an overview
Glycogenoses

There are a number of glycogen-storage disorders, or glycogenoses, which often affect muscle, the commonest of which are acid-maltase deficiency (AMD, or Pompe's disease) and McArdle's disease (also discussed in specific entries). Here a list of the glycogen-storage disorders with their specific enzyme defects and clinical features is given. Most are autosomal recessive, with the exception of type IX (Bresolin's disease) and some forms of type VIII; and possibly some autosomal-dominant forms of type V (McArdle's disease). Most show elevated creatine kinase levels when symptomatic, and have a myopathic EMG. Defective enzyme may be assayed in muscle in most cases, and sometimes also in other tissues such as leukocytes and fibroblasts.

- Type I: von Gierke's disease, glycogen-storage disease (GSD) I

  Enzyme defect: four subtypes, 1a–1d, result from glucose-6-phosphatase (G6P) deficiency; deficiency of G6P transporter 1 produces a similar phenotype. Genetic linkage to chromosome 1p21 and 11, respectively.

  Inheritance: autosomal recessive.

  Clinical phenotype: hepatomegaly, renal enlargement, infantile hypotonia; raised lipids, low glucose, ketoacidosis. Does not affect skeletal muscle.

- Type II: AMD, Pompe's disease, GSD II

  Enzyme defect: acid α-glucosidase (acid-maltase).

  Inheritance: autosomal recessive.

  Clinical phenotype: variable. _Infantile_: cardiomegaly and heart failure, +/− hepatosplenomegaly, macroglossia, firm muscles. _Late-infantile/juvenile (Smith's disease)_: proximal muscle weakness, +/− respiratory difficulty, large calves. _Adult (Engel's disease)_: proximal muscle weakness (slowly progressive), respiratory failure.

- Type III: Cori–Forbes disease, GSD III, debranching enzyme deficiency

  Enzyme defect: glycogen debrancher enzyme deficiency in liver +/− muscle. Genetic linkage to chromosome 1p21.

  Inheritance: autosomal recessive.

  Clinical phenotype: infantile presentation may resemble von Gierke's; progressive skeletal myopathy of childhood and adolescence with hypotonia and contractures; creatine kinase sometimes elevated; liver involvement gradually improves; high protein diet may be helpful.

- Type IV: Andersen disease, GSD IV

  Enzyme defect: branching enzyme. Genetic linkage to chromosome 3.

  Inheritance: autosomal recessive.

  Clinical phenotype: infantile or childhood failure to thrive, growth retardation, hypotonia and wasting with contractures, hepatosplenomegaly. More benign forms in later life. One form of polyglucosan body disease is allelic.

- Type V: McArdle's disease, GSD V (*q.v.*)

    Enzyme defect: myophosphorylase deficiency. Genetic linkage to chromosome 11.

    Inheritance: autosomal recessive; some cases may be autosomal dominant.

    Clinical phenotype: exercise-induced muscle cramps, sometimes leading to marked creatine kinase elevation, rhabdomyolysis, myoglobinuria, and acute renal failure; no organomegaly.
- Type VI: Hers disease, GSD VI

    Enzyme defect: hepatic phosphorylase. Genetic linkage to chromosome 14.

    Inheritance: autosomal recessive.

    Clinical phenotype: hepatosplenomegaly, growth retardation, hypoglycaemia; no myopathy.
- Type VII: phosphofructokinase (PFK) deficiency, Tarui disease, GSD VII (*q.v.*)

    Enzyme defect: muscle PFK. Genetic linkage to chromosome 1.

    Inheritance: autosomal recessive.

    Clinical phenotype: as for McArdle's disease.
- Type VIII: Hug's disease, Ohtani's disease, GSD VIII

    Enzyme defect: phosphorylase B kinase.

    Inheritance: autosomal recessive, some X-linked.

    Clinical phenotype: as for McArdle's disease but no "second wind phenomenon"; + organomegaly.
- Type IX: Bresolin's disease, GSD IX

    Enzyme defect: phosphoglycerate kinase. Genetic linkage to chromosome Xq13.

    Inheritance: X-linked recessive.

    Clinical phenotype: as for McArdle's disease but no "second wind phenomenon"; + organomegaly.
- Type X: Tonin's disease, GSD X

    Enzyme defect: phosphoglycerate mutase. Genetic linkage to chromosome 7p12–p13.

    Inheritance: autosomal recessive.

    Clinical phenotype: as for McArdle's disease but no "second wind phenomenon"; adult onset.
- Type XI: Tsujino's disease, GSD XI

    Enzyme defect: lactic dehydrogenase. Genetic linkage to chromosome 11.

    Inheritance: autosomal recessive.

    Clinical phenotype: as for McArdle's disease.
- Type XII: Kreuder's disease, GSD XII

    Enzyme defect: aldolase. Genetic linkage to chromosome 16q22–q24.

    Reference Maertens P, Dyken PR. Storage diseases: neuronal ceroid-lipofuscinoses, lipidoses, glycogenoses, and leukodystrophies. In: Goetz CG (ed.). *Textbook of Clinical Neurology* (2nd edition). Philadelphia: Saunders, 2003: 601–628.

    Other relevant entries Acid-maltase deficiency; McArdle's disease; Tarui disease.

■ GM1 gangliosidosis – see Gangliosidoses: an overview

■ GM2 gangliosidosis – see Gangliosidoses: an overview; Sandhoff's disease; Tay–Sachs disease

■ Gnathostomiasis

Nematode infection (*Gnathostoma sphingerum*) occurring in Asia, causing fever, subcutaneous swellings, eosinophilia, subarachnoid haemorrhage, myelitis, encephalitis.

Other relevant entry Helminthic diseases.

■ Godot syndrome

The name Godot syndrome has been used (after Beckett's play *Waiting for Godot*) to describe anxiety provoked by a fear of upcoming events, seen for example in Alzheimer's disease. Such anxiety may confound repeated assessment of cognitive function.

Reference Larner AJ, Doran M. Broader assessment needed for treatment decisions in AD. *Progress in Neurology and Psychiatry* 2002; **6**(3): 5–6.

■ Godtfredsen's syndrome

Godtfredsen's syndrome refers to combined abducens (VI) nerve and hypoglossal (XII) nerve palsies seen in the context of nasopharyngeal carcinoma; trigeminal numbness may also be counted part of the syndrome. The combination may occur with other clival lesions, particularly tumours, although occasionally lesions within the lower brainstem or meninges may produce this clinical picture.

Reference Keane JR. Combined VIth and XIIth cranial nerve palsies: a clival syndrome. *Neurology* 2000; **54**: 1540–1541.

■ Goldberg syndrome – see Sialidoses: an overview

■ Goldenhar syndrome, Goldenhar–Gorlin syndrome
Oculoauriculovertebral dysplasia

This is an autosomal-dominant or -recessive condition, usually affecting males, in which there is:

Facial asymmetry (unilateral hypoplasia).
Ocular anomalies: bilateral epibulbar dermoid or lipodermoid at the lateral corneoscleral junction; coloboma.
Preauricular tags; $+/-$ conductive hearing deficit.

Malformation (especially hemivertebrae) of the (upper) spine; occasionally scoliosis.

Mental retardation.

+/− cardiac, pulmonary anomalies.

The prognosis is generally good.

Other relevant entries Dermoid; Hallermann–Streiff syndrome; Treacher–Collins syndrome.

◼ Goltz syndrome
Focal dermal hypoplasia

A rare, possibly X-linked-dominant, condition of females characterized by areas of dermal atrophy, hernia of adipose tissue; skeletal anomalies (syndactyly, kyphoscoliosis); malposition and hypoplasia of teeth and nails; and ocular anomalies (coloboma, aniridia, microphthalmos). It enters the differential diagnosis of incontinentia pigmenti (Bloch–Sulzberger syndrome).

◼ Gonyalgia paraesthetica

Gonyalgia paraesthetica follows damage to the infrapatellar branch of the saphenous nerve, causing numbness and paraesthesia over the patella. It usually develops insidiously after trauma to the knee.

Other relevant entries Entrapment neuropathies; Neuropathies: an overview.

◼ Gorlin–Goltz syndrome – see Naevoid basal cell carcinoma syndrome

◼ Gourmand syndrome

This is an eating disorder in which there is a preoccupation with food and a preference for fine eating. It is associated with pathology in the right anterior part of the brain (tumour, vascular, epilepsy, trauma). There are often associated neuropsychological features such as impaired spatial memory, conceptual thinking, and visual perception (hemispatial neglect). It may be a disorder of impulse control.

Reference Regard M, Landis T. "Gourmand syndrome": eating passion associated with right anterior lesions. *Neurology* 1997; **48**: 1185–1190.

Other relevant entry Eating disorders.

◼ Gowers' manoeuvre, Gowers' sign

Gowers observed that boys with proximal lower limb weakness due to Duchenne muscular dystrophy (DMD) used their hands to rise from the ground, initially to push up and so raise the rump and straighten the legs (hence the American appellation of "butt-first manoeuvre"), then to raise the trunk by pushing on the legs ("climbing up oneself"). The sign may occur in any cause of proximal lower limb weakness, not just DMD.

Gowers' name is also associated with a manoeuvre to stretch the sciatic nerve and hence exacerbate sciatic symptoms.

Other relevant entries Duchenne muscular dystrophy; Sciatica.

■ Gradenigo's syndrome
Gradenigo–Lannois syndrome

Gradenigo's syndrome is characterized by facial pain, particularly in the first division of the trigeminal nerve, and diplopia due to sixth cranial nerve palsy, associated with disease at the apex of the petrous temporal bone where the abducens nerve is closely related to the trigeminal nerve. Causes include inflammation (petrositis, possibly spreading from a local infection such as otitis or mastoiditis), tumours (cholesteatoma, chordoma, meningioma, nasopharyngeal carcinoma, metastatic disease), and skull base fracture.

Other relevant entries Cranial nerve disease: VI: Abducens nerve; Facial pain: differential diagnosis.

■ Graefe's sign

Graefe's, or von Graefe's, sign refers to the lid lag seen on looking down which occurs in thyroid eye disease. A pseudo-Graefe's sign, characterized by retraction or elevation of the upper eyelid, medial rotation of the eye, and pupillary constriction on attempted downgaze or adduction, is seen following aberrant regeneration of the oculomotor nerve.

Other relevant entries Cranial nerve disease: III: Oculomotor nerve; Thyroid disease and the nervous system.

■ Granulomatous angiitis – see Isolated angiitis of the central nervous system

■ Graves' disease – see Thyroid disease and the nervous system

■ Greenfield's disease – see Metachromatic leukodystrophy

■ Gregg syndrome – see Rubella

■ Grisel syndrome

As originally described by Grisel, this is the name given to non-traumatic atlanto-axial subluxation, leading to torticollis, associated with inflammatory processes in the neck. Fever and torticollis may be seen in children with upper respiratory tract infection, pharyngitis, tonsillitis, cervical lymphadenopathy, but a recent study found that atlanto-axial subluxation was in fact rare in this syndrome.

References Grisel P. Enucleation de l'atlas et torticollis nasopharyngien. *Presse Medicale* 1930; **38**: 50–53.

Meuze WC, Taha ZM, Bashir EM. Fever and acquired torticollis in hospitalized children. *Journal of Laryngology and Otology* 2002; **116**: 280–284.

Other relevant entries Dystonia: an overview; Spasmodic torticollis.

Guam amyotrophic lateral sclerosis

The very high incidence of motor neurone disease (MND) amongst the Chamorro people on the Pacific island of Guam has been known since the mid-1940s. Similar foci are found on the Kii peninsula of Japan and amongst the Auyu and Jakai people of south-western New Guinea.

Clinically the condition is like MND found elsewhere in the world. However, there is a frequent familial occurrence, common co-occurrence of parkinsonism–dementia complex (PDC), and an association with an unusual linear retinopathy known as Guam retinal pigment epitheliopathy (GRPE).

The cause of this disease is unknown. It was hypothesized that it related to the ingestion of a putative neurotoxin, β-methylamino-L-alanine (BMAA), found in seeds of the false sago palm, *Cycas circinalis*, which form part of the staple diet. This idea is now questioned, and the role of genetic factors more favoured. Pathologically the brains of many individuals with Guam ALS show the neurofibrillary tangles typically seen in PDC.

Reference Morris HR, Al-Sarraj S, Schwab C *et al*. A clinical and pathological study of motor neurone disease on Guam. *Brain* 2001; **124**: 2215–2222.

Other relevant entries Guam parkinsonism–dementia complex; Motor neurone diseases: an overview.

Guam parkinsonism–dementia complex
Lytico–Bodig • Parkinsonism–dementia complex (PDC) of Guam

A form of parkinsonism associated with a severe progressive dementia occurs in high frequency on the island of Guam among the Chamorro population.

Clinically there is:

Parkinsonism: rigidity, bradykinesia; +/− resting tremor.
Dementia: memory impairment, disorientation, difficulty with calculation; this may be the presenting feature, or occur in isolation.

These features may co-occur with amyotrophic lateral sclerosis.

Neuropathologically there is brain atrophy. The morphological hallmark microscopically is the large number of neurofibrillary tangles seen in hippocampus, entorhinal cortex, amygdala, basal forebrain, and neocortex; the immunohistochemical and ultrastructural features are identical to those seen in Alzheimer's disease. Neuronal loss in the substantia nigra and locus coeruleus is prominent in cases with parkinsonism. Eosinophilic rod-like bodies (Hirano bodies) may also be seen but amyloid plaques, congophilic angiopathy, and Lewy bodies are not seen.

The cause of this disease is not known. Whether it shares common risk factors with, or is independent of, the amyotrophic lateral sclerosis prevalent on Guam and with which it often co-occurs, remains uncertain.

Reference Perl DP. Amyotrophic lateral sclerosis/parkinsonism–dementia complex of Guam. In: Esiri MM, Morris JH (eds). *The Neuropathology of Dementia*. Cambridge: CUP, 1997: 194–203.

Other relevant entries Alzheimer's disease; Dementia: an overview; Guam amyotrophic lateral sclerosis; Parkinsonian syndromes, parkinsonism.

■ Guillain–Barré syndrome

Acute inflammatory demyelinating polyradiculopathy (AIDP) • Landry–Guillain–Barré syndrome

Pathophysiology First described in 1859 by Landry (and possibly earlier, by Wardrop), but named after the description by Guillain, Barré, and Strohl in 1916, this is a relatively common acute neuropathy, often following an infective illness (e.g. *Campylobacter jejuni* enteritis, *Mycoplasma pneumoniae*, cytomegalo virus (CMV), and Epstein–Barr virus (EBV)). A number of variants are described, but most usually this is a monophasic demyelinating poly(radiculo)neuropathy, the pathogenesis of which is thought to be autoimmune attack directed against antigens in myelin, perhaps as a cross reaction to antigens in infective agents. Anti-GM1 antibodies are found in ~50% of cases, although these may be epiphenomenal. Disruption of normal nerve impulse conduction ensues. Recovery is slow, but often substantial if the patient can be adequately supported during the acute phase, when respiratory and cardiac problems may occur. Immune modulatory therapy (plasma exchange, intravenous immunoglobulin, IVIg) speeds recovery. Acute inflammatory demyelinating polyradiculopathies may be classified as follows:

Acute post-infectious demyelinating polyradiculoneuropathy (classical Guillain–Barré syndrome, GBS).

Acute post-infectious axonal polyradiculoneuropathy (AMSAN, axonal GBS).

Pure motor GBS (acute motor axonal neuropathy, AMAN; Chinese paralytic syndrome).

Acute sensory ataxic neuropathy (ASAN).

Miller Fisher syndrome, MFS (*q.v.*): ophthalmoplegia, ataxia, areflexia.

Relapsing inflammatory demyelinating polyradiculoneuropathy: relapsing over weeks and months with increasing disability at each relapse.

Subacute demyelinating polyradiculoneuropathy: patient continues to deteriorate after 4 weeks but <8 weeks (by definition this is not GBS).

Chronic inflammatory demyelinating polyradiculoneuropathy (CIDP): symptoms progress for >8 weeks.

Clinical features: history and examination

- Antecedent illness: gastrointestinal, respiratory; may not always be a feature of the history.
- Back pain in 30–50% of cases involving the lower back +/− thighs and buttocks; abdominal pain may also occur, sometimes of sufficient severity to be confused with an acute abdomen and leading to laparotomy/laparoscopy.
- Ascending numbness and weakness, with areflexia.
- Cranial nerve involvement with bulbar and facial weakness in about 50% of cases.
- Ophthalmoplegia: especially in the MFS.
- Weakness may involve the respiratory muscles, leading to insidious onset of respiratory failure; hence monitoring of vital capacity is crucial.
- Sphincter abnormalities occur in 10–20% of cases with involvement of the external urethral sphincter.
- Autonomic instability and autonomic failure may occur: labile blood pressure and cardiac arrhythmias (hence need for monitoring), with gastric paresis.
- Progression of sensorimotor dysfunction reaches a plateau in most patients after 2 weeks, and improvement starts within 4 weeks. Progression beyond 4 weeks falls outside the definition of GBS and into subacute IDP and CIDP.

Investigations and diagnosis *Bloods*: usually unremarkable; look for evidence of infection (*Campylobacter* serology); anti-ganglioside antibodies, probably of more relevance in variants (Miller Fisher: GQ1b; ASAN: GD1b).

Imaging: not usually indicated.

CSF: characteristically there is a raised protein, which may take a few days to develop, in the absence of cellular reaction (*dissociation albuminocytologique*). CSF leukocytosis sometimes occurs, but if >50 cells/μl, other diagnoses should be considered. Oligoclonal bands identical to those in serum may be found.

Neurophysiology: abnormalities on EMG/NCS depend on when the study is done relative to the disease onset. No abnormalities may be seen in studies performed very early in disease course. The typical picture is of evidence of proximal and distal demyelination with absent F waves. Occasionally a purely axonal picture is seen.

Nerve biopsy: rarely needed, unless there is clinical suspicion of vasculitis. Monitor VC, ECG.

Differential diagnosis Other acute neuropathies include:

Lyme disease
porphyria
vasculitic and non-systemic vasculitic neuropathy (especially systemic lupus erythematosus, SLE)
HIV disease

paraneoplastic neuronopathy

lead poisoning

poliomyelitis

botulism (if there is ophthalmoplegia)

Brainstem stroke.

Hysteria.

Treatment and prognosis Supportive treatment: best nursed on intensive therapy unit (ITU) or high dependency unit (HDU).

Monitor vital capacity: if <1 l, elective ventilation may be needed.

Monitor cardiac rhythm: if heart block, arrhythmia, pacemaker may be required.

Specific therapy: plasma exchange and IVIg (0.4 g/kg/day for 5 days) have been shown equally effective in GBS (oral or intravenous steroids probably not helpful but this is currently being re-evaluated). IVIg is simplest to give.

About 10% have permanently disability as a result of GBS (e.g. require an aid for walking).

About 5% of patients die from GBS.

The worse prognostic groups are the elderly, those with severe rapid onset GBS requiring early ventilation, and those with axonal loss on nerve conduction studies.

References Hughes RAC. *Guillain–Barré Syndrome*. London: Springer-Verlag, 1990.

Parry GJ. *Guillain–Barré Syndrome*. New York: Thieme, 1993.

Schonberger LB, Bregman DJ, Sullivan-Bolyai JZ *et al.* Guillain–Barré syndrome following vaccination in the national influenza immunization program, United States, 1976–1977. *American Journal of Epidemiology* 1979; **110**: 105–123.

Other relevant entries Chronic inflammatory demyelinating polyradiculoneu-ropathy; Gangliosides and neurological disorders; Miller Fisher syndrome; Neuropathies: an overview.

■ Guinea worm infection – see Dracunculiasis

■ Gulf War syndrome

Veterans of the 1991 Gulf War from both the USA and UK have presented with a variety of non-specific symptoms, including fatigue and weakness, and some have developed motor neurone disease. There is a question as to whether any, or all, of these might be due to exposure to drugs (pyridostigmine) or nerve gas agents (sarin) or toxins (depleted uranium) during the conflict. Some authors have reported finding electrophysiological evidence of peripheral nerve problems in veterans, but this has not been confirmed. As yet, no definitive explanation for the symptoms experienced by ex-servicemen is forthcoming, and the issue is unfortunately clouded by political and legal (and psychological ?) ramifications.

Gunn phenomena

Marcus Gunn phenomena

Two phenomena are associated with the name of the ophthalmologist Robert Marcus Gunn:

- Pupillary sign: this refers to the pupillary response to light when there is damage to the retina and/or optic nerve, the affected eye showing a reduced direct light response but a normal consensual response. Thus swinging the light stimulus from one eye to the other causes a paradoxical dilatation of the pupil in the affected eye ("swinging flashlight sign"). In addition there is a failure to sustain pupillary constriction to a continuous light stimulus.
- Jaw winking: this is a congenital abnormality in which a ptotic eyelid retracts transiently when the jaw is opened or moved from side to side. The converse of this (inverse Marcus Gunn phenomenon) is occasionally seen.

Reference Rowland LP. Marcus Gunn and Möbius syndromes. In: Rowland LP (ed.). *Merritt's Textbook of Neurology* (9th edition). Baltimore: Williams & Wilkins, 1995: 533–534

Other relevant entries Cranial nerve disease: II: Optic nerve; Marin–Amat syndrome.

Gustatory sweating – see Frey's syndrome

Guttmann's sign

Guttmann's sign is facial vasodilatation with nasal congestion, occurring as a feature of autonomic disturbance in the context of high spinal cord lesions.

Gynaecomastia

Gynaecomastia, inappropriate breast development in males, may be observed in various clinical situations, including some neurological diseases:

- Chronic liver disease.
- Excessive pituitary prolactin release secondary to impaired dopamine release from the hypothalamus due to local tumour or treatment with dopaminergic antagonist drugs (e.g. anti-psychotic medications).
- Kennedy's syndrome (X-linked bulbospinal neuronopathy).
- Klinefelter's syndrome.
- POEMS syndrome.

Hh

■ **Habit spasms – see Tics**

■ **Haemangioblastoma – see Von Hippel–Lindau disease**

■ **Haematoma: an overview**

A haematoma is a focal collection of blood, forming a space-occupying lesion. Blood may be arterial or venous in origin, the former tending to have a more acute presentation. Bleeding may occur at various locations within the nervous system, with varying neurological presentation:

- Cerebral haematoma: see Intracerebral haemorrhage (ICH).
- Spinal cord haematoma (haematomyelia): rare compared to cerebral haemorrhage; common causes are trauma, vascular malformations, anticoagulation (see Spinal cord vascular diseases).
- Epidural or extradural haematoma: located between dura and bone, these may be cranial or, less often, spinal.

  Cranial: most commonly follows head trauma in parietal or temporal area, causing tearing of blood vessels, most often the middle meningeal artery; less often there is a dural venous tear. A history of brief unconsciousness associated with the trauma, followed by a lucid period of hours or a day (or with venous bleeding, several days or a week) followed by increasing drowsiness, aphasia, seizures, and coma, is typical. Skull X-ray may show a temporoparietal fracture; CT will show the haematoma. If the patient is unconscious, or the level of consciousness is deteriorating, urgent surgical decompression is required.

  Spinal: may produce spinal cord and/or cauda equina compression; sudden onset of neck or back pain is followed by sensorimotor deficit, progressing to paraplegia or quadriplegia. MRI is imaging modality of choice, followed by surgical decompression.

- Subdural haematoma (*q.v.*):
  Cranial > spinal.

  Other relevant entries Intracerebral haemorrhage; Paraparesis: acute management and differential diagnosis; Spinal cord vascular diseases; Subdural haematoma.

■ **Haematomyelia – see Spinal cord vascular diseases**

■ **Haemochromatosis**

Primary (hereditary) haemochromatosis is an autosomal-recessive disorder of iron overload, causing pathological deposition of iron in liver parenchyma and pancreas, with symptoms of hepatocellular dysfunction, diabetes mellitus and arthralgia. Primary neurological problems are rare, but peripheral neuropathy and dementia have been reported on occasion. Their exact relationship to the biochemical abnormality, if any, remains unclear.

References Hermann W, Guenther P, Clark D, Wagner A. Polyneuropathy in idiopathic haemochromatosis. *Journal of Neurology* 2002; **249**: 1316–1317.

■ Haemorrhagic leukoencephalitis – see Acute disseminated encephalomyelitis

■ Haemosiderosis – see Superficial siderosis of the central nervous system

■ Hallermann–Streiff syndrome

Hallermann–Streiff syndrome, or oculomandibulodyscephaly with hypotrichosis, is characterized by:

  prominent brow, parietal bones;
  beaked, large nose;
  mandibular hypoplasia;
  congenital cataracts, microphthalmia;
  sparse, thin hair;
  thin skin;
  slight mental retardation;
  +/– short stature.

It may be mistaken for other oculoauriculocephalic syndromes such as Treacher–Collins, or Goldenhar.

Other relevant entries Goldenhar syndrome, Goldenhar–Gorlin syndrome; Treacher–Collins syndrome.

■ Hallervorden–Spatz disease, Hallervorden–Spatz syndrome
Pantothenate kinase associated neurodegeneration (PKAN)

Pathophysiology An autosomal-recessive disorder associated with iron accumulation in the basal ganglia and neurodegeneration.

Clinical features: history and examination
- Early-onset (before age 20 years) progressive dystonia.
- Intellectual impairment (frontal subcortical type).
- Pigmentary retinopathy.
- Choreoathetosis.

- Pyramidal signs.
- Optic atrophy.

Investigations and diagnosis *Bloods, CSF, neurophysiology*: normal.

Imaging: MRI T$_2$-weighted scans show decreased signal intensity in the pallidal nuclei with central hyperintensity, the "eye-of-the-tiger" sign.

Neurogenetics: mutations in the pantothenate kinase (PANK) gene on chromosome 20p13 in some but not <u>all</u> cases.

Neuropsychology: frontal subcortical-type deficits: bradyphrenia, reduced verbal fluency, judgement difficulties, attentional impairment; memory preserved.

Differential diagnosis

Neuroacanthocytosis.

Neuroferritinopathy.

Treatment and prognosis No specific treatment. Symptomatic treatment of dystonia. Death usually occurs after 5–20 years of disease.

References Halliday W. The nosology of Hallervorden–Spatz disease. *Journal of the Neurological Sciences* 1995; **134**: 84–91.

Hayflick SJ, Westaway SK, Levinson B *et al.* Genetic, clinical, and radiographic delineation of Hallervorden–Spatz syndrome. *New England Journal of Medicine* 2003; **348**: 33–40.

Zhou B, Westaway SK, Levinson B, Johnson MA, Gischier J, Hayflick SJ. A novel pantothenate kinase gene is defective in Hallervorden–Spatz syndrome. *Nature Genetics* 2001; **28**: 345–349.

Other relevant entries Dystonia an overview; Neuroacanthocytosis; Neuroferritinopathy.

■ Hallgren's syndrome

An early onset cerebellar ataxia with retinal degeneration and deafness.

Other relevant entry Cerebellar disease: an overview.

■ HAM – see HTLV-1 myelopathy

■ Hamartoma – see Cowden's disease; Gelastic epilepsy; Hypothalamic disease: an overview

■ Hand–Schüller–Christian disease – see Langerhans cell histiocytosis

■ Handcuff neuropathy – see Cheiralgia paraesthetica

Handlebar palsy – see Ramsay Hunt syndrome (3); Ulnar neuropathy

Hansen's disease – see Leprosy

"Happy puppet syndrome" – see Angelman syndrome

Hard + E syndrome – see Walker–Warburg syndrome

Harding's disease

Harding's disease is the name given to a syndrome of multiple sclerosis-like illness associated with Leber's-related mutations of mitochondrial DNA (especially at base pair 11 778, typically seen in Leber's hereditary optic neuropathy). Clinically there is demyelination of the central nervous system (CNS) with disproportionate involvement of the optic nerves.

> **Reference** Harding AE, Sweeney MG, Miller DH *et al.* Occurrence of a multiple sclerosis-like illness in women who have a Leber's hereditary optic neuropathy mitochondrial DNA mutation. *Brain* 1992; **115**: 979–989.

> **Other relevant entries** Leber's hereditary optic neuropathy; Mitochondrial disease: an overview; Multiple sclerosis; Optic neuritis.

Harlequin syndrome

Loss of thermoregulatory flushing and sweating on one side of the face without miosis and ptosis due to local autonomic dysfunction, most usually from an ipsilateral cervical pre- or postganglionic sympathetic deficit.

> **Other relevant entries** Holmes–Adie syndrome; Ross syndrome.

HARP syndrome

The syndrome of *h*ypoprebetalipoproteinaemia, *a*canthocytosis, *r*etinitis pigmentosa, and *p*allidal degeneration is called HARP syndrome. Orofacial dystonia is particularly prominent. It is related to Bassen–Kornzweig disease (abetalipoproteinaemia), and may also be confused with Hallervorden–Spatz syndrome.

> **Reference** Orrell RW, Amrolia PJ, Heald A *et al.* Acanthocytosis, retinitis pigmentosa and pallidal degeneration: a report of three patients, including the second reported case of hypoprebetalipoproteinemia (HARP syndrome). *Neurology* 1995; **45**: 487–492.

> **Other relevant entries** Abetalipoproteinaemia; Bassen–Kornzweig disease; Hallervorden–Spatz disease, Hallervorden–Spatz syndrome; Neuroacanthocytosis.

■ Harris's syndrome – see Cluster headache

■ Hartnup's disease

This autosomal-recessive inborn error of metabolism causes a defect in the transport of neutral amino acids in kidney and gut with consequent deficiency of niacinamide and a clinical syndrome reminiscent of pellagra (skin rash), with progressive ataxia, $+/-$ optic atrophy, dystonia, pyramidal signs, tremor, delirium. The urine contains large amounts of neutral, monamino-monocarboxylic amino acids, which are decreased in plasma. Many subjects with aminoaciduria are asymptomatic (Hartnup's disorder). Treatment is with oral nicotinamide, with or without a high protein diet.

Other relevant entries Aminoacidopathies; Pellagra.

■ Hashimoto's encephalopathy

A diffuse encephalopathy may occur in association with Hashimoto's thyroiditis with elevated antithyroglobulin antibody titres: patients may be hyper- hypo-, or euthyroid. Clinically, there may be a subacute confusional state, stroke-like episodes, focal deficits, seizures (myoclonic, partial complex, generalized tonic–clonic), and neuropsychological impairment. CSF may show elevated protein. Although uncommon, identification is important since the condition is steroid sensitive.

References Barker R, Zajicek J, Wilkinson I. Thyrotoxic Hashimoto's encephalopathy. *Journal of Neurology, Neurosurgery and Psychiatry* 1996; **60**: 234.

Shaw PJ, Walls TJ, Newman PK, Cleland PG, Cartlidge NEF. Hashimoto's encephalopathy: a steroid-responsive disorder associated with high anti-thyroid antibody titers. Report of 5 cases. *Neurology* 1991; **41**: 228–233.

Other relevant entries Encephalopathies: an overview; Thyroid disease and the nervous system.

■ "Haw River" syndrome – see Dentatorubral–Pallidoluysian atrophy

■ Headache: an overview

Pathophysiology Headache is the commonest reason for patient consultation in the general neurology outpatient clinic, accounting for around 20% of all consultations. The vast majority of such headaches are benign, although most patients have an underlying concern that their headache reflects a brain tumour. Diagnosis is usually possible on the basis of history and examination alone. The precise causes of head pain remain uncertain, but are presumably related to fibres of the trigeminal system innervating the dura.

Essentially headaches may be divided into migraine (*q.v.*) and tension-type headache, the latter having a tendency to chronicity. The current (1988) classification of headache suggested by the International Headache Society encompasses:

Migraine

Tension-type headache: episodic, chronic

Cluster headache and chronic paroxysmal hemicrania

Headache associated with head trauma

Headache associated with vascular disorders

Headache associated with non-vascular intracranial disorders

Headache associated with substances and their withdrawal

Headache associated with non-cephalic infection

Headache associated with metabolic abnormality

Headache or facial pain associated with disorders of cranium, neck, eyes, ears, nose, sinuses, teeth, mouth or other facial or cranial structures

Cranial neuralgias, nerve trunk pain, deafferentation pain

Other types of headache or facial pain

Headache not classifiable.

Whilst all these categories may need to be borne in mind when seeing a patient with headache, the vast majority will have tension-type headache, especially in the out-patient setting.

Clinical features: history and examination

- Tension-type headache: episodic or chronic head pain, generally lasting all day for days or weeks (>50% of the time = chronic daily headache), often worse as the day goes on; no postural features. May be described as generalized aching, especially bifrontal, on the vertex, at the back, with superimposed localized stabbing sensations. A pressure-type sensation on top of the head and/or a band-like compression or vice around the head is common. Headache may have been intermittently present for months or years; short duration of headache symptoms should increase index of suspicion for symptomatic cause.

- Enquire for features of raised intracranial pressure: headache worse with recumbency, morning headache, nausea and vomiting, visual obscurations (particularly alarming).

- Although rare, giant cell arteritis or temporal arteritis should always be thought of since it may cause blindness and is treatable: therefore enquire for jaw claudication, weight loss, and palpate temporal arteries.

- History of medication use: searching for evidence of medication overuse or medication-maintained headache (*q.v.*).

- Features most predictive of migraine when compared to tension-type headache are: nausea, photophobia, phonophobia, exacerbation by physical activity.

Investigations and diagnosis Diagnosis is essentially clinical, that is, based on the history (as in psychiatric diseases). Examination is usually normal. Unexpected findings (e.g. papilloedema) mandate further imaging.

The role of hypertension in the genesis of headaches is debated, but certainly it should be adequately controlled.

Check ESR if there is a possibility of giant cell arteritis.

In our technology-obsessed age, many headache patients (and their general practitioners) expect a brain scan (rather than a clinical diagnosis from a practitioner skilled in the art); opinion is divided as to whether one should accede to or resist these expectations. The patient's desire to "put my mind at ease" by having a scan may backfire if incidental abnormalities are found: the obligation to inform the patient of these may serve only to increase anxiety.

Differential diagnosis Medication overuse headache.

Treatment and prognosis Patient (and general practitioner) education is important, by means of an explanation of the headache, its non-serious nature, and its amenability to treatment.

Analgesia may be effected with simple analgesia, such as aspirin or paracetamol, or with non-steroidal anti-inflammatory preparations. Long-term, and opiate, analgesia is best avoided because of the risk of inducing medication overuse headache. Amitriptyline given for some months is an option.

Resistant headache may mandate referral to a pain clinic. The role of underlying psychological and psychiatric issues in headache maintenance is debated (generally neurologists think these important, patients do not), likewise how they are best addressed.

References Headache Classification Committee of the International Headache Society. Classification and diagnostic criteria for headache disorders, cranial neuralgias and facial pain. *Cephalalgia* 1988; **8(suppl 7)**: 1–96.

Smetana GW. The diagnositc value of historical features in primary headache syndromes: a comprehensive review. *Archives of Internal Medicine* 2000; **160**: 2729–2737.

Other relevant entries Cluster headache; Coital cephalgia, Coital headache; Cough headache; Erythrocyanotic headache; "Exploding head syndrome"; Facial pain: differential diagnosis; Giant cell arteritis; Hypnic headache; Idiopathic intracranial hypertension; Medication overuse headache; Migraine; Subarachnoid haemorrhage; SUNCT syndrome; Thunderclap headache.

■ Hearing loss: differential diagnosis

Hearing loss may be conductive or sensorineural. Sensorineural hearing loss with accompanying neurological signs may suggest a neurological syndrome causing deafness, rather than isolated disease of the cochlear apparatus. Hearing impairment may not be the most notable feature in some of these conditions. The differential diagnosis of hearing loss is broad, including:

- Inherited disorders:
    Alport's syndrome
    Alström's syndrome
    Behr's syndrome

Brown–Vialetto–Van Laere syndrome

Canavan's syndrome

Charcot–Marie–Tooth disease (types 4D, 2, 2X)

Cockayne's syndrome

Flynn–Aird syndrome

Friedreich's ataxia

GM1 gangliosidosis

Herrmann disease

Jervell–Lange–Nielsen (prolonged QT) syndrome

Jeune–Tommasi syndrome

Krabbe's disease

Latham–Monro disease

Lannois–Bensaude disease

Lemieux–Neemeh disease

Leopard syndrome

Lichtenstein–Knorr disease

Mannosidoses

May–White syndrome

Mitochondrial diseases (especially A3243G mutation; cochlear hearing loss)

Möbius syndrome

Mohr–Tranebjaerg syndrome

Mucopolysaccharidoses: Hurler, Hunter, Morquio

Norrie disease

Nyssen–van Bogaert syndrome

Oculodentodigital dysplasia syndrome

Osuntokun syndrome

Pendred's syndrome

Primrose syndrome

Refsum's disease

Richards–Rundle syndrome

Rosenberg–Bergstrom syndrome

Rosenberg–Chutorian syndrome

Small's disease

Sylvester disease

Tay–Sachs disease

Telfer's syndrome

Tunbridge–Paley syndrome

Usher's syndrome

Wolfram syndrome

Xeroderma pigmentosa

- Acquired disorders
    Infection
        Intrauterine CMV, rubella

Meningococcal disease
Ramsay Hunt syndrome
Syphilis

Inflammatory/Vasculitic
Cogan's syndrome
Gradenigo's syndrome
Susac syndrome
Vogt–Koyanagi–Harada syndrome
Wegener's granulomatosis

Metabolic
Kernicterus
Schilder's disease
Schindler's disease
Strachan's syndrome
Superficial siderosis

Structural
Apert's syndrome
Cholesteatoma
Fibrous dysplasia
Glomus jugulare tumour
Klippel–Feil anomaly
Paget's disease of bone
Van Buchem's syndrome
Vestibular schwannoma

- Ménière's disease.

Clinical features: history and examination/investigations and diagnosis/differential diagnosis/treatment and prognosis/other relevant entries See individual entries, including Cogan's syndrome (2); Ramsay Hunt syndrome (2).

▓ Heatstroke

The cardinal features of exertional heatstroke are:

Loss of consciousness of variable duration (*cf.* commoner condition of heat exhaustion, where there is no loss of consciousness).
Hyperthermia despite vigorous sweating.

Recognized complications include:

Rhabdomyolysis, myoglobinuria, acute renal failure.
Hepatocellular damage, acute hepatic failure.
Abnormal haemostasis (with or without liver injury).

The syndrome is most often seen in the context of unaccustomed exercise in hot climates (e.g. unconditioned military recruits, novice runners, and pilgrims to Mecca).

There may be an underlying metabolic myopathy akin to that responsible for malignant hyperthermia.

Treatment involves reduction of body temperature by cooling: fanning and tepid sponging encourages convective and evaporative heat loss; plunging into ice water is not recommended because the cutaneous vasoconstriction will inhibit, rather than promote, heat loss. Pharmacotherapy with dantrolene, which blocks sarcoplasmic reticulum calcium release channels to uncouple muscle excitation and contraction, may be useful. If mechanical ventilation is required, paralysis with non-depolarizing neuromuscular blocking agents may help control muscle heat generation.

Neurological sequelae in the survivors of heatstroke include cerebellar syndromes and spinal cord lesions with motor neurone loss. Peripheral neuropathy following hyperpyrexia has also been described. The take home message is that "neurones are quickly cooked".

Other relevant entries Critical illness polyneuropathy; Malignant hyperthermia; Rhabdomyolysis.

■ Heavy metal poisoning

Various metals may have adverse, toxic effects on nervous system structure and function, whether due to inadvertent exposure or therapeutic use. All are rare. These include (in alphabetical order):

- Aluminium: encephalopathy, "dialysis dementia"
- Arsenic: neuropathy: axonal degeneration in chronic poisoning, GBS-like (+ / − encephalopathy with pericapillary encephalorrhagia, or brain purpura) with acute poisoning; both accompanied by gastrointestinal symptoms
- Bismuth: myoclonic encephalopathy
- Gold: acute or subacute sensorimotor neuropathy; myokymia
- Lead (see individual entry for further details)
- Manganese (see individual entry for further details)
- Mercury:
    Inorganic/elemental: mild sensorimotor peripheral neuropathy; may sometimes resemble motor neurone disease; tremor (often circumoral); personality change: timidity, seclusion, secretiveness (erethism, "Mad Hatter syndrome")
    Organic (e.g. Minamata disease): paraesthesiae, sensory ataxia, visual field constriction
- Thallium: neuropathy, alopecia
- Tin: organic tin compounds may cause seizures, muscle weakness, raised intracranial pressure
    References Playford RJ, Matthews CH, Campbell MJ *et al*. Bismuth induced encephalopathy caused by tri potassium dicitrato bismuthate in a patient with chronic renal failure. *Gut* 1990; **31**: 359–360.

Windebank AJ. Heavy metals and neurological disease. In: Evans RW, Baskin DS, Yatsu FM (eds). *Prognosis of Neurological Disorders*. New York: OUP, 1992: 571–576.

Other relevant entries Encephalopathies: an overview; Lead and the nervous system; Manganese poisoning, Manganism; Neuropathies: an overview; Renal disease and the nervous system.

Heerfordt syndrome – see Sarcoidosis

Heidenhein variant – see Creutzfeldt–Jakob disease; Prion disease: an overview

HELLP syndrome – see Eclampsia; Fatty acid oxidation disorders

Helminthic diseases

Pathophysiology Helminths are multicellular metazoan parasites, with complex life cycles involving human and animal hosts at different stages of development.

Helminths causing CNS disease may be classified as:

- Cestodes (tapeworms): cysticercosis, echinococcosis, sparganosis; diphyllobothriasis (indirectly through vitamin B_{12} deficiency);
- Nematodes (roundworms): strongyloidiasis, trichinosis, onchocerciasis, angiostrongyliasis, gnathostomiasis, ascariasis, dracunculiasis, toxocariasis;
- Trematodes (flukes): schistosomiasis, paragonimiasis.

Clinical features: history and examination/investigations and diagnosis/differential diagnosis/treatment and prognosis See individual entries.

References Awasthi S, Bundy DAP, Savioli L. Helminthic infections. *British Medical Journal* 2003; **327**: 431–433.

Nishimura K, Hung T. Current views on geographic distribution and modes of infection of neurohelminthic diseases. *Journal of the Neurological Sciences* 1997; **145**: 5–14.

Salata RA, King CH, Mahmoud AAF. Parasitic infections of the central nervous system. In: Aminoff MJ (ed). *Neurology and General Medicine. The Neurological Aspects of Medical Disorders* (2nd edition). New York: Churchill Livingstone, 1995: 811–839.

Other relevant entries Cysticercosis; Echinococcosis; Gnathostomiasis; Paragonimiasis; Schistosomiasis; Strongyloidiasis; Trichinosis.

Hemiataxia–Hypaesthesia syndrome – see Thalamic syndromes

Hemiatrophy–Hemiparkinsonism

A rare syndrome of early onset hemiparkinsonism with hemiatrophy, the latter usually unnoticed by the patient, often with unilateral dystonia, which may respond to levodopa. Early birth injury (trauma, hypoxia) may be responsible (hence secondary parkinsonism); MRI may show hemiatrophy of contralateral cortex.

Reference Klawans HL. Hemiparkinsonism as a late complication of hemiatrophy: a new syndrome. *Neurology* 1981; **31**: 625–628.

Other relevant entries Parkinsonian syndromes, Parkinsonism; Parry–Romberg syndrome.

■ Hemiballismus, Hemichorea

Hemiballismus is an involuntary hyperkinetic movement disorder in which there are large amplitude, vigorous ("flinging") irregular movements of the limbs, which may show a loss of normal muscular tone (hypotonia), on one side of the body. Hemiballismus overlaps clinically with hemichorea ("violent chorea"); the term *hemiballismus–hemichorea* is sometimes used to reflect this overlap.

Hemiballismus is most often associated with lesions of the contralateral subthalamic nucleus of Luys or its efferent pathways, although occasionally it is associated with lesions of the caudate, putamen, globus pallidus, lentiform nucleus, thalamus, and precentral gyrus; and even with ipsilateral lesions. Pathologically, vascular events (ischaemia, haemorrhage) are the commonest associated lesion but space-occupying lesions (tumour, arteriovenous malformation), inflammation (encephalitis, systemic lupus erythematosus, post-streptococcal), demyelination, metabolic causes (hyperosmolar non-ketotic hyperglycaemia [HONKS]), infection (toxoplasmosis in AIDS), drugs (oral contraceptives, phenytoin, levodopa, neuroleptics) and head trauma have also been reported.

Hemiballismus of vascular origin usually improves spontaneously, but drug treatment with neuroleptics (haloperidol, pimozide, sulpiride) may be helpful. Other drugs which are sometimes helpful include tetrabenazine, reserpine, clonazepam, clozapine, and sodium valproate.

Other relevant entry Chorea.

■ Hemibasal syndrome – see Garcin syndrome

■ Hemibulbar syndrome – see Babinski–Nageotte syndrome

■ Hemifacial spasm

Pathophysiology Hemifacial spasm is an involuntary, painless, dyskinetic (not dystonic) movement disorder, characterized by contractions of muscles on one side of the face, sometimes triggered by eating or speaking, and exacerbated by fatigue or emotion. The movements may result from compression of the facial (VII) nerve, usually at the root entry zone, often by a tortuous anterior or posterior inferior cerebellar artery (hence a neurovascular compression syndrome). Other causes include intrapontine lesions (e.g. demyelination), mass lesions (tumour, arteriovenous malformation) located anywhere from the facial nucleus to the stylomastoid foramen, and following a Bell's palsy. Some cases remain idiopathic. Posterior fossa lesions contralateral to the hemifacial spasm (i.e. false localizing) have occasionally been reported.

Clinical features: history and examination

- Twitching movements around the eye or the angle of the mouth, sometimes described as a pulling sensation. Movements may continue during sleep. Patients often find the movements embarrassing because it attracts the attention of onlookers.
- Paradoxical elevation of the eyebrow, as orbicularis oris contracts and the eye closes, may be seen; this synkinesis ("Babinski's other sign") is not reproducible by will.

Investigations and diagnosis Diagnosis is essentially clinical. If movements are not evident when the patient attends clinic, suggest relatives/friends make a home video.

Imaging: MRI may be undertaken to exclude symptomatic lesions.

Differential diagnosis

Oromandibular dystonia.

Focal epilepsies may give rise to facial twitching.

Facial myokymia: "creeping flesh".

Fasciculation of facial muscles as in Kennedy's syndrome.

Treatment and prognosis Symptomatic lesions (e.g. tortuous vessel) may be amenable to surgical resection/correction.

For idiopathic hemifacial spasm, or patients declining surgery, botulinum toxin injections are the treatment of choice. These need to be repeated about every 3 months.

References Barker FG, Jannetta PJ, Bissonette DJ *et al.* Microvascular decompression for hemifacial spasm. *Journal of Neurosurgery* 1995; **82**: 201–210.

Devoize JL. "The other" Babinski sign: paradoxical raising of the eyebrow in hemifacial spasm. *Journal of Neurology, Neurosurgery and Psychiatry* 2001; **70**: 516.

Elston JS. Botulinum toxin treatment of hemifacial spasm. *Journal of Neurology, Neurosurgery and Psychiatry* 1986; **49**: 827–829.

Other relevant entries Botulinum toxin therapy; Bell's palsy; Cranial nerve disease: VII: Facial nerve; Facial myokymia; Neurovascular compression syndromes.

▓ Hemimedullary syndrome – see Babinski–Nageotte syndrome

▓ Hepatic encephalopathy

Portal-systemic encephalopathy

Pathophysiology Liver disease is one of the commonest causes of encephalopathy seen in hospital practice. Hepatic encephalopathy may occur in the context of:

- acute liver failure (fulminant hepatocellular failure), for example in acute viral hepatitis, Wilson's disease, or drug-induced hepatocellular necrosis; due to failure of hepatic detoxifying functions; or

- acute decompensation of chronic liver disease (acute-on-chronic, e.g. cirrhosis); due to the production of ammonia and other related compounds. Decompensation to encephalopathy may be precipitated by drugs, gastrointestinal (especially oesophageal variceal) bleeding, increased dietary protein, infection, constipation.

Clinical features: history and examination
- Encephalopathy: suggestive features may be asterixis (can occur in other forms of encephalopathy), hepatic fetor.
- Stigmata of chronic liver disease may be evident (jaundice, caput medusae, telangiectasia, ascites).

Investigations and diagnosis *Bloods*: FBC (for anaemia), clotting screen, electrolytes, glucose (need to exclude hypoglycaemia), liver function tests, serum ammonia level; serum copper and caeruloplasmin in young individual with otherwise unexplained acute hepatic failure, + blood film (for haemolysis), to exclude Wilson's disease. Infection screen including blood cultures.

Urine: culture.

Other: ascitic tap for infection.

EEG: may show various abnormalities depending on the degree of encephalopathy, including triphasic complexes.

Imaging: MRI may show pallidal abnormality.

Differential diagnosis Other causes of encephlaopathy.

Treatment and prognosis In acute decompensation, reverse any precipitants; avoid sedative drugs, restrict dietary protein whilst administering lactulose, vigorously treat any infection; oesophageal variceal bleeding may necessitate sclerotherapy.

In acute (fulminant) hepatic failure, full supportive care is required. Some causes gradually improve, but in others liver transplantation may be the only hope of survival.

Recurrent bouts of hepatic encephalopathy may give rise to non-Wilsonian hepatocerebral degeneration with fixed neurological deficits such as dementia, dysarthria, gait ataxia, extrapyramidal features +/− myelopathy.

> **Reference** Lockwood AH. Hepatic encephalopathy and other neurological disorders associated with gastrointestinal disease. In: Aminoff MJ (ed). *Neurology and General Medicine. The Neurological Aspects of Medical Disorders* (2nd edition). New York: Churchill Livingstone, 1995: 247–266.

> **Other relevant entries** Encephalopathies: an overview; Non-Wilsonian hepatocerebral degeneration; Wilson's disease.

Hepatocerebral degeneration

Hepatocerebral degeneration may be:
- Hereditary: Wilson's disease.
- Acquired: Non-Wilsonian hepatocerebral degeneration (NWHCD).

> **Other relevant entries** Non-Wilsonian hepatocerebral degeneration; Wilson's disease.

■ Hepatolenticular degeneration – see Wilson's disease

■ Hereditary cerebral haemorrhage with amyloidosis, Dutch type – see Alzheimer's disease; Amyloid and the nervous system: an overview; Cerebral amyloid angiopathy

■ Hereditary cerebral haemorrhage with amyloidosis, Icelandic type – see Amyloid and the nervous system: an overview; Cerebral amyloid angiopathy

■ Hereditary fructose intolerance

Several hereditary disorders of fructose metabolism exist, including hereditary fructose intolerance (HFI), hereditary fructosuria, and fructose-1,6-diphosphatase deficiency.

- HFI is due to a defect in the enzymatic activity of fructose bisphosphate aldolase and may present with severe hypoglycaemia and fits with vomiting, failure to thrive, hepatorenal disease and aversion to fructose-containing foods (e.g. fruits). It can be diagnosed by measuring the specific enzyme activities and challenging the patient to a fructose load in hospital. However, the intravenous fructose tolerance test is not without hazard, and has now been largely superseded by genetic diagnosis of mutations in the gene encoding aldolase. The presence of non-glucose reducing substances in the urine is a clue to the diagnosis (also seen in galactosaemia); there is also lactic acidosis.
- Hereditary fructosuria is asymptomatic and due to a defect in the enzyme fructokinase.
- Fructose-1,6-diphosphatase deficiency presents with fasting hypoglycaemia, an encephalopathy with fits, and a metabolic acidosis. It may be difficult to distinguish from glycogen-storage disease type I (von Gierke's disease) since hepatomegaly is common to both, but response to glucagon is found only in fructose-1,6-diphosphatase deficiency.

All of these disorders can be treated by avoidance of dietary fructose. When such a diet is followed no long-term sequelae occur.

> **Reference** Cross NCP, Cox TM. Molecular analysis of aldolase B genes in the diagnosis of hereditary fructose intolerance. *Quarterly Journal of Medicine* 1989; **73**: 1015–1020.

> **Other relevant entries** Galactosaemia; Glycogen-storage disorders: an overview.

■ Hereditary haemorrhagic telangiectasia – see Osler–Weber–Rendu syndrome

■ Hereditary motor and sensory neuropathy

Pathophysiology The classification of hereditary neuropathies proposed by Dyck and Lambert in 1968 included the category of hereditary motor and sensory neuropathies (HMSN). These were later subdivided according to those with motor nerve conduction velocities below or above 38 m/s (types I and II respectively, also known as Charcot–Marie–Tooth types I and II). The clinical classification of HMSN now encompasses seven groups, viz.:

HMSN I (CMT-I)
HMSN II (CMT-II)
HMSN III: Déjerine–Sottas syndrome (*q.v.*)
HMSN IV: Refsum's disease (*q.v.*)
HMSN V: HMSN + spastic paraparesis
HMSN VI: HMSN with optic atrophy
HMSN VII: HMSN with retinitis pigmentosa

Types I and II are the most common.

The HMSN classification is being superseded to some extent by the increasingly detailed molecular genetic definition of hereditary neuropathies; for further details of molecular genetics, see entry on Charcot–Marie–Tooth (CMT) disease.

Clinical features: history and examination

- Slowly progressive distal muscle weakness and atrophy: small foot muscles, peroneal muscles, hands, forearms.
- Distal, usually symmetrical, sensory deficits; positive sensory symptoms such as paraesthesiae make the diagnosis unlikely.
- Foot deformities: pes cavus, claw (or hammer) toes.
- Diminished tendon reflexes.
- Family history.
- In HMSN types I and II males are more likely to be symptomatic, and severely affected, whereas females are more often asymptomatic.

Investigations and diagnosis *Neurophysiology*: EMG/NCS: nerve conduction velocities may be severely reduced (HMSN I or CMT-I, demyelinating neuropathy), or normal or only slightly reduced (HMSN II or CMT-II, predominantly axonal neuropathy). Sensory nerve action potentials severely reduced or not recordable. EMG of distal muscles often shows chronic denervation.

Nerve biopsy: variable according to subtype.

Neurogenetics: increasingly useful in defining these syndromes.

Differential diagnosis

Distal spinal muscular atrophy.
HMSN I: CIDP; Friedreich's ataxia if ataxia also present.
HMSN II: idiopathic axonal polyneuropathy.

Treatment and prognosis

No specific treatment with the exception of Refsum's disease (*q.v.*).
Patients seldom become wheelchair bound.

References Dyck PJ, Lambert EH. Lower motor and primary sensory neurone diseases with peroneal muscular atrophy. I. Neurologic, genetic and electrophysiologic findings in hereditary polyneuropathies. *Archives of Neurology* 1968; **18**: 603–618.

Harding AE, Thomas PK. The clinical features of hereditary motor and sensory neuropathy types I and II. *Brain* 1980; **103**: 259–280.

Other relevant entries Charcot–Marie–Tooth disease; Déjerine–Sottas syndrome; Friedreich's ataxia; Neuropathies: an overview; Refsum's disease.

▓ Hereditary motor neuropathy – see Spinal muscular atrophy

▓ Hereditary neuralgic amyotrophy – see Neuralgic amyotrophy

▓ Hereditary neuropathy with liability to pressure palsies
Tomaculous neuropathy

This autosomal-dominant condition manifests, usually between the ages of 20 and 40 years, with painless focal peripheral lesions, often following minimal trauma or compression, including carpal tunnel syndrome, common peroneal nerve palsy, and brachial plexopathy. Symptoms gradually improve over weeks to months. A slowly progressive neuropathy similar to Charcot–Marie–Tooth disease type 1 may develop.

Neurophysiologically there is slowing of nerve conduction velocity, prolonged distal motor latencies, and conduction blocks. Pathologically nerves show characteristic swellings or tomacula ("sausages") with signs of demyelination and remyelination. Neurogenetic studies have revealed deletions of chromosome 17p11.2 encompassing the peripheral myelin protein 22 (PMP22 gene; region duplicated in CMT-1A), and other cases resulting from point mutations of this gene have also been reported, suggesting genetic homogeneity, although the exact pathogenesis is unknown.

References Andersson PB, Yuen E, Parko K, So YT. Electrodiagnostic features of hereditary neuropathy with liability to pressure palsies. *Neurology* 2000; **54**: 40–44.

Chance P, Alderson M, Leppig K *et al.* DNA deletion associated with hereditary neuropathy with liability to pressure palsies. *Cell* 1993; **72**: 143–151.

Other relevant entries Brachial plexopathies; Carpal tunnel syndrome; Charcot–Marie–Tooth disease; Neuralgic amyotrophy; Neuropathies: an overview.

▓ Hereditary sensory and autonomic neuropathy

Hereditary sensory and autonomic neuropathies are, as their name implies, characterized by autonomic and sensory disturbance. Five variants are described in the classification suggested by Dyck:

- HSAN type I: autosomal-dominant, onset second decade; distal pain, painless ulcerations, sensory deficit mainly affecting pain and temperature sensation; nerve biopsy shows axonal loss affecting small fibres more severely. Linked to chromosome 9q22.1–q22.3. One form linked to a point mutation in the gene encoding serine-palmitoyltransferase-1 (SPTLC1).

- HSAN type II: autosomal-recessive, onset in infancy; acroparaesthesiae, distal injury and Charcot joint formation, pan-sensory loss. No chromosomal linkage yet mapped. Some cases of "congenital insensitivity to pain" may be examples of HSAN type II.
- HSAN type III: familial dysautonomia, Riley–Day syndrome (*q.v.*); autosomal recessive; most cases associated with mutations in the inhibitor of kappa light polypeptide gene (IKBKAP) gene.
- HSAN type IV: "congenital insensitivity to pain and anhidrosis" (CIPA); autosomal recessive; very early onset with unexplained fever, anhidrosis, self-mutilating behaviour and mental retardation; nerve biopsy shows almost complete loss of unmyelinated fibres. Caused by mutations in the neurotrophin-receptor tyrosine kinase 1 (NTRK1) gene, previously known as trkA, which encodes a receptor for nerve growth factor (NGF).
- HSAN type V: clinically similar to type IV, but less severe; autosomal recessive; small myelinated fibres lost in nerve biopsies, unmyelinated fibres well preserved. Also caused by mutations in the neurotrophin-receptor tyrosine kinase 1 (NTRK1) gene.

Reference Kuhlenbäumer G, Young P, Hünermund G, Ringelstein B, Stögbauer F. Clinical features and molecular genetics of hereditary peripheral neuropathies. *Journal of Neurology* 2002; **249**: 1629–1650.

Other relevant entries Congenital insensitivity to pain; Neuropathies: an overview; Riley–Day syndrome.

■ Hereditary spastic paraparesis
Hereditary spastic paraplegia

Hereditary spastic paraparesis or paraplegia (HSP) is the name given to a heterogeneous group of inherited motor system disorders, characterized by lower limb spasticity and weakness (spasticity usually more predominant). This may be:

- Pure: spasticity, weakness, mild diminution of lower limb vibration sensation $+/-$ proprioception
- Complicated: HSP $+/-$ seizures, dementia, amyotrophy, extrapyramidal signs, and peripheral neuropathy.

Most HSP is inherited as an autosomal-dominant condition (*ca.* 70%), but autosomal-recessive and X-linked modes of inheritance have been described. Various genetic loci, labelled SPG (for "spastic gait"), have been defined, and mutations in certain genes identified, that is, those encoding the proteins spastin, paraplegin, cell adhesion molecule (L1-CAM), proteolipid protein gene (PLP) and spartin. It is likely that further loci and genetic mutations will be defined.

Gene	Locus	Inheritance	Clinical classification	Protein
SPG1	Xq28	X-linked		L1-CAM
SPG2	Xq22	X-linked		PLP
SPG3a	14q11–q21	Dominant	Pure	Atlastin
SPG4	2p22	Dominant	Pure	Spastin
SPG5a	8p12–q13	Recessive		
SPG6	15q11.1	Dominant	Pure	
SPG7	16q24.3	Recessive		Paraplegin
SPG8	8q23–q24	Dominant	Pure	
SPG9	10q23.3–q24.1	Dominant	Pure	
SPG10	12q13	Dominant	Pure	
SPG11	15q13–q15	Recessive		
SPG12	19q13	Dominant	Pure	
SPG13	2q24–q34	Dominant	Pure	
SPG14	3q27–q28	Recessive	Complicated	
SPG16	Xq11.2	X-linked		
SPG17	11q12–q14	Dominant	Complicated	
SPG19		Dominant		
SPG20	13q12.3	Recessive	Complicated	Spartin

Other forms of HSP with additional neurological features include:

Behr's syndrome
Charlevoix–Saguenay syndrome (ARSACS)
Kjellin syndrome
Mast syndrome
Sjögren–Larsson disease

(see individual entries for further details).

Clinical features: history and examination

- Variable date of onset, usually in early adulthood with stiffness of legs and difficulty walking, with or without backache and lumbar lordosis.
- Clinically, spasticity is out of proportion to weakness. Arms, sensation, and sphincter function are generally normal.
- In the "complicated" variants, other features may develop, including seizures, dementia, amyotrophy, extrapyramidal signs, peripheral neuropathy.
- Asymptomatic family members may have upper motor neurone signs.
- Although the clinical picture of HSP may be uniform, symptom onset and severity may vary between and within families linked to the same genetic locus.

Investigations and diagnosis

Usually unremarkable.

Imaging: MRI spinal cord normal; may show slight atrophy.

CSF: acellular, no oligoclonal bands; may be slightly elevated protein.

Electrophysiology: central motor conduction time may be prolonged.

Differential diagnosis Other causes of myelopathy, for example

Multiple sclerosis
MND, Primary lateral sclerosis (PLS)
HTLV-1 myelopathy

Krabbe's disease has been reported to present in this way.
SPG2 is allelic with Pelizaeus–Merzbacher disease (PMD).

Treatment and prognosis Slow progression is typical, but patients generally remain ambulant for many years.

Symptomatic treatment of spasticity: baclofen, tizanidine, dantrolene; intrathecal baclofen; physiotherapy.

Genetic counselling to family.

References McDermott CJ, White K, Bushby K *et al.* Hereditary spastic paraparesis: a review of new developments. *Journal of Neurology, Neurosurgery and Psychiatry* 2000; **69**: 150–160.

Tallaksen CME, Dürr A, Brice A. Recent advances in hereditary spastic paraplegia. *Current Opinion in Neurology* 2001; **14**: 457–463.

Other relevant entries Charlevoix–Saguenay syndrome; Mitochondrial disease: an overview; Myelopathy: an overview; Pelizaeus–Merzbacher disease; Sjögren–Larsson disease; Troyer syndrome.

◼ Hermansky–Pudlak syndrome – see Albinism

◼ HERNS

HERNS is *h*ereditary *e*ndotheliopathy with *r*etinopathy, *n*ephropathy and *s*troke, an autosomal-dominant condition linked to chromosome 3p21 in which both cerebral and retinal vessels are affected. Clinically there is early progressive visual loss, focal neurological deficits, dementia and headache, along with renal insufficiency and proteinuria. It resembles others cerebroretinal vasculopathies linked to 3p21 but with the additional renal features.

Reference Jen J, Cohen AH, Yue Q *et al.* Hereditary endotheliopathy with retinopathy, nephropathy and stroke (HERNS). *Neurology* 1997; **49**: 1322–1330.

◼ Heroin

Heroin use may be associated with various neurological sequelae, including:

Spinal cord syndrome: acute paraplegia: hypotensive, toxic, anterior spinal artery syndrome; chronic myelopathy.
Cerebral vasculitis.
Peripheral neuropathy, mononeuropathy, plexopathy.
Seizures.

■ Herpes simplex encephalitis

Pathophysiology The herpes simplex virus (HSV) is the commonest cause of encephalitis, most usually (90%) due to HSV-1; HSV-2 affects neonates and the immunocompromised. The recognition of HSE is crucial since early and appropriate treatment has been shown to reduce mortality and morbidity significantly. However, HSE may present in various ways and investigations in the early stages can be normal, thus a high index of suspicion is needed. In case of doubt, antiviral therapy with aciclovir should be started prior to diagnostic confirmation.

Viral invasion of the brain (source uncertain, possibly via spread from olfactory pathways or trigeminal ganglia, possibly *de novo* infection rather than reactivation of latent viral infection) causes characteristic pathological changes: acute necrotizing encephalitis of orbitofrontal and temporal lobes, $+/-$ insular and cingulate cortices, $+/-$ overlying meningitis; may be asymmetric. Uncal herniation may be seen in fatal cases. Microscopically there is neuronophagia, perivascular inflammatory infiltrates, glial nodules and intranuclear Cowdry type A inclusion bodies. Immunostaining reveals HSV antigen in brain tissue.

Clinical features: history and examination HSE may present in various ways, ranging from a dramatic vascular-type onset to a more chronic indolent disease. Typically, however, patients present with:

- Prodrome: fever, headache, malaise, anorexia $+/-$ behavioural changes.
- Confusion, clouding of consciousness, coma.
- Seizures: focal, generalized.
- Aphasia, mutism.
- $+/-$ meningism, focal motor weakness, brainstem encephalitic picture.

The advent of highly sensitive CSF polymerase chain reaction (PCR) for the diagnosis of HSE has revealed a variety of unusual presentations of HSV infection, including:

- Mild or subacute encephalitis.
- Psychiatric presentations.
- Brainstem encephalitis.
- Benign recurrent meningitis (of Mollaret type).
- Myelitis (HSV-2).

Investigations and diagnosis *Bloods*: usually normal.

Imaging: CT scan is often normal. MRI is modality of choice, showing focal oedema in the medial temporal lobe, orbital surface of the frontal lobe, insular and cingulate cortex, sometimes asymmetrically, with gadolinium enhancement; occasionally MRI may be normal. SPECT may show (non-specific) focal hypoperfusion.

CSF: may be normal but in most cases is under raised pressure with a lymphocytic pleocytosis (10–200 cells/mm^3) $+/-$ increased red cell count (or xanthochromia) with a raised protein (0.6–6.0 g/l) but a normal glucose level. CSF PCR for HSV is a highly specific and sensitive test for confirming the diagnosis; false negatives may be encountered in early (<48 hours) or late (>10 days) disease.

Neurophysiology: EEG: invariably abnormal; shows a non-specific disorganized and slow background rhythm in the early stages; epileptiform abnormalities such as high voltage periodic lateralizing epileptiform discharges (PLEDs) may appear later. A normal prolonged EEG should raise doubts as to the diagnosis of HSE.

Brain biopsy for confirmation of disease was once popular, particularly in the USA and Europe, but is now seldom required following the advent of CSF PCR for HSV and aciclovir therapy; it is reserved for atypical cases or where a tumour in the temporal lobe is considered part of the differential diagnosis.

Differential diagnosis

Other viral encephalitides, especially CMV (*cf.* treatment with ganciclovir).

Sagittal sinus thrombosis.

Meningitis.

Vasculitis, small vessel vasculopathy or conventional vascular event in temporal lobe.

Hashimoto's encephalopathy.

Wernicke's encephalopathy.

Paraneoplastic (limbic) encephalitis.

Brain tumour (e.g. glioma).

Poorly controlled temporal lobe epilepsy.

Subdural empyaema.

Acute disseminated encephalomyelitis (ADEM).

Treatment and prognosis Aciclovir (10 mg/kg intravenously every 8 hours) should be given as soon as the diagnosis is contemplated (i.e. before confirmation) for 10–14 days; relapse rate is lower with 14 days treatment. In immunocompromised patients, 21 days treatment may be given. Monitoring CSF PCR for HSV may assist with decision-making concerning the duration of treatment.

Symptomatic treatment: anticonvulsants if seizures complicate the clinical course; supportive intensive therapy unit (ITU) care may be required, including ventilation.

Early treatment greatly improves survival and reduces long-term complications.

Mortality of untreated cases is 70–80%, falling to 20–30% in cases where treatment is given. The outlook is best in patients treated early, the young, and those with GCS > 6 at onset of treatment.

The major morbidity results from ongoing epilepsy, cognitive deficits (especially anterograde memory deficits, i.e. amnesia) and behavioural problems.

Recurrence is reported.

References Cinque P, Cleator GM, Weber T *et al.* The role of laboratory investigation in the diagnosis and management of patients with suspected herpes simplex encephalitis: a consensus report. *Journal of Neurology, Neurosurgery and Psychiatry* 1996; **61**: 339–345.

Kennedy PGE, Chaudhuri A. Herpes simplex encephalitis. *Journal of Neurology, Neurosurgery and Psychiatry* 2002; **73**: 237–238.

■ Herpes zoster and postherpetic neuralgia
Shingles

Pathophysiology Herpes zoster or shingles develops in patients years (usually decades) after primary varicella zoster virus (VZV) infection as chickenpox. Virus lies dormant in neurones of sensory ganglia, prior to reactivation, sometimes in the context of systemic cancer, immunodeficiency, or trauma, although a precipitating cause is not identified in most cases. Around 10% of herpes zoster cases are complicated by postherpetic neuralgia, a persistent pain in the distribution of the previous zoster rash: this may be burning or paroxysmal and lancinating.

Clinical features: history and examination

- Herpes zoster:

    Sharp, burning pain in dermatomal distribution.

    Followed by rash: macular, becoming vesicular, in dermatomal distribution.

    Some cases lack a rash: zoster sine herpete.

    Usually unilateral, involving a single dermatome.

    Distribution: trunk > head (typically first division of the trigeminal nerve) > limbs.

    Recovery over weeks: residual dermatomal hypo- or hyperalgesia.

- Complications:

    virus may spread to:

    Eye: herpes zoster ophthalmicus (HZO).

    Anterior roots, motor nerves: radiculitis.

    Spinal cord: myelitis.

    Brain: encephalomyelitis.

    - Involvement of the geniculate ganglion leads to geniculate herpes or Ramsay Hunt syndrome.
    - HZO may be followed by contralateral hemiparesis about 2 months after rash, presumed due to a granulomatous angiitis.
    - Postherpetic neuralgia: pain for >1 year in distribution of prior herpes zoster; often disabling pain.

Investigations and diagnosis Clinical history and examination usually adequate Complications may necessitate imaging, electrophysiology, CSF analysis to exclude other causes.

Differential diagnosis Herpes zoster *per se* unlikely to be mistaken (unless zoster sine herpete).

Complications: consider differential diagnosis of radiculopathy, myelitis, encephalomyelitis.

Treatment and prognosis Herpes zoster: simple analgesics: local measures. Aciclovir in immunocompromised patient. Zoster immune globulin of doubtful efficacy. Steroids controversial.

Postherpetic neuralgia: agents for neuropathic pain: amitriptyline, gabapentin, carbamazepine, fluphenazine, capsaicin cream, transcutaneous electrical nerve stimulator (TENS); despite which pain may persist.

References Gnann JW Jr, Whitley RJ. Herpes zoster. *New England Journal of Medicine* 2002; **347**: 340–346.

Johnson RW, Dworkin RH. Treatment of herpes zoster and postherpetic neuralgia. *British Medical Journal* 2003; **326**: 748–750.

Other relevant entry Varicella zoster virus and the nervous system.

▮ Herrmann disease

A dominantly inherited syndrome of hearing loss, diabetes mellitus, photomyoclonus, mental deterioration and nephropathy.

Other relevant entries Hearing loss: differential diagnosis; Lemieux–Neemeh syndrome; Renal disease and the nervous system.

▮ Hers' disease – see Glycogen-storage disorders: an overview

▮ Hertwig–Magendie syndrome
Skew deviation

This refers to an acquired, non-paretic, vertical misalignment of the eyes, of supranuclear origin, causing vertical diplopia. There is downward and inward rotation of one eye, with upward and outward rotation of the other, associated with nystagmus. The associated lesion involves the brainstem tegmentum, anywhere between the diencephalon and medulla. Various patterns of skew deviation may be described, of possible localizing value.

Reference Brandt Th, Dieterich M. Different types of skew deviation. *Journal of Neurology, Neurosurgery and Psychiatry* 1991; **54**: 549–550.

▮ Heterotopia

Heterotopias are malformations of the cerebral cortex due to disordered neuronal migration during embryogenesis. These may be classified as:

- Subependymal or periventricular
    Periventricular nodular heterotopia (e.g. BPNH).
    Periventricular laminar/ribbon heterotopia.

- Subcortical heterotopia
    Large subcortical heterotopia with abnormal cortex, hypogenetic corpus callosum.
    Single subcortical heterotopic nodule.
    Excessive single neurones in white matter.
- Band heterotopia (double cortex syndrome): demarcated layer of neurones in white matter; mostly sporadic but may be associated with mutations in the doublecortin (DCX) gene on Xq22.3–q23 or, less frequently, LIS1 gene on chromosome 17p13.3.

These conditions may manifest with seizures, +/− mental and developmental delay. They are best identified with MRI.

References Barkovich AJ, Kuzniecky R, Jackson GG *et al*. Classification system for malformations of cortical development. *Neurology* 2001; **57**: 2168–2178.

D'Agostino MD, Bernasconi A, Das S *et al*. Subcortical band heterotopia (SBH) in males: clinical imaging and genetic findings in comparison with females. *Brain* 2002; **125**: 2507–2522.

Other relevant entries Agenesis of the corpus callosum; Bilateral nodular periventricular heterotopia; Lissencephaly.

■ Hexosaminidase deficiency – see Gangliosidoses: an overview; Sandhoff disease; Tay–Sachs disease

■ Hindbrain headache – see Chiari malformations; Cough headache; Headache: an overview

■ Hirayama disease – see Monomelic amyotrophy

■ Histidinaemia – see Aminoacidopathies: an overview

■ Histiocytosis – see Erdheim–Chester disease

■ Histiocytosis X – see Langerhans cell histiocytosis

■ Histoplasmosis

A fungal infection causing a chronic non-specific meningitis, seldom identified from the CSF; culture from extraneural sites may be possible.

Other relevant entry Meningitis: an overview.

■ HIV/AIDS and the nervous system

Pathophysiology   The HIV retrovirus is neurotropic, rendering the whole neuraxis vulnerable to damage. Furthermore, the immunosuppression of AIDS may be associated with opportunistic CNS infection and the emergence of neoplastic disease. Multiple pathologies may coexist, an important point in management.

Clinical features: history and examination

- Seroconversion
    Encephalitis
    Aseptic meningitis
    Myelitis
    Cauda equina syndrome
    Guillain–Barré syndrome
    Myositis

Up to 10% of patients may present with a neurological disorder at seroconversion

- Complications of HIV infection

    Opportunistic infection
    Toxoplasmosis, causing cerebral abscess, encephalitis
    Cryptococcosis, causing meningitis
    Progressive multifocal leukoencephalopathy (PML)
    Cytomegalovirus, causing retinitis, encephalitis, mononeuritis multiplex,
        cauda equina syndrome
    Tuberculosis: TB meningitis, tuberculoma

    Tumours
    Primary CNS lymphoma

    HIV-related disorders
    Dementia
    Vacuolar myelopathy
    Distal sensory polyneuropathy
    Polymyositis

    Nutritional disorders
    Vitamin B_{12} deficiency
    Wernicke–Korsakoff's syndrome (WKS)

    Drug-related toxicity
    Mitochondrial myopathy (zidovudine)
    Peripheral neuropathy

    Stroke
    Ischaemic: embolic, thrombotic
    Haemorrhagic: thrombocytopenia, vasculitis

- Clinical neurological disorders associated with HIV infection include:
    Meningitis
    Viral: HIV related, herpes simplex, Varicella
    Bacterial: *Mycobacteria, Listeria, Streptococcus pneumoniae*, syphilis

Fungal: cryptococcosis
Aseptic
Encephalopathy
Myelopathy
   vacuolar myelopathy
Radiculopathy
   especially lumbosacral, cauda equina syndrome
Neuropathy
   sensory, sensorimotor, autonomic; cranial (Bell's palsy); multiple
     mononeuropathy
Myopathy

Investigations and diagnosis A high index of clinical suspicion may be required to determine that a particular neurological syndrome is related to HIV seroconversion. In established HIV infection, diagnosis may be simpler.

Bloods: HIV test after appropriate counselling, if not already done; CD4 count is helpful, since different neurological syndromes occur at different counts: toxoplasmosis, cryptococcosis < $200/mm^3$; CMV < $50/mm^3$.

Imaging: CNS mass lesions may reflect abscess (toxoplasmosis), lymphoma, TB.

CSF: often mild pleocytosis in neurologically normal HIV patients; in context, may require PCR for viruses, TB; indian ink staining, cryptococcal antigen.

Neurophysiology: EMG/NCS for peripheral neuropathies, myopathy/myositis

Biopsy: may be indicated for cerebral mass lesion(s).

Differential diagnosis Extremely broad, that is, dependent on context, differential diagnosis of meningitis, encephalopathy, dementia, neuropathy, myopathy.

In an HIV positive patient with any evidence of focal signs, seizures, headache, or altered mental status, imaging may reveal focal lesions. In this circumstance, the differential diagnosis encompasses toxoplasmosis, primary CNS lymphoma, tuberculoma, PML, or cryptococcoma. If lesions are multiple, then it is probably reasonable to give treatment for toxoplasmosis for a period of 2–6 weeks, with clinical and radiological re-evaluation; if there is no improvement, then biopsy may be considered, although the alternative pathologies (lymphoma, PML) are unlikely to be treatable. For a single lesion with negative toxoplasma serology, biopsy is indicated.

Treatment and prognosis See individual entries for specific conditions (e.g. toxoplasmosis, PML).

For HIV infection *per se*, HAART (highly active antiretroviral therapy), a combination of nucleoside and non-nucleoside reverse transcriptase inhibitors and protease inhibitors which reduces "virus load" (HIV RNA), has been shown to reduce significantly the incidence of opportunistic infections and prolong survival in AIDS-related PML.

References Berger JR. AIDS and the nervous system. In: Aminoff MJ (ed). *Neurology and General Medicine. The Neurological Aspects of Medical Disorders* (2nd edition). New York: Churchill Livingstone, 1995: 757–778.

Cohen BA. Neurologic complications in AIDS. In: Biller J (ed). *Practical Neurology* (2nd edition). Philadelphia: Lippincott Williams & Wilkins, 2002: 574–592.

Harrison MJG, McArthur JC. *AIDS and Neurology*. Edinburgh: Churchill Livingstone, 1995.

Manji H. Neurological manifestations. In: Adler MW (ed). *ABC of AIDS* (5th edition). London: BMJ Books, 2001: 42–45.

Report of a Working Group of the American Academy of Neurology AIDS Task Force. Nomenclature and research case definitions for neurologic manifestations of human immunodeficiency virus-type 1 (HIV-1) infection. *Neurology* 1991; **41**: 778–785.

Other relevant entries Cryptococcosis; Dementia: an overview; Lymphoma; Meningitis: an overview; Progressive multifocal leukoencephalopathy; Toxoplamosis; Tuberculosis and the nervous system.

Hodgkin's disease

Neurological associations of this localized or systemic lymphomatous condition include:

Spinal cord compression
Sesnory neuronopathy (paraneoplastic); CIDP; cranial nerve palsies
Cerebral/spinal cord vasculitis (rare)
Consequences of immunosuppression (e.g. PML).

Other relevant entries Lymphoma; Vasculitis.

Hoffman's syndrome

Hypothyroidism may be accompanied by a proximal myopathy. Hoffmann's syndrome refers to enlargement of affected muscles, which may demonstrate myxoedema, local mounding when percussed.

Other relevant entries Kocher–Débre–Sémélaigne syndrome; Thyroid disease and the nervous system.

Holmes–Adie syndrome
Adie's tonic pupil

The Holmes–Adie syndrome refers to the association of a Holmes–Adie pupil with other neurological features:

Holmes–Adie, or tonic, pupil: enlarged pupil, usually unilateral (hence causing anisocoria), unresponsive to a phasic light stimulus in a darkened environment, but slowly responsive to a tonic light stimulus. Accommodation reaction is preserved, hence there is light-near pupillary dissociation. The pupil shows denervation supersensitivity, constricting with application of dilute (0.2%) pilocarpine, indicating a peripheral lesion.

+/− loss of lower limb tendon reflexes (especially ankle jerks).

+/− impaired corneal sensation.

+/− chronic cough.

+/− localized or generalized anhidrosis, sometimes with hyperhidrosis (Ross syndrome).

The syndrome is much commoner in women.

Reference Martinelli P. Holmes–Adie syndrome. *Lancet* 2000; **356**: 1760–1761.

Other relevant entries Cranial nerve disease: II: Optic nerve; Cranial nerve disease: III: Oculomotor nerve; Ross syndrome.

■ Holmes syndrome

An early onset cerebellar ataxia with hypogonadism.

Other relevant entry Cerebellar disease: an overview.

■ Holmes's tremor – see Tremor: an overview

■ Holocarboxylase deficiency – see Biotin-responsive encephalopathy

■ Holoprosencephaly

In this cerebral malformation, the hemispheres are fused in the midline. Three varieties are delineated:

- Alobar holoprosencephaly: single, midline, telencephalic ventricle; no corpus callosum;
- Semilobar holoprosencephaly: incomplete interhemispheric fissure posteriorly; frontal lobes fused; no corpus callosum;
- Lobar holoprosencephaly: the least severe variety, with well-formed hemispheres linked by band of cortex at frontal pole, incompletely formed corpus callosum.

Developmental delay and mental retardation, refractory seizure disorder, hydrocephalus, and endocrine pituitary problems (e.g. diabetes insipidus) often accompany holoprosencephaly. Concurrent midline facial dysplasias may give a clue to the presence of holoprosencephaly at birth. There may also be malformations of the viscera and musculoskeletal system.

MRI demonstrates the variants of holoprosencephaly; EEG is abnormal with multifocal spikes or hypsarrhythmia.

Recognized associations include Patau syndrome (trisomy 13) and Smith–Lemli–Opitz syndrome.

Reference Kobori JA, Herrick MK, Urich H. Arhinencephaly. *Brain* 1987; **110**: 237–260.

Other relevant entries Agenesis of the corpus callosum; Patau syndrome; Smith–Lemli–Opitz syndrome.

■ Homocystinuria
Cystathionine β-synthase deficiency

Pathophysiology Accumulation of homocystine, a dimer of homocysteine, is associated with dysmorphism. The commonest cause is an autosomal-recessive inborn error of metabolism resulting from deficiency of cystathionine β-synthase (CBS). Homocystinuric syndromes with abnormalities of folate or vitamin B_{12} metabolism with or without methylmalonic aciduria are also described.

Clinical features: history and examination

- Learning disability: moderate.
- Psychiatric problems; psychosis rare.
- Lens dislocation (downward; *cf.* Marfan's syndrome: upward); myopia, retinal detachment, secondary glaucoma.
- Osteoporosis, especially spine; thoracic scoliosis.
- Marfanoid habitus, but no true arachnodactyly, and no cardiac abnormalities.
- Cerebral arterial or venous thrombosis (may also have peripheral arterial, venous and coronary thrombosis).
- $+/-$ seizures.
- Occasionally associated with dystonia, possibly due to vascular damage in the basal ganglia.

Investigations and diagnosis *Bloods*: plasma amino acids show raised methionine; homocystine and mixed disulphides are also present. Fibroblast enzyme analysis shows reduced activity of cystathionine β-synthase.

Urine: amino acid analysis shows elevated homocystine.

Neurogenetics: mutations in cystathionine β-synthase gene, mapping to chromosome 21q22.3: most are missense, many are private; common mutations are I278T associated with pyridoxine responsiveness, and G307S, associated with pyridoxine unresponsiveness.

Differential diagnosis Marfan's syndrome; other causes of "young stroke".

Treatment and prognosis Biochemical abnormalities may be normalized with large doses of pyridoxine (250–500 mg/day) in about half of patients; CBS requires pyridoxine as a prosthetic group for catalytic activity. Pyridoxine 500–1000 mg/day should be given for several weeks before a patient is deemed pyridoxine unresponsive.

Methionine-restricted diet supplemented with betaine is recommended. Folate repletion may be necessary.

Symptomatic treatment of vascular syndromes.

Without treatment, patients die from thromboembolic complications. Outlook is better in pyridoxine-responsive patients.

Reference Kraus JP, Janosik M, Kozich V *et al.* Cystathionine β-synthase mutations in homocystinuria. *Human Mutation* 1999; **13**: 362–375.

Other relevant entries Aminoacidopathies: an overview; Cerebrovascular disease: arterial; Marfan's syndrome.

▓ Hopkins' syndrome
Asthmatic amyotrophy

Cases of a poliomyelitis-like syndrome with onset following asthma attacks have been described as Hopkins' syndrome. Most have occurred in children, but adult cases are described. There is a flaccid monoparesis, sometimes with sensory and/or pyramidal involvement, with denervation on EMG studies. The picture suggests widespread involvement of the spinal cord. HyperIgEaemia, with allergen-specific IgE, is reported. Enteroviral infection has been suspected as a cause of both the asthma exacerbation and the neurological syndrome.

Reference Horiuchi I, Yamasaki K, Osoegawa M *et al.* Acute myelitis after asthma attacks with onset after puberty. *Journal of Neurology, Neurosurgery and Psychiatry* 2000; **68**: 665–668.

Other relevant entries Japanese encephalitis; Motor neurone diseases: an overview; Myelitis; Poliomyelitis.

▓ Horner's syndrome
Bernard–Horner syndrome • Oculosympathetic paresis

Pathophysiology Impaired ocular sympathetic innervation results in Horner's syndrome. The sympathetic pathway is long, extending from the ipsilateral diencephalon to the cervicothoracic spinal cord, then back up to the eye via the superior cervical ganglion, the internal carotid artery, and the ophthalmic (first) division of the trigeminal (V) nerve. Hence, a wide variety of pathological processes, spread across a large anatomical area, may cause a Horner's syndrome, although many examples remain idiopathic.

Recognized causes include:

carotid aneurysm, carotid artery dissection: often painful;
brainstem/cervical cord disease (vascular, demyelination, syringomyelia);
Pancoast tumour;
malignant cervical lymph nodes;
involvement of T1 fibres, for example in T1 radiculopathy, or lower trunk brachial plexopathy;
cluster headache;
congenital.

Clinical features: history and examination The features of Horner's syndrome are:

> partial ptosis: weakness of Müller's muscle;
> miosis: due to the unopposed action of the parasympathetically innervated
>   sphincter pupillae muscle;

These are usually the most evident signs which bring the patient to medical attention. In addition there may be:

> +/− anhidrosis: loss of sweating (if the lesion is distal to the superior cervical
>   ganglion);
> +/− enophthalmos: retraction of the eyeball (seldom measured).
> +/− heterochromia iridis: different colour of the iris on the affected side (if the
>   lesion is congenital);
> +/− elevation of the inferior eyelid due to a weak inferior tarsal muscle ("reverse
>   ptosis" or "upside-down ptosis").

Dependent on cause, there may be additional neurological features (e.g. with carotid artery dissection and Pancoast tumour).

Investigations and diagnosis Determining whether the lesion causing a Horner's syndrome is pre- or postganglionic may be done by applying to the eye 1% hydroxyamphetamine hydrobromide, which releases noradrenaline into the synaptic cleft, which dilates the pupil if Horner's syndrome results from a preganglionic lesion. However, this is not particularly helpful in determining cause, whereas accompanying neurological features are: contralateral hemiparesis would mandate investigation for carotid dissection (MRI, MRA, angiography), and this is probably sensible for any painful Horner's syndrome of acute onset. Arm symptoms and signs in a smoker mandate a chest radiograph for Pancoast tumour.

If the Horner's syndrome is isolated and painless, then no investigation may be required. In this situation, a symptomatic cause is seldom identified despite investigation. Syringomyelia presenting with isolated Horner's syndrome has been reported.

Differential diagnosis Unilateral miosis may be mistaken for contralateral mydriasis if ptosis is subtle, leading to suspicion of a partial oculomotor nerve palsy on the "mydriatic" side. Observation of anisocoria in the dark will help here, since increased anisocoria indicates a sympathetic defect (normal pupil dilates) whereas less anisocoria suggests a parasympathetic lesion. Applying to the eye 10% cocaine solution will also diagnose a Horner's syndrome if the pupil fails to dilate after 45 minutes in the dark (normal pupil dilates).

Treatment and prognosis Treatment of cause where possible, although once developed Horner's syndrome is generally not reversible. Functional consequences are few, but it may cause cosmetic complaint.

Other relevant entries Pancoast's syndrome; Pourfour du Petit syndrome; Raeder's paratrigeminal syndrome.

■ Horton's headache, Horton's neuralgia – see Cluster headache

■ Horton's syndrome – see Giant cell arteritis

■ HTLV-1 myelopathy

HTLV-1-associated myelopathy (HAM) • Tropical spastic paraparesis (TSP)

Pathophysiology Infection with human T-lymphotropic virus type I (HTLV-1) may cause a chronic progressive myelopathy, seen most often in Japan and equatorial Africa and South America, and more often in women. The virus is transmitted via breast milk, sexual intercourse, and exposure to contaminated blood products (e.g. hypodermic needles).

Clinical features: history and examination

- Symptoms:
  - Leg weakness
  - Backache
  - Painful legs
  - Paraesthesiae
  - Bladder symptoms
- Signs:
  - Leg spasticity
  - Walking difficulty/inability
  - Urinary frequency
  - Sensory loss

Investigations and diagnosis *Bloods*: serology for HTLV-1: ELISA, PCR; blood film may show atypical lymphocytes with convoluted nuclei (flower cells).

Imaging: spinal cord MRI is usually normal; brain MRI may show white matter lesions.

CSF: lymphocytic pleocytosis, elevated protein common; glucose normal; oligoclonal bands common; antibodies to HTLV-1 may be found in CSF.

Electrophysiology: lower limb somatosensory evoked potential (SSEPs) may show increased latency, due to central pathology.

Differential diagnosis Other causes of spastic paraparesis (e.g. multiple sclerosis, hereditary spastic paraparesis and lathyrism).

Treatment and prognosis

No specific treatment currently available; steroids are not helpful.

Symptomatic treatment for spasticity along with bladder care.

Prevention, by attention to mode of spread, is possible.

> **Reference** Engstrom JW. HTLV-I infection and the nervous system. In: Aminoff MJ (ed). *Neurology and General Medicine. The Neurological Aspects of Medical Disorders* (2nd edition). New York: Churchill Livingstone, 1995: 779–790.
>
> **Other relevant entries** Hereditary spastic paraparesis; Multiple sclerosis.

◼ Hughes syndrome – see Antiphospholipid (antibody) syndrome

◼ Hug's disease – see Glycogen-storage disorders: an overview

◼ Human immunodeficiency virus – see HIV/AIDS and the nervous system

◼ Humeroperoneal myopathy – see Emery–Dreifuss muscular dystrophy

◼ Hunter's syndrome
Mucopolysaccharidosis type II (MPS II)

This mucopolysaccharidosis is caused by deficiency of iduronate-2-sulphatase, resulting in increased deposition and urinary excretion of dermatan sulphate and heparan sulphate. Unlike other MPS it is an X-linked-recessive trait, linked to Xq27/28. Clinically there is coarsened facies, short stature, deafness, mental retardation and hepatosplenomegaly, but unlike Hurler's disease corneal clouding and gibbus deformity seldom if ever occur; moreover, the onset is later, at 2–5 years of age. Diarrhoea and limb and scapular cutaneous nodular thickening are common. The disease is of variable severity: survival may be until the second or third decade in the milder cases, death occurring from cardiac and respiratory compromise.

Other relevant entries Hurler's disease; Mucopolysaccharidoses.

◼ Huntington's disease
Huntington's chorea

Pathophysiology This autosomal-dominant disorder causing a movement disorder and cognitive dysfunction most often results from a defect in the coding region of the gene encoding huntingtin (IT15) on the short arm of chromosome 4, namely an expansion of a CAG trinucleotide repeat. Exactly how this genetic change brings about clinical disease is still uncertain, but anticipation with increasing repeat length is seen.

Clinical features: history and examination
- Personality change: irritability, apathy, depression, schizophrenia-like features
- Movement disorder: chorea, initially transient, often progresses to continuous athetotic and dystonic movement; patient unable to feed, dress, toilet; gait disorder may also be evident. Juvenile cases may present with parkinsonism (Westphal variant).
- Cognitive disorder: subcortical-type dementia.
- Family history of movement disorder, dementia, suicide, may be suggestive.

Investigations and diagnosis *Bloods*: unremarkable.

Imaging: CT/MRI may demonstrate caudate atrophy, with dilatation of frontal horns of lateral ventricles (box-like appearance of ventricles); decreased signal may be seen in globus pallidus and putamen on T_2-weighted MR scans; SPECT/PET may show decreased caudate/striatal perfusion and glucose metabolism.

EEG: normal early on; low voltage with poorly developed or absent α-rhythm may be seen in symptomatic cases.

Neurogenetics: CAG trinucleotide repeat expansion in the IT15 gene is the diagnostic test, but requires pretest counselling about implications. Recently genetic heterogeneity in HD has been noted, perhaps 6% of clinically diagnosed patients lacking an expansion in IT15; some of these patients have been found to harbour mutations (trinucleotide repeat expansion) in the genes encoding JPH3 or TBP, or an insertion in the octapeptide coding region of the prion protein gene.

Pathology: brain atrophy, particularly marked in striatum and caudate nucleus. Loss of spiny neurones in the basal ganglia. Brain intranuclear aggregates suggest that abnormal protein handling is a feature of the disease, whether pathogenetic or epiphenomenal.

Differential diagnosis The choreiform disorder is often characteristic, but other causes of chorea may have to be excluded (e.g. neuroacanthocytosis, DRPLA); ditto young onset parkinsonism. Benign hereditary chorea is also autosomal dominant but the absence of dementia means it is unlikely to be mistaken for HD. HD-like phenotype has also been noted in some families with mutations in the prion protein gene and some forms of autosomal-dominant cerebellar ataxia (ADCA).

Familial dementias (e.g. familial Alzheimer's disease) may be considered, but neuropsychological profile is different and movement disorder absent.

Treatment and prognosis No specific curative treatment is currently available. Mitochondrial disorders can occasionally look like HD. The possibility of nerve cell transplantation is also being investigated.

Symptomatic treatment for the movement disorders may include sulpiride or tetrabenazine. Cognitive and behavioural deficits are difficult to manage; the latter may mandate haloperidol or newer "atypical" neuroleptics such as risperidone or olanzapine. Depression may be treated with SSRIs.

Genetic counselling is important in affected families. Support may also be obtained from patient organizations.

Prognosis from onset to death is around 15–20 years. In some patients there is serious risk of suicide.

References Harper PS, Bates GP, Jones L (ed). *Huntington's Disease* (3rd edition). London: Saunders, 2002.

Rosser AE, Barker RA, Harrower T *et al.* Unilateral transplantation of human primary fetal tissue in four patients with Huntington's disease: NEST-UK safety report ISRCTN no. 36485475. *Journal of Neurology, Neurosurgery and Psychiatry* 2002; **73**: 678–685.

Stevanin G, Fujigasaki H, Lebre A-S *et al*. Huntington's disease-like phenotype due to trinucleotide repeat expansions in the *TBP* and *JPH3* genes. *Brain* 2003; **126**: 1599–1603.

Other relevant entries Autosomal-dominant cerebellar ataxia; Benign hereditary chorea; Chorea; Dementia: an overview; Dentatorubral–pallidoluysian atrophy; Prion disease: an overview; Trinucleotide repeat disorders.

■ Hurler's disease
Mucopolysaccharidosis type I-H (MPS I-H)

Pathophysiology This prototypical mucopolysaccharidosis, an autosomal-recessive trait linked to chromosome 4p16.3, results from a defect in the lysosomal enzyme α-L-iduronidase, resulting in increased deposition and urinary excretion of dermatan sulphate and heparan sulphate. Scheie's syndrome (MPS I-S) results from an identical biochemical defect but the phenotype is less severe. An overlap syndrome (MPS I-H/S, Hurler–Scheie syndrome) is recognized.

Clinical features: history and examination
- Normal at birth.
- Macrocephaly, developmental delay.
- Recurrent upper respiratory tract infections in first year.
- Coarsened facies: frontal bossing, hypertelorism, open mouth with macroglossia, flat nasal bridge.
- Thick coarse hair.
- Short stature: skeletal deformities = dysostosis multiplex; gibbus spinal deformity, broad short hands.
- Hepatosplenomegaly.
- +/− hydrocephalus.
- +/− corneal clouding, glaucoma.
- +/− deafness.
- Progressive mental deterioration.
- Angina pectoris.

Investigations and diagnosis
Diagnosis based on clinical phenotype.
Urine: increased dermatan sulphate and heparan sulphate.

Differential diagnosis The Hurler phenotype may have various causes, including MPS I-H:

Mucolipidoses:
  Types I (sialidosis type II); II (I-cell disease); III (pseudo-Hurler's disease); and IV.
Mannosidosis (α and β).
Fucosidosis.
Aspartylglucosaminuria.

The differentiation is made, in part, by the absence of mucopolysacchariduria in these disorders.

GM1 gangliosidosis.

Treatment and prognosis
No specific treatment known.
Course is of gradual progression; death from respiratory or cardiac causes by age 10 years is usual.

Other relevant entries Fucosidosis; Gangliosidoses: an overview; Mannosidoses; Mucopolysaccharidoses; Mucolipidoses; Pseudo-Hurler's syndrome.

■ Hurst's disease – see Acute disseminated encephalomyelitis; Encephalomyelitis: differential diagnosis

■ Hutchinson–Gilford syndrome – see Progeria

■ Hydatid disease – see Echinococcosis

■ Hydrocephalus

Pathophysiology Hydrocephalus may be defined as an increase in the production and/or circulation, or impaired absorption, of CSF within the skull. This may be caused by:

Increased CSF production (e.g. choroid plexus papilloma).
Obstruction to CSF flow between secretion from the choroid plexuses and absorption in the arachnoid villi in the sagittal sinus (e.g. posterior fossa tumour, aqueduct stenosis, Chiari malformations).
Impaired CSF absorption due to inflammation (e.g. meningitis) or sagittal sinus thrombosis.

Hydrocephalus may be classified as:
• Obstructive (internal, non-communicating, tension): obstruction of CSF circulation.
• Communicating (external, non-obstructive): disturbed formation or absorption of CSF.
  Hereditary or familial forms of hydrocephalus are described, most commonly an X-linked-type associated with aqueduct stenosis; this may be associated with mutations in the gene encoding the neural cell adhesion molecule L1-CAM.
  Autosomal-recessive and, rarely, autosomal-dominant, forms of hydrocephalus have also been described.

Clinical features: history and examination
• Infantile: large head, prominent scalp veins, "setting sun" eye sign; increased intracranial pressure slight or absent due to the deformability of the skull; seizures, spastic lower limbs; may have impaired cognition.

- Post-infantile: signs of raised intracranial pressure conspicuous if obstructive hydrocephalus: headache, nausea, vomiting, papilloedema; cranial nerve palsies (VI, VII = false-localizing signs) may occur.

Investigations and diagnosis May be clinically obvious in infancy.

Imaging may be required in adulthood: CT/MRI good for showing obstructive dilated ventricles; MRI better for defining any obstructive lesion.

Differential diagnosis Radiologically it is important to distinguish ventricular enlargement due to *ex vacuo* brain atrophy from communicating hydrocephalus, for example in patients with cognitive decline where normal pressure hydrocephalus may be suspected.

"Pseudohydrocephalus" in Silver–Russell syndrome.

Treatment and prognosis Of cause where possible. Shunting to relieve pressure may be necessary. Third ventriculostomy may be an alternative in certain circumstances.

References Chalmers RM, Andreae L, Wood NW, Durai-Raj RV, Casey AT. Familial hydrocephalus. *Journal of Neurology, Neurosurgery and Psychiatry* 1999; **67**: 410–411.

Gjerris F. Hydrocephalus and other disorders of cerebrospinal fluid circulation. In: Bogousslavsky J, Fisher M (eds). *Textbook of Neurology*. Boston: Butterworth-Heinemann, 1998: 655–674.

Rosenthal A, Jouet M, Kenwrick S. Aberrant splicing of neural cell adhesion molecule L1 mRNA in a family with X-linked hydrocephalus. *Nature Genetics* 1992; **2**: 107–112.

Other relevant entries Alexander's disease; Canavan's disease; Normal pressure hydrocephalus; Silver–Russell syndrome.

Hydrophobia – see Rabies

Hyperekplexia

Hyperekplexia is an involuntary movement disorder in which there is pathological exaggeration of the startle response, usually to sudden unexpected (often auditory) stimuli.

The hyperekplexias may be classified as:

- Primary

    Major form: autosomal-dominant disorder with hyperekplexia and hypertonia, manifested as a hesitant and wide-based gait, and hypnagogic myoclonic jerks. Some families demonstrate a mutation in the α_1-subunit of the inhibitory glycine-receptor gene.

    Minor form: excessive startle triggered by acute febrile illness in childhood or stress in adult life.

- Secondary/symptomatic

    Perinatal ischaemic–hypoxic encephalopathy.

    Brainstem or thalamic lesions.

    Drugs (e.g. cocaine and amphetamines).

    Tourette syndrome.

Clonazepam may be helpful in primary hyperekplexias.

Reference Wilkins DE, Hallett M, Wess MM. Audiogenic startle reflex of man and its relationship to startle syndromes. A review. *Brain* 1986; **109**: 561–573.

Other relevant entry Startle syndromes.

■ Hypereosinophilic syndrome

Suggested diagnostic criteria for this rare syndrome are:

- Persistent eosinophilia ($>1500/mm^3$);
- No evidence of parasitic infection or other recognized cause of eosinophilia;
- Signs and symptoms of organ involvement or dysfunction caused by eosinophil infiltration or another mechanism.

The latter may include involvement of the following organs:

- Heart: conduction disturbance, congestive failure;
- Vascular system: Raynaud's phenomenon; splinter haemorrhages;
- Lung: pulmonary infiltrates and asthma;
- Blood: anaemia, hypergammaglobulinaemia;
- Nervous system: polymyositis-like picture ("eosinophilic polymyositis"); mono-myositis; stroke.

The differential diagnosis encompasses necrotizing vasculitides such as polyarteritis nodosa and Churg–Strauss syndrome, but tissue biopsies provide no evidence to confirm these diagnoses, whereas inflammatory infiltrates with prominent eosinophilic infiltration are found.

Despite the unknown aetiology, the syndrome often responds dramatically to steroids, although the long-term outlook is not good, dependent on organ involvement.

Reference Weller PF, Bubley GJ. The idiopathic hypereosinophilic syndrome. *Blood* 1994; **83**: 2759–2779.

Other relevant entries Churg–Strauss syndrome; Eosinophilic myopathy.

■ Hyperkalaemic periodic paralysis – see Channelopathies: an overview; Periodic paralysis

■ Hyperosmolar non-ketotic syndrome – see Diabetes mellitus and the nervous system; Hemiballismus, Hemichorea

■ Hyperostosis cranialis generalisata – see Van Buchem's syndrome

◾ Hyperostosis cranialis interna

An inherited syndrome, probably autosomal dominant, characterized by intracranial hyperostosis and osteosclerosis of the calvaria and skull base (hence a craniotubular hyperostosis) causing cranial nerve entrapment, usually recurrent facial nerve palsy, and, less often, impaired smell, taste, vision, and cochleovestibular symptoms.

Reference Manni JJ, Scaf JJ, Huygen PLM, Cruysberg JRM, Verhagen WIM. Hyperostosis cranialis interna: a new hereditary syndrome with cranial-nerve entrapment. *New England Journal of Medicine* 1990; **322**: 450–454.

Other relevant entries Fibrous dysplasia; Paget's disease.

◾ Hyperoxaluria

Deficiency of alanine glyoxalate aminotransferase, with resulting hyperoxaluria, nephrocalcinosis and renal failure, may be complicated by a painful peripheral neuropathy of combined axonal and demyelinating type.

◾ Hypersomnia, Hypersomnolence – see Sleep Disorders: an overview

◾ Hypertension and the nervous system

Pathophysiology Most hypertension remains "essential", that is, the ultimate causes are unknown. If resistant to treatment, and particularly in young individuals, possible renal (e.g. renal artery stenosis) or endocrine (e.g. Cushing's syndrome, Conn's syndrome and phaeochromocytoma) contributors to hypertension may be sought. If inadequately treated, hypertension may have various adverse effects on the nervous system.

Clinical features: history and examination

- Hypertension *per se* may be associated with headache, dizziness.
- Hypertension is a modifiable risk factor for both ischaemic and haemorrhagic stroke; and both vascular dementia and Alzheimer's disease. There is a log–linear relationship between usual diastolic blood pressure and stroke throughout the normal range.
- Hypertensive encephalopathy: headache, seizures, focal neurological deficits, papilloedema with retinal haemorrhages and exudates, as well as renal and cardiac impairment; occurs in the context of uncontrolled (may be malignant) hypertension. Search for an underlying cause is mandatory and treatment with anti-hypertensive agents is needed.
- Chronic encephalopathy (Binswanger's disease): may develop in patients with hypertension: picture is of a subcortical dementia, may be in association with other motor deficits.
- Risk factor for microangiopathic sixth (abducens) and third (oculomotor) nerve palsies.

Investigations and diagnosis *Bloods*: electrolytes (especially for hypokalaemia); renal function; may need to assay cortisol.

Urine: for red cells; presence may suggest ongoing end-organ damage (malignant hypertension); collection for creatinine clearance; may need to assay urinary vanillylmandelic acid (VMA) or catecholamines (phaeochromocytoma)

Imaging:

Brain CT/MRI may show evidence of subcortical infarcts, lacunar state.

Renal: may show small kidney, underperfused.

CXR: Heart enlargement.

Echocardiography: left ventricular hypertrophy.

ECG: left ventricular hypertrophy, strain pattern.

Treatment and prognosis

Of cause where possible.

Symptomatic treatment includes β-blockers, ACE inhibitors, calcium channel antagonists, diuretics.

Prognosis related to how effective blood pressure control is.

Other relevant entries Binswanger's disease; Cerebrovascular disease: arterial; Cranial nerve disease: III: Oculomotor nerve; Cranial nerve disease: VI: Abducens nerve; Dementia: an overview; Eclampsia; Encephalopathies: an overview; Intracerebral haemorrhage; Lacunar syndromes; Renal disease and the nervous system; Vascular dementia.

■ Hyperviscosity syndrome – see Bing–Neel syndrome

■ Hypnic headache
"Alarm clock" headache • *Solomon's syndrome*

A rare syndrome, mostly seen in the elderly and predominating in women, in which pulsating headache wakes the patient at the same time on most nights, with associated nausea. Unlike cluster headache, the pain is generalized and there are no autonomic features. The headache lasts about 30 minutes (range 5–180) and may occur up to three times per night. There are no associated clinical signs. The clinical description differs from "exploding head syndrome" although both occur at night. The headache may respond to lithium carbonate, indomethacin, or caffeine (as in coffee) taken before retiring.

Reference Dodick DW, Mosek AC, Campbell JK. The hypnic ("alarm clock") headache syndrome. *Cephalalgia* 1998; **18**: 152–156.

Other relevant entries Cluster headache; "Exploding head syndrome"; Headache: an overview.

■ Hypobetalipoproteinaemia

Familial hypobetalipoproteinaemia is an autosomal-dominant condition, which in its homozygous state is clinically indistinguishable from abetalipoproteinaemia.

In the heterozygous state the disease is often asymptomatic. The defect is an abnormal synthetic rate, and hence lower concentration, of betalipoproteins. As a result there are secondary reductions in the levels of VLDL and LDL and so plasma cholesterol and triglyceride levels are reduced. Malabsorption is uncommon as chylomicrons are formed.

Other relevant entry Abetalipoproteinaemia.

▓ Hypochondriasis – see Somatoform disorders

▓ Hypoglossal nerve palsy – see Cranial nerve disease: XII: Hypoglossal nerve

▓ Hypokalaemic periodic paralysis – see Channelopathies: an overview; Periodic paralysis

▓ Hypomelanosis of Ito – see Incontinentia pigmenti (Achromians)

▓ Hypophysitis – see Lymphocytic hypophysitis

▓ Hypopituitarism – see Pituitary disease and apoplexy

▓ Hypoprebetalipoproteinaemia – see HARP syndrome

▓ Hypothalamic disease: an overview

Pathophysiology The hypothalamus has key roles in neuroendocrine and autonomic function, and also in controlling circadian and seasonal rhythms and sleep–wake cycles. Clinical clues to the involvement of the hypothalamus in disease processes include disorders of temperature regulation, sleep regulation, water balance, caloric balance, reproductive function, emotional behaviour and affect.

Disease of the hypothalamic region may be the consequence of various pathological processes:

Inflammatory, infiltrative: sarcoidosis; Langerhans cell histiocytosis; multiple sclerosis (rare).
Neoplastic: hamartoma, post-pituitary surgery.
Infection: Whipple's disease.

Clinical features: history and examination
• Temperature regulation: hypothermia (e.g. spontaneous periodic hypothermia), hyperthermia.

- Sleep regulation: hypersomnia (narcolepsy, Kleine–Levin syndrome), insomnia (Whipple's disease).
- Seizures: "diencephalic", gelastic.
- Water balance: diabetes insipidus, syndrome of inappropriate ADH secretion (SIADH), disturbance of thirst/water balance.
- Caloric balance: obesity, hyperphagia (Prader–Willi syndrome; Laurence–Moon syndrome, Bardet–Biedl syndrome; Kleine–Levin syndrome); emaciation (anorexia nervosa; diencephalic [Russell's] syndrome).
- Endocrine function: precocious puberty (hypothalamic hamartoma); gonadal underdevelopment (Prader–Willi syndrome; Froehlich's syndrome), gynaecomastia.
- Emotional affect: rage reactions, fear, disinhibition, apathy.
- Abnormal growth: dwarfism, gigantism.
(See individual entries for further details.)

Investigations and diagnosis *Bloods*: dependent on context, may need to assay electrolytes (water balance), hormones (disorders of growth, gonadal development, caloric balance).

Imaging: MRI is modality of choice for structural change in hypothalamus.

Treatment and prognosis Of cause, where established.

Reference Brazis PW, Masdeu JC, Biller J. *Localization in clinical neurology* (4th edition). Philadelphia: Lippincott Williams & Wilkins, 2001: 387–402.

Other relevant entries Autonomic failure; Diabetes insipidus; Diencephalic syndrome; Dwarfism; Eating disorders; Emotional lability: differential diagnosis; Froehlich's syndrome; Gelastic seizures; Gigantism; Kleine–Levin syndrome; Narcolepsy, narcoleptic syndrome; Pituitary disease and apoplexy; Septo-optic dysplasia; Sleep disorders: an overview; Spontaneous periodic hypothermia; Syndrome of inappropriate ADH secretion; Whipple's disease.

■ Hypoxanthine phosphoribosyltransferase deficiency – see Lesch–Nyhan disease

■ Hysteria – see Somatoform disorders

Ii

■ I-cell disease
Mucolipidosis type II (ML type II)

This condition results from deficiency or dysfunction of N-acetylglucosamine (or acetylglucosaminyl) phosphotransferase, as in mucolipidosis type III (pseudo-Hurler's disease), and is linked to chromosome 4q. Clinically the phenotype is severe (*cf.* pseudo-Hurler's disease) with developmental delay, poor growth, skeletal abnormalities (kyphoscoliosis, lumbar gibbus), gingival hypertrophy, subcutaneous nodules, and hepatosplenomegaly, with death occurring around 4–8 years of age usually from cardiopulmonary failure.

Other relevant entries Mucolipidoses; Pseudo-Hurler's syndrome.

■ Idiopathic cranial polyneuropathy

A syndrome characterized by subacute, constant, facial pain, often retro-orbital, followed by multiple cranial nerve palsies, often developing suddenly, including (in order of frequency) III, IV, VI; V; VII; IX–XII. I and VIII are spared. All investigations for a cause of cranial polyneuropathy are negative. The syndrome responds to steroids, and may be related to orbital pseudotumour ("Tolosa–Hunt syndrome").

Reference Juncos JL, Beal MF. Idiopathic cranial polyneuropathy: a fifteen-year experience. *Brain* 1987; **110**: 197–211.

Other relevant entries Cranial polyneuropathy; Tolosa–Hunt syndrome.

■ Idiopathic hyperCKaemia

This term was coined for persistently elevated serum levels of creatine kinase (CK) in apparently healthy individuals. A number of such individuals will harbour sub-clinical neuromuscular disease which may be elucidated by muscle biopsy, but some remain entirely normal, thereby meriting the diagnosis of "idiopathic hyperCKaemia". Cases with mutations of the caveolin 3 (CAV3) gene have been described, a condition which is allelic with rippling muscle disease and limb-girdle muscular dystrophy type 1C.

Reference Prelle A, Tancredi L, Sciacco M *et al.* Retrospective study of a large population of patients with asymptomatic or minimally symptomatic raised serum creatine kinase levels. *Journal of Neurology* 2002; **249**: 305–311.

Other relevant entries Limb-girdle muscular dystrophy; Rippling muscle disease.

■ Idiopathic hypersomnia
Essential hypersomnolence

This name has been given to a syndrome characterized by excessive daytime somnolence with episodes of sleep for which no cause, such as narcolepsy or obstructive sleep apnoea syndrome, can be found. There is no associated cataplexy or sleep paralysis, and although the condition runs in families there is no obvious HLA association (*cf.* narcolepsy). Confusional arousal ("sleep drunkenness") may be a feature. Reports of preceding Epstein–Barr virus infection, Guillain–Barré syndrome and HIV infection have appeared. It may be difficult to distinguish from narcolepsy, usually affecting young adults, but sleep studies show no sleep onset rapid eye movement (REM). The condition is lifelong, and may be very disabling.

Besides other sleep disorders, it is important to exclude a hypothalamic lesion and depression in these patients, since these diagnoses open other therapeutic approaches.

Other relevant entries Hypothalamic disease: an overview; Narcolepsy, Narcoleptic syndrome; Sleep disorders: an overview.

■ Idiopathic intracranial hypertension

Benign intracranial hypertension (BIH) • Meningitis serosa • Pseudotumour cerebri

Pathophysiology Idiopathic intracranial hypertension (IIH) was first described by Quincke in 1897 as "meningitis serosa". It is a relatively common neurological condition in which there is raised CSF pressure, usually with papilloedema, but normal brain imaging; there is no central nervous system (CNS) mass lesion (hence another appellation, "pseudotumour cerebri") or hydrocephalus. Cerebral venous thrombosis, most often of the sagittal sinus, can produce a similar picture.

The aetiopathogenesis of IIH is not understood. Some form of obstruction of CSF outflow, either at the arachnoid villi or in the dural venous sinuses is suspected. Risk factors include female sex (F : M = 4–10 : 1), reproductive age, menstrual irregularity, obesity, recent weight gain and hypertension. Various other associations have been described, including vitamin A deficiency and toxicity, and drug use including corticosteroids, oral contraceptives, tetracycline, nitrofurantoin, and nalidixic acid.

The papilloedema consequent on raised CSF pressure may cause loss of vision if untreated (hence "benign" is an inappropriate epithet). There have been no randomized-controlled trials of any of the various medical and surgical treatment modalities. Joint follow-up by neurologist and ophthalmologist may be the optimal management.

Clinical features: history and examination Modified Dandy's criteria for the diagnosis of IIH are:

- Signs and symptoms of raised intracranial pressure:

    Headache, +/− nausea, vomiting and visual obscurations; the latter are characteristically described as momentary loss ("greying out") of vision bilaterally, often on standing up or bending over. They are probably due to reduced perfusion of the optic nerve head.

    Papilloedema, which is usually bilateral and can be chronic in appearance; very occasionally patients with IIH have no papilloedema.

    Visual field mapping shows enlargement of the blind spot, often with constricted peripheral fields. The visual acuity may be normal, impairment developing later (hence not a good test to monitor disease).

- No localizing neurological signs with the exception of sixth nerve palsy (unilateral, bilateral, with diplopia).
- Normal neuroimaging (small ventricles, empty sella allowed).

- Raised CSF pressure ($>250\,mmH_2O$) with normal composition.
- Exclusion of primary structural or systemic cause of raised intracranial pressure (e.g. venous sinus thrombosis, hyperviscosity, right heart failure).

Occasionally patients complain of a number of other minor symptoms including neck stiffness, tinnitus, paraesthesia and joint pains.

Rarely, there are other false-localizing signs in IIH (e.g. facial nerve palsy).

Investigations and diagnosis *Bloods*: usually normal; abnormalities in the thrombophilia screen have been described even in the absence of sagittal sinus thrombosis.

Imaging: generally normal, an empty sella may be observed. CT $+/-$ MRV may be done to exclude other causes for the papilloedema. MRI may be indicated to exclude a chronic meningitic process in some cases.

CSF: to measure the opening pressure and exclude meningitis process.

Differential diagnosis

Space-occupying lesion.

Sagittal or lateral sinus thrombosis.

Meningitic process; either chronic inflammatory or malignant.

Hydrocephalus.

Malignant hypertension.

Bilateral optic neuritis.

Obstructive sleep apnoea syndrome.

Treatment and prognosis Medical therapy: in patients with headache only, weight loss and diuretics (e.g. acetazolamide 250 mg tds) $+/-$ analgesia are recommended, as is monitoring of visual fields.

Surgical therapy: if there are visual symptoms, or progressive visual field loss, then surgical intervention may be undertaken. Options include ventriculoperitoneal shunting or optic nerve sheath defenestration. Repeated lumbar punctures (LPs) are also an option, often unpopular, but may have a place in pregnancy when diuretics are contraindicated.

None of these treatments has been submitted to a randomized-controlled trial.

Natural history of IIH is for 25% of cases to remit spontaneously after the first LP.

References Corbett JJ. Idiopathic intracranial hypertension. In: Kennard C (ed.). *Recent Advances in Clinical Neurology 8*. Edinburgh: Churchill Livingstone, 1995: 51–71.

Lueck CJ, McIlwaine GG. Idiopathic intracranial hypertension. *Practical Neurology* 2002; **2**: 262–271.

Round R, Keane JR. The minor symptoms of increased intracranial pressure. 101 cases with benign intracranial hypertension. *Neurology* 1988; **38**: 1461–1464.

Other relevant entries Behçet's disease; Cerebrovascular disease: venous; Cranial nerve disease: II: Optic nerve; Empty sella syndrome; Headache: an overview; Meningitis: an overview; Multiple sclerosis; Obstructive sleep apnoea syndrome.

■ Idiopathic late-onset cerebellar ataxia

Progressive cerebellar ataxia without a family history is quite common; involvement of other central and/or peripheral nervous structures may also occur. The disease is usually relentlessly though slowly progressive, most patients eventually losing the ability to walk independently. Investigation is usually unrewarding, other than to exclude other causes of ataxia. Imaging shows some degree of cerebellar and brainstem atrophy and excludes other causes such as a posterior fossa mass lesion or hydrocephalus. Thyroid function tests, vitamin B_{12}, and tests to exclude bronchial, ovarian or breast malignancy, should be undertaken.

The suggestion that some of these patients have cerebellar atrophy secondary to gluten sensitivity, with or without enteropathy (coeliac disease: small bowel villous atrophy) has been made. So-called gluten ataxia is worth looking for, since potentially treatable (gluten-free diet) though probably uncommon. Some idiopathic late-onset cerebellar ataxia (ILOCA) patients may have the cerebellar presentation of multiple system atrophy (MSA) but this may only become apparent at postmortem; these patients may decline more quickly than those with ILOCA.

Reference Bürk K, Bösch S, Müller CA *et al.* Sporadic cerebellar ataxia associated with gluten sensitivity. *Brain* 2001; **124**: 1013–1019.

Other relevant entries Autosomal-dominant cerebellar ataxia; Cerebellar disease: an overview; Coeliac disease (gluten-sensitive enteropathy); Multiple system atrophy.

■ Idiopathic Parkinson's disease – see Parkinson's disease

■ Idiopathic recurrent stupor – see Transient unresponsiveness of the elderly

■ Idiopathic torsion dystonia – see Dystonia: an overview; Primary torsion dystonia

■ Idiot savant syndrome – see Savant syndrome

■ Iduronidase deficiency – see Hurler's disease; Scheie's syndrome

■ Iduronate-2-sulphatase deficiency – see Hunter's syndrome

■ Ilioinguinal neuropathy

Lesions of the ilioinguinal nerve, arising from the L1 and sometimes the L2 spinal roots, cause burning and stabbing pain in the inguinal region which may radiate to the genitalia and the hip. In the recumbent position, the hip is kept slightly flexed and medially rotated. Due to their proximity, the iliohypogastric and genitofemoral nerves are also often affected. The cremasteric reflex may be absent. Surgery is probably the commonest cause of neuropathy. L1 radiculopathy enters the differential diagnosis, as does primary hip joint pathology.

Other relevant entries Genitofemoral neuropathy; Neuropathies: an overview.

▓ Imerslund–Grasbeck syndrome
Cubulin deficiency

A rare condition, possibly autosomal recessive, characterized by:
- Megaloblastic anaemia.
- Proteinuria.
- Neurological features: spasticity, ataxia, brain atrophy.

The syndrome responds to parenteral vitamin B_{12} therapy, and is thought to result from a defective uptake of intrinsic factor–vitamin B_{12} complexes in the terminal ileum due to defects in a specific receptor, cubulin.

Reference Salameh MM, Benda RW, Mohdi AA. Reversal of severe neurological abnormalities after vitamin B_{12} replacement in the Imerslund–Grasbeck syndrome. *Journal of Neurology* 1991; **238**: 349–350.

Other relevant entry Vitamin B_{12} deficiency.

▓ Immunosuppressive therapy and diseases of the nervous system

Familiarity with immunosuppressive therapies is of great importance to the practising neurologist since these agents may:
- be required for the treatment of neurological disease, especially of inflammatory/immunological aetiology; sometimes there is a reasonable evidence base to support such intervention;
- predispose to neurological disease: opportunistic infection; malignancy.

Therapeutic options include:

Steroids: prednisolone, methylprednisolone.

"Steroid sparing agents" (e.g. azathioprine, cyclophosphamide).

Other immunosuppressive agents: methotrexate, ciclosporin, FK506 (tacrolimus), interferons, CAMPATH-1H.

Intravenous immunoglobulin (IVIg).

Plasma exchange.

Total body irradiation.

Immunosuppressive treatment is frequently used in the management of:

Multiple sclerosis

Myasthenia gravis.

Inflammatory neuropathies and myopathies: Guillain–Barré syndrome (GBS), chronic inflammatory demyelinating polyneuropathy (CIDP), polymyositis.

Inflammatory diseases which may affect the nervous system: sarcoidosis, SLE, Behçet's disease, giant cell arteritis, Wegener's granulomatosis.

Immunosuppressive treatment is also frequently used empirically, in diseases of uncertain aetiology, or where no other treatment is known.

Opportunistic diseases of the nervous system which may emerge in the context of immunocompromise include:

Infection
  Toxoplasmosis
  Progressive multifocal leukoencephalopathy (PML)
  Cryptococcosis
  Brain abscess.
Tumours
  Lymphoma.

(See individual entries for further details).

Reference Wiles CM, Brown P, Chapel H *et al.* Intravenous immunoglobulin in neurological disease: a specialist review. *Journal of Neurology, Neurosurgery and Psychiatry* 2002; **72**: 440–448.

Other relevant entries Ataxia telangiectasia; Common variable immunodeficiency; Guillain–Barré syndrome; HIV/AIDS and the nervous system; Kawasaki disease.

■ Inclusion body myositis

Pathophysiology This is perhaps the most common acquired myopathy of middle-aged and elderly patients, especially men (F : M = 1 : 5), often presenting with isolated quadriceps weakness. Although classified with the inflammatory myopathies, its pathogenesis is uncertain; it is resistant to immunosuppressive therapy. The resemblance of muscle histology to certain of the features seen in Alzheimer's disease brain prompts the suggestion that this may be a degenerative condition with an inflammatory component.

Clinical features: history and examination

- Weakness, often of quadriceps; distal weakness also seen (e.g. finger flexors, ankle dorsiflexors); involvement often asymmetric. Individual muscles may seem to be "picked out".
- Dysphagia.
- +/− concurrent autoimmune disorder: for example Sjögren's syndrome.

Investigations and diagnosis *Bloods*: creatine kinase may be moderately elevated.
Neurophysiology: EMG/NCS: myopathic, fibrillation potentials, positive sharp waves.
Muscle biopsy: diagnostic test, showing endomysial inflammatory infiltrates, predominantly of T-cell origin, rimmed vacuoles, eosinophilic cytoplasmic inclusions, ragged red fibres, A β-amyloid within or next to vacuoles; filaments of phosphorylated τ-protein in cytoplasm or nuclei on electron microscopy.

Differential diagnosis

Other inflammatory myopathies: polymyositis, dermatomyositis.
Absence of sensory features makes neuropathic conditions (e.g. brachial, lumbar plexopathy) unlikely.

Treatment and prognosis No specific therapy shown to be of benefit; immunosuppression [steroids, intravenous immunoglobulin (IVIg)] often tried.

> **Reference** Askanas V, Engel WK. Inclusion body myositis and myopathies: different aetiologies, possibly similar pathogenic mechanisms. *Current Opinion in Neurology* 2002; **15**: 525–531.

> **Other relevant entries** Alzheimer's disease; Dermatomyositis; Immunosuppressive therapy and diseases of the nervous system; Myositis; Polymyositis.

■ Incontinentia pigmenti (achromians)

Bloch–Sulzberger syndrome ● Hypomelanosis of Ito

A neurocutaneous syndrome, third only to neurofibromatosis and tuberous sclerosis in frequency, yet rare; possibly a disorder of neuroblast migration. It may manifest with dermatological, neurological, skeletal, and ocular features:

- Hypopigmented/depigmented streaks or whorls in the skin, following the lines of Blaschko (best seen using Woods light).
- Cerebral and cerebellar developmental abnormalities: mental retardation, seizures.
- Arteriovenous malformations.
- Tumours: medulloblastoma, choroid plexus papilloma.
- Dental dysplasia, conical teeth.
- Alopecia.

In most cases it is due to a large-scale deletion of exons in the NEMO gene.

> Symptomatic treatment for seizures is possible.

> **Other relevant entries** Goltz syndrome; Phakomatosis.

■ Infantile spasms – see West's syndrome

■ Infection and the nervous system: an overview

Pathophysiology Infection of the nervous system may produce inflammatory change, either directly or as a consequence of infection (postinfectious, parainfectious), at different sites:

Brain: encephalitis
Meninges: meningitis
Spinal cord: myelitis
Nerve roots: radiculitis

Plexi: plexitis
Peripheral nerves: neuritis
Muscle: myositis
Combinations: for example meningoencephalitis, encephalomyelitis

Focal or localized infection may occur in the form of an abscess (*q.v.*):

Intraparenchymal: cranial, spinal cord;
Parameningeal spaces:
    Epidural/extradural: cranial, spinal
    Subdural: cranial/spinal.

Microbial agents responsible for infection may be:

Bacterial: for example
    Pyogenic bacteria: *Streptococcus, Meningococcus, Haemophilus influenzae*, etc.
    Toxin producing bacteria: botulism, tetanus, diphtheria
    Zoonoses: brucellosis, anthrax
    Enteric bacteria: Campylobacter, Whipple's disease
    Mycobacteria: TB, leprosy
    Spirochaetes: syphilis, borreliosis
    Rickettsia
    Respiratory pathogens: mycoplasma
    Actinomycetes: Nocardia, Actinomycosis.
Viral: for example
    Herpesviruses: Herpes simplex, Epstein–Barr virus (EBV), cytomegalovirus
        (CMV), Varicella zoster virus (VZV)
    Rabies
    Poliovirus
    Arboviruses
    Measles
    Rubella
    Retroviruses : HIV, HTLV-1.
Fungal: for example
    Cryptococcus
    Coccidiodomycosis
    Histoplasmosis
    Candidosis
    Aspergillosis
    Mucormycosis.
Protozoal/parasitic: for example
    Malaria
    Toxoplasmosis

Trypanosomiasis

Helminths.

Clinical features: history and examination See individual entries for further details.

Investigations and diagnosis If an infective aetiology for neurological disease is suspected, then confirmation may be achieved by:

Bloods: some organisms may be identified by culture; serology for specific organism: paired samples with changing titres of antibodies may be required for some diagnoses. PCR is highly sensitive and specific for some organisms.

Urine: some organisms may be cultured from urine.

CSF: specific staining methods (Gram, Ziehl–Nielsen, indian ink); culture; PCR.

Tissue: in some circumstances, tissue may be required for diagnosis.

Occasionally, despite best efforts, organisms may not be identified. Therapeutic response to empirical therapy may sometimes be the only evidence in favour of an infective aetiology (e.g. tuberculosis).

Immunosuppression increases susceptibility to infection, and some inherited metabolic diseases seem particularly associated with certain infective complications (e.g. *E. coli* sepsis in infants with galactosaemia): dependent on context, additional investigations to seek underlying immunosuppressive or metabolic disorders may be required.

Differential diagnosis Other inflammatory, non-infectious, disorders may mainfest in similar ways, for example connective tissue diseases, sarcoidosis; paraneoplasia.

Treatment and prognosis Of cause where identified, although occasionally "best guess" treatment may be given before investigation if index of suspicion is high (e.g. meningococcal meningitis, herpes simplex encephalitis), or empirical therapy may be given when no microbial diagnosis forthcoming (e.g. tuberculosis).

Reference Roos KL. Central nervous system infections. In: Biller J (ed.). *Practical Neurology* (2nd edition). Philadelphia: Lippincott Williams & Wilkins, 2002: 562–573.

Other relevant entries Abscess: an overview; Aseptic meningitis; "Atypical pneumonias" and the nervous system; Encephalitis: an overview; Encephalomyelitis: differential diagnosis; Galactosaemia; Helminthic disease; Herpes simplex encephalitis; HIV/AIDS and the nervous system; Immunosuppressive therapy and diseases of the nervous system; Meningitis: an overview; Myelitis: an overview; Myositis; Parameningeal infection; Rickettsial diseases; Tuberculosis and the nervous system.

■ Infectious mononucleosis and the nervous system – see Epstein–Barr virus infection and the nervous system

◼ Infective endocarditis – see Endocarditis and the nervous system

◼ Inflammatory bowel disease and the nervous system – see Gastrointestinal disease and the nervous system

◼ Inherited metabolic diseases and the nervous system
Neurometabolic disorders

Progressive diseases of the nervous system as a result of inborn errors of metabolism are individually rare but collectively common. They most usually present in infancy, with developmental slowing or regression, acute or chronic encephalopathy, stroke-like episodes, myopathy, seizure disorder, movement disorder, or some combination thereof. Metabolic acidosis, sometimes lactic acidosis or ketoacidosis, may be a prominent feature. Hepatocellular dysfunction and cardiomyopathy may also occur. Dysmorphism, classically associated with "metabolic-storage disorders", may also be present, along with visceromegaly, skin changes, and radiologically evident bone changes. A family history of sudden infant death or unexplained illness may also raise clinical suspicion.

The number of possible diagnoses, and hence the appropriate investigations to be considered, is large, requiring the input of someone familiar with the art.

Within this category may be included:

Aminoacidopathies (*q.v.*): for example
  Phenylketonuria, Homocystinuria, Tyrosinaemia
  Maple syrup urine disease; Urea cycle enzyme disorders.
Organic acidopathies (*q.v.*): for example
  Canavan's disease
  Glutaric aciduria.
Mitochondrial disorders (*q.v.*): for example
  Pyruvate carboxylase (PC) deficiency
  Pyruvate dehydrogenase (PDH) deficiency
  Respiratory chain defects: Leigh's disease, Leber's hereditary optic neuropathy
    (LHON), Kearns–Sayre syndrome (KSS), MELAS, MERRF, MNGIE
  Fatty acid oxidation defects (*q.v.*).
Peroxisomal disorders (*q.v.*): for example
  Zellweger syndrome
  Adrenoleukodystrophy (X-ALD)
  Refsum's disease.
Lysosomal disorders (*q.v.*): for example
  Mucopolysaccharidoses
  Mucolipidoses

Sialidoses
Niemann–Pick disease
Gaucher's disease
Gangliosidoses
Neuronal ceroid lipofuscinoses.
DNA repair defects: for example
Cockayne syndrome
Xeroderma pigmentosa
Ataxia telangiectasia.
Metals: for example
Wilson's disease, Menkes' disease, Hallervorden–Spatz disease.
Lipoproteins: for example
Abetalipoproteinaemia, Tangier disease.
Transport defects: for example
Lowe syndrome, Hartnup's disease.
Leukodystrophies (q.v.): for example
Metachromatic leukodystrophy, Pelizaeus–Merzbacher disease.
Carbohydrate disorders: for example
Galactosaemia, Hereditary fructose intolerance.
Porphyrias (q.v.).

**Clinical features: history and examination/investigations and diagnosis/
differential diagnosis/treatment and prognosis** See individual entries for further
details.

   References Clarke JTR. *A Clinical Guide to Inherited Metabolic Diseases* (2nd edition). Cambridge: CUP, 2002.

   Gray RG, Preece MA, Green SH *et al.* Inborn errors in metabolism as a cause of neurological disease in adults: an approach to investigation. *Journal of Neurology, Neurosurgery and Psychiatry* 2000; **69**: 5–12.

   Lyon G, Adams RD, Kolodny EH. *Neurology of Hereditary Metabolic Diseases of Children* (2nd edition). New York: McGraw-Hill, 1996.

   Swanson PD. Diagnosis of inherited metabolic disorders affecting the nervous system. *Journal of Neurology, Neurosurgery and Psychiatry* 1995; **59**: 460–470.

Other relevant entries Aminoacidopathies: an overview; Fatty acid oxidation defects; Gangliosidoses: an overview; Leukodystrophies: an overview; Lysosomal-storage disorders: an overview; Metabolic-storage disorders: an overview; Mitochondrial disease: an overview; Organic acidopathies; Peroxisomal disorders: an overview; Porphyria; Sialidoses: an overview; Urea cycle enzyme defects.

■ **Inner ear disease – see Vestibular disorders: an overview**

▓ Insomnia

Total insomnia of long duration, or agrypnia, may occur in a number of conditions, including:

Prion disorders: fatal familial insomnia; sporadic fatal insomnia.
Autoimmune conditions: Morvan's syndrome; relapsing–remitting agrypnia.
Trauma: brainstem, thalamus.
Von Economo's disease.
Trypanosomiasis.
Delirium tremens.

However, probably the commonest cause of patient complaint of insomnia is poor sleep hygiene. A sleep disorder resulting in daytime somnolence should be considered.

Other relevant entries Fatal familial insomnia; Morvan's syndrome; Sleep disorders: an overview.

▓ Internuclear ophthalmoplegia

Ataxic nystagmus • Medial longitudinal fasciculus syndrome

Internuclear ophthalmoplegia consists of:
• ipsilateral weakness of eye adduction;
• contralateral nystagmus of the abducting eye (ataxic or dissociated nystagmus);
• preserved convergence.

These abnormalities may be obvious with examination of pursuit eye movements, but may be better seen when testing reflexive saccades or optokinetic responses, the adducting eye "lagging" behind the abducting eye. Internuclear ophthalmoplegia (INO) may be unilateral or bilateral, asymptomatic or, rarely, may cause diplopia, oscillopsia, or a skew deviation. The patho-anatomical substrate is the medial longitudinal fasciculus, a pathway linking the nuclei of cranial ocular motor nerves (III, IV, VI).

Causes of INO include:
• multiple sclerosis (particularly in young patients)
• cerebrovascular disease (particularly in older patients)
• Wernicke–Korsakoff's syndrome
• encephalitis
• trauma
• paraneoplasia.

Pseudo-internuclear ophthalmoplegia may occur in myasthenia gravis.

Other relevant entries Cranial nerve disease: III: Oculomotor; Cranial nerve disease: VI: Abducens; Multiple sclerosis; Myasthenia gravis; Ophthalmoplegia; Wernicke–Korsakoff's syndrome.

■ Intervertebral disc prolapse

Pathophysiology With increasing age, the intervertebral discs become increasingly dehydrated and liable to herniate into the spinal canal and/or intervertebral foramina, especially in the cervical and lumbar regions, with resultant myelopathy and/or radiculopathy. Concurrent spondylotic change is frequent, although seldom the cause of neurological symptoms and signs *per se*.

Disc prolapse may be (in order of frequency):

- Posterolateral/paracentral: compressing nerve roots in lateral recess of spinal canal.
- Lateral/foraminal: nerve root compressed against vertebral pedicle in intervertebral foramen.
- Central: unusual because posterior longitudinal ligament reinforces this area, hence has to be ruptured for disc to prolapse in this direction; may cause cord or cauda equina syndrome; former may present with sudden urinary incontinence with paucity of other neurological findings.

In terms of frequency, roots affected by disc prolapse are lumbar > cervical >> thoracic.

Clinical features: history and examination Prolapse leading to root compression produces a syndrome of:

Pain: in radicular distribution (e.g. sciatica); knife-like, aggravated by actions which raise intraspinal pressure (coughing, sneezing, straining at stool).

Sensory impairment/loss: in dermatomal distribution.

Motor features: weakness in the affected myotome, $+/-$ depression or loss of reflex subserved by affected root.

Investigations and diagnosis *Imaging*: MRI is modality of choice to visualize herniated disc material and bony anatomy; CT-myelography is an option (e.g. patients too large for MR scanner, claustrophobic individuals).

Neurophysiology: EMG/NCS: EMG fibrillation potentials in two or more muscles innervated by the same root, preferably via different peripheral nerves, and no abnormalities in muscles innervated by rostral and caudal neighbours of affected root is diagnostic; especially true for C5, C7, C8. However, fibrillation potentials take 2–3 weeks to develop, so not useful in the acute situation. Sensory nerve action potentials are preserved in radiculopathies (*cf.* plexopathy, peripheral neuropathy).

CSF: protein may be elevated; not essential if MRI available.

Differential diagnosis Other causes of limb pain, sensory impairment, weakness: plexopathy, diabetic polyradiculoneuropathy ("diabetic amyotrophy"), focal nerve entrapment syndrome (e.g. carpal tunnel syndrome).

Treatment and prognosis Conservative treatment: rest, analgesia, gentle exercise; cervical collar for cervical radiculopathy.

Surgery: indicated if cauda equina syndrome (may be urgent especially if presentation is with loss of sphincter function); severe and/or progressive neurological deficit; severe pain continues after 4–6 weeks of conservative treatment.

Reference McCormick PC. Intervertebral discs and radiculopathy. In: Rowland LP (ed.). *Merritt's Textbook of Neurology* (9th edition). Baltimore: Williams & Wilkins, 1995: 447–455.

Other relevant entries Cervical cord and root disease; Low back pain: an overview; Lumbar cord and root disease; Myelopathy: an overview; Radiculopathies: an overview; Sciatica.

▉ Intracerebral haemorrhage

Pathophysiology Haemorrhage accounts for around 15% of all strokes (*cf.* 80% ischaemic), and is commoner in men than women. Mortality remains high, as does morbidity. Search for a potential cause is important because this may determine treatment.

Recognized causes of intracerebral haemorrhage include:

Head trauma (may be occult).
Hypertension: common sites are basal ganglia, thalamus, pons, cerebellum, lobar.
Haemorrhagic transformation of ischaemic stroke.
Aneurysm: usually saccular, but consider also mycotic (infective endocarditis).
Vascular malformations: arteriovenous malformations, cavernous angioma.
Moyamoya.
Drugs: amphetamines, cocaine, Ecstasy.
Tumour: primary, metastasis.
Cerebral amyloid angiopathy.
Vasculitis: primary; secondary to drugs, infection (herpes zoster, HIV).
Cerebral venous (sinus) thrombosis.
Bleeding diathesis: thrombocytopenia, haemophilia, sickle-cell disease; therapeutic anticoagulation: risk factors are intensity of anticoagulation, age, hypertension, insulin-dependent diabetes mellitus, leukoaraiosis.

Clinical features: history and examination Although there are no completely reliable clinical criteria to distinguish cerebral haemorrhage from cerebral ischaemia, the possibility of the former should be considered if there is:

Sudden onset (simplistically: bleed = event; atherothrombosis = process)
Intense headache
Accompanying features: nausea, vomiting, prostration
Disturbed consciousness.

Investigations and diagnosis *Imaging*: immediate CT is usually adequate to diagnose intracerebral haemorrhage; may need to be repeated if there is further clinical deterioration (rebleed, hydrocephalus).

Additional investigations are aimed at ascertaining cause and/or managing the consequences:

Bloods: FBC, ESR, electrolytes, glucose, clotting studies; urgent INR if receiving warfarin; arterial blood gases if hypoxia or respiratory failure suspected; blood cultures if infective endocarditis suspected.

Imaging: MRI: for age of haemorrhage; MRA, catheter angiography: possible aneurysms, vasculitis.

Urine: levels of recreational drugs.

Other: echocardiography if infective endocarditis suspected; brain biopsy if vasculitis suspected.

Differential diagnosis Ischaemic stroke.

Treatment and prognosis

Acute:

ABC of life support; oxygen for hypoxia; correct hyper- or hypoglycaemia, thrombocytopenia if profound; reverse excessive therapeutic anticoagulation.

Monitor vital signs, neurological signs.

Control arterial hypertension: labetalol, nitroprusside, hydralazine, enalapril.

Treat raised intracranial pressure.

Surgical evacuation: indications not certain, other than cerebellar haemorrhage compressing the brainstem or obstructing CSF pathways. Ventricular shunt for secondary hydrocephalus.

Cause-specific treatment: clipping of aneurysms; anticoagulation may be favoured for cerebral venous thrombosis even in the presence of cerebral haemorrhage.

Reference Adams Jr HP, Shoaib MA. Hemorrhagic cerebrovascular disease. In: Biller J (ed.). *Practical Neurology* (2nd edition). Philadelphia: Lippincott Williams & Wilkins, 2002: 456–468.

Other relevant entries Cerebral amyloid angiopathy; Cerebrovascular disease: arterial; Cerebrovascular disease: venous; Hydrocephalus; Hypertension and the nervous system; Moyamoya.

■ Intracranial vascular malformations: an overview

A wide terminology has been applied to vascular malformations, and not always in a standardized way. A recent classification draws a clear distinction between: "malformations" in which there is normal endothelial cell turnover, and growth, if it occurs at all, is by hypertrophy; and haemangiomas, in which endothelial hyperplasia occurs. In arteriovenous malformations (AVM), there is a tangled anastomosis of vessels, whereas in an arteriovenous fistula (AVF) there is a direct high flow connection between artery and vein. Malformations and fistulas may be in the brain parenchyma or in the dura.

- Benign proliferating vascular anomalies
    Haemangioma.
- Non-proliferating vascular anomalies
    Capillary malformation: telangiectasis.
    Venous malformation: developmental venous anomaly.
    Cavernous malformation: cavernoma.
    Arterial malformation: angiodysplasia, aneurysm.
    Arteriovenous shunting: brain AVM, brain AVF, dural AVF, vein of Galen AVF.
    Mixed malformations.

Reference Chaloupka JC, Huddle DC. Classification of vascular malformations of the central nervous system. *Neuroimaging Clinics of North America* 1998; **8**: 295–321.

Other relevant entries Arteriovenous malformations of the brain; Spinal cord vascular diseases.

Intravascular lymphomatosis – see Angioendotheliomatosis

Isaacs syndrome – see Neuromyotonia

Ischaemic optic neuropathy

Pathophysiology Ischaemic optic neuropathy may be described as anterior or posterior.
- Anterior ischaemic optic neuropathy:
    causes subacute monocular visual loss; it may be non-arteritic(ischaemic, atheromatous) or arteritic (giant cell arteritis) in origin. The main difference between the two forms is age at onset, arteritic ischaemic optic neuropathy (ION) being a disease of the elderly. There is a high risk of involvement of the contralateral eye within 2 years (*ca.* 40%).
- Posterior ischaemic optic neuropathy:
    less common; retrobulbar optic nerve infarction most often occurs in the context of severe perioperative hypotension, although embolism and migraine are sometimes implicated.

Clinical features: history and examination
- Painless visual loss, either subacute +/− stepwise, but occasionally sudden (more likely with arteritic cause).
- Systemic symptoms (headache, tender scalp, jaw claudication, aching shoulders and hips, weight loss, fever, night sweats) may suggest arteritic cause.
- Visual field defect: central scotoma, altitudinal defect, inferior nasal quadrantic field defect; relative afferent pupillary defect may be present.
- Fundoscopy: acute optic disc swelling (oedema), may be sectoral rather than general, +/− haemorrhage, followed by atrophy; pseudo-Foster–Kennedy syndrome may be seen if there is previous involvement of contralateral eye.

- Risk factors: of vascular disease; anatomical predisposition: low hypermetropic eyes with small optic discs with low cup-disc ratio ("the disc at risk").

Investigations and diagnosis *Bloods*: ESR, CRP to exclude arteritic cause. Biopsy of temporal artery to exclude giant cell arteritis.

Differential diagnosis

Optic neuritis: disc haemorrhages less common than in ION.

Optic nerve compression.

Leber's hereditary optic neuropathy (LHON).

Treatment and prognosis Arteritic cases: treatment as for giant cell arteritis, viz. prednisolone 80–120 mg/day, usually resolves symptoms.

Non-arteritic cases: reduce intraocular pressure to increase optic nerve head perfusion with oral or topical carbonic anhydrase inhibitors; identify and treat vascular risk factors; steroids are also often given although there is no strong evidence of efficacy.

There may be no or incomplete improvement in vision.

There is a high risk of involvement of the contralateral eye within 2 years; no prophylactic treatment known, other than control of risk factors.

> **Reference** Hayreh SS. Anterior ischemic optic neuropathy. *Archives of Neurology* 1981; **38**: 675–678.

> **Other relevant entries** Giant cell arteritis; Leber's hereditary optic neuropathy; Visual loss: differential diagnosis.

■ Isolated angiitis of the central nervous system
Primary angiitis of the central nervous system (PACNS)

Pathophysiology A very rare granulomatous angiitis, confined to the central nervous system (hence "isolated"), affecting small leptomeningeal, cortical and spinal blood vessels. It may on occasion be associated with herpes zoster infection and lymphoma.

Clinical features: history and examination
- Subacute encephalopathy: headache, confusion, cognitive decline.
- Seizures.
- Stroke: ischaemia > haemorrhage.
- +/− myelopathy.
- +/− radiculopathy.
- Systemic symptoms (rare): fever.

Investigations and diagnosis *Bloods*: may be raised ESR.

Imaging: often normal or non-specific; angiography non-specific.

CSF: may show raised protein, lymphocytosis.

Tissue required for diagnosis: meningeal + cortical biopsy.

Differential diagnosis Sarcoidosis may cause a very similar angiitis.

Treatment and prognosis Immunosuppression is usually given, but efficacy is uncertain. Cases of spontaneous resolution have been claimed. More usually death occurs in weeks or months.

References Hankey GJ. Isolated angiitis/angiopathy of the central nervous system. *Cerebrovascular Diseases* 1991; **1**: 2–15.

Schmidley JW. *Central Nervous System Angiitis*. Boston: Butterworth-Heinemann, 2000.

Other relevant entries Cerebrovascular disease: arterial; Sarcoidosis.

■ Isovaleric acidaemia

A disorder of organic acid metabolism, due to a defect in isovaleryl–CoA dehydrogenase, often presenting in the first few weeks of life with:

- Encephalopathy + metabolic acidosis
- Peculiar odour, likened to sweaty feet
- Hyperammonaemia, reduced plasma carnitine, increased glycine
- Neutropenia, thrombocytopenia
- Ketonuria
- Urine organic acid analysis shows a typical, diagnostic pattern.

Clinically the condition may be indistinguishable from other disorders of organic acid metabolism such as methylmalonic aciduria and propionic aciduria.

Treatment is with dietary restriction of isoleucine, valine, methionine and threonine, with carnitine and glycine supplementation. Death within the first year is common.

Other relevant entries Methylmalonic acidaemia; Organic acidopathies; Propionic acidaemia.

Jj

■ Jackson's syndrome

This is the eponym given to a syndrome involving homolateral cranial nerves X, XI, and XII, usually by an extramedullary lesion before the nerve roots leave the skull, which causes paresis of palate, pharynx, larynx, trapezius, sternocleidomastoid, and tongue. It may be differentiated from the syndromes of Schmidt (no XII involvement), Tapia (no XI involvement), Collet–Sicard (additional IX involvement), and Villaret (additional IX and cervical sympathetic involvement).

Other relevant entries Cranial polyneuropathy; Jugular foramen syndrome.

■ Jacksonian fit

Partial seizures arising in the precentral gyrus may manifest as jerking movements which progress, or "march", from one part of the body to another as the abnormal electrical discharge spreads over the motor strip homunculus, a phenomenon first described by Hughlings Jackson. For example, a seizure commencing in the hand may pass sequentially up the arm and down the leg, or one beginning in the foot may pass up the leg and down the arm, following the cortical representation of these structures. The march may take some time, a clue in differentiating Jacksonian fits from the briefer but morphologically similar events which originate in the supplementary motor area.

Such seizures with focal origin mandate cerebral imaging in search of a focal lesion.

Other relevant entry Epilepsy: an overview.

▥ Jadassohn's naevus phakomatosis – see Epidermal naevus syndrome

▥ Jamaican neuritis – see Strachan's syndrome

▥ Jansky–Bielchowsky disease – see Neuronal ceroid lipofuscinosis

▥ Janz syndrome – see Juvenile myoclonic epilepsy

▥ Japanese encephalitis

Pathophysiology Japanese encephalitis (formerly known as Japanese type B encephalitis) is a typical example of the zoonotic arboviral encephalitides, all of which produce similar symptoms and signs but differ in their animal reservoir, vector of infection, geographical distribution, and seasonal appearance.

Japanese encephalitis is caused by an RNA flavivirus which has its reservoir in pigs, birds (heron, egrets), cows, and buffalo, and is spread by mosquitoes, most commonly *Culex* (typically *C. tritaenorrhyncus*) but also *Anopheles*. It causes disease epidemics in the monsoon months in Asia. Young children and adolescents are most at risk of infection.

After the mosquito bite, there is a systemic viraemia, the neurotropic virus entering the central nervous system (CNS) via vascular endothelium, causing a meningoencephalitic illness characterized pathologically by grey and white matter involvement, neuronolysis, T-cell inflammation, and early intrathecal IgM antibody synthesis. There is a significant mortality and morbidity.

Clinical features: history and examination

- Few infected individuals develop encephalitis. The incubation period is 1–2 weeks.
- *Prodromal phase*: headache, malaise, fever, anorexia, vomiting; lasts 2–3 days.
- *Acute encephalitic phase*: altered consciousness, seizures, meningism (variable) +/– focal neurological deficits; cranial nerve palsies, papilloedema,

both rare; lasts 2–4 days. A poliomyelitis-like illness, with flaccid paralysis, has been reported, which may meet the clinical case definition of Guillain–Barré syndrome.

- *Early recovery stage/defervescence*: lasts 7–10 days.
- *Convalescent stage*: 1–2 months or longer.

Investigations and diagnosis *Bloods*: polymorphonuclear leukocytosis with lymphopenia. Rising antibody titres in serum are the diagnostic test. Virus may be isolated.

Imaging: CT/MRI is usually normal; may show low-density lesions.

CSF: leukocytosis, initially neutrophilia, then lymphocytosis. Glucose normal, protein raised. Virus may be isolated.

EEG: generalized slowing $+/-$ spikes.

Pathology: brain biopsy, post-mortem: circumvascular necrolysis, microglial infiltration.

Differential diagnosis

Other viral encephalitides.

Pyogenic, tuberculosis (TB) meningitis.

Other bacterial and fungal infections.

Cerebral malaria.

Febrile convulsions.

Reye's syndrome.

Herpes simpex encephalitis.

Poliomyelitis, Guillain–Barré syndrome.

Treatment and prognosis Supportive therapy only.

Fatality rate: 5–50%. Neurological sequelae in up to a third of patients, especially the very young and old, usually consisting of seizures, cognitive impairment, ataxia, paralysis (poliomyelitis-like picture), and parkinsonism. Personality change.

Prevention is the best treatment: options include eradication of the mosquito vector and vaccination of at risk individuals or animal reservoirs. All are difficult to achieve.

References Bu'lock FA. Japanese B virus encephalitis in India – a growing problem. *Quarterly Journal of Medicine* 1986; **60(233)**: 825–836.

Solomon T, Dung NM, Kneen R, Gainsborough M, Vaughn DW, Khanh VT. Japanese encephalitis. *Journal of Neurology, Neurosurgery and Psychiatry* 2000; **68**: 405–415.

Other relevant entries Encephalitis: an overview; Malaria; Meningitis: an overview; Tuberculosis and the nervous system.

Jeavons syndrome
Eyelid myoclonia with absences

A reflex idiopathic generalized epilepsy syndrome characterized by the triad of:
- eyelid myoclonia with or without absences;
- eye closure-induced seizures, EEG paroxysms, or both;
- photosensitivity.

Eyelid myoclonia, marked jerking of the eyelids, is the clinical hallmark, with or without brief absence seizures lasting a few seconds. Generalized tonic–clonic seizures may occur, myoclonic jerks are rare. Investigations are normal with the exception of the EEG which shows brief high amplitude generalized discharges related to eye closure. Concurrent video may show the eyelid myoclonia with or without absences. Eyelid myoclonia may be confused with facial tics, eye closure in other forms of idiopathic generalized epilepsy, and eyelid jerking in typical absence seizures or juvenile myoclonic epilepsy. Treatment with sodium valproate, with or without clonazepam or ethosuximide, is probably most effective.

Although distinctive, Jeavons syndrome does not feature in the current ILAE classification of epileptic seizures.

References Duncan JS, Panayiotopoulos CP (eds). *Eyelid Myoclonia with Absences*. London: John Libbey, 1996.

Jensen syndrome – see Mohr–Tranebjaerg syndrome

Jerking stiff man syndrome – see Stiff people: an overview

Jervell–Lange–Nielsen syndrome – see Prolonged QT syndromes

Jeune–Tommasi syndrome

One of the syndromes of hearing loss and ataxia, accompanied by mental retardation and pigmentary skin changes, with an autosomal-recessive pattern of inheritance.

Other relevant entries Hearing loss: differential diagnosis; Lichtenstein–Knorr syndrome; Richards–Rundle syndrome.

Jolliffe syndrome – see Pellagra

Joseph disease – see Machado–Joseph disease

Joubert's syndrome

This is a congenital inherited (autosomal-recessive) cerebellar ataxia; additional features include episodic hyperpnoea or panting tachypnoea, abnormal eye movements $+/-$ ocular abnormalities, and mental retardation. Pathologically there is dysgenesis of the cerebellar vermis.

References Joubert M, Eisenring JJ, Robb JP *et al*. Familial agenesis of the cerebellar vermis. *Neurology* 1969; **19**: 813–825.

Other relevant entries Cerebellar disease: an overview; Gillespie's syndrome; Paine's syndrome.

■ Jugular foramen syndrome

Skull base lesions at or around the jugular foramen may involve various combinations of the glossopharyngeal (IX), vagus (X), and accessory (XI) cranial nerves.

The clinical features are:

- ipsilateral weakness and atrophy of sternocleidomastoid and trapezius due to accessory nerve involvement (atrophy may be the more evident, hence the importance of palpating the muscle bellies);
- dysphagia, dysphonia, palatal droop, impaired gag reflex; ipsilateral reduced taste sensation on the posterior third of the tongue, and anaesthesia of the posterior third of the tongue, soft palate, pharynx, larynx, and uvula, due to glossopharyngeal and vagus nerve involvement.

The term may sometimes be used synonymously with Vernet's syndrome.

Recognized causes of a jugular foramen syndrome include:

skull base trauma/fracture,
glomus jugulare and nasopharyngeal tumours,
inflammatory/infective collection at the skull base (e.g. sarcoidosis),
ischaemia.

The differential diagnosis includes a variety of other syndromes involving the lower cranial nerves (IX–XII), with or without involvement of the sympathetic chain. These include:

- Collet–Sicard syndrome: IX, X, XI, XII; retroparotid space-occupying lesions, either intra- or extracranial.
- Villaret's syndrome: IX, X, XI, XII + sympathetic chain (i.e. Collet–Sicard syndrome + sympathetic palsy) +/− facial nerve (VII); retropharyngeal or retroparotid space-occupying lesions.
- Lannois–Jouty syndrome: IX, X, XI, XII; skull base lesion.
- Mackenzie syndrome: IX, X, XI, XII + Horner's syndrome: retroparotid space tumour.
- Jackson's syndrome: X, XI, XII; may be intraparenchymal (medulla) and usually intracranial before nerve fibres leave the skull.
- Schmidt's syndrome: X, XI; usually intracranial lesion, before nerve fibres leave the skull.
- Tapia syndrome: X, XII +/− XI, sympathetic.
- Avellis syndrome: brainstem syndrome with X involvement.
- Garcin syndrome: all cranial nerves on one side.

Fractures of the skull base which extend to the jugular foramen with paralysis of IX, X, and XI may go by the name of Siebenmann's syndrome.

The definition of particular eponymous syndromes is perhaps of little importance for management, which will be based on MRI findings.

Other relevant entries Cranial polyneuropathy; Collet–Sicard syndrome; Vernet's syndrome; Villaret's syndrome.

■ Jumping Frenchman of Maine – see Startle syndromes

■ Juvenile dystonic lipidosis – see Niemann–Pick disease

■ Juvenile myoclonic epilepsy
Janz syndrome

Pathophysiology A subtype of idiopathic generalized epilepsy with onset usually between 8 and 20 years of age. A genetic linkage to chromosome 6 has been suggested, but is disputed.

Clinical features: history and examination

- Myoclonic jerks, especially in the morning, of variable intensity ranging from simple twitching ("flying saucer syndrome") to falls; consciousness not impaired.
- Generalized tonic–clonic seizures, especially in the morning, after waking.
- Typical absences may also occur, usually prior to myoclonic jerks.
- Myoclonic and tonic–clonic attacks may be precipitated by alcohol and sleep deprivation.
- Normal intelligence.
- First degree relatives often have a seizure disorder.

Investigations and diagnosis *EEG*: generalized spikes, 4–6 Hz spike and wave, and multiple spike ("polyspike") discharges.

Treatment and prognosis Sodium valproate is the drug of choice for both seizures and myoclonus. The syndrome does not remit, so treatment is generally lifelong. For those not controlled by valproate, options include lamotrigine and levetiracetam.

References Grunewald RA, Panayiotopoulos CP. Juvenile myoclonic epilepsy.
A review. *Archives of Neurology* 1993; **50**: 594–598.

Renganathan R, Delanty N. Juvenile myoclonic epilepsy: under-appreciated and under-diagnosed. *Postgraduate Medical Journal* 2003; **79**: 78–80.

Schmitz B, Sander T (eds). *Juvenile Myoclonic Epilepsy: The Janz Syndrome.*
Petersfield: Wrightson, 2000.

Other relevant entries Epilepsy: an overview; Myoclonus.

Kk

■ Kahlbaum's syndrome – see Catatonia

■ Kallmann's syndrome
Olfactogenital dysplasia • X-linked hypogonadotrophic hypogonadism

An X-linked syndrome of:

congenital anosmia: congenital absence or hypoplasia of primary-receptor neurones;
hypogonadotrophic hypogonadism.

Clinically there may also be mirror movements.

Brain imaging may show arhinencephaly.

> **Reference** Mayston MJ, Harrison LM, Quinton R, Stephens JA, Krams M,
> Bouloux P-MG. Mirror movements in X-linked Kallmann's syndrome. I.
> A neurophysiological study. *Brain* 1997; **120**: 1199–1216.

> **Other relevant entries** Arhinencephaly; Cranial nerve disease: I: Olfactory nerve.

◼ Kanner syndrome – see Autism, autistic disorder

◼ Kawasaki's disease

This is an acute febrile disease of childhood characterized by:

  conjunctival injection;
  dry lips, "strawberry tongue";
  cervical lymphadenopathy;
  Polymorphic skin rash;
  $+/-$ pancarditis, coronary arteritis.

Neurological features may include:

  aseptic meningitis;
  hemiplegic stroke;
  encephalopathy;
  facial palsy.

Pathologically, Kawasaki's disease is an acute systemic inflammatory vasculitis. Anti-endothelial cell antibodies may be found in the serum, which may be pathogenic for vascular injury. Whatever, treatment with intravenous immunoglobulin (IVIg) is of therapeutic benefit, and this is one of the few conditions deemed to have class I evidence for efficacy of IVIg.

> **Reference** Nadeau SE. Neurologic manifestations of systemic vasculitis.
> *Neurologic Clinics* 2002; **20**: 123–150.

> **Other relevant entries** Immunosuppressive therapy and diseases of the nervous
> system; Vasculitis.

◼ Kearns–Sayre syndrome
Oculocraniosomatic syndrome

Pathophysiology Kearns–Sayre syndrome (KSS) is a mitochondrial disease usually caused by large rearrangements of the mitochondrial genome. Its clinical features overlap in some ways with the chronic progressive external ophthalmoplegia (CPEO) phenotype, but onset is earlier.

Clinical features: history and examination Features deemed by some authorities as invariable are:

onset before 15 or 20 years of age;
ophthalmoplegia;
retinal pigmentary degeneration.

Other features include:

cerebellar dysfunction;
cardiac conduction deficits (often heart block);
raised CSF protein.

These six features have been seen as defining criteria by some authors. Other features may also be present, suggesting overlap with other mitochondrial disorders. The term "ophthalmoplegia plus" has sometimes been used:

+ / − psychomotor regression;
+ / − sensorineural deafness;
+ / − short stature;
+ / − lactic acidosis;
+ / − seizures;
+ / − cardiomyopathy (may be delayed for years);
+ / − diabetes mellitus;
+ / − calcification of the basal ganglia.

Investigations and diagnosis *Bloods*: raised lactate.
Imaging: degenerative change may be seen, for example cerebellar atrophy; calcification of the basal ganglia.
CSF: raised lactate, protein.
Neurophysiology: EEG – a variety of abnormalities may be seen.
ECG: for evidence of cardiac conduction disorder.
Muscle biopsy: ragged red fibres on Gomori trichrome stain; cytochrome-*c* oxidase deficiency.
Neurogenetics: deletions within mtDNA may be found in a wide variety of tissues.
Others: ophthalmology consultation for fundus photography, ERG; audiometry.
Differential diagnosis Other mitochondrial disorders.
Treatment and prognosis No specific treatment. Supportive treatment only, for example pacemaker for heart block, anti-epileptic drugs for seizures.

Reference Bindoff L, Brown G, Poulton J. Mitochondrial myopathies. In: Emery AEH (ed.). *Diagnostic Criteria for Neuromuscular Disorders* (2nd edition). London: Royal Society of Medicine Press, 1997: 85–90.

Other relevant entries Basal ganglia calcification; Chronic progressive external ophthalmoplegia; Mitochondrial disease: an overview.

■ Kennedy's syndrome
X-linked bulbospinal neuronopathy (XLBSN)

Pathophysiology A pure lower motor neurone, X-linked-recessive, syndrome with onset in the third to fifth decades, it was the first neurological condition demonstrated to result from a trinucleotide repeat expansion, in the androgen-receptor gene.

Clinical features: history and examination

- Hand and pelvic muscles may be affected first, with bulbar features thereafter, possibly after a long latent period; alternatively dysarthria and dysphagia may predate limb weakness by years. Tendon reflexes lost.
- No upper motor neurone signs.
- Fasciculations: limb, tongue, facial muscles.
- Postural tremor of the arms may be seen.
- Gynaecomastia (60–90%); hypogonadism, testicular atrophy, infertility.
- Diabetes mellitus (10–20%).
- Respiratory muscle weakness rare.

Investigations and diagnosis *Bloods*: elevated creatine kinase, up to 10 times normal; no consistent changes in sex hormone levels.

> *Neurophysiology*:
>
> EMG/NCS: motor studies show chronic lower motor neurone change; + absent or diminished sensory nerve action potentials.
>
> Sensory evoked potentials: may be abnormal, despite absence of sensory signs.
>
> Central motor conduction time: normal.
>
> *Neurogenetics*: CAG expansion in exon 1 of androgen-receptor gene.

Differential diagnosis Often misdiagnosed as motor neurone disease; prolonged survival may lead to revision of this misdiagnosis.

Adult-onset spinal muscular atrophy.

Hereditary sensorimotor neuropathy.

Limb girdle dystrophy.

Facioscapulohumeral (FSH) dystrophy.

Treatment and prognosis No specific treatment although there is some recent evidence suggesting that "anti-androgen" therapies may have some neuroprotective effects. Usually only slowly progressive, with survival to seventh or eighth decade. Rapid onset of disability may occur.

> **Reference** La Spada AR, Wilson EM, Lubahn DB *et al.* Androgen receptor gene mutations in X-linked spinal and bulbar muscular atrophy. *Nature* 1991; **352**: 77–79.

> **Other relevant entries** Motor neurone diseases: an overview; Trinucleotide repeat diseases.

■ Kernicterus
Bilirubin encephalopathy

Elevated blood levels of unconjugated bilirubin in the neonatal period are able to cross the immature blood–brain barrier to cause an encephalopathy with paroxysmal extensor spasms, evolving to an extrapyramidal disorder with supranuclear vertical gaze palsy and deafness. Pathologically the brain is stained canary yellow, with widespread neuronal degeneration and secondary astrocytosis, in basal ganglia, cerebellum and hippocampus. The condition has been particularly associated with haemolytic disorders such as erythroblastosis fetalis and pyruvate kinase deficiency. Awareness of the hazards of unconjugated bilirubinaemia to the developing nervous system and vigorous treatment of neonatal jaundice, as well as prophylaxis for erythroblastosis fetalis, have made kernicterus a rare condition now.

▨ Kernohan's syndrome
Crus syndrome • Kernohan–Woltman syndrome • Notch syndrome

Raised intracranial pressure as a result of an expanding supratentorial lesion (e.g. tumour, subdural haematoma) may cause herniation of brain tissue through the tentorium into the subtentorial space, putting pressure on the midbrain. If the midbrain is shifted against the contralateral margin (free edge) of the tentorium, the cerebral peduncle on that side may be compressed, resulting in a hemiparesis which is ipsilateral to the supratentorial lesion (and hence may be considered "false localizing").

There may also be an oculomotor nerve palsy ipsilateral to the lesion, which may be partial (unilateral pupil dilatation).

References Cohen AR, Wilson J. Magnetic resonance imaging of Kernohan's notch. *Neurosurgery* 1990; **27**: 205–207.

Kernohan JW, Woltman HW. Incisura of the crus due to contralateral brain tumor. *Archives of Neurology and Psychiatry* 1929; **21**: 274–287.

▨ Kiloh–Nevin syndrome – see Anterior interosseous syndrome

▨ Kinky hair disease – see Menkes' disease

▨ Kinsbourne's syndrome – see Paraneoplastic syndromes

▨ Kitamura syndrome – see Periodic paralysis; Thyroid disease and the nervous system

▨ Kjellin's syndrome

An autosomal-recessive syndrome, sometimes classified with the hereditary spastic parapareses, comprising:

  spastic paraparesis;
  cerebellar dysarthria + upper limb ataxia;
  pigmentary macular degeneration, not usually giving rise to visual loss;

+/− distal wasting;

+/− dementia.

The fundal appearances may resemble those of Stargardt disease.

If ophthalmoplegia is also present, the name Barnard–Scholz syndrome may be given, although the cases reported by the latter authors lacked spastic paraparesis.

Other relevant entry Hereditary spastic paraparesis.

■ Kleine–Levin syndrome

This rare sleep disorder occurs typically in adolescence, more often in males, and is characterized by episodes of hypersomnolence and bulimia lasting days (usually 4–7) to weeks, in which the patient may sleep 16–18 hours per day and eat voraciously on awakening. Cycles occur every few months. Other behavioural features include hypersexuality, altered mood, hallucinations, and memory impairment. The multiple sleep latency test shows pathological sleepiness, but unlike narcolepsy there is no REM sleep at sleep onset. Lithium and sodium valproate may be useful in the management. The condition seems to remit in adulthood.

Other relevant entries Eating disorders; Sleep disorders: an overview.

■ Klinefelter's syndrome

This chromosomal dysgenetic syndrome occurs only in males, with the karyotype 47XXY (or XXYY). There is characteristic dysmorphology comprising wide arm span, sparse facial and body hair, gynaecomastia, small testicles (i.e. poor sexual development, androgen deficiency), mild mental retardation, and a high incidence of psychosis, asthma, and diabetes mellitus. Both Leydig cells and seminiferous tubules are affected and patients are infertile. Complement pathway deficiency (C3 or C3b inhibitor) leading to exhaustion of the alternative pathway is an associated feature.

■ Klippel–Feil anomaly

The Klippel–Feil anomaly consists of abnormality of the cervical vertebrae which may be malformed or fused (congenital synostosis), creating a short neck with limited movement, sometimes with compromise of the cervical spinal cord or roots. Mirror movements may be seen. This may occur in isolation or be associated with other developmental anomalies, such as Mullerian duct aplasia (absent vagina and uterus), renal aplasia, other bony defects (cervicothoracic somite dysplasia), deafness, and gastrointestinal defects. One form is linked to chromosome 5q11.2.

References Thomsen MN, Schneider U, Weber M, Johannisson R, Neithard FU. Scoliosis and congenital anomalies associated with Klippel–Feil syndromes types I–III. *Spine* 1997; **22**: 396–401.

■ Klippel–Trénaunay–Weber syndrome

In this syndrome, a vascular malformation of the spinal cord is associated with a cutaneous vascular naevus, which may be associated with hypertrophy of connective tissues and bone (haemangiectatic hypertrophy) affecting fingers or a whole limb, and underdevelopment of other parts. Additional features may include ocular abnormalities, visceromegaly, mental retardation, and seizures.

Other relevant entries Cobb syndrome; Spinal cord vascular diseases.

■ Klumpke's paralysis

Déjerine–Klumpke palsy or paralysis • Inferior plexus paralysis

This describes a lower brachial plexus lesion involving fibres from the C8/T1 roots, as a consequence of which there is weakness of the small hand muscles and flexors of the hand, causing a claw hand. There may additionally be a Horner's syndrome, and trophic changes in the hand and fingers.

Causes of Klumpke's paralysis include trauma (road traffic accident, obstetric trauma, post-sternotomy for cardiac surgery, electrical injury), pressure from a cervical rib, and Pancoast's (pulmonary sulcus) tumour.

Other relevant entries Brachial plexopathies; Erb's palsy, Erb–Duchenne palsy; Horner's syndrome; Pancoast's syndrome.

■ Klüver–Bucy syndrome

The Klüver–Bucy syndrome is a neurobehavioural syndrome observed following bilateral temporal lobectomy, initially described in monkeys and subsequently in man. The characteristic features, not all of which may be present, are:

visual agnosia (e.g. misrecognition of others), also known as psychic blindness;
hyperorality;
hyperphagia, binge eating;
hypermetamorphosis;
hypersexuality;
emotional changes: apathy; loss of fear, rage reactions.

Recognized causes of Klüver–Bucy syndrome include:

bilateral temporal lobectomy;
post-ictal: in the context of previous unilateral temporal lobectomy;
Pick's disease;
Alzheimer's disease: especially hyperorality and hyperphagia, but it is rare to have all the features.

References Anson JA, Kuhlman DT. Post-ictal Klüver–Bucy syndrome after temporal lobectomy. *Journal of Neurology, Neurosurgery and Psychiatry* 1993; **56**: 311–313.

Klüver H, Bucy P. Preliminary analysis of functions of the temporal lobes in monkeys. *Archives of Neurology and Psychiatry* 1939; **42**: 979–1000.

Other relevant entry Emotional lability: differential diagnosis.

■ Kocher–Débre–Sémélaigne syndrome

Generalized enlargement or hypertrophy of the muscles may be seen in infants with hypothyroidism ("infant Hercules"), which resolves with replacement therapy.

Other relevant entries Hoffman's syndrome; Thyroid disease and the nervous system.

■ Kohlmeier–Degos disease

Degos disease • Malignant atrophic papulosis

A very rare cause of cerebral and spinal cord (and gut) ischaemic events due to endothelial proliferation in small arteries, along with characteristic skin lesions consisting of crops of painless, occasionally itchy, pinkish papules on the trunk and limbs which heal as circular porcelain-white scars (atrophic papulosis).

Reference Subbiah P, Wijdicks E, Muenter M *et al*. Skin lesion with a fatal neurologic outcome (Degos' disease). *Neurology* 1996; **46**: 636–640.

Other relevant entry Cerebrovascular disease: arterial.

■ Kojewnikoff's syndrome, Kozhevnikov syndrome – see Rasmussen's encephalitis, Rasmussen's syndrome

■ Konzo

Mantakassa

Pathophysiology A symmetrical spastic paraparesis occurring in epidemics in Central Africa. Believed to be a consequence of poisoning with cyanide (an inhibitor of the mitochondrial enzyme cytochrome oxidase) through the consumption of insufficiently processed roots of cassava (*Manihot esculenta*), a food staple in rural communities. Concurrent low sulphur intake may also be important in pathogenesis, since this may contribute to impaired detoxification of cyanide. Symptoms may develop very acutely, sometimes in <1 hour, always within 1 week.

Clinical features: history and examination

- Spastic gait, hyperreflexia, clonus.
- Flexion contractures of the legs.
- Disturbances of vision, eye movements.
- Spastic dysarthria and bulbar symptoms.

Investigations and diagnosis Dietary history.

Few others reported.

MRI: normal,

Transcranial magnetic stimulation: failed.

Differential diagnosis Lathyrism.

Treatment and prognosis No specific or symptomatic therapy reported. After some initial improvement, disability remains unchanged over many years. Second episodes have been reported.

> **Reference** Rosling H, Tylleskar T Konzo. In: Shakir RA, Newman PK, Poser CM (eds). *Tropical Neurology* London: Saunders, 1996: 353–364.

> **Other relevant entries** Lathyrism; Motor neurone diseases: an overview.

▓ Körber–Salus–Elschnig syndrome

This describes convergence–retraction nystagmus, in which adducting saccades (medial rectus contraction) occur spontaneously or on attempted upgaze, often accompanied by retraction of the eyes into the orbits. This is associated with mesencephalic lesions of the pretectal region (e.g. pinealoma). The term may be used interchangeably with Parinaud's syndrome or pretectal syndrome.

> **Other relevant entry** Parinaud's syndrome.

▓ Korsakoff's psychosis – see Wernicke–Korsakoff's syndrome

▓ Krabbe–Weber–Dimitri disease – see Sturge–Weber syndrome

▓ Krabbe's disease, Krabbe's leukodystrophy

Galactosylceramide lipidosis • Globoid cell leukodystrophy

Pathophysiology This is an autosomal-recessive leukodystrophy in which there is a deficiency of the lysosomal enzyme galactocerebroside β-galactosidase (GALC), resulting from mutations in the GALC gene at chromosome 14q24.3–q32.1. Storage of galactosylceramide within multinucleated macrophages of the CNS white matter forms globoid cells. Destruction of oligodendroglia results from the action of psychosine, a metabolite of galactocerebroside.

Clinical features: history and examination Three types distinguished by age at onset:

- Infantile: within first 6 months of life; commonest variant; central nervous system (CNS) and peripheral nervous system (PNS) demyelination causes implacable irritability, spasticity, opisthotonos, ataxia, seizures; hypotonia, weakness, areflexia; +/− optic atrophy, cortical blindness, hearing loss; no organomegaly.
- Late-infantile/juvenile form: onset between ages 2 and 10 years: ataxia prominent in young children, spasticity commoner in older children; bulbar palsy; dementia in children with younger onset.
- Adult form: after 10 years of age; may present as an hereditary spastic paraparesis without neuroimaging abnormalities.

Investigations and diagnosis *Bloods*: white cell or fibroblast enzyme analysis.

Imaging: MRI may show progressive demyelination periventricularly and in centrum semiovale with sparing of subcortical U-fibres, but can be normal in the early stages of disease; MRS may show diffuse increases in white matter choline resonances, without change in N-acetyl aspartate levels, consistent with myelin breakdown.

Neurophysiology: EMG/NCS: peripheral nerve demyelination; may be normal in later onset variants.

CSF: raised protein especially in infantile forms.

Other: ophthalmology opinion, ERG; audiometry.

Neurogenetics: mutations in GALC gene.

Differential diagnosis Other leukodystrophy.

Treatment and prognosis

Progressive psychomotor decline leading to quadriplegia; death within a few years.

Bone marrow transplantation may reverse the neurological manifestations.

References Krivit W, Shapiro EG, Perters C *et al*. Hematopoietic stem-cell transplantation in globoid cell leukodystrophy. *New England Journal of Medicine* 1998; **338**: 1119–1126.

Wenger DA, Rafi MA, Luzi P. Molecular genetics of Krabbe disease (globoid cell leukodystrophy): diagnostic and clinical implications. *Human Mutation* 1997; **10**: 268–279.

Other relevant entries Leukodystrophies: an overview; Lysosomal-storage disorders: an overview.

▇ Kufs' disease – see Neuronal ceroid lipofuscinosis

▇ Kugelberg–Welander syndrome

"Arrested Werdnig–Hoffmann disease" • SMA Type III

This refers to an autosomal-recessive, childhood onset, proximal spinal muscular atrophy, akin to type I (Werdnig–Hoffmann disease) but with later age at onset (up to 15 years) and generally better prognosis.

Clinically, in addition to proximal limb weakness of variable severity, there may be facial weakness, tongue wasting, weak intercostal muscles, widespread muscle fasciculation, and areflexia. Lordosis, scoliosis, and contractures may occur.

Diagnosis is by means of electrophysiology, +/− muscle biopsy.

Hexosaminidase deficiency enters the differential diagnosis.

Prognosis is very variable but survival to the fifth or sixth decade may occur. Although there is no specific treatment, the management of skeletal deformity, a major source of morbidity, is important.

Other relevant entry Spinal muscular atrophy.

▨ Kuru

Kuru is the prototypical prion disease, seen in the Fore people of the Eastern highlands of New Guinea, who perfomed ritual cannibalism of their dead, including consumption of the brain. This was particularly reserved for women and children, in whom this neurodegenerative condition occurred, characterized pathologically by spongiosis and the occurrence of kuru plaques. The condition is now extremely rare, following the cessation of cannibalism in this tribal group in the 1950s, but occasional new cases occur, suggesting that an extremely long incubation time is possible in this disorder, which may have implications for other prion diseases such as variant Creutzfeldt–Jakob disease in which, unlike sporadic CJD, kuru-type plaques may be seen.

References Gajdusek DC. Unconventional viruses and the origin and disappearance of kuru. *Science* 1977; **197**: 943–960.

Zigas V. *Laughing Death: The Untold Story of Kuru*. Clifton NJ: Humana, 1990.

Other relevant entries Creutzfeldt–Jakob disease; Prion disease: an overview; Variant Creutzfeldt–Jakob disease.

Ll

▨ L-2-hydroxyglutaric acidaemia

This rare autosomal-recessive inborn metabolic error may result in mental retardation, pyramidal and extrapyramidal signs, ataxia with cerebellar atrophy, seizures, and cardiomyopathy. Onset is most often in infancy but adult presentations with migraine and with tremor have been reported. There may be macrocephaly. There is organic acidaemia with hyperlysinaemia, and increased L-2-hydroxyglutaric acid in urine, plasma, and CSF. MRI shows subcortical leukoencephalopathy.

References Barth PG, Hoffmann GF, Jaeken J *et al*. L-2-hydroxyglutaric acidemia: a novel inherited neurometabolic disease. *Annals of Neurology* 1992; **32**: 66–71.

Fujitake J, Ishikawa Y, Fujii H *et al*. L-2-hydroxyglutaric aciduria: two Japanese adult cases in one family. *Journal of Neurology* 1999; **246**: 378–382.

▨ Labyrinthitis – see Vestibular neuritis

▨ Lactate dehydrogenase deficiency

Glycogen-storage disease (GSD) type XI • Tsujino's disease

Deficiency of lactate dehydrogenase (LDH), inherited as an autosomal-recessive condition, causes an incomplete block of glycolysis with resultant exercise intolerance, muscle cramps, and exercise-induced myoglobinuria.

Other relevant entries Cramps; Glycogen-storage disorders: an overview; Myopathy: an overview.

■ Lactic acidosis

Accumulation of lactate, the end product of anaerobic glucose metabolism, occurs when production exceeds use, as in anaerobic exercise, or pathological states, such as ischaemia–hypoxia, hepatocellular failure, and uncontrolled diabetes mellitus ("type A lactic acidosis"); there may be an increase in the lactate to pyruvate (L/P) ratio. In inherited metabolic diseases, lactic acidosis may be associated with increased pyruvate production or decreased oxidation of pyruvate (normal or increased L/P ratio). Care is needed in the measurement of venous blood lactate, since false elevations may occur with use of a tourniquet, delay in analysing the sample, and inadequate mixing of blood with fluoride in the collecting tube. Arterial or CSF samples may overcome some of these difficulties. Fasting samples are required for the measurment of pyruvate.

Examples of conditions associated with lactic acidosis include:

- Pyruvate carboxylase (PC) deficiency.
- Pyruvate dehydrogenase (PDH) deficiency.
- Mitochondrial disorders (e.g. MELAS, Leigh's disease).
- Disorders of gluconeogenesis
    Glycogen-storage disease (GSD) type I.
    Hereditary fructose intolerance (HFI).
    PEPCK deficiency.
- Fatty acid oxidation defects.
- Biotin metabolism defects: biotinidase deficiency, holocarboxylase deficiency.
- Methylmalonic acidaemia.
    (See individual entries for further details.)

Hence confirmation of lactic acidosis without obvious cause should initiate a search for metabolic disorders, which may necessitate analysis of blood glucose, amino acids and ammonia, urinary organic acids, plus other studies (MRI, muscle biopsy, fibroblast enzymatic studies).

Other relevant entry Mitochondrial disease: an overview.

■ Lacunar syndromes

The lacunar syndromes were originally described by Miller Fisher on the basis of pathological findings. Although the term may also be used for clinical–radiological syndromes, associated with small, deep vascular lesions of the corona radiata, internal capsule, thalamus, cerebral peduncle, and pons, the term "small, deep infarct" is preferred. Sometimes a clinically defined "lacunar syndrome" may be associated with an infarct in the territory of one of the major cerebral arteries.

Typically, there are no cortical (aphasia, visual deficit) or brainstem (diplopia, crossed deficits) features in lacunar syndromes. They are presumed to reflect occlusion of small perforating arteries due to degenerative vascular disease, often in the context of hypertension.

Although a variety of lacunar syndromes have been proposed, the four principal types are:

- Pure motor stroke, pure motor hemiplegia (*ca.* 50%):

     Unilateral motor deficit affecting face, upper limb, lower limb; although there may be sensory symptoms there are no sensory signs. There may be a flurry of preceding transient ischaemic attacks (TIAs) (the capsular warning syndrome). The lesion is usually in the internal capsule or pons, sometimes the corona radiata or cerebral peduncle, rarely in the medullary pyramid.

- Pure sensory stroke (*ca.* 5%):

     Symptoms of sensory loss, with or without sensory signs, in the same distribution as for pure motor stroke; the lesion is usually in the thalamus.

- Sensorimotor stroke (*ca.* 35%):

     Pure motor stroke with sensory signs in the affected parts; the lesion is usually in the thalamus or internal capsule but may be in the corona radiata or pons.

- Ataxic hemiparesis: includes "dysarthria–clumsy hand syndrome" and homolateral ataxia with crural paresis (*ca.* 10%):

     A combination of corticospinal and ipsilateral cerebellar dysfunction; the lesion is usually in the pons, internal capsule, or cerebral peduncle.

Although debate continues about the utility of such a clinical classification with the advent of neuroimaging, many neurologists continue to find these syndromes clinically useful.

References Bamford J. Lacunar syndromes – are they still worth diagnosing? In: Donnan G, Norrving B, Bamford J, Bogousslavsky J (eds). *Subcortical Stroke* (2nd edition). Oxford: OUP, 2002: 161–174.

Fisher CM. Ataxic hemiparesis. A pathologic study. *Archives of Neurology* 1978; **35**: 126–128.

Fisher CM. Pure sensory stroke and allied conditions. *Stroke* 1982; **13**: 434–447.

Other relevant entry Cerebrovascular disease: arterial.

Lafora body disease

An autosomal-recessive syndrome of progressive myoclonic epilepsy, usually presenting between 6 and 20 years of age, although later onset and protracted course have been described. Besides epileptic seizures (frequently focal occipital attacks), the clinical picture includes personality change and progressive dementia. The characteristic finding is of Lafora bodies, round basophilic periodic acid–Schiff (PAS)-positive intracellular inclusions of 3–30 μm diameter, in central nervous system (CNS) neurones and in the excretory ducts of eccrine or apocrine sweat glands; they may also be seen in skin, liver, and muscle biopsies, although all may produce negative findings. Prognosis is generally poor, with death occurring within a few years.

Other relevant entry Progressive myoclonic epilepsy.

▓ Laing myopathy
Early-adult-onset distal myopathy type 3

Unlike the Nonaka and Miyoshi forms of early-adult-onset distal myopathy, Laing myopathy is an autosomal-dominant condition, characterized clinically by distal weakness in the anterior compartment of the legs, weak neck flexors, and distal finger extensors, with mild (up to three times) elevation of creatine kinase. Muscle biopsy pathology shows myopathic changes without rimmed vacuoles (*cf.* Nonaka myopathy). Linkage is to chromosome 14q11.

> **Reference** Laing NG, Laing BA, Meredith C *et al.* Autosomal dominant distal myopathy: linkage to chromosome 14. *American Journal of Human Genetics* 1995; **56**: 422–427.

> **Other relevant entries** Distal muscular dystrophy; Distal myopathy; Miyoshi myopathy; Nonaka myopathy.

▓ Lake's disease – see Neuronal ceroid lipofuscinosis

▓ Lambert–Eaton myasthenic syndrome

Pathophysiology A rare syndrome of fluctuating muscle weakness with autonomic features, of autoimmune aetiology, due to antibodies directed against presynaptic P/Q-type voltage-gated calcium channels (VGCC). There is an association with underlying, sometimes occult, malignant disease, particularly small-cell lung carcinoma.

Clinical features: history and examination
- Proximal limb weakness, legs > arms (difficulty with stairs, rising from sitting).
- Fatigue, fluctuation of symptoms; improvement with sustained or repeated exercise.
- Autonomic dysfunction: xerophthalmia, xerostomia.
- +/− myalgia, muscle stiffness, distal paraesthesia, erectile dysfunction.
- Depressed or absent tendon reflexes, may be elicited following sustained muscular contraction.
- Other autoimmune disorders, such as thyroid disease, may develop.

Investigations and diagnosis *Bloods*: antibodies to VGCC in >85% of patients.
Neurophysiology: EMG/NCS: low amplitude Compound Motor Action Potentials (CMAPs), decrement to slow rates of stimulation, but facilitation after brief exercise.
Imaging: to search for underlying neoplasm, especially chest. Malignancy may remain occult for many years.

Differential diagnosis
Myasthenia gravis.
Weakness and areflexia may be mistaken for Guillain–Barré syndrome.

Treatment and prognosis Symptomatic therapy: weakness may be improved with cholinesterase inhibitors, or 3,4-diaminopyridine (3,4-DAP); immunosuppression is sometimes used; xerophthalmia may be treated with hypromellose eye drops.

Specific treatment of underlying neoplasm, if found.

Reference O'Neill JH, Murray NM, Newsom-Davis J. The Lambert–Eaton myasthenic syndrome. A review of 50 cases. *Brain* 1988; **111**: 577–596.

Other relevant entries Myasthenia gravis; Neuromuscular junction diseases: an overview.

■ Lance–Adams syndrome
Post-anoxic (action) myoclonus

Lance–Adams syndrome is the name given to myoclonic jerking observed after brain hypoxia, for example in the context of resuscitation from respiratory and cardiac arrest. Survivors may be left with action myoclonus, presumably of cortical origin, which may range in severity from mild to disabling. Pharmacotherapy with clonazepam, sodium valproate, piracetam, and baclofen may be tried, sometimes in combination. The movements may initially be confused with epileptic seizures, but consciousness is preserved.

Reference Lance JW, Adams RD. The syndrome of intention or action myoclonus as a sequel to hypoxic encephalopathy. *Brain* 1963; **86**: 111–136.

Other relevant entries Myoclonus; Posthypoxic syndromes.

■ Landau–Kleffner syndrome
Acquired epileptic aphasia

This unusual syndrome of childhood is characterized by acquired aphasia, with a reduction in spontaneous speech, behavioural, and psychomotor disturbances. Boys are affected twice as often as girls. Typically language development is normal for several years until there is loss of comprehension or use of language; the main deficit seems to be a verbal auditory agnosia. The condition may also present with seizures of various types, generalized and focal, although some patients never suffer seizures. A fluctuating course may occur, with remissions and exacerbations. Structural brain imaging is normal, although functional imaging may show temporal lobe abnormalities. EEG abnormalities may include multifocal sharp and slow waves, mainly in posterior temporal foci, which may intensify during slow-wave sleep.

Seizures and EEG abnormalities often remit in teenage. Treatment with anti-epileptic medications may be undertaken in those with frequent seizures, or to reduce EEG abnormalities in the belief that these are responsible for the linguistic (and other) symptoms. Steroids may be used if anti-epileptic therapy fails. Ultimate prognosis is variable: some normalize completely, others are left with permanent sequelae which may be severe; seizures may continue, often infrequently.

References Panayiotopoulos CP. *A Clinical Guide to Epileptic Syndromes and Their Treatment: Based on the New ILAE Diagnostic Scheme*. Chipping Norton: Bladon, 2002: 81–85.

Paquier PF, Van Dongen HR, Loonen CB. The Landau–Kleffner syndrome or "acquired aphasia with convulsive disorder": long-term follow-up of six children and a review of the recent literature. *Archives of Neurology* 1992; **49**: 354–359.

Other relevant entries Agnosia; Aphasia; Epilepsy: an overview.

■ Landouzy–Déjerine dystrophy – see Facioscapulohumeral muscular dystrophy

■ Landry–Guillain–Barré–Strohl syndrome – see Guillain–Barré syndrome

■ Langerhans cell histiocytosis
Histiocytosis X

Pathophysiology This rare granulomatous disorder has a broad clinical spectrum, ranging from solitary eosinophilic granuloma of bone to aggressive multisystem disease (Letterer–Siwe disease); Hand–Schüller–Christian disease is a form intermediate between these extremes. Lesions may be solitary, multiple, or systemic, affecting bone, parenchymatous organs, lymph nodes, or skin. Pathophysiologically there is a clonal (non-malignant) proliferation of a subgroup of histiocytes bearing the Langerhans cell phenotype, most convincingly demonstrated by the presence on electron microscopy of Birbeck (Langerhans cell) granules. Langerhans cell histiocytosis (LCH) is generally a disease of childhood, but the neurological manifestations afflict an older age group, of juveniles and young adults.

Clinical features: history and examination Neurological features may affect:

- Hypothalamic–hypophyseal axis: diabetes insipidus, endocrine dysfunction.
- Extrahypothalamic lesions are rare, but may manifest as seizures, focal signs, or raised intracranial pressure (either from mass lesion or dural involvement leading to venous sinus thrombosis).
- In some cases a cerebellar syndrome can be seen.

Investigations and diagnosis *Imaging*: MR may show tumour-like parenchymal or dural masses or diffuse infiltration; intense enhancement with gadolinium.
Tissue biopsy: bone, skin, brain is diagnostic.

Differential diagnosis Other causes of hypothalamic–hypophyseal disease, for example sarcoidosis; Erdheim–Chester disease.

Treatment and prognosis

Very variable, dependent on extent of disease.

Solitary lesions may be treated with surgery, $+/-$ radiation.

Multiple lesions require chemotherapy $+/-$ radiation.

Reference Hund E, Steiner HH, Jansen O, Sieverts H, Sohl G, Essig M. Treatment of cerebral Langerhans cell histiocytosis. *Journal of the Neurological Sciences* 1999; **171**: 145–152.

Other relevant entries Diabetes insipidus; Erdheim–Chester disease; Rosai–Dorfman disease.

▓ Lannois–Bensaude disease

Madelung's disease ● Multiple symmetric lipomatosis

A syndrome of symmetrical lipomata of the neck and shoulders, with sparing of the buttocks and legs, associated in up to 80% of patients with axonal sensorimotor polyneuropathy, and sometimes deafness. Abnormalities of complex IV and multiple mitochondrial DNA deletions have been observed.

Reference Naumann M, Schalke B, Klopstock T *et al.* Neurological multisystem manifestation in multiple symmetric lipomatosis: a clinical and electrophysiological study. *Muscle and Nerve* 1995; **18**: 693–698.

▓ Lannois–Jouty syndrome

Paresis of cranial nerves IX, X, XI, XII due to a lesion of the skull base. The clinical features are similar to those of Collet–Sicard syndrome and Mackenzie syndrome (*q.v.*).

Other relevant entry Jugular foramen syndrome.

▓ Laron dwarfism – see Dwarfism

▓ Latah – see Startle syndromes

▓ Lateral medullary syndrome

Wallenberg's syndrome

Pathophysiology The lateral medullary syndrome most often results from infarction of a wedge-shaped area of the lateral medulla following occlusion of the intracranial vertebral artery (e.g. associated with vertebral artery dissection) or of the posterior inferior (PICA) or anterior inferior cerebellar artery (AICA), but the clinical syndrome may also occur in association with demyelination, neoplasm, haematoma, and trauma.

Clinical features: history and examination

- Nausea, vomiting, vertigo, oscillopsia: reflects involvement of vestibular nuclei.
- Contralateral hypoalgesia, thermoanaesthesia: spinothalamic tract involvement.
- Ipsilateral facial hypoalgesia, thermoanaesthesia, + facial pain: trigeminal spinal nucleus and tract involvement.
- Horner's syndrome: descending sympathetic tract involvement; +/− ipsilateral hypohidrosis of the body.

- Ipsilateral ataxia of limbs: involvement of olivocerebellar/spinocerebellar fibres, inferior cerebellum.
- Dysphagia, dysphonia, impaired gag reflex (hoarseness said to be commoner in PICA syndrome).
- +/− eye movement disorders, including nystagmus, abnormalities of ocular alignment (skew deviation, ocular tilt reaction, environmental tilt), smooth pursuit and gaze holding, and saccades.
- +/− hiccup.
- +/− tinnitus, hearing loss, facial weakness (said to be commoner in AICA syndrome).

Investigations and diagnosis The clinical picture is usually diagnostic. Investigations aim to establish cause.

Imaging: MR is the modality of choice; MRA to evaluate vertebral and posterior inferior cerebellar arteries may be undertaken.

Differential diagnosis Unlikely to be mistaken for other brainstem disorders: inflammatory, central pontine myelinolysis.

Treatment and prognosis Dependent on cause. Antiplatelet agents (aspirin, clopidogrel) may be considered as secondary prophylaxis for ischaemic causes; vertebral artery dissection may indicate anticoagulation.

> **Reference** Sacco RL, Freddo L, Bello JA, Odel JG, Onesti ST, Mohr JP. Wallenberg's lateral medullary syndrome. Clinical–magnetic resonance imaging correlations. *Archives of Neurology* 1993; **50**: 609–614.

> **Other relevant entries** Brainstem vascular syndromes; Cerebrovascular disease: arterial; Medial medullary (infarction) syndrome; Vertebral artery dissection.

■ Latham–Monro disease

A syndrome of congenital deafness and epilepsy, apparently autosomal recessive.
> **Other relevant entry** Hearing loss: differential diagnosis.

■ Lathyrism
Neurolathyrism

Pathophysiology A non-progressive spastic paraparesis endemic in Ethiopia, India, Bangladesh, Nepal, and China, believed to be a result of consumption of the chickling pea, *Lathyrus sativus*. The toxin was initially thought to be the non-protein amino acid β-oxalyl-amino-L-alanine (BOAA). Unlike the irreversible clinical syndrome, BOAA administration produces a reversible anterior horn cell syndrome in monkeys.

Clinical features: history and examination
- Spastic paraparesis of acute, subacute, or, rarely, chronic insidious onset.
- +/− pain, cramps, in lumbosacral, waist, thigh area.
- Sensory and autonomic features may occur but are unusual.

Investigations and diagnosis

Dietary history.

No specific investigations yet reported.

Differential diagnosis

Konzo (in Africa).

Tropical spastic paraparesis.

Motor neurone disease.

Cord compression.

Treatment and prognosis No specific treatment. Deficits permanent; muscle atrophy, contractures may develop.

> **Reference** Tekle-Haimanot R. Lathyrism. In: Shakir RA, Newman PK, Poser CM
> (eds). *Tropical Neurology*. London: Saunders, 1996: 365–374.

> **Other relevant entries** Konzo; Motor neurone diseases: an overview.

▓ Laughing madness – see Fou rire prodromique

▓ Laurence–Moon syndrome
Laurence–Moon–Bardet–Biedl syndrome

A syndrome of mental retardation, obesity, hypogenitalism, and retinitis pigmentosa. It may overlap with Bardet–Biedl syndrome (hence Laurence–Moon–Bardet–Biedl syndrome), polydactyly being common in the latter.

> **Other relevant entries** Bardet–Biedl syndrome; Retinitis pigmentosa.

▓ Lead and the nervous system
Plumbism

Pathophysiology Lead may have a variety of effects on the nervous system. Ingestion may be occupational (metal workers) or in children following consumption of lead-based paints. Organic lead exposure is usually related to tetraethyl lead, the anti-knock compound in petrol.

Clinical features: history and examination

- Inorganic
    Adults: motor peripheral neuropathy (especially wrist drop from radial nerve palsy; foot drop).

    Children: subacute encephalopathy +/− anaemia: seizures, ataxia, raised intracranial pressure.

- Organic
    Irritability, confusion, psychosis (hallucinations), myoclonus, ataxia (peripheral neuropathy not reported).

Other possible consequences include toxic optic neuropathy, auditory, and vestibular symptoms.

Low level lead exposure in children may produce developmental cognitive and behavioural problems; the safe level of lead exposure remains a subject of debate.

Investigations and diagnosis Index of clinical suspicion is probably the most important factor in establishing diagnosis.

Bloods: anaemia, basophilic stippling of erythrocytes on blood film; serum lead concentration may be measured to assess recent exposure but the best measure of chronic exposure is free erythrocyte protoporphyrin level.

Imaging: lead lines in the epiphyseal plates of the long bones may be seen in children.

Neurophysiology: EMG/NCS: motor nerve conduction velocities slowed in those with neuropathic presentation.

Nerve biopsy: loss of large myelinated axons, paranodal demyelination.

Differential diagnosis

Of neuropathy: porphyria.

Other causes of subacute encephalopathy.

Treatment and prognosis

Removal from source of lead.

Chelation therapy.

Neurobehavioural features persist.

> **Reference** Rubens O, Logina I, Kravale I *et al*. Peripheral neuropathy in chronic occupational inorganic lead exposure: a clinical and electrophysiological study. *Journal of Neurology, Neurosurgery and Psychiatry* 2001; **71**: 200–204.
>
> **Other relevant entry** Porphyria.

■ Leber's hereditary optic neuropathy

Pathophysiology A mitochondrial disorder characterized by subacute blindness due to retinal ganglion cell degeneration. Around 95% of cases are associated with one of three mutations of the mitochondrial genome encoding proteins of complex I, but clinical expression shows incomplete penetrance and marked gender bias (M > F).

Clinical features: history and examination

- Onset usually in adolescence, early adulthood.
- Bilateral subacute loss of central vision (central scotoma) due to focal degeneration of the retinal ganglion cell layer and optic nerve; telangiectatic microangiopathy and swelling of nerve fibre layer around optic disc may be evident on fundoscopy acutely. Some recovery of vision may occur.
- +/− cardiac conduction defects.
- Some patients with the typical LHON mutation G11778A evolve to a multiple sclerosis-like clinical picture (Harding's syndrome).

Investigations and diagnosis *Neurogenetics*: most usual associated mutations are G3460A, G11778A, and T14484C in the mitochondrial genome.

Differential diagnosis

Optic neuritis.

Ischaemic optic neuropathy.

Treatment and prognosis No specific treatment. Low vision aids.

> **Reference** Man PY, Turnbull DM, Chinnery PF. Leber hereditary optic neuropathy. *Journal of Medical Genetics* 2002; **39**: 162–169.

> **Other relevant entries** Harding's syndrome; Ischaemic optic neuropathy; Mitochondrial disease: an overview; Multiple sclerosis.

▓ Leeuwenhoek's disease

The Dutchman Anthony van Leeuwenhoek, the seventeenth century pioneer of microscopy, also described a respiratory myoclonus (diaphragmatic flutter) in himself, epigastric pulsation and fullness associated with rhythmic activity of the inspiratory muscles not in time with the pulse.

> **Other relevant entry** Myoclonus.

▓ Legionnaires' disease

Pathophysiology The organism *Legionella pneumophila* lives in water and is transmitted to humans via airborne droplets. It may be found in air conditioning systems and often causes small epidemics of disease. It causes an "atypical pneumonia", so called because of the prominent extrapulmonary symptoms, including neurological features.

Clinical features: history and examination
- Incubation period 2–10 days.
- Symptoms

    respiratory: cough, often non-productive;

    systemic: fever, myalgia;

    gastrointestinal: frequent; nausea, vomiting, diarrhoea (25–50%);

    neurological (*ca.* 50% of patients)

    encephalopathy: greater than expected on the basis of metabolic disturbance; ranges from mild confusion to coma;

    ataxia;

    peripheral neuropathy: predominantly a motor axonopathy;

    cranial neuritis: especially sixth cranial nerve.

Investigations and diagnosis *Bloods*: leukocytosis, raised ESR, hyponatraemia, hypophosphataemia; serology for *L. pneumophila*.

Urine: antigen test.

Imaging:

CXR: pneumonia; lobar infiltrates may be diffuse or interstitial; pleural effusion. CT/MRI.

CSF: elevated protein (5%), pleocytosis (20%).

Neurophysiology: EEG, EMG/NCS if indicated.

Differential diagnosis Other "atypical pneumonias": watery diarrhoea, hyponatraemia point to Legionnaires' disease.

Treatment and prognosis Supportive treatment.

Antibiotics: erythromycin 1 g qds for 10 days then 500 mg qds for a further 10 days; alternatives are doxycycline, ciprofloxacin, co-trimoxazole, clarithromycin.

7% die despite appropriate treatment and apparent immunocompetence.

References Johnson JD, Raff MJ, Van Arsdall JA. Neurologic manifestations of Legionnaires' disease. *Medicine (Baltimore)* 1984; **63**: 303–310.

Stout JE, Yu VL. Legionellosis. *New England Journal of Medicine* 1997; **337**: 682–687.

Other relevant entries "Atypical pneumonias" and the nervous system; Infection and the nervous system: an overview.

■ Leigh's disease, Leigh's syndrome
Subacute necrotizing encephalomyelopathy

Pathophysiology Leigh's disease is a metabolic disorder of mitochondrial function which may be inherited as an autosomal-recessive, X-linked, or maternal condition, associated with mutations in mitochondrial genes or in nuclear genes encoding mitochondrial proteins. The phenotype is heterogeneous, as is the age of onset. It has been associated with defects in complex I (NADH dehydrogenase), complex IV (cytochrome-*c* oxidase), and complex V, as well as pyruvate carboxylase (PC) deficiency and pyruvate dehydrogenase (PDH) deficiency. Basal ganglia, brainstem, and cerebellum are the areas primarily affected.

Clinical features: history and examination

Heterogeneous: onset in infancy, childhood, or adulthood

- feeding difficulties (poor sucking), failure to thrive: 1st or 2nd year of life;
- recurrent episodes of apnoea, ataxic breathing, tachypnoea;
- oculomotor abnormalities: ophthalmoplegia, retinitis pigmentosa;
- relapsing acute encephalopathy;
- seizures;
- psychomotor retardation, regression: progressive cerebral degeneration;
- early hypotonia, later spasticity;
- ataxia;
- neuropathy;
- *n*eurogenic weakness, *a*taxia, and *r*etinitis *p*igmentosa (NARP) syndrome;
- +/− cardiomyopathy;
- +/− multifocal myoclonus.

Investigations and diagnosis *Bloods*: persistent lactic acidosis, although sometimes it is difficult to know whether this reflects a primary defect in lactic acid metabolism or the consequence of uncontrolled seizure activity. Glucose, ammonia usually normal.

Urine: organic acids usually normal.

Imaging: destructive lesions in brainstem, basal ganglia, thalamus, usually symmetrical; white matter T_2 signal hyperintensity (may suggest leukodystrophy).

CSF: raised lactate; less likely to be spuriously elevated than plasma lactate.
EEG: background slowing, typical of encephalopathy.
Muscle biopsy: for mitochondrial features, mtDNA analysis.
Pathology: similar to thiamine deficiency, but mammillary bodies spared.

Differential diagnosis Other causes of lactic acidosis with seizures: Alpers disease, mitochondrial encephalomyopathies, metabolic encephalopathies, hepatic failure.

Treatment and prognosis No effective treatment. Supportive care: ventilation, feeding, treatment of infection, anti-epileptic drugs when appropriate. Biotin, thiamine, coenzyme Q10 may be tried.

The disease pursues a variable course, with periods of partial recovery and acute deterioration, but is inevitably fatal.

> **Reference** Van Erven PMM, Cillessen JPM, Eekhoff EMW *et al.* Leigh syndrome, a mitochondrial encephalo(myo)pathy. *Clinical Neurology and Neurosurgery* 1987; **89**: 217–230.

> **Other relevant entries** Alpers disease; Lactic acidosis; Mitochondrial disease: an overview; NARP syndrome; Pyruvate carboxylase deficiency; Pyruvate dehydrogenase deficiency.

■ Lemierre's syndrome

Fusobacterium infection of the head and neck may cause fever, rigors, oropharyngeal and neck pain and swelling, headache, thrombophlebitis of the internal jugular vein, and metastatic abscesses.

> **Reference** Tan NCK, Tan DYL, Tan LCS. An unusual headache: Lemierre's syndrome. *Journal of Neurology* 2003; **250**: 245–246.

■ Lemieux–Neemeh syndrome

A syndrome of hereditary hearing loss, possibly autosomal recessive, with chronic sensorimotor polyneuropathy and nephritis.

> **Other relevant entries** Hearing loss: differential diagnosis; Renal disease and the nervous system.

■ LEMS – see Lambert–Eaton myasthenic syndrome

■ Lennox–Gastaut syndrome

Pathophysiology This severe epileptic syndrome of childhood (onset age 1–8 years, 60% boys) may be cryptogenic or symptomatic: recognized causes include perinatal brain injury, following encephalitis, focal cerebral lesion, or tuberous sclerosis. A prior history of infantile spasms (West's syndrome) is not uncommon. However, some have questioned whether Lennox–Gastaut is a genuine "syndrome" or simply a non-specific developmental response to brain damage.

Clinical features: history and examination There is a characteristic triad of:

- seizures: multiple types, intractable

    tonic

    atonic (astatic)

    atypical absence

    +/− myoclonic

    +/− tonic–clonic

    +/− epileptic falls (drop attacks)

    +/− episodes of non-convulsive status.

    Seizures are often refractory to anti-epileptic treatment. As a consequence of poor seizure control, memory may be impaired. Mental deterioration may occur ("epileptic encephalopathy").

- Cognitive and behavioural abnormalities; may predate seizure onset.
- EEG with diffuse slow spike and waves and paroxysms of fast activity.

Investigations and diagnosis *Neurophysiology*: EEG: various changes include slow background rhythms, generalized (bilateral) slow (<2.5 Hz) spike and wave discharges, generalized fast paroxysmal spike activity (>10 Hz), and other multifocal abnormalities.

Imaging: often unrewarding, although sometimes a structural brain lesion is discovered which may be amenable to surgical removal (despite bilateral EEG findings).

Pathology: variable.

Differential diagnosis Other intractable seizure disorders. Unlikely to be mistaken for Rasmussen's syndrome because of absence of focal neurological signs. EEG also fairly typical.

Treatment and prognosis

Difficult.

Sodium valproate is good for all seizure types.

Clonazepam for myoclonic seizures.

Phenytoin for tonic attacks.

+ various other anti-epileptic drugs, with variable effect; carbamazepine may exacerbate absence seizures.

Corticosteroids may be tried, likewise a ketogenic diet.

Polytherapy frequent (with attendant risks thereof).

Outlook poor; perhaps 10% make a full recovery; otherwise moderate to severe disability with epilepsy persists.

References Niedermeyer E, Degen R (eds). The Lennox–Gastaut syndrome. *Neurology and Neurobiology, vol. 45.* New York: Alan R Liss, 1988.

Panayiotopoulos CP. *A Clinical Guide to Epileptic Syndromes and Their Treatment: Based on the New ILAE Diagnostic Scheme.* Chipping Norton: Bladon, 2002: 70–80.

Other relevant entries Epilepsy: an overview; Tuberous sclerosis; West's syndrome.

■ LEOPARD syndrome

A neurocutaneous syndrome, autosomal dominant, characterized by:

*L*entigines over the whole body
*E*lectrocardiographic conduction defects
*O*cular hypertelorism, triangular-shaped face
*P*ulmonary stenosis
*A*bnormal genitalia
*R*etarded growth
*D*eafness: congenital, sensorineural.

Other relevant entries Hearing loss: differential diagnosis; Phakomatosis.

■ Leprosy
Hansen's disease

Pathophysiology Infection with the acid-fast bacillus *Mycobacterium leprae* remains a common cause of morbidity and mortality globally, though rare in the West. Spread is by aerosol or skin-to-skin transmission. A spectrum of disease is recognized dependent on the degree of host immunological/inflammatory reaction to the bacilli, ranging from tuberculoid (paucibacillary) through borderline to lepromatous (multibacillary). Neurological features may be seen at either end of the disease spectrum, and in association with reversal reactions encountered during treatment.

Clinical features: history and examination Neurological features include:

- Tuberculoid leprosy (vigorous tissue-mediated immune response to *M. leprae*):
  Anaesthetic skin lesions: erythematous or hypopigmented macular skin lesions, clearly demarcated, are often the earliest sign of disease, and generally show impairment of light touch and pin prick sensation and anhydrosis; nerve damage due to local epithelioid granulomata. Tend to self-heal. Local major nerves may demonstrate nerve thickening, especially ulnar, peroneal, with sensorimotor deficits in the area innervated by the thickened nerve.

- Lepromatous leprosy (little evidence of tissue-mediated immune response to *M. leprae*):
  Organisms proliferate in cool body parts, leading to widespread symmetrical involvement of skin reminiscent of a distal sensory neuropathy (although palms of hands and soles of feet may be spared); other sites (anterior chamber of eye, tip of nose, ears, malar area) also involved; moreover tendon reflexes are preserved.

- Borderline leprosy: features fall somewhere between tuberculoid and lepromatous.
  Change in immunity, either occurring spontaneously or, more commonly, in response to treatment may cause acute deterioration in neurological features (erythema nodosum leprosum), with neuritis, iritis, and orchitis.

Investigations and diagnosis The diagnostic test is the demonstration of acid-fast bacilli in skin smears; however, most of the disease is paucibacillary in which case skin smears are negative.

Lepromin skin testing: positive in TT, negative in LL.

Differential diagnosis Painless injury may also be seen in syringomyelia, tabes dorsalis, and congenital insensitivity to pain (probably a form of hereditary sensory neuropathy).

Treatment and prognosis

Prevention: vaccination with BCG.

Drug treatment to eradicate *M. leprae*: dapsone, rifampicin $+/-$ clofazimine.

Treatment of leprosy reactions, which may be more devastating than the disease itself: steroids, thalidomide, clofazimine.

Rehabilitation: cosmetic surgery.

References Jardin MR, Antunes SLG, Santos AR *et al.* Criteria for diagnosis of pure neural leprosy. *Journal of Neurology* 2003; **250**: 806–809.

Lockwood DNJ, Reid AJC. The diagnosis of leprosy is delayed in the United Kingdom. *Quarterly Journal of Medicine* 2001; **94**: 207–212.

Malin AS, Waters MFR, Shehade SA, Roberts MM. Leprosy in reaction: a medical emergency. *British Medical Journal* 1991; **302**: 1324–1326.

Sabin TD, Swift TR. Neurological complications of leprosy. In: Aminoff MJ (ed.). *Neurology and General Medicine. The Neurological Aspects of Medical Disorders* (2nd edition). New York: Churchill Livingstone, 1995: 717–729.

Other relevant entry Neuropathies: an overview.

■ Leptospirosis
Weil's disease

Zoonotic infection with Gram-negative spirochaetes of the genus *Leptospira*, from direct or indirect exposure to urine of infected rodents or domestic animals, may cause a biphasic illness, initially with pyrexia, myalgia, meningism, and headache. Disease is often subclinical or mild, but an aseptic meningitis may be found, or the organism may be recovered from CSF (or blood). Jaundice and renal failure may also occur (Weil's disease). Following the acute illness there may rarely be neurological complications such as encephalitis, myelitis, optic neuritis, or peripheral neuritis, thought to be immune mediated since the organism can no longer be isolated. Treatment is with penicillin or tetracyclines.

Other relevant entry Aseptic meningitis.

■ Lermoyez syndrome – see Ménière's disease

■ Lesch–Nyhan disease
X-linked hypoxanthine phosphoribosyltransferase (HPRT) deficiency

Pathophysiology This syndrome of severe learning disability and self-mutilation results from deficiency of the purine salvage enzyme HPRT, an X-linked disorder due to mutations in the HPRT gene on chromosome Xq26. The phenotype is variable, with a milder condition resulting from partial HPRT deficiency. Genotype : phenotype correlations provide no indication that specific disease features associate with specific mutations.

Clinical features: history and examination
- Choreoathetosis, dystonia.
- Psychomotor retardation.
- Compulsive self-mutilation: biting lips, cheeks, fingers.
- Partial deficiency: gouty arthritis, nephrolithiasis; neurological features in 20%: cerebellar ataxia, mild learning disability, no self-mutilation.

Investigations and diagnosis *Bloods*: increased uric acid; specific enzyme assay may be performed with leukocytes, fibroblasts.

Urine: increased uric acid.

Neurogenetics: analysis of HPRT gene.

Differential diagnosis
Cerebral palsy.
Glutaric aciduria type I.
Neuroacanthocytosis.

Treatment and prognosis Allopurinol may help the arthritis and nephrolithiasis, but there is no specific treatment for the neurological features.

> **References** Caskey CT, Rossiter BJF. HPRT deficiency: Lesch–Nyhan syndrome and gouty arthritis. In: Conneally PM (ed.). *Molecular Basis of Neurology*. Boston: Blackwell Scientific, 1993: 129–145.
>
> Jinnah HA, De Gregorio L, Harris JC, Nyhan WL, O'Neill JP. The spectrum of inherited mutations causing HPRT deficiency: 75 new cases and a review of 196 previously reported cases. *Mutation Research* 2000; **463**: 309–326.

> **Other relevant entries** Glutaric aciduria; Neuroacanthocytosis.

▥ Letterer–Siwe disease – see Langerhans cell histiocytosis

▥ Leukodystrophies: an overview

The leukodystrophies are a heterogeneous group of disorders, having in common a non-inflammatory dysmyelinating neuropathology. The advent of neuroimaging has perhaps made these conditions easier to recognize, yet they remain rare. They are most often diseases of childhood, but occasionally may be diagnosed in young adults. Peripheral nerve involvement may also occur. The specific biochemical defects causing some of these conditions are known. See individual entries for further details.

Classification may be according to inheritance pattern:
- Autosomal recessive
    metachromatic leukodystrophy (MLD)
    Austin disease

Krabbe (globoid cell) disease

Canavan disease.

- Sex linked

  adrenoleukodystrophy (X-ALD)

  Pelizaeus–Merzbacher disease (PMD).

- Others

  Alexander's disease

  18q syndrome

  Cockayne syndrome

  Schilder's disease

  Leukodystrophy with ovarian dysgenesis.

Leukodystrophies may also be described as orthochromatic or sudanophilic, an ill-defined group including PMD.

Differential diagnosis

Vascular encephalopathies: CADASIL, homocystinuria.

Mitochondrial encephalopathies.

Vanishing white matter disease.

Others: cerebrotendinous xanthomatosis (CTX); Refsum's disease, phenylketonuria (PKU).

> **References** Baumann N, Turpin J-C. Adult-onset leukodystrophies. *Journal of Neurology* 2000; **247**: 751–759.
>
> Berger J, Moser HW, Forss-Petter S. Leukodystrophies: recent developments in genetics, molecular biology, pathogenesis and treatment. *Current Opinion in Neurology* 2001; **14**: 305–312.

■ Levine–Critchley syndrome – see Neuroacanthocytosis

■ Lewis Sumner syndrome

Multifocal *a*cquired *d*emyelinating *s*ensory *a*nd *m*otor neuropathy (MADSAM) ● Multifocal chronic inflammatory demyelinating polyneuropathy (CIDP)

The nosological relationship of MADSAM to multifocal motor neuropathy – distinct entity or variant with sensory features – remains a matter of debate. The condition is steroid responsive.

Other relevant entry Multifocal motor neuropathy.

■ Lewy body disease: an overview

Dementia with Lewy bodies (DLB) ● Diffuse Lewy body disease (DLBD) ● Lewy body variant (LBV)

Lewy bodies are eosinophilic neuronal inclusions, found in various neurological disorders including classically idiopathic Parkinson's disease where they are found in the cell bodies of surviving substantia nigra neurones. These inclusions are also immunopositive for the protein α-synuclein (hence these conditions may be labelled as synucleinopathies). A clinicopathological spectrum of diseases associated with Lewy body pathology has been described, in which the regional distribution of pathology determines phenotype, for example in DLB the pathology is predominantly cortical rather than affecting the basal ganglia, and in pure autonomic failure (PAF) the autonomic ganglia are most affected. Hence in this spectrum may be included:

Idiopathic Parkinson's disease; Parkinson's disease with dementia
DLB
PAF
Lewy body dysphagia
Incidental Lewy body disease
Multiple system atrophy (MSA).

Overlap syndromes may be encountered, for example DLB presenting as PAF or MSA.

References Ince PG, Perry EK, Morris CM. Dementia with Lewy bodies. A distinct non-Alzheimer dementia syndrome? *Brain Pathology* 1998; **8**: 299–324.

Larner AJ, Mathias CJ, Rossor MN. Autonomic failure preceding dementia with Lewy bodies. *Journal of Neurology* 2000; **247**: 229–231.

Other relevant entries Dementia with Lewy bodies; Multiple system atrophy; Parkinson's disease; Pure autonomic failure; Synucleinopathy.

Lhermitte–Duclos disease

A slowly evolving mass lesion of the cerebellum of uncertain pathogenesis, which may be associated with macrocephaly, raised intracranial pressure, learning disability, and developmental delay. Pathologically the lesion contains granule, Purkinje, and glial elements. It has been variously labelled as a hamartoma (possibly related to Cowden disease), a dysplastic gangliocytoma, a neoplasm, or a malformation. The growth potential is small, and the prognosis good.

Reference Vinchon M, Blond S, Lejeune JP *et al.* Association of Lhermitte–Duclos and Cowden disease: report of a new case and review of the literature. *Journal of Neurology, Neurosurgery and Psychiatry* 1994; **57**: 699–704.

Other relevant entry Cowden disease.

Li–Fraumeni syndrome

The Li–Fraumeni syndrome is a rare hereditary (autosomal-dominant) disorder of familial and intraindividual clustering of malignancies, specifically:

- sarcoma before the age of 45 years, $+/-$ premenopausal breast carcinoma, brain tumours (e.g. glioma), leukaemias, adrenocortical carcinoma (in children), epithelial, or mesenchymal tumours;
- a first degree relative with carcinoma before the age of 45 years;
- a first or second-degree relative with carcinoma before the age of 45 years or sarcoma at any age.

Hence the condition is heterogeneous with respect to clinical features and age at onset.

Germline mutations in the coding region of the tumour suppressor gene p53 are found in 50–70% of cases.

Reference Chompret A. The Li–Fraumeni syndrome. *Biochimie* 2002; **84**: 75–82.

Other relevant entries Glioma; Tumours: an overview.

■ Lichtenstein–Knorr syndrome

One of the syndromes of hearing loss and ataxia, with an autosomal-recessive pattern of inheritance.

Other relevant entries Hearing loss: differential diagnosis; Jeune–Tommasi syndrome; Richards–Rundles syndrome.

■ Lightning injury – see Electrical injuries and the nervous system

■ Limb-girdle muscular dystrophy

Pathophysiology Limb-girdle muscular dystrophy (LGMD) forms the most heterogeneous group of muscular dystrophies, with some 15 genetic types defined to date, some autosomal-recessive (which tend to be clinically more severe, and more common), some autosomal dominant. Cardiac involvement is prominent in some. Inter- and intrafamilial heterogeneity may be seen.

The following LGMD types are recognized:

Type	Chromosome linkage	Abnormal protein
Autosomal dominant		
1A	5q	Myotilin
1B	1q	Lamin A/C
1C	3p	Caveolin
1D	6q	?
1E	7q	?
1F	2q	?
Autosomal recessive		
2A	15q	Calpain 3
2B	2p	Dysferlin
2C	13q	γ-sarcoglycan
2D	17q	α-sarcoglycan (adhalin)
2E	4q	β-sarcoglycan
2F	5q	δ-sarcoglycan
2G	17q	Telethonin
2H	9q	?
2I	19q	Fukutin-related

Some of these conditions are allelic (e.g. LGMD 1B with autosomal-dominant/autosomal-recessive Emery–Dreifuss muscular dystrophy); LGMD 2B with Miyoshi myopathy; LGMD 1C with idiopathic hyperCKaemia and rippling muscle disease.

Clinical features: history and examination

- Wasting and weakness of limb girdle musculature; no facial weakness; cognitive function normal
- +/− cardiac involvement: types 1B, 1D, 2C, 2E, 2F.
- +/− respiratory muscle involvement.

Investigations and diagnosis *Bloods*: creatine kinase of around 1000 IU/l or more. *EMG*: myopathic.

Neurogenetics: has helped with the classification of LGMD, but about 70% of patients presenting with this clinical phenotype still currently elude molecular diagnosis.

Other: cardiac evaluation (ECG) may be indicated, as may a muscle biopsy.

Differential diagnosis Other causes of proximal limb weakness, including:

X-linked dystrophies (Duchenne, Becker).
Facioscapulohumeral (FSH) dystrophy.
Acid-maltase deficiency, other metabolic myopathy.
Bethlem myopathy.

Treatment and prognosis No specific treatment.

Reference Bushby KMD. Making sense of the limb-girdle muscular dystrophies. *Brain* 1999; **122**: 1403–1420.

Other relevant entries Bethlem myopathy; Congenital muscular dystrophies; Dysferlinopathy; Emery–Dreifuss muscular dystrophy; Idiopathic hyperCKaemia; Miyoshi myopathy; Muscular dystrophies: an overview; Proximal weakness; Rippling muscle disease; Sarcoglycanopathy.

■ Limb shaking

"Limb shaking" episodes are recurrent, involuntary, irregular movements described by patients as shaking, trembling, twitching, or flapping. They are associated with severe stenosis or occlusion of the contralateral carotid artery, with exhausted intracranial vasomotor reactivity: hence these are transient ischaemic attacks (TIAs) in the carotid territory reflecting haemodynamic failure. These episodes may be mistaken for simple partial epileptic seizures. The differential diagnosis of unilateral limb shaking also includes Parkinson's disease.

References Baquis GD, Pessin MS, Scott RM. Limb shaking – a carotid TIA. *Stroke* 1985; **16**: 444–448.

Baumgartner RW, Baumgartner I. Vasomotor reactivity is exhausted in transient ischaemic attacks with limb shaking. *Journal of Neurology, Neurosurgery and Psychiatry* 1998; **65**: 561–564.

Other relevant entries Carotid artery disease; Transient ischaemic attack.

■ Limbic encephalitis

A syndrome of impairment of recent memory, often accompanied by anxiety and depression, which may be subacute or chronic in its onset. In addition, there may be other neurological features, such as seizures, hypersomnia, hallucinations. CSF may show pleocytosis and raised protein. Brain imaging may be normal or there may be medial temporal lobe abnormalities.

Limbic encephalitis is usually a complication of underlying malignancy, hence a paraneoplastic syndrome, particularly in association with small-cell lung cancer but also reported with other carcinomas and Hodgkin's disease. A non-paraneoplastic variant with serum antibodies directed against voltage-gated potassium channels (VGKC) has also been reported, which may respond to steroids, intravenous immunoglobulin (IVIg), and plasma exchange.

Reference Alamowitch S, Graus F, Uchuya M *et al.* Limbic encephalitis and small cell lung cancer – clinical and immunological features. *Brain* 1997; **120**: 923–938.

Other relevant entries Amnesia, Amnesic syndrome; Encephalitis: an overview; Memory; Paraneoplastic syndromes.

■ Lingual dystonia – see Oromandibular dystonia

■ Lipogranulomatosis – see Farber's lipogranulomatosis

■ Lissencephaly

Lissencephaly is a disorder of neuronal migration and cortical lamination resulting in a smooth cerebral cortex without convolutions (agyria). There may be areas of pachygyria, abnormally large and poorly formed gyri; and polymicrogyria, excessively numerous and abnormally small gyri. This may occur as a consequence of non-genetic disturbances of neuroepithelial proliferation or neuroblast migration, or may be seen in genetic diseases, viz.:

- Type I, classical: cerebral cortex remains smooth or has a cobblestone appearance; histologically there is four-layered cortex; may be associated with deletions or mutations of the LIS1 gene on chromosome 17p13 as in Miller–Dieker syndrome; a sporadic, dysmorphic variant also exists.
- Type II, cobblestone: poorly laminated cortex, smooth cerebrum with may be a few poorly formed sulci, histologically showing disorganized and disoriented neurones; may be seen in Walker–Warburg syndrome and related congenital muscular dystrophies.

These malformations may be associated with limited survival, with the clinical accompaniment of seizures, poor temperature regulation, apnoeic attacks, and failure to thrive.

Reference Pilz D, Stoodley N, Golden JA. Neuronal migration, cerebral cortical development, and cerebral cortical anomalies. *Journal of Neuropathology and Experimental Neurology* 2002; **61**: 1–11.
Other relevant entries Heterotopia; Walker–Warburg syndrome.

■ Little's disease

This name is sometimes given to that variety of cerebral palsy characterized by spastic diplegia or diparesis, which may cause scissoring (adductor spasm) of the legs and preclude ambulation. Intelligence and speech are usually unimpaired; there may be some hand clumsiness. Perinatal brain ischaemia, particularly in watershed zones, is the commonest cause.

Other relevant entry Cerebral palsy, Cerebral palsy syndromes.

■ Liver disease and the nervous system

Liver dysfunction (abnormal liver-related blood tests) may be seen in the context of neurological disease for various reasons, which are not necessarily mutually exclusive (i.e. may occur in combination):

- Liver dysfunction causing nervous system dysfunction:
    Alcohol and the nervous system (e.g. hepatic encephalopathy)
    Some cases of delirium
    Non-Wilsonian hepatocerebral degeneration.
- Pathological process simultaneously affecting liver and nervous system, including inherited metabolic disorders with hepatic presentation:
    Alcohol and the nervous system
    Alpers disease
    Antiphospholipid antibody syndrome (hepatic venous thrombosis)
    Behçet's disease (hepatic venous thrombosis)
    Central pontine myelinolysis
    Gaucher's disease types I and III
    Glycogen-storage diseases (GSD)
    Haemochromatosis
    Heatstroke
    Lafora body disease
    Leigh's disease
    Medium-chain acyl-CoA dehydrogenase (MCAD) deficiency
    Metastatic disease
    Niemann–Pick disease (type C)
    Organic acidopathies
    Peroxisomal disorders
    Reye's syndrome

Sarcoidosis

Strychnine poisoning

Thrombotic thrombocytopenic purpura

Tyrosinaemia type I

Urea cycle enzyme defects

Wilson's disease and a range of infections.

- Drugs used to treat neurological conditions, secondarily affecting the liver:

  Anti-epileptic medications

  Anti-tuberculous therapy

  Anti-immune therapy.

Liver biopsy may still occasionally be useful in diagnosing a neurological disease, especially "storage" disorders (Gaucher's disease, metachromatic leukodystrophy (MLD), Wolman's disease), Wilson's disease, sarcoidosis.

Liver transplantation is associated with a gamut of neurological complications: iatrogenic mononeuropathies, rhabdomyolysis, quadriplegia, posterior leukoencephalopathy syndrome.

Liver transplantation may be "curative" for certain neurological diseases, in terms of reversing the metabolic defect, although pre-existing neurological deficits may not be reversed, including Wilson's disease, familial amyloid polyneuropathies, tyrosinaemia.

Reference Wijdicks EF, Litchy WJ, Wiesner RH, Krom RA. Neuromuscular complications associated with liver transplantation. *Muscle and Nerve* 1996; **19**: 696–700.

Other relevant entries See individual entries; Immunosuppressive therapy and diseases of the nervous system.

■ Locked-in syndrome
De-efferented state • Pseudocoma

Pathophysiology Locked-in syndrome refers to a condition in which a patient is mute and motionless yet awake, alert, aware of self and able to perceive sensory stimuli. This most often results from basilar artery thrombosis, sometimes heralded by laughter (*fou rire prodromique*) causing bilateral ventral pontine infarction or haemorrhage, but may also occur with pontine tumours, and central pontine myelinolysis; rare causes include tentorial herniation, Guillain–Barré syndrome, and myasthenia gravis. These lesions interrupt descending motor pathways, resulting in a state of de-efferentation, but spare the reticular formation, hence wakefulness is preserved.

Clinical features: history and examination

- Usually acute onset: infarct, haemorrhage.
- Awake, alert; mute, motionless.
- Able to cooperate with examination; that is, can blink to command, and answer yes/no (two blinks/one blink) if instructed.
- Horizontal eye movements often impaired > vertical eye movements, eyelid movements.

Investigations and diagnosis *Imaging*: MRI is modality of choice to demonstrate ventral pontine lesion; if infarction, angiography may be undertaken to see if basilar artery thrombosed. Catheter angiography also presents an opportunity for local thrombolysis.

Neurophysiology: EEG: reflects patient's state of wakefulness.

PET scanning may help reveal cortical activation confirming locked in state (*cf.* persistant vegetative state)

Differential diagnosis

Abulia.

Akinetic mutism.

Catatonia.

Coma.

Vegetative state.

Treatment and prognosis Of cause, where identified.

If ischaemia/infarction is identified early, attempts to recanalize the basilar artery with local or systemic thrombolysis have been undertaken, with variable outcome in terms of degree of recovery; the risk is that ventral pontine infarction will be converted to haemorrhage. Once established, the deficits are permanent; the anguish of survivors, alert but unable to move and able to communicate only with blinking or eye movements, cannot be imagined. One survivor has "written" an account.

References Bauby J-D. *The Diving-Bell and the Butterfly*. London: Fourth Estate, 1997.

Patterson JR, Grabois M. Locked-in syndrome: a review of 139 cases. *Stroke* 1986; **17**: 758–764.

Other relevant entries Brainstem vascular syndromes; Central pontine myelinolysis; Cerebrovascular disease: arterial; *Fou rire prodromique*.

■ Long thoracic nerve palsy

The long thoracic nerve of Bell originates from the motor roots of C5, C6, and often C7, descends through the medial scalenus muscle and dorsal to the brachial plexus, and along the medial axillary wall to innervate the serratus anterior muscle. Long thoracic nerve palsy results in weakness of serratus anterior, manifest as winging of the scapula (scapula alata), either at rest or when elevating the upper arm (e.g. pushing against a wall with arms slightly flexed at elbows). The absence of other symptoms (sensory) and signs differentiates it from C6 and C7 root lesions. The commonest causes are neuralgic amyotrophy and trauma (e.g. rucksack paralysis, chest wall surgery), and it has also been reported with borreliosis. Spontaneous recovery is the rule.

Reference Staal A, Van Gijn J, Spaans F. *Mononeuropathies: Examination, Diagnosis and Treatment*. London: WB Saunders, 1999: 19–21.

Other relevant entries Neuralgic amyotrophy; Rucksack paralysis.

■ Lou Gehrig's disease – see Motor neurone disease

■ Louis–Bar disease, Louis–Bar syndrome – see Ataxia telangectasia

■ Louping ill – see Arbovirus disease

■ Low back pain: an overview

Pathophysiology Low back pain, with or without radiation to the leg(s), is an extremely common clinical problem; in most instances, degenerative disease of the bony and ligamentous spinal column is to blame. For the neurologist referred a patient with low back pain, the issue is to determine whether compromise of the spinal cord and/or spinal roots is contributing, that is, lumbosacral radiculopathy, lumbar canal stenosis.

Clinical features: history and examination Features which suggest a cause other than mechanical for low back pain include:

- No history of trauma
- Pain at night
- Fever: consider infection
- Leg pain, weakness, sensory disturbance
- Sphincteric symptoms.

Symptoms and signs correlating with radiological (MR) evidence of lumbosacral nerve root compression include:

- Leg pain > back pain
- Dermatomal pain
- Pain exacerbated by coughing, sneezing, straining at stool
- Paroxysmal pain
- Pain on straight leg raising
- Limb paresis, reflex loss
- Finger-floor distance >25 cm on bending to touch floor with fingers.

Investigations and diagnosis

Imaging:

Plain radiology may disclose mechanical factors (fracture, tumour, ankylosing spondylitis); but degenerative osteoarthritic change is increasingly frequent with age even without symptoms, so of doubtful diagnostic value, especially in the older age group.

MR: definitive investigation for lumbar spinal cord and lumbosacral nerve root compression; myelography +/− CT may still be required if patient is intolerant of MR.

Bone scan may be undertaken if malignant disease suspected.

EMG/NCS: may show evidence of radiculopathy.

CSF: seldom required, unless malignant root infiltration suspected on clinical +/− radiological grounds (cytology).

Differential diagnosis
Musculoskeletal problems

Post-traumatic, fracture
Osteoarthritis
Spondylolisthesis (slippage of one vertebral body over another)
Scoliosis
Ankylosing spondylitis
Bony tumours: primary, metastatic
Infection: epidural space, discitis.

Cord/root tumours: ependymoma, chordoma, neurofibroma.
Vascular insufficiency (claudication) more likely to cause exercise-related leg pain, not back pain.

Treatment and prognosis Of cause, where identified. Lumbar cord compression, lumbosacral nerve root compression and lumbar canal stenosis may all mandate surgical intervention. Low back pain without neurological features requires analgesia.

> **Reference** Nelson PB. Approach to the patient with low back pain, lumbosacral radiculopathy, and lumbar stenosis. In: Biller J (ed.). *Practical Neurology* (2nd edition). Philadelphia: Lippincott Williams & Wilkins, 2002: 282–288.

> **Other relevant entries** Ankylosing spondylitis and the nervous system; Cauda equina syndrome and conus medullaris disease; Discitis; Failed back syndrome; Lumbar cord and root disease; Radiculopathies: an overview; Sciatica; Spinal stenosis.

▪ Low conus syndrome – see Tethered cord syndrome

▪ Low pressure headache – see Spontaneous intracranial hypotension

▪ Lowe syndrome
Oculocerebrorenal syndrome

This sex-linked-recessive inherited metabolic disease manifests clinically as:

Severe mental retardation,
Delayed physical development,
Myopathy,
Congenital glaucoma or cataract.

Biochemically there is generalized aminoaciduria of Fanconi type with renal tubular acidosis and rickets. MR brain imaging shows white matter involvement.

A defect in phosphatidylinositol-4,5-bisphosphate 5-phosphatase may be the ultimate cause, leading to impaired Golgi apparatus function, with impaired intestinal and renal tubular transport of lysine (+ arginine).

The main differential diagnosis is Zellweger syndrome.

Death is usually from renal failure.

Other relevant entries Zellweger syndrome.

■ Lowenberg–Hill syndrome – see Pelizaeus–Merzbacher disease

■ Lower-half headache – see Sphenopalatine (ganglion) neuralgia

■ Lubag – see Dystonia: an overview; X-linked dystonia–parkinsonism syndrome

■ Luft disease
Euthyroid hypermetabolism

An extremely rare mitochondrial disorder with defective coupling of oxidation and phosphorylation, characterized clinically by early childhood onset of heat intolerance, hyperthermia, excessive sweating, polyphagia, polydipsia, and mild generalized fatiguable weakness. Basal metabolic rate is elevated but thyroid function tests are normal. ECG shows sinus tachycardia; EMG shows features of myopathy. Muscle biopsy shows ragged red fibres, increased oxidative enzymes, and accumulations of mitochondria which may have enlarged and tightly packed cristae. Isolated mitochondria show a maximal respiratory rate, even in the absence of ADP, indicating a loss of respiratory control. Chloramphenicol has been reported of benefit in one patient.

References DiMauro S, Bonilla E, Zeviani M, Nakagawa M, DeVivo DC. Mitochondrial myopathy. *Annals of Neurology* 1985; **17**: 521–538.

Luft R, Ikkos D, Palmieri G *et al.* A case of severe hypermetabolism of nonthyroid origin with a defect in the maintenance of mitochondrial respiratory control: a correlated clinical, biochemical and morphological study. *Journal of Clinical Investigation* 1962; **41**: 1776–1804.

Other relevant entry Mitochondrial disease: an overview.

■ Lumbar cord and root disease
Lumbar myelopathy • Lumbar radiculopathy

Pathophysiology Although only a small percentage of patients with low back pain have compromise of spinal cord or nerve roots, nonetheless these conditions are common and need to be considered in all patients presenting with low back pain.

Clinical features: history and examination

- *Myelopathy*:

  History

  Pain may or may not be a feature

  Complaint of limb weakness, giving way, dragging, tripping

  May be sphincter involvement, especially if intramedullary lesion

  Examination

  Upper motor neurone signs: spasticity, pyramidal pattern of weakness (flexors > extensors), hyperreflexia, Babinski sign

- *Radiculopathy*:

  History

  Leg pain usually > back pain

  Dermatomal pain

  Paroxysmal pain, increased by coughing, sneezing, straining at stool

  Examination

  Pain on straight leg raising (Lasègue's sign)

  Paresis appropriate to root

  Reflex loss appropriate to root

  Finger-floor distance on bending to touch floor with fingers >25 cm

- *Specific roots*:

  L1 (rare): inguinal sensory symptoms +/− lower abdominal paresis (internal oblique, transverse muscles).

  L2: sensory symptoms over anterior thigh; +/− weak thigh adduction, flexion, eversion, leg extension; depressed cremasteric reflex.

  L3: sensory symptoms over lower anterior thigh and medial knee; +/− weak thigh adduction, flexion, eversion, leg extension; +/− depressed (patellar) knee reflex.

  L4: low back, buttock, anterior thigh and leg pain; sensory disturbance on knee and medial leg; +/− weak leg extension, foot dorsiflexion and inversion; +/− depressed (patellar) knee reflex.

  L5 (common): low back, buttock, lateral thigh and anterolateral calf pain; sensory disturbance on lateral leg, dorsomedial foot, hallux; weak glutei, knee flexion, foot dorsiflexion and plantarflexion, inversion (*cf.* common peroneal nerve palsy) and eversion; knee and ankle reflexes spared.

  S1 (common): low back, buttock, lateral thigh and calf pain; sensory disturbance on little toe, lateral foot, sole of foot; +/− weak hip extension, knee flexion, foot plantarflexion; depressed ankle (Achilles) reflex.

  S2–S5: sensory disturbances on calf, posterior thigh, buttocks, perianal region; +/− sphincteric control impaired.

  More than 80% of lumbar disc herniations involve L5 or S1.

Investigations and diagnosis   *Bloods*: glucose to exclude diabetes.

Imaging: MR modality of choice for lumbar cord and root lesions, compression.

EMG/NCS: may confirm presence of radiculopathy.

Differential diagnosis

Other causes of low back pain.

Peripheral mononeuropathies may be confused, for example common peroneal nerve palsy with L5 radiculopathy; lumbosacral plexopathy with multiple radiculopathies.

Treatment and prognosis Surgical decompression may be required to prevent further neurological deterioration; reversal of neurological deficits already present cannot be guaranteed.

> **References** Nelson PB. Approach to the patient with low back pain, lumbosacral radiculopathy, and lumbar stenosis. In: Biller J (ed.). *Practical Neurology* (2nd edition). Philadelphia: Lippincott Williams & Wilkins, 2002: 282–288.
>
> Vroomen PCAJ, de Krom MCTFM, Wilmink JT, Kester ADM, Knottnerus JA. Diagnostic value of history and physical examination in patients suspected of lumbosacral nerve root compression. *Journal of Neurology, Neurosurgery and Psychiatry* 2002; **72**: 630–634.

> **Other relevant entries** Arachnoiditis; Cauda equina syndrome and conus medullaris disease; Cervical cord and root disease; Diabetes mellitus and the nervous system; Intervertebral disc prolapse; Low back pain: an overview; Lumbosacral plexopathies; Mononeuritis multiplex, Mononeuropathy multiplex; Myelopathy: an overview; Neuropathies: an overview; Radiculopathies: an overview; Sciatica; Spinal stenosis.

■ Lumbosacral plexopathies

Pathophysiology Various causes of lumbosacral plexopathy are recognized, as for brachial plexopathy. These include:

Idiopathic

Infection: influenza, varicella zoster; anogenital herpes simplex type 2 infection

Drug abuse: heroin

Vasculitis

Tumour infiltration

Compression: pelvic fracture, surgery; psoas haematoma in bleeding diathesis

Hereditary neuropathy with liability to pressure palsies (HNLPP)

Radiation plexopathy.

Clinical features: history and examination

- Pain, often of abrupt onset and severe; anterior thigh with upper plexus lesions; buttock, posterior thigh with lower plexus involvement. Pain not aggravated by movement (*cf.* radiculopathy).
- Muscle weakness; pattern dependent on level and extent of plexus involvement; reflex diminution, loss.
- Limb paraesthesia.
- Some causes may be obvious from history.

Investigations and diagnosis *Bloods*: FBC, ESR; glucose, electrolytes, LFTs, syphilis serology, auto-antibodies.

Imaging: CT/MRI of lumbar spine and plexus.

CSF: cell count, protein, glucose, oligoclonal bands, cytology.

Neurophysiology: EMG/NCS: changes are often diffuse and patchy which may assist in differentiation from radiculopathy; paraspinal muscles are normal with plexopathy (*cf.* radiculopathy); lower limb sensory nerve action potentials are spared in radiculopathy.

Differential diagnosis

Radiculopathy: acute disc prolapse, diabetic.

Mononeuropathy multiplex

Sacral myeloradiculitis (Elsberg syndrome)

Mononeuropathies of lower limbs

Treatment and prognosis

Of cause, where possible.

Idiopathic lumbosacral plexopathy may be responsive to steroids or other immuno-suppressive therapy.

Prognosis is thought poorer than for brachial plexopathy, especially if there is distal weakness.

Reference Russell JW, Windebank AJ. Brachial and lumbar neuropathies. In: McLeod JG (ed.). *Inflammatory Neuropathies*. London: Baillière Tindall, 1994: 173–191.

Other relevant entries Brachial plexopathies; Lumbar cord and root disease; Mononeuritis multiplex, Mononeuropathy multiplex; Neuropathies: an overview; Radiculopathies: an overview; Sciatica.

■ Lyme disease – see Borreliosis

■ Lymphocytic hypophysitis

Pathophysiology A rare inflammatory disorder of the pituitary gland, affecting particularly women in the peripartum period.

Clinical features: history and examination

- Prolactin hypersecretion
- Anterior pituitary hormone failure
- Diabetes insipidus unusual ("infundibulohypophysitis").
- May extend to suprasellar region, cavernous sinus, causing neuro-ophthalmological signs
- +/− coexisting autoimmune disorders.

Investigations and diagnosis *Bloods*: prolactin, thyroid function, LH, FSH.

Imaging: MRI: pituitary mass lesion; thickened stalk; peripheral enhancement.

Pathology: anterior pituitary tissue with lymphocytic (T- and B-cells) infiltrate, foci of infarction and necrosis, cavitation; no granulomata, caseation. Surrounding interstitial reactive fibrosis.

Differential diagnosis Non-functioning pituitary adenoma: may be impossible to distinguish on clinical and radiological grounds.

Other pituitary masses: craniopharyngioma, Rathke's pouch remnant, metastasis.

Treatment and prognosis Spontaenous recovery may occur; hormone replacement may be required. Expanding lesion with visual signs may require surgery.

> **Reference** Farah J, Rossi M, Foy PM, Macfarlane IA. Cystic lymphocytic hypophysitis, visual field defects and hypopituitarism. *International Journal of Clinical Practice* 1999; **53**: 643–644.

Other relevant entries Craniopharyngioma; Pituitary disease and apoplexy.

■ Lymphoma

Pathophysiology Primary lymphoma of the central nervous system (CNS) accounts for around 1% of all CNS tumours, but its incidence has increased in recent years, both among immunosuppressed (e.g. post-transplantation, HIV positive) and apparently immunocompetent individuals, the latter for reasons that are not clear. Most lymphomas are of B-cell lineage.

Neurological features may occur with systemic and/or localized lymphomatous deposits of Hodgkin's or non-Hodgkin's types.

Clinical features: history and examination

- Parenchymal: headache, disturbance of higher cortical function, focal signs such as cranial nerve palsies.
- Meningeal: lumbosacral radiculitis, cauda equina syndrome.
- Ocular: vitreous lymphoma.
- Subacute motor neuronopathy.
- Sensory neuropathy, presumed paraneoplastic.
- Recognized predisposing immunodeficiency states/disease associations of lymphoma:
    HIV/AIDS
    Organ transplantation
    Wiskott–Aldrich syndrome
    Systemic lupus erythematosus
    Sarcoidosis
    Sjögren's syndrome
    Isolated angiitis of the nervous system
    Idiopathic thrombocytopenic purpura
    Ataxia telangiectasia
    Coeliac disease (gluten-sensitive enteropathy).

Investigations and diagnosis *Bloods*: may show monoclonal gammopathy.

Imaging: brain CT/MRI: space-occupying lesion(s), may be central location (basal ganglia, corpus callosum); paraventricular site, abutting ependymal surface, is characteristic, and may explain capacity for CSF spread; supratentorial > infratentorial, may be symmetrical lesions. Focal meningeal deposits. Usually enhance homogeneously with contrast. Lesions may shrink with steroids. Imaging features may be suggestive but not diagnostic.

CSF: cytology/immunocytochemistry for lymphoma cells; may have raised protein, reduced glucose.

Biopsy: diagnostic test.

Other: CT/MR abdomen/thorax seldom required, ditto bone marrow; consider HIV test if risk factors (following appropriate counselling).

Differential diagnosis Other CNS mass lesions: glioma.

Treatment and prognosis Lymphomatous mass lesions may shrink with empirical steroid therapy, giving a false sense of security ("inflammatory lesion"), for which reason biopsy of all mass lesions is advocated by some.

Most effective regime of radiotherapy/chemotherapy not yet decided.

References De Angelis LM. Primary central nervous system lymphoma. *Journal of Neurology, Neurosurgery and Psychiatry* 1999; **66**: 699–701.

O'Neill BP, Illig JJ. Primary central nervous system lymphoma. *Mayo Clinic Proceedings* 1989; **64**: 1005–1020.

Other relevant entries HIV/AIDS and the nervous system; Hodgkin's disease; Paraneoplastic syndromes; Subacute motor neuronopathy; Tumours: an overview.

Lysosomal-storage disorders: an overview

Conditions resulting from lysosomal enzyme disorders may be classified as follows:

- Mucopolysaccharidoses
    - Type I: Hurler and Scheie disease
    - Type II: Hunter disease
    - Type III: Sanfilippo disease
    - Type IV: Morquio disease
    - Type VI: Maroteaux–Lamy disease
    - Type VII: Sly disease.
- Mucolipidoses
    - Type I: Infantile sialidosis
    - Type II: I-cell disease
    - Type III: pseudo-Hurler's polydystrophy
    - Type IV.
- Glycoproteinoses
    - Galactosialidosis
    - Fucosidosis
    - α-, β-mannosidosis
    - Aspartylglycosaminuria
    - Pycnodysostosis.
- Sphingolipidoses
    - GM1 gangliosidosis
    - GM2 gangliosidosis: Tay–Sachs, Sandhoff
    - Metachromatic leukodystrophy (MLD); Multiple sulphatase deficiency (Austin syndrome)

Krabbe's disease
Fabry's disease
Niemann–Pick disease, types A–C
Schindler's disease
Farber lipogranulomatosis
Gaucher disease, type I.
- Neuronal ceroid lipofuscinoses
    Infantile: Santavuori–Haltia
    Late infantile: Jansky–Bielschowsky
    Juvenile: Vogt–Spielmeyer
    Adult: Kufs disease.
- Other lysosomal enzyme disorders
    Acid lipase deficiency (Wolman's disease, cholesterol ester-storage disease)
    Glycogenosis II (Pompe's disease)
    Sialic acid-storage disease (infantile form, Salla disease).
- Aminoacidopathy
    Cystinosis.

Clinical features: history and examination/Investigations and diagnosis/Differential diagnosis See individual entries.

Treatment and prognosis See individual entries.

Bone marrow transplantation may be an option for some of these disorders.

> **References** Krivit W, Peters C, Shapiro EG *et al.* Bone marrow transplantation as
> effective treatment of central nervous system disease in globoid cell leukodystro-
> phy, metachromatic leukodystrophy, adrenoleukodystrophy, mannosidosis,
> fucosidosis, aspartylglucosaminuria, Hurler, Maroteaux–Lamy, and Sly syndromes,
> and Gaucher disease type III. *Current Opinion in Neurology* 1999; **12**: 167–176.
>
> Pastores GM, Kolodny EH. Lysosomal storage disorders. In: Noseworthy JH (ed.).
> *Neurological Therapeutics: Principles and Practice*. London: Dunitz, 2003: 1484–1498.
>
> **Other relevant entries** Mucolipidoses; Mucopolysaccharidoses; Neuronal ceroid
> lipofuscinosis; Sanfilippo disease; Sialidoses.

■ Lytico–bodig – see Guam parkinsonism–dementia complex

Mm

■ Machado–Joseph disease
Azorean disease

This autosomal dominant condition, which is common among those of Portuguese
or Azorean descent, is characterized by progressive cerebellar ataxia, parkinsonism,
dystonia, eyelid retraction with bulging eyes, and bulbar fasciculation. Considerable

variation within and between families is noted. Classified phenotypically within the category of autosomal-dominant cerebellar ataxia (ADCA) type I, its genetic basis was subsequently shown to be mutation of a gene at chromosome 14q32.1, a tri-nucleotide (CAG) expansion (normal 13–44; abnormal 65–84 repeats) affecting expression of the ataxin 3 protein. Hence Machado–Joseph disease is now classified as spinocerebellar ataxia (SCA) type 3.

Other relevant entries Autosomal-dominant cerebellar ataxia; Cerebellar diseae: an overview; Spinocerebellar ataxia.

Mackenzie syndrome

Paresis of cranial nerves IX, X, XI, XII +/− Horner's syndrome due to a retroparotid space tumour at the skull base. The clinical features are similar to those of Collet–Sicard syndrome and Lannois–Jouty syndrome (*q.v.*).

Other relevant entry Jugular foramen syndrome.

Madelung's disease – see Lannois–Bensaude disease

"Mad Hatter syndrome" – see Heavy metal poisoning

MADSAM – see Lewis Sumner syndrome

Malaria

Pathophysiology A diffuse encephalopathy, termed cerebral malaria, occurs in 0.5–1% of cases of infection with the protozoan parasite *Plasmodium falciparum*. The pathophysiology of cerebral malaria is uncertain, and is probably multifactorial, related to sequestration of parasitized erythrocytes in cerebral vessels, with cerebral ischaemia, immune-mediated damage, intravascular thrombosis, cerebral hypoxia, and hypoglycaemia. The role of raised intracranial pressure from cerebral oedema is uncertain, since steroids have a detrimental effect on outcome.

Clinical features: history and examination
- Prodromal systemic illness: fever, arthralgia, abdominal and muscle pain, tachyp-noea (duration hours to weeks).
- Encephalopathy: coma, fever, convulsions.
- Headache, meningism, delirium.
- Focal signs: aphasia, hemiparesis, ataxia, ophthalmoplegia.
- Chorea, tremor, rigidity.
- Bruxism.

Investigations and diagnosis *Bloods*: films, thick and thin, to look for parasites.
Imaging: CT/MRI brain: may show brain swelling, or be normal.
CSF: often normal, but may show raised pressure, pleocytosis, raised protein, raised lactate.

Differential diagnosis

Bacterial meningitis

Viral encephalitides

Heat stroke

Babesiosis is a malaria-like illness caused by a protozoan parasite and transmitted by tick bite, occurring in north-eastern and western United States.

Treatment and prognosis Untreated, cerebral malaria is uniformly fatal within 72 hours.

Treatment: IV quinine (high dose) or artemeter; 50% dextrose for hypoglycaemia +/− anticonvulsants (phenobarbitone); steroids not helpful, in fact deleterious.

Prevention: chemoprophylaxis during travel to endemic areas.

Sequelae: hemiplegia, aphasia, cerebellar ataxia, cortical blindness, psychosis. (Neurological syndromes may follow other types of malaria infection: see Postmalaria neurological syndromes.)

References Newton CRJC, Hien TT, White N. Cerebral malaria. *Journal of Neurology, Neurosurgery and Psychiatry* 2000; **69**: 433–441.

Warrell DA. Cerebral malaria. In: RA Shakir, PK Newman, CM Poser (eds). *Tropical Neurology*. London: Saunders, 1996: 213–245.

Other relevant entry Postmalaria neurological syndromes.

■ Malignant hyperthermia

Pathophysiology A syndrome characterized by hyperthermia, rhabdomyolysis and high mortality, reflecting an autosomal dominantly inherited susceptibility to the effects of general anaesthetic agents. Uncontrolled skeletal muscle metabolism related to malfunction of the sarcoplasmic reticulum calcium channel, or ryanodine receptor, is the ultimate cause.

Clinical features: history and examination During/following general anaesthesia, especially with agents such as halothane, succinylcholine:

Hyperthermia (hyperpyrexia), up to 43°C.

Metabolic acidosis.

Tachycardia.

Muscle rigidity (e.g. trismus).

Disseminated intravascular coagulation.

Coma, death.

Family history of adverse reactions to general anaesthetic agents.

Patients with Duchenne muscular dystrophy and central core disease may be predisposed to develop malignant hyperthermia.

Investigations and diagnosis *Bloods*: very high creatine kinase + other muscle enzymes; hyperkalaemia, metabolic acidosis, renal failure.

Urine: myoglobinuria.

Neurogenetics: mutations in ryanodine-receptor gene on chromosome 19 (the central core disease phenotype, characterized by myopathy, is also associated with mutations in this gene).

Differential diagnosis Neuroleptic malignant syndrome has similar clinical features but a slower onset.

Treatment and prognosis Discontinue anaesthesia. Supportive care: correction of acid–base disorder, ventilation if necessary, intravenous fluids, +/− steroids.

Dantrolene is specific therapy since it uncouples excitation and contraction by preventing calcium release from the sarcoplasmic reticulum.

Fatality may occur despite full supportive care.

Screening of relatives of patients suffering malignant hyperthermia may be undertaken.

Reference Quane KA, Healy JM, Keating KE *et al*. Mutations in the ryanodine-receptor gene in central core disease and malignant hyperthermia. *Nature Genetics* 1993; **5**: 51–55.

Other relevant entries Central core disease; Channelopathies: an overview; Duchenne muscular dystrophy; Neuroleptic malignant syndrome.

Malignant meningitis – see Meningeal carcinomatosis; Meningitis: an overview

Malignant neuroleptic syndrome – see Neuroleptic malignant syndrome

Malingering

Malingering may be defined as the false and fraudulent simulation or exaggeration of physical or mental disease or defect, performed in order to obtain money or drugs, or to evade duty or criminal responsibility, or for other reasons that may be readily understood by an objective observer from the individual's circumstances, rather than from learning the individual's psychology. The last rider is included to preclude the need to establish whether or not the patient has insight into what is happening (i.e. are actions wilful, or involuntary).

The exaggeration of neurological symptoms, or at least a lack of correlation between reported symptoms and what is observed clinically, is not uncommon in the neurology clinic. However, it may be better to label such phenomena as "neurologically unexplained symptoms" rather than use such a charged term as malingering.

Reference Halligan PW, Bass C, Oakley DA. *Malingering and Illness Deception*. Oxford: OUP, 2003.

Other relevant entries Ganser phenomenon; Ganser syndrome.

Manganese poisoning, manganism

Miners of manganese ore are at risk of poisoning from inhalation and ingestion of manganese particles. This may cause an early confusional–hallucinatory state, or a later parkinsonian syndrome, with or without dystonia, corticobulbar and corti-cospinal signs, and psychiatric features. Axial rigidity and dystonia similar to Wilson's disease may occur. Dystonic symptoms may respond to levodopa, parkinsonian signs generally do not.

References Calne DB, Chu NS, Huang CC, Lu CS, Olanow W. Manganism and idio-pathic parkinsonism: similarities and differences. *Neurology* 1994; **44**: 1583–1586.

Huang C-C, Chu N-S, Lu C-S *et al*. Long-term progression in chronic manganism. *Neurology* 1998; **50**: 698–700.

Other relevant entries Parkinsonian syndromes, parkinsonism; Wilson's disease.

Man-in-a-barrel syndrome

This name has been applied to the clinical syndrome of brachial diplegia with preser-vation of brainstem function and of muscle strength in the legs. This may occur as a result of bilateral borderzone infarcts in the territories between the anterior and mid-dle cerebral arteries ("watershed infarction"), as a consequence of cerebral hypoper-fusion. A similar clinical picture has also been reported with cerebral metastases, and with acute central cervical cord lesions, for example after severe hyperextension injury, or after unilateral vertebral artery dissection causing anterior cervical spinal cord infarction. Flail arm syndrome, a variant of motor neurone disease, produces a neurogenic man-in-a-barrel syndrome.

Reference Sage JI, van Uitert RL. Man-in-the-barrel syndrome. *Neurology* 1986; **36**: 1102–1103.

Other relevant entry Flail arm syndrome.

Mannosidoses

Pathophysiology α- and β-mannosidosis are inherited disorders of glycoprotein degradation. α-mannosidosis is a rare autosomal-recessive disorder due to a defi-ciency of the lysosomal enzyme α-mannosidase, whereas β-mannosidosis is a very rare condition resulting from β-mannosidase deficiency, both resulting in accumula-tion of mannose-containing oligosaccharides.

Clinical features: history and examination
- *α-mannosidosis*: infantile (Type I) and juvenile (Type II) forms may be distinguished.
    Chronic encephalopathy with developmental delay; psychomotor retardation. Early sensorineural hearing loss.

Lenticular and corneal opacity.

"Storage facies" = coarsening of facial features.

Dysostosis multiplex.

Hepatomegaly.

$+/-$ kyphoscoliosis.

Susceptibility to upper respiratory infections.

- *β-mannosidosis*:

    Mental retardation, hearing loss, seizures.

    Cases reported have been heterogeneous with respect to neurological features, including behavioural changes, quadriplegia, seizures, and peripheral neuropathy.

Investigations and diagnosis Both: enzyme deficiency may be demonstrated in fibroblasts, leukocytes, plasma.

α-mannosidosis:

Bloods: smears may show translucent vacuoles in 20–90% of lymphocytes and coarse granulations in polymorphonuclear leukocytes.

Urine: excessive amounts of mannose-containing oligosaccharides on thin layer chromatography.

Imaging: mild dysostosis multiplex (beaking of the vertebral bodies).

β-mannosidosis:

Bloods: no leukocyte inclusions.

Urine: excessive amounts of mannose-containing oligosaccharides on thin layer chromatography.

Differential diagnosis Other disorders of glycoprotein degradation:

Fucosidosis

Aspartylglycosaminuria

Sialidoses.

Mucopolysaccharidosis

Mucolipidosis.

Treatment and prognosis No specific treatment. Usually fatal within 4–6 years.

Oral zinc therapy and bone marrow transplantation has been attempted in α-mannosidosis without success.

References Levade T, Graber D, Flurin V *et al*. Human β-mannosidase deficiency associated with peripheral neuropathy. *Annals of Neurology* 1994; **35**: 116–119.

Niemann S, Beck M, Seidel G, Spranger J, Vieregge P. Neurology of adult α-mannosidosis. *Journal of Neurology, Neurosurgery and Psychiatry* 1996; **61**: 116–117.

Other relevant entries Fucosidosis; Lysosomal-storage diseases: an overview.

■ Maple syrup urine disease
Branched-chain ketoaciduria • Leucine encephalopathy

Pathophysiology An autosomal recessively inherited inborn error of metabolism, branched-chain acyl-CoA dehydogenase (BCKAD) deficiency, resulting in passage of urine with a sweet, maple syrup-like, odour. Neonatal screening may be used to ensure early diagnosis and hence avoid acute metabolic deterioration.

Clinical features: history and examination
- Usually presents in the newborn period as an acute encephalopathy; milder variants may present later.
- Chronic failure to thrive.
- Psychomotor retardation.
- Drowsiness, anorexia, vomiting herald decompensation.
- Hypertonicity, opisthotonos.
- Seizures: myoclonic or clonic.
- Fluctuating course between lucidity and coma.
- Raised intracranial pressure.
- Infection: often misdiagnosed as sepsis or meningitis: associated infections may trigger protein catabolism, leading to coma.
- No dysmorphism, liver disease.
- Intermittent ataxia: mild or intermittent variants.

Investigations and diagnosis *Bloods*: no hyperammonaemia or metabolic acidosis; key test is plasma amino acid analysis which shows marked elevations of branched-chain amino acids (BCAA) leucine, isoleucine and valine: diagnostic of maple syrup urine disease (MSUD). Blood glucose usually normal, may be mild hypoglycaemia.

Urine: 2,4-dinitrophenylhydrazine test positive (non-specific); positive for ketones, α-ketoacids (specifically α-ketoisocaproic acid, α-ketoisovaleric acid and α-keto-β-methyl-valeric acid, derivatives of leucine, valine and isoleucine, respectively), organic acids.

Imaging: acutely may see brain swelling, oedema, white matter attenuation; may subside with appropriate treatment.

Neurophysiology: EEG: characteristic "comb-like" sharp wave pattern may be seen in newborn; may improve with treatment.

Neurogenetics: BCKAD is a multienzyme complex (subunits E1, E2, E3); mutations in all subunits are recorded.

Pathology: structural brain changes akin to those in phenylketonuria, viz. fewer cortical layers, ectopic foci of neuroblasts, abnormal dendritic development.

Differential diagnosis Other causes of neonatal coma: urea cycle disorders, organic aciduria, fatty acid oxidation disorders, non-ketotic hyperglycinaemia. Phenylketonuria. Sepsis, meningitis.

Treatment and prognosis Aggressive measures to lower plasma leucine are undertaken, some form of dialysis.

Lipid and glucose intravenously to reduce protein breakdown.

Specific amino acid solutions without BCAA are available for parenteral nutrition. Nonetheless, acute presentation, delayed diagnosis, may result in fatal outcome. Chronic management requires a careful balance of providing sufficient BCAA for growth without causing excess levels; monitoring of BCAA levels is required, excess may manifest with dermatitis (scalded skin syndrome).

Thiamine supplementation, L-carnitine.

With adequate treatment outlook is good (normal IQ, school performance).

References Peinemann F, Danner DJ. Maple syrup urine disease 1954–1993. *Journal of Inherited Metabolic Disease* 1994; **17**: 3–15.

Uziel G, Savoiardo M, Nardocci N. CT and MRI in maple syrup urine disease. *Neurology* 1988; **38**: 486–488.

Other relevant entries Organic acidopathies; Phenylketonuria.

Marburg disease

Marburg described an acute monophasic demyelinating encephalitis leading to death within weeks to months. This may reflect a malignant monophasic presentation of multiple sclerosis or, possibly, the acute haemorrhagic leukoencephalitic subtype (Hurst's disease) of acute disseminating encephalomyelitis (ADEM).

Reference Marburg O. Die sogenannte "akute multiple Sklerose" (Encephalomyelitis periaxialis scleroticans). *Jahrb Psychiat Neurol* 1906; **27**: 211–312.

Other relevant entries Acute disseminated encephalomyelitis; Multiple sclerosis.

Marchiafava–Bignami syndrome

Marchiafava–Bignami syndrome or disease is a rare neurological complication of chronic alcoholism characterized by lesions in the corpus callosum (and sometimes elsewhere, such as the putamen) causing an interhemispheric disconnection syndrome with combinations of apraxia, agraphia, and Balint's syndrome. Patients may present with coma, regarded as a poor prognostic sign. The role of thiamine treatment is controversial, concurrent thiamine deficiency is not uncommon in chronic alcoholics but whether this plays a pathogenetic role in the callosal lesions is not known. Recovery with or without thiamine supplements is recorded.

Other relevant entries Alcohol and the nervous system: an overview; Disconnection syndromes.

Marcus Gunn phenomena – see Gunn phenomena

Marfan syndrome

Pathophysiology An autosomal-dominant disorder of connective tissue producing a typical body habitus, first described by the French paediatrician Antonin Marfan in

1896. Abraham Lincoln and Sergei Rachmaninov are claimed as famous sufferers. Linkage to chromosome 15q21.1 led to the identification of the mutant gene encoding fibrillin-1. More than 100 mutations have now been identified.

Clinical features: history and examination

- Skeletal: tall stature; high-arched palate; arachnodactyly; scoliosis, chest wall deformity, acetabular protrusion, joint hypermobility, dural ectasia.
- Cardiac: aortic dilatation, aortic dissection; aortic regurgitation, mitral valve prolapse.
- Ophthalomological: myopia, ectopia lentis.
- Neurological: young stroke (secondary to cardiac problems); arachnoid diverticula; spontaneous intracranial hypotension (low pressure headache); subarachnoid haemorrhage.
- Family history of similarly affected relatives (although *ca*. 25% of cases result from new spontaneous mutations).

Investigations and diagnosis

Diagnosis usually possible on clinical picture and family history.

ECG, echocardiogram: for cardiac status.

Ophthalmology opinion, slit lamp: for lens abnormalities.

Neurogenetics: mutation in the fibrillin gene on chromosome 15.

Differential diagnosis Homocystinuria: may produce a similar body habitus but ectopia lentis does not occur; mental retardation would also be more suggestive of homocystinuria.

Stickler's syndrome.

Treatment and prognosis No specific treatment. Attention to cardiovascular status may reduce risk of cerebrovascular events.

References Aburawi EH, O'Sullivan J, Hasan A. Marfan's syndrome: a review. *Hospital Medicine* 2001; **62**: 153–157.

Robinson PN, Godfrey M. The molecular genetics of Marfan syndrome and related microfibrillopathies. *Journal of Medical Genetics* 2000; **37**: 9–25.

Other relevant entries Collagen vascular disorders and the nervous system: an overview; Homocystinuria; Spontaneous intracranial hypotension; Subarachnoid haemorrhage.

■ Marin–Amat syndrome
Inverse Marcus Gunn phenomenon

This synkinetic syndrome consists of involuntary eyelid closure on jaw opening (*cf.* jaw winking, or the Marcus Gunn phenomenon, in which congenital ptosis improves with jaw opening, chewing or swallowing).

The Marin–Amat syndrome is thought to result from aberrant regeneration of the facial (VII) nerve, for example after a Bell's palsy.

Reference Rana PVS, Wadia RS. The Marin–Amat syndrome: an unusual facial synkinesia. *Journal of Neurology, Neurosurgery and Psychiatry* 1985; **48**: 939–941.

Other relevant entries Bell's palsy; Cranial nerve disease: VII: Facial nerve; Gunn phenomena.

■ Marinesco–Sjögren syndrome

An autosomal-recessive ataxia syndrome of unknown aetiology, onset usually before age 20 years, comprising:

• Ataxia.
• Cataracts.
• Mental retardation.
• Short stature.
• Delayed sexual development.

Hence similar to Gillespie's syndrome, except cataracts rather than aniridia.

Other relevant entries Cerebellar disease: an overview; Gillespie's syndrome.

■ Markesbery–Griggs/Udd myopathy
Late-adult-onset distal myopathy type 2

Weakness in the anterior compartment of the legs is the presenting feature, usually after age 40 years, with spread to distal upper extremities and sometimes proximally. Creatine kinase is modestly elevated, EMG shows myopathic features. Biopsy shows a vacuolar myopathy. The condition is linked to chromosome 2q.

Other relevant entries Distal muscular dystrophy, Distal myopathy; Welander's myopathy.

■ Maroteaux–Lamy disease
Mucopolysaccharidosis type VI (MPS VI)

Deficiency of arylsulphatase B (N-acetylgalactosamine-4-sulphatase), linked to chromosome 5q13.3, is responsible for this mucopolysaccharidosis of which mild, intermediate and severe varieties are described. Increased urinary excretion of dermatan sulphate is found. Clinically there is a typical Hurler phenotype (corneal clouding, hepatosplenomegaly, short stature). Hydrocephalus secondary to pachymeningitis is common, and peripheral nerve entrapment syndromes may occur. Death is usually from heart failure.

Other relevant entries Hurler's disease; Mucopolysaccharidoses.

■ Martin–Bell syndrome – see Fragile X syndrome

■ MASA syndrome

This rare syndrome of *m*ental retardation, *a*phasia, *s*pastic paraplegia, and *a*dducted thumbs results from mutations in the gene encoding the neural cell adhesion molecule L1.

> **Reference** Jouet M, Rosenthal A, Armstrong G *et al*. X-linked spastic paraplegia (SPG1), MASA syndrome and X-linked hydrocephalus result from mutations in the L1 gene. *Nature Genetics* 1994; **7**: 402–407.
>
> **Other relevant entries** Hereditary spastic paraparesis; Hydrocephalus.

■ Mast syndrome

An autosomal-recessive disorder observed in the Amish community, with onset in the second decade of life, consisting of paraplegia, dysarthria, dementia and athetosis.

> **Reference** Cross HE, McKusick VA. The Mast syndrome: a recessively inherited form of pre-senile dementia with motor disturbances. *Archives of Neurology* 1967; **16**: 1–13.
>
> **Other relevant entry** Hereditary spastic paraparesis.

■ May–White syndrome

A syndrome comprising:
- Late-onset autosomal-dominant cerebellar ataxia.
- Deafness.
- Myoclonus.
- Peripheral neuropathy.
- $+/-$ generalized tonic–clonic seizures.

Maternal transmission in some reported families suggested this might be a mitochondrial disorder, a supposition confirmed by the finding of the myoclonic epilepsy with ragged red fibres (MERRF) mutation at nucleotide 8344 of the mitochondrial genome in some cases; others have a C insertion at position 7472.

Autopsy findings include loss of Purkinje and dentate nuclear cells with atrophy of cerebellar white matter.

> **Other relevant entries** Cerebellar disease: an overview; MERRF syndrome; Mitochondrial disease: an overview.

■ McArdle's disease
Glycogen-storage disease (GSD) type V • Myophosphorylase deficiency

Pathophysiology Myophosphorylase deficiency is an inborn error of metabolism which typically presents in early adulthood with muscle cramps induced by intense exercise, reflecting a defect in the glycolytic pathway. With brief periods of rest, moderate levels of activity can be resumed without pain, the "second wind phenomenon", presumably due to a metabolic switch to fatty acid oxidation to provide muscle energy. Most cases are autosomal-recessive but autosomal-dominant transmission has been seen in a few families.

Clinical features: history and examination

- Intense exercise induces muscle cramps, causing exercise intolerance, and sometimes leading to rhabdomyolysis, myoglobinuria and acute renal failure.
- Permanent proximal muscle weakness may develop.

Investigations and diagnosis

Bloods: marked creatine kinase elevation during cramps, may also be elevated at rest; urea and creatinine to look for renal failure.

Ischaemic forearm exercise test: no accumulation of lactic acid as in normals; exaggerated increase in plasma ammonium.

Urine: may appear pink (wine-coloured); myoglobin.

Neurogenetics: R49X is the commonest mutation found in the gene encoding myophosphorylase.

Phosphorus magnetic resonance spectroscopy: absence of normal fall in intramuscular pH with exercise, due to impaired lactate production.

Muscle biopsy: accumulation of glycogen, absence of phosphorylase staining.

Differential diagnosis

Muscle phosphofructokinase deficiency (glycogen-storage disease type VII, Tarui disease).

Myoadenylate deaminase deficiency.

Carnitine palmitoyltransferase type II (CPT II) deficiency..

Lactate dehydrogenase (LDH) deficiency.

Phosphoglycerate kinase deficiency.

Phosphoglycerate mutase deficiency.

Treatment and prognosis

No specific treatment. Branched-chain amino acid supplements have been advocated but there is no controlled evidence for efficacy.

References Hilton-Jones D. McArdle's disease. *Practical Neurology* 2001; **1**: 122–125.

McArdle B. Myopathy due to a defect in muscle glycogen breakdown. *Clinical Science* 1951; **10**: 13–33.

Other relevant entries Cramps; Glycogen-storage disorders: an overview; Myoadenylate deaminase deficiency; Myopathy: an overview; Phosphoglycerate kinase deficiency; Tarui disease.

■ McCune–Albright syndrome

Polyostotic fibrous dysplasia

Progressive fibrous dysplasia of the skull and long bones causes bone pain, fractures, and cranial nerve palsies. Brown pigmented patches are also seen on the skin, and endocrine abnormalities such as precocious puberty may occur. Pituitary tumours may also feature.

Other relevant entries Fibrous dysplasia; Pituitary disease and apoplexy.

■ McLeod's syndrome
Benign X-linked myopathy with acanthocytes

McLeod's syndrome is an X-linked condition in which there is a weak expression of the immunogenic Kell antigens on erythrocytes in the absence of the otherwise ubiquitous surface antigen Kx. Clinically this may occur in asymptomatic individuals (first detected in blood donors), but may also be associated with raised levels of serum creatine kinase, with or without a myopathy, amyotrophy, or involuntary movements, and acanthocytes (~25% of the erythrocytes).

Other relevant entries Abetalipoproteinaemia; Neuroacanthocytosis.

■ Medial longitudinal fasciculus syndrome – see Internuclear ophthalmoplegia

■ Medial medullary (infarction) syndrome
Déjerine anterior bulbar syndrome

Infarction of the medial part of the medulla, in the vertebrobasilar circulation, causes the following clinical picture:

- Hemiparesis, sparing the face, contralateral to the infarct: due to involvement of the pyramid.
- Hemisensory loss of posterior column type (position, vibration), contralateral to the infarct: due to involvement of the medial lemniscus.
- Weakness of the tongue with atrophy and fibrillation, ipsilateral to the infarct: due to involvement of the hypoglossal nerve.
- +/− neuro-ophthalmological signs: upbeat nystagmus.

Medial medullary infarcts classified by MRI appearances may sometimes be associated with pure hemiparesis ("incomplete syndrome").

Medial medullary infarction is occasionally bilateral (causing quadriparesis, bilateral sensory loss, dysphagia, dysarthria, and dysphonia), and may occur with lateral medullary infarction to produce the hemimedullary syndrome of Babinski–Nageotte.

Verterbal artery atherosclerosis and branch atheromatous disease of the penetrating arteries are the main causes.

Reference Kumral E, Afsar N, Kirbas D, Balkir K, Özdemirkiran T. Spectrum of medial medullary infarction: clinical and magnetic resonance findings. *Journal of Neurology* 2002; **249**: 85–93.

Other relevant entries Babinski–Nageotte syndrome; Brainstem vascular syndromes; Cerebrovascular disease: arterial; Lateral medullary syndrome.

▓ Median neuropathy

Pathophysiology The median nerve may be compressed or damaged in the carpal tunnel, the commonest of the entrapment neuropathies, and between the heads of the pronator teres muscle; the anterior interosseous branch may be selectively compressed.

Clinical features: history and examination

- Motor: weakness of median innervated muscles: lateral lumbricals, opponens pollicis, abductor pollicis brevis, flexor pollicis brevis; long finger and wrist flexors, with the exception of flexor carpi ulnaris and third and fourth flexor digitorum profundis (innervated by the ulnar nerve); weak pronator teres, pronator quadratus; no reflex changes expected.

- Sensory: loss on ventral aspect of hand, thumb, index, middle, and half of ring finger (palmar cutaneous branch); tips of dorsal aspects of thumb, index, middle, and half ring finger (digital nerves).

  Tinel and Phalen's signs may be evident in carpal tunnel compression of the median nerve.

Investigations and diagnosis *Neurophysiology*: EMG/NCS: may identify reduced amplitude CMAP in median innervated muscles and reduced or absent *Sensory Nerve Action Potentials* (SNAPs). Local slowing of nerve conduction, with or without evidence of denervation and/or reinnervation in EMG of abductor pollicis brevis, are found in carpal tunnel syndrome. Abnormalities beyond median nerve territory may refute a diagnosis of mononeuropathy.

Differential diagnosis Radiculopathy, brachial plexopathy: clinical features unlikely to be mistaken.

Treatment and prognosis Of cause where possible.

> **Reference** Staal A, Van Gijn J, Spaans F. *Mononeuropathies: Examination, Diagnosis and Treatment*. London: WB Saunders, 1999: 49–68.

> **Other relevant entries** Anterior interosseous syndrome; Carpal tunnel syndrome; Entrapment neuropathies: an overview; Neuropathies: an overview; Pronator teres syndrome.

▓ Medication overuse headache

Analgesia-induced headache • Medication-maintained headache

A number of medications prescribed for tension-type or migraine headache may, if used repeatedly, exacerbate or maintain headache, having previously been helpful. Examples include ergotamine and sumatriptan for migraine, narcotic analgesics, and probably most commonly mild analgesics (aspirin or paracetamol + narcotic, caffeine, benzodiazepine, barbiturate) given for tension-type headache. The result is constant headache of waxing and waning severity, often causing nocturnal waking, briefly relieved by further doses of medication, hence creating a vicious cycle. Weaning from medication may be difficult since headache will inevitably worsen on cessation of medication; withdrawal may necessitate hospitalization.

Reference Olesen J. Analgesic headache. *British Medical Journal* 1995; **310**: 479–480.

Other relevant entries Headache: an overview; Migraine.

Medium-chain acyl-CoA dehydrogenase deficiency

Pathophysiology Medium-chain acyl-CoA dehydrogenase (MCAD) deficiency is the commonest inherited disorder of fatty acid oxidation. Failure of mitochondrial fatty acid β-oxidation means that fatty acids cannot be utilized appropriately; urine ketone concentrations are low. Neurological or hepatic presentations follow, not metabolic acidosis.

Clinical features: history and examination

- Intercurrent illness may precipitate decompensation in a previously healthy child, with: anorexia, vomiting, drowsiness and lethargy, progressing to stupor and coma.
- Sudden unexpected death may occur, perhaps as a result of cardiac arrhythmia although there is no cardiomyopathy.
- Recurrence of such episodes may be a feature of the history, as may a positive family history.
- Clinically there is hypotonia and hepatomegaly.

Investigations and diagnosis *Bloods*: hepatocellular dysfunction, hypoketotic hypo-glycaemia, and hyperammonaemia during acute episodes; acylcarnitines in plasma may be elevated even in asymptomatic periods.

Urine: organic acid analysis may show large amounts of dicarboxylic acids (adipic, suberic, sebacic), although analysis may be normal when the child is well.

Neurogenetics: mutation screening may be helpful since >90% of cases are accounted for by one mutant allele.

Differential diagnosis Reye syndrome; other disorders of fatty acid oxidation; carnitine palmitoyltransferase II (CPT II) deficiency.

Treatment and prognosis Early treatment with glucose, before all laboratory tests return, may be life saving.

Other relevant entries Fatty acid oxidation disorders; Reye syndrome.

Medulloblastoma

Medulloblastoma is the most commonly diagnosed primitive neuroectodermal tumour, typically occurring in the posterior fossa, in the paediatric age group, with slight male preponderance.

Presentation is with raised intracranial pressure, +/− focal brainstem signs.

Metastasis may occur throughout the craniospinal axis, and to sites outside the neuraxis such as bone, lymph nodes, lung, pleura, liver, breast (poor prognostic feature).

Treatment is by maximal surgical resection and radiotherapy, both local and to the rest of the neuraxis, with around 50% 10-year survival. Recurrences may be treated with multidrug chemotherapy regimes.

Reference Garton GR, Schomberg PJ, Scheithauer BW *et al.* Medulloblastoma: prognostic factors and outcome of treatment – review of Mayo Clinic experience. *Mayo Clinic Proceedings* 1990; **65**: 1077–1086.

Other relevant entries Naevoid basal cell carcinoma syndrome; Primitive neuroectodermal tumours.

■ Meige's syndrome

Pathophysiology A movement disorder affecting the face with blepharospasm and oromandibular dystonia, characterized as a cranial focal or segmental dystonia. Incomplete syndromes may occur.

Clinical features: history and examination

- Blepharospasm.
- Oromandibular dystonia: involuntary mouth opening, jaw clenching, tongue protrusion, dysarthria, dysphagia.
- +/− spasmodic dysphonia.
- +/− torticollis.

Investigations and diagnosis Usually idiopathic; investigations may be undertaken to exclude other, secondary, causes (see Dystonia: an overview).

Differential diagnosis Neuroacanthocytosis, Lesch–Nyhan syndrome, may produce involuntary facial dyskinesia, as may tardive dyskinesia syndromes.

Treatment and prognosis Botulinum toxin injections may be used to control symptoms.

Reference Tolosa ES, Klawans HL. Meige's disease: clinical form of facial convulsion, bilateral and medial. *Archives of Neurology* 1979; **36**: 635–637.

Other relevant entries Blepharospasm; Botulinum toxin therapy; Brueghel syndrome; Dystonia: an overview; Oromandibular dystonia; Spasmodic dysphonia; Spasmodic torticollis.

■ Melanoma

This tumour originating from neural crest tissues, most commonly skin, is usually malignant and may give rise to cerebral metastases, even when a primary origin may not be evident. Metastases are often multiple and may be associated with significant oedema on neuroimaging.

Familial cases of melanoma occur, and may be associated with cerebral or optic gliomas.

Other relevant entries Meningeal carcinomatosis; Metastatic disease and the nervous system; Tumours: an overview.

▓ MELAS syndrome

Pathophysiology The syndrome of *m*itochondrial *e*ncephalomyopathy, *l*actic *a*cidosis, and *s*troke-like episodes (MELAS) usually presents in middle to late childhood, although cases presenting in the fifth or sixth decade have been reported. Clinical heterogeneity is the norm. Various mutations of the mitochondrial genome have been associated with this clinical syndrome, with a particular "hot spot" at nucleotide 3243; the mitochondrial complex I ND5 gene may be another.

Clinical features: history and examination

- Psychomotor delay, growth failure, short stature.
- Headaches (migrainous), vomiting (sometimes exercise induced).
- Seizures: many types, including recurrent episodes of epilepsia partialis continua and generalized convulsive status epilepticus; non-convulsive status has also been described.
- Hemiparesis: may be alternating.
- Visual field defects, blindness.
- Muscle weakness.
- +/− sensorineural deafness.
- +/− movement disorders: jaw tremor.
- +/− renal tubular dysfunction.
- +/− diabetes mellitus.
- +/− cardiomyopathy.

No ophthalmoplegia, retinal degeneration, cerebellar dysfunction, or myoclonus is reported in "pure" MELAS, but some overlap with the features of Kearns–Sayre syndrome and chronic progressive external ophthalmoplegia may occur.

Investigations and diagnosis *Bloods*: lactic acidosis, especially during periods of acute encephalopathy, but may be normal between episodes of decompensation; lactate/pyruvate (L/P) ratio may be helpful.

Imaging: CT/MRI brain shows patchy cortical abnormalities of ischaemic origin, not conforming to the boundaries of arterial territories; these changes may therefore represent focal areas of metabolic disorder.

CSF: elevated protein, lactate; lactate/pyruvate (L/P) ratio.

Neurophysiology: EEG: various abnormalities, but seldom focal changes.

Muscle biopsy: histochemical studies for ragged red fibres (not always seen); electron microscopy; biochemical studies.

Neurogenetics: most commonly associated with mutation at nucleotide 3243 of the mitochondrial genome (although mutations at this nucleotide may be associated with other phenotypes such as Chronic progressive external ophthalmoplegia (CPEO), Myoclonic epilepsy with ragged red fibres (MERRF), myopathy alone). Mutations at nucleotides 3250, 3271 also reported.

Differential diagnosis

<u>*Childhood acute encephalopathy, seizures*</u>: Alpers disease, Leigh's disease.

Other mitochondrial multisystem disorders.

<u>Adult</u>: progressive, relapsing disorders (e.g. multiple sclerosis).

Treatment and prognosis There is currently no specific treatment for MELAS: coenzyme Q10, idebenone may be tried. Acute deteriorations merit full supportive care, since marked recovery may occur. However, overall prognosis is poor.

References Hammans SR, Sweeney MG, Hanna MG, Brockington M, Morgan Hughes JA, Harding AE. The mitochondrial DNA transfer RNA Leu (UUR) A→G (3243) mutation. A clinical and genetic study. *Brain* 1995; **118**: 721–734.

Liolitsa D, Rahman S, Benton S, Carr LJ, Hanna MG. Is the mitochondrial complex I ND5 gene a hot-spot for MELAS causing mutations? *Annals of Neurology* 2003; **53**: 128–132.

Montagna P, Gallassi R, Medori R *et al*. MELAS syndrome: characteristic migrainous and epileptic features and maternal transmission. *Neurology* 1988; **38**: 751–754.

Pavlakis SG, Phillips PC, DiMauro S, DeVivo DC, Rowland LP. Mitochondrial myopathy, encephalopathy, lactic acidosis and stroke like episodes: a distinctive clinical syndrome. *Annals of Neurology* 1984; **16**: 481–488.

Other relevant entries Chronic progressive external ophthalmoplegia; Kearns–Sayre syndrome; MERRF syndrome; Mitochondrial disease: an overview.

▨ Melioidosis

Infection with the Gram-negative organism *Buckholderia pseudomallei* is a common cause of sepsis in east Asia and northern Australia, to which diabetics are peculiarly susceptible. The cardinal clinical feature is abscess formation in the lung, liver, spleen, and skeletal muscle, but about 4% of Australian patients present with a brainstem encephalitis.

Reference White NJ. Melioidosis. *Lancet* 2003; **361**: 1715–1722.

Other relevant entries Abscess: an overview; Diabetes mellitus and the nervous system; Encephalitis: an overview.

▨ Melkersson–Rosenthal syndrome

Classical Melkersson–Rosenthal syndrome consists of the triad of:
- Recurrent facial palsy
- Orofacial swelling/oedema
- Fissured tongue (lingua plicata).

Monosymptomatic presentations of this syndrome are common, for example as cheilitis granulomatosa. The condition is characterized histologically by non-caseating granulomata. No controlled trials have been performed in this rare syndrome; for the neurological features steroids may be of benefit, although surgical intervention (facial nerve decompression) has also been reported.

Other relevant entry Cranial nerve disease: VII: Facial nerve.

■ Memory

Pathophysiology Memory is not a unitary function, although the term is often used as such by the laity. Neuropsychologists distinguish different types of memory processes, viz.

- Explicit (declarative) memory
    Short-term (working) memory = selective attention: visual, spatial
        subcomponents.
    Long-term memory
        Episodic/autobiographical (events): defects may be anterograde (i.e. learning
            new material) or retrograde (i.e. recalling already learned material)
        Semantic (facts).
- Implicit (non-declarative, procedural) memory
    Conditioning
    Priming
    Motor skills.

For clinical neurologists, it is explicit memory function which is of most interest. The different components of memory may be selectively affected by disease processes:

Working memory: acute confusional state, delirium; frontal damage.
Episodic memory: amnesia, amnesic syndrome: early Alzheimer's disease, transient
    global amnesia; sequela of herpes simplex encephalitis.
Semantic memory: semantic dementia; later stages of Alzheimer's disease (in
    addition to episodic memory deficit).

Investigations and diagnosis The subcomponents of memory may be tested with relatively specific tests, for example:

Working memory: digit span; 30 to 1 backwards, months of year/days of week back-
    wards.
Episodic memory: amnesia, amnesic syndrome: learning new name and address;
    Warrington (Camden) Recognition Memory Test.
Semantic memory: Pyramids and Palm Trees test.

Differential diagnosis Complaint of memory disorder without neuropsychological evidence of cognitive function deficit is not uncommon. In these cases, there may be underlying affective disorder (anxiety, depression) and/or sleep disturbance, or drug-induced effects. Some patients without these features may be labelled "worried well" but it is best to keep an open mind about such individuals as some go on to develop frank deficits with time; "purely subjective memory impairment" is an alternative term.

Treatment and prognosis See entries for individual conditions.

References Baddeley AD, Wilson BA, Watts FN (eds). *Handbook of Memory
    Disorders*. Chichester: Wiley, 1995.

Hodges JR, Greene JDW. Disorders of memory. In: Kennard C (ed.). *Recent Advances in Clinical Neurology 8*. Edinburgh: Churchill Livingstone, 1995: 151–169.

Kopelman MD. Disorders of memory. *Brain* 2002; **125**: 2152–2190.

Other relevant entries Alzheimer's disease; Amnesia, Amnesic syndrome; Dementia: an overview; Dementia with Lewy bodies; Delirium; Frontotemporal dementia; Herpes simplex encephalitis; Semantic dementia; Transient global amnesia; Vascular dementia; Wernicke–Korsakoff's syndrome.

▓ Ménière's disease
Idiopathic endolymphatic hydrops

Pathophysiology A disorder of the inner ear characterized by the triad of fluctuating hearing loss, tinnitus, and vertigo, associated with endolymphatic hydrops. The underlying mechanism is uncertain but the aural symptoms are thought to be a consequence of endolymphatic hydrops and the episodic vertigo to follow rupture of the endolymph (potassium-rich) into the perilymph (potassium-poor) with resultant potassium intoxication of vestibular hair cells and increased firing rate in the vestibular nerve, which is then compensated for concurrent with resolution of vertigo. The condition may evolve with time to constant ringing tinnitus and bilateral sensorineural hearing loss.

Clinical features: history and examination

- Aural symptoms: tinnitus, sensorineural hearing loss, fullness or pressure sensation in the ear, typically lasting hours to weeks. They may improve after the vertigo spell (Lermoyez syndrome).
- Vestibular symptoms: episodic, recurrent vertigo, usually lasting minutes to hours. Mild disequilibrium may persist for a few days.
- Neurological examination is normal but tuning fork tests suggest sensorineural hearing loss.

Investigations and diagnosis Ménière's disease remains a clinical diagnosis with no definitive diagnostic test, but the following investigations may help to confirm the diagnosis or refute other possible diagnoses.

Bloods: to exclude other causes of endolymphatic hydrops (see Differential Diagnosis).

Vestibular testing: reduced vestibular responses on caloric testing.

Audiometry: low frequency sensorineural hearing loss.

Imaging: MRI: may be indicated in unilateral hearing loss to exclude acoustic nerve tumour (schwannoma, meningioma).

Neurophysiology: brainstem auditory evoked responses: may be indicated in unilateral hearing loss to exclude acoustic nerve tumour.

Differential diagnosis The triad is characteristic, but alternative (symptomatic) causes of endolymphatic hydrops should be considered (e.g. viral infection, head trauma, vascular insufficiency, syphilis, autoimmune inner ear disease, hypothyroidism, abnormal glucose metabolism).

Acoustic nerve tumours may need to be excluded.

Treatment and prognosis Acute episodes: vertigo is usually brief and does not require treatment, but anti-emetic and vestibular suppressant medications may be given.

Low-salt diet and diuretics (e.g. hydrochlorothiaziade and triamterene) may treat the underlying endolymphatic hydrops. Reduction of caffeine intake and stress levels is also recommended.

Following acute episodes, hearing loss and tinnitus may become permanent and progressive, with abnormal loudness recruitment and diplacusis. This may reflect permanent damage and loss of hair cells.

Surgical approaches include endolymphatic sac surgery, vestibular nerve section, and labyrinthectomy, none of which affect the hearing problem, for which cochlear implantation may be suitable.

The condition becomes bilateral, usually within 2 years, in 5–50% of patients.

Reference Saeed SR. Diagnosis and treatment of Ménière's disease. *British Medical Journal* 1998; **316**: 368–372.

Other relevant entries Hearing loss: differential diagnosis; Vertigo; Vestibular disorders: an overview.

■ Meningeal carcinomatosis
Carcinomatous meningitis • Leptomeningeal metastasis • Malignant meningitis

Pathophysiology Dissemination of tumour cells throughout the leptomeninges may occur with metastatic spread of many different tumours but breast, lung, and gastrointestinal adenocarcinomas, melanoma, and leukaemias are the commonest. Clinically the condition resembles meningitis.

Clinical features: history and examination

- Headache; may reflect meningism and/or the development of hydrocephalus.
- Backache.
- Cranial nerve palsies, may be multiple: III, IV, VI, V, VII, VIII.
- Radiculopathy, especially of cauda equina.
- Confusional state.

Investigations and diagnosis *CSF*: almost always abnormal: lymphocytic pleocytosis; cytology may show malignant cells (may need to repeat CSF analysis if clinical suspicion high but cytology initially negative); hypoglycorrhachia; raised pressure; elevated protein concentration; may also look for tumour markers in CSF, such as lactate dehydrogenase, β_2-microglobulin, carcinoembryonic antigen.

Imaging: CT/MRI may show hydrocephalus; MRI + gadolinium may show enhancement on surface of nerve roots, spinal cord; may be abnormal despite non-diagnostic CSF.

Differential diagnosis Infective meningitis, particularly bacterial or fungal.

Treatment and prognosis

Systemic disease status should be considered in treatment decisions.

Craniospinal irradiation, focused on most symptomatic areas.

Intrathecal chemotherapy: for example methotrexate; ventricular catheter with subcutaneous (Ommaya) reservoir may be used for drug delivery.

Combination therapy.

Better response of leukaemia/lymphoma as opposed to other solid tumours.

> **References** Baiges-Octavio JJ, Huerta-Villanueva M. Meningeal carcinomatosis [in Spanish]. *Revista de Neurologia* 2000; **31**: 1237–1241.
>
> Fischer-Williams M, Bosanquet FD, Daniel PM. Carcinomatosis of the meninges. *Brain* 1955; **78**: 42–58.
>
> **Other relevant entries** Meningitis: an overview; Metatstatic disease and the nervous system.

■ Meningioma

Meningioma is a common tumour of the central nervous system, with a predilection for certain sites which determines the clinical features: olfactory groove, falx, parasagittal region, sphenoid bone, spinal cord. They are commoner in women (especially cord tumours). Meningioma may occur in the context of inherited syndromes, such as neurofibromatosis. Imaging studies generally show a well-circumscribed lesion, with a dural attachment, with usually uniform post-contrast enhancement. Generally they are slow-growing and benign tumours, amenable to complete resection with excellent prognosis, although recurrence may occur. Occasionally malignant meningioma with anaplastic features occurs, necessitating closer follow-up.

> **Other relevant entries** Cowden's disease; Glioma; Neurofibromatosis; Rosai–Dorfman disease; Tumours: an overview.

■ Meningitis: an overview

Pathophysiology Meningitis is inflammation of the meninges. This may have various aetiologies, including:

Infective

    Bacterial

        Meningococcus

        Haemophilus influenzae

        Pneumoccocus

        Gram-negative organisms

        Streptococcus

Listeria
Tuberculosis
Viral
Enterovirus
Coxsackie
HIV
HSV (probably includes Mollaret's meningitis)
Fungal
Cryptococcus
Coccidiodomycosis
Histoplasmosis
Parasitic
Amoebae: Naegleria, Acanthamoeba
Angiostrongylus (eosinophilic meningitis).
Aseptic (*q.v.*)
Infiltrative: neoplastic, carcinomatous
Chemical: for example blood from subarachnoid haemorrhage, leak from epidermoid cysts, rupture of parasitic cysts (e.g. echinococcosis).

(See individual entries for further details).

Clinical features: history and examination

Pace of onset may vary from acute to subacute; occasionally chronic.

Clinical features are common to all types, but of variable severity, including:

- Fever, malaise, irritability
- Headache
- Photophobia
- Neck stiffness (nuchal rigidity): Kernig's sign, Brudzinski's sign
- Vomiting
- Confusion
- +/− epileptic seizures
- +/− systemic infection
- +/− focal signs: hemiparesis, aphasia.

The typical signs may be absent in:

Very young and very old patients
Immunocompromised patients
Overwhelming infection.

Index of clinical suspicion must be accordingly raised in these groups.

Investigations and diagnosis
Imaging: to exclude subarachnoid haemorrhage, focal lesions (e.g. abscess and subdural empyema).

CSF: for opening pressure, cell count, protein, glucose, Gram stain, Ziehl–Nielsen stain, culture; indian ink stain, cryptococcal antigen may be appropriate in some situations. CSF PCR for viral agents.

Differential diagnosis

Infective:

Encephalitis

Cerebral abscess

Subdural empyema

Septicaemia.

Non-infective:

Inflammatory disorders: SLE, Behçet's disease, sarcoidosis, angiitis, Vogt–Koyanagi–Harada syndrome

Subarachnoid haemorrhage

Migraine

Drug-induced meningitis

Brain tumour

Sagittal sinus thrombosis.

Treatment and prognosis Of cause, when possible. However, prompt administration of "best guess" antibiotics before a microbiological diagnosis is made may be life-saving in some forms of bacterial meningitis (e.g. meningococcal).

Antimicrobial therapy appropriate for viruses, fungi, parasites.

Supportive care; hydration, ventilation.

Anti-epileptic drugs if seizures occur; prophylaxis may be appropriate in some forms of bacterial meningitis. Steroids also recommended in certain instances.

Mortality highest in infants, elderly.

References Anderson M. Meningitis. In: Donaghy M (ed.). *Brain's Diseases of the Nervous System* (11th edition). Oxford: OUP, 2001: 1097–1116.

Tunkel AR. *Bacterial Meningitis*. Philadelphia: Lippincott Williams & Wilkins, 2001.

Other relevant entries Aseptic meningitis; Encephalitis: an overview; Meningeal carcinomatosis; Meningococcal disease; Mollaret's meningitis; Subarachnoid haemorrhage; Subdural empyema; Tuberculosis and the nervous system; Vogt–Koyanagi–Harada syndrome.

▓ Meningococcal disease

Pathophysiology The Gram-negative aerobic diplococci of *Neisseria meningitidis* may be classified into several serogroups according to immunological reactivity of capsular polysaccharides (e.g. A,B,C,W,Y). The human nasopharynx is the only natural reservoir, from which organisms are transmitted by aerosol or secretions. Recognized risk factors for developing disease include:

immunodeficiency (of antibody-dependent, complement-mediated immune lysis), for example asplenia, properdin deficiency, terminal complement component deficiency; possibly HIV infection;

low socioeconomic status (possibly related to crowding);

exposure (active or passive) to tobacco smoke;

crowded living conditions (e.g. military recruits, university students).

Clinical features: history and examination Infection with *N. meningitidis* may produce various clinical syndromes:

- Meningococcal meningitis
- Meningococcal bacteraemia
- Meningococcaemia: purpura fulminans, Waterhouse–Friederichsen syndrome
- Respiratory tract infection
    Pneumonia
    Epiglottitis
    Otitis media
- Focal infection (uncommon)
    Conjunctivitis
    Septic arthritis
    Urethritis
    Purulent pericarditis
- Chronic meningococcaemia: intermittent fever, rash, arthralgia, headache.

Investigations and diagnosis *Bloods*: serology with ELISA.

CSF: Gram-negative diplococci; polymerase chain reaction (PCR).

Culture of the organism from blood, CSF; culture from the nasopharynx is non-specific since many individuals harbour the organism as a commensal.

Differential diagnosis Other causes of meningitis (e.g. *Streptococcus pneumoniae*), pneumonia.

Treatment and prognosis Antibiotics: most strains are sensitive to penicillin, but because the differential diagnosis of meningitis includes *Streptococcus pneumoniae*, which is often penicillin-resistant, cephalosporins and vancomycin are often used. In epidemics in developing countries, treatment with a single intramuscular dose of chloramphenicol in an oily suspension has been effective.

Treatment should be initiated early: if the index of clinical suspicion for meningococcal meningitis is high (e.g. child with fever and purpuric rash), then "best guess" antibiotics should be administered immediately, prior to hospital transfer and further investigations.

Household contacts of index cases are those at highest additional risk of developing disease, and should receive chemoprophylaxis as soon as possible (e.g. with rifampicin, ciprofloxacin).

Despite treatment with appropriate antibiotics and optimal medical care there is still a substantial mortality (*ca.* 10%). Up to 20% of survivors have sequelae such as hearing loss, neurological disability, or loss of limb(s).

Vaccines with efficacy against various serogroups are available for at-risk populations.

Reference Rosenstein NE, Perkins BA, Stephens DS, Popovic T, Hughes JM. Meningococcal disease. *New England Journal of Medicine* 2001; **344**: 1378–1388.

Other relevant entries HIV/AIDS and the nervous system; Meningitis: an overview.

■ Meningocoele, Meningomyelocoele – see Spina bifida

■ Menkes' disease

Menkes' kinky/steely hair disease • Trichopoliodystrophy

Pathophysiology An X-linked-recessive neurodegenerative disease of children, first described 1962, due to a defect in copper metabolism. Linkage to chromosome Xq13.3 eventually led to the identification of the mutant gene, ATP7A, a copper transporting ATPase which catalyses the ATP-dependent transfer of copper to intracellular compartments or to the extracellular space. Occipital horn syndrome is a milder, allelic, condition. Deficient activity of copper requiring enzymes may explain many of the clinical features, for example dopamine β-hydroxylase (autonomic abnormalities), cytochrome-c oxidase (hypotonia, weakness), lysyl oxidase (arterial, connective tissue features), tyrosine hydroxylase (lack of pigmentation), and copper–zinc superoxide dismutase (oxidative stress, cytotoxicity).

Clinical features: history and examination
- Presentation 2–3 months of age.
- Impaired brain development: extensive focal degeneration of cortical grey matter; developmental arrest, clinical seizures and deterioration of neurological function, multifocal myoclonic jerks; pale optic discs.
- Hypothermia, poor feeding, impaired weight gain
- Connective tissue abnormalities: metaphyseal spurring of bones, diaphyseal periosteal reaction; bone fractures frequent. In occipital horn syndrome, characteristic ossified occipital "horns" may be seen, as well as clavicular and long bone morphological changes.
- Cerebral blood vessels: elongated, tortuous.
- Hair: colourless, friable; microscopically pili torti (twisted) and trichorrhexis nodosa (hair shaft fractures).
- Recurrent infections.

Investigations and diagnosis *Bloods*: low copper and caeruloplasmin (may be elevated in other tissues such as fibroblasts, intestinal mucosa, kidney).
Imaging: CT/MRI cortical atrophy, subdural effusions, tortuous enlarged intracranial vessels.
Neurophysiology: EEG: multifocal spike and slow-wave activity.
CSF: normal.

Differential diagnosis Characteristic hair changes unlikely to be mistaken. Bone fractures and subdural collections, along with failure to thrive, may suggest a diagnosis of child neglect/abuse.

Treatment and prognosis Untreated the condition is lethal; death before age 3 years is usual. Survival is longer in occipital horn syndrome, sometimes into the third decade but with marked physical and cognitive disabilities.

Copper therapy instituted before 2 months of age has been reported to prevent neuronal degeneration in some cases.

References Kodama H, Murata Y, Kobayashi M. Clinical manifestations and treatment of Menkes disease and its variants. *Pediatrics International* 1999; **41**: 423–429.

Tumer Z, Moller LB, Horn N. Mutation spectrum of ATP7A, the gene defective in Menkes disease. *Advances in Experimental Medicine and Biology* 1999; **448**: 83–95.

Other relevant entries Occipital horn syndrome; Wilson's disease.

■ MEPOP syndrome – see MNGIE syndrome

■ Meralgia paraesthetica
Bernhardt–Roth syndrome • Lateral femoral cutaneous neuropathy

Pathophysiology Sensory impairment in the distribution of the lateral cutaneous nerve of the thigh, or lateral femoral cutaneous nerve, is one of the commonest entrapment neuropathies, producing the syndrome of meralgia paraesthetica. Arising from the L2–L3 spinal nerves, this cutaneous nerve passes under the lateral border of the inguinal ligament and supplies a variable area on the anterolateral thigh. Entrapment is most commonly at the level of the inguinal ligament although occasionally retroperitoneal pathology may injure the nerve.

Clinical features: history and examination
• Motor: no features.
• Sensory: pain, numbness, crawling sensation, over anterolateral thigh.

Investigations and diagnosis Diagnosis can usually be established on clinical grounds alone. EMG may be used in atypical cases to detect involvement of muscles which would refute the diagnosis of meralgia paraesthetica.

Differential diagnosis
Femoral neuropathy.
Lumbosacral plexopathy.
L2 radiculopathy.

Other relevant entries Entrapment neuropathies; Femoral neuropathy; Neuropathies: an overview.

■ Mercury poisoning – see Heavy metal poisoning

■ MERRF syndrome
Fukuhara syndrome

Pathophysiology The syndrome of *m*yoclonic *e*pilepsy and *r*agged *r*ed *f*ibres is a mitochondrial disease with onset usually in childhood or adolescence (before 20 years of age). It results from point mutations in the mitochondrial genome, most commonly at nucleotide 8344 (hence allelic with NARP).

Clinical features: history and examination
• Seizures: myoclonic.
• Cerebellar dysfunction.

- Action-induced polymyoclonus.
- Psychomotor delay, growth failure, short stature.
- $+/-$ sensorineural deafness.
- $+/-$ weakness, hypotonia (myopathy).
- No ophthalmoplegia, retinal degeneration, cortical blindness, hemiparesis, renal tubular dysfunction, diabetes mellitus.

Investigations and diagnosis *Bloods*: lactic acidosis, especially during periods of acute encephalopathy, but may be normal between episodes of decompensation; lactate/pyruvate (L/P) ratio may be helpful.

Imaging: CT/MRI brain shows patchy cortical abnormalities of ischaemic origin, not conforming to the boundaries of arterial territories; leukoencephalopathy.

CSF: elevated protein, lactate; L/P ratio.

Muscle biopsy: histochemical studies for ragged red fibres; electron microscopy; biochemical studies.

Neurogenetics: most commonly associated with mutation at nucleotide 8344 of the mitochondrial genome.

Differential diagnosis Other causes of progressive myoclonic epilepsy (*q.v.*), mitochondrial disease.

Treatment and prognosis No specific treatment; symptomatic treatment of seizures (e.g. clonazepam). Coenzyme Q10, riboflavin may be tried.

> **Reference** DiMauro S, Hirano M, Kaufmann P *et al*. Clinical features and genetics of myoclonic epilepsy with ragged red fibres. *Advances in Neurology* 2002; **89**: 217–229.

> **Other relevant entries** May–White syndrome; MELAS syndrome; Mitochondrial disease: an overview; Progressive myoclonic epilepsy.

■ Meryon's disease – see Duchenne's muscular dystrophy

■ Metabolic myopathies – see Myopathy: an overview

■ Metabolic-storage disorders: an overview

With increasingly sophisticated definition of the metabolic disturbance leading to substrate accumulation, this categorization is less used nowadays. A common consequence of inborn errors of metabolism is dysmorphism, with characteristic ("storage") facies, organomegaly (especially hepatosplenomegaly) and sometimes bone changes (dysostosis multiplex).

Within the category of metabolic-storage diseaeses may be included:
- Lysosomal-storage disorders (*q.v.*)
    Mucopolysaccharidoses
    Mucolipidoses
    Glycoproteinoses

Sphingolipidoses

Neuronal ceroid lipofuscinoses

Other lysosomal enzyme disorders: Wolman's disease, Pompe's disease

- Peroxisomal disorders (*q.v.*)

    Zellweger syndrome

    Pseudo-Zellweger syndrome

    Neonatal adrenoleukodystrophy

    Infantile Refsum's disease

    Rhizomelic chondrodysplasia punctata

- Mitochondrial disorders (*q.v.*)

    Electron transport chain defects

    Pyruvate dehydrogenase (PDH) deficiency

    Glutaric aciduria type II

- Other biosynthetic defects

    Smith–Lemli–Opitz syndrome

    Homocystinuria

    Menkes' disease

    Sjögren–Larsson syndrome.

Due to the lack of dysmorphic features, glycogen-storage diseases (*q.v.*) are not typically included in this rubric.

Other relevant entries Glycogen-storage disorders: an overview; Inherited metabolic diseases and the nervous system; Lysosomal-storage disorders: an overview; Mitochondrial disease: an overview; Peroxisomal disorders: an overview.

■ Metachromatic leukodystrophy
Arylsulphatase A deficiency

Pathophysiology An autosomal-recessive disease characterized biochemically by an accumulation of sulphatides (sulphogalactosylceramides), classically due to deficiency of the lysosomal hydrolase arylsulphatase A (also known as cerebroside sulphate sulphatase) associated with mutations in the arylsulphatase A gene on chromosome 22q13.31. The normal catalytic function of arylsulphatase A requires a sphingolipid activator protein saposin B, deficiency of which may be associated with mutations in the prosaposin gene on chromosome 10q21. Genetic and clinical heterogeneity (age of onset, phenotype) is a feature of metachromatic leukodystrophy (MLD), but central nervous system (CNS) and peripheral nervous system (PNS) demyelination is invariable.

Clinical features: history and examination Different forms are recognized according to age at onset, itself inversely correlated with residual enzyme activity:

- Late infantile, classical, MLD (Greenfield's disease): onset 12–30 months

    Difficulty walking; flaccid paresis with absent tendon reflexes (neuropathy). Mental regression, dysarthria.

Bulbar, pseudobulbar palsy; optic atrophy, quadriparesis.
Seizures (late).

- Juvenile MLD (Scholz's disease): onset 3–10 years
  Similar to late-infantile MLD, but emotional disturbance or dementia (e.g. declining school performance) may be initial symptom; gait disorder, tremor, nystagmus (cerebellar and upper motor neurone).
- Adult MLD: onset around 30 years
  Psychiatric disorder which may be misdiagnosed as schizophrenia or manic–depressive disease; progressive dementia; truncal ataxia, hyperreflexia, seizures; no clinical signs of peripheral neuropathy.

If there are additional sulphatase deficiencies (as in Austin disease), symptoms relevant to them may be evident (e.g. ichthyosis, mucopolysaccharidosis).

Investigations and diagnosis *Bloods*: standard haematology and biochemistry normal. Reduced arylsulphatase A activity in leukocytes or fibroblasts found in the classical form; pseudodeficiency is an autosomal-recessive trait in which enzyme activity is diminished in the absence of neurological disease. Normal activity may be seen in some cases of MLD in which there is a genetic deficiency of sulphatide activator protein (sphingolipid activator protein B, saposin B).

Imaging: CT/MRI: diffuse demyelination, bilateral, symmetrical; may temporarily be limited to periventricular regions.

Urine: sulphatiduria.

CSF: elevated protein.

Neurophysiology:

EMG/NCS: slowed nerve conduction velocities
VER, SSEP delayed in adult form.

Pathology: metachromasia of stored substances = sulphatides: brain, peripheral nerve (segmental demyelination and remyelination), liver, kidney, spleen.

Neurogenetics: numerous mutations in the arylsulphatase A gene on chromosome 22 are described (hence biochemical studies remain important for diagnosis); prosaposin mutations in patients with normal arylsulphatase A activity (allelic to saposin C deficiency causing Gaucher's disease).

Differential diagnosis

Psychiatric features may resemble schizophrenia.

Imaging features: other leukodystrophies.

Adult-onset disease may be mistaken for multiple sclerosis if ataxia prominent.

Treatment and prognosis No specific treatment; bone marrow transplantation has been tried without conspicuous success. Natural history is of slow but relentless progression to death: infantile form within about 5 years, juvenile form may live 20 years or more.

Reference Polten A, Fluharty AL, Fluharty CB *et al*. Molecular basis of different forms of metachromatic leukodystrophy. *New England Journal of Medicine* 1991; **324**: 18–22.

Other relevant entries Austin disease; Leukodystrophies: an overview.

■ Metal toxicity – see Heavy metal poisoning

■ Metastatic disease and the nervous system

Pathophysiology Metastasis must be considered in any patient with known malignancy developing new neurological symptoms and in the differential diagnosis of any cerebral mass lesion or spinal root or cord compression; metastasis to vertebral column, with resultant spinal root or cord compression, is commoner than metastasis to the spinal cord *per se*.

Common sources of brain metastases include:

Lung
Breast
Melanoma
Unknown.

Common sources of vertebral metastases include:

Lung
Breast
Thyroid
Prostate.

Spread of malignancy along CSF pathways may present with malignant meningitis (meningeal carcinomatosis, *q.v.*) or root infiltration.

Clinical features: history and examination *Cerebral metastasis* may present with
- Seizure: focal $+/-$ secondary generalization.
- Focal signs: weakness, ataxia, sensory features, behavioural change.
- Headache: if raised intracranial pressure.

Vertebral column metastasis may present with
- Focal signs: weakness, sensory features suggestive of intramedullary myelopathy; acute cord compression.

Investigations and diagnosis *Imaging*: CT/MRI may be diagnostic.
Biopsy: may sometimes be required for brain lesions, especially if isolated with no known primary.
Other: search for primary may be necessary; focus should be on lung.

Differential diagnosis
Other cranial/spinal mass lesions: tumour, abscess, haematoma, cyst.
Other causes of spinal root/cord compression: especially spondylotic radiculopathy, myelopathy.

Treatment and prognosis Short-term symptomatic treatment with steroids indicated, $+/-$ symptomatic treatment for headache, emesis.
Local radiotherapy, especially in context of cord compression, single brain metastasis.

Whole brain irradiation for multiple metastases.

Systemic chemotherapy for multiple metastases of chemoresponsive tumour (e.g. breast, small-cell lung tumour, germ-cell tumours).

Surgery probably not indicated if active cancer elsewhere; no improvement in survival.

References Fetell MR. Metastatic tumors. In: Rowland LP (ed.). *Merritt's Textbook of Neurology* (9th edition). Baltimore: Williams & Wilkins, 1995: 395–405.

Posner JB. *Neurologic Complications of Cancer*. Philadelphia: Davis, 1995.

Other relevant entries Lymphoma; Meningeal carcinomatosis; Myelopathy: an overview; Paraneoplastic syndromes; Tumours: an overview.

Methanol poisoning

Methanol (methyl alcohol) poisoning produces drowsiness, headache, nausea, vomiting, visual blurring, dyspnoea and cyanosis; it may progress to delirium and coma. Blindness is the most common symptom and may persist after recovery from acute intoxication: there is reduced visual acuity, central scotoma and constriction of the peripheral fields. Methanol may produce a toxic parkinsonism. Treatment of acute poisoning is by means of gastric lavage, adminstration of alkali, and ethanol (antagonizes oxidation of methanol to formaldehyde and formic acid in the liver).

Methylenetetrahydrofolate reductase deficiency

A rare inborn error of metabolism of folic acid, presenting either as an acute infantile syndrome of hiccups, hypotonia, myoclonic seizures, apnoeic attacks, impaired leukocyte function with bacterial and fungal infection, with death at 3–4 months of age if untreated; or a more indolent late-infantile form with seizures, progressive pyramidal and cerebellar signs and cognitive decline. Hypomethioninaemia is the key laboratory finding; neutropenia may also be found. Management is to provide adequate methionine, as betaine and methionine supplements, with monitoring to avoid high levels of homocysteine in the blood.

Methylmalonic acidaemia

A disorder of organic acid metabolism, due to a defect in methylmalonyl-CoA mutase (classical methylmalonic acidaemia, MMA), often presenting in the first few weeks of life with

- Encephalopathy + severe metabolic acidosis.
- Mucocutaneous candidiasis.
- $+/-$ seizures: clonic, myoclonic.
- Facial dysmorphism: high forehead, triangular mouth, epicanthal folds.

- Increased muscle tone (*cf.* hypotonia in propionic acidaemia).
- Basal ganglia infarcts may occur.
- Hyperammonaemia, reduced plasma carnitine, increased glycine; moderate hypoglycaemia.
- Neutropenia, thrombocytopenia.
- Ketonuria.
- Urine organic acid analysis shows a typical, diagnostic, pattern: massive methyl-malonic aciduria.

Clinically the condition may be indistinguishable in the newborn from other disorders of organic acid metabolism such as propionic aciduria and isovaleric aciduria. Homocystinuria enters the differential diagnosis (basal ganglia infarcts, methyl-malonic acidaemia).

Acutely, bicarbonate is used to control acidosis, plus intravenous fluids to remove methylmalonic acid. Long-term treatment is with dietary restriction of isoleucine, valine, methionine and threonine, with carnitine supplementation and metronidazole.

Methylmalonyl-CoA mutase requires cobalamin (vitamin B_{12}) for activity: defects of intramitochondrial processing or adenosylation of cobalamin may cause milder MMA than complete enzyme deficiency. It responds to pharmacological doses of vitamin B_{12}.

Whereas most infants used to die, prognosis is now good if methylmalonic acid levels can be successfully managed.

Other relevant entries Homocystinuria; Isovaleric acidaemia; Organic acidopathies; Propionic acidaemia; Vitamin B_{12} deficiency.

■ Meyer–Betz disease

Recurrent myoglobinuria of unknown cause, presumably reflecting undiagnosed or undefined metabolic myopathy.

Other relevant entry Rhabdomyolysis.

■ Micturition syncope – see Syncope

■ Midbrain syndrome (dorsal) – see Parinaud's syndrome

■ Migraine

Pathophysiology The precise pathophysiology of migraine is still debated, but probably involves an alteration of blood flow in the cerebral vessels, such that intracranial vessels are constricted and extracranial vessels are dilated; a wave of spreading electrical depression over the cortex, first observed in animals by Leao in 1944, may be significant in the genesis of the progressive focal neurological signs. A family history of migraine is common, suggesting genetic risk factors, and in one variant (familial hemiplegic migraine) deterministic mutant genes have been identified. Migraine is commoner in women, suggested a role for hormonal factors.

Clinical features: history and examination A number of variants of migraine are described. Generally, migraine is characterized by an episodic headache, usually severe, often but not exclusively unilateral (*cf.* cluster headache), throbbing in character, often accompanied by nausea and vomiting, such that the patient wishes to lie still (*cf.* cluster headache) and rest, avoiding light (photophobia) and noise (phonophobia). Headache often improves with sleep.

- Migraine with aura: preceded by visual disturbances: flashing spots, lines, jagged edges (fortification spectra, teichopsia), for perhaps 20–30 minutes; followed by headache, with gradual build up in intensity. Tingling, sensory complaints, or heaviness on one side of the face or body are not uncommon; this is not the same as familial hemiplegic migraine.
- Migraine without aura: no preceding visual disturbance.
- Migraine without headache (migraine equivalent, acephalgic migraine): an aura not followed by headache.
- Familial hemiplegic migraine (FHM), cerebellar migraine: transient hemiparesis associated with migraine headache; associated mutations have been defined, in brain-specific neuronal voltage-gated calcium channel α_1-subunit gene (CACNA1A) at 19q13.1 (hence a channelopathy, allelic with spinocerebellar ataxia type 6 and episodic ataxia type 2), and in ATP1A2 at 1q23.
- Basilar (artery) migraine: bilateral visual disturbances followed by paraesthesiae of lips, hands and feet, dysarthria and diplopia, occipital headache, $+/-$ impairment of consciousness. Features thought suggestive of posterior circulation ischaemia.
- Status migrainosus: recurrent episodes of migraine headache without recovery from previous episode; rare.
- Abdominal migraine: cyclical vomiting of childhood may be a migraine equivalent.
- Retinal migraine: occurrence of photopsia, monocular field defects (altitudinal) and blindness, occurring with migraine headache.
- Ophthalmoplegic migraine (*q.v.*): now better characterized as a focal variant of demyelinating neuropathy.
- Facial migraine, lower-half migraine, Sluder's neuralgia, sphenopalatine (ganglion) neuralgia: episodic pain of ear, nose, neck.
- Migrainous infarction, migrainous stroke: may be defined as: a stroke occurring in a patient with a past medical history of migraine; no other identified cause for stroke; cortical infarction, stroke occurring in the context of a migraine headache; or an aura lasting >7 days. Migraine *per se* may be a risk factor for stroke, but not of as a great a magnitude as other modifiable factors: smoking and oral contraceptive pill use.

Investigations and diagnosis Diagnosis is essentially clinical, that is, based on history and examination.

Bloods: Migraine is associated with a range of autoimmune disorders, so some would advocate PRC, ESR, clotting, ANA, anti-cardiolipin antibodies as baseline tests.

Imaging: CT/MR has no diagnostic role, but may be used to rule out other possibilities in the differential (e.g. subarachnoid haemorrhage). Previous suggestions that consistently unilateral headaches might be associated with an underlying arteriovenous malformation have not been borne out by systematic studies.

CSF: may be performed to exclude meningitis.

Neurogenetics: FHM is a channelopathy, seek specific mutations.

Differential diagnosis Other types of headache: cluster headache, episodic tension-type headache, medication overuse headache; subarachnoid haemorrhage, meningitis.

Migraine without headache may be erroneously labelled as TIA.

Treatment and prognosis Identify/avoid trigger factors: sleep deprivation, dietary triggers; stop smoking.

Acute therapy: aspirin, triptans, non-steroidal anti-inflammatory agents may be used. Potential for excess triptan consumption to lead to medication overuse headache (*q.v.*). Vomiting and impaired gastrointestinal motility may reduce absorption of oral medication; concurrent use of an anti-emetic, or administration by parenteral route (nasal spray, injection) may be required.

Prophylactic therapy: options include propranolol, pizotifen, amitriptyline, sodium valproate, cyproheptadine, methysergide (6 months only, monitor for pleuroperitoneal fibrosis).

In women, headaches may be more evident at times of hormonal change, for example menarche, menopause, oral contraceptive pill use; may improve or remit during pregnancy.

Rarely a permanent hemiparesis develops in FHM, or as a consequence of migrainous stroke.

References Ducros A, Tournier-Lasserve E, Bousser M-G. The genetics of migraine. *Lancet Neurology* 2002; **1**: 285–293.

Ferrari MD. Migraine. *Lancet* 1998; **351**: 1043–1051.

Lipton RB, Scher AI, Kolodner K, Liberman J, Steiner TJ, Stewart WF. Migraine in the United States: epidemiology and patterns of health care use. *Neurology* 2002; **58**: 885–894.

Silberstein S. Practice parameter: Evidence-based guidelines for migraine headache (and evidence-based review). *Neurology* 2000; **55**: 754–762.

Silberstein S, Goadsby PJ, Lipton RB. Management of migraine: an algorithmic approach. *Neurology* 2000; **55 (suppl 2)**: S46–S52.

Other relevant entries Cluster headache; Headache: an overview; Medication overuse headache; Ophthalmoplegic migraine; Sphenopalatine (ganglion) neuralgia.

■ Migrainous neuralgia – see Cluster headache

■ Migrant sensory neuritis – see Wartenberg's neuropathy

Mild cognitive impairment

Pathophysiology In the continuum between normal and abnormal cognitive function, there are individuals with cognitive impairment with respect to others matched for age and education, who are destined to develop dementia but are not yet demented; these individuals may be labelled as having mild cognitive impairment (MCI). MCI is a subject of great current interest, as it is hoped that intervention at this stage of the illness might prevent further decline (i.e. dementia).

Clinical features: history and examination Suggested clinical criteria are:

Memory complaint (preferably corroborated by an informant).
Objective memory impairment.
Intact general cognition.
Essentially preserved activities of daily living.
Not demented.

MCI is heterogeneous. Distinctions may be drawn between
- Amnestic MCI, thought to be a harbinger of Alzheimer's disease (AD).
- Multiple domain MCI: may reflect AD, vascular dementia, or normal aging.
- Single non-memory domain MCI: may reflect vascular dementia, dementia with Lewy bodies, frontotemporal dementia, primary progressive aphasia.

Investigations and diagnosis As for dementia syndromes; MCI destined to become AD may show selective hippocampal shrinkage.

Differential diagnosis Besides dementia syndromes, MCI patients may have affective disorder (e.g. depression) or normal aging.

Treatment and prognosis

Perhaps 10–15% of patients with MCI convert to dementia each year.
No specific treatment yet known. Risk factors for known dementia syndromes may be addressed.

> **References** Golomb J, Kluger A, Garrard P, Ferris S. *Clinician's Manual on Mild Cognitive Impairment*. London: Science Press, 2001.
>
> Petersen RC (ed.). *Mild Cognitive Impairment. Aging to Alzheimer's disease*. Oxford: OUP, 2003.
>
> **Other relevant entries** Alzheimer's disease; Dementia: an overview; Dementia with Lewy bodies; Frontotemporal dementia; Primary progressive aphasia; Vascular dementia.

Millard–Gubler syndrome

Pathophysiology Millard–Gubler syndrome is a brainstem vascular syndrome following pontine infarction, with crossed paralysis.

Clinical features: history and examination
- Lateral rectus paralysis (involvement of abducent nerve fascicles).

- Ipsilateral facial paresis (lower motor neurone type).
- Contralateral hemiplegia sparing the face (pyramidal tract involvement).

Investigations and diagnosis MRI to confirm diagnosis of brainstem stroke.

Differential diagnosis

Raymond syndrome (alternating abducens hemiplegia): no ipsilateral facial paresis. Foville syndrome.

Treatment and prognosis Acute care on a stroke unit. Early aspirin. Secondary prophylaxis (control of risk factors: hypertension, hypercholesterolaemia).

> **Reference** Silverman IE, Lui GT, Galetta SL. The crossed paralyses. The original brain-stem syndromes of Millard–Gubler, Foville, Weber and Raymond–Céstan. *Archives of Neurology* 1995; **52**: 635–638.

> **Other relevant entries** Brainstem vacular syndromes; Cerebrovascular disease: arterial; Foville's syndrome; Raymond syndrome, Raymond–Céstan syndrome.

■ Miller–Dieker syndrome – see Lissencephaly

■ Miller Fisher syndrome

Pathophysiology A monophasic inflammatory disorder, thought to be a variant of Guillain–Barré syndrome (GBS), which may be associated with the presence of antibodies directed against the ganglioside GQ1b. There may be preceding respiratory or gastrointestinal (*Campylobacter*) infection. Whether the disorder has a central, peripheral or combined origin has been debated.

Clinical features: history and examination

- Ophthalmoplegia, causing diplopia; may progress to complete immobilization of the eyes; +/− ptosis, pupillary sphincter paralysis.
- Ataxia: gait > limb clumsiness.
- Areflexia.
- +/− peripheral neuropathy; paraesthesia; oropharyngeal, facial weakness; dysautonomia.

Investigations and diagnosis *Bloods*: Anti-GQ1b antibody seems to correlate with the presence of ophthalmoplegia.

CSF: protein elevated in the majority of cases.

Neurophysiology: EMG/NCS: most studies show demyelinating peripheral neuropathy, with reduced sensory nerve action potential amplitudes and lesser degrees of slowing.

Imaging: cases with CT/MRI evidence of central lesions occur, but whether these are necessary for the clinical signs is less certain.

Differential diagnosis Guillain–Barré syndrome.

Bickerstaff's brainstem encephalitis: exact relationship uncertain, both may be associated with anti-GQ1b antibody. Purists would say that Bickerstaff's brainstem encephalitis (BBE) presents with drowsiness which is never a feature of Miller Fisher syndrome (MFS).

Botulism.

Diphtheritic neuropathy.

Treatment and prognosis No clinical trials of treatment modalities are reported, perhaps because of the infrequency of the condition, but by analogy with GBS treatment with plasma exchange or intravenous immunoglobulin seems reasonable. Most patients recover, although relapsing cases have been described.

References Chiba A, Kusunoki S, Shimizu T, Kanazawa I. Serum IgG antibody to ganglioside GQ1b is a possible marker of Miller Fisher syndrome. *Annals of Neurology* 1992; **31**: 677–679.

Fisher M. An unusual variant of acute idiopathic polyneuritis (syndrome of ophthalmoplegia, ataxia, and areflexia). *New England Journal of Medicine* 1956; **255**: 57–65.

Ropper AH. Miller Fisher syndrome and other acute variants of Guillain–Barré syndrome. In: McLeod JG (ed.). *Inflammatory neuropathies*. London: Baillière Tindall, 1994: 95–106.

Other relevant entries Bickerstaff's brainstem encephalitis; Gangliosides and neurological disorders; Guillain–Barré syndrome.

■ Mills' syndrome, Mills' variant

Mills described a slowly progressive ascending or descending hemiplegia in 1900, which was ascribed to a primary degeneration of the corticospinal pyramidal pathways. The entity has remained controversial, since other disease processes might produce a similar clinical picture, for example brain tumour, cervical spine or cervico-occipital abnormalities, pontine lesions, small lacunar infarcts, multiple sclerosis. In more recent times, it has been suggested that Mills' syndrome is in fact a variant of primary lateral sclerosis, itself a form of motor neurone disease characterized by upper motor neurone signs only.

Reference Gastaut J-L, Bartolomei F. Mills' syndrome: ascending (or descending) progressive hemiplegia: a hemiplegic form of primary lateral sclerosis? *Journal of Neurology, Neurosurgery and Psychiatry* 1994; **57**: 1280–1281.

Other relevant entries Motor neurone diseases: an overview; Primary lateral sclerosis.

■ Minamata disease – see Heavy metal poisoning

■ Minicore–multicore disease

Multicore disease

This congenital myopathy, which may be sporadic, autosomal dominant or recessive, produces generalized weakness in infancy with little or no progression. Diaphragmatic weakness and respiratory failure may occur, simulating nemaline myopathy. The name relates to multiple cores in muscle fibres, unlike those in central core disease.

Other relevant entry Congenital muscle and neuromuscular disorders: an overview.

■ Mitochondrial disease: an overview
Mitochondrial cytopathies • Mitochondriopathies

Pathophysiology Diseases due to defects in the function of the mitochondrial electron transport chain show marked clinical heterogeneity. Their inheritance may be autosomal-recessive, autosomal-dominant, X-linked, or mitochondrial (matrilineal), depending on whether they result from mutations in nuclear genes which encode mitochondrial respiratory chain proteins, or in the small mitochondrial DNA (mtDNA) genome. They may manifest as multisystem diseases, affecting both central and peripheral nervous systems. Whether these should be "lumped" or "split" is still a subject of debate; certain it is that overlap between syndromes occurs.

Mitochondrial dysfunction has also been implicated in other neurodegenerative diseases such as Parkinson's disease, Alzheimer's disease, Huntington's disease and motor neurone disease. A number of conditions have now been shown to be due to mutations in nuclear encoded mitochondrial non-respiratory chain proteins, for example Friedreich's ataxia, Wilson's disease, hereditary spastic paraparesis linked to chromosome 16 (paraplegin mutations), Mohr–Tranebjaerg syndrome. These disorders could also legitimately be labelled "mitochondrial diseases".

Clinical features: history and examination The clinical phenotype is very heterogeneous.

Common features:
- Persistent lactic acidosis
- Myopathy (weakness, hypotonia)
- Failure to thrive, short stature
- Psychomotor retardation, dementia
- Seizures.

Other neurological features often encountered:
- Ophthalmoplegia
- Retinal pigmentary degeneration
- Cerebellar ataxia
- Myoclonus
- Sensorineural hearing loss
- Stroke-like episodes
- Peripheral neuropathy
- Cognitive impairment
- Raised CSF protein.

Other non-neurological features often encountered:

- Cardiomyopathy
- Diabetes mellitus
- Renal tubular dysfunction, Fanconi syndrome
- Respiratory abnormalities (tachypnoea, periodic apnoea)
- Gastrointestinal hypomotility, pseudo-obstruction
- Hypoparathyroidism.

Despite this heterogeneity, some reasonably distinct syndromes have been described (see individual entries for details), viz.

Chronic progressive external ophthalmoplegia (CPEO)
Kearns–Sayre syndrome (KSS)
Leber's hereditary optic neuropathy (LHON)
Leigh's disease, Leigh's syndrome
Luft disease
MELAS syndrome
MERRF syndrome
MNGIE syndrome
NARP syndrome
Pyruvate carboxylase (PC) deficiency
Pyruvate dehydrogenase (PDH) deficiency
Wolfram syndrome.

Investigations and diagnosis *Bloods*: persistent lactic acidosis (but beware of false positives with this test; CSF is more reliable).

Imaging: MR: cerebellar atrophy or non-vascular territory strokes or basal ganglia lesions.

Electrophysiology: SSEP: cortical hyperexcitability; abnormal ERGs; ECG for cardiac rhythm abnormalities.

CSF: increased protein, lactate.

Muscle biopsy: histochemical studies with the Gomori trichrome stain may show subsarcolemmal aggregations of mitochondria as ragged red fibres (although these may occur in some other myopathies, and with normal aging); fibres deficient in cytochrome oxidase staining may also be seen. Electron microscopy may show abnormal mitochondrial cristae with paracrystalline inclusions of variable morphology. Extraction of mitochondria may allow biochemical studies showing deficient respiratory chain function.

Neurogenetics: identification of mitochondrial DNA deletions, point mutations.

Differential diagnosis Although the gestalt may make diagnosis obvious, it may be necessary, dependent on the clinical presentation, to consider other causes of young stroke, myopathy, ophthalmoplegia, seizures. Other hereditary metabolic disorders may be considered.

Occasional cases with many clinical features suggestive of mitochondrial disease but in which no mitochondrial defect is found ("pseudomitochondrial disease") have been presented.

Treatment and prognosis There is currently no specific treatment for mitochondrial diseases. Symptomatic and supportive care (e.g. for seizures, diabetes and cardiac involvement) is the mainstay of management. Creatine may be helpful for muscle symptoms.

References Bindoff L, Brown G, Poulton J. Mitochondrial myopathies. In: Emery AEH (ed.). *Diagnostic Criteria for Neuromuscular Disorders* (2nd edition). London: Royal Society of Medicine Press, 1997: 85–90.

Chinnery PF, Elliott C, Green GR *et al*. The spectrum of hearing loss due to mitochondrial DNA defects. *Brain* 2000; **123**: 82–92.

DiMauro S, Schon EA. Mitochondrial respiratory-chain diseases. *New England Journal of Medicine* 2003; **348**: 2656–2668.

Johns DR. Mitochondrial DNA and disease. *New England Journal of Medicine* 1995; **333**: 638–644.

Leonard JV, Schapira AHV. Mitochondrial respiratory chain disorders I: mitochondrial DNA defect. *Lancet* 2000; **355**: 299–304.

Leonard JV, Schapira AHV. Mitochondrial respiratory chain disorders II: neurodegenerative disorders and nuclear gene defects. *Lancet* 2000; **355**: 389–394.

Schmiedel J, Jackson S, Schäfer J, Reichmann H. Mitochondrial cytopathies. *Journal of Neurology* 2003; **250**: 267–277.

Other relevant entries Chronic progressive external ophthalmoplegia; Friedreich's ataxia; Hereditary spastic paraparesis; Kearns–Sayre syndrome; Lactic acidosis; Leber's hereditary optic neuropathy; Leigh's disease, Leigh's syndrome; Luft disease; MELAS syndrome; MERRF syndrome; MNGIE syndrome; Mohr–Tranebjaerg syndrome; NARP syndrome; Pseudomitochondrial disease; Pyruvate carboxylase deficiency; Pyruvate dehydrogenase deficiency; Wilson's disease; Wolfram syndrome.

■ Mitochondrial encephalomyopathy, lactic acidosis, and stroke-like episodes – see MELAS syndrome

■ Mitochondrial neurogastrointestinal encephalopathy syndrome – see MNGIE syndrome

■ Mixed connective tissue disease
Sharp's syndrome

A disorder in which there is overlap of features from more than one collagen vascular or rheumatic disorder, such as systemic sclerosis, systemic lupus erythematosus, Sjögren's syndrome, and polymyositis. Antinuclear antibody is positive with a speckled pattern, high levels of antibodies directed against extractable nuclear antigens (ENA) are found, particularly nuclear ribonucleoprotein (nRNP), and rheumatoid factor (RhF) may be positive.

As with other collagen vascular disorders, neurological features may occur, affecting >50% of patients in one series, including:

- Aseptic meningitis.
- Seizures.
- Psychosis.
- Trigeminal neuralgia.
- Sensory neuropathy.
- Stroke (small vessel vasculitis).

References Bennett RM, Bong DM, Spargo BH. Neuropsychiatric problems in mixed connective tissue disease. *American Journal of Medicine* 1978; **65**: 955–962.

Nadeau S. Neurologic manifestations of connective tissue disease. *Neurologic Clinics* 2002; **20**: 151–178.

Other relevant entries Aseptic meningitis; Polymyositis; Sjögren's syndrome; Systemic lupus erythematosus and the nervous system; Systemic sclerosis; Trigeminal neuralgia.

■ Miyoshi myopathy

Early-adult-onset distal myopathy type 2

An autosomal-recessive distal muscular dystrophy usually of early-onset (<30 years), common in Japan, characterized by muscle wasting and weakness in a predominantly distal distribution (e.g. the posterior compartment of the legs), although intrafamilial phenotypic variation does occur. Creatine kinase is elevated (>10 times normal). Muscle biopsy pathology shows dystrophic changes without rimmed vacuoles (*cf.* Nonaka myopathy). Linkage is to chromosome 2p, and mutations within the gene encoding dysferlin have been identified. Hence this is a dysferlinopathy, and allelic with limb-girdle muscular dystrophy type 2B.

Reference Nakagawa M, Matsuzaki T, Suehara M *et al.* Phenotypic variation in a large Japanese family with Miyoshi myopathy with nonsense mutation in exon 19 of dysferlin gene. *Journal of the Neurological Sciences* 2001; **184**: 15–19.

Other relevant entries Distal muscular dystrophy, Distal myopathy; Dysferlinopathy; Limb-girdle muscular dystrophy; Nonaka myopathy.

■ MNGIE syndrome

Mitochondrial encephalomyopathy with polyneuropathy, ophthalmoplegia and pseudo-obstruction (MEPOP) • Mitochondrial neurogastrointestinal encephalopathy syndrome • Myoneurogastrointestinal encephalopathy

A rare mitochondrial disorder, generally beginning in childhood. The clinical features include:

- Gastrointestinal dysmotility: diarrhoea, intestinal pseudo-obstruction (may lead to laparotomy), malabsorption;

- Ophthalmoplegia: almost invariant; +/− ptosis.
- Progressive leukodystrophy: cognitive impairment, dementia.
- Myopathy.
- Peripheral neuropathy: sensorimotor polyneuropathy.

Ragged red fibres are prominent on muscle biopsy.

The pattern of inheritance may be maternal, autosomal recessive or autosomal dominant. Depletion and/or multiple deletions of mitochondrial DNA have been observed in some families; defective electron transport chain activity affecting complex IV (cytochrome-*c* oxidase) has also been observed. Autosomal-recessive disease is associated with mutations in the gene encoding thymidine phosphorylase (TP), and there is reduced leukocyte TP activity.

Abetalipoproteinaemia enters the differential diagnosis, but there is no retinopathy or acanthocytosis in MNGIE. There is no specific treatment, only supportive care. Death usually occurs in the fourth decade.

Reference Nishino I, Spinazzola A, Papadimitriou A *et al*. Mitochondrial neurogastrointestinal encephalomyopathy: an autosomal recessive disorder due to thymidine phosphorylase mutations. *Annals of Neurology* 2000; **47**: 792–800.

Other Relevant entry Mitochondrial disease: an overview.

■ Möbius syndrome
Congenital facial diplegia

The clinical features of this syndrome are
- Congenital facial diplegia.
- Bilateral sixth nerve (abducens) palsies.
- +/− dysarthria, dysphagia, hearing loss.
- +/− mental retardation.

The syndrome may be evident in the neonatal period as poor sucking and lack of facial expression, but if the facial paralysis is incomplete diagnosis may not be made until later. Unlike other causes of facial paralysis, the lower face is often less severely affected than the upper face, with more difficulty closing the eyes than moving the lips. The syndrome may have more than one cause, including agenesis of brainstem motor neurones or aplasia of ocular muscles. The differential diagnosis includes congenital myotonic muscular dystrophy or facioscapulohumeral dystrophy. Other anomalies may coexist (e.g. Poland anomaly).

Reference Rowland LP. Marcus Gunn and Möbius syndromes. In: Rowland LP (ed.). *Merritt's Textbook of Neurology* (9th edition). Baltimore: Williams & Wilkins, 1995: 533–534.

Other relevant entries Cranial nerve disease: VI: Abducens nerve; Cranial nerve disease: VII: Facial nerve; Poland anomaly.

■ Moersch–Woltman syndrome – see Stiff people: an overview

■ Mohr–Tranebjaerg syndrome

A sex-linked syndrome of sensorineural deafness and dystonia, sometimes accompanied by blindness, fractures, and mental retardation. Linkage to chromosome Xq21.3–Xq22 was followed by identification of mutations in a gene named deafness/dystonia peptide (DDP) gene. Mutations in the same gene have been identified in Jensen syndrome (opticoacoustic nerve atrophy and dementia), hence the conditions are allelic. In one mutation, female carriers may show dystonic features.

> **Reference** Swerdlow RH, Wooten GF. A novel deafness/dystonia peptide gene
> mutation that causes dystonia in female carriers of Mohr–Tranebjaerg syndrome.
> *Annals of Neurology* 2001; **50**: 537–540.

> **Other relevant entries** Dystonia: an overview; Mitochondrial disease: an overview.

■ Mollaret meningitis

A rare syndrome of recurrent aseptic meningitis, as originally described with a distinctive CSF cytology featuring large mononuclear (Mollaret) cells. For long classified as idiopathic, in recent years use of the polymerase chain reaction has identified herpes simplex virus type 2 (HSV-2) in CSF of many cases, without necessarily a prior history of genital herpes. These findings suggest that antiviral therapy such as aciclovir might be appropriate.

A similar syndrome of recurrent aseptic meningitis may be caused by rupture of dermoids or epidermoids into the CSF.

> **Other relevant entries** Aseptic meningitis; Dermoid; Epidermoid; Herpes simplex
> encephalitis; Meningitis: an overview.

■ Monge disease – see Altitude sickness

■ Moniliasis – see Candidiasis

■ Monoclonal gammopathies

Paraproteins are present in about 1% of the general population, often without clinical correlate, but in a much greater percentage of patients with a peripheral neuropathy, perhaps 10%. In a few of these, there is an underlying malignancy (myeloma, lymphoma) or amyloidosis, but most have a "monoclonal gammopathy of undetermined significance" (MGUS). Follow up to see whether a malignancy emerges is suggested.

The neuropathy associated with MGUS is typically sensory, affecting lower limbs more than upper, and slowly progressive over years. Neurophysiological studies show features of both axonal and demyelinating involvement. Neuropathies associated with IgM, IgG and IgA may be heterogeneous, since IgM has been reported not to respond to plasma exchange. Other immunosuppressive agents such as prednisolone, azathioprine, cyclophosphamide and ciclosporin have been tried in these cases, sometimes with success.

References Dyck PJ, Low PA, Windebank AJ *et al.* Plasma exchange in polyneuropathy associated with monoclonal gammopathy of undetermined significance. *New England Journal of Medicine* 1991; **325**: 1482–1486.

Notermans NC, Franssses H, Eurelings M *et al.* Diagnostic criteria for demyelinating polyneuropathy associated with monoclonal gammopathy. *Muscle and Nerve* 2000; **23**: 73–79.

Other relevant entries Neuropathies: an overview; Paraproteinaemic neuropathies.

■ Monomelic amyotrophy
Chronic asymmetric spinal muscular atrophy (CASMA) ● Hirayama disease

A syndrome of neurogenic muscular wasting, affecting a single limb (arm > leg), commoner in men, usually occurring in the second to fourth decades. The wasting progresses for a year or 2, then seems to arrest. EMG/NCS shows chronic partial denervation, MRI may show asymmetry of the spinal cord. This is thought to be a localized form of spinal muscular atrophy, but it must be remembered that monomelic atrophy may sometimes be the presenting feature of motor neurone disease.

Reference Kiernan MC, Lethlean AK, Blum PW. Monomelic amyotrophy: non progressive atrophy of the upper limb. *Journal of Clinical Neuroscience* 1999; **6**: 353–355.

Other relevant entries Motor neurone disease; Spinal muscular atrophy.

■ Mononeuritis multiplex, Mononeuropathy multiplex
Multiple mononeuropathy

Involvement of several peripheral (and cranial) nerves over a period of days to weeks, causing patchy sensorimotor deficits and pain, is the characteristic of mononeuritis multiplex, or mononeuropathy multiplex since the aetiology is not always inflammatory. Electrophysiological studies confirm the patchy nature of the process, which may progress to become more like polyneuropathy.

Recognized causes include:
- Vasculitis
    Polyarteritis nodosa
    Churg–Strauss syndrome
    Rheumatoid arthritis
    Systemic lupus erythematosus
    Wegener's granulomatosis
    Giant cell arteritis
    Behçet's disease.

- Infections
    Meningococcal septicaemia
    Infective endocarditis
- Diabetes
- Sarcoidosis
- Neurofibromatosis
- Haematological disorders
    Leukaemia, Lymphoma
    Paraproteinaemia.

Treatment and prognosis are related to cause, where established.

Reference Staal A, Van Gijn J, Spaans F. *Mononeuropathies: Examination, Diagnosis and Treatment.* London: WB Saunders, 1999: 169–173.

Other relevant entries Lumbosacral plexopathies; Neuropathies: an overview; Polyarteritis nodosa; Vasculitis.

■ Morquio's syndrome

Mucopolysaccharidosis type IV (MPS IV)

This uncommon MPS, of which two biochemical variants are recognized, A and B, is transmitted as an autosomal-recessive trait, linked respectively to chromosomes 16q24 and 3. Type A results from deficiency of N-acetylgalactosamine-6-sulphatase, type B from β-galactosidase deficiency (i.e. type B is allelic with GM1 gangliosidosis). Both result in increased urinary concentrations of keratan sulphate (*cf.* all other MPS: dermatan and heparan sulphate). Type B is generally milder than type A.

Clinically there is skeletal deformity resulting in short stature and hyperextensible joints; cervical instability and cord compression is common, and often causes death. Progressive deafness may occur.

Facies are only mildly coarsened.

Intelligence is normal (unless compromised by the development of hydrocephalus).

Other relevant entries Gangliosidoses: an overview; Mucopolysaccharidoses.

■ Morton's metatarsalgia

Pain in the sole of the foot, constant aching plus paroxysms of lancinating pain, due to compression of a digital nerve neuroma between the heads of the metatarsals (second/third, third/fourth). Pressure over the neuroma on the sole of the foot may reproduce the symptoms. The neuroma may be amenable to surgical resection.

■ Morvan's syndrome

Morvan's fibrillary chorea

In 1890, Morvan described a syndrome of myokymia, muscle pain, hyperhidrosis, severe insomnia (agrypnia) and hallucinations. As myokymia, perhaps more appropriately termed neuromyotonia (Isaacs' syndrome), has been shown to be associated with auto-antibodies directed against presynaptic voltage-gated potassium channels (VGKC), it was logical to look for these antibodies in Morvan's syndrome, which may be characterized as neuromyotonia with central nervous system (CNS) involvement. Other features reported in cases with high titres of VGKC antibodies include CSF oligoclonal bands and a neurohormonal profile showing elevated noradrenaline and cortisol with absent circadian rhythms of melatonin and prolactin (as seen in the prion disorder fatal familial insomnia). Clinical improvement with plasma exchange has been reported. There may be an underlying neoplasm (i.e. this may be a paraneoplastic syndrome).

References Barber PA, Anderson NE, Vincent A. Morvan's syndrome associated with voltage-gated K$^+$ channel antibodies. *Neurology* 2000; **54**: 771–772.

Liguori R, Vincent A, Clover L *et al*. Morvan's syndrome: peripheral and central nervous system and cardiac involvement with antibodies to voltage-gated potassium channels. *Brain* 2001; **124**: 2417–2426.

Other relevant entries Fatal familial insomnia; Neuromyotonia; Paraneoplastic syndromes.

■ Moschowitz syndrome – see Thrombotic thrombocytopenic purpura

■ Motor neurone disease
Amyotrophic lateral sclerosis (ALS) • Lou Gehrig's disease

Pathophysiology A disorder of both upper and lower motor neurones causing muscle wasting and weakness, with gradual and inexorable decline of function leading to death. Motor neurone disease (MND) remains one of the most feared diagnoses in neurological practice because of its dismal prognosis, although some patients do survive many years. Aetiology remains uncertain, although deterministic genes have been identified in some of the 10% of cases in which the disease is inherited as an autosomal-dominant condition. Mutations in the copper–zinc superoxide dismutase (Cu/Zn-SOD) gene suggested a possible pathophysiological role for oxidative stress.

Clinical features: history and examination Diagnostic criteria exist, but essentially the diagnosis requires:

- Evidence (clinical, electrophysiological, neuropathological) of lower motor neurone degeneration.
- Evidence (clinical) of upper motor neurone degeneration.
- Progressive spread of symptoms and signs.
- Absence of electrophysiological, pathological or neuroimaging evidence of other disease process(es) that might better explain the observed signs.
- Sensory loss and early sphincter dysfunction would argue against the diagnosis.

The criteria propose a number of diagnostic categories (Clinically definite, Clinically probable, Clinically probable–laboratory supported, Clinically possible) which are helpful for clinical trials. Clinically definite MND is defined by UMN and LMN signs in three regions.

Older clinical classifications enumerated variants such as progressive bulbar palsy, progressive muscular atrophy, indicating where the brunt of the initial clinical problem was, but it is recognized that these all reflect the same underlying disease. Symmetrical wasting and weakness of the arms without, or with only minimal, leg and bulbar involvement has been labelled the flail arm syndrome, and may correspond to what was previously called Vulpian–Bernhardt syndrome.

Recognized types and patterns of MND may be listed as sporadic MND, genetically determined MND, and MND plus syndromes, for example with parkinsonism, frontal-type dementia ("motor neurone disease dementia").

Investigations and diagnosis *Bloods*: creatine kinase may be modestly elevated; depending upon the patients age, additional tests may be undertaken to exclude other cause of a motor neurone disease, for example hexosaminidase deficiency (white cell enzymatic assays), spinal muscular atrophy (SMN gene mutations). If there is a family history suggesting autosomal-dominant inheritance, look for mutations in Cu/Zn-SOD gene.

Neurophysiology: EMG/NCS: evidence of denervation, particularly significant if found in clinically normal muscles, distant from clinically symptomatic areas.

Imaging: MRI of the cervical spine may be undertaken to exclude multiple compressive radiculopathies as a cause for upper limb wasting, weakness, fasciculation.

CSF: may be performed to look for evidence of inflammatory change (oligoclonal bands); very rarely, motor neurone diseases responding to immunosuppression have been reported.

Muscle biopsy: sometimes performed to confirm neurogenic change, and/or exclude inflammatory (and potentially treatable) myopathy.

Differential diagnosis

Other motor neurone diseases (*q.v.*).

Multiple radiculopathies +/− myelopathy

Treatment and prognosis No curative treatment. Natural history is one of progressive decline, often leading to respiratory failure, aspiration, and death. Occasional long-term survivors, sometimes >15 years.

Riluzole may prolong life for 3–6 months, and is licensed for the treatment of MND.

Many other negative trials: for example branched-chain amino acids, creatine monohydrate.

Supportive therapy is of the greatest importance: physiotherapy, occupational therapy (including home modifications such as grab rails, banisters, stair-lift, bed hoist, walk-in shower, downstairs bedroom), speech therapy. Access to appropriate financial benefits.

The issues of respiratory support (nasal CPAP, nocturnal intermittent positive-pressure ventilation) and assisted feeding (percutaneous endoscopic gastrostomy or jejunostomy) should be addressed, preferably sometime before their institution becomes necessary, particularly before respiratory failure requires urgent intervention. Some patients and families will want such interventions, others not.

References Brooks BR, Miller RG, Swash M, Munsat TL. El Escorial revisited: revised criteria for the diagnosis of amyotrophic lateral sclerosis. *Amyotrophic Lateral Sclerosis and other Motor Neuron Disorders* 2000; **1**: 293–299.

Leigh PN, Swash M (eds). *Motor Neuron Disease: Biology and Management.* London: Springer-Verlag, 1995.

Li TM, Day SJ, Alberman E, Swash M. Differential diagnosis of motoneurone disease from other neurological conditions. *Lancet* 1986; **2**: 731–733.

Miller RG, Rosenberg JA, Gelinas DF *et al.* Practice parameter: the care of the patient with amyotrophic lateral sclerosis (an evidence-based review): report of the Quality Standards Subcommittee of the American Academy of Neurology. *Neurology* 1999; **52**: 1311–1323.

Traynor BJ, Codd MB, Corr B, Forde C, Frost E, Hardiman OM. Clinical features of amyotrophic lateral sclerosis according to the El Escorial and Airlie House diagnostic criteria: a population-based study. *Archives of Neurology* 2000; **57**: 1171–1176.

Other relevant entries Flail arm syndrome; Motor neurone diseases: an overview; Neuropathies: an overview.

■ Motor neurone diseases: an overview
Motor neuronal diseases

Motor neurone diseases may be classified clinically on the basis of whether disease is localized to the upper motor neurones, lower motor neurones, or both.

- Combined upper and lower motor neurone involvement
    Motor neurone disease (MND)/amyotrophic lateral sclerosis (ALS)
        Sporadic
        Familial (adult onset; juvenile onset).
- Pure upper motor neurone involvement
    Primary lateral sclerosis (PLS)
    Hereditary spastic paraparesis (HSP)
    Lathyrism
    Konzo.
- Pure lower motor neurone involvement
    Spinal muscular atrophy (SMA):
        Proximal hereditary motor neuronopathy, for example Werdnig–Hoffmann, Kugelberg–Welander types
        Hereditary bulbar palsy (e.g. Fazio–Londe, Brown–Vialetto–Van Laere)
        Focal/segmental variants: monomelic amyotrophy, O'Sullivan–McLeod syndrome
    X-linked bulbospinal neuronopathy (Kennedy's syndrome)
    Hexosaminidase deficiency
    Multifocal motor neuropathies

Poliomyelitis, postpolio syndrome

Postirradiation syndrome.

See individual entries for further details.

References Donaghy M. The motor neurone diseases. In: Donaghy M (ed.). *Brain's Diseases of the Nervous System* (11th edition). Oxford: OUP, 2001: 443–460.

World Federation of Neurology Classification Subcommittee. Classification of neuromuscular diseases. *Journal of the Neurological Sciences* 1988; **86**: 333–360.

Other relevant entries Motor neurone disease; Spinal muscular atrophy.

■ Motor neuropathies – see Neuropathies: an overview

■ Moyamoya

This is an occlusive vasculopathy of uncertain aetiology, most commonly seen in the Japanese. It may present in childhood as a syndrome of recurrent cerebral ischaemia and infarction, associated with cognitive impairment, headache, and seizures; or in adulthood with recurrent cerebral or subarachnoid haemorrhage. Radiologically there is severe stenosis or occlusion of one or both distal internal carotid arteries, sometimes extending to the circle of Willis, with fine anastomotic (telangiectatic) collateral vessels developing from perforating and pial arteries at the base of the brain (basal cerebral *rete mirabile*), orbital and ethmoidal branches of the external carotid artery, and leptomeningeal vessels. These vessels are the source of haemorrhage in cases presenting in adulthood, and may be visualized at angiography as a "puff of smoke" or "haze", from the Japanese term for which the syndrome takes its name.

Although often idiopathic, recognized associations and symptomatic causes of moyamoya include:

- basal meningeal/nasopharyngeal infection,
- vasculitis,
- irradiation,
- trauma,
- fibromuscular dysplasia,
- sickle-cell disease,
- neurofibromatosis.

Atheromatous disease very rarely produces a moyamoya picture; presumably the extensive collateralization can only develop during childhood.

Treatment is uncertain. Drug treatment with steroids, calcium channel blockers, and antiplatelet drugs has produced variable results; anticoagulation is not helpful. Surgical revascularization is advocated by some authorities, for example with superficial temporal artery to middle cerebral artery anastomosis, or simply by apposition of the temporalis muscle to the surface of the brain (arterial myosynangiosis).

Other relevant entries Cerebrovascular disease: arterial; Fibromuscular dysplasia.

Mucolipidoses

The mucolipidoses are uncommon lysosomal-storage diseases, inherited as autosomal-recessive traits, in which both mucopolysaccharides and lipids accumulate in lysosomes, giving a clincal picture akin to both the mucopolysaccharidoses and the GM1 gangliosidoses. The four mucolipidoses may be classified as follows:

Type I: Sialidosis (*q.v.*)
Type II: I-cell disease (*q.v.*)
Type III: Pseudo-Hurler's polydystrophy (*q.v.*)
Type IV: Berman's mucolipidosis

Diagnosis should be considered in any child with a Hurler phenotype (with the exception of type IV) but without excessive urinary mucopolysaccharide excretion. Diagnosis is confirmed by enzymatic analysis of fibroblasts.

See individual entries for types I–IV.

References Lyon G, Adams RD, Kolodny EH. *Neurology of Hereditary Metabolic Diseases of Children* (2nd edition). New York: McGraw-Hill, 1996: 161–165.

Maertens P, Dyken PR. Storage diseases: neuronal ceroid-lipofuscinoses, lipidoses, glycogenoses, and leukodystrophies. In: Goetz CG (ed.). *Textbook of Clinical Neurology* (2nd edition). Philadelphia: Saunders, 2003: 601–628.

Other relevant entries Berman's mucolipidosis; I-cell disease; Lysosomal-storage disorders: an overview; Mucopolysaccharidoses; Pseudo-Hurler's syndrome; Sialidoses: an overview; Sialidosis.

Mucopolysaccharidoses

Pathophysiology The mucopolysaccharidoses (MPS) are hereditary lysosomal-storage diseases in which enzyme deficiencies lead to pathological accumulation and urinary excretion of mucopolysaccharides. All varieties exhibit a period of normal development followed by regression of mental and motor function. The MPS may be classified as follows:

Type I: Hurler's syndrome (I-H), Scheie's syndrome (I-S) and an overlap syndrome (I-H/S)
Type II: Hunter's syndrome
Type III: Sanfilippo disease (types A, B, C, D)
Type IV: Morquio disease (types A and B)
Type VI: Maroteaux–Lamy disease
Type VII: Sly disease
Type VIII: De Ferrante syndrome

Multiple sulphatase deficiency (Austin disease) may be included in the classification.

Chronic encephalopathy may dominate the presentation, but in some it is the non-neurological features which predominate (e.g. MPS 1H, II, VII).

See individual entries for details.

Investigations and diagnosis Clinical phenotype is supplemented by:

Blood: enzymatic assay on cultured fibroblasts or white cells is diagnostic test.

Urine: for mucopolysaccharides, thin layer chromatography is required: dermatan sulphate (Types I-H, I-S, II, VI, VII); heparan sulphate (Types I-H, I-S, II, III, IVB, VII); and keratan sulphate (Types IVA, IVB).

Radiology: dysostosis multiplex.

Differential diagnosis

Mucolipidoses.

GM1 gangliosidoses.

Treatment and prognosis Reduced life expectancy common to all MPS. No specific treatment currently available, although bone marrow transplantation may help if performed early. Enzyme replacement therapy is also undergoing investigation.

References Krivit W, Peters C, Shapiro EG *et al.* Bone marrow transplantation as effective treatment of central nervous system disease in globoid cell leukodystrophy, metachromatic leukodystrophy, adrenoleukodystrophy, mannosidosis, fucosidosis, aspartylglucosaminuria, Hurler, Maroteaux–Lamy, and Sly syndromes, and Gaucher disease type III. *Current Opinion in Neurology* 1999; **12**: 167–176.

Lyon G, Adams RD, Kolodny EH. *Neurology of Hereditary Metabolic Diseases of Children* (2nd edition). New York: McGraw-Hill, 1996: 151–161.

Maertens P, Dyken PR. Storage diseases: neuronal ceroid-lipofuscinoses, lipidoses, glycogenoses, and leukodystrophies. In: Goetz CG (ed.). *Textbook of Clinical Neurology* (2nd edition). Philadelphia: Saunders, 2003: 601–628.

Wraith JE. The mucopolysaccharidoses: a clinical review and guide to management. *Archives of Disease in Childhood* 1995; **72**: 263–267.

Other relevant entries Lysosomal-storage disorders: an overview; Mucolipidoses.

■ Mucormycosis
Phycomycosis • Zygomycosis

Infection with the fungus *Mucorales* spreads from the nasal turbinates and paranasal sinuses to the retro-orbital space, causing proptosis, ophthalmoplegia and peri-orbital oedema, and to the brain causing haemorrhages infarction; vasculitis has also been reported. Infection is a complication of diabetes mellitus (esp. acidosis), drug abuse, and may also occur in the context of leukaemia and lymphoma. Necrotic eschar replacing the nasal mucosa is a highly suggestive sign. Malignant invasive infection is often rapidly fatal, although recovery may occur with correction of risk factors and administration of intravenous amphotericin.

Reference Brotman D, Taege A, Ruggieri P, Kinkel PR. Acute ophthalmoplegia. *Lancet* 2003; **361**: 930.

Other relevant entry Diabetes mellitus and the nervous system.

■ Multicore disease – see Minicore–multicore disease

■ Multifocal motor neuropathy

Multifocal motor neuropathy with conduction block (MMNCB)

Pathophysiology A neuropathy of probable autoimmune pathogenesis, characterized electrophysiologically by conduction block, running a chronic course and commoner in women (M : F = 1 : 3), generally with onset in the second to fifth decades. It is important to identify multifocal motor neuropathy (MMN) since the condition does respond to intravenous immunoglobulin (IVIg).

Clinical features: history and examination

- Early: gradually evolving weakness in territory of single peripheral nerve (e.g. radial, median, ulnar), hence asymmetric, with little or no wasting.
- Progression: involvement of other sites in upper and lower limbs, such that confluent involvement may develop; denervation atrophy frequent.
- + muscle cramp, fatigue, twitching/fasciculation; occasionally true muscle hypertrophy.
- Tendon reflexes variable: lost, normal, or brisk!
- Although sensory nerves are classically spared, sensory symptoms and signs may sometimes occur (differential diagnosis = Lewis Sumner syndrome, MADSAM).

Investigations and diagnosis *Bloods*: creatine kinase, serum IgM may be slightly elevated; anti-GM1 anti-ganglioside antibodies present in 50% of cases (absence unhelpful).

Neurophysiology: EMG/NCS: hallmark is the finding of conduction block away from usual sites of nerve entrapment; block is variably defined but suggests a reduction in CMAP amplitude (>10%) and increase in duration (<20%) when stimulating from adjacent sites; chronic neurogenic change with fasciculation may be seen in the later stages.

CSF: elevated protein in one-third of cases; cell count normal.

Imaging: MRI: may show increased signal intensity on T_2-weighted images in parts of the brachial plexus.

Nerve biopsy: rarely required, to differentiate MMN from nerve tumour or vasculitis; must biopsy a motor or mixed nerve, which may show demyelination, onion bulb formation and axonal atrophy.

Differential diagnosis

- Early: solitary or multiple mononeuropathy.
- Late:
    CIDP
    Motor neurone disease
    Spinal muscular atrophies
    Other motor neuropathies: lead, hereditary neuropathy with liability to pressure palsies.

Treatment and prognosis Mild cases may require no treatment. Benefit has been clearly demonstrated with IVIg (e.g. 2 g/kg over 3–5 days) but the effect wanes over a few months such that repeated courses may be necessary. Neither steroids nor plasma exchange are helpful but there may be a role for cyclophosphamide.

References Nobile-Orazio E. Multifocal motor neuropathy. *Journal of Neuro-immunology* 2001; **115**: 4–18.

Willison H, Mills K. Multifocal motor neuropathy. *Practical Neurology* 2002; **2**: 298–301.

Other relevant entries Lewis Sumner syndrome; Neuropathies: an overview.

▓ Multi-infarct dementia – see Vascular dementia

▓ Multiphasic disseminated encephalomyelitis – see Acute disseminated encephalomyelitis

▓ Multiple endocrine neoplasia – see Pituitary disease and apoplexy

▓ Multiple sclerosis
Disseminated sclerosis

Pathophysiology A common inflammatory demyelinating disorder of central nervous system (CNS) white matter, believed to reflect immune attack on the myelin-oligodendrocyte complex. The ultimate causes of this process are unknown, but may include non-specific viral infection, and possibly, trauma (controversial). Genetic predisposition is related to human leukocyte antigen (HLA) types and possibly other genes relating to immune function. Epidemiology confirms greater risk further from the equator.

Clinical features: history and examination Phenotype is very diverse. The old requirement for episodes of demyelination disseminated in space and time has been superseded with the advent of MRI which may demonstrate spatial dissemination at time of single (initial) attack.

Typical presentations include:
- Clinically isolated syndromes
    Optic neuritis
    Transverse myelitis/myelopathy (usually partial rather than complete)
    Disseminated encephalomyelitis (ADEM).
- Cerebellar ataxia.

However, virtually any focal sensory and/or motor presentation may occur. Internuclear ophthalmoplegia (INO) in a young patient is highly suggestive.

Pattern of disease varies with time:

Relapsing–remitting (RRMS) disease: common in early stages, relapses followed by full or almost full recovery.

Secondary progressive: RRMS often evolves with time into a slowly progressive disorder, with or without superimposed acute relapses.

Primary progressive: occasionally disease is unremitting from the outset.

Variants are recognized (*q.v.*):

Balò's concentric sclerosis.
Marburg disease, Marburg syndrome.
Schilder's disease.

Investigations and diagnosis *Bloods*: non-contributory.

Imaging: MRI is modality of choice to display multiple white matter lesions, both clinically relevant and clinically silent; most usually periventricular in location, lesions often oriented away from axis of ventricles; brainstem lesions, especially cerebellar white matter; spinal cord lesions (usually only one vertebra in longitudinal extent). Enhancement with gadolinium, indicative of blood–brain barrier breakdown, in newer lesions, other (older) lesions non-enhancing. Interval scan (6 months) may show development and regression of lesions. Various MR criteria for the diagnosis of multiple sclerosis (MS) have been suggested.

VERs: typically delayed waveform after optic neuritis, even in clinically silent cases.

CSF: oligoclonal bands in majority (>95%), although non-specific, may occur in other inflammatory CNS diseases.

Differential diagnosis Monophasic illness: clinically isolated syndromes, acute disseminated encephalomyelitis.

Other relapsing–remitting disorders: inflammatory (e.g. sarcoidosis, Behçet's); structural (cavernous haemangioma).

Primary progressive disease: other myelopathies.

Treatment and prognosis Benign disease (single relapse, or relapses separated by years or decades), without acquisition of neurological disability, requires no specific treatment.

Treatment, when required, remains largely symptomatic: intravenous methylprednisolone probably hastens recovery from an acute relapse, oral high dose steroids possibly also help.

So-called disease-modifying drugs (interferons, glatiramer) have been shown to reduce relapse rate by one-third (as have other immunosuppressive agents such as azathioprine), but whether this translates into longer-term prevention of disability remains an open question, trials to date having been inconclusive. Interferons may reduce the risk of conversion of clinically isolated syndrome to MS. Other immunomodulatory drugs such as CAMPATH-1H may modify disease but at risk of other immune-mediated disorders (Graves' disease).

With the development of fixed disability, such as limb spasticity or bladder dysfunction, symptomatic treatments may be appropriate: baclofen, tizanidine for spasticity, oxybutynin, clean intermittent self-catheterization for bladder dysfunction. Physiotherapy, occupational therapy, speech therapy may have much to offer at this stage of the disease.

Cognitive decline ("white matter" or subcortical-type dementia) may develop.

References Barnes MP. Multiple sclerosis. In: Greenwood RJ, Barnes MP, McMillan TM, Ward CD (eds). *Handbook of Neurological Rehabilitation* (2nd edition). Hove: Psychology Press, 2003: 533–552.

Compston A, Coles A. Multiple sclerosis. *Lancet* 2002; **359**: 1221–1231.

Compston A, Ebers G, Lassmann H, McDonald I, Matthews B, Wekerle H. *McAlpine's Multiple Sclerosis* (3rd edition). London: Churchill Livingstone, 1998.

Feinstein A. *The Clinical Neuropsychiatry of Multiple Sclerosis*. Cambridge: Cambridge University Press, 1999.

McDonald WI, Compston A, Edan G *et al.* Recommended diagnostic criteria for multiple sclerosis: guidelines from the International Panel on the Diagnosis of Multiple Sclerosis. *Annals of Neurology* 2001; **50**: 121–127.

Noseworthy JH, Lucchinetti C, Rodriguez M, Weinshenker BG. Multiple sclerosis. *New England Journal of Medicine* 2000; **343**: 938–952.

Scolding N. Multiple sclerosis. In: Scolding N (ed.). *Immunological and Inflammatory Disorders of the Central Nervous System*. Oxford: Butterworth-Heinemann, 1999: 21–73.

Other relevant entries Acute disseminated encephalomyelitis; Balò's concentric sclerosis; Clinically isolated syndromes; Devic's disease, Devic's syndrome; Internuclear ophthalmoplegia; Marburg disease; Optic neuritis; Schilder's disease; Transverse myelitis, transverse myelopathy.

■ Multiple sulphatase deficiency – see Austin disease

■ Multiple symmetric lipomatosis – see Lannois–Bensaude disease

■ Multiple system atrophy
Multisystem atrophy

Pathophysiology A sporadic neurodegenerative disorder with autonomic, parkinsonian, cerebellar and pyramidal features that may occur in any combination. For this reason, subtypes have been defined according to the presenting neurological feature:

MSA-P: parkinsonism.

MSA-C: cerebellar (includes cases previously labelled olivopontocerebellar atrophy, OPCA).

MSA-M: mixed, combination of neurological features (includes striatonigral degeneration).

Autonomic features are integral to the diagnosis; Shy–Drager syndrome was once used to label such patients. Some patients diagnosed with isolated autonomic failure evolve to multiple system atrophy (MSA); likewise some idiopathic late-onset cerebellar ataxias (ILOCA) eventually prove to be MSA. It is difficult to differentiate MSA-P from idiopathic Parkinson's disease (PD) in the early stages but clues come from early bladder symptoms and lack of sustained response to levodopa.

Oligodendroglial intracytoplasmic argyrophilic inclusions (GCI) containing α-synuclein are the specific pathological feature; hence MSA may be considered a synucleinopathy. There is neuronal loss and gliosis in the striatum, substantia nigra, locus ceruleus, pontine nuclei, cerebellum (Purkinje cells), and inferior olivary nuclei; and in the spinal cord intermediolateral columns and Onuf's nucleus.

The condition is slightly commoner in males; its prevalence is less than that of progressive supranuclear palsy (PSP). In Europe the parkinsonian form predominates; the reverse is true in Japan.

Clinical features: history and examination

- Parkinsonism

  Akinetic-rigid syndrome;

  Tremor: postural > rest > action; postural tremor is often jerky and irregular, exaggerated by tapping the hand (i.e. stimulus-sensitive myoclonus); pill-rolling rest tremor rare.

- Dysautonomia

  Erectile failure (early)

  Urinary incontinence (neurogenic bladder, urge incontinence early)

  Syncope, presyncope

  Urinary retention

  Faecal incontinence (rare).

- Cerebellar syndrome

  Limb ataxia > gait; intention tremor

  Dysarthria: atypical, "strangled", dystonic

  Dysphagia

  Stridor

  Antecollis.

- Cognition generally believed to be preserved, but occasional cases with cognitive dysfunction akin to PSP have been presented. Some MSA presentations have "evolved" to dementia with Lewy Bodies.

Investigations and diagnosis Diagnosis is essentially clinical.

Imaging: MRI hypointensity in putamen, +/− juxtaposed slit-like T_2 hyperintensity; velar atrophy ("hot cross bun sign") is suggestive but may occur in other conditions; it is thought to be due to loss of pontine neurones and myelinated transverse pontocerebellar fibres with preservation of corticospinal tracts.

Sphincter EMG: denervation previously thought to be diagnostic of MSA but may also be seen in advanced PD, PSP.

Clonidine test: administration of clonidine fails to elicit the rise in growth hormone levels seen in normals, PD, and primary autonomic failure (PAF) (peripheral autonomic involvement); claimed to be sensitive and specific, but not all authorities agree.

Other: otorhinolaryngology consult for vocal cord visualization.

Differential diagnosis

Autonomic features: may be difficult to separate MSA from PAF.

MSA-P: very difficult to differentiate from PD in early stages.

MSA-C: ILOCA.

Treatment and prognosis Progressive disease; tends to progress more quickly than PD.

MSA-P: there is poor or no response to levodopa; if the latter, then the medication should be withdrawn, since it may exacerbate orthostatic hypotension. Levodopa-induced dyskinesias may occur in MSA, as in PD but is relatively unusual. Dopamine agonists, amantadine may also be tried. Focal dystonias may be treated with botulinum toxin, but not antecollis (may cause or exacerbate dysphagia).

Dysautonomia:

Orthostatic hypotension
  Head-up bed tilt
  Elastic stockings
  Increased salt intake
  Fludrocortisone, ephedrine, midodrine.
Postprandial hypotension
  octreotide.
Bladder
  Oxybutynin for detrusor hyperreflexia
  Desmopressin for nocturnal polyuria
  Intermittent self-catheterization for retention, increased residual volume.
Erectile failure
  sildenafil (Viagra), intracavernosal papaverine, penile prosthesis.

References Gilman S, Low PA, Quinn N *et al*. Consensus statement on the diagnosis of multiple system atrophy. *Journal of the Autonomic Nervous System* 1998; **74**: 189–192.

Quinn N. Multiple system atrophy. In: Marsden CD, Fahn S (eds). *Movement Disorders 3*. Oxford: Butterworth-Heinemann, 1994: 262–281.

Wenning GK, Ben-Shlomo Y, Magalhaes M *et al*. Clinical features and natural history of multiple system atrophy. An analysis of 100 cases. *Brain* 1994; **117**: 835–845.

Other relevant entries Autonomic failure; Cerebellar disease: an overview; Idiopathic late-onset cerebellar ataxia; Lewy body disease: an overview; Parkinsonian syndromes, parkinsonism; Parkinson's disease; Progressive supranuclear palsy; Pure autonomic failure; Synucleinopathy.

■ Munchausen's syndrome, Munchausen's syndrome by proxy

Pathophysiology Patients with Munchausen's syndrome are characterized by simulated illness, often supported by a plausible and dramatic history, often with previous multiple investigations and surgery, in whom the history is later found to be false. If the false history is provided on behalf of another, who is then subjected to multiple investigations (e.g. a child), this is called Munchausen's syndrome by proxy (MSBP).

Clinical features: history and examination Features which may alert the clinician to the possibility of Munchausen's syndrome include:

- Evidence of falsified physical and/or psychological symptoms/signs.
- Evidence of falsification of past personal and medical history; use of aliases.
- Multiple presentations to various hospital casualty departments, often out of hours (when junior staff only available).
- Unexplained scars, self-inflicted or from previous surgery.
- No fixed address; few social contacts.
- Personality disorder: especially histrionic, borderline.
- Medical or paramedical background, hence working knowledge of medical symptoms, investigations.

Investigations and diagnosis A high index of clinical suspicion is probably the most important factor for early diagnosis, before multiple, unnecessary, investigations are undertaken.

Covert surveillance (e.g. video recording) has been advocated for the detection of Munchausen's syndrome by proxy.

Differential diagnosis

Somatization.

Hypochondriasis.

Psychotic states with hypochondriacal delusion.

Substance abuse.

Malingering.

Treatment and prognosis Behaviour tends to be chronic, although with phases of quiescence. Confrontation is usually met with denial and self-discharge from hospital, and patients generally do not wish to engage with psychiatric treatments, exacerbated by the (commonly observed) peripatetic lifestyle. Whether such patients are detainable under the Mental Health Act 1983 is controversial.

In the case of MSBP, removal of a child at risk from (usually) its mother may be necessary, as well as psychiatric assessment of the responsible parent.

References Asher R. Munchausen's syndrome. *Lancet* 1951; **i**: 339–341 [also in Avery Jones F (ed.). *Richard Asher Talking Sense.* Edinburgh: Churchill Livingstone, 1986: 170–179].

Enoch MD, Ball HN. *Uncommon Psychiatric Syndromes* (4th edition). London: Arnold, 2001: 111–133.

Meadow R. Munchausen syndrome by proxy. The hinterland of child abuse. *Lancet* 1977; **ii**: 343–345.

Other relevant entries Malingering; Psychiatric disorders and neurological disease.

■ Murray valley encephalitis – see Arbovirus disease; Encephalitis: an overview

■ Muscle–eye–brain disease

Muscle–eye–brain syndrome of Santavuori

A form of congenital muscular dystrophy, with autosomal-recessive inheritance, linked to chromosome 1p32–34 and a defect in the protein glycosyltransferase. It is characterized by eye abnormalities in addition to neuronal migration defects. Clinical features are mental retardation, severe myopia, retinal dysplasia, cataracts and optic atrophy, but children are usually able to stand and walk. Survival to the second decade is common, occasionally to adulthood.

Other relevant entries Congenital muscular dystrophy; Walker–Warburg syndrome.

■ Muscular dystrophies: an overview

Pathophysiology Muscular dystrophies are myogenic disorders causing progressive muscle wasting and weakness of variable distribution (generally symmetrical) and severity. They are hereditary degenerative diseases of muscle, without a neuropathic abnormality.

The following conditions may be classified as muscular dystrophies (see individual entries for further details):

- Duchenne muscular dystrophy (DMD), Becker muscular dystrophy (BMD) = dystrophinopathies
- Emery–Dreifuss muscular dystrophy (EMD)
- Congenital muscular dystrophy (CMD)
- Facioscapulohumeral (FSH) muscular dystrophy
- Scapuloperoneal muscular dystrophy
- Limb girdle muscular dystrophy (LGMD)
- Distal myopathies
- Oculopharyngeal muscular dystrophy (OPMD).

Investigations and diagnosis *Bloods*: many are associated with raised creatine kinase, DMD from birth.

Neurophysiology: EMG: myopathic; excludes neurogenic cause for weakness.

Muscle biopsy: variation in fibre size, fibre necrosis, macrophage invasion; inflammatory changes may be prominent (e.g. FSH, LGMD type 2B) sufficient to cause confusion with polymyositis; rimmed vacuoles may be seen (e.g. OPMD, some distal myopathies) as may nuclear inclusions (OPMD). Immunohistochemistry may show absence or deficiency of certain proteins (e.g. dystrophin, sarcoglycans, dysferlin).

Neurogenetics: certain diseases are allelic:

Dystrophin: DMD, BMD
Lamin A: EMD (autosomal-dominant, autosomal-recessive), LGMD type 1B, Dunnigan partial lipodystrophy, progeria
Dysferlin: LGMD type 2B, Miyoshi-type distal myopathy
Caveolin 3: LGMD type 1C, rippling muscle disease, idiopathic hyperCKaemia.

References Emery AEH (ed.). *The Muscular Dystrophies*. Oxford: OUP, 2002. Emery AEH. The muscular dystrophies. *Lancet* 2002; **359**: 687–695.
Other relevant entries See individual entries; Myopathy: an overview.

■ Musculocutaneous neuropathy

Mononeuropathy of the musculocutaneous nerve, which arises from the lateral cord of the brachial plexus is uncommon, it may follow shoulder dislocation or trauma.

Clinical features: history and examination
- Motor: weak arm flexion due to involvement of biceps and brachialis muscles; biceps reflex may be reduced or normal.
- Sensory: loss over lateral forearm (lateral cutaneous nerve of the forearm).

Investigations and diagnosis *EMG/NCS*: reduced lateral cutaneous nerve of the forearm SNAP; EMG changes confined to muscles innervated by musculocutaneous nerve.

Differential diagnosis C5 radiculopathy.

Other relevant entry Neuropathies: an overview.

■ Mutism

Mutism is an absence of speech output. Unlike aphasia or aphonia, mutism carries the implication of no effort or attempt on the part of the patient to articulate, merely a persisting silence despite the efforts of interlocutors to engage the patient in conversation.

Mutism may result from:
- psychiatric disease:
    schizophrenia;
    affective disorders, with or without catatonia;
    elective mutism in childhood.

- neurological disease, in which case other neurological signs are often present:

  akinetic mutism;

  dementia syndromes, especially frontal lobe dementia, late stages of primary
    progressive aphasia, progressive loss of speech output with orofacial dyspraxia;

  encephalopathy (toxic/drug induced/metabolic);

  damage to Broca's area, supplementary motor area; severe pseudobulbar palsy,
    bilateral thalamic damage;

  cerebellar mutism: rare, following midline cerebellar surgery in children.

In neurological disorders there may be, in addition to mutism, difficulty initiating
movements, completing motor sequences, or inhibition of appropriate responses.

References Altshuler LL, Cummings JL, Mills MJ. Mutism: review, differential diagnosis and report of 22 cases. *American Journal of Psychiatry* 1986; **143**:
    1409–1414 (erratum: *American Journal of Psychiatry* 1987; **144**: 542).

Ersahin Y, Mutluer S, Cagli S, Duman Y. Cerebellar mutism: report of seven cases
  and review of the literature. *Neurosurgery* 1996; **38**: 60–66.

Other relevant entries Aphasia; Aphonia.

■ Myasthenia gravis
Erb–Goldflam disease

Pathophysiology Although probably first described by Thomas Willis in the seventeenth century, myasthenia gravis was so named by Jolly in 1895. It is characterized
by fatiguable weakness of striated muscles, with a predilection for the extraocular,
bulbar and proximal limb musculature. The autoimmune nature of myasthenia
gravis (MG) was postulated in the 1960s, borne out by the strong association with
thymic hyperplasia and thymoma, other autoimmune disorders, especially thyrotoxicosis but also rheumatoid arthritis, systemic lupus erythematosus (SLE) and
polymyositis, and the identification of auto-antibodies directed against nicotinic
acetylcholine receptors in a large percentage of cases. Whether these antibodies are
pathogenic or merely markers of a disease process is debated. Both symptomatic
treatment, with anticholinesterases, and disease-modifying treatment, with
immunomodulatory therapies and thymectomy, is possible.

Clinical Features: history and examination
- Onset is usually insidious; commonest age of presentation is 10–30 years old in
  women and 50–70 years old in men.
- The typical presentation is with ocular symptoms and signs: variable ptosis and
  diplopia, worse at the end of the day and better after sleep, with asymmetric
  involvement of extraocular muscles on examination, with ptosis, frontalis overactivity and bilateral weakness of orbicularis oculi (which is almost pathognomonic
  for this condition). Test for fatiguability of both eye movements (e.g. ask patient to
  fixate in a non-primary position) and ptosis (i.e. looking up). In *ca.* 10% of patients
  MG remains clinically restricted to ocular muscles.

- Other cranial musculature may be involved, commonly the facial and bulbar muscles, causing fatiguable dysarthria and dysphagia. It is always advisable to check swallowing function in patients with MG, as they are at risk of aspiration.
- Proximal weakness is common in MG and again needs to be tested after exercise (e.g. lifting the arms up and down 20 times). The neck flexors are especially vulnerable to the disease process. Occasionally predominantly distal limb weakness may occur.
- Sensory loss, sphincter disturbance and loss of reflexes are not features of MG; muscle atrophy is rarely seen.
- Certain drugs may interfere with neurotransmission at the neuromuscular junction and worsen, or even induce, the clincal features of, MG. Examples include:

Antibiotics: streptomycin, neomycin, gentamicin, tetracyclines, ciprofloxacin.
Cardiovascular drugs: lidocaine, procainamide, quinine, quinidine, propranolol, oxprenolol.
Anti-rheumatic drugs: chloroquine, D-penicillamine.
Psychotropic drugs: lithium, chlorpromazine.
Anti-epileptic drugs: phenytoin.
Others: corticosteroids, interferon-α, succinylcholine, d-tubocurarine; anticholinergics?

Investigations and Diagnosis *Bloods*: routine haematology and biochemistry usually all normal; need to check thyroid function tests. Acetylcholine-receptor (AChR) antibodies are found in 85% of patients with generalized MG and 60% of patients with purely ocular involvement. The titre is not correlated with disease severity, but very high levels may be suggestive of an underlying thymoma. In addition, anti-striated muscle (or anti-myosin) antibodies are found in some patients with MG, and when present suggest a thymoma. AChR antibodies are only occasionally seen in other conditions (e.g. SLE, primary biliary cirrhosis, Satoyoshi syndrome). Presumably pathogenic antibodies directed at other neuromuscular junction proteins (anti-MuSK, anti-titin) have been identified in some patients with MG who have negative AChR antibodies.

Neurophysiology: EMG/NCS: routine studies show a decremental response to repetitive nerve stimulation in 60% of cases. Single fibre studies (SFEMG) demonstrate increase jitter and intermittent block in 99% of cases, although the technique is operator dependent. These abnormal findings are not normally affected by acetyl-cholinesterase medication.

Tensilon test: undertaken with the patient lying down with full resuscitation facilities to hand. A clear end-point needs to be established (e.g. degree of ptosis, strength of particular muscle group). Failure to define accurately the end-point will produce an equivocal test response. The procedure varies slightly from one neurologist to another:

Give the patient 0.6 mg atropine intravenously.
Give test dose of 2 mg tensilon intravenously and monitor if any response.
If no adverse reaction give remaining 8 mg of tensilon; a positive response is usually evident within 1 minute and lasts for 3–4 minutes.

Confirmation that the drug has produced an effect may be forthcoming if fasciculations are seen, especially in the periorbital musculature, and if there is watering of the eyes.

If a negative result is obtained and the suspicion of MG is strong, a double dose (20 mg) tensilon test can be given with care, or alternatively a neostigmine test.

Ice test: for ptosis, holding an ice cube over the eyelid aponeurosis for 2–5 minutes may produce objective improvement, consistent with the clinical observation that some myasthenic patients improve in the cold.

Sleep test: the clinical observation that ptosis improves with rest or sleep has been operationalized into a test for MG.

Imaging: CT or MRI of the chest is necessary, in order to assess whether there is thymic enlargement or tumour.

Spirometry: vital capacity should be checked, since symptoms of impending respiratory failure may be few. If the vital capacity is <1 l in a weak patient, elective ventilation should be contemplated.

Differential diagnosis There is usually no difficulty in diagnosing cases of generalized MG.

In cases with restricted ocular involvement, mitochondrial and thyroid disease should be considered; posterior fossa lesions have also been reported to mimic the ocular features of MG.

Other conditions that can occasionally cause confusion are polymyositis, Lambert–Eaton myasthenic syndrome (LEMS), oculopharyngeal muscular dystrophy (OPMD), polyneuritis cranialis and motor neuropathies.

Treatment and prognosis

- Symptomatic

    Anticholinesterase drugs: for example pyridostigmine (Mestinon); enhance the efficacy of endogenous acetylcholine by inhibiting its enzymatic breakdown. Usually start at a low dose (e.g. pyridostigmine 30 mg tds) and titrate upwards according to efficacy and side-effects (maximum ~90 mg six times a day). Side-effects include blurred vision and gastrointestinal upset; the latter may be treated with buscopan. Overdosage can produce cholinergic crisis, which can resemble a myasthenic crisis, but in the former the pupils are classically small. If in doubt a tensilon test can be done in the ITU, the tensilon will improve a myasthenic crisis but will worsen a cholinergic crisis.

Preparation	Oral dose (mg)	Intravenous equivalent (mg)	Intramuscular equivalent (mg)	Duration of action
Mestinon	60	2	2	3–4 hours
Neostigmine	15	0.5	1.5	2–3 hours

- Disease modifying:

  Immunosuppressive therapy; various options, of which steroids are most often used.

  Prednisolone is introduced at a low dose and increased slowly, since some patients initially deteriorate on high-dose steroid therapy (some neurologists pursue a policy of hospitalization for introduction of steroids). A standard regime would be 10 mg on alternate days, increasing by 10 mg a week to a maintenance dose of between 60–80 mg of prednisolone every other day. Around 75% of patients will improve markedly with this therapy and a further 15% will have a moderate improvement in their condition. Once the patient has been stabilized the prednisolone dose may be slowly reduced to a level that controls the disease process. If long-term steroid use is required, osteoporosis prophylaxis should be started. Ocular disease may be completely controlled with alternate day steroids.

  If rapid introduction of high-dose steroids is required this should be done in hospital, often in conjunction with plasma exchange.

  Azathioprine may be used as a steroid sparing agent, but it may take 4–6 months before it takes effect. The usual starting dose is 50 mg/day, increasing to a maintenance dose of 150 mg/day. FBC and LFTs should be monitored, weekly for 8 weeks and thereafter every 3 months. Dose reduction or discontinuation may be required if the WCC drops below 3.5×10^9 or LFTs become abnormal.

  Plasma exchange may be used acutely in MG patients with threatened respiratory failure. It is highly effective, but repeated use may catalyse the production of AChR antibodies. Intravenous immunoglobulin appears to have a similar clinical effect.

  Other treatments which have been tried include methotrexate, cyclophosphamide, and ciclosporin.

  Thymectomy was pioneered before the autoimmune nature of MG was understood. It is mandatory in patients with thymoma, and strongly recommended in patients <40 years old with positive AChR antibodies (see table below). In these cases a third are cured, a third improve and a third are unchanged.

	Early onset: <40 years old	Thymoma: any age	Late onset: >40 years old	Seronegative: any age
Thymus	Hyperplastic	Thymoma	Atrophy (normally)	Atrophy (normally)
AChR antibodies	+++	++	+	−
Symptoms	Generalized	Generalized	Generalized/ Ocular	Generalized/ Ocular
Role of surgery	1/3 remit within 2 years of thymectomy	Mandatory but often does not improve symptoms	Doubtful value	Doubtful value

The greatest risk of morbidity and mortality from MG is during the first year.

10–15% of cases of MG improve spontaneously.

Younger-onset patients tend to run a more benign course.

If MG remains confined to the eyes for >2 years, there is only a 15% chance of it becoming generalized.

> **References** Gronseth GS, Barohn RJ. Practice parameter: thymectomy for auto-immune myasthenia gravis (an evidence-based review): report of the Quality Standards Subcommittee of the American Academy of Neurology. *Neurology* 2000; **55**: 7–15.
>
> Kaeser HE. Drug-induced myasthenic syndromes. *Acta Neurologica Scandinavica* 1984; **70**(suppl 100): 39–47.
>
> **Other relevant entries** Botulism; Channelopathies: an overview; Congenital myasthenic syndromes; Lambert–Eaton myasthenic syndrome; Neuromuscular junction diseases: an overview.

◼ Myasthenic syndrome – see Lambert–Eaton myasthenic syndrome

◼ Mycobacterial infection – see Leprosy; Tuberculosis and the nervous system

◼ Mycoplasma

Pathophysiology Infection with *Mycoplasma pneumoniae* causes an "atypical pneumonia" which may be complicated by constitutional symptoms including a variety of neurological features.

Clinical features: history and examination Mycoplasma tends to affect young adults, often occurring in epidemics although sporadic cases are recognized.

Symptoms:

- Respiratory: pneumonia, tracheobronchitis or pharyngitis, with persistent cough.
- Systemic: fever, headache, myalgia.
- Neurological (*ca.* 10% of patients)
   - Encephalitis, meningitis or meningoencephalitis
   - Ataxia
   - Peripheral neuropathy
   - Transverse myelitis +/– ADEM; MS-like presentation
   - Bullous myringitis (5%).

Investigations and diagnosis *Bloods*: leukocytosis, raised ESR, +/– cold agglutinins; positive serology for *M. pneumoniae*.

Imaging:

CXR: pneumonia.

CT/MRI: white matter changes suggestive of ADEM or MS may be seen.

Differential diagnosis

Other causes of pneumonia with associated neurological features.

Other causes of meningoencephalitis.

Treatment and prognosis Supportive treatment.

Antibiotics: erythromycin 0.5 g tds for 14–21 days or doxycyline 100 mg bd for 14–21 days.

Recovery is often complete but occasional patients with tranverse myelitis or central nervous system (CNS) involvement fail to recover.

> **References** Francis DA, Brown A, Miller DH, Wiles CM, Bennett ED, Leigh N. MRI appearances of the CNS manifestations of Mycoplasma pneumoniae: a report of two cases. *Journal of Neurology* 1988; **235**: 441–443.
>
> Ogata S, Kitamoto O. Clinical complications of Mycoplasma pneumoniae disease: central nervous system. *Yale Journal of Biology and Medicine* 1983; **56**: 481–486.

Other relevant entry "Atypical pneumonias" and the nervous system.

■ Mycotic aneurysm – see Endocarditis and the nervous system

■ Myelitis: an overview

Inflammatory disease of the spinal cord may produce a myelopathy; this may be acute or subacute, complete or partial (e.g. Brown–Séquard syndrome). A wide variety of aetiologies is recognized:

- Primary/Idiopathic: clinically isolated syndrome ("transverse myelitis"), may be harbinger of multiple sclerosis.
- Secondary: post-infectious (e.g. varicella, EBV, mycoplasma, Brucella).
    Post-vaccination (e.g. influenza).
    Multiple sclerosis, neuromyelitis optica (Devic's syndrome).
    Sarcoidosis.
    Collagen vascular diseases: systemic lupus erythematosus (SLE), Sjögren's syndrome, antiphospholipid antibody syndrome, giant cell arteritis.

Clinical features: history and examination/investigations and diagnosis/differential diagnosis/treatment and prognosis See individual entries.

> **References** Andersen O. Myelitis. *Current Opinion in Neurology* 2000; **13**: 311–316.
>
> Bakshi R, Kinkel PR, Mechtler LL *et al*. Magnetic resonance imaging findings in 22 cases of myelitis: comparison between patients with and without multiple sclerosis. *European Journal of Neurology* 1998; **5**: 35–48.

Other relevant entries Acute disseminated encephalomyelitis; Antiphospholipid (antibody) syndrome; Brucellosis; Devic's disease, Devic's syndrome; Epstein–Barr virus and the nervous system; Giant cell arteritis; Multiple sclerosis; Myelopathy: an overview; Sarcoidosis; Sjögren's syndrome; Systemic lupus erythematosus and the nervous system; Transverse myelitis, transverse myelopathy.

Myeloma – see Amyloid and the nervous system: an overview; Monoclonal gammopathies; Paraproteinaemic neuropathies; POEMS syndrome; Renal disease and the nervous system.

Myelopathy: an overview

Pathophysiology Myelopathy is a disorder of the spinal cord. Myelopathies may be characterized as intrinsic or intramedullary (lesions are always intradural), or extrinsic or extramedullary (lesions may be intradural or extradural). It may be possible to differentiate intramedullary from extramedullary lesions on clinical grounds, although this distinction is never absolute because of clinical overlap.

Pathologies recognized to cause myelopathy include:
- Intrinsic:

    inflammatory disease: myelitides; multiple sclerosis, other causes of transverse myelitis (complete or partial), for example viral infection, HTLV-1 infection, HIV-related vacuolar myelopathy (often discovered incidentally at post-mortem), tabes dorsalis;

    tumour: primary, secondary;

    syringomyelia;

    infarction, for example anterior spinal artery syndrome;

    metabolic causes: vitamin B_{12} deficiency producing subacute combined degeneration of the cord, adrenoleukodystrophy (adrenomyeloneuropathy).
- Extrinsic:

    prolapsed disc, osteophyte bar;

    tumour (primary, secondary);

    arteriovenous malformation/haematoma;

    abscess.

Clinical features: history and examination
- Intrinsic/intramedullary myelopathy: dependent on the extent to which the cord is involved, the following features may occur: some pathologies have a predilection for posterior columns, central cord, *etc.*

    Motor: lower motor neurone signs may be prominent and diffuse; upper motor neurone signs tend to occur late (spastic paraparesis below level of lesion).

A combination of upper and lower motor neurone signs is much more likely to reflect intrinsic than extrinsic pathology;

Sensory: symptoms of central (funicular) pain may occur; dissociated sensory loss (spinothalamic > dorsal column involvement, or *vice versa*), suspended sensory loss, and sacral sparing are characteristic of intramedullary lesions; a Brown–Séquard syndrome may occur. Vibratory sensibility is more often affected than proprioception;

Sphincters: bladder involvement common, often early and slow to recover.

- Extrinsic/extramedullary myelopathy:

Motor: sequential spastic paraparesis below the level of the lesion; upper motor neurone signs occur early; lower motor neurone signs are unusual and have a segmental (radicular) distribution if present;

Sensory: symptoms of pain may be radicular (e.g. secondary to a neurofibroma) or vertebral (e.g. secondary to neoplastic or inflammatory processes); sensory signs are not usually marked until the later stages, and all modalities are often involved. A Brown–Séquard syndrome may be commoner in extrinsic than intrinsic myelopathies;

Sphincters: may have bladder urgency, impotence.

Investigations and diagnosis *Bloods*: dependent on context, may require FBC, vitamin B_{12}, auto-antibodies, serology for HIV, HTLV-1, syphilis, EBV; very long-chain fatty acids.

Imaging: MR is often helpful in defining the cause of myelopathy.

CSF: may be required, for cell count, protein, glucose, oligoclonal bands, serology.

Differential diagnosis See individual entries.

Treatment and prognosis Of cause, where identified. See individual entries for more details.

References Rowland LP, McCormick PC. Cervical spondylotic myelopathy. In: Rowland LP (ed.). *Merritt's Textbook of Neurology* (9th edition). Baltimore: Williams & Wilkins, 1995: 455–459.

Tartaglino LM, Flanders AE, Rapoport RJ. Intramedullary causes of myelopathy. *Seminars in Ultrasound, CT, and MRI* 1994; **15**: 158–188.

Other relevant entries Brown–Séquard syndrome; Cauda equina syndrome and conus medullaris disease; HIV/AIDS and the nervous system; HTLV-1 myelopathy; Intervertebral disc prolapse; Multiple sclerosis; Myelitis: an overview; Paraparesis: acute management and differential diagnosis; Quadriplegia: an overview; Transverse myelitis, transverse myelopathy.

■ Myoadenylate deaminase deficiency

Myoadenylate deaminase deficiency (MADD) is a common inherited metabolic defect, resulting from mutations in the AMPD1 gene, with heterogeneous clinical phenotype, ranging from asymptomatic to mild exercise-induced myalgia and cramps (which enters the differential diagnosis of McArdle's disease). In the ischaemic forearm exercise test, creatine kinase may be elevated, there is a normal lactate response but no increase in ammonium. Distinctions have been drawn between primary MADD, resulting from homozygous mutation of the AMPD1 gene, and secondary or acquired MADD in which non-genetic factors, such as the presence of another neuromuscular disease, lead to discovery of MADD, perhaps due to the carrier state; heterozygous mutations of AMPD1 are present in 20% of Westerners.

References Fishbein WN. Primary, secondary, and coincidental types of myoad-enylate deaminase deficiency. *Annals of Neurology* 1999; **45**: 547–548.

Sabina RL. Myoadenylate deaminase deficiency. A common inherited defect with heterogeneous clinical presentation. *Neurologic Clinics* 2000; **18**: 185–194.

Other relevant entries McArdle's disease; Tarui disease.

▪ Myoclonic epilepsy – see Progressive myoclonic epilepsy

▪ Myoclonic epilepsy and ragged red fibres – see MERRF syndrome

▪ Myoclonus

Pathophysiology Myoclonus is "shock-like" involuntary muscle jerking, which may be rhythmic or irregular.

Pathophysiologically myoclonus may be characterized as:

- Cortical.
- Subcortical or reticular.
- Segmental (e.g. palatal and spinal).
- Propriospinal.

Electrophysiological recordings are required to make such distinctions.

A wide variety of pathological processes may manifest with myoclonus. The *aetiological differential diagnosis* of myoclonus includes:

- Physiological, for example "sleep starts" (hypnic jerks);
- Essential: in the absence of any other abnormality of the CNS;
- Epileptic: as a manifestation of idiopathic epilepsy;
- Symptomatic: of other neurological diseases, of which there are many, including:
    anoxic brain injury (Lance–Adams syndrome);
    vascular lesions;
    neoplasia;
    encephalopathies: especially of metabolic origin, but also toxic, viral, paraneoplastic, mitochondrial;
    degenerations: basal ganglia (e.g. multiple system atrophy, corticobasal degeneration), spinocerebellar;

malabsorption syndromes (coeliac disease, Whipple's disease);

storage disorders, for example Lafora body disease, Tay–Sachs disease, sialidosis;

dementias: Alzheimer's disease (usually late), Creutzfeldt–Jakob disease (usually early); not frontotemporal dementia.

Clinical features: history and examination Myoclonic jerks may be classified clinically as focal, multifocal, or generalized. Multiple irregular asynchronous myoclonic jerks may be termed polymyoclonus. Furthermore, myoclonus may be characterized as:

Spontaneous

Action: following voluntary action, for example asking the patient to reach out to touch the examiner's hand;

Reflex, stimulus sensitive: jerks produced by somaesthetic stimulation of a limb.

According to aetiology, other neurological signs may be present.

Investigations and diagnosis In light of the broad differential diagnosis of myoclonus, many investigations may be undertaken to establish the cause (see individual entries for details).

Differential diagnosis Myoclonus must be differentiated from other hyperkinetic involuntary movement disorders including: chorea, tic, tremor, and certain peripheral nerve disorders (fasciculation, myokymia).

Treatment and prognosis Drugs useful in the symptomatic treatment of myoclonus include clonazepam, sodium valproate, primidone, and piracetam. These may need to be given in combination to suppress severe action myoclonus.

Prognosis is according to cause: see individual entries.

References Barker R. Myoclonus. *Advances in Clinical Neuroscience and Rehabilitation* 2003; **3**(5): 20, 22.

Marsden CD, Hallett M, Fahn S. The nosology and pathophysiology of myoclonus. In: Marsden CD, Fahn S (eds). *Movement Disorders*. London: Butterworth, 1982: 196–248.

Obeso JA, Artieda J, Rothwell JC, Day B, Thompson P, Marsden CD. The treatment of severe action myoclonus. *Brain* 1989; **112**: 765–777.

Other relevant entries Andermann syndrome (2); Chorea; Juvenile myoclonic epilepsy; Lance–Adams syndrome; Leeuwenhoek disease; Mitochondrial disease: an overview; Myoclonus–dystonia syndrome; Opsoclonus; Prion disease: an overview; Progressive encephalomyelitis with rigidity and myoclonus; Progressive myoclonic epilepsy; Startle syndromes.

■ Myoclonus–dystonia syndrome

This autosomal-dominant condition is characterized by:

- Brief, alcohol-responsive, myoclonic jerks: neck and arms affected more than legs, gait.

- +/− cervical/brachial dystonia.
- +/− psychiatric features: obsessive–compulsive disorder, panic attacks, alcohol dependence.
- Imaging (MRI) is normal.
- Mutations in a gene on chromosome 7 encoding ε-sarcoglycan have been demonstrated.

Reference Asmus F, Zimprich A, Tezenas du Montcel S *et al*. Myoclonus–dystonia syndrome: ε-sarcoglycan mutations and phenotype. *Annals of Neurology* 2002; **52**: 489–492.

Other relevant entries Alcohol and the nervous system: an overview; Dystonia: an overview; Myoclonus; Obsessive–compulsive disorder; Sarcoglycanopathy.

■ Myofascial pain syndrome – see Fibromyalgia syndrome

■ Myoglobinuria – see Rhabdomyolysis

■ Myokymia

The term myokymia may be used to describe involuntary, spontaneous, wave-like, undulating, flickering movements within a muscle, movements which may be likened to a "bag of worms". Clinically myokymia may need to be distinguished from fasciculations.

Electrophysiologically myokymia corresponds to regular groups of motor unit discharges, of peripheral nerve origin, hence peripheral nerve hyperexcitability. Myokymia is thus related to neuromyotonia and stiffness, since there may be concurrent impairment of muscle relaxation and a complaint of muscle cramps.

Electrophysiological evidence of myokymia may be helpful in the assessment of a brachial plexopathy, since this is found in radiation-induced, but not neoplastic, lesions.

Reference Thompson PD. Stiff people. In: Marsden CD, Fahn S (eds). *Movement Disorders 3*. Boston: Butterworth, 1994: 373–405.

Other relevant entries Brachial plexopathies; Cramps; Episodic ataxias; Facial myokymia; Morvan's syndrome; Neuromyotonia; Stiff people: an overview; Superior oblique myokymia.

■ Myopathy: an overview

Myopathy is a disease of muscle. Myopathies may be classified according to location (proximal versus distal), but more usually they are classified according to aetiology:

Inflammatory (myositis, *q.v.*; polymyositis, dermatomyositis)
Muscular dystrophy (*q.v.*)

Myotonic dystrophy (*q.v.*)

Non-dystrophic myotonias, periodic paralyses

Congential myopathies (*q.v.*; central core, nemaline, myotubular)

Metabolic myopathies:

Carbohydrate metabolism (e.g. McArdle's disease)

Lipid metabolism (e.g. carnitine palmitoyltransferase deficiency)

Mitochondrial myopathy

Malignant hyperthermia

Endocrine myopathies: Steroid myopathy, thyroid myopathies.

Toxin/drug-induced myopathies: ethanol, statins

Clinical features: history and examination

- History: look for evidence of muscle pain, weakness; distribution, diurnal pattern; myotonia.

Preceding illness, drug exposure.

Family history of muscle disease.

- Examination: muscle wasting, tone, power (distribution of weakness); reflexes.
- Other systems: especially skin, heart (concurrent cardiomyopathy).

Investigations and diagnosis *Bloods*: muscle-related enzymes: creatine kinase +/− aldolase, LDH.

Neurophysiology: EMG/NCS: myopathic change.

Muscle biopsy: often diagnostic: weak but not atrophic muscle is probably best target.

For specific diagnoses, additional investigations may be required (e.g. other blood tests, lumbar puncture). Neurogenetics is increasingly useful as loci and mutations are defined.

Differential diagnosis

Neuromuscular junction disease (e.g. myasthenia gravis).

Motor neuropathies (e.g. multifocal motor neuropathy with conduction block).

Motor neuronopathy (e.g. motor neurone disease).

Other causes of weakness: neuropathy, radiculopathy.

Treatment and prognosis See individual entries.

References Finsterer J, Stollberger C. Cardiac involvement in primary myopathies. *Cardiology* 2000; **94**: 1–11.

Mandler RN. Myopathy. In: Biller J (ed.). *Practical Neurology* (2nd edition). Philadelphia: Lippincott Williams & Wilkins, 2002; 623–641.

Other relevant entries Channelopathies: an overview; Congenital muscle and neuromuscular disorders: an overview; Congenital muscular dystrophies; Distal muscular dystrophy, Distal myopathy; Dystrophia myotonica; Endocrinology and the nervous system; Malignant hyperthermia; Mitochondrial disease: an overview; Motor neurone disease; Motor neurone diseases: an overview; Multifocal motor neuropathy; Muscular dystrophies: an overview; Myasthenia gravis; Myositis; Myotonia and myotonic disorders; Neuropathies: an overview; Periodic paralysis; Proximal weakness; Thyroid disease and the nervous system.

■ Myophosphorylase deficiency – see Glycogen-storage disorders: an overview; McArdle's disease

■ Myositis

The myositides are inflammatory disorders of muscle. These may be classified as:
- Infective
    Bacterial
        Pyomyositis: muscle abscess due to *Staphylococcus aureus*
        Borreliosis (Lyme disease)
        Clostridia perfringens
        Mycobacteriae: *tuberculosis, leprae*
    Viral
        Influenza
        HIV
        HTLV-1
        Coxsackievirus B: pleurodynia (devil's grip, Bornholm disease) may be accompanied by an inflammatory myopathy
    Parasitic
        Trichinosis
        Toxoplasmosis (may be more severe in context of AIDS)
        Cysticercosis
        Echinococcosis
    Fungal
        Candida (rare)
- Idiopathic
    Polymyositis
    Dermatomyositis
    Inclusion body myositis
    [Polymyalgia rheumatica]
- Other
    Eosinophilic myositis
    Sarcoid myositis.

Inflammatory changes may be seen in muscle biopsies in conditions not typically thought inflammatory, for example facioscapulohumeral (FSH) dystrophy, metabolic myopathies, and in normals following vigorous exertion.

Clinical features: history and examination/Investigations and diagnosis/treatment and prognosis See individual entries.

Differential diagnosis Non-inflammatory myopathies.

> **Reference** Mandler RN. Myopathy. In: Biller J (ed.). *Practical Neurology* (2nd edition). Philadelphia: Lippincott Williams & Wilkins, 2002: 623–641.

> **Other relevant entries** Borreliosis; Cysticercosis; Dermatomyositis; Echinococcosis; HIV/AIDS and the nervous system; Inclusion body myositis;

Myopathy: an overview; Polymyositis; Sarcoidosis; Trichinosis; Tuberculosis and the nervous system.

■ Myositis ossificans

Fibrodysplasia ossificans progressiva

An extremely rare autosomal-dominant disorder characterized by progressive ossification of muscle tissue, beginning in childhood and affecting the muscles of the neck, back, shoulder and pelvic girdles. Muscles are painful, tender to touch, and become progressively stiffer and restricted in their range of movement. Although the diaphragm is not affected by ossification, restriction of thoracic movement may lead to respiratory compromise and death.

Heterotopic ossification of muscle occurs more commonly in the context of trauma (myositis ossificans traumatica), sometimes associated with repeated minor (occupational) trauma, such as thigh adductors (horse riding) and pectoralis and deltoid (drilling).

Reference Kaplan FS, Delatycki M, Gannon FH *et al*. Fibrodysplasia ossificans progressiva. In: Emery AEH (ed.). *Neuromuscular Disorders: Clinical and Molecular Genetics*. New York: John Wiley, 1998: 289–321.

■ Myotonia and myotonic syndromes

Pathophysiology Myotonia is a stiffness of muscle, with difficulty in relaxing muscle following voluntary contraction. This may give rise to symptoms of cramp or stiffness. Typically this improves with repeated muscle use ("warm-up phenomenon"); in paramyotonia, a related condition, stiffness is precipitated and exacerbated by exercise and cold. Such stiffness may have various causes:

* Myogenic
  Dystrophic myotonias
    Dystrophia myotonica (DM; myotonic dystrophy type 1, DM1)
    Proximal myotonic myopathy (PROMM, Ricker's disease,
      Thornton–Griggs–Moxley disease; myotonic dystrophy type 2, DM2)
  Non-dystrophic myotonias
    Channelopathies
      Myotonia congenita: Thomsen (autosomal dominant), Becker (autosomal
        recessive)
      Myotonia fluctuans
      Periodic paralysis: hypokalaemic, hyperkalaemic, thyrotoxic
      Paramyotonia congenita
      Potassium-aggravated myotonia
      Schwartz–Jampel syndrome (chondrodystrophic myotonia)
      Andersen's syndrome.

- Neurogenic

    Neuromyotonia (*q.v.*).

Investigations and diagnosis EMG reveals myotonic discharges with prolonged twitch relaxation phase; discharges typically wax and wane, producing a characteristic "dive bomber" effect on the audio recording.

Neurogenetics: increasingly useful in diagnosis.

See individual entries.

Differential diagnosis Myotonias need to be differentiated from pseudomyotonia, slow muscle relaxation not accompanied by myotonic EMG discharges, for example in hypothyroidism with "hung-up" tendon reflexes (Woltman's sign), Brody's disease. Muscle rigidity is also a feature of malignant hyperthermia.

Treatment and prognosis See individual entries.

References Cannon SC. Myotonia and periodic paralysis: disorders of voltage-gated ion channels. In: Noseworthy JH (ed.). *Neurological Therapeutics: Principles and Practice*. London: Dunitz, 2003: 2365–2377.

Lehmann-Horn F, Rüdel R. Hereditary nondystrophic myotonias and periodic paralyses. *Current Opinion in Neurology* 1995; **8**: 402–410.

Mankodi A, Thornton CA. Myotonic syndromes. *Current Opinion in Neurology* 2002; **15**: 545–552.

Ptacek LJ, Johnson KJ, Griggs RC. Genetics and physiology of the myotonic muscle disorders. *New England Journal of Medicine* 1993; **328**: 482–489.

Other relevant entries Andersen's syndrome; Brody's disease; Channelopathies: an overview; Dystrophia myotonica; Malignant hyperthermia; Myotonia congenita; Periodic paralysis; Potassium-aggravated myotonia; Proximal myotonic myopathy; Schwartz–Jampel syndrome; Thyroid disease and the nervous system.

▓ Myotonia congenita

Pathophysiology Hereditary myotonic syndromes may be either autosomal dominant or recessive:

    Thomsen disease: autosomal dominant.
    Becker disease: autosomal recessive.
    Myotonia levior: autosomal dominant.

In recent times these disorders have been shown to be allelic, all linked to chromosome 7q32, resulting from mutations in the gene encoding chloride ion channels, hence channelopathies.

Clinical features: history and examination

- Myotonia: severe (Thomsen, Becker), mild (levior); appears after exercise, sometimes with emotional stress or pregnancy; warm-up phenomenon may be evident (i.e. better after repeated contractions).

- Pain in muscle may occur after prolonged activity but spasm *per se* is painless.
- Weakness not evident.
- Percussion myotonia.
- Muscle hypertrophy (especially Becker).
- No other features of myotonic dystrophy (e.g. frontal balding, cataracts, endocrine changes).
- No cardiac involvement.

Investigations and diagnosis *Bloods*: mild increase in creatine kinase may be observed during attacks; serum K^+ during and between attacks is normal.

Neurogenetics: mutations in chloride ion-channel (CLCN1) gene at chromosome 7q32.

Differential diagnosis Dystrophia myotonica.

Autosomal-dominant myotonia congenita may be confused with potassium-aggravated myotonia (indeed some cases reported as Thomsen's disease have been shown to harbour sodium channel gene mutations typical of potassium-aggravated myotonia); myotonia fluctuates in the latter.

Treatment and prognosis Myotonia may be treated with mexilitene, quinidine sulphate, procainamide, or phenytoin.

> **Reference** Zhang J, George AL Jr, Griggs RC *et al*. Mutations in the human skeletal muscle chloride channel gene (CLCN1) associated with dominant and recessive myotonia congenita. *Neurology* 1996; **47**: 993–998.

> **Other relevant entries** Channelopathies: an overview; Dystrophia myotonica; Myotonia and myotonic syndromes; Potassium-aggravated myotonia.

■ Myotonia fluctuans

An autosomal-dominant myotonic syndrome of:
- Fluctuating severity (*cf.* myotonia congenita).
- Delayed onset exercise-induced myotonia (*cf.* myotonia congenita: reduced myotonia with exercise; paramyotonia: immediate onset exercise-induced myotonia).
- No effect from cooling (*cf.* paramyotonia).
- Increased myotonia with K^+ load (*cf.* hyperkalaemic periodic paralysis: weakness with K^+ load).

> **Reference** Lennox G, Purves A, Marsden D. Myotonia fluctuans. *Archives of Neurology* 1992; **49**: 1010–1011.

> **Other relevant entries** Myotonia and myotonic syndromes; Paramyotonia; Periodic paralysis.

■ Myotonia permanens – see Potassium-aggravated myotonia

■ Myotonic dystrophy – see Dystrophia myotonica; Myotonia and myotonic syndromes; Proximal myotonic myopathy

- **Myotubular myopathy** – see Centronuclear myopathy

- **Myriachit** – see Startle syndromes

- **Myxoedema** – see Thyroid disease and the nervous system

Nn

Naegleria

Along with Acanthamoeba, this protozoan, *Naegleria fowleri*, is one of the causes of primary amoebic meningoencephalitis, most often affecting children who have been swimming in infected water; the presentation mimics that of acute bacterial meningitis. Examination of CSF may reveal motile trophozoites. Prognosis is poor, with death within 1 week the norm. Amphotericin (systemic, intrathecal) is the treatment most usually given, although miconazole, rifampicin, doxycycline, chloramphenicol may be tried.

Other relevant entry Acanthamoeba.

Naevoid basal cell carcinoma syndrome
Basal cell naevus syndrome • Gorlin–Goltz syndrome

This condition of uncertain inheritance (autosomal dominant, autosomal recessive) is characterized by skin, bone, and central nervous system (CNS) abnormalities, with a tendency to develop neoplastic change. The skin shows increased sensitivity to X-irradiation. Features include:

- Skin

    Basal cell carcinoma, affecting head, neck, upper trunk; 15% develop before puberty
    Small epidermal depressions (pits) in the palms and soles, which may undergo
        malignant change

- Bone

    Odontogenic cysts of the jaw, which are usually asymptomatic
    Frontoparietal bossing
    Kyphoscoliosis

- CNS

    Posterior fossa tumours, for example medulloblastoma; falx calcification, agenesis of the corpus callosum, occasionally mental retardation.

Monitoring for neoplastic change is appropriate.

Reference Gorlin R. Nevoid basal cell carcinoma syndrome. In: Gomez MR (ed.). *Neurocutaneous Diseases: A Practical Approach*. London: Butterworth, 1987: 67–79.

■ Naffziger's syndrome – see Thoracic outlet syndromes

■ Narcolepsy, Narcoleptic syndrome
Gélineau's syndrome

Pathophysiology Narcolepsy is a disorder of excessive daytime sleepiness with "sleep attacks", usually beginning in adolescence or young adulthood. Some authors require features in addition to narcolepsy to establish the diagnosis, specifically cataplexy, sleep paralysis, and hypnagogic (and/or hypnapompic) hallucinations. The syndrome or complex is closely associated with certain human leukocyte antigen (HLA) antigens, and has been linked with mutations in a gene encoding the protein orexin or hypocretin, lower levels of which are found in CSF of narcoleptics compared to normals. Disturbed aminergic mechanisms in rapid eye movement (REM) sleep seem to be the underlying pathogenesis.

Clinical features: history and examination The core clinical tetrad consists of:

- Excessive daytime sleepiness, sleep attacks: irresistible desire to fall asleep, often in inappropriate circumstances, such as when driving, eating, talking; brief naps (10–20 minutes) which refresh the patient (*cf.* obstructive sleep apnoea syndrome [OSAS]). May present with poor school performance. Variable frequency, persist throughout life.
- Cataplexy: transient episodes of weakness or even frank paralysis (atonia), causing falls, often precipitated by strong emotion (laughter, anger).
- Sleep paralysis: a sensation of paralysis during the transition between sleep and waking, often with inability to speak; frightening.
- Hypnagogic/hypnapompic hallucinations: frightening visual, auditory or movement perceptions which reflect dreaming whilst awake.

Additional features which may occur include:

insomnia (with the preceding four, may constitute the narcoleptic pentad);
complaints of poor memory;
depression;
automatic behaviours.

Investigations and diagnosis *Bloods*: normal (*cf.* OSAS); strong HLA linkage, to DR2, DQw15.

CSF: low levels of the hypothalamic peptide hypocretin (orexin).

Polysomnography: short sleep latency; early onset of REM sleep; reduced sleep efficiency.

Multiple sleep latency test (MLST): usually performed the day after overnight polysomnography: should show excessive sleepiness with at least two REM-onset sleep periods; a labour-intensive investigation, essentially requires an observer to be with the patient for a whole day.

Neurogenetics: testing for mutations in the hypocretin/orexin gene available in specialist centres; eventually may obviate the need for MLST.

Differential diagnosis Other causes of excessive daytime somnolence (e.g. OSAS); this is commoner, generally has a later onset, and results in sleep episodes which are not refreshing; idiopathic central nervous system (CNS) hypersomnolence, Kleine–Levin syndrome.

Episodes of loss of consciousness (e.g. epilepsy).

Chronic fatigue syndrome.

Treatment and prognosis For narcolepsy, options include:

modafinil (200–800 mg/day);

mazindol (2–8 mg/day);

methylphenidate;

dexamphetamine (5–60 mg/day; NB abuse potential).

For cataplexy, fluoxetine (20–60 mg/day), clomipramine, and other antidepressants may be tried.

References Scammell TE. The neurobiology, diagnosis, and treatment of narcolepsy. *Annals of Neurology* 2003; **53**: 154–166.

Taheri S, Zeitzer JM, Mignot E. The role of hypocretins (orexins) in sleep regulation and narcolepsy. *Annual Review of Neuroscience* 2002; **25**: 283–313.

Zeman A, Douglas N, Aylward R. Narcolepsy mistaken for epilepsy. *British Medical Journal* 2001; **322**: 216–218.

Other relevant entries Cataplexy; Epilepsy: an overview; Obstructive sleep apnoea syndrome; Sleep disorders: an overview.

■ NARP syndrome

NARP syndrome, an acronym for *n*eurogenic weakness, *a*taxia, and *r*etinitis *p*igmentosa, is a mitochondrial disorder most commonly resulting from a point mutation at base pair 8993 (T8993G) of the mitochondrial genome. Besides the clinical features encapsulated in the name, there may also be psychomotor regression, seizures, diabetes mellitus, cardiomyopathy, and lactic acidosis. Clinical expression is variable; some patients have a Leigh-type syndrome.

Reference Holt IJ, Harding AE, Petty RK *et al*. A new mitochondrial disease associated with mitochondrial DNA heteroplasmy. *American Journal of Human Genetics* 1990; **46**: 428–433.

Other relevant entries Leigh's disease, Leigh's syndrome; Mitochondrial disease: an overview; Retinitis pigmentosa.

■ Nasu–Hakola disease
Membranous lipodystrophy • Polycystic lipomembranous osteodysplasia • Presenile dementia with bone cysts

An autosomal-recessive disorder characterized by large-scale destruction of cancellous bone and presenile dementia.

In the 20s, bone cysts cause pain and swelling of wrists and ankles, the cysts filled with triglycerides, fractures may occur. In the 30s, cognitive decline and epileptic seizures develop. MRI reveals frontal myelin loss and massive gliosis ("sclerosing leukoencephalopathy").

Families have been identified with deletions of chromosome 19q13.1 which partially encompass the *DAP12* gene; point mutations and single base deletions have been identified in this gene in other families, but not in all, suggestive of genetic heterogeneity.

Reference Kondo T, Takahashi K, Kohara N *et al.* Heterogeneity of presenile dementia with bone cysts (Nasu–Hakola disease). Three genetic forms. *Neurology* 2002; **59**: 1105–1107.

Other relevant entry Dementia: an overview.

■ NEAD – see Pseudoseizures

■ Neck–tongue syndrome

In the neck–tongue syndrome, sudden turning of the head results in pain in the upper neck and occiput accompanied by numbness of the ipsilateral half of the tongue; lingual pseudo-athetosis may also occur. It is thought to be due to irritation of the second cervical dorsal root, which carries proprioceptive fibres from the tongue via the hypoglossal nerve and its communication with the second root. Pseudo-athetosis may reflect lingual de-afferentation.

Reference Orrell RW, Marsden CD. The neck–tongue syndrome. *Journal of Neurology, Neurosurgery and Psychiatry* 1994; **57**: 348–352.

Other relevant entries Cranial nerve disease: XII: Hypoglossal nerve; Facial pain: differential diagnosis.

■ Necrotizing myelopathy

Diseases of the spinal cord which can cause tissue necrosis, with or without secondary cavity (syrinx) formation, include:
- Spinal dural arteriovenous fistula (Foix–Alajouanine syndrome).
- Malignancy: primary, metastatic.
- Paraneoplasia.
- Devic's disease (neuromyelitis optica); Vernant's disease.
- Post-vaccination syndrome.
- Idiopathic disease.

Reference Kim RC. Necrotizing myelopathy. *American Journal of Neuroradiology* 1991; **12**: 1084–1086.

Other relevant entries Devic's disease, Devic's syndrome; Foix–Alajouanine syndrome; Myelopathy: an overview; Spinal cord diseases: an overview; Syringomyelia and syringobulbia; Vernant's disease.

■ Necrotizing polymyopathy – see Rhabdomyolysis

■ Nemaline myopathy

Pathophysiology An inherited myopathy with both autosomal-dominant and, more commonly, autosomal-recessive forms, with variable clinical phenotype but typical histological findings of granules or rods of filamentous material (*nema* = thread, in Greek). Mutations in a number of genes have been associated with nemaline myopathy, hence routine genetic testing is not possible.

Clinical features: history and examination

- Variable phenotype:

    <u>Birth</u>: floppy infant, feeding difficulty, $+/-$ respiratory muscle involvement.

    <u>Childhood</u>: delayed motor milestones; weak face, tent-shaped mouth, high-arched palate, nasal voice, diffuse limb weakness, usually proximal > distal.

    <u>Adult</u>: facial and proximal weakness, dropped head syndrome, respiratory involvement.

- $+/-$ cardiomyopathy.
- $+/-$ kyphoscoliosis.
- Once diagnosis is made, respiratory function should be monitored for insidious onset of hypoventilation.

Investigations and diagnosis *Bloods*: unremarkable; normal or only slightly elevated creatine kinase.

EMG/NCS: non-specific myopathic EMG.

Muscle biopsy: hallmark is nemaline rods in the subsarcolemmal region, staining red with the Gomori trichrome method. Nemaline rods can be secondary phenomena in other disorders. Type 1 fibre predominance, selective atrophy of type 1 fibres, deficiency of type 2b fibres.

Neurogenetics: deterministic mutations have been identified in genes encoding the proteins nebulin, α-actin, α-tropomyosin 3, slow skeletal muscle troponin T, and β-tropomyosin (TPM2).

Differential diagnosis Other congenital myopathies.

Treatment and prognosis Progression of weakness is typically slow. Hypoventilation may require nocturnal positive-pressure ventilation. Scoliosis may require surgery.

References Ryan MM, Schnell C, Strickland CD *et al*. Nemaline myopathy: a clinical study of 143 cases. *Annals of Neurology* 2001; **50**: 312–320.

Wallgren-Pettersson C. Nemaline and myotubular myopathies. *Seminars in Pediatric Neurology* 2002; **9**: 132–144.

Other relevant entries Congenital muscle and neuromuscular disorders: an overview; Myopathy: an overview; Respiratory failure; Scoliosis.

■ Neoplastic angioendotheliomatosis – see Angioendotheliomatosis

■ Neuralgic amyotrophy

Brachial plexus neuritis • Idiopathic brachial plexopathy • Parsonage–Turner syndrome

Pathophysiology A painful syndrome of brachial plexopathy, often following an upper respiratory tract infection or immunization and thought to be immune mediated. Exercise, such as carrying a heavy rucksack, may also be a precipitating factor. Familial forms are also described: hereditary neuralgic amyotrophy (HNA) is linked to chromosome 17q25 (i.e. distinct from hereditary neuropathy with liability to pressure palsies, which may also manifest with isolated brachial plexopathy); these patients may have mild dysmorphic features (epicanthic folds, hypertelorism).

Clinical features: history and examination

- Abrupt onset of severe arm pain (may be confused with cardiac ischaemia or acute cervical disc prolapse), usually unilateral, worse with movement of the arm, followed by weakness of the arm, more usually proximal than distal, involving selectively or in combination muscles innervated by the axillary, suprascapular, long thoracic, radial, musculocutaneous, and anterior interosseous nerves. Wasting may be marked and extremely focal. Reflexes may be lost. Sensory loss or paraesthesia may occur but are minor features in comparison to the motor deficit.
- Diaphragmatic weakness may occur, with possible respiratory compromise.
- Bilateral symptoms occur in ~25% of cases, with the involvement being sequential rather than simultaneous in onset. Neuralgic amyotrophy may be recurrent in perhaps 5% of cases.

Investigations and diagnosis *Neurophysiology*: EMG/NCS: early in the course no abnormalities may be evident, but 7–10 days after the onset of weakness axonal injury is evident in the distribution of the specific nerves affected and fibrillation potentials are seen in weak muscles and even in some clinically normal muscles.

Differential diagnosis Pain may mimic a musculoskeletal disorder, or ischaemic cardiac pain.

Focal onset may be confused with mononeuropathy, radiculopathy.

Other causes of brachial plexopathy, although none are associated with such an acute onset of pain (metastatic infiltration of the plexus has a slower onset).

Treatment and prognosis Natural history of improvement but very slow, up to 2–3 years. Wasting, weakness and reflex loss may persist. No effective treatment is known.

References Staal A, Van Gijn J, Spaans F. *Mononeuropathies: Examination, Diagnosis and Treatment*. London: WB Saunders, 1999: 153–157.

Tsairis P, Dyck PJ, Mulder DW. Natural history of brachial plexus neuropathy. Report on 99 patients. *Archives of Neurology* 1972; **27**: 109–117.

Brachial plexopathies; Hereditary neuropathy with liability to pressure palsies; Long thoracic nerve palsy; Rucksack paralysis; Wartenberg's neuropathy.

■ Neurally mediated syncope – see Syncope

■ Neuraminidase deficiency – see Sialidosis

■ Neuroacanthocytosis

Acanthocytosis • Choreoacanthocytosis • Familial amyotrophic chorea–acanthocytosis • Levine–Critchley syndrome

Pathophysiology Acanthocytes are red blood cells with a crenellated, spiky membrane, which are found in a number of conditions including abetalipoproteinaemia, hypobetalipoproteinaemia and the McLeod syndrome (areflexia and myopathy). Neuroacanthocytosis is a rare autosomal-recessive condition linked to chromosome 9q21 and mutations in a gene encoding chorein. The presence of acanthocytes is not associated with lipoprotein abnormalities but is associated with neurological disease. The clinical entity of an hereditary movement disorder associated with acanthocytes and no biochemical abnormality was first reported in the 1960s, most notably by Critchley and Levine. The disease is characterized by abnormal movements, variable cognitive impairment, a motor neuropathy and epileptic fits.

The underlying defect is unknown. Pathological findings are of:

- CNS: severe neuronal loss in the striatum and to a lesser extent the globus pallidus, thalamus, substantia nigra, and anterior horns of the spinal cord, with relative sparing of the cerebral cortex;
- PNS: axonal degeneration and demyelination.

Clinical features: history and examination

- Rare; autosomal-recessive inheritance; M = F.
- Onset usually age 10–40 years (mean age of onset ~32 years).
- Movement disorder: especially orofacial dyskinesias which frequently produce mutilating injuries to the lips and tongue. In addition the patient can develop motor and vocal tics, lingual and oral action dystonia, chorea, and even parkinsonism. Relatively few cases have been described without a movement disorder.
- Cognitive disorder: tends to be progressive, may ultimately lead to dementia. However the extent and progression of cognitive deficits is very variable; there may be psychiatric symptoms.
- Motor neuropathy with amyotrophy and reduced tendon jerks.
- Epileptic fits.

Investigations and diagnosis *Bloods*: film should show at least 10% acanthocytes on three fresh blood films with normal lipoprotein and vitamin E concentrations. Creatine kinase may be raised.

Imaging: CT/MRI/PET: all may show a degree of striatal atrophy and hypometabolism. In addition frontal cortical hypometabolism has been seen in some patients.

CSF: usually normal.

Neurophysiology:

EMG/NCS: may show a predominantly axonal motor neuropathy.

Evoked potentials: usually normal.

EEG: may be abnormal, but often non-specific with background slowing only.

Neuropsychology: often impaired, especially on tests sensitive to frontal lobe function.

Neurogenetics: trinucleotide repeat disorders, Huntington's disease (HD) and dentatorubral–pallidoluysian atrophy (DRPLA), may be excluded on genetic testing.

Differential diagnosis On clinical features:

HD.

DRPLA.

Organic acidaemias.

Gilles de la Tourette syndrome.

Cerebral vasculitis.

On haematological features:

Abetalipoproteinaemia, hypobetalipoproteinaemia.

McLeod syndrome.

Treatment and prognosis Treatment of abnormal movements and epileptic fits is symptomatic. The disease tends to run a progressive course, but the speed of progression is highly variable (~5–30 years).

References Hardie RJ, Pullon HW, Harding AE *et al*. Neuroacanthocytosis. A clinical, haematological and pathological study of 19 cases. *Brain* 1991; **114**: 13–49.

Rinne JO, Daniel SE, Scaravilli F, Pires M, Harding AE, Marsden CD. The neuropathological features of neuroacanthocytosis. *Movement Disorders* 1994; **9**: 297–304.

Stevenson VL, Hardie RJ. Acanthocytosis and neurological disorders. *Journal of Neurology* 2001; **248**: 87–94.

Ueno S, Maruki Y, Nakamura M *et al*. The gene encoding a newly discovered protein, chorein, is mutated in chorea–acanthocytosis. *Nature Genetics* 2001; **28**: 121–122.

Other relevant entries Abetalipoproteinaemia; Benign hereditary chorea; Chorea: an overview; Dystonia: an overview; Huntington's disease;

Hypobetalipoproteinaemia; McLeod syndrome; Organic acidopathies; Parkinsonian syndromes, parkinsonism; Tourette syndrome; Vitamins and the nervous system.

■ Neuroaxonal dystrophy

Infantile neuroaxonal dystrophy • Seitelberger disease

Pathophysiology This is a rare autosomal-recessive condition, relentlessly progressive and invariably fatal, presenting usually within the first 3 years of life, with eosinophilic spheroids of swollen axoplasm in brain and spinal cord.

Clinical features: history and examination

- Psychomotor deterioration.
- Hypotonia, hyperreflexia, Babinski signs: many children never achieve independent walking (motor disorder may progress from legs to arms).
- Never acquire normal language.
- Progressive visual loss with optic atrophy.
- +/− seizures (rare), myoclonus, extrapyramidal signs, ataxia, nystagmus, sensory deficits in legs, urinary retention.
- Terminal spasticity, pseudobulbar signs, decerebrate rigidity.

Investigations and diagnosis *Bloods*: normal.

Imaging: CT normal; MRI diffuse cerebellar atrophy with hyperintense cerebellar cortex.

CSF: normal.

Neurophysiology:

EEG: may see characteristic high amplitude fast rhythms (16–22 Hz), although EEG changes may be non-specific or absent.

EMG/NCS: denervation, but conduction velocities normal.

Biopsy: skin and conjunctival nerves show characteristic axonal spheroids.

Differential diagnosis Late-onset cases may be indistinguishable from Hallervorden–Spatz disease, and some authorities consider them to be the same condition.

Treatment and prognosis No specific treatment; vegetative state, death by 3–8 years.

Reference Aicardi J, Castelein P. Infantile neuroaxonal dystrophy. *Brain* 1979; **102**: 727–748.

Other relevant entries Hallervorden–Spatz disease, Hallervorden–Spatz syndrome.

■ Neurobehçet's disease – see Behçet's disease

■ Neuroblastoma

This tumour of neural elements, a CNS primitive neuroectodermal tumour (PNET), is one of the most common solid tumours seen in children. It is consistently associated with deletion of the short arm of chromosome 1; a possible tumour suppressor gene may be located at 1p36.1. Adrenal medulla and sympathetic ganglia are the most common locations, but cerebral and olfactory (esthesioneuroblastoma) tumours may also occur. Differentiated neuroblastoma or neurocytoma is a variant, usually found in the lateral ventricles, with a good prognosis.

Although only a small proportion of children with neuroblastoma develop the opsoclonus–myoclonus syndrome (Kinsbourne's syndrome), an underlying neuroblastoma is found in about 50% of children with opsoclonus–myoclonus syndrome: those with a tumour have a better prognosis. In cases with tumour, which may be demonstrated by CT of thorax and abdomen, there may be elevated urinary catecholamines.

Other relevant entries Esthesioneuroblastoma; Opsoclonus; Primitive neuroecto-dermal tumours; Tumours: an overview.

◼ Neuroborreliosis – see Borreliosis

◼ Neurobrucellosis – see Brucellosis

◼ Neurocutaneous syndrome – see Phakomatosis

◼ Neurocysticercosis – see Cysticercosis

◼ Neurocytoma – see Neuroblastoma

◼ Neuroenteric cyst – see Cysts: an overview

◼ Neuroferritinopathy

Mutations in the gene encoding ferritin light polypeptide (FTL) have been identified in families with phenotypically heterogeneous movement disorders, including dystonia, chorea, and akinetic-rigid syndrome. There is associated cystic degeneration of the caudate and lentiform nuclei, and ferritin deposition in the brain, particularly the globus pallidus. Disordered brain iron metabolism may thus be implicated in neurodegeneration and movement disorders.

References Chinnery PF, Curtis AR, Fey C *et al*. Neuroferritinopathy. *Journal of Neurology, Neurosurgery and Psychiatry* 2002; **73**: 213 (abstract 1).

◼ Neurofibromatosis
Von Recklinghausen's disease

Pathophysiology A common, autosomal-dominant, neurocutaneous syndrome characterized by tumours arising from nerves (neurofibroma, neuroma) and café-au-lait spots, with a wide spectrum of severity. A distinction is made between:

- Neurofibromatosis type 1 (NF-1) = peripheral type, von Recklinghausen's disease;
- Neurofibromatosis type 2 (NF-2) = central type (much rarer than NF-1);
- Localized forms = segmental neurofibromatosis.

Clinical features: history and examination *Diagnostic criteria for NF-1*: two or more of

- café-au-lait macules, ≥ 6;
- axillary or inguinal freckling;
- two or more dermal fibromas;
- a plexiform neurofibroma;
- first degree relative with NF-1;
- optic nerve glioma;
- two or more Lisch nodules (=melanocytic, brown, hamartomas of the iris; 100% of patients);
- distinctive osseous lesion such as sphenoid dysplasia or thinning of the long bone cortex, with or without pseudo-arthrosis.

Diagnostic criteria for NF-2:

- bilateral acoustic neuromas (=vestibular schwannoma);
- first-degree relative with NF-2;
- unilateral acoustic neuroma, neurofibroma, glioma, meningioma, schwannoma, early lens opacity.

Segmental neurofibromatosis:

- neurofibromas, café-au-lait spots, limited to one segment of the body; there may be underlying intra-thoracic or intra-abdominal neurofibromas.
  - +/− kyphoscoliosis.
  - +/− hypertension (1% phaeochromocytoma; renal artery stenosis).
  - +/− epilepsy.
  - +/− thoracic, abdominal pain from neurofibromas.
  - Risk factor for subarachnoid haemorrhage.

Investigations and diagnosis Diagnosis is essentially clinical
Neurogenetics:

NF-1: mutations in neurofibromin gene, chromosome 17q11.2.

NF-2: mutations in the merlin or schwannomin gene, chromosome 22q12; tumour suppressor gene; may also be mutated in cases of sporadic acoustic neuroma, meningioma.

Imaging: for identification and monitoring of intracranial tumours; increased incidence of aqueduct stenosis in NF-1.

Differential diagnosis Unlikely to be mistaken; some overlap with Proteus syndrome. Café-au-lait spots in Noonan syndrome, Watson syndrome.

Treatment and prognosis No specific treatment. Monitoring for intracranial tumours, optic nerve tumours, with surgical intervention if appropriate. Shunting of aqueduct stenosis only if symptomatic. Symptomatic treatment of epilepsy, pain.

Monitor blood pressure: screen for phaeochromocytoma, renal artery stenosis if hypertensive.

Malignant brain tumours may reduce life expectancy.

References Huson SM, Harper PS, Compston DAS. Von Recklinghausen's neurofibromatosis. A clinical and population study in SE Wales. *Brain* 1988; **111**: 1355–1381.

Martuza RL, Eldridge R. Neurofibromatosis 2. *New England Journal of Medicine* 1988; **318**: 684–688.

North K. Neurofibromatosis type 1. *American Journal of Medical Genetics* 2000; **97**: 119–127.

Wallace MR, Collins FS. Neurofibromatosis. In: Conneally PM (ed.). *Molecular Basis of Neurology*. Boston: Blackwell Scientific, 1993: 161–180.

Other relevant entries Phakomatosis; Subarachnoid haemorrhage; Vestibular schwannoma.

■ Neuroleptic malignant syndrome

Malignant catatonia • Malignant neuroleptic syndrome

Pathophysiology A syndrome associated, in most cases, with the use of neuroleptic drugs: a similar phenomenon may be seen with sudden withdrawal of levodopa in patients with Parkinson's disease, and descriptions of "lethal catatonia" from the pre-neuroleptic era seem similar. Loss of dopaminergic drive in the basal ganglia has been suggested as a mechanism, although other neurotransmitters may also be implicated. Some authorities classify this syndrome as a malignant form of catatonia, responsive to the same treatments as catatonia.

Clinical features: history and examination Characteristic features are:

- hyperpyrexia,
- hypertonus,
- fluctuating level of consciousness;
- autonomic disturbances: labile blood pressure, tachycardia.
- History of neuroleptic drug use.

Investigations and diagnosis *Bloods*: raised creatine kinase, lactate dehydrogenase is typical.

Imaging: no diagnostic features; pre-existing or concurrent organic brain disease (e.g. vascular change) is recognized to be a predisposing factor.

CSF: normal.

Differential diagnosis Hypertonicity may suggest an akinetic-rigid syndrome but the acute onset is against this.

Treatment and prognosis Full supportive treatment: hydration; may require sedation, intubation and ventilation.

Dopamine agonists (e.g. bromocriptine) sometimes tried.

Lorazepam, ECT, as used for catatonia, may also be helpful in NMS.

References Buckley PF, Hutchinson M. Neuroleptic malignant syndrome. *Journal of Neurology, Neurosurgery and Psychiatry* 1995; **58**: 271–273.

Guze BH, Baxter LR. Neuroleptic malignant syndrome. *New England Journal of Medicine* 1985; **313**: 163–166.

Larner AJ, Smith SC, Farmer SF. "Non-neuroleptic malignant" syndrome. *Journal of Neurology, Neurosurgery and Psychiatry* 1998; **65**: 613.

Other relevant entries Catatonia; Drug-induced movement disorders; Parkinsonian syndromes, parkinsonism.

■ Neuromuscular junction diseases: an overview

Defects of neurotransmission at the neuromuscular junction underlie the pathogenesis of a variety of disorders:

- Myasthenia gravis
    juvenile and adult forms;
    neonatal myasthenia;
    congenital myasthenic syndromes (*q.v.*);
    drug-induced myasthenia (e.g. following penicillamine therapy).
- Lambert–Eaton myasthenic syndrome (LEMS).
- Neuromyotonia
- Botulism.
- Antibiotic-induced neuromuscular blockade: aminoglycosides, polypeptide antibiotics.

Other relevant entries Arthrogryposis multiplex congenita; Botulism; Congenital myasthenic syndromes; Lambert–Eaton myasthenic syndrome; Myasthenia gravis.

■ Neuromyelitis optica – see Devic's disease, Devic's syndrome

■ Neuromyotonia

Isaacs syndrome • Peripheral nerve hyperexcitability

Pathophysiology Neuromyotonia is continuous muscle activity of peripheral nerve origin, persisting after proximal nerve block or general anaesthesia but abolished by depolarizing muscle relaxants and neuromuscular blocking agents. The clinical associations of neuromyotonia – paraneoplastic and autoimmune conditions – first suggested its autoimmune aetiology, subsequently confirmed by the discovery of antibodies to voltage-gated potassium channels (VGKC) in the serum of some affected patients.

Clinical features: history and examination

- Muscle twitching at rest: myokymia, a wave-like rippling or a "bag of worms" below the skin.

- Cramps: may be triggered by voluntary or induced muscle contraction.
- Impaired muscle relaxation: pseudomyotonia; no percussion myotonia (*cf.* dystrophia myotonica).
- Muscle stiffness, muscle hypertrophy.
  - $+/-$ excessive sweating;
  - $+/-$ mild muscle weakness;
  - $+/-$ paraesthesia;
  - $+/-$ absent tendon reflexes.

Neuromyotonia may occur in isolation, and may remit spontaneously, or be a feature of other conditions such as episodic ataxia type I, or hereditary motor and sensory neuropathy.

Associations include thymoma, myasthenia gravis, vitiligo, lymphoma, Hashimoto's thyroiditis and penicillamine treatment.

An ocular variant is also described, in which spontaneous spasm in extraocular muscles may follow prolonged voluntary activation of specific muscles; this rare syndrome commonly follows irradiation for pituitary tumour but has also been reported in association with internal carotid artery aneurysm or alcohol consumption. Carbamazepine may help symptoms.

Investigations and diagnosis *Bloods*: specific test is VGKC antibody assay.

Neurophysiology: EMG: spontaneous continuous single motor unit discharges (doublet, triplet or multiplet) at high intraburst frequency (30–300 Hz). Fibrillation potentials and fasciculations are often present. Electrical stimulation of the nerve typically leads to increased spontaneous activity (after-discharges).

Search for underlying causes, especially thymoma, myasthenia gravis, lymphoma.

Differential diagnosis Electrophysiological findings are quantitatively rather than qualitatively different from those seen in Denny–Brown, Foley (cramp–fasciculation) syndrome.

Stiff man syndrome also results from continuous motor activity, involving spinal interneuronal networks.

Treatment and prognosis Neuromyotonia occurring in isolation may remit spontaneously. Muscle weakness is usually mild. Anticonvulsants such as phenytoin, carbamazepine, sodium valproate, and lamotrigine may suppress neuronal repetitive firing. Immunotherapy, including plasma exchange, may be appropriate for acquired neuromyotonia. Underlying causes may influence prognosis (e.g. small-cell lung carcinoma), treatment of which may have little effect on neuromyotonia.

References Ezra E, Spalton D, Sanders MD, Graham EM, Plant GT. Ocular neuromyotonia. *British Journal of Ophthalmology* 1996; **80**: 350–355.

Hart IK, Maddison P, Newsom-Davis J, Vincent A, Mills KR. Phenotypic variants of autoimmune peripheral nerve hyperexcitability. *Brain* 2002; **125**: 1887–1895.

Hart IK, Waters C, Vincent A *et al.* Autoantibodies detected to expressed K^+ channels are implicated in neuromyotonia. *Annals of Neurology* 1997; **48**: 238–246.

Isaacs H. A syndrome of continuous muscle-fibre activity. *Journal of Neurology, Neurosurgery and Psychiatry* 1961; **24**: 319–325.

Maddison P. Neuromyotonia. *Practical Neurology* 2002; **2**: 225–229.

Other relevant entries Cramps; Denny–Brown, Foley syndrome; Dystrophia myotonica; Episodic ataxias; Morvan's syndrome; Myasthenia gravis; Myotonia and myotonic disorders; Stiff people: an overview.

■ Neuronal ceroid lipofuscinosis
Batten's disease

Pathophysiology The neuronal ceroid lipofuscinoses (NCLs) are a group of neurodegenerative disorders characterized by the accumulation of autofluorescent inclusion bodies in neurones and other tissues. A number of forms are recognized. Initially these were characterized according to age of onset, for example:

Infantile (INCL)/Santavuori–Haltia disease/Finnish type.
Late-infantile (LINCL)/early childhood/Jansky–Bielschowsky type.
Juvenile (JNCL)/Vogt–Spielmeyer or Spielmeyer–Sjögren type.
Adult/Kufs' disease.

Inheritance is autosomal recessive, with the exception of the adult form which may show autosomal-dominant inheritance. Eight genetic loci have currently been mapped and mutant genes identified encoding lysosomal enzymes or putative membrane proteins. With the increasing understanding of the genetic basis of these conditions, a revised classification has been suggested:

Type	Linkage	Mutant enzyme
NCL1 (Santavuori/acute infantile/"Finnish form")	1p32	Palmitoyl-protein thioesterase 1 (PPT1)
NCL2 (Bielschowsky/acute late infantile)	11p15	Tripeptidyl peptidase 1 (TPP1)
NCL3 (Batten/juvenile chronic)	16p12	Battenin
NCL4 (Kufs/adult)	AR or AD	Not known
NCL5 (Finnish variant/childhood)	13q22	Not known
NCL6 (Lake's/late infantile)	15q21–q23	Linclin
NCL7 (Turkish variant/late infantile)	AR	Not known
NCL8 (Northern epilepsy/juvenile)	8p23	lysosomal membrane protein

Clinical features: history and examination

- NCL1

  Psychomotor collapse from >3 months after birth onwards

  Motor dysfunction: knitting hyperkinesia, pyramidal, extrapyramidal
  signs, +/− myoclonus

  Retinal degeneration: brown discolouration of macula, optic atrophy

  Mental retardation

  +/− Epilepsy, refractory

- NCL2

  onset seldom before age 4 years

  progressive refractory seizure disorder

  mental deterioration

  visual loss: retinal artery attenuation, macular granular degeneration

- NCL3

  Onset 5–15 years

  Visual dysfunction, progressing to blindness

  Psychosis, slow cognitive decline

  Seizures

  Motor dysfunction: pyramidal, extrapyramidal, +/− myoclonus.

  Progression to vegetative state

- NCL4

  onset second to third decade

  Type A: Seizures: often myoclonic

  Type B: Psychiatric, cognitive features, progressive spasticity, rigidity, ataxia,
  choreoathetosis

  Vision preserved: no retinal changes (ditto NCL8).

Investigations and diagnosis *Bloods*: no specific abnormalities.

Urine: raised dolichols in urinary sediment (disputed by some authors).

Imaging: atrophy; may be selective to cerebellum in some variants.

Neurophysiology:

EEG: may show epileptogenic pattern

ERG: diminution or loss (not NCL4, NCL8)

VER: large responses to slow rates of flicker (especially NCL2)

SSEP: may be exaggerated responses.

Biopsy: rectal mucosa, skin biopsy, endothelial cells, blood lymphocytes, conjunctival
cells, may show typical inclusion bodies/cytosomes:

Fingerprint inclusions: NCL 3, 4, 5, 6, 7

Curvilinear inclusion bodies: NCL 2; atypical in NCL 5, 6, 7, 8

Granular osmiophilic deposit (GROD): NCL1; may be seen in NCL4

Rectilinear bodies: NCL 4, 5, 6, 7, 8.

Lipofuscin bodies are not diagnostic.

Neurogenetics: tests available for mutations in genes encoding lysosomal enzyme palmitoyl-protein thioesterase (PPT1; NCL1), lysosomal enzyme tripeptidyl peptidase (TPP1; NCL2).

Differential diagnosis

Gangliosidoses and sphingomyelinoses may need to be differentiated.

Kufs: other causes of progressive myoclonic epilepsy.

Treatment and prognosis No specific treatment currently available. Bone marrow transplantation has been attempted, without conspicuous success.

Symptomatic control of seizures (valproate), dystonia, myoclonus.

NCL1: death at 8–13 years of age.

References Bennett MJ, Hofmann SL. The neuronal ceroid-lipofuscinoses (Batten disease): a new class of lysosomal storage diseases. *Journal of Inherited Metabolic Disease* 1999; **22**: 535–544.

Berkovic SF, Carpenter S, Andermann F *et al*. Kufs' disease: a critical reappraisal. *Brain* 1988; **111**: 27–62.

Wisniewski KE, Kida E, Golabek AA, Kaczmarski W, Connell F, Zhong N. Neuronal ceroid lipofuscinoses: classification and diagnosis. *Advances in Genetics* 2001; **45**: 1–34.

Other relevant entries Dementia: an overview; Lysosomal-storage disorders: an overview; Progressive myoclonic epilepsy.

Neuropathies: an overview

Pathophysiology Pathological processes affecting the peripheral nerves may be classified in various ways:

Course
    Time course of evolution: acute, subacute, chronic.
Anatomy
    principal locus of pathology within the nerve trunk: axon, myelin sheath;
    principal fibre type affected: motor, sensory, autonomic; mixed;
    distribution: mononeuropathy, mononeuritis multiplex, polyneuropathy.
Inherited or acquired.

- Course
    Acute
        Guillain–Barré syndrome (GBS);
        acute sensory ataxic neuropathy (ASAN);
        acute motor axonal neuropathy (AMAN) = axonal variant of GBS;
        acute post-infectious axonal polyradiculoneuropathy (AMSAN, axonal GBS).
    Subacute
    Chronic
        Chronic inflammatory demyelinating polyneuropathy (CIDP).
        Many cryptogenic neuropathies of later life.

- Anatomy: axonal/demyelinating
    - Axonal
        - Trauma
        - Malignancy
        - Critical illness polyneuropathy
        - Toxins: especially thallium, organophosphates
        - Acute axonal form of GBS = AMAN.
    - Demyelinating
        - GBS
        - CIDP
        - Paraprotein-associated demyelinating neuropathy (PDN)
        - Post-immunization neuropathy
        - Diphtheritic neuropathy
        - Infectious mononucleosis; hepatitis; HIV.
- Anatomy: motor/sensory/autonomic
    - Motor
        - Multifocal motor neuropathy (MMN) with conduction block
    - Sensory
        - Acute sensory ataxic neuropathy (ASAN)
        - Cryptogenic sensory neuropathy of elderly patients
        - Hereditary sensory (and autonomic) neuropathies
        - Pure sensory variant of CIDP (rare).
    - Autonomic
        - GBS may be predominantly or exclusively autonomic; amyloid neuropathy
        - Mixed.
- Anatomy: mononeuropathy, mononeuritis multiplex, polyneuropathy
    - Mononeuropathy
        - Arm and trunk
            - Dorsal scapular nerve
            - Long thoracic nerve
            - Suprascapular nerve
            - Axillary nerve
            - Musculocutaneous nerve
            - Radial nerve
            - Median nerve
            - Ulnar nerve.
        - Leg
            - Iliohypogastric, ilioinguinal nerves
            - Genitofemoral nerve
            - Lateral cutaneous nerve of thigh
            - Posterior cutaneous nerve of thigh
            - Femoral nerve
            - Obturator nerve

Gluteal nerve
Sciatic nerve
Tibial nerve
Peroneal nerve
Sural nerve.
Neuronopathy
Motor
Anterior horn cell disease.
Sensory (=ganglionopathy)
Paraneoplastic sensory neuronopathy.
(with or without anti-Hu antibodies).
Sjögren's syndrome.
Mononeuritis multiplex, Mononeuropathy multiplex (q.v.).
Polyneuropathy: for example diabetes mellitus, vitamin B_{12} deficiency,
drug/toxin induced.
- Inherited/hereditary
Inherited neuropathies
Hereditary motor and sensory neuropathies (HMSN; q.v.);
Charcot–Marie–Tooth (CMT) disease (q.v.)
Hereditary sensory and autonomic neuropathies (HSAN; q.v.)
Familial amyloid neuropathies (FAP; q.v.)
Spinocerebellar syndromes (e.g. Friedreich's ataxia)
Fabry's disease.
- Acquired
Inflammatory: Vasculitic, for example polyarteritis nodosa (PAN); rheumatoid
arthritis; systemic lupus erythematosus (SLE); Wegener's granulomatosis,
Sjögren's syndrome, non-systemic vasculitic neuropathy.
Metabolic/nutritional: diabetes, uraemia, vitamin B_{12} deficiency, porphyria,
amyloidosis.
Infective: leprosy, borreliosis (Lyme disease), syphilis, HIV.
Drug/toxin induced: alcohol induced, cisplatin, pyridoxine, lead, nitrofurantoin,
isoniazid, arsenic, mercury, thallium.
Granulomatous: sarcoidosis.
Infiltrative: amyloid; malignancy.
Cryptogenic sensory neuropathy of elderly patients.

Clinical features: history and examination

- Pace of onset (acute, subacute, chronic).
- Predisposing/precipitating factors: diabetes, drug use, recent infection (especially
gastrointestinal infection).
- Careful family history, with examination of other family members if possible.
- Motor
weakness appropriate to single nerve (mononeuropathy);
patchy weakness appropriate to several nerves (mononeuropathy multiplex);

distal > proximal weakness $+/-$ distal reflex loss (polyneuropathy).

- Sensory

  Focal sensory loss appropriate to a single nerve (mononeuropathy);

  Patchy loss suggestive of involvement of several different cutaneous nerve territories (mononeuropathy multiplex);

  Distal "glove and stocking" loss (polyneuropathy);

  Predominantly pain and temperature sensory loss in some neuropathies (e.g. Tangier disease); ganglionopathies may have marked proprioceptive loss leading to sensory ataxia (which may be mistaken for a cerebellar syndrome).

- Autonomic

  Vomiting, diarrhoea, impotence; cardiac arrhythmia.

- Other features of specific diseases, for example ataxia in spinocerebellar ataxias, sicca syndrome in Sjögren's syndrome.

Investigations and diagnosis Many investigations may be performed in an attempt to discover the cause of a peripheral neuropathy. Not all are required in every case; particular circumstances may dictate the most appropriate. The importance of diabetes mellitus cannot be overestimated. Despite extensive investigation, an aetiological cause remains elusive in many cases, often >50% of cases although some centres claim a better rate of diagnosis.

Bloods:

  Haematology: FBC, ESR, vitamin B_{12}, cryoglobulins.

  Biochemistry: glucose (fasting, $+/-$ HbA$_{1c}$, oral glucose tolerance test), urea and electrolytes, liver function tests, CRP, immunoglobulins, serum angiotensin converting enzyme (ACE), porphyria screen, serum lead.

  Serology: auto-antibody profile including ANA, ANCA, ENA, rheumatoid factor, *Borrelia* serology, hepatitic serology, anti-ganglioside antibodies (GD1b in acute sensory axonal neuropathy [ASAN], GQ1b in Miller Fisher syndrome), anti-neuronal antibodies (anti-Hu antibodies in paraneoplastic neuronopathy).

Urine:

  Microscopy: for active sediment.

  Biochemistry: porphyrins, ALA and phorphobilinogen; 24-hour urine for heavy metals.

Faeces:

  Biochemistry: faecal porphyrins.

  Culture: for *Campylobacter jejuni* infection.

Neurophysiology: EMG/NCS: often unhelpful in the early stages of an acute neuropathy, but generally reliable for differentiating established axonal from demyelinating neuropathy, and mononeuropathy from mononeuritis multiplex and polyneuropathy. Changes may be confined to sensory evaluation (e.g. reduced or absent sensory nerve action potentials) in pure sensory neuropathy, or to motor evaluation (e.g. reduced CMAP amplitude) in pure motor neuropathy. Conduction block should be sought in a purely motor neuropathy.

Imaging: may include chest X-ray (CXR), chest/abdominal/pelvic CT/MRI, as well as cranial and spinal cord imaging, looking for amyloid, malignancy, and CNS lesions.

CSF: cell count, protein (may be very high in GBS, CIDP), glucose, oligoclonal bands, ACE, cytology.

Nerve biopsy: may need to be considered if diagnosis not forthcoming from other investigations, especially if the patient is deteriorating rapidly and/or vasculitis is a possible diagnosis. Selective fibre loss may suggest diagnosis (e.g. reduction of unmyelinated fibres in HSAN type IV, or of small myelinated fibres in HSAN types II, V). Amyloid infiltration.

Differential diagnosis Neuropathies should be differentiated from plexopathies and radiculopathies (may sometimes coexist, as in acute inflammatory radiculoneuropathies).

Acute peripheral weakness mimicking neuropathy may occur in:

Hypokalaemia.

"Spinal shock" or extensive spinal cord damage with areflexia and hypotonia; this may also be seen in vascular events involving the lower brainstem.

Neuromuscular junction dysfunction (e.g. botulism).

Treatment and prognosis

Dependent on cause.

Cryptogenic neuropathies in the elderly tend not to progress rapidly and seldom take people off their legs.

References Dyck PJ, Thomas PK, Griffin JW, Low PA, Podulso JF (eds). *Peripheral Neuropathy* (3rd edition). Philadelphia: WB Saunders, 1995.

Ginsberg L, King R, Orrell R. Nerve biopsy. *Practical Neurology* 2003; **3**: 306–312.

Kuhlenbäumer G, Young P, Hünermund G, Ringelstein B, Stögbauer F. Clinical features and molecular genetics of hereditary peripheral neuropathies. *Journal of Neurology* 2002; **249**: 1629–1650.

McLeod JG. Investigation of peripheral neuropathy. *Journal of Neurology, Neurosurgery and Psychiatry* 1995; **58**: 274–283.

Mumenthaler M, Schliack H, Mumenthaler M, Goerke H. *Peripheral Nerve Lesions: Diagnosis and Treatment*. New York: Thieme, 1990.

Pareyson D. Diagnosis of hereditary neuropathies in adult patients. *Journal of Neurology* 2003; **250**: 148–160.

Staal A, Van Gijn J, Spaans F. *Mononeuropathies: Examination, Diagnosis and Treatment*. London: WB Saunders, 1999.

Stewart JD. *Focal Peripheral Neuropathies* (3rd edition). Philadelphia: Lippincott Williams & Wilkins, 2000.

Other relevant entries Autonomic failure; Charcot–Marie–Tooth disease; Diabetes mellitus and the nervous system; Drug-induced neuropathies; Familial amyloid polyneuropathies; Friedreich's ataxia; Gangliosides and neurological disorders; Heavy metal poisoning; Hereditary motor and sensory neuropathy; Hereditary sensory and autonomic neuropathy; Paraneoplastic syndromes; Radiculopathies: an overview; Refsum's disease; Renal disease and the nervous system; Riley–Day syndrome; Sjögren's syndrome; Spinal cord disease: an overview; Strachan's syndrome; Vitamin B_{12} deficiency; Wartenberg's neuropathy.

■ Neurosarcoidosis – see Sarcoidosis

■ Neuro-Sweet disease – see Sweet's syndrome

■ Neurosyphilis – see Syphilis

■ Neurovascular compression syndromes

Several disorders of uncertain aetiology are postulated to result from compression of cranial nerves by vascular loops, causing aberrant transmission of nerve impulses as a result of local demyelination. Examples include:

- trigeminal neuralgia (Vth cranial nerve);
- hemifacial spasm (VIth cranial nerve);
- superior oblique myokymia (IVth cranial nerve);
- vascular cross compression of the eighth cranial nerve (=disabling positional vertigo, vestibular paroxysmia).

■ Nevin–Jones syndrome – see Creutzfeldt–Jakob disease

■ Niemann–Pick disease
Juvenile dystonic lipidosis

Pathophysiology An inherited metabolic disorder of variable phenotype. Types A and B result from deficiency of the lysosomal enzyme acid sphingomyelinase (hence, primary sphingomyelinosis), mapped to chromosome 11p, whereas type C results from a defect in cellular trafficking of cholesterol allowing lysosomal accumulation of unesterified cholesterol, hence it is biochemically and genetically distinct from types A and B.

Clinical features: history and examination

- Type A (infantile form):
   Linked to chromosome 11p15
   Massive hepatosplenomegaly in the first few months of life
   Later neurological problems: failure to thrive, chronic encephalopathy, cherry red macular spot, normal eye movements, psychomotor regression (rarely achieve sitting balance), seizures
   Respiratory problems: pulmonary interstitial disease.

- Type B (non-neuropathic)
  - Linked to chromosome 11p15
  - Hepatosplenomegaly
  - Pulmonary infiltration
  - $+/-$ minor bone lesions
  - May have mild ataxia
- Type C:
  - Autosomal recessive: type NPC1 linked to mutations on chromosome 18q11 (NPC1 gene), type NPC2 to chromosome 14q24 (HE1 gene).
  - May present in infancy or early childhood as an hepatic syndrome, or in later childhood as a progressive neurodegenerative disease with:
    - Progressive gait disturbance, dystonia
    - Dysarthria
    - Emotional lability
    - Intellectual regression
    - Supranuclear gaze palsy with impaired vertical saccadic eye movements
    - Ataxia
    - Extrapyramidal signs
    - Seizures
    - Cataplexy
    - Mild hepatosplenomegaly
- Type D (Nova Scotia variant):
  - Allelic variant of NPC1
  - Early onset hepatosplenomegaly
  - Neurological features as for type C
  - Protracted course, survival into adulthood.

Investigations and diagnosis *Bloods*: liver-related blood tests may be mildly abnormal.

Imaging: skeletal radiographs usually normal; chest radiograph commonly shows diffuse reticular infiltration.

Bone marrow biopsy: smears show foamy-storage histiocytes (suggestive but not pathognomonic, also occur in sialidosis) and sea-blue histiocytes in type C (may be absent).

Other: measure enzyme activity in leukocytes or fibroblasts: sphingomyelinase activity almost absent in type A. Filipin staining of cultured skin fibroblasts in type C.

Brain: neurofibrillary tangles in hippocampus in type C; in type A excessive sphingomyelin, and gangliosides GM2 and GM3.

Differential diagnosis Type A: Gaucher disease, neurological involvement later in NPD.

Type B: Gaucher disease type 1.

Treatment and prognosis

No specific treatment, supportive only.

Type A usually die by age 5 years.

Type B at risk of respiratory infection, otherwise normal life expectancy.

References Carstea ED, Morris JA, Coleman KG *et al*. Niemann–Pick C1 disease gene: homology to mediators of cholesterol homeostasis. *Science* 1997; **277**: 228–231.

Fink JK, Filling-Katz MR, Sokol J *et al*. Clinical spectrum of Niemann–Pick disease type C. *Neurology* 1989; **39**: 1040–1049.

Other relevant entries Emotional lability: differential diagnosis; Gaucher's disease; Sialidosis.

Night terrors – see Pavor nocturnus

Nocardiosis

Nocardia species are aerobic actinomycetes; filamentous, weakly Gram-positive, bacteria, spread from soil by inhalation, which cause localized or disseminated infections, the latter often involving the central nervous system (CNS), most particularly in immunocompromised individuals. Pulmonary disease may seed via the bloodstream to the brain as multiple abscesses, often multiloculated, causing space occupation, raised intracranial pressure, focal deficits and epilepsy. The abscesses are clinically and radiologically identical to abscesses of different aetiology, diagnosis relying on identification of the organism in pus from a stereotactic biopsy. Meningitis may also occur. Treatment is with sulphonamides + trimethoprim, minocycline, imipenem or aminoglycoside, despite which mortality remains high (30–60%).

Other relevant entries HIV/AIDS and the nervous system; Immunosuppressive therapy and diseases of the nervous system.

Nonaka myopathy
Early-adult-onset distal myopathy type 1

An autosomal-recessive distal muscular dystrophy usually of early-onset characterized by muscle wasting and weakness in a predominantly distal distribution (e.g. the anterior compartment of the legs, causing foot drop and steppage gait; hand and finger weakness may also be present). Creatine kinase is elevated (<10 times normal). Muscle biopsy shows a vacuolar myopathy (*cf.* Miyoshi myopathy); vacuoles are rimmed and have nuclear or cytoplasmic inclusions (15–18 nm filaments). Linkage is to chromosome 9p.

Reference Nonaka I, Sunohara N, Ishiura S, Satoyoshi E. Familial distal myopathy with rimmed vacuole and lamellar (myeloid) body formation. *Journal of the Neurological Sciences* 1981; **51**: 141–155.

Other relevant entries Distal muscular dystrophy, Distal myopathy; Laing myopathy; Miyoshi myopathy.

Non-convulsive status epilepticus – see Status epilepticus

■ Non-epileptic seizures – see Pseudoseizures

■ Non-ketotic hyperglycinaemia
Glycine encephalopathy

A metabolic defect in the glycine cleavage system leads to compromise of serine synthesis and elevated blood, urine, CSF, and tissue levels of glycine. With onset of protein feeding, infants develop poor feeding, lethargy, hypotonia, myoclonic seizures, hiccups, and apnoea. Progressive encephalopathy leads to early death. With greater residual enzyme activity presentation may be later, with mild mental retardation, hiccups, and myoclonic seizures. MRI may show brain atrophy, abnormal myelination, +/− absent corpus callosum. Attempts to lower glycine levels (high-dose benzoate therapy, haemodialysis, exchange transfusion) may be life saving but neurological sequelae (mental retardation, seizures, myoclonus) are common.

Other relevant entry Aminoacidopathies: an overview.

■ Non-Wilsonian hepatocerebral degeneration

This condition is characterized by fixed or progressive neurological deficits, including dementia, dysarthria, gait ataxia, intention tremor, and choreoathetosis, reflecting cerebral degeneration in the context of repeated episodes of hepatic encephalopathy; individually such episodes may be reversible but there seems to be a cumulative effect on neural tissue. Spinal cord damage with spastic paraparesis may also occur. Pathologically the brain shows microcavitary degenerative changes in layers V and VI of the cortex, underlying white matter, basal ganglia and cerebellum. Intranuclear PAS positive inclusions may be seen, as are abnormalities in spinal cord tracts. Some authors have doubted the existence of this condition as a separate entity.

Reference Victor M, Adams RD, Cole M. The acquired (non-Wilsonian) type of chronic hepatocerebral degeneration. *Medicine (Baltimore)* 1965; **44**: 345–395.
Other relevant entry Hepatic encephalopathy.

■ Noonan syndrome

An autosomal-dominant congenital dysmorphic syndrome, occurring mainly in girls, characterized by congenital heart defects, short stature, ptosis, antimongolian eye slant, low hairline, cubitus valgus, high-arched palate, hypertelorism; neurologically there may be seizures, mental retardation, and sensorineural hearing loss. Café-au-lait spots may also be seen.

Other relevant entries Neurofibromatosis; Turner's syndrome.

■ Normal pressure hydrocephalus

Pathophysiology Although the term "normal pressure hydrocephalus" was coined by Adams and colleagues in 1965, it is likely that similar cases had been described prior to this. The classical picture is the clinical triad of gait difficulty, urinary symptoms, and dementia (cognitive decline) in association with communicating hydrocephalus. This may be primary or idiopathic, or secondary to some defined disease process, such as subarachnoid haemorrhage, basal meningitis, or a disorder causing raised CSF protein concentration. The exact incidence of the condition, its pathogenesis, and the optimal treatment still remain subjects of debate, but it does seem to be commoner in the elderly. Some authors advocate abolition of the term in favour of "chronic hydrocephalus".

Clinical features: history and examination

- Clinical triad:

    gait difficulty, sometimes labelled "apraxia" or "magnetic gait";

    urinary symptoms;

    cognitive decline: although described as dementia in the original accounts, the commoner picture is of subcortical deficits (increased forgetfulness, inertia, reduced attention, mental slowness); NPH may not in fact be a true cause of "reversible dementia".

- No rest tremor; no clinical benefit from levodopa.

Investigations and diagnosis *Imaging*: CT/MRI: hydrocephalus, communicating in type; the presence of normal-sized Sylvian fissures and cortical sulci may increase suspicion of NPH (*cf. ex vacuo* atrophy). Evans index (=maximum width of frontal horns/maximum width to inner tables of the skull) >0.3 is in keeping with the diagnosis of NPH. Proton-density MRI may show periventricular hyperintensity suggesting transependymal flow. Isotope cisternography has been used to demonstrate impaired CSF absorption but is not a reliable predictor of response to shunting.

CSF: may show raised protein, oligoclonal bands; single pressure measurements are typically normal but prolonged intracranial pressure monitoring may show mild elevations or episodic appearance of high pressure b waves. The place of CSF infusion studies remains to be clarified. The CSF tap test or Fisher's test (removal of 20–30 ml of CSF, with assessment of gait +/− cognitive function before and after) may be helpful, clinical improvement suggesting that shunting will be beneficial (although this has never been systematically investigated).

Differential diagnosis Cerebrovascular disease may produce a similar clinical picture, and in elderly patients there may be incidental atrophy causing *ex vacuo* ventricular dilatation; however, cortical sulci and the Sylvian fissures are usually widened too. Subdural haematoma and degenerative dementias may produce a similar picture.

Treatment and prognosis Ventriculoperitoneal shunting (not ventriculo-atrial, or lumboperitoneal) in carefully selected cases can be beneficial. Good response occurs in those with:

Identified aetiology

Predominantly gait abnormalities with little or no cognitive deficit

Substantial improvement with the CSF tap test

Normal-sized Sylvian fissures, cortical sulci

Minimal white matter change.

If there are contraindications to surgery, medical therapy with acetazolamide or repeated lumbar punctures may be undertaken.

References Adams RD, Fisher CM, Hakim S *et al.* Symptomatic occult hydrocephalus with "normal" cerebrospinal fluid pressure. *New England Journal of Medicine* 1965; **273**: 117–126.

Bret P, Guyotat J, Chazal J. Is normal pressure hydrocephalus a valid concept in 2002? A reappraisal in five questions and proposal for a new designation of the syndrome as "chronic hydrocephalus". *Journal of Neurology, Neurosurgery and Psychiatry* 2002; **73**: 9–12.

Vanneste JA. Diagnosis and management of normal pressure hydrocephalus. *Journal of Neurology* 2000; **247**: 5–14.

Other relevant entries Dementia: an overview; Hydrocephalus; Subdural haematoma.

▪ Normokalaemic periodic paralysis – see Channelopathies: an overview; Periodic paralysis

▪ Norrie disease
Norrie–Warburg syndrome ● Oculoacousticocerebral degeneration

This X-linked-recessive disorder is characterized by:
- Congenital blindness: degenerative, proliferative dysplasia of neuroretina
- Progressive sensorineural deafness (one-third)
- Mental retardation (half)
  +/– cataplexy, abnormal REM sleep organization.

The mutant gene, NDP, is located at Xp11.2, its product is norrin. Complete deletion of the gene results in an absence of platelet monoamine oxidase-B, which may explain the cataplexy and abnormal rapid eye movement (REM) sleep organization.

Reference Vossler DG, Wyler AR, Wilkus RJ, Gardner-Walker G, Vleck BW. Cataplexy and monoamine oxidase deficiency in Norrie disease. *Neurology* 1996; **46**: 1258–1261.

Other relevant entries Cataplexy; Coats' disease; Sleep disorders: an overview.

▪ Notalgia paraesthetica

A condition of unknown aetiology characterized by a burning sensation, paraesthesia and itching over an area at the medial edge of scapula. It is entirely benign and may wax and wane over the years. The territory involved encompasses the dorsal branches of roots T2–T6.

References Knight R. Notalgia paraesthetica. *Practical Neurology* 2001; **1**: 56–57.

Pleet AB, Massey EW. Notalgia paresthetica. *Neurology* 1978; **28**: 1310–1312.

Other relevant entry Entrapment neuropathies.

■ Nothnagel's syndrome

Ophthalmoplegia–ataxia syndrome

This brainstem vascular syndrome affecting the midbrain is characterized by:

- an ipsilateral oculomotor nerve palsy; and
- contralateral cerebellar ataxia;
- +/− trochlear nerve palsy, nystagmus, and sensory loss.

It may thus be differentiated from Benedikt's syndrome, Claude's syndrome, and Weber's syndrome on clinical grounds although the underlying pathogenesis (occlusion of a penetrating branch of the posterior cerebral artery to the midbrain, less commonly to basilar artery involvement) is similar.

Reference Liu GT, Crenner CW, Logigian EL *et al.* Midbrain syndromes of Benedikt, Claude and Nothnagel: setting the record straight. *Neurology* 1992; **42**: 1820–1822.

Other relevant entries Benedikt's syndrome; Brainstem vascular syndromes; Cerebrovascular disease: arterial; Claude's syndrome; Weber's syndrome.

■ "Numb and clumsy hands" syndrome

A syndrome of "numb and clumsy hands" has been described with midline cervical disc protrusions at the C3/C4 level, that is well above the segments supplying the hand and hence a false-localizing sign. Concurrent with numbness of fingertips and palms, there may be a tightening sensation at mid-thoracic level. With the availability of MRI of the cervical cord, the responsible lesion is unlikely to be overlooked.

Reference Nakajima M, Hirayama K. Midcervical central cord syndrome: numb and clumsy hands due to midline cervical disc protrusion at the C3–C4 intervertebral level. *Journal of Neurology, Neurosurgery and Psychiatry* 1995; **58**: 607–613.

Other relevant entries Cervical cord disease; Foramen magnum lesions, foramen magnum syndrome.

■ Numb cheek, numb chin syndrome

Numb chin syndrome (Roger's sign) is an isolated neuropathy affecting the mental branch of the mandibular division of the trigeminal (V) nerve, causing pain, swelling, and numbness of the lower lip, chin and mucous membrane inside the lip. This is usually a sign of metastatic spread of cancer to the jaw.

Numb cheek syndrome, involving the cheek, upper lip, upper incisors and gingiva, is due to involvement of the infraorbital portion of the maxillary division of the trigeminal nerve, usually by an infiltrating malignancy.

References Campbell WW Jr. The numb cheek syndrome: a sign of infraorbital neuropathy. *Neurology* 1986; **36**: 421–423.

Furukawa T. Numb chin syndrome in the elderly. *Journal of Neurology, Neurosurgery and Psychiatry* 1990; **53**: 173.
Other relevant entry Cranial nerve disease: V: Trigeminal nerve.

Nyssen–van Bogaert syndrome
Optico-cochleo-dentate syndrome

A rare neurological condition characterized by loss of vision (optic atrophy), sensori-neural deafness and ataxia, with characteristic neuropathological changes comprising pigmented macrophages and astrocytes.

Reference Larnaout A, Ben-Hamida M, Hentati F. A clinicopathological observation of Nyssen–van Bogaert syndrome with second motor neuron degeneration: two distinct clinical entities. *Acta Neurologica Scandinavica* 1998; **98**: 452–457.
Other relevant entry Hearing loss: differential diagnosis.

Nystagmus: an overview

Pathophysiology Nystagmus, or talantropia, is an involuntary to-and-fro movement of the eyeballs, of which there are many varieties. It is usually bilateral, but occasionally may be unilateral, as in internuclear ophthalmoplegia (INO). The pathophysiological underpinnings are diverse, but all involve brainstem nuclei and tracts which control eye movements and gaze holding, especially the III, IV and VI cranial nerve nuclei, paramedian pontine reticular formation, vestibular nuclei, medial longitudinal fasciculus, central tegmental tract, cerebellar connections to these structures, interstitial nucleus of Cajal, and nucleus prepositus hypoglossi. The nature of the nystagmus may permit inferences about the precise location of pathology.

Clinical features: history and examination Nystagmus may be classified in various ways. Observations should be made in the nine cardinal positions of gaze for direction, amplitude and beat frequency of nystagmus. Nystagmus may be abortive or sustained in duration.

Waveform:

- Pendular (undulatory): eye movements are more or less equal in amplitude and velocity (sinusoidal oscillations) about a central (null) point. This is often congenital, in which case it is known simply as congenital nystagmus; acquired causes include multiple sclerosis and brainstem infarctions.
- Jerk: at least one of the directions of eye movement is slow (slow phase; <40°/sec) followed by a rapid, corrective, saccadic movement in the opposite direction (fast phase) for which direction the nystagmus is named. However, since it is the slow phase which is pathological, it is more eloquent concerning anatomical substrate. The intensity of jerk nystagmus may be classified by a three point scale:

    first degree: present when looking in the direction of the fast phase;

second degree: present in the neutral position;

third degree: present when looking in the direction of the slow phase (i.e. present in all directions of gaze).

Direction:

- Horizontal: common
- Torsional: usually accompanies horizontal nystagmus of peripheral vestibular (labyrinthine) origin.
- Vertical: rare:

Downbeat: seen with structural lesions of the cervico-medullary junction, midline cerebellum and floor of the fourth ventricle, but also with more diffuse cerebellar disease;

Upbeat: of less-localizing value than downbeat, upbeat nystagmus may occur with pontomesencephalic, pontomedullary, and even caudal medullary lesions (infarct, inflammation); bow-tie nystagmus is probably a variant of upbeat nystagmus.

Anatomy/Aetiology

- Vestibular

Peripheral: unidirectional (directed to side opposite lesion), and more pronounced when looking in direction of the fast phase (i.e. first degree), usually with a rotatory component and associated with vertigo. Tends to fatigue, and usually transient. Nystagmus of peripheral vestibular origin is typically reduced by fixation (hence these patients hold their heads still) and enhanced by removal of visual fixation (in the dark, with Frenzel's lenses).

Central: unidirectional or multidirectional, first, second or third degree; typically sustained and persistent. There may be other signs of central pathology (e.g. cerebellar signs, upper motor neurone signs). Not affected by removal of visual fixation.

- Cerebellar/brainstem: commonly gaze-evoked due to a failure of gaze-holding mechanisms. It may be unidirectional with unilateral cerebellar lesion (e.g. vascular disease) in which case it typically occurs when the eyes are looking in the direction of the lesion (*cf.* peripheral vestibular nystagmus); multidirectional nystagmus of cerebellar origin may occur in multiple sclerosis, drug/toxin exposure, cerebellar degenerations.
- Ataxic/dissociated: in abducting >> adducting eye, as in internuclear ophthalmoplegia and pseudo-internuclear ophthalmoplegia.
- Periodic alternating: primary position nystagmus, almost always in the horizontal plane, which stops and then reverses direction every minute or so; 4–5 minutes observation may be required to see the whole cycle; localizing value similar to downbeat nystagmus (structural lesions of the cervico-medullary junction, midline cerebellum and floor of the fourth ventricle, but also with more diffuse cerebellar disease).

- Convergence–retraction (Körber–Salus–Elschnig syndrome): adducting saccades (medial rectus contraction), occurring spontaneously or on attempted upgaze, often accompanied by retraction of the eyes into the orbits, associated with mesencephalic lesions of the pretectal region (e.g. pinealoma).
- See-saw: a disconjugate cyclic movement of the eyes, comprising elevation and intorsion of one eye while the other eye falls and extorts, followed by reversal of these movements; may be congenital (e.g. with albinism, retinitis pigmentosa) or acquired (mesodiencephalic or lateral medullary lesions, e.g. brainstem stroke, head trauma, syringobulbia).

It should be remembered that some types of nystagmus are physiological:

- Optokinetic nystagmus (OKN; e.g. looking out of a moving railway carriage);
- Induced by vestibular stimuli (e.g. merry-go-round; caloric testing);
- Nystagmoid jerks: in extremes of lateral or vertical gaze (end-point nystagmus, a form of gaze-evoked nystagmus).

Investigations and diagnosis If nystagmus is thought pathological, the following investigations may be undertaken, aimed principally at defining the underlying pathology. The commonest are demyelination, vascular disease, tumour, neurodegenerative disorders of cerebellum and/or brainstem, metabolic causes (e.g. Wernicke–Korsakoff's syndrome), paraneoplasia, drugs (alcohol, phenytoin, barbiturates, sedative–hypnotic drugs), toxins, and epilepsy.

Video-oculography or infrared oculography, to characterize the waveform of nystagmus (saw-tooth, exponential) is available only in specialist centres.

Imaging: MRI is investigation of choice for brainstem pathology.

Vestibular testing: may be used if a vestibular origin for nystagmus is suspected.

Audiometry.

EEG.

Differential diagnosis Nystagmus should be distinguished from other involuntary eye movements, especially saccadic fixation instabilities such as square-wave jerks, ocular flutter, and opsoclonus (*q.v.*).

Treatment and prognosis Of underlying condition where identified.

Symptomatic treatment of nystagmus may not be pressing unless it is associated with oscillopsia.

Pendular nystagmus may respond to anticholinesterases, consistent with its being a result of cholinergic dysfunction.

Periodic alternating nystagmus responds to baclofen: See-saw nystagmus may respond to baclofen, clonazepam, or alcohol.

References Janssen JC, Larner AJ, Morris H, Bronstein AM, Farmer SF. Upbeat nystagmus – clinicoanatomical correlation. *Journal of Neurology, Neurosurgery and Psychiatry* 1998; **65**: 380–381.

Leigh RJ, Zee DS. *The Neurology of Eye Movements* (3rd edition). New York: OUP, 1999.

Lopez LI, Bronstein AM, Gresty MA, Du Boulay EPG, Rudge P. Clinical and MRI correlates in 27 patients with acquired pendular nystagmus. *Brain* 1996; **119**: 465–472.

Lueck CJ. A simple guide to nystagmus. *Hospital Medicine* 2000; **61**: 544–546, 548–549.

Serra A, Leigh RJ. Diagnostic value of nystagmus: spontaneous and induced ocular oscillations. *Journal of Neurology, Neurosurgery and Psychiatry* 2002; **73**: 615–618.

Other relevant entries Albinism; Benign paroxysmal positional vertigo; Cerebellar disease: an overview; Congenital nystagmus; Körber–Salus–Elschnig syndrome; Opsoclonus; Oscillopsia; Periodic alternating nystagmus; Vertigo; Wernicke–Korsakoff's syndrome.

Oo

■ Obesity–hypoventilation syndrome – see Pickwickian syndrome

■ Obsessional slowness

Obsessional slowness is a feature in some patients with obsessive–compulsive disorder, characterized by difficulty initiating goal-directed action and suppressing intrusive or perseverative behaviour. Washing and eating may be extremely slow because of rituals, checking behaviour, and compulsions. These patients may have subtle neurological signs such as cogwheel rigidity and tics, such that the condition may be confused with other akinetic-rigid (parkinsonian) syndromes. Dysfunction in a frontal basal ganglia loop is implicated in pathogenesis, and PET scanning has demonstrated hypermetabolism in orbital frontal, premotor, and mid-frontal cortex.

Reference Hymas N, Lees A, Bolton D, Epps K, Head D. The neurology of obsessional slowness. *Brain* 1991; **114**: 2203–2233.

Other relevant entries Obsessive–compulsive disorder; Parkinsonian syndromes, parkinsonism.

■ Obsessive–compulsive disorder

Obsessive–compulsive disorder (OCD) is defined as:

• The presence of obsessions or compulsions or both, on most days for a period of at least 2 weeks.

• Obsessions and compulsions share the following features:
    acknowledged as arising from the mind of the patient and not from outside,
    repetitive and unpleasant,
    resisted (at least one successfully),
    carrying out the obsessive thought or compulsive act is not in itself pleasurable.

There is probably a spectrum of OC-related disorders, including hypochondriasis, body dysmorphic disorder, trichotillomania, tic disorders, and depersonalization disorder. There may also be overlap, for example, up to 30% of patients with OCD manifest tics and many patients with Gilles de la Tourette syndrome fulfil diagnostic criteria for OCD. Similar phenomena may also follow streptococcal infection in children (PANDAS syndrome).

Pharmacotherapy with serotonin reuptake inhibitors (clomipramine) or selective serotonin reuptake inhibitors (SSRI) such as fluoxetine, fluvoxamine, sertraline, paroxetine, and citalopram, is often effective in treating obsessions and compulsions. Dopamine antagonists may also be required for refractory cases or those with additional tics (pimozide, haloperidol). These observations have engendered the view that dysfunction in serotoninergic and dopaminergic pathways may be central to these conditions, and functional imaging has indicated elevated levels of metabolic activity in orbitofrontal cortex and caudate nucleus which normalizes with treatment.

Reference Fineberg N, Marazziti D, Stein DJ (eds). *Obsessive Compulsive Disorder: A Practical Guide.* London: Martin Dunitz, 2001.

Other relevant entries Obsessional slowness; PANDAS syndrome; Somatoform disorders; Tourette syndrome.

▪ Obstructive hydrocephalus – see Hydrocephalus

▪ Obstructive sleep apnoea syndrome
Sleep apnoea/hypopnoea syndrome (SAHS)

Pathophysiology Critical narrowing of the upper airway during sleep, due to reduced muscle tone, leads to increased resistance to the flow of air, and partial obstruction results in apnoea, hypopnoea, and loud snoring. A gradation exists between the normal sleep-related increase in upper airway resistance, through upper airway resistance syndrome (UARS; subtle airflow limitation with nocturnal arousals), to obstructive sleep apnoea syndrome (OSAS). Sleep is restless due to successive episodes of apnoea, which are relieved by brief arousals from sleep, with excessive daytime somnolence in consequence. Risk factors for the development of OSAS include narrow anteroposterior pharyngeal diameter, obesity, high alcohol intake, and male sex. The condition is associated with increased cardiovascular and cerebrovascular morbidity and mortality and an increased risk of road traffic accidents.

Clinical features: history and examination Excessive daytime somnolence.

• Neurological features

"loss of consciousness" (falling asleep in inappropriate circumstances)

personality change

cognitive decline

morning headache with features of raised intracranial pressure; may simulate idiopathic intracranial hypertension (IIH).

- History from a bed partner, regarding snoring, apnoeas, and daytime sleepiness may be helpful in establishing the diagnosis.
- Examination may reveal obesity (increased body mass index; collar size), stridor at rest, narrow pharyngeal anteroposterior diameter, short thick neck, enlarged tonsils (ENT referral may be appropriate), asterixis, hypertension. Papilloedema may occur.
- History of alcohol intake.

Investigations and diagnosis *Bloods*: may have raised haemocrit as a consequence of nocturnal hypoxaemia; arterial blood gases during the night may confirm hypoxaemia although this is intermittent.

Sleep studies: either formal nocturnal polysomnography or overnight oximetry (may be done at home), looking for dips in oxygen saturation associated with heart rate rise. Severity of OSAS may be measured by apnoea/hypopnoea index (AHI), or respiratory disturbance index (RDI), calculated as the number of apnoeas/hypopnoeas per hour of sleep on polysomnography: AHI or RDI of 10–20 = mild, 20–50 = moderate, and >50 = severe disease. With pulse oximetry, a desaturation index (DI) may be calculated as the number of desaturations (decrease in oxygen saturation by ≥4%) per hour of sleep or, if the recording is unattended, per time of recording; DI ≥ 5 may be used to define sleep-disordered breathing.

Other measures (subjective rating scales) may be used including the Epworth Sleepiness Scale, Stanford Sleepiness Scale, and the Sleep–Wake Activity Inventory.

Differential diagnosis Other causes of excessive daytime somnolence; narcolepsy generally occurs in a younger age group than OSAS and is less common; the absence of associated features of the narcoleptic syndrome (cataplexy, hypnagogic hallucinations, sleep paralysis) may assist in differential diagnosis. Narcoleptics usually feel refreshed after waking from a sleep attack, whereas OSAS patients generally feel drowsy and fatigued on awakening.

Loss of consciousness may be confused with epilepsy.

Morning headache may be confused with raised intracranial pressure; headache and papilloedema with no other localizing signs may be mistaken for IIH.

Cognitive decline may be mistaken for other causes of dementia.

Depression and chronic fatigue syndrome.

Treatment and prognosis Weight loss (dietary advice; in extreme circumstances bariatric surgery).

Reduced alcohol consumption.

Assisted nocturnal intermittent positive-pressure ventilation (CPAP, NIPPY) is very effective in relief of symptoms.

In selected cases, laryngeal surgery such as tonsillectomy or uvulopalatopharyngoplasty may be appropriate.

Modafinil is now licensed for the treatment of OSAS (as well as narcolepsy).

Cardiovascular and cerebrovascular morbidity and mortality is increased in patients with OSAS; and because of the daytime somnolence, there is a six-fold increase in the risk of road traffic accidents; hence the importance of establishing the diagnosis and treating appropriately.

References Douglas NJ. Obstructive sleep apnoea and stroke. *Advances in Clinical Neuroscience and Rehabilitation* 2003; **2(6)**: 14–16.

Larner AJ. Obstructive sleep apnoea syndrome presenting in a neurology outpatient clinic. *International Journal of Clinical Practice* 2003; **57**: 150–152.

Stradling JR. Sleep apnoea syndromes. In: Brewis RAL, Corrin B, Geddes DM, Gibson GJ (eds). *Respiratory Medicine* (2nd edition). London: WB Saunders, 1995: 973–1005.

Other relevant entries Idiopathic intracranial hypertension; Narcolepsy, Narcoleptic syndrome; Pickwickian syndrome; Sleep disorders: an overview.

■ Obturator neuropathy

Pathophysiology Isolated obturator neuropathy is unusual, most commonly being associated with pelvic masses or obturator hernias.

Clinical features: history and examination
- Motor: weak hip adduction (adductor magnus, longus, brevis); no reflex loss.
- Sensory: loss along the medial upper thigh.

Obturator neuropathy may occur in the context of pelvic or hip fracture, benign and malignant pelvic masses. Pelvic and rectal examinations may be appropriate to ascertain a cause.

Investigations and diagnosis EMG/NCS may help in confirming or, if electrophysiological changes are more widespread than clinical findings, refuting the diagnosis.

Differential diagnosis Lumbosacral plexopathy.

L3–L4 radiculopathy (look for weak hip flexors, knee extensors; patellar reflex loss).

Reference Staal A, Van Gijn J, Spaans F. *Mononeuropathies: Examination, Diagnosis and Treatment.* London: WB Saunders, 1999: 109–111.

Other relevant entry Neuropathies: an overview.

■ Occipital horn syndrome

This X-linked disorder which is characterized by skeletal dysplasia, including occipital horns and skin changes, has been known as X-linked cutis laxa and as Ehlers–Danlos syndrome type IX. However, it is now known to result from mutations in the same gene (ATP7A), and hence is allelic with, Menkes' disease, its phenotype being milder than in Menkes.

Other relevant entries Ehlers–Danlos syndrome; Menkes' disease.

■ Occipital neuralgia
Arnold's neuralgia

Attacks of jabbing pain in the posterior part of the scalp, extending up to the coronal suture, the territory of the occipital nerves (greater occipital nerve, from the dorsal ramus of C2; lesser occipital nerve, from the ventral ramus of C2), and associated with local hypoesthesia or dysaesthesia; usually unilateral but may be bilateral. There may be tenderness over the affected nerve, and pain may radiate to the frontal region. Causes include trauma, injury, inflammation, or compression of the nerves (the greater occipital nerve runs through the aponeurosis of trapezius); because C2 does not pass through an intervertebral foramen it is relatively immune to entrapment or compression by disc herniation and spondylosis. Intramedullary causes (upper cervical cavernous angioma) have also been reported. Suggested treatments include local injection of the nerves with local anaesthetic +/− steroids, or systemic non-steroidal anti-inflammatory drugs, carbamazepine, or gabapentin.

Other relevant entry Facial pain: differential diagnosis.

■ Occupational dystonias
Task-specific dystonias

A number of dystonia syndromes have been described which are associated with certain occupations or activities, for example:

Writer's cramp
Auctioneer's jaw
Musician's dystonia: playing various musical instruments, for example fingers with piano, hand with violin, drum; mouth with brass, woodwind
Typists: hand
Sport: "the yips", golf, darts.

References Altenmüller E. Focal dystonia: advances in brain imaging and understanding of fine motor control in musicians. *Hand Clinics* 2003; **19**: 523–538.
Scolding NJ, Smith SM, Sturman S, Brookes GB, Lees AJ. Auctioneer's jaw: a case of occupational oromandibular hemidystonia. *Movement Disorders* 1995; **10**: 508–509.
Other relevant entries Botulinum toxin therapy; Dystonia: an overview; Writer's cramp.

■ Ocular myasthenia – see Myasthenia gravis

■ Ocular neuromyotonia – see Neuromyotonia

■ Oculocerebrorenal syndrome – see Lowe syndrome

■ Oculocraniosomatic syndrome – see Mitochondrial disease: an overview

■ Oculodentodigital dysplasia syndrome

This rare autosomal-dominant condition affects development of the face, eyes, limbs, and dentition.

Neurological complications include:

Gaze palsy, squinting, nystagmus
Spasticity
Sphincter problems
Visual loss, blindness
Hearing loss
Ataxia
Muscle weakness
Paraesthesia.

MRI may show:

Subcortical white matter lesions
Basal ganglia changes.

Reference Loddenkemper T, Grote K, Evers S, Oelerich M, Stögbauer F. Neurological manifestations of the oculodentodigital dysplasia syndrome. *Journal of Neurology* 2002; **249**: 584–595.

■ Oculogyric crisis

Oculogyric crisis describes acute upward and lateral displacement of the eye, which is thought to be a dystonia of the ocular muscles. The eye movement disorder may be accompanied by a disorder of attention, with obsessive or persistent thoughts.

Oculogyric crisis is a feature of symptomatic (secondary) dystonias, rather than idiopathic (primary) dystonias, for example:

* neuroleptic-induced dystonia (commonest cause): may be acute or chronic (tardive);
* post-encephalitic dystonia (e.g. encephalitis lethargica).

It has also been described with Wilson's disease, neuroleptic malignant syndrome, and organophosphate poisoning. Lesions within the lentiform nuclei have been recorded in cases with oculogyric crisis.

Treatment of acute neuroleptic-induced oculogyric crisis is with parenteral benzodiazepines or anticholinergic agents such as procyclidine, benztropine, or trihexyphenidyl.

Reference Kim JS, Kim HK, Im JH, Lee MC. Oculogyric crisis and abnormal magnetic resonance imaging signals in bilateral lentiform nuclei. *Movement Disorders* 1996; **11**: 756–758.

Other relevant entries Drug-induced movement disorders; Dystonia: an overview.

■ Oculomotor nerve palsy – see Cranial nerve disease: III: Oculomotor nerve

■ Oculopalatal myoclonus – see Eight-and-a-half syndrome; Myoclonus

■ Oculopharyngeal muscular dystrophy

Pathophysiology An inherited (usually autosomal-dominant) disorder of voluntary muscle with characteristic phenotype and unusually late onset (fifth to sixth decade), occurring most frequently in French-Canadians. The genetic basis of this condition has been defined as a stable trinucleotide repeat sequence encoding polyalanine in the gene encoding poly(A)-binding protein II (PAB II) on chromosome 14q.

Clinical features: history and examination

- Bilateral ptosis.
- Dysphagia, cachexia.
- Ophthalmoplegia, but diplopia rare.
- +/− Proximal limb weakness (shoulder, pelvis).
- Positive family history.

Investigations and diagnosis *Bloods*: creatine kinase normal.

Neurophysiology: EMG: myopathic (non-specific).

Muscle biopsy: rimmed vacuoles in sarcoplasm; intranuclear filamentous/tubular inclusions (<10% of muscle nuclei); +/− mitochondrial morphological changes.

Neurogenetics: expansion of the GCG trinucleotide repeat in exon 1 of the PAB II gene: normal = 6, 7; abnormal = 8–13 repeats.

Differential diagnosis

Myasthenia gravis.

Mitochondrial disease.

Inclusion body myositis.

Treatment and prognosis No specific treatment; nasogastric tube or percutaneous endoscopic gastrostomy (PEG) for dysphagia, nutrition; corrective surgery for ptosis.

References Brais B, Bouchard J-P, Xie Y-G *et al*. Short GCG expansions in the PAB2 gene cause oculopharyngeal muscular dystrophy. *Nature Genetics* 1998; **18**: 164–167.

Hill ME, Creed GA, McMullan TF *et al*. Oculopharyngeal muscular dystrophy: phenotypic and genotypic studies in a UK population. *Brain* 2001; **124**: 522–526.

Tomé FMS, Fardeau M. Nuclear inclusions in oculopharyngeal muscular dystrophy. *Acta Neuropathologica (Berlin)* 1980; **49**: 85–87.

Victor M, Hayes R, Adams RD. Oculopharyngeal muscular dystrophy: a familial disease of late life characterized by dysphagia and progressive ptosis of the eyelids. *New England Journal of Medicine* 1962; **207**: 1267–1272.

Other relevant entries Mitochondrial disease: an overview; Muscular dystrophies: an overview; Trinucleotide repeat diseases.

■ Ohtahara's syndrome
Early infantile myoclonic encephalopathy

A syndrome of myoclonic seizures beginning before 3 months of age, associated with a serious underlying disorder, such as an inborn error of metabolism. Partial seizures, tonic spasms, and generalized tonic–clonic seizures may follow the myoclonic seizures. EEG shows a burst-suppression pattern. MRI often shows severe abnormalities of brain development. Seizures are refractory to most anti-epileptic drugs; sodium valproate, and clonazepam are most often used, carbamazepine may exacerbate seizures. Morbidity and mortality are high. Survival may be associated with evolution of clinical and EEG pattern to that of West's syndrome and, eventually, to Lennox–Gastaut features. It is suggested that Ohtahara's syndrome may be the earliest age-related specific epileptic reaction of the developing brain to heterogeneous insults, similar to West's and Lennox–Gastaut syndromes at later stages of brain maturity.

Reference Yamatogi Y, Ohtahara S. Early-infantile epileptic encephalopathy with suppression-bursts, Ohtahara syndrome: its overview referring to our 16 cases. *Brain and Development* 2002; **24**: 13–23.

Other relevant entries Epilepsy: an overview; Lennox–Gastaut syndrome; West's syndrome.

■ Ohtani's disease – see Glycogen-storage disorders: an overview

■ Olfactory nerve disease – see Cranial nerve disease: I: Olfactory nerve

■ Olfactory neuroblastoma – see Esthesioneuroblastoma

■ Oligodendroglioma

This tumour, a subtype of glioma, accounting for perhaps 5% of all gliomas, typically develops during childhood or early adulthood (20–40 years old), and is more common in men (M : F = 2 : 1). Typically oligodendrogliomas are found in cerebral hemispheres, usually presenting with seizures. Imaging may show an intraparenchymal lesion, which may be partially calcified, but with little mass effect or oedema. The tumours are slowly progressive and may transform into anaplastic oligodendrogliomas. Positive immunostaining for glial fibrillary acidic protein (GFAP) is usual.

Other relevant entries Glioma; Tumours: an overview.

■ Olivopontocerebellar atrophy – see Autosomal-dominant cerebellar ataxia; Cerebellar disease: an overview; Multiple system atrophy

■ Ollier disease

A chondrodysplasia of the long bones which may also cause optic nerve compression and ophthalmoplegia.

■ Onchocerciasis
River blindness

Infection with the filarial nematode *Onchocerca volvulus* is a common cause of blindness. The parasites are transmitted by blackflies (*Simulium*) near rushing streams or rivers, in Central and West Africa and Latin America. Penetration of the eye by microfilariae may cause conjunctivitis, keratitis, uveitis, choreoretinitis, and optic atrophy. Slit-lamp examination may show microfilariae in the anterior chamber. Ivermectin, given as a single oral dose, kills microfilariae, and has been shown to reduce the incidence of blindness in endemic areas.

Other relevant entries Helminthic diseases; Visual loss: differential diagnosis.

■ Ondine's curse – see Sleep disorders: an overview

■ One-and-a-half syndrome

Pathophysiology The one-and-a-half syndrome is a disorder of eye movement due to a brainstem lesion of the pontine tegmentum, usually inflammatory or vascular in origin. It is characterized by homolateral horizontal gaze palsy and internuclear ophthalmoplegia (INO), the only preserved horizontal eye movement being abduction in the contralateral eye. Vertical eye movements and convergence are spared. A vertical one-and-a-half syndrome has also been described with thalamo-mesencephalic infarction.

Clinical features: history and examination

- Symptoms
    Diplopia, blurred vision, oscillopsia.
- Diagnostic signs
    Ipsilateral horizontal gaze palsy due to involvement of the abducens (VI) nerve
        nucleus or the adjacent paramedian pontine reticular formation
    INO due to involvement of the medial longitudinal fasciculus.
- Associated signs:
    Gaze-evoked upbeat/downbeat nystagmus
    Skew deviation
    Cranial nerve palsies: V, VII (="eight-and-a-half syndrome"), VIII, IX
    Horner's syndrome
    Weakness, spasticity, upgoing plantars
    Ataxia
    Sensory deficits (may be suspended).
- Vertical one-and-a-half syndrome
    Vertical upgaze palsy
    Monocular paresis of downgaze, either ipsilateral or contralateral to the
        lesion.

Investigations and diagnosis *Imaging*: ideally with MRI: reveals a brainstem lesion (vascular, demyelination, tumour) usually within the pontine tegmentum.
CSF: for oligoclonal bands if demyelination suspected.
Electro-oculography (optional).

Differential diagnosis The commonest causes are demyelination, particularly in young patients, whereas in the older age group brainstem ischaemia is the likely cause.

A pseudo-one-and-a-half syndrome may occur in myasthenia gravis.

Treatment and prognosis Dependent on cause: acute demyelination may require steroids; aspirin for secondary prophylaxis of brainstem ischaemia; consider anti-coagulation in vertebral artery dissection.

References Pierrot-Deseilligny C, Chain F, Serdaru M *et al*. The "one-and-a-half" syndrome. Electro-oculographic analyses of five patients with deductions about the physiological mechanisms of lateral gaze. *Brain* 1981; **104**: 665–699.

Wall M, Wray SH. The one-and-a-half syndrome. A unilateral disorder of the pontine tegmentum: a study of 20 cases and a review of the literature. *Neurology* 1983; **33**: 971–980.

Other relevant entries Brainstem vascular syndromes; Cranial nerve disease: VI: Abducens nerve; Eight-and-a-half syndrome; Internuclear ophthalmoplegia.

Opalski's syndrome

The submedullary syndrome of Opalski, first described in 1946, consists of:
- an ipsilateral hemiplegia in association with
- a lateral medullary (Wallenberg) syndrome.

The syndrome follows a vascular event in the medulla, sometimes a vertebral artery occlusion, below the decussation of the pyramids (*cf.* Babinski–Nageotte syndrome).

Reference Montaner J, Alvarez-Sabín J. Opalski's syndrome. *Journal of Neurology, Neurosurgery and Psychiatry* 1999; **67**: 688–689.

Other relevant entries Babinski–Nageotte syndrome; Brainstem vascular syndromes; Cerebrovascular disease: arterial; Lateral medullary syndrome.

Ophthalmoplegia

Ophthalmoplegia is a weakness or paralysis of the musculature of the eye resulting in limitation of eye movements. Internal and external ophthalmoplegia may be distinguished:
- Internal ophthalmoplegia: impairment of pupillary and ciliary muscle function, resulting in iridoplegia. May be seen in an oculomotor (III) nerve palsy.

- External ophthalmoplegia: weakness of the extraocular muscle function, which may result in diplopia. This may be due to pathology anywhere from central nervous system (CNS) to extraocular muscles *per se*:

    Supranuclear: for example progressive supranuclear palsy, abetalipoproteinaemia.

    Nuclear, internuclear: for example internuclear ophthalmoplegia (INO), Möbius syndrome.

    Cranial nerve palsy: III, IV, VI, or combinations thereof.

    Neuromuscular junction: myasthenia gravis.

    Extraocular muscles: for example oculopharyngeal muscular dystrophy (OPMD), chronic progressive external ophthalmoplegia (CPEO), thyroid ophthalmopathy.

The term "ophthalmoplegia plus" has been used to denote the combination of progressive external ophthalmoplegia with additional symptoms and signs, indicative of brainstem, pyramidal, endocrine, cardiac, muscular, hypothalamic, or auditory system involvement, as in mitochondrial disease.

Other relevant entries Chronic progressive external ophthalmoplegia; Internuclear ophthalmoplegia; Oculopharyngeal muscular dystrophy.

◼ Ophthalmoplegic migraine

Ophthalmoplegic migraine is a very rare condition characterized by recurrent attacks of severe unilateral headache followed by an oculomotor (third) nerve palsy, usually complete, usually beginning in childhood, and without evidence for a parasellar lesion such as an aneurysm. Some cases may be steroid responsive. Although previously classified as a variant of migraine, it may be better characterized as a recurrent demyelinating neuropathy, since MRI shows swelling of the cisternal segment of the oculomotor nerve with contrast enhancement, especially during symptomatic periods, which slowly improves as symptoms remit.

References Doran M, Larner AJ. MRI findings in ophthalmoplegic migraine: nosological implications. *Journal of Neurology* 2004; **251**: 100–101.

Mark AS, Casselman J, Brown D, Sanchez J, Kolsky M, Larsen TC 3rd, Lavin P, Ferraraccio B. Ophthalmoplegic migraine: reversible enhancement and thickening of the cisternal segment of the oculomotor nerve on contrast-enhanced MR images. *American Journal of Neuroradiology* 1998; **19**: 1887–1891.

Other relevant entries Cranial nerve disease: III: Oculomotor nerve; Migraine.

◼ Opisthotonos – see Decerebrate rigidity, decorticate rigidity; Drug-induced movement disorders

◼ Opportunistic infection – see HIV/AIDS and the nervous system; Immunosuppressive therapy and diseases of the nervous system

■ Opsoclonus

Saccadomania

Opsoclonus is an eye movement disorder characterized by involuntary bursts of polydirectional saccades, sometimes with a horizontal preference. Unlike square-wave jerks, opsoclonic movements have no intersaccadic interval.

Opsoclonus reflects mesencephalic or cerebellar disease affecting the omnipause cells which exert tonic inhibition of the burst neurones which generate saccades, although occasional normal individuals can voluntarily induce opsoclonus.

Recognized causes of opsoclonus include:

- paraneoplasia: opsoclonus–myoclonus syndrome ("dancing eyes, dancing feet") is most commonly associated with small-cell lung cancer but it may also occur in association with breast cancer in which case onconeural antibodies (anti-Ri, or type 2 anti-neuronal nuclear antibodies [ANNA-2]) may be detected in serum and CSF; children with neuroblastoma may also have opsoclonus (Kinsbourne's syndrome) which may be steroid responsive;
- postinfectious: a monophasic disorder following respiratory or gastrointestinal infection, which generally remits spontaneously;
- intraparenchymal (especially mesencephalic) lesions, for example tumour, demyelination, sarcoidosis, metabolic/toxic encephalopathy.

Reference Digre KB. Opsoclonus in adults. *Archives of Neurology* 1986; **43**: 1165–1175.
Other relevant entries Myoclonus; Neuroblastoma; Paraneoplastic syndromes.

■ Optic atrophy

Optic atrophy is pallor of the optic nerve head, visualized by ophthalmoscopy, as a consequence of loss of axons in the optic nerve and/or gliotic change within the damaged nerve. The temporal disc may appear pale in a normal fundus, so that optic atrophy can only be confidently diagnosed when there is also nasal pallor.

The appearance of optic atrophy is non-specific with respect to aetiology, it being the end stage of a variety of pathological processes which may primarily affect:

retina,
optic nerve,
optic chiasm,
optic tract.

Hence, if a preceding pathology is not known, imaging to exclude a compressive lesion is considered mandatory.

Optic atrophy may be categorized according to cause:

- Hereditary: autosomal-dominant optic atrophy, autosomal-recessive optic atrophy, Leber's hereditary optic neuropathy (LHON), other mitochondrial disorders; Behr's syndrome.
- Macular dystrophies

- Deficiency: tobacco–alcohol amblyopia; vitamin B_{12} deficiency
- Drug induced: for example ethambutol, isoniazid and chloroquine
- Demyelination
- Glaucoma
- Chronic papilloedema, optic nerve compression.

Older texts draw a distinction between primary optic atrophy and secondary, consecutive or sequential optic atrophy, but these distinctions are no longer favoured.

Other relevant entries Behr's syndrome; Cranial nerve disease: II: Optic nerve; Rosenberg–Chutorian syndrome.

■ Optic neuritis
Retrobulbar neuritis

Pathophysiology Inflammation within the optic nerve may occur in isolation, or be the harbinger of an underlying cerebral inflammatory disorder such as multiple sclerosis (MS). The advent of MRI means that prediction of future neurological problems in patients with a clinically isolated optic neuritis may more easily be made, although whether, in the absence of any meaningful intervention which can be made in light of this knowledge, this represents an "advance" remains open to question.

Clinical features: history and examination

- Pain in, around and behind eye. Especially noticeable with eye movement. Usually unilateral, although bilateral cases do occur, often with a disparity between the severity with which each eye is affected (*cf.* acute disseminated encephalomyelitis, ADEM).
- Reduced visual acuity; gradually worse over hours or days; natural history is of gradual improvement although full recovery may not occur; impairment of colour vision (as tested with pseudo-isochromatic plates) may remain.
- Other clinical features of underlying neurological disease: MS, sarcoidosis.
- Recurrence occurs in up to 1/4, and carries increased risk for development of MS.

Investigations and diagnosis *Neurophysiology*: visual evoked potentials/responses (VEPs/VERs): increased latency with relatively preserved waveform is highly suggestive of optic neuritis.

Imaging: MRI can visualize optic nerves, and show swelling and focal increased signal, especially in optic neuritis; MRI may also show inflammatory lesions elsewhere, which if periventricular may suggest a diagnosis of MS.

CSF: may show oligoclonal bands; if so, increased risk of progression to MS.

If appropriate, investigations to confirm or refute the diagnosis of sarcoidosis may be undertaken (*q.v.*).

Differential diagnosis

Structural lesions of optic nerve (usually more gradual onset).

Ischaemic optic neuropathy usually has a more acute onset.

Devic's syndrome (neuromyelitis optica).

Leber's hereditary optic neuropathy (LHON).

Toxic amblyopia.

ADEM: especially if bilateral, in young person, with other neurological features.

Treatment and prognosis Acute use of intravenous steroids (e.g. intravenous methyl-prednisolone, 1 g/day for 3–5 consecutive days) is frequently used, and may hasten recovery, without impacting on the natural history of any underlying disease especially if there is a lot of pain, bilateral involvement, or marked loss of visual activity.

β-interferon may reduce the speed of conversion of clinically isolated lesions to MS, but there is no evidence that it actually prevents MS from developing.

References Hess RF, Plant GT (eds). *Optic Neuritis*. Cambridge: CUP, 1986.

Jacobs LD, Beck RW, Simon JH *et al*. Intramuscular interferon β-1a therapy initiated during a first demyelinating event in multiple sclerosis. CHAMPS Study Group. *New England Journal of Medicine* 2000; **343**: 898–904.

Optic Neuritis Study Group. The 5-year risk of MS after optic neuritis. Experience of the Optic Neuritis Treatment Trial. *Neurology* 1997; **49**: 1404–1413.

O'Riordan JI, Thompson AJ, Kingsley DPE *et al*. The prognostic value of brain MRI in clinically isolated syndromes of the CNS. *Brain* 1998; **121**: 495–503.

Other relevant entries Acute disseminated encephalomyelitis; Devic's disease, Devic's syndrome; Harding's disease; Ischaemic optic neuropathy; Leber's hereditary optic neuropathy; Multiple sclerosis; Sarcoidosis.

▓ Optic neuropathy – see Cranial nerve disease: II: Optic nerve

▓ Orbital apex syndrome

A lesion at the orbital apex may involve several cranial nerves, causing:

• External ophthalmoplegia: III, IV, VI
• Sensory deficit in face: V, ophthalmic division
• Visual deficit: II (peripheral, central field defects, papilloedema, optic atrophy).

Clearly, there is clinical overlap with the cavernous sinus syndrome and the superior orbital fissure syndrome.

Other relevant entry Cavernous sinus disease.

▓ Orbital myositis

An acute inflammatory process localized to the extraocular muscles, causing orbital pain worse with eye movement, redness of the conjunctiva adjacent to muscle insertions, diplopia caused by restriction of ocular movement, proptosis, and eyelid oedema. The patient feels systemically unwell, and the ESR is raised. Orbital imaging helps to differentiate orbital myositis from other causes of orbital inflammation such as pseudotumour. The condition seems to resolve spontaneously although steroids may hasten recovery. Underlying connective tissue disease is seldom defined.

References Dua HS, Smith FW, Singh AK, Forrester JV. Diagnosis of orbital myositis by nuclear magnetic resonance imaging. *British Journal of Ophthalmology* 1987; **71**: 54–57.

Spoor TC, Hartel WC. Orbital myositis. *Journal of Clinical Neuro-ophthalmology* 1983; **3**: 67–74.

Other relevant entry Myositis.

■ Orbital pseudotumour – see Orbital tumours; Tolosa–Hunt syndrome

■ Orbital tumours

Pathophysiology Mass lesions within the orbit may be divided into:

- Intraconal: within the cone of the extraocular muscles.
- Extraconal.

This division provides some clue as to underlying pathology.

Periorbital lesions may sometimes impinge on orbital structures.

Clincal features: history and examination

- *Intraconal*: forward displacement of the globe (proptosis), $+/-$ impairment of visual acuity, diplopia, optic disc swelling; scirrhous breast tumour metastases may cause tethering and enophthalmos.
- *Extraconal*: upward or downward displacement of the globe.

Investigations and diagnosis *Imaging*: MRI is modality of choice, $+/-$ fat-suppression sequences; angiography if vascular lesion suspected.

Biopsy: if histological diagnosis required to facilitate planning of appropriate treatment; need to exclude a vascular lesion before undertaking biopsy.

Differential diagnosis

Intraconal

Tumour

Primary: optic nerve sheath meningioma, optic nerve glioma, lymphoma
Secondary: metastasis (breast, lung, prostate).

Vascular

Cavernous haemangioma, varices.

Extraconal

Tumour

Primary: orbital rhabdomyosarcoma; dermoid, mucocele
Inflammatory: orbital pseudotumour: Wegener's granulomatosis, "Tolosa–Hunt syndrome".

Treatment and prognosis Of specific cause: some may be amenable to resection (e.g. cavernous haemangioma); others may be left (e.g. varices). Steroids are treatment of choice for inflammatory masses. Resection plus enucleation of the eye may be necessary in some cases.

Other relevant entries Tolosa–Hunt syndrome; Tumours: an overview.

■ Organic acidopathies

Pathophysiology Disorders of organic acid metabolism, evident as organic aci-daemias and/or organic aciduria, are inborn errors of metabolism with a broad clinical spectrum, featuring not only metabolic acidosis but disorders of heart, liver, kidney, and nervous system.

Diagnosis is usually straightforward due to accumulation of metabolites proximal to the enzyme defect, which being water soluble may be detected in plasma and urine.

Clinical features: history and examination
See entries for specific conditions.
- Metabolic acidosis + encephalopathy.
- Liver dysfunction, failure.
- +/− neutropenia, predisposition to pyogenic infection.
- +/− dystonia, seizures, myopathy, hypotonia.
- +/− cardiomyopathy.

Investigations and diagnosis *Bloods*: increased anion gap (>25 mmol/l); hyperam-monaemia; hypoglycaemia.

Urine: organic acid analysis: specific pattern is often key to making diagnosis.

Differential diagnosis
Classification

Amino acid metabolism

> Maple syrup urine disease (MSUD)
> Methylmalonic acidaemia
> Propionic acidaemia
> Isovaleric acidaemia
> 3-Hydroxy-3-methylglutaryl-CoA (HMG-CoA) lyase deficiency
> Glutaric aciduria (GA) type I
> Multiple carboxylase deficiency
> 3-Oxothiolase deficiency
> 3-Methylcrotonic aciduria
> 3-Methylglutaconic acidaemia
> 4-Hydroxybutyric aciduria.

Krebs cycle

> Fumaric aciduria/fumarase deficiency.

Fatty acid metabolism

> Dicarboxylic aciduria
>> medium chain acyl-CoA dehydrogenase (MCAD) deficiency
>> long-chain fatty acyl-CoA dehydrogenase (LCAD) deficiency
> Ethylmalonic aciduria, for example short-chain acyl-CoA dehydrogenase (SCAD) deficiency
> 3-hydroxydicarboxylic aciduria
> GA type II.

Adventitious or spurious causes of an abnormal organic aciduria should be borne in mind, such as intestinal bacterial infection or overgrowth, use of certain medications.

Treatment and prognosis Dietary restriction of particular amino acids, often with carnitine supplementation to restore free coenzyme A (CoA) levels and to facilitate excretion of organic acids. Glycine in large oral doses may also enhance excretion of organic acids (e.g. in isovaleric acidaemia).

Liver transplantation has been undertaken in certain organic acidopathies (e.g. propionic acidaemia).

References DiDonato S, Uziel G. Organic acidurias. In: Rowland LP (ed.). *Merritt's Textbook of Neurology* (9th edition). Baltimore: Williams & Wilkins, 1995: 582–584.

Gascon GG, Ozand PT. Aminoacidopathies and organic acidopathies, mitochondrial enzyme defects, and other metabolic errors. In: Goetz CG (ed.). *Textbook of Clinical Neurology* (2nd edition). Philadelphia: Saunders, 2003: 629–664.

Lehotay D, Clarke JTR. Organic acidurias and related abnormalities. *Critical Reviews in Clinical Laboratory Sciences* 1995; **32**: 377–429.

Other relevant entries Carnitine deficiency; Fatty acid oxidation disorders; Glutaric aciduria; Isovaleric acidaemia; Medium chain acyl-CoA dehydrogenase deficiency; Methylmalonic acidaemia; Propionic acidaemia.

■ Ornithine transcarbamoylase deficiency

Ornithine transcarbamoylase (OTC), encoded by a gene on the short arm of the X-chromosome, catalyses the condensation of intramitochondrial ornithine, an analogue of the amino acid lysine, with carbamoylphosphate to produce citrulline. OTC deficiency, the commonest of the urea cycle enzyme defects (UCED), presents in boys in the newborn period with an acute encephalopathy; stroke-like episodes may occur. OTC deficiency is characterized biochemically by severe hyperammonaemia and accumulation of carbamoylphosphate. The latter diffuses to the cytosol where orotic acid and orotidine are produced, increased concentrations of which are found in the urine. Citrulline biosynthesis is defective resulting in low plasma levels of citrulline.

Female carriers of OTC deficiency may be symptomatic: feeding problems, failure to thrive, intermittent ataxia, intermittent encephalopathy; may precede an acute (and sometimes) fatal encephalopathy.

Other relevant entries Sex-linked forms of inherited metabolic diseases; Urea cycle enzyme defects.

■ Ornithosis – see Psittacosis

■ Orofaciodigital syndromes

A heterogeneous group, comprising >10 syndromes, characterized by:
- oral malformations,
- facial anomalies,
- digital anomalies.

Intracranial abnormalities such as cysts may also be found.

Orofaciodigital (OFD) I (Papillon–Leage syndrome, Psaume syndrome): X-linked-dominant syndrome, occurring mostly in females.

OFD II (Mohr syndrome): autosomal recessive, with median cleft lip, polylobed tongue, absence of medial incisors, polydactyly of hands and feet.

OFD IV (Mohr–Majewski syndrome).

OFD VI (Varadi syndrome, Papp–Varadi syndrome).

Oromandibular dystonia
Lingual dystonia

Oromandibular dystonia involves the lower face and tongue, and may manifest as jaw clenching, forced jaw opening (gaping), or involuntary tongue protrusions, with or without dysphagia and dysarthria. It is often exacerbated by talking and eating. The combination of oromandibular dystonia with blepharospasm is termed Meige's syndrome.

Like other forms of cranial dystonia, such as blepharospasm, oromandibular dystonia may respond to botulinum toxin injections, although such treatment is not recommended for isolated lingual dystonia because of the risk of inducing bulbar weakness.

Other relevant entries Botulinum toxin therapy; Dystonia: an overview; Meige's syndrome.

Oroya fever – see Bartonellosis

Orphan diseases

Rare conditions are occasionally labelled as "orphan diseases". A definition of this term has been proposed, namely diseases with a prevalence of <5 cases per 10 000 of the population. Accepting this definition, many neurological disorders fall into this category.

Orthochromatic leukodystrophy – see Leukodystrophies: an overview

Orthostatic hypotension – see Autonomic failure; Pure autonomic failure

Orthostatic syncope – see Syncope

Orthostatic tremor – see Primary orthostatic tremor

■ Ortner syndrome
Cardiovocal syndrome

Dysphonia due to left recurrent laryngeal nerve dysfunction caused by an enlarged left atrium.

■ Oscillopsia

Oscillopsia is the blurring, jumping, or oscillation of the visual representation of the environment during active or passive head movement due to excessive slip of images on the retina ("retinal slip") as a consequence of acquired bilateral loss of vestibular function and hence loss of the vestibulo-ocular reflexes (VOR).

This may be tested for clinically by: recording visual acuity whilst the head is passively shaken horizontally, a drop of three to seven lines of acuity versus performance with the head still, suggests a loss of VOR (the dynamic illegible E test); and by observing the optic disc with an ophthalmoscope as the head is gently shaken, as the disc moving with the head is seen if VOR are lost. Vestibular testing will also demonstrate bilateral loss of vestibular function.

Other recognized causes of oscillopsia include:
- acquired nystagmus,
- superior oblique myokymia,
- other ocular oscillations.

Oscillopsia does not occur in congenital nystagmus, nor in opsoclonus, presumably due to the operation of the visual-suppression mechanism which normally operates during saccadic eye movements.

Oscillopsia may be treated with clonazepam; if due to acquired pendular nystagmus anticholinesterases or alcohol may help.

Reference Leigh RJ. Oscillopsia: impaired vision during motion in the absence of the vestibulo-ocular reflex. *Journal of Neurology, Neurosurgery and Psychiatry* 1998; **65**: 808.

Other relevant entries Nystagmus: an overview; Superior oblique myokymia.

■ Osler–Weber–Rendu Syndrome
Familial telangiectasia • Hereditary haemorrhagic telangiectasia (HHT) • Rendu–Osler–Weber syndrome

An autosomal-dominant condition characterized by telangiectasia in the skin, mucous membranes, gastrointestinal tract, genitourinary system, and occasionally the nervous system. The vascular lesions are of various sizes and have a tendency to bleed, gastrointestinal and genitourinary lesions sometimes leading to iron-deficiency anaemia.

Neurological complications include:

- Brain or spinal cord angiomas; may present acutely with haemorrhage, or with insidious focal features from gradual enlargement or repeated small haemorrhages.
- Cerebral abscess as a consequence of pulmonary fistulae.

Embolization of angiomas may be possible.

Reference Shovlin CL, Guttmacher AE, Buscarini E *et al*. Diagnostic criteria for hereditary hemorrhagic telangiectasia (Rendu–Osler–Weber syndrome). *American Journal of Medical Genetics* 2000; **91**: 66–67.

Other relevant entries Abscess: an overview; Phakomatosis.

▨ Osmotic demyelination syndrome – see Central pontine myelinolysis

▨ Ossification of the posterior longitudinal ligament

Pathophysiology Ossification of the posterior longitudinal ligament of the spine has been recognized as a cause of myelopathy in Japan for many years, but only in more recent times has a similar condition been identified in the West. It is commoner in men, the peak age of onset is in the sixth decade, and its cause remains unknown although it may occur in association with diffuse idiopathic skeletal hyperostosis (DISH), spondylosis, and ankylosing spondylosis.

Clinical features: history and examination

- May be asymptomatic.
- Most commonly affects the cervical spine causing a spastic quadriparesis; may be progressive or acute, may cause quadriplegia.

Investigations and diagnosis *Imaging*: ossification of the posterior longitudinal ligament may be evident with plain radiography of the cervical spine, myelography, or MRI.

Differential diagnosis Other causes of spastic quadriplegia, especially compressive cervical spondylotic myelopathy.

Treatment and prognosis Some cases progress, others improve spontaneously or with surgical intervention.

Reference Trojan DA, Pouchot J, Pokrupa R *et al*. Diagnosis and treatment of ossification of the posterior longitudinal ligament of the spine: report of eight cases and literature review. *American Journal of Medicine* 1992; **92**: 296–306.

Other relevant entries Ankylosing spondylitis and the nervous system; Cervical cord and root disease; Diffuse idiopathic skeletal hyperostosis; Myelopathy: an overview; Quadriplegia: an overview.

■ Osteitis deformans – see Paget's disease

■ Osteogenesis imperfecta

This inherited connective tissue disorder due to a quantitative or qualitative defect in collagen synthesis resulting in bone fragility is clinically very variable with respect to age of onset and number of fractures, which in turn influences walking ability and prognosis. In addition to cardiac and respiratory consequences of bone fractures and deformity, a number of neurological features have been reported:

- Spinal deformity
- Basilar impression/invagination
- Impaired hearing (sensorineural)
- Cerebrovascular associations (occasional)
    Carotico-cavernous fistula (CCF)
    Moyamoya disease
    Cerebral aneurysms.

Treatment of the underlying bone disease with growth hormone and bisphosphonates has been attempted. Symptomatic treatment of neurological complications may be required.

Other relevant entries Ehlers–Danlos syndrome; Marfan syndrome; Pseudo-xanthoma elasticum.

■ Osteomalacia

Osteomalacia may be associated with proximal myopathy as well as bone pain and skeletal problems. Creatine kinase level is usually normal, EMG and muscle biopsy are myopathic.

Other relevant entries Myopathy: an overview; Proximal weakness; Renal disease and the nervous system.

■ Osteopetrosis – see Albers–Schönberg disease

■ O'Sullivan–McLeod syndrome

A rare form of distal spinal muscular atrophy (SMA), of autosomal-recessive or autosomal-dominant inheritance, causing slowly progressive wasting of the hands. Electrophysiological studies may confirm anterior horn cell disease, and focal changes have on occasion been seen on MRI of the anterior horns of the spinal cord at a level appropriate to the wasting.

Reference Petiot P, Gonon V, Froment JC, Vial C, Vighetto A. Slowly progressive spinal muscular atrophy of the hands (O'Sullivan–McLeod syndrome): clinical and magnetic resonance imaging presentation. *Journal of Neurology* 2000; **247**: 654–655.

Other relevant entry Spinal muscular atrophy.

■ Osuntokun's syndrome

This rare syndrome of hearing loss and indifference to pain sensation is characterized clinically by:

- Auditory imperception: hearing intact, but difficulty comprehending the spoken word (verbal auditory agnosia?).
- Congenital indifference to pain: reduced pain and temperature sensation; light touch, proprioception; vibration normal.

No specific investigations have been described as assisting with the diagnosis. The condition may represent a sensory neuropathy akin to hereditary sensory neuropathy (especially hereditary sensory and autonomic neuropathy (HSAN) types II, IV, and V). There is no specific treatment; hearing aids are not helpful. Protection against trophic damage is important.

> **Reference** Osuntokun BO, Odeku EL, Luzzato L. Congenital pain asymbolia and auditory imperception. *Journal of Neurology, Neurosurgery and Psychiatry* 1968; **31**: 291–296.

> **Other relevant entries** Congenital insensitivity to pain; Hereditary sensory and autonomic neuropathy; Neuropathies: an overview.

■ Othello syndrome

A psychiatric illness in which the dominant symptom is a delusional belief in the infidelity of the spouse or sexual partner; this may occur in isolation or in the context of an already established psychotic illness. Males are more often affected than females.

> **Reference** Enoch MD, Ball HN. *Uncommon Psychiatric Syndromes* (4th edition). London: Arnold, 2001: 50–73.

> **Other relevant entry** Psychiatric disorders and neurological disease.

■ Otolithic catastrophe of Tumarkin – see Tumarkin's otolithic crisis

■ Overlap syndrome

The concurrence of an inflammatory myopathy (polymyositis, dermatomyositis) with a connective tissue disease (Sjögren's syndrome, systemic sclerosis, SLE).

> **Other relevant entries** Dermatomyositis; Systemic sclerosis.

Pp

■ Paget's disease
Osteitis deformans

Pathophysiology A disorder of bone, with a predilection for the skull and vertebral column, characterized by increased bone turnover with excessive osteoclastic resorption and disorganized new bone formation. Bone pain is often the major symptom although the condition is frequently asymptomatic, coming to light as the explanation for an elevated blood level of alkaline phosphatase. A variety of neurological complications secondary to the bony pathology may occur. It predominantly affects the older population. Aetiology is not known; there may be a combination of genetic and environmental factors (paramyxovirus infection of osteoclasts has been demonstrated in some cases).

Clinical features: history and examination

- Bone:
    - Pain: stretching of periosteum over enlarging bone, fractures (especially long bones)
    - Deformity
    - Malignancy (rare): osteosarcoma, chondrosarcoma, fibrosarcoma, giant cell tumour.
- Cardiac:
    - High output failure.
- Neurological:
    - Cranial nerve palsies, due to foraminal entrapment: VIII (deafness), II (optic atrophy), V, VII.
    - Basilar invagination: lower cranial nerve palsies (X, XII); normal pressure hydrocephalus (gait disorder, sphincter incontinence, frontal-subcortical type of cognitive decline); high cervical cord compression, syringomyelia secondary to skull base Paget's.
    - Extradural myelopathy, secondary to disease in several adjacent vertebrae affecting bodies, pedicles, and laminae.

Investigations and diagnosis *Bloods*: raised alkaline phosphatase reflects disease activity; calcium, phosphate normal unless the patient has been immobile.

Urine: hydroxyproline levels reflect osteoclastic activity.

Imaging:

Plain radiology (skull, spine) for typical bone changes: irregular bone thickening, areas of resorption; widening of diploic spaces in skull with osteolytic and osteosclerotic areas giving "cotton wool"-like appearance.

CT/MRI: for hydrocephalus, skull base change; MRI for cord compression.

Radioisotope scanning (Tc^{99m}): may be helpful in determining extent and activity of disease.

Differential diagnosis Other causes of isolated or combined cranial nerve palsies, myelopathy.

Treatment and prognosis Treatment of Paget's: diphosphonates (e.g. etidronate) reduce osteoclastic activity; calcitonin inhibits bone resorption.

Symptomatic treatment: NSAIDs for pain; repeated lumbar puncture or shunting for hydrocephalus; posterior decompression for cord compression.

References Chen J-R, Rhee RS, Wallach S, Avramides A, Flores A. Neurologic distribution in Paget disease of bone: response to calcitonin. *Neurology* 1979; **29**: 448–457.

Hamdy RC. Clinical features and pharmacologic treatment of Paget's disease. *Endocrinologic and Metabolic Clinics of North America* 1995; **24**: 421–436.

Klein RM, Norman A. Diagnostic procedures for Paget's disease. Radiologic, pathologic and laboratory testing. *Endocrinologic and Metabolic Clinics of North America* 1995; **24**: 437–450.

Other relevant entries Cranial polyneuropathy; Myelopathy: an overview; Normal pressure hydrocephalus (NPH).

▓ Paine's syndrome

Paine's syndrome is an X-linked-recessive condition characterized by ataxia, mental retardation and microcephaly. It enters the differential diagnosis of congenital inherited ataxic disorders along with Joubert's syndrome and Gillespie's syndrome.

Other relevant entries Cerebellar disease: an overview; Gillespie's syndrome; Joubert's syndrome.

▓ Painful legs and moving toes

Pathophysiology A condition of unknown aetiology manifesting as deep, chronic, poorly localized pain, usually within the feet or legs, with involuntary writhing movements of the digits. Pain predates movements, sometimes by years. The syndrome may on occasion be associated with nerve root or spinal cord lesions.

Clinical features: history and examination
- Gnawing, aching, twisting pain, deep in an extremity (usually lower leg and foot, maybe toes); unilateral or bilateral; sometimes relieved by activity.
- Involuntary writhing movements of toes (1–2 Hz); maybe temporarily suppressed by voluntary effort.
- Absence of abnormal sensory or motor neurological signs.
- A painless variant ("painless legs and moving toes") is also described, as is a similar syndrome in the upper limbs ("painful arms and moving fingers").

Investigations and diagnosis *Neurophysiology*: EMG/NCS to exclude a nerve root lesion.

Imaging: MRI spinal cord to exclude intrinsic lesions.

Differential diagnosis Restless legs syndrome.

Treatment and prognosis There is no specific treatment. Symptomatic treatment with agents useful for dysaesthesia (amitriptyline, carbamazepine, TENS, lumbar sympathetic blockade) may be tried. The symptoms usually continue indefinitely.

References Dressler D, Thompson PD, Gledhill RF, Marsden CD. The syndrome of painful legs and moving toes. *Movement Disorders* 1994; **9**: 13–21.

Nathan PW. Painful legs and moving toes: evidence on the site of the lesion. *Journal of Neurology, Neurosurgery and Psychiatry* 1978; **41**: 934–939.

Spillane JD, Nathan PW, Kelly RE, Marsden CD. Painful legs and moving toes. *Brain* 1971; **94**: 541–556.

Other relevant entry Restless legs syndrome.

■ Palatal myoclonus – see Myoclonus

■ Palinopsia

Pathophysiology Palinopsia is the perseveration of visual images. It is suggestive of an occipitoparietal lesion, either structural (e.g. infarct) or functional (e.g. seizures, substance abuse), although it has been reported in normal individuals.

Clinical features: history and examination Patients report persistence or recurrence of multiple visual images after the stimulus has been removed.

On examination a left homonymous hemianopia may be found.

Investigations and diagnosis *Imaging*: CT/MRI to exclude right occipitoparietal lesion.

Neurophysiology: EEG to exclude right occipitoparietal focus.

Differential diagnosis Visual hallucinations, for example Charles Bonnet syndrome if in conjunction with visual field defect.

Treatment and prognosis No specific treatment; may be self-limiting.

References Michel EN, Troost BT. Palinopsia: cerebral localization with CT. *Neurology* 1980; **30**: 887–889.

Pomeranz HD, Lessell S. Palinopsia and polyopia in the absence of drugs or cerebral disease. *Neurology* 2000; **54**: 855–859.

Other relevant entries Charles Bonnet syndrome; Top of the basilar syndrome.

■ Pallido-ponto-nigral degeneration

Pallido-ponto-nigral degeneration (PPND) is a form of frontotemporal dementia with parkinsonism linked to chromosome 17 caused by mutations within the τ-gene.

Other relevant entries Dementia: an overview; Tauopathy.

■ Panayiotopoulos syndrome

This idiopathic childhood epilepsy syndrome is characterized by a susceptibility to seizures with autonomic features, accompanied by occipital or extraoccipital spikes on the EEG. The seizures most often occur during sleep, often with vomiting; there may in addition be pallor, mydriasis, cardiorespiratory, gastrointestinal and thermoregulatory alterations, incontinence and hypersalivation. Attacks may last minutes to hours (autonomic status) and may be associated with unresponsiveness (ictal syncope) mimicking encephalitis. Behavioural disturbance and headache are common at onset; the eyes may deviate to one side or the child may stare ahead. A generalized convulsion may occur at the end of the seizure. EEG may show multifocal spikes, which may be occipital. The condition is benign, with remission common within 2 years of onset. Hence, treatment with anti-epileptic drugs is generally unnecessary.

References Ferrie CD, Grunewald RA. Panayiotopoulos syndrome: a common and benign childhood epilepsy. *Lancet* 2001; **357**: 821–823.

Koutroumanidis M. Panayiotopoulos syndrome. *British Medical Journal* 2002; **324**: 1228–1229.

Other relevant entries Benign epilepsy syndromes; Epilepsy: an overview.

▣ Pancerebellar syndrome – see Cerebellar disease: an overview

▣ Pancoast's syndrome

Pathophysiology Tumour in the lung apex or superior sulcus, usually a squamous cell carcinoma, may involve the lower cervical and upper thoracic spinal nerves, the sympathetic chain, and in the later stages may invade the spinal cord causing compression. This may occur in the absence of pulmonary symptoms.

Clinical features: history and examination
- Pain in the arm (inner aspect), behind the upper part of the scapula.
- Numb hand, inner arm (T1, T2).
- Weakness of hand muscles, +/− triceps.
- Horner's syndrome +/− warm dry ipsilateral hand if stellate ganglion involved (stellate ganglion syndrome).
- +/− spinal cord compression, paraplegia.
- +/− recurrent laryngeal nerve palsy, unilateral vocal cord paresis, weak ("bovine") cough.
- +/− superior vena cava syndrome.
- Late cough, haemoptysis, dyspnoea.

Investigations and diagnosis *Imaging*: Chest X-ray, CT, MRI: neurological symptoms may predate radiological evidence of tumour.

Cytology: sputum, bronchoscopic washings, fine needle aspiration.

Neurophysiology: EMG/NCS: root, brachial plexus lesion.

Differential diagnosis

Cervical radiculopathy.

Spinal cord metastasis.

Treatment and prognosis Treatment of tumour; symptomatic treatment of arm pain.

References Arcasoy SM, Jett JR. Superior pulmonary sulcus tumors and Pancoast's syndrome. *New England Journal of Medicine* 1997; **337**: 1370–1376.

Attar S, Krasna MJ, Sonett JR *et al.* Superior sulcus (Pancoast) tumor: experience with 105 patients. *Annals of Thoracic Surgery* 1998; **66**: 193–198.

Pancoast HK. Superior pulmonary sulcus tumor: tumor characterized by pain, Horner's syndrome, destruction of bone and atrophy of hand muscles. *Journal of the American Medical Association* 1932; **99**: 1391–1396.

Other relevant entries Horner's syndrome; Paraparesis: acute management and differential diagnosis; Stellate ganglion syndrome.

■ PANDAS syndrome

PANDAS is an acronym for *p*aediatric *a*utoimmune *n*europsychiatric *d*isorders *a*ssociated with *s*treptococcal infections. Suggested criteria for the diagnosis are:

- obsessive–compulsive disorder or tic disorder;
- prepubertal symptom onset (mean onset 6–7 years);
- episodic course of symptom severity, often with relapsing–remitting pattern;
- association with Gram-positive β-haemolytic streptococcal infection, often pharyngitis or upper respiratory tract infection;
- association with neurological abnormalities.

The condition often has an acute and dramatic onset. Exacerbations may also be triggered by Gram-positive β-haemolytic streptococcal infections. Psychiatric co-morbidities include emotional lability, anxiety, rituals, cognitive decline, oppositional behaviours, and motor hyperactivity. Its relationship to Sydenham's chorea and encephalitis lethargica is currently of great interest.

Reference Swedo SE, Leonard HL, Garvey M *et al.* Pediatric autoimmune neuropsychiatric disorders associated with streptococcal infections: clinical description of the first 50 cases. *American Journal of Psychiatry* 1998; **155**: 264–271.

Other relevant entries Emotional lability: differential diagnosis; Obsessive–compulsive disorder; Sydenham's chorea.

■ Pandysautonomia

Pandysautonomia is characterized by pre- and post-ganglionic lesions of both the sympathetic and parasympathetic pathways. This may be:

Congenital
Acquired:
    acute (e.g. after a viral infection such as infectious mononucleosis);
    subacute (e.g. the "autonomic-only" form of Guillain–Barré syndrome);
    chronic (e.g. pure autonomic failure, multiple system atrophy, certain hereditary neuropathies).

Clinical features include:
- Visual blurring; pupillary areflexia.
- Orthostatic hypotension.
- Cardiac arrhythmia.
- Abdominal pain, diarrhoea, vomiting, constipation, ileus, pseudo-obstruction.

Response to intravenous immunoglobulin has been reported in idiopathic pandysautonomia.

> **Reference** Heafield MT, Gammage MD, Nightingale S, Williams AC. Idiopathic dysautonomia treated with intravenous immunoglobulin. *Lancet* 1996; **347**: 28–29.

> **Other relevant entries** Autonomic failure; Guillain–Barré syndrome; Immunosuppressive therapy and diseases of the nervous system.

■ Panencephalitis – see Encephalitis: an overview

■ Pantokinate kinase associated neurodegeneration – see Hallervorden–Spatz syndrome

■ PARA syndrome

*P*rogressive *a*symmetrical *r*igidity and *a*praxia (the so-called PARA syndrome) are common to all the suggested diagnostic criteria of corticobasal degeneration (CBD).

> **Other relevant entry** Corticobasal degeneration.

■ Paraganglioma – see Glomus jugulare tumour

■ Paragonimiasis

Infection with trematodes of the *Paragonimus* species (oriental lung fluke), following ingestion of larval metacercaria in raw or undercooked freshwater crustaceans or water plants, may lead to pulmonary disease or, with aberrant fluke migration, cerebral disease. Cyst, abscess, and granuloma formation may occur as a consequence of host reaction to worms and eggs, manifesting clinically as acute or chronic encephalitis with seizures and focal neurological signs. Brain haemorrhage, infarction, space-occupying lesions, raised intracranial pressure, papilloedema, and optic atrophy may occur. Oral praziquantel is the treatment of choice.

> **Other relevant entries** Helminthic disease; Schistosomiasis.

■ Paralysis agitans – see Parkinson's disease

■ Parameningeal infection

Parameningeal infection may occur in the following spaces:

Epidural or extradural: between dura and bone; spinal > cranial.
Subdural: between dura and arachnoid.

Such processes may induce a meningeal reaction and meningism.

Other relevant entries Abscess: an overview; Infection and the nervous system: an overview; Subdural empyema.

■ Paramyotonia

Eulenburg's disease • Paramyotonia congenita

Pathophysiology Paramyotonia is similar to myotonia, that is, there is abnormal muscle relaxation following voluntary or induced contraction, but differs ("paradoxical myotonia") in that repetitive muscle use leads to an increased delay in relaxation (*cf.* myotonia). Paramyotonia congenita is a channelopathy affecting the α-subunit of the sodium channel. Hyperkalaemic periodic paralysis, K^+-aggravated myotonia and hypokalaemic periodic paralysis may result from mutations in the same gene (allelic heterogeneity, phenotype divergence).

Clinical features: history and examination

- Abnormal muscle relaxation, especially in face and forearms: repeated forced eye closure may lead to persistent closure for a minute or so.
- Symptoms worsened by cooling.

Investigations and diagnosis *Neurophysiology*: EMG: muscle cooling leads to electrical inexcitability (contracture).

Neurogenetics: sodium channel gene (SCN4A) mutations at chromosome 17q23–q25 (as in hyperkalaemic periodic paralysis, potassium-aggravated myotonia, and rare cases of hypokalaemic periodic paralysis).

Differential diagnosis Other myotonic syndromes, periodic paralyses.

Treatment and prognosis Avoid repeated forced muscle contraction, cold exposure.

References Davies NP, Eunson LH, Gregory RP, Mills KR, Morrison PJ, Hanna MG. Clinical, electrophysiological, and molecular genetic studies in a new family with paramyotonia. *Journal of Neurology, Neurosurgery and Psychiatry* 2000; **68**: 504–507.

Ebers GC, George AL, Barchi RL *et al*. Paramyotonia congenita and hyperkalaemic periodic paralysis are linked to the adult muscle sodium channel gene. *Annals of Neurology* 1991; **30**: 810–816.

Other relevant entries Channelopathies: an overview; Episodic ataxia; Myotonia and myotonic syndromes; Periodic paralysis.

■ Paraneoplastic syndromes

Pathophysiology Paraneoplastic disorders are rare non-metastatic manifestations of cancer, the symptoms of which usually precede those of the underlying malignancy. Paraneoplastic syndromes are thought to be autoimmune phenomena, in which neurological dysfunction is triggered by immune responses directed against antigens on distant tumour cells. Devastating though the neurological syndromes may be (they are often rapidly progressive), the autoimmune responses may hold the tumour in check. Detection of the underlying tumour may be difficult with conventional imaging techniques, and it may be several years before a tumour is located; sometimes only at postmortem is a tumour found. Primary treatment of the tumour generally does not lead to remission of the neurological syndrome. Immune modulatory therapy may sometimes be helpful.

Clinical features: history and examination A number of paraneoplastic neurological syndromes are described, including:

- Cerebral:
    Encephalomyelitis (+/− sensory neuronopathy)
    Limbic encephalitis (+/− sensory neuronopathy).
- Cerebellar/brainstem:
    Cerebellar degeneration
    Opsoclonus/myoclonus ("dancing eyes, dancing feet", Kinsbourne's syndrome)
    Brainstem encephalitis.
- Eye:
    Cancer-associated retinopathy.
- Peripheral nerves:
    Paraneoplastic sensory neuropathy
    Paraneoplastic motor neuropathy.
- Neuromuscular junction:
    Lambert–Eaton myasthenic syndrome (LEMS)
    Thymoma-associated myasthenia gravis.
- Muscle:
    Dermatomyositis.

Investigations and diagnosis Other causes of these clinical syndromes need to be excluded (see under individual entries), which may require imaging (MRI), CSF analysis, EEG, ERG.

Anti-neuronal antibodies may be helpful in establishing the diagnosis of a paraneoplastic syndrome, although these may be epiphenomenal rather than pathogenetic. Moreover, false positives and negatives occur; referral to a specialist laboratory is required.

Site of pathology	Clinical syndrome	Common associated malignancy	Antibody
Brain, brainstem	Limbic encephalitis, brainstem encephalitis	SCLC	Anti-Hu
	Limbic encephalitis, brainstem encephalitis	Testis	Ma2, Ta
	Cerebellar degeneration	SCLC	Anti-Hu
	Cerebellar degeneration	Breast, ovary	Anti-Yo
	Cerebellar degeneration	Hodgkin's disease	Tr
	Opsoclonus/myoclonus	Breast	Anti-Ri
			(*Continued*)

Site of pathology	Clinical syndrome	Common associated malignancy	Antibody
Retina	Retinopathy	SCLC	Anti-CAR
Dorsal root ganglia	Sensory neuronopathy	SCLC	Anti-Hu
Neuromuscular junction	LEMS	SCLC	Voltage-gated calcium channels (VGCCs)
	Myasthenia gravis	Thymoma	AChR
Muscle	Dermatomyositis	many	–

A search for underlying malignancy is often undertaken: [^{18}F] fluoro-2-deoxyglucose PET (FDG-PET) scanning may be helpful in these circumstances, due to its excellent spatial resolution (of the order of 6–8 mm). However, whether identification of the tumour has therapeutic implications is uncertain, since treatment of the tumour *per se* may not influence the neurological syndrome.

Differential diagnosis Other causes of these clinical syndromes (see under individual entries). A non-paraneoplastic limbic encephalitis with serum voltage-gated potassium channel (VGKC) antibodies, which may respond to steroids, IVIg, and plasma exchange, has been described.

Treatment and prognosis No specific treatment. IVIg has been tried sometimes with apparent benefit. Course is usually progressive and may be rapidly so (e.g. cerebellar syndrome). Very occasionally remission may occur with successful treatment of the underlying tumour.

References Dalmau J, Gultekin HS, Posner JB. Paraneoplastic neurologic syndromes: pathogenesis and physiopathology. *Brain Pathology* 1999; **9**: 275–284.

Giometto B, Taraloto B, Graus F. Autoimmunity in paraneoplastic neurological syndromes. *Brain Pathology* 1999; **9**: 261–273.

Grant R. What the general neurologist needs to know about the paraneoplastic syndromes. *Practical Neurology* 2002; **2**: 318–327.

Scaravilli F, An SF, Groves M, Thom M. The neuropathology of paraneoplastic syndromes. *Brain Pathology* 1999; **9**: 251–260.

Sutton I, Winer JB. The immunopathogenesis of paraneoplastic neurological syndromes. *Clinical Science* 2002; **102**: 475–486.

Other relevant entries Cerebellar disease: an overview; Dermatomyositis; Lambert–Eaton myasthenic syndrome; Limbic encephalitis; Myoclonus; Neuromyotonia; Neuropathies: an overview; Opsoclonus.

■ Paraparesis: acute management and differential diagnosis

Pathophysiology Paraparesis is weakness of the lower limbs; paraplegia is a total weakness, or "paralysis". Paraparesis may result from structural or functional interruption of upper motor neurone (corticospinal, vestibulospinal, reticulospinal, and other extrapyramidal tracts) or lower motor neurone pathways. In the acute stages, differential diagnosis may be difficult on clinical grounds alone, necessitating neuroimaging and neurophysiological assessment.

Clinical features: history and examination

- Acute: flaccidity, areflexia; urinary retention; this may be of lower motor neurone origin, for example acute neuropathy of Guillain–Barré type, in which lower limb weakness in a so-called "pyramidal distribution" (flexors > extensors) may be observed; or of upper motor neurone origin (e.g. "spinal shock").
- Chronic: upper motor neurone lesions evolve to a syndrome characterized by hypertonia, spasticity, sustained clonus, hyperreflexia, loss of abdominal and cremasteric reflexes, and Babinski's sign. There may also be enhanced flexion defence reflexes ("flexor spasms") with hip and knee flexion, ankle and toe dorsiflexion, which are often painful. These flexor responses may develop into a fixed flexion deformity with secondary contractures ("paraplegia in flexion"). "Paraplegia in extension", with extension at the hip and knee, may be seen with incomplete or high spinal cord lesions.

Investigations and diagnosis Acute paraplegia mandates emergency investigation with spinal cord imaging, preferably MRI, to exclude compression which may require surgical intervention. Other lesions are also demonstrated by this modality, although some arteriovenous malformations may be overlooked; myelography is indicated if there is a high index of clinical suspicion for this diagnosis.

Differential diagnosis Recognized causes of paraparesis include:

- Upper motor neurone lesions:

    Traumatic section of the cord.

    Cord compression from intrinsic or extrinsic mass lesion, for example tumour, metastasis, abscess, empyema, haematoma (epidural, subdural).

    Inflammatory lesions: acute transverse myelitis of viral origin, multiple sclerosis, neuromyelitis optica (Devic's syndrome), systemic lupus erythematosus, Behçet's disease, giant cell arteritis (rare).

    Structural lesions: tethered cord syndrome, arteriovenous malformation, rarely parasagittal meningioma.

    Metabolic: Hereditary spastic paraparesis (HSP), adrenoleukodystrophy (X-ALD), subacute combined degeneration of the cord (usually mild).

- Lower motor neurone lesions:

    Acute or chronic neuropathies (Guillain–Barré syndrome, chronic inflammatory demyelinating polyneuropathy).

Treatment and prognosis Treatment of cause where possible.

Prevention of flexor spasms which are often provoked by skin irritation/ulceration, constipation, bladder infection, and poor nutrition. Physiotherapy.

Spasticity: baclofen, tizanidine, dantrolene, diazepam; botulinum toxin injections for focal spasticity.

Reference Johnston RA. Acute spinal cord compression. In: RAC Hughes (ed.). *Neurological Emergencies* (2nd edition). London: BMJ Publishing Group, 1997: 272–294.

Other relevant entries Adrenoleukodystrophy; Arachnoiditis; Guillain–Barré syndrome; Haematoma: an overview; Hereditary spastic paraparesis; Myelopathy: an overview; Quadriplegia: an overview; Spina bifida; Spinal cord trauma; Spinal cord vascular diseases; Tethered cord syndrome.

■ Paraproteinaemic neuropathies
Paraprotein-associated demyelinating neuropathy (PDN)

Pathophysiology Peripheral neuropathy, usually of demyelinating type, may occur in conditions associated with a serum paraprotein, such as myeloma, Waldenström's macroglobulinaemia, and monoclonal gammopathy of undetermined significance (MGUS, especially of IgM subtype). The paraprotein is thought to be pathogenetically relevant in at least some of these cases since it may be demonstrated bound to nerve in biopsy specimens. Various antibody specificities have been reported, with antibodies against myelin-associated glycoprotein (MAG) being common. Plasma exchange may be helpful in these conditions. In other situations a paraprotein may be no more than a marker for an underlying inflammatory process, such as vasculitis or amyloidosis, or entirely incidental to the neuropathy.

Clinical features: history and examination
MGUS:
- Sensory symptoms: feet, hands
- Symmetrical distal wasting, weakness
- Pain
- Action/postural tremor (3.5–6.5 Hz) – especially IgM
- Ataxia, probably sensory
- +/− fasciculation.

Commoner in men.

Investigations and diagnosis *Bloods*: Paraprotein detected by serum electrophoresis; quantitative immunoglobulins; serum immunofixation (in MGUS, IgM > IgG > IgA; usually κ light chain); raised ESR, CRP, viscosity.

CSF: may show increased protein and matched monoclonal band with serum.

Imaging: skeletal survey to look for myeloma (osteolytic, osteosclerotic).

Bone marrow examination: myeloma, Waldenström's macroglobulinaemia, MGUS.

Neurophysiology: EMG/NCS: commonest finding is slowing of nerve conduction velocities suggesting demyelinating process (IgM usually demyelinating), but axonal changes are also reported (IgA, IgG may be demyelinating or axonal).

Nerve biopsy: demyelination, loss of myelinated fibres; immunocytochemistry may demonstrate IgM on myelin.

Characterization of specificity of auto-antibodies, for example MAG, sulfatide, SGPG, GM1 (especially multifocal motor neuropathy with conduction block); available in specialist centres only. Around 50% of IgM cases are anti-MAG positive, yet paradoxically response to plasma exchange is better with IgA and IgG.

Differential diagnosis

Myeloma, especially osteosclerotic type (plasmacytoma).

Waldenström's macroglobulinaemia.

MGUS.

POEMS syndrome.

Other demyelinating neuropathies: genetic (hereditary sensory and motor neuropathies), chronic inflammatory demyelinating neuropathy (CIDP), vasculitic neuropathy.

Treatment and prognosis Steroids alone are ineffective; chlorambucil, cyclophosphamide, plasma exchange may be helpful.

Irradiation of isolated osteosclerotic myelomatous bone lesions may be curative.

References Steck AJ, Erne B, Gabriel JM, Schaeren-Wiemers N. Paraproteinaemic neuropathies. *Brain Pathology* 1999; **9**: 361–368.

Thomas PK, Willison HJ. Paraproteinaemic neuropathy. In: McLeod JG (ed.). *Inflammatory Neuropathies*. London: Baillière Tindall, 1994: 129–147.

Other relevant entries Monoclonal gammopathies; Neuropathies: an overview; POEMS syndrome; Tremor: an overview.

■ Parasomnias

Pathophysiology Parasomnias are non-epileptic phenomena associated with sleep. Most are benign and commoner in childhood. Their recognition is important in order to avoid inappropriate investigation and to reassure patients (and parents).

Clinical features: history and examination

- History from a bed partner may be crucial in making a diagnosis.
- Myoclonus: hypnic/pompic jerks; sensory starts
- Confusion: night terrors (pavor nocturnus)
- Talking in sleep (somniloquy)
- Bruxism
- Sleep paralysis
- Nightmares
- Sleep walking (somnambulism)
- *R*apid *e*ye *m*ovement (REM) sleep *b*ehaviour *d*isorder (RBD).

Investigations and diagnosis Polysomnography may be undertaken in specialist centres to determine whether events occur during REM sleep (e.g. nightmares, sleep paralysis) or non-REM sleep (e.g. sleep walking, night terrors, talking in sleep, bruxism). Such monitoring may also confirm the presence of myoclonus (hypnic/pompic jerks, sensory starts).

Differential diagnosis

Periodic movements of sleep (sometimes seen as a feature of restless legs syndrome). Jerks may be mistaken for nocturnal seizures.

Isolated sleep paralysis may be mistaken as an indication of narcolepsy.

Treatment and prognosis Explanation is often sufficient. Prognosis is very good, although sleep walking can lead to self-injury. Benzodiazepines are largely unsuccessful. Clomipramine has been tried in sleep paralysis. Serotonin reuptake inhibitors may be helpful.

References Parkes JD. *Sleep and Its Disorders*. London: Saunders, 1985.

Shneerson JM. *Handbook of Sleep Medicine*. Oxford: Blackwell Science, 2000.

Other relevant entries Bruxism; Narcolepsy, narcoleptic syndrome; Restless legs syndrome; Sleep disorders: an overview.

▪ Parathyroid disorders and the nervous system – see Basal ganglia calcification; Endocrinology and the nervous system; Parkinsonian disorders, parkinsonism

▪ Paratonia – see *Gegenhalten*

▪ Paratrigeminal syndrome of Raeder – see Raeder's paratrigeminal syndrome

▪ Parinaud's syndrome

Dorsal midbrain syndrome • Periaqueductal grey matter syndrome • Pretectal syndrome • Sylvian aqueduct syndrome

Pathophysiology Dorsal midbrain lesions affecting the pretectum and posterior commissure interfere with conjugate eye movements in the vertical plane. The key anatomical substrates, damage to which causes the syndrome, are probably the interstitial nucleus of Cajal and the nucleus of the posterior commissure and their projections. Pineal tumours are probably the commonest cause of this syndrome.

Clinical features: history and examination

- Eye movements:

    Paralysis of vertical gaze, especially upgaze: Bell's phenomenon may be spared.

    Loss of convergence; convergence spasm may cause slow abduction ("midbrain pseudo-sixth").

    Skew deviation.

    Convergence–retraction nystagmus (Körber–Salus–Elschnig syndrome); sometimes downbeat nystagmus.

- Eyelids:

    Lid retraction (Collier's sign) or ptosis (ventral extension of lesion).

- Pupils:

    Mydriasis.

    Loss of pupillary light reflexes (light-near dissociation).

Investigations and diagnosis *Imaging*: MRI of midbrain.

Differential diagnosis Other causes of vertical gaze paresis, for example hydrocephalus in infants, progressive supranuclear palsy, Wolfram syndrome.

Treatment and prognosis Pineal tumours may be amenable to resection.

> **Reference** Parinaud H. Paralysie des mouvements associés des yeux. *Archives de Neurologie, Paris* 1883; **5**: 145–172.

> **Other relevant entries** Körber–Salus–Elschnig syndrome; Pineal tumours; Top of the basilar syndrome; Tumours: an overview; Wolfram syndrome.

■ Parkinsonian syndromes, parkinsonism
Extrapyramidal syndromes

Pathophysiology Although idiopathic Parkinson's disease is by far the commonest cause of parkinsonism, a number of other syndromes characterized by parkinsonism (akinesia, rigidity) have been described, sometimes under the rubric of "Parkinson's plus syndromes" due to additional clinical features not evident in idiopathic Parkinson's disease. These syndromes are poorly, if at all, responsive to levodopa preparations and they tend to progress more quickly. Although most of these syndromes reflect an underlying neurodegenerative process, parkinsonism resulting from remediable structural, inflammatory or metabolic disease of the nervous system does occur.

Clinical features: history and examination

- Akinesia, rigidity present, but tremor less common than in idiopathic Parkinson's disease.
- Marked unilateral apraxia, pyramidal signs may suggest corticobasal degeneration (CBD).
- Supranuclear gaze palsy, early falls, may suggest progressive supranuclear palsy (PSP).
- Early visual hallucinations, fluctuations, and dementia suggests dementia with Lewy bodies (DLB); dementia may be the presenting feature of CBD.
- Autonomic features (orthostatic hypotension), cerebellar syndrome may suggest multiple system atrophy (MSA).

Investigations and diagnosis See individual entries. Since Wilson's disease is potentially treatable, this diagnosis must not be missed and hence it is advisable to check copper and caeruloplasmin levels and perform slit-lamp examination for Kayser–Fleischer rings in all patients presenting with parkinsonism below the age of 50 years.

Differential diagnosis

Idiopathic Parkinson's disease.

PSP, Steele–Richardson–Olszewski syndrome.

MSA with predominant parkinsonism (MSA-P).

CBD.

Drug/toxin-induced parkinsonism, especially related to neuroleptic use; neuroleptic malignant syndrome (NMS); manganese poisoning, carbon disulphide, carbon monoxide, cyanide; MPTP.

Wilson's disease.

DLB.

Post-encephalitic parkinsonism (encephalitis lethargica, Von Economo's disease).

Huntington's disease (HD), especially juvenile-onset form (Westphal variant).

Subcortical cerebrovascular disease ("arteriosclerotic parkinsonism").

Normal pressure hydrocephalus (NPH).

Post-traumatic parkinsonism, dementia pugilistica.

Guam parkinsonism–dementia complex.

Systemic lupus erythematosus, Sjögren's syndrome.

Hypoparathyroidism.

Tumour-associated parkinsonism: a debatable entity: a cerebral tumour and PD may be incidental, although some reports of parkinsonism "responding" to tumour removal have been published.

Treatment and prognosis Largely unresponsive to levodopa preparations. Wilson's disease mandates chelation therapy. See under individual entries for appropriate symptomatic treatments.

> **Reference** Oertel WH, Quinn NP. Parkinsonism. In: Brandt T, Caplan LR, Dichgans J, Diener HC, Kennard C (eds). *Neurological Disorders: Course and Treatment.* San Diego: Academic Press, 1996: 715–772.

> **Other relevant entries** Apraxia; Carbon monoxide poisoning; Corticobasal degeneration; Cyanide poisoning; Drug-induced movement disorders; Encephalitis lethargica; Guam parkinsonism–dementia complex; Huntington's disease; Lewy body disease: an overview; Manganese poisoning, manganism; Multiple system atrophy; Neuroleptic malignant syndrome; Normal pressure hydrocephalus; Parkinson's disease; Progressive supranuclear palsy; Sjögren's syndrome; Systemic lupus erythematosus and the nervous system; Wilson's disease.

■ Parkinsonism–dementia complex of Guam – see Guam parkinsonism–dementia complex

■ Parkinson's disease
Idiopathic Parkinson's disease • Paralysis agitans

Pathophysiology An idiopathic disorder characterized by slowness in the initiation and performance of movement (hypokinesia, akinesia, bradykinesia) with limb resistance to passive movement (rigidity) and sometimes tremor, most usually at rest. First described by James Parkinson in 1817 as "paralysis agitans" (a misnomer), the condition is due at least in part to depletion of dopamine in the striatum due to death of nigral dopaminergic neurones with loss of the nigrostriatal pathway. Most patients respond well initially to dopamine replacement therapy but response fluctuations become troublesome as the disease progresses. Dementia may develop.

A number of genetic loci have been defined associated with autosomal-dominant or autosomal-recessive Parkinson's disease, including α-synuclein parkin and PINKI. Exactly how mutations in these genes lead to the clinical syndrome awaits definition.

Clinical features: history and examination The classical triad (not all of which need be present at onset) consists of:

- Akinesia/hypokinesia: slowness or inability to initiate voluntary movement; bradykinesia, slowness in the performance of voluntary movement, is also present.
- Rigidity: involuntary resistance to passive limb movement which is consistent throughout the range of joint movement (*cf.* spasticity) and for this reason sometimes known as "leadpipe rigidity"; a jerky quality ("cogwheeling") may be evident due to superimposed tremor.
- Tremor: typically a 4–6 Hz "pill-rolling" rest tremor of the hand, although a postural tremor (especially with walking) may predate this.
- Some would add postural instability as a key feature (hence a tetrad).
- Symptoms and signs are typically unilateral at onset, gradually spreading to involve the other side.
  Other features which may be seen include:
- Stooped posture; reduced arm swing on walking; difficulty turning; falls only occur in later stages [*cf.* progressive supranuclear palsy (PSP)]
- Pain in rigid muscles
- Micrographia, progressively more evident as writing continues ("slow micrographia")
- Hypomimia, poverty of facial expression, "mask-like" facies
- Hypophonia, monotonic voice
- Sialorrhoea
- Seborrhoea
- Hypometric saccadic eye movements
- Impaired olfactory sense
- Limb dystonia (late)
- Cognitive impairments (late): "Parkinson's disease dementia" (PD-D).

Investigations and diagnosis The diagnosis remains clinical, but problematic: post-mortem studies indicate that only 80% of patients diagnosed in life with idiopathic Parkinson's disease by experienced neurologists have the typical pathological features. Atypical features should prompt consideration of other parkinsonian syndromes, for example early falls consider progressive supranuclear palsy. In patients under 50 years of age, checking blood copper and caeruloplasmin to exclude Wilson's disease is appropriate, since there is specific treatment for this condition which, if missed, produces irreversible effects. Prompt and satisfactory response to levodopa preparations is suggestive of the diagnosis of Parkinson's disease, but may also be seen in some other parkinsonian syndromes.

Rare families with PD should be screened for mutations in the α-synuclein and parkin genes, especially in young onset cases (<30 yrs old) for parkin.

Post-mortem pathology shows macroscopic depigmentation of the substantia nigra, and microscopic depletion of dopaminergic cells with eosinophilic inclusions (Lewy bodies) in those remaining.

Differential diagnosis Other parkinsonian syndromes, viz.

PSP, Steele–Richardson–Olszewski syndrome
Multiple system atrophy (MSA) with predominant parkinsonism (MSA-P)
Corticobasal degeneration (CBD)
Drug-induced parkinsonism, especially related to neuroleptic and anti-emetic use; neuroleptic malignant syndrome
Wilson's disease
Dementia with Lewy bodies (DLB)
Post-encephalitic parkinsonism (encephalitis lethargica, Von Economo's disease)
Huntington's disease (HD), especially juvenile-onset form
Subcortical cerebrovascular disease ("arteriosclerotic parkinsonism")
Normal pressure hydrocephalus (NPH)
Post-traumatic parkinsonism, dementia pugilistica
Systemic lupus erythematosus, Sjögren's syndrome
Hypoparathyroidism.

Treatment and prognosis Levodopa preparations, in combination with peripheral dopa-decarboxylase inhibitors, remain the "gold standard" for the treatment of Parkinson's disease. They are the most reliable medications to produce motor benefit (especially for the akinesia and rigidity, less reliably for tremor), but their prolonged use is associated with development of motor fluctuations (dyskinesias) which can become intrusive and disabling. For this reason, deferring their use is recommended, particularly in young patients (i.e. those judged likely to survive >10 years with the disease), in favour of dopamine agonists. Monotherapy with dopamine agonists in newly diagnosed patients results in fewer dyskinesias at the cost of slightly less good motor improvement. Selegeline, a monoamine oxidase B inhibitor, is another option for early treatment; early claims that it had a neuroprotective effect are difficult to substantiate in view of its undoubted symptomatic effects. Amantadine is sometimes used as early monotherapy. Anticholinergics such as benzhexol may be helpful for tremor but their use is not advised in patients with confusion (likewise dopamine agonists).

When response fluctuations with levodopa set in, they are initially predictable (end of dose or wearing-off effects, peak dose dyskinesias) and may be ameliorated by fractionation of levodopa doses. The catechol-O-methyl transferase (COMT) inhibitor entacapone prolongs the action of levodopa by inhibiting inappropriate metabolism, and is useful for the treatment of wearing-off effects. Addition of dopamine agonists to a levodopa regime may enhance motor benefit and allow reduction of total levodopa dose with reduction in dyskinesias. When response fluctuations become unpredictable (on–off phenomenon, yo-yoing), treatment is difficult and the patient may have to choose between mobility with dyskinesia or immobility: most prefer the former. The dopamine agonist apomorphine, given as an intermittent or continuous subcutaneous injection, may help in this situation. Stereotactic surgery, once popular for tremor, has recently enjoyed a renaissance, with lesions or stimulators being applied to the thalamus, pallidum or subthalamic nucleus. Although still at an experimental stage, such surgery might become more widespread in the future. Thalamotomy seems particularly helpful for tremor, pallidotomy for dyskinesia (and dystonia), and subthalamic stimulation for akinesia and bradykinesia. A prior positive response to dopaminergic therapy is necessary for functional neurosurgery to be beneficial.

References Bhatia K, Brooks DJ, Burn DJ *et al*. Guidelines for the management of Parkinson's disease. The Parkinson's Disease Consensus Working Group. *Hospital Medicine* 1998; **59**: 469–480.

Foltynie T, Sawcer S, Brayne C, Barker RA. The genetic basis of Parkinson's disease. *Journal of Neurology, Neurosurgery and Psychiatry* 2002; **73**: 363–370.

Gardner-Thorpe C. *James Parkinson 1755–1824*. Exeter: A Wheaton & Co. Ltd, 1987.

Hughes AJ, Ben-Shlomo Y, Daniel SE, Lees AJ. What features improve the accuracy of clinical diagnosis in Parkinson's disease: a clinicopathologic study. *Neurology* 1992; **42**: 1142–1146.

Marsden CD. Parkinson's disease. In: Wiles CM (ed.). *Management of Neurological Disorders*. London: BMJ Publishing Group, 1995: 179–203.

Olanow CW, Watts RL, Koller WC. An algorithm (decision tree) for the management of Parkinson's disease (2001): treatment guidelines. *Neurology* 2001; **56 (suppl 5)**: S1–S88.

Quinn N, Bhatia K. Functional neurosurgery for Parkinson's disease. *British Medical Journal* 1998; **316**: 1259–1260.

Schapira AHV. Parkinson's disease. *British Medical Journal* 1999; **318**: 311–314.

Other relevant entries Corticobasal degeneration; Dementia with Lewy bodies; Dystonia: an overview; Encephalitis lethargica; Huntington's disease; Lewy body disease: an overview; Multiple system atrophy; Normal pressure hydrocephalus; Parkinsonian syndromes, parkinsonism; Progressive supranuclear palsy; Sjögren's syndrome; Systemic lupus erythematosus and the nervous system; Wilson's disease.

■ Parkinson's plus

This terminology is sometimes used to describe patients with an extrapyramidal syndrome with additional neurological abnormalities which may point towards a specific parkinsonian syndrome, for example:

- Cerebellar signs: multiple system atrophy (MSA-C).
- Autonomic features: MSA (although autonomic features may occur in Parkinson's disease).

- Pyramidal signs: corticobasal degeneration (CBD).
- Oculomotor features: progressive supranuclear palsy (PSP).
- Cognitive features: dementia with Lewy bodies (DLB).

■ Parkinson's syndrome

Parkinson's syndrome of unilateral abducens (VI) nerve palsy and ipsilateral Horner's syndrome localizes pathology to that part of the cavernous sinus where the sympathetic fibres to the eye briefly join the abducens nerve as they pass from the pericarotid plexus to the ophthalmic branch of the trigeminal nerve.

> **Reference** Silva MN, Saeki N, Hirai S, Yamaura A. Unusual cranial nerve palsy caused by cavernous sinus aneurysms. Clinical and anatomical considerations reviewed. *Surgical Neurology* 1999; **52**: 148–149.

> **Other relevant entries** Cavernous sinus disease; Cranial nerve disease: VI: Abducens nerve; Horner's syndrome.

■ Paroxysmal dyskinesias
Paroxysmal dystonias

Pathophysiology Involuntary movement disorders occurring in brief bursts lasting seconds to hours may be designated as paroxysmal or episodic; some are provoked by movement (kinesigenic). These conditions may be idiopathic (familial or sporadic), symptomatic, or psychogenic in origin. The term encompasses paroxysmal kinesigenic choreoathetosis (PKC)/dystonia and paroxysmal non-kinesigenic dystonia/choreoathetosis (PDC). Other involuntary movement disorders which are both paroxysmal/episodic and dyskinetic are not usually considered under this rubric (e.g. hyperekplexia, tics, stereotypies, Sandifer's syndrome). Hereditary paroxysmal dyskinesias may be channelopathies.

Clinical features: history and examination
- PKC/dystonia
     dystonic postures, chorea, athetosis, ballism; unilateral or bilateral;
     attacks last seconds to 5 minutes;
     frequency of attacks: up to 100 per day;
     triggered by sudden movement, startle, hyperventilation;
     no alteration of consciousness;
     mostly idiopathic or familial; may be symptomatic (e.g. multiple sclerosis);
     sensitive to anticonvulsants;
     may be autosomal dominant or autosomal recessive; past history of febrile fits.
- PDC
As for PKC but:

     longer attacks (2 minutes to 4 hours);
     lower frequency (maximum three per day);
     not triggered by movement;

precipitated by stress, alcohol, caffeine, excitement, fatigue, exercise;
symptomatic causes include endocrine dysfunction (hypoparathyroidism,
hyperthyroidism, hypoglycaemia); structural brain injury, infection;
not sensitive to anticonvulsants;
mostly autosomal dominant.

Paroxysmal exertion-induced dyskinesia/dystonia has also been
described, +/− rolandic epilepsy, writer's cramp.

Investigations and diagnosis

Video attack if possible.

Keep attack diary to look for triggers, precipitants; attack frequency, duration.

Investigate for symptomatic causes, for example endocrine tests, brain imaging.

Differential diagnosis Paroxysmal dystonic features may occur in some symptomatic
dystonias:

Metabolic disorders
Hypoparathyroidism
Thyrotoxicosis
Hartnup's disease
Pyruvate decarboxylase deficiency
D-glyceric acidaemia.
Degenerative conditions (rarely)
Parkinson's disease
Progressive supranuclear palsy (PSP).
Cerebral palsy
Drug induced.

Other conditions which may masquerade as paroxysmal dystonia include:

Focal epilepsy
Hyperekplexia
Tetany
Hysteria
Transient ischaemic attacks
Tonic spasms of MS.

Treatment and prognosis PKC is sensitive to anticonvulsants, for example carbamazepine; symptomatic PKC/PDC may respond to treatment of cause.

References Demirkiran M, Jankovic J. Paroxysmal dyskinesias: clinical features and
classification. *Annals of Neurology* 1995; **38**: 571–579.

Fahn S. The paroxysmal dyskinesias. In: Marsden CD, Fahn S (eds). *Movement
Disorders 3*. Oxford: Butterworth-Heinemann, 1994: 310–345.

Houser MK, Soland VK, Bhatia KP, Quinn NP, Marsden CD. Paroxysmal kinesigenic
choreoathetosis: a report of 26 patients. *Journal of Neurology* 1999; **246**: 120–126.

Other relevant entries Channelopathies: an overview; Episodic ataxias;
Hyperekplexia; Periodic paralysis.

■ Paroxysmal nocturnal haemoglobinuria

This haematological disorder causing intravascular haemolysis and thrombocytopenia may be complicated by cerebral arterial and venous thrombosis.

Other relevant entries Cerebrovascular disease: arterial; Cerebrovascular disease: venous.

■ Parry–Romberg syndrome
Facial hemiatrophy • Hemifacial atrophy

Pathophysiology A clinically and aetiologically heterogeneous syndrome characterized by hemifacial atrophy, sometimes with ipsilateral intracerebral abnormalities producing neurological features. Usually it begins in adolescence or early-adult life, but late-onset cases are also reported. The syndrome may result from maldevelopment of autonomic innervation or vascular supply, or be an acquired feature following trauma or a consequence of linear scleroderma (morphoea). A genetic basis has been suggested, but discordance in monozygotic twins has been observed.

Clinical features: history and examination
- Hemifacial atrophy, especially subcutaneous tissues; may involve bone, brain.
- +/− ipsilateral limb/trunk atrophy.
- Neurological manifestations:
    Hemiparesis
    Hemianopia
    Focal seizures
    Cognitive impairment.
- Dermatological manifestations:
    Coup de sabre
    Circumscribed alopecia; achromia/hyperchromia of hair
    Telangiectatic naevus.

In its most advanced state, the face is gaunt, the skin thin and wrinkled, the hair white or absent and the sebaceous glands atrophic whilst the muscles are unaffected.

Investigations and diagnosis Examination of old photographs to confirm change in facial appearance.
Bloods: markers for scleroderma, for example SCL70, anti-ds DNA, anti-centromere.
In the presence of neurological features:

Imaging: may reveal ipsilateral cerebral atrophy.
Neurophysiology: EEG: focal epileptiform abnormalities.
Autonomic function testing: for example of pupil, facial sweating.

Differential diagnosis Congenital hemiatrophy (usually of whole body) secondary to *in utero* insult or birth injury.

Treatment and prognosis No specific treatment; symptomatic treatment of seizures. In extreme cases, cosmetic surgery may be appropriate.

References Hensiek AE, Hawkes CH. Late presentations of Parry–Romberg syndrome. *Journal of Neurology, Neurosurgery and Psychiatry* 1999; **67**: 839.

Larner AJ, Bennison DP. Some observations on the aetiology of progressive hemifacial atrophy ("Parry–Romberg syndrome"). *Journal of Neurology, Neurosurgery and Psychiatry* 1993; **56**: 1035–1036.

Other relevant entry Systemic sclerosis.

Parsonage–Turner syndrome – see Brachial plexopathies; Neuralgic amyotrophy

Partington syndrome

This congenital dysmorphic syndrome is characterized by low birth weight, short stature, skin pigmentation, facial weakness and delayed closure of the fontanelles, and also enters the differential diagnosis of hereditary dystonia.

Patau syndrome
Trisomy 13

Pathophysiology A chromosomal dysgenetic syndrome producing trisomy of chromosome 13. It occurs in about 1:2000 live births, and is more common in boys.

Clinical features: history and examination

- Typical facies: hypo- or hypertelorism, mongoloid eye slant, microphthalmia or anophthalmia, cleft lip and palate, sloping forehead.
- Holoprosencephaly, severe mental retardation; microcephaly; seizures; hypotonia, hypertonia.
- Optic nerve coloboma.
- Impaired hearing.
- Polydactyly.
- Cryptorchidism.
- Cardiac (80%) and renal (30–50%) anomalies.

Investigations and diagnosis *Imaging*: Brain: may show holoprosencephaly, agenesis of the corpus callosum, and cerebellar anomalies.

Imaging: for cardiac and renal anomalies.

Differential diagnosis Unlikely to be mistaken for Meckel's syndrome.

Treatment and prognosis No specific treatment; symptomatic control of seizures. Death in early childhood, in the majority before the age of 1 year.

Reference Patau K, Smith DW, Therman E, Inhorn SL, Wagner HP. Multiple congenital anomaly caused by an extra autosome. *Lancet* 1960; **1**: 790–793.

Other relevant entries Agenesis of the corpus callosum; Down syndrome; Holoprosencephaly.

■ Patent foramen ovale

Patent foramen ovale (PFO) may be associated with neurological disease, principally stroke due to paradoxical embolism. Divers are at particular risk. Isolated PFO does not seem to increase the risk of recurrent stroke unless it is associated with an atrial septal aneurysm.

An association has also been reported between PFO and transient global amnesia but remains to be corroborated.

References Klotzsch C, Sliwka U, Berlit P, Noth J. An increased frequency of patent foramen ovale in patients with transient global amnesia: analysis of 53 consecutive patients. *Archives of Neurology* 1996; **53**: 504–508.

Mas JL, Arquizan C, Lamy C, Zuber M, Cabanes L, Derumeaux G, Coste J. Recurrent cerebrovascular events associated with patent foramen ovale, atrial septal aneurysm, or both. *New England Journal of Medicine* 2001; **345**: 1740–1746.

Other relevant entries Cerebrovascular disease: arterial; Transient global amnesia.

■ Pavor nocturnus
Night terrors • Sleep terrors

This common parasomnia of slow-wave sleep begins in childhood and may persist into adulthood. There is abrupt arousal in the first part of the night, with intense autonomic and motor symptoms, including loud piercing screams, and the patient appears confused and frightened. In the morning, the patient has no recollection of the event. Many patients have concurrent sleep walking (somnambulism) and a positive family history. Pharmacotherapy is of limited efficacy, options including:

- Hypnotics (e.g. zopiclone);
- Benzodiazepines (e.g. clonazepam);
- Selective serotonin reuptake inhibitors (SSRIs) (e.g. fluoxetine);
- Neuroleptics.

Other relevant entry Parasomnias.

■ Payne syndrome
Rowland–Payne syndrome

A syndrome comprising:
- Phrenic nerve palsy

- Ipsilateral Horner's syndrome
- Ipsilateral vocal cord paresis.

This results from metastatic disease to the neck, usually from breast carcinoma, involving the phrenic nerve, sympathetic chain, and recurrent laryngeal nerve.

> **Reference** Payne CME. Newly recognized syndrome in the neck: Horner's syndrome with ipsilateral vocal cord and phrenic nerve palsies. *Journal of the Royal Society of Medicine* 1981; **74**: 814–818.

■ Pearson's syndrome – see Kearns–Sayre syndrome; Mitochondrial disease: an overview

■ Pelizaeus–Merzbacher disease

Sudanophilic leukodystrophy • Tigroid leukoencephalopathy

Pathophysiology An X-linked-recessive disorder of myelin due to deficiency of proteolipid protein (PLP) usually presenting in the first months of life with a combination of a movement disorder and intellectual decline. Various forms have been described (connatal, classic, transitional, late-onset). More than 60 point mutations in the PLP gene have been identified, accounting for 15–20% of cases; duplication of a portion of the X-chromosome containing the PLP gene may account for another 50–75% of cases. Deletion mutations have also been reported. One of the X-linked forms of hereditary spastic paraparesis (SPG2) is allelic. Patients with the clinical phenotype of Pelizaeus–Merzbacher disease (PMD) but normal PLP gene have been identified, suggesting that other regulatory genes may also be involved in disease pathogenesis.

Clinical features: history and examination

Variable:
- Eye movement disorder: nystagmus (pendular, rotatory, chaotic)
- Head tremor
- Laryngeal stridor
- Choreoathetosis
- Pyramidal signs
- Intellectual decline
- Microcephaly
- Cerebellar ataxia
- Seizures (occasional)
- Optic atrophy (late)
- +/− pes cavus, kyphoscoliosis.

An adult form of PMD known as Lowenberg–Hill syndrome has been described, with autosomal-dominant inheritance.

Investigations and diagnosis *Bloods*: usually normal.

Imaging: MRI may show diffuse symmetrical white matter abnormalities (low intensity on T_1, high intensity on T_2) reflecting dysmyelination.

Neurophysiology:

Evoked potentials: BSAEP, somatosensory evoked potential (SSEP), abnormal; Visual evoked potential (VEP) variably abnormal.

EEG: non-specifically abnormal.

Brain biopsy: patchy dysmyelination, reduced numbers of oligodendrocytes. Absence of myelin in some (Seitelberger variant, neonatal onset).

Neurogenetics: linked to Xq22; point mutations, duplications in PLP gene.

Differential diagnosis Cockayne's syndrome.

Other leukodystrophies.

Spasmus nutans (usually benign).

Treatment and prognosis No specific treatment. Prognosis is uniformly fatal, although survival into the third decade is recorded.

References Garbern J, Cambi F, Shy M, Kamholz J. The molecular pathogenesis of Pelizaeus–Merzbacher disease. *Archives of Neurology* 1999; **56**: 1210–1214.

Seitelberger F. Neuropathology and genetics of Pelizaeus–Merzbacher disease. *Brain Pathology* 1995; **5**: 267–273.

Other relevant entries Alexander's disease; Apraxia; Cockayne's syndrome; Hereditary spastic paraparesis; Leukodystrophies: an overview; Spasmus nutans.

■ Pellagra

Pathophysiology The syndrome of pellagra is often remembered as "dermatitis, diarrhoea, and dementia", although not all these features need be present. It has been thought that pellagra results from a deficiency of niacin (nicotinic acid and nicotinamide). Niacin is found in many foodstuffs (plants, meat, fish) and may be synthesized *in vivo* from the amino acid tryptophan. However, deficiency of other water-soluble vitamins of the B group and possibly tryptophan may also contribute to the pathogenesis of pellagra. Dietary deficiency is now rare, occurring only in areas where maize is the staple diet (southern Africa, India). Other risk factors include prolonged isoniazid therapy without pyridoxine supplementation, Hartnup's disease, chronic alcoholism with malnutrition (in which situation an encephalo-pathic syndrome may occur), general malabsorption, very low protein diets, and the carcinoid syndrome.

Clinical features: history and examination

- Dermatological:
    Dermatitis of skin exposed to sunlight (e.g. Casal's necklace or collar); if chronic, thickening, dryness, and pigmentation may be seen.
- Gastroenterological:
    Commonly diarrhoea but sometimes constipation; glossitis, angular stomatitis, nausea, vomiting.

- Neurological: confined to chronic disease.

   Depression, apathy, hallucinations, psychosis, irritability, insomnia, delirium, impaired consciousness (the encephalopathy of pellagra may be referred to as Jolliffe syndrome).

   $+/-$ extrapyramidal features, cerebellar signs, myelopathy, polyneuropathy, optic atrophy, tremor.

Investigations and diagnosis No specific investigations. Careful dietary history may be necessary; plus investigations for secondary causes (e.g. malabsorption, carcinoid syndrome) if other symptoms and signs suggest.

Pathological findings reported include chromatolysis of large neurones of the motor cortex ("central neuritis" of Adolph Meyer).

Differential diagnosis Deficiency of other water-soluble vitamins of the B group, for example riboflavin, pyridoxine, thiamine, and possibly also of tryptophan. Rash may resemble that seen in Hartnup's disease.

Treatment and prognosis Treatment with niacin alone is often not effective, suggesting the possibility of other deficiencies contributing to the syndrome. Response to nicotinic acid/nicotinamide is better, but it is usual to give vitamin B complex to try to cover other deficiencies. Increasing the protein content of the diet may also be helpful.

Cerebral symptoms and signs may not be completely reversible.

References Coates M. Pellagra. In: Cox FEG (ed.). *The Wellcome Trust Illustrated History of Tropical Diseases*. London: Wellcome Trust, 1996: 398–405.

Langworthy OR. Lesions of the central nervous system characteristic of pellagra. *Brain* 1931; **54**: 291–302.

Serdaru M, Hausser-Hauw C, Laplane D *et al.* The clinical spectrum of alcoholic pellagra encephalopathy. *Brain* 1988; **111**: 829–842.

Other relevant entries Alcohol and the nervous system: an overview; Beriberi; Hartnup's disease; Vitamin deficiencies and the nervous system; Wernicke–Korsakoff's syndrome.

■ PEMA syndrome (of Guiraud), PES syndrome

Names sometimes given to distinctive clinical symptom constellations typically seen in frontal lobe degenerations, and rare in Alzheimer's disease:

PEMA = palilalia, echolalia, mutism, and amimia.
PES = palilalia, echolalia, and stereotypy.

Other relevant entries Alzheimer's disease; Dementia: an overview; Pick's disease.

■ Pendred's syndrome

Congenital hypothyroidism, hearing loss, and vestibular dysfunction.

Other relevant entries Hearing loss: differential diagnosis; Thyroid disease and the nervous system.

■ Perimesencephalic haemorrhage – see Subarachnoid haemorrhage

■ Periodic alternating nystagmus

Periodic alternating nystagmus is a horizontal jerk nystagmus, which damps or stops for a few seconds and then reverses direction. Eye movements may need to be observed for up to 5 minutes to see the whole cycle. Periodic alternating nystagmus may be congenital or acquired, if the latter then its localizing value is similar to that of downbeat nystagmus (with which it may coexist), especially for lesions at the cervico-medullary junction (e.g. Chiari malformation). Treatment of the associated lesion may be undertaken, otherwise periodic alternating nystagmus usually responds to baclofen, hence the importance of correctly identifying this particular form of nystagmus.

> **Reference** Halmagyi GM, Rudge P, Gresty MA *et al.* Treatment of periodic alternating nystagmus. *Annals of Neurology* 1980; **8**: 609–611.

> **Other relevant entries** Chiari malformations; Nystagmus: an overview.

■ Periodic limb movement disorder, periodic limb movements of sleep – see Restless legs syndrome

■ Periodic paralysis

Pathophysiology Periodic paralyses are autosomal-dominant inherited disorders characterized by attacks of weakness, of variable frequency and duration, and with differing precipitants. These disorders were previously classified according to con-current serum potassium ion concentrations as hyperkalaemic (Gamstorp's disease, adynamia episodica hereditaria), hypokalaemic or, rarely, normokalaemic. With the advent of molecular genetic techniques, all these disorders have been shown to result from mutations in genes encoding ion-channel proteins: hyperkalaemic periodic paralysis (PP) results from sodium channel mutations, hypokalaemic PP from muta-tions in the L-type calcium channel gene, potassium channel gene, or even the same sodium channel gene implicated in hyperkalaemic PP. Normokalaemic PP also is associated with sodium channel mutations and hence is a variant of hyperkalaemic PP; at the end of paralytic attacks, serum K^+ may fall, giving a false impression of the concentration during an attack.

These disorders manifest phenotype divergence or allelic heterogeneity: mutations in the sodium channel gene SCN4A may cause hyperkalaemic PP, potassium-aggra-vated myotonia, paramytonia congenita, and even hypokalaemic PP.

Clinical features: history and examination Attacks of limb muscle weakness usually begin in childhood; ocular and respiratory muscles are spared, and consciousness preserved.

	Hyperkalaemic PP	Hypokalaemic PP
Inheritance	Autosomal dominant	Autosomal dominant
Penetrance	100%	100% male, 50% female
Chromosomal location(s):	17q23–q25	1q31–q32
Gene:	SCN4A (sodium channel)	CACNA1S (calcium channel) [SCN4A (sodium channel), KCNE3 (potassium channel)]
Age of onset:	Early childhood to second decade	Early childhood, 60% before age 16, as late as third decade
Time of attacks:	Morning	Night, early morning
Provoking factors:	Rest after exercise Fasting Oral K^+ intake	Strenuous physical activity Carbohydrate rich meal High sodium intake
Duration of attacks:	10 minutes to 1 hour	Hours to days
Clinical features:	Weakness longer and more severe in hypokalaemic PP as compared to hyperkalaemic PP; no myotonia in hypokalaemic PP; females with hypokalaemic PP may present with a late-onset proximal myopathy.	

Investigations and diagnosis *Bloods*: K^+ level during an attack (sent immediately to laboratory to avoid haemolysis and false reading; often missed). Nowadays, if the diagnosis is suspected clinically, sending blood to a reference laboratory for mutation analysis is appropriate. Concurrent thyroid function tests (association with thyrotoxicosis may be known as Kitamura syndrome).

Neurophysiology: EMG/NCS: decrement in compound muscle action potential amplitude after a period of sustained exercise is characteristic.

Differential diagnosis Thyrotoxic PP: especially in Orientals with onset in adulthood; otherwise clinically indistinguishable from hypokalaemic PP.

Treatment and prognosis Avoid recognized precipitating factors.

Many patients with hyperkalaemic PP benefit from treatments which prevent hyperkalaemia (i.e. prophylaxis for weakness): thiazide diuretics, β-adrenoreceptor agonists (e.g. salbutamol); carbonic anhydrase inhibitors (e.g. acetazolamide, dichlorphenamide) may also help.

If present (hyperkalaemic PP), myotonia may be treated with mexiletine.

Frequency and severity of attacks diminish with age.

A progressive vacuolar myopathy may develop.

Reference Kullman DM. The neuronal channelopathies. *Brain* 2002; **125**: 1177–1195.

Other relevant entries Channelopathies: an overview; Episodic ataxias; Myotonia and myotonic disorders; Paramyotonia; Potassium-aggravated myotonia; Thyroid disease and the nervous system.

■ Perisylvian syndrome

Developmental Foix–Chavany–Marie syndrome

Pathophysiology A limited and localized developmental brain injury, thought to be ischaemic in origin, involving the perisylvian regions of the brain, causing facial weakness, and speech problems. Some cases may be related to loss of a monochorionic twin in early pregnancy.

Clinical features: history and examination

- Pregnancy history: loss of twin.
- Developmental delay.
- Cognitive deficits, although comprehension may be relatively preserved.
- Pseudobulbar symptoms:
     abnormal tongue movements (side to side, $+/-$ protrusion)
     voluntary orofacial paresis (emotional movements preserved)
     variable dysarthria
     dysphagia
     drooling may be prominent
     absent gag reflex
     brisk jaw jerk.
- Seizures, onset age 6–12 months.
- Pyramidal signs.

Investigations and diagnosis *Imaging*: MRI: bilateral perisylvian atrophy with cortical malformations (polymicrogyria).

Differential diagnosis Worster-Drought Syndrome: some cases originally labelled as such (before the advent of neuroimaging) may in fact represent the perisylvian syndrome, although Worster-Drought's cases did not have seizures or mental retardation.

Foix–Chavany–Marie syndrome/opercular syndrome.

In patients labelled as "cerebral palsy" in whom bulbar or oromotor dysfunction is prominent, this diagnosis needs to be considered.

Treatment and prognosis

Speech therapy.

Symptomatic control of seizures; if intractable, surgery may be indicated (commissurotomy).

> **Reference** Kuzniecky R, Andermann F, Guerrini R and the CBPS Multicenter Collaborative Study. Congenital bilateral perisylvian syndrome: a study of 31 patients. *Lancet* 1991; **341**: 608–612.

> **Other relevant entries** Cerebral palsy, cerebral palsy syndromes; Foix–Chavany–Marie syndrome; Worster-Drought Syndrome (2).

■ Pernicious anaemia – see Vitamin B$_{12}$ deficiency

Peroneal muscular atrophy – see Charcot–Marie–Tooth syndrome; Hereditary motor and sensory neuropathy; Neuropathies: an overview

Peroneal neuropathy

Common peroneal nerve palsy

Pathophysiology The common peroneal nerve is the lateral division of the sciatic nerve, comprising fibres from the L4 to S2 spinal roots. It branches from the sciatic nerve within the popliteal fossa, giving rise to sural and lateral cutaneous sensory branches before winding around the head of the fibula where it is particularly vulnerable to compression injury. Beyond the tendinous arch formed by the peroneus longus muscle, it divides into the superifical peroneal nerve, which supplies the peroneus longus and brevis, and the deep peroneal nerve which innervates tibialis anterior, extensor hallucis longus, and extensor digitorum longus muscles, then via its terminal portion extensor digitorum brevis.

Clinical features: history and examination

- Motor: foot drop (weak tibialis anterior, extensor hallucis longus, and extensor digitorum longus causing weak ankle dorsiflexion, ankle eversion and toe dorsiflexion; ankle inversion and foot plantar flexion spared, *cf.* L5 radiculopathy); often no reflex loss although the ankle jerk may be lost.
- Sensory: minimal; anterolateral lower leg, dorsum of foot.

Investigations and diagnosis *EMG/NCS*: may identify site and extent of axonal injury, and distinguish peroneal neuropathy from L4 to L5 radiculopathy.

Differential diagnosis Other causes of lower motor neurone (floppy) foot drop (*q.v.*):

lumbar radiculopathy

lumbosacral plexopathy

sciatic neuropathy involving lateral division only.

References Katirji B. Peroneal neuropathy. *Neurologic Clinics* 1999; **17**: 567–591.

Staal A, Van Gijn J, Spaans F. *Mononeuropathies: Examination, Diagnosis and Treatment*. London: WB Saunders, 1999: 133–141.

Other relevant entries Foot drop: differential diagnosis; Lumbar cord and root disease; Neuropathies: an overview; Sciatic neuropathy; Tibial neuropathy.

Peroxisomal disorders: an overview

Pathophysiology Peroxisomes are subcellular organelles, dysfunction of which produces a heterogeneous group of multisystem disorders, usually with neonatal or childhood onset:

- Zellweger syndrome
- Pseudo-Zellweger syndrome
- Neonatal adrenoleukodystrophy

- Infantile Refsum's disease
- Rhizomelic chondrodysplasia punctata.

Peroxisomes may be absent (e.g. Zellweger syndrome), lack a particular enzyme (e.g. X-linked adrenoleukodystrophy) or have defective enzymes (e.g. Zellweger-like syndrome, Refsum's disease). Accumulation of very long-chain fatty acids (VLCFAs) in tissues and plasma is a feature of most of these disorders. Genetic testing for some variants (all X-linked or autosomal recessive) is now available. Neurological features may or may not be present.

Clinical features: history and examination

- Broad phenotype: features which raise the possibility of a peroxisomal disorder in neonates or infants include:

    Seizures
    Craniofacial dysmorphology
    Psychomotor retardation
    Sensorineural hearing impairment
    Peripheral neuropathy
    Ocular abnormalities: congenital cataract, retinitis pigmentosa, abnormal ERG
    Hypotonia
    Hepatomegaly, hepatocellular dysfunction
    Renal cysts.

Investigations and diagnosis If a peroxisomal disorder is suspected, liaison with specialist units/laboratories for advice regarding investigations is recommended. Investigations may include:

    Plasma VLCFAs
    +/− phytanic acid, pristanic acid, pipecolic acid, bile acids
    Red blood cell plasmalogens
    Study of cultured fibroblasts to identify enzymatic basis of syndrome
    Synacthen test
    Liver biopsy
    Neurogenetics
    Brain imaging
    Neurophysiology: EEG, EMG/NCS, ERG, Evoked potentials.

Differential diagnosis See individual entries.

Treatment and prognosis Pharmacological induction of peroxisomes, for example with sodium 4-phenylbutyrate, has been suggested on the basis of successful *in vivo* animal studies.

References McGuinness MC, Wei H, Smith KD. Therapeutic developments in peroxisome biogenesis disorders. *Expert Opinion on Investigational Drugs* 2000; **9**: 1985–1992.

Moser HW, Raymond GV. Genetic peroxisomal disorders: why, when, and how to test. *Annals of Neurology* 1998; **44**: 713–715.

Powers JM, Moser HW. Peroxisomal disorders: genotype, phenotype, major neuropathologic lesions, and pathogenesis. *Brain Pathology* 1998; **8**: 101–120.

Theil AC, Schutgens RBH, Wanders RJA, Heymans HSA. Clinical recognition of patients affected by a peroxisomal disorder: a retrospective study in 40 patients. *European Journal of Paediatrics* 1992; **151**: 117–120.

Other relevant entries Adrenoleukodystrophy; Allgrove's syndrome; Refsum's disease; Zellweger syndrome.

■ Perry syndrome

A very rare autosomal-dominant parkinsonian syndrome with associated mental depression, apathy, central hypoventilation, and weight loss. Parkinsonism may be levodopa responsive but the other features are not. The respiratory problems may require tracheostomy and home ventilation. The condition does not seem to be linked to mutations in the α-synuclein gene.

Other relevant entry Parkinsonian syndromes, parkinsonism.

■ Persistent vegetative state – see Vegetative states

■ Pfeiffer syndrome
Acrocephalosyndactyly V • Thanatophoric dysplasia

Pathophysiology An autosomal-dominant syndrome of premature closure of cranial sutures, with cutaneous syndactylies. The condition has been linked to mutations in the gene encoding fibroblast growth factor-receptor 1 and 2 (FGFR), some of which are identical to those found in Crouzon syndrome.

Clinical features: history and examination

- Acrobrachicephaly (tower skull) or turribrachicephaly ("clover leaf skull", kleeblattschädel); raised intracranial pressure.
- Hypertelorism, divergent strabismus, antimongoloid palpebral fissures
- Radiohumeral, radioulnar synostoses.
- Large thumbs with deviating terminal phalanges; large first toes.
- Low set ears.
- Irregularly aligned teeth.
- Mental development usually normal.
- +/− cortical dysgenesis.

Investigations and diagnosis *Imaging*: shows typical skull abnormalities; MRI may show cortical dysgenesis.

Neurophysiology:

EEG: may show abnormalities beyond those expected from raised intracranial pressure alone, suggesting presence of cortical dysgenesis.

Visual evoked potentials (VEPs): may be absent.

Differential diagnosis Other acrocephalosyndactyly syndromes.

Treatment and prognosis No specific treatment. Death usual within days of birth. Symptomatic treatment of raised intracranial pressure.

References Pfeiffer RA. Dominant erbliche Akrocephalosyndaktylie. *Z, Kinderheild*. 1964; **90**: 301–320.

Schell V, Hehr A, Feldman GJ *et al*. Mutations in FGFR1 and FGFR2 cause familial and sporadic Pfeiffer syndrome. *Human Molecular Genetics* 1995; **4**: 323–328.

Other relevant entries Apert syndrome; Carpenter syndrome; Craniostenosis; Saethre–Chotzen syndrome.

■ Phaeochromocytoma – see Erythrocyanotic headache; Hypertension and the nervous system; Neurofibromatosis; Pure autonomic failure; Von Hippel–Lindau disease

■ Phakomatosis

Congenital ectodermosis • Neurocutaneous syndrome

Phakomatoses are hereditary disorders involving ectodermal structures [central nervous system (CNS), eyes, skin], which evolve slowly during childhood and adolescence, and show a tendency to hamartoma formation (benign tumour-like developmental lesions, which may undergo malignant transformation).

The disorders encompassed by this category include:

- Neurofibromatosis
- Tuberous sclerosis.

A number of conditions characterized by cutaneous angiomatosis with CNS abnormalities, including:

- Sturge–Weber syndrome
- Von Hippel–Lindau (VHL) disease
- Ataxia telangiectasia (Louis–Bar syndrome)
- Fabry's disease
- Osler–Weber–Rendu syndrome.

These conditions are usually set apart from other diseases involving skin and brain in which ectodermal malformations (often haemangiomas) develop *in utero* rather than in childhood and adolescence, although both may be encompassed under the rubric of "neurocutaneous syndrome". Within the latter group are conditions such as:

- Bloch–Sulzberger syndrome (incontinentia pigmenti)
- Blue rubber bleb naevus syndrome
- Epidermal naevus syndrome
- Sjögren–Larsson syndrome

- Rothmund–Thomson syndrome
- Xeroderma pigmentosum.

Other conditions with neurological and non-haemangiomatous dermatological features may also be labelled as neurocutaneous syndromes, for example Cowden's disease, Leopard syndrome, Lesch–Nyhan syndrome, Parry–Romberg syndrome, pseudoxanthoma elasticum, Sweet's syndrome, Weber–Christian disease.

Neurofibromatosis, tuberous sclerosis, and VHL disease probably result from mutations in tumour suppressor genes, as in retinoblastoma. A loss of heterozygosity in tumour cells suggests a "two-hit" mechanism in tumour pathogenesis.

Clinical features: history and examination/investigations and diagnosis/differential diagnosis/treatment and prognosis See individual entries.

> **References** Berg BO. Neurocutaneous syndromes. In: Aminoff MJ (ed.). *Neurology and General Medicine. The Neurological Aspects of Medical Disorders* (2nd edition). New York: Churchill Livingstone, 1995: 201–218.
>
> Grant R. Neurocutaneous syndromes. In: Donaghy M (ed.). *Brain's Diseases of the Nervous System* (11th edition). Oxford: OUP, 2001: 585–599.
>
> Miller VS, Roach ES. Neurocutaneous syndromes. In: Bradley WG, Daroff RB, Fenichel GM, Marsden CD (eds). *Neurology in Clinical Practice* (3rd edition). Boston: Butterworth-Heinemann, 2000: 1665–1700.

> **Other relevant entries** Ataxia telangiectasia; Blue rubber bleb naevus syndrome; Fabry's disease; Incontinentia pigmenti (achromians); Lesch–Nyhan syndrome; Neurofibromatosis; Osler–Weber–Rendu syndrome; Parry–Romberg syndrome; Pseudoxanthoma elasticum; Rothmund–Thomson syndrome; Sjögren–Larsson syndrome; Sturge–Weber syndrome; Tuberous sclerosis; Von Hippel–Lindau disease; Weber–Christian disease; Wyburn–Mason disease; Xeroderma pigmentosum and related conditions.

▓ Phenylalanine hydroxylase deficiency – see Phenylketonuria

▓ Phenylketonuria
Phenylalanine hydroxylase deficiency

Pathophysiology An autosomal-recessive disorder of amino acid metabolism, caused by deficiency of the hepatic enzyme phenylalanine hydroxylase (PAH), the resultant metabolic block leading to hyperphenylalaninaemia. Effective neonatal screening for this disorder, and treatment with a phenylalanine-free diet, has made complications from this condition rare.

Clinical features: history and examination *Of the untreated condition*:
- Developmental delay from about 2 months of age, $+/-$ persistent vomiting
- Mental retardation
- Hyperkinesia

- Psychosis
- Seizures (25%; myoclonic)
- Microcephaly
- Pyramidal/extrapyramidal signs unusual despite central nervous system (CNS) involvement
- Musty smell
- Fair complexion, eczematoid lesions.

Investigations and diagnosis

Bloods: phenylalanine >1.2 mmol/l (NR < 0.15 mmol/l).

Liver biopsy for enzyme assay.

Neurophysiology: EEG: diffusely abnormal.

Imaging: MRI: symmetrical periventricular white matter changes in parieto-occipital region; changes may regress with resumption of exclusion diet.

Neurogenetics: many point mutations in the PAH gene, located at chromosome 12q22–q24.1, have been described, resulting in differing degrees of residual enzyme activity.

Differential diagnosis Clinical features: adrenoleukodystrophy, multiple sclerosis. Childhood mental retardation: fragile X syndrome, homocystinuria. Raised serum phenylalanine: biopterin deficiency.

Treatment and prognosis Restriction of phenylalanine intake; although unpalatable, the diet is most effective if commenced before the end of the first month of life [hence the importance of neonatal screening for phenylketonuria (PKU)].

Monitoring of blood phenylalanine levels may be helpful to check compliance. Prognosis is very good if treatment is initiated in the first month of life.

References Eisensmith RC, Woo SLC. Phenylketonuria. In: Conneally PM (ed.). *Molecular Basis of Neurology*. Boston: Blackwell Scientific, 1993: 181–198.

Thompson AJ, Tillotson S, Smith I *et al*. Brain MRI changes in phenylketonuria. Association with dietary status. *Brain* 1993; **116**: 811–821.

Other relevant entries Aminoacidopathies: an overview; Biopterin deficiency; Hartnup's disease; Maple syrup urine disease.

▓ Phosphoenolpyruvate carboxykinase deficiency

The enzyme phosphoenolpyruvate carboxykinase (PEPCK) is important in gluconeogenesis. PEPCK in the mitochondrial and cytosolic compartments catalyses the conversion of oxaloacetate, produced by the carboxylation of pyruvate, to phosphoenolpyruvate which is then converted to glucose by a series of steps which mirror those of glycolysis. PEPCK deficiency is a very rare hereditary disorder of gluconeogenesis resulting in severe hypoglycaemia, lactic acidosis, hepatomegaly, renal tubular dysfunction, hypotonia, and deteriorating liver function. Steatosis and inflammatory change may be seen on liver biopsy. Diagnosis may be established by measuring enzyme activity in fibroblasts.

■ Phosphofructokinase deficiency – see Tarui disease

■ Phosphoglycerate kinase deficiency
Bresolin's disease • Glycogen-storage disease (GSD) type IX

Deficiency of this glycolytic pathway enzyme, encoded by a gene at Xq13 and hence an X-linked-recessive trait, produces a phenotype similar to that of myophosphorylase deficiency, along with haemolytic anaemia, mental retardation and seizures.

Other relevant entries Glycogen-storage disorders: an overview; McArdle's disease.

■ Phosphoglycerate mutase deficiency
Tonin's disease • Glycogen-storage disease (GSD) type X

Deficiency of this enzyme, encoded by a gene at 7p12–p13, produces a phenotype similar to that of myophosphorylase deficiency, with attacks of muscle pain and myoglobinuria; there may also be high levels of uric acid with gout.

Other relevant entries Glycogen-storage disorders: an overview; McArdle's disease.

■ Phosphorylase deficiency – see McArdle's disease

■ Phycomycosis – see Mucormycosis

■ Phytanic acid-storage disease – see Refsum's disease

■ Pick's disease
Focal lobar atrophy • Frontotemporal dementia (FTD) • Frontotemporal lobar degeneration • Pick complex • Primary progressive aphasia (PPA) • Semantic dementia (SD)

Pathophysiology Pick originally presented (1892) a report of focal cerebral atrophy, affecting predominantly frontal and/or temporal lobes. It was not until 1911 that Alzheimer described the microscopic pathological changes in these cases which subsequently became known as Pick bodies and Pick cells. Latterly it became apparent that focal atrophy could occur with different pathological changes. Hence, debate as to what should be included under the rubric of "Pick's disease" continues, the extreme positions being represented by those who accept only Pick body positive focal lobar atrophy (almost impossible to predict from clinical findings alone), and those who accept lobar atrophy independent of the pathological findings.

Clinical features: history and examination Depending on the precise definition accepted, the clinical phenotype of Pick's disease may be very broad, encompassing:

- Behavioural disorder (frontal lobe degeneration): restlessness, aggression, wandering.
- Language disorder:
  non-fluent: primary progressive aphasia (PPA)
  fluent: semantic dementia (SD).

Overlap between these entities tends to develop with prolonged follow-up.

Investigations and diagnosis *Neuropsychology*: may show focal deficits in frontal lobe tasks (frontal lobe degeneration), or language function, which deteriorate with sequential testing.

Imaging: CT/MRI may show focal atrophy; may be unilateral; functional imaging (SPECT/PET) may show reduced perfusion/metabolism of the frontal +/− temporal lobes, may be asymmetric.

Neurophysiology: EEG: tends to remain normal in frontotemporal dementia (*cf.* Alzheimer's disease).

CSF: may show an elevated protein, non-specific.

Differential diagnosis The behavioural disorder may be confused with mania. Although frontal deficits occur in Alzheimer's disease they tend to develop *pari passu* with the other features (amnesia, visuospatial problems) rather than in advance of them.

Treatment and prognosis No specific treatment. Behavioural features may be helped with carbamazepine.

> **References** Hodges J. Pick's disease: its relationship to progressive aphasia, semantic dementia and frontotemporal dementia. In: O'Brien J, Ames D, Burns A (eds). *Dementia* (2nd edition). London: Arnold, 2000: 747–758.
>
> Kertesz A, Munoz DG (eds). *Pick's Disease and Pick Complex*. New York: Wiley, 1998.
>
> Snowden JS, Neary D, Mann DMA. *Fronto-Temporal Lobar Degeneration: Fronto-Temporal Dementia, Progressive Aphasia, Semantic Dementia*. New York: Churchill Livingstone, 1996.
>
> **Other relevant entries** Alzheimer's disease; Dementia: an overview; Frontotemporal dementia; Primary progressive aphasia; Progressive subcortical gliosis (of Neumann); Semantic dementia.

■ Pickwickian syndrome
Obesity–hypoventilation syndrome

Pathophysiology A syndrome of somnolence, hypoventilation, and episodic apnoea in obese children, named for a character (Joe, the fat boy) who appeared in Charles Dickens's *Posthumous Papers of the Pickwick Club* (1836–1837). The associated ruddy complexion and dropsy are also mentioned by Dickens (although other authors suspect Joe may have suffered from Prader–Willi syndrome, a diencephalic tumour, or the consequences of a head injury). Pickwickian syndrome represents a very advanced form of obstructive sleep apnoea syndrome (OSAS).

Clinical features: history and examination

- Excessive daytime somnolence.
- Apnoeic episodes during sleep; snoring.
- Obesity.
- Narrow anteroposterior pharyngeal diameter.
- Limited diaphragm movement secondary to fat accumulation.
- +/− right heart failure.
- +/− bilateral optic disc oedema.

Investigations and diagnosis *Sleep study* (pulse oximetry, nocturnal polysomnography) to monitor apnoeic episodes, oxygen desaturation during snoring.
Blood: polycythaemia.

Differential diagnosis OSAS.

Treatment and prognosis Nocturnal intermittent positive-pressure ventilation; weight loss.

References Burwell CS, Robin ED, Whaley RD, Bickelmann AG. Extreme obesity associated with alveolar hypoventilation – a Pickwickian syndrome. *American Journal of Medicine* 1956: **21**: 811–818.

Gastaut H, Tassinari CA, Duron B. Polygraphic study of the episodic diurnal and nocturnal (hypnic and respiratory) manifestations of the Pickwick syndrome. *Brain Research* 1966; **1**: 167–186.

Other relevant entries Obstructive sleep apnoea syndrome; Prader–Willi syndrome; Sleep disorders: an overview.

■ Pierre Robin syndrome
First pharyngeal arch syndrome

Pathophysiology A fairly common developmental dysmorphic syndrome, possibly autosomal recessive, characterized by the triad of lower jaw hypoplasia, cleft palate, and glossoptosis. This may occur in isolation, the Pierre Robin triad, or as a component of a more widespread syndrome, Pierre Robin syndrome or complex.

Clinical features: history and examination

- Microcephaly without craniostenosis.
- Symmetrical lower jaw hypoplasia causing chin recession; micrognathia leads to retroglossia and glossoptosis; narrowing of the airway may cause stridor, hypoxia.
- Cleft palate.
- Flat nasal bridge, low set ears.
- +/− bulging of upper rib cage.
- Mental retardation: ?secondary to brain anomaly, hypoxia.
- Short stature (bent bones, short limbs).
- +/− congenital heart disease.

Investigations and diagnosis Diagnosis by clinical appearance at birth.

Differential diagnosis Clinical picture is typical.

Treatment and prognosis Maintenance of airway, oxygen to prevent hypoxia; tracheostomy as a last resort.

Surgery to cleft palate, lower jaw.

> **Reference** McKenzie J. The first arch syndrome. *Developmental Medicine and Child Neurology* 1966; **8**: 55–66.

> **Other relevant entry** Treacher Collins syndrome.

■ Pineal tumours

Numerous tumour types may arise within the pineal gland. The clinical presentation may be with Parinaud's syndrome (*q.v.*), diabetes insipidus, or hydrocephalus.

Tumours may be:

Parenchymal:
  Pineocytoma
  Parenchymal tumour with intermediate differentiation
  Pineoblastoma (resembles primitive neuroectodermal tumour).
Germ-cell tumours (*q.v.*): germinoma, teratoma, etc.
Glioma.
Metastases (e.g. lung).
Cysts: simple, dermoid, epidermoid.

Although tumour markers may give the diagnosis (e.g. for certain germ-cell tumours), biopsy or surgery may be necessary to identify tumour type precisely.

> **Reference** Hirato J, Nakazato Y. Pathology of pineal region tumors. *Journal of Neuro-oncology* 2001; **54**: 239–249.

> **Other relevant entries** Germ-cell tumours; Germinoma; Parinaud's syndrome; Primitive neuroectodermal tumour; Teratoma.

■ Piriformis syndrome

Pathophysiology A syndrome of gluteal and leg pain ascribed to entrapment of the sciatic nerve by the piriformis muscle as it passes beneath it, beyond the sciatic notch. Few rigorous case reports support the existence of this syndrome: at best it is very unusual.

Clinical features: history and examination
- Unilateral gluteal pain, $+/-$ leg pain along back of thigh, calf.
- Localized tenderness over piriformis muscle (may also be found in patients with plexopathy or lumbosacral radiculopathy).
- Absent or asymmetric ankle jerk.
- Sensory abnormalities along the lateral aspect of the foot, fifth toe.

Investigations and diagnosis *Neurophysiology*: EMG/NCS: absent or low amplitude sural sensory nerve action potential; prolonged or dispersed tibial nerve F waves;

abnormal H reflex; normal lower limb nerve conduction velocities. Denervation potentials in gastrocnemius +/− hamstring (i.e. as in other causes of sciatic neuropathy).

Imaging: CT/MRI of lumbosacral region: normal.

Differential diagnosis Other causes of proximal sciatic neuropathy:

L5–S1 disc herniation
Intrapelvic compressive lesion: carcinoma, lymphoma
Pelvic bone lesion: sarcoma, metastasis
Idiopathic lumbosacral plexopathy
Intraneural neurofibroma
Diabetic ischaemic neuropathy.

Treatment and prognosis Surgical decompression may, theoretically, be appropriate.

Reference Al-Memar AY, Hudson N, Thomas G, Hughes P, Wimalaratna HSK. The piriformis syndrome: a sciatic nerve entrapment. *Journal of Neurology, Neurosurgery and Psychiatry* 1997; **62**: 210.

Other relevant entries Entrapment neuropathies; Neuropathies: an overview; Sciatic neuropathy.

Pisa syndrome

The so-called "Pisa syndrome" is a rare extrapyramidal side-effect caused by neuroleptic medications, characterized by twisting and bending of the upper thorax, neck and head, to one side. Tilting symptoms occurring bilaterally may be labelled as "metronome Pisa syndrome".

Pituitary disease and apoplexy

Pathophysiology Disease of the pituitary gland, most usually an adenoma, may produce both local effects, due to compression of adjacent neurological structures (most commonly the optic chiasm), and distant effects due to endocrinological changes. Infarction of an adenoma which has outgrown its blood supply leads to the syndrome of pituitary apoplexy, an acute medical emergency. Ischaemic necrosis of the pituitary gland, occurring most often in the postpartum period (Sheehan's syndrome), can cause panhypopituitarism.

Occasionally pituitary tumours may occur in the context of familial syndromes:

- Multiple endocrine neoplasia (MEN) type 1: autosomal dominant; parathyroid, endocrine pancreas, and pituitary tumours (especially prolactinoma); linked to chromosome 11q13;
- Carney complex: skin and cardiac myxoma; testicular, adrenal, and pituitary tumours;
- McCune–Albright syndrome (*q.v.*).

Clinical features: history and examination

- Local:

  Chiasmal compression: bitemporal hemianopia, junctional scotoma of Traquair (pre-chiasmal compression)

  Optic atrophy, visual failure

  Headache

  Ocular palsies (extension to cavernous sinus)

  Seizures (extension to temporal lobe)

  Somnolence, diabetes insipidus (hypothalamic extension)

  CSF rhinorrhoea.

- Distant (endocrine):

  Prolactinoma: secondary amenorrhoea, thin skin

  Adrenocorticotropic hormone (ACTH) (Cushing's disease): myopathy, hypertension, osteoporosis, striae

  GH: gigantism, acromegaly

  LH, FSH (rare)

  TSH (rare).

- Apoplexy:

  Acute headache

  Visual loss

  Ophthalmoplegia (parasellar extension)

  Drowsiness/coma (diagnosis may be difficult if pituitary tumour not previously diagnosed).

  Panhypopituitarism (Simmonds syndrome): may follow tumour, apoplexy.

Investigations and diagnosis *Bloods*: prolactin (majority of functioning tumours, 60–70%); GH, ACTH, LH, FSH, TSH.

Imaging: CT: enlarged, eroded sella turcica; MRI shows extent of tumour, relation to optic nerves, other local structures; in apoplexy, MRI shows infarction of tumour with or without haemorrhage above the sella.

Visual field mapping: to document visual field defects.

CSF: in apoplexy shows pleocytosis +/− subarachnoid haemorrhage.

Differential diagnosis Visual field changes may be confused with those secondary to craniopharyngioma.

Apoplexy: intracerebral or subarachnoid haemorrhage, encephalitis or meningitis, eclampsia, idiopathic thunderclap headache.

Treatment and prognosis Medical: prolactinoma: dopamine agonists (bromocriptine, cabergoline); acromegaly: octreotide.

Surgical: excision: trans-sphenoidal approach, transcranial if suprasellar extension.

Apoplexy: acute medical emergency: dexamethasone +/− surgery.

References Brougham M, Heusner AP, Adams RD. Acute degenerative changes in adenomas of the pituitary body – with special reference to pituitary apoplexy. *Journal of Neurosurgery* 1950; **7**: 421–439.

Link MJ, Pollock BE. Diagnosis and treatment of pituitary tumors. In: Noseworthy
    JH (ed.). *Neurological Therapeutics: Principles and Practice*. London: Dunitz,
    2003: 724–736.

Reid RL, Quigley ME, Yen SSC. Pituitary apoplexy: a review. *Archives of Neurology*
    1985; **42**: 712–719.

Other relevant entries Carney complex; Cavernous sinus disease;
    Craniopharyngioma; Endocrinology and the nervous system; Gigantism;
    McCune–Albright syndrome; Ophthalmoplegia; Optic atrophy; Subarachnoid
    haemorrhage; Thunderclap headache; Thyroid disease and the nervous system.

▓ Pleurodynia – see Myositis

▓ Plexopathy – see Brachial plexopathies; Lumbosacral plexopathies; Neuropathies: an overview

▓ Plumbism – see Lead and the nervous system

▓ Plumboporphyria

In this rare inherited condition, lead exposure within accepted safety limits precipi-
tates porphyric neuropathy (especially wrist drop), due to an underlying deficiency
of the enzyme δ-aminolaevulinic acid dehydratase (ALAD).

Reference Dyer J, Garrick DP, Ingus A, Pye IF. Plumboporphyria (ALAD deficiency)
    in a lead worker: a scenario for potential diagnostic confusion. *British Journal of
    Industrial Medicine* 1993; **50**: 1119–1121.

Other relevant entries Neuropathies: an overview; Porphyria.

▓ POEMS syndrome
Crow–Fukase syndrome

Pathophysiology A rare multisystem disorder, commoner in men, characterized by
osteosclerotic myeloma (plasmacytoma) with a circulating monoclonal protein, and
peripheral neuropathy. Immunopathogenesis is uncertain but the condition does
improve following disappearance of the M protein.

Clinical features: history and examination

- POEMS is an acronym for the chief clinical features:

    P = polyneuropathy: demyelinating, predominantly motor, type; cranial nerves
        typically spared, although papilloedema may occur in up to 60%;

    O = organomegaly: hepatosplenomegaly;

    E = endocrinopathy: gynaecomastia and impotence in males; secondary amenor-
        rhoea in females; diabetes mellitus; hypothyroidism;

M = M-protein, usually λ-light chains, IgM, IgA;

S = skin changes: hyperpigmentation, hypertrichosis, skin thickening.

+ / − cardiomyopathy, pleural effusion, peripheral oedema, ascites.

- Castlemann disease (angiofollicular lymphoid hyperplasia, a diffuse B-cell dyscrasia as opposed to a focal myelomatous lesion) may also be associated with a syndrome of POEMS type.

Investigations and diagnosis

Bloods: M protein with λ-light chains.

CSF: raised protein.

Imaging: skeletal survey to identify sclerotic lesions.

Biopsy: of sclerotic lesion, to confirm plasmacytoma.

Differential diagnosis

Myeloma.

Chronic inflammatory demyelinating polyneuropathy (CIDP), other demyelinating neuropathy (e.g. paraprotein-associated demyelinating neuropathy).

Treatment and prognosis There is no report of spontaneous remission or stabilization without treatment. Single lesions may be surgically excised or irradiated; improvement may not be apparent for several months thereafter. Medical treatment with prednisolone and melphalan has also been used, and autologous stem-cell transplantation has been tried. A report of benefit with tamoxifen has appeared.

References Enevoldson TP, Harding AE. Improvement in the POEMS syndrome after administration of tamoxifen. *Journal of Neurology, Neurosurgery and Psychiatry* 1992; **55**: 71–72.

Jaccord A, Royer B, Bordessoule D, Brouet JC, Fermand JP. High-dose therapy and autologous blood stem cell transplantation in POEMS syndrome. *Blood* 2002; **99**: 3057–3059.

Other relevant entries Monoclonal gammopathies; Neuropathies: an overview; Paraproteinaemic neuropathies.

Poland anomaly

This is the absence of the pectoral muscle, with or without radial ray abnormalities in the upper limb. It may occur in conjunction with Möbius syndrome, hence Poland–Möbius syndrome, which may be familial.

Other relevant entry Möbius syndrome.

Poliodystrophy – see Alpers disease; Menkes' disease

Poliomyelitis

Pathophysiology Infection with poliovirus (a small RNA enterovirus) is usually asymptomatic or non-specific, but occasionally paralytic disease, resulting from the neurotropic properties of the virus, may be devastating or fatal. Children are particularly vulnerable. Vaccination programmes have greatly reduced the frequency of the disease in developed countries, although occasional cases in vaccine recipients or their unvaccinated family members are still reported.

Clinical features: history and examination

- Incubation: 3–35 days.

    Malaise, sore throat, gastrointestinal upset, headache, vomiting, fever; meningeal irritation, low back pain.

- Neurological illness:

    Aseptic lymphocytic meningitis, followed by flaccid paralysis (proximal > distal, legs > arms), often asymmetric, +/− muscle pain, tenderness; areflexia (involvement of anterior horn cells), atrophy, +/− fasciculation.

    Involvement of cranial nerve nuclei (10–15%), causing bulbar weakness, facial weakness less often.

    Respiratory failure (bulbar involvement).

    Autonomic involvement: hyper- or hypohidrosis, systemic hypertension (less commonly hypotension), urinary retention.

    Definite sensory loss very rare but documented (dorsal root ganglia involvement).

    Extraocular muscles not involved.

    Rarely encephalitic illness.

- 10% fatality rate in acute paralytic illness.
- Scoliosis developed in virtually all patients contracting paralytic polio before the pubertal growth spurt.

Investigations and diagnosis *Bloods*: serology for polio virus.

CSF: increased cell count, initially polymorphonuclear cells, later a pleocytosis; raised protein occurs late.

Microbiology: stool culture for virus; pharyngeal swab for virus culture less often positive.

Neurophysiology: EMG: usually normal in the acute stage, later shows changes typical of anterior horn cell disease (fasciculations, fibrillations).

Pathology: degeneration of anterior horn cells of the spinal cord, motor and sensory cranial nerve nuclei, layers III and V of motor cortex, thalamus, cerebellar vermis.

Differential diagnosis Bulbar symptoms: myasthenia gravis.

Flaccid paralysis: Guillain–Barré syndrome, acute intermittent porphyria, other viral infections (Coxsackie A and B, enterovirus EV70, 71); Japanese encephalitis and other arboviruses are reported to produce a similar acute syndrome on occasion.

Treatment and prognosis

No specific treatment.

Monitor respiratory status, supportive treatment of respiratory failure (ventilation if need be).

In the acute phase, some muscles recover quickly, but paralysis at 1 month is permanent.

A motor neurone disease developing 20 years or so after an attack of polio has been reported, but late deterioration may have many other causes (see entry on postpolio syndrome).

Prevention with oral live attenuated (Sabin) vaccine: leads to excretion of virus in stools from which the non-immune can become infected.

References Gould T. *A Summer Plague – Polio and Its Survivors*. Newhaven: Yale University Press, 1995.

Kidd D, Williams AJ, Howard RS. Poliomyelitis. *Postgraduate Medical Journal* 1996; **72**: 641–647.

Wood M, Anderson M. *Neurological Infections*. London: WB Saunders, 1988: 487–502.

Other relevant entries Guillain–Barré syndrome; Japanese encephalitis; Motor neurone disease; Motor neurone diseases: an overview; Porphyria; Postpolio syndrome.

■ Polyarteritis nodosa
Systemic necrotizing vasculitis

Pathophysiology Classical polyarteritis nodosa (cPAN) is a necrotizing vasculitis of small- and medium-sized arteries, especially affecting branch points and sometimes resulting in aneurysmal dilatation. Similar to Churg–Strauss syndrome, it may overlap with microscopic polyangiitis (mPAN). Although it may present with systemic and renal features, neurological complications may also occur.

Clinical features: history and examination

- Fever, weight loss, malaise.
- Kidney: hypertension, vasculitis, glomerulonephritis.
- Skin rash.
- Gastrointestinal features.
- Cardiac features.
- Lungs unaffected (*cf.* Churg–Strauss syndrome).
- Neurological features:

    Peripheral nervous system (PNS): ca. *60% affected*:

    Peripheral neuropathy:

    Mononeuritis multiplex: peripheral or cranial (V, VII, VIII)

    Distal polyneuropathy

    Cutaneous neuropathy

    Radiculopathy uncommon.

    Central nervous system (CNS): ca. *20% affected*:

    Global: headache, aseptic meningitis; dementia, psychosis, encephalopathy, depression, mania.

    Focal: stroke-like syndromes causing aphasia, hemiparesis, visual field defects; rarely chorea, parkinsonism, cranial nerve involvement, cerebellar ataxia; spinal cord syndromes including infarction/necrosis, acute transverse myelopathy.

Investigations and diagnosis *Bloods*: hepatitis B serology may be positive; ANCA usually negative (*cf.* microscopic polyangiitis); PAN has been reported as a paraneoplastic consequence of hairy cell leukaemia.

Imaging: CT/MRI may show cerebral atrophy, focal/multifocal infarction, haemorrhage (all non-specific); renal angiography may show presence of microaneurysms which may assist diagnosis.

CSF: raised pressure, protein, and cell count (lymphocytic pleocytosis in aseptic meningitis).

Neurophysiology:

EMG: always abnormal with clinically apparent PNS disease (axonal neuropathy most common) and often abnormal in asymptomatic patients, suggesting subclinical disease.

EEG: generalized slowing in encephalopathic patients.

Nerve biopsy: vasculitis of epineural blood vessels, nerve infarction.

Differential diagnosis Other vasculitic syndromes; important to distinguish from microscopic polyangiitis.

Treatment and prognosis CNS involvement in PAN is the second commonest cause of death after renal disease. Vigorous treatment is therefore indicated with corticosteriods and cyclophosphamide +/− ivIg.

Reference Nadeau SE. Neurologic manifestations of systemic vasculitis.
Neurologic Clinics 2002; **20**: 123–150.

Other relevant entries Churg–Strauss syndrome; Encephalopathies: an overview; Mononeuritis multiplex, Mononeuropathy multiplex; Neuropathies: an overview; Vasculitis.

◼ Polycystic kidney disease – see Renal disease and the nervous system; Subarachnoid haemorrhage

◼ Polycythaemia rubra vera

A myeloproliferative disease with increased red cell mass and blood volume, resulting in erythrocytosis (raised haematocrit) and increased blood viscosity, which may be associated with transient ischaemic attacks and thrombotic strokes, less commonly with cerebral haemorrhage, chorea.

Other relevant entries Cerebrovascular disease: arterial; Chorea; Sydenham's chorea.

◼ Polyglucosan body disease

Pathophysiology Adult polyglucosan body (PGB) disease has a broad phenotype, with onset in the fifth to seventh decades, and a positive family history in about a third. It is characterized by accumulation of PGBs, composed of abnormally branched glycogen (amylopectin), in the central and peripheral nervous system. PGB are also seen in Lafora body disease, type IV glycogenosis, and can occur incidentally with ageing (corpora amylacea).

Clinical features: history and examination

- Gait disorder, sphincter problems, sensory complaints, mixture of upper and lower motor neurone signs, cognitive decline, psychiatric features.
- Peripheral (axonal) neuropathy.
- Dementia (of frontal type).
- Neurogenic bladder.
- Upper motor neurone signs.
- +/− amyotrophy, cerebellar signs, optic atrophy, extrapyramidal syndrome.

Investigations and diagnosis Essentially a tissue diagnosis, all other investigations produce non-specific findings.

Neurophysiology: EMG/NCS: diffuse axonal neuropathy, denervation.

Imaging: CT/MRI: extensive white matter abnormalities.

Neuropsychology: subcortical-type picture (slowness, problem solving difficulties, impaired abstract reasoning).

Tissue biopsy:

Nerve biopsy: PGB are large rounded intra-axonal inclusions, especially in myelinated fibres, up to 30 μm in diameter, metachromatic with toluidine blue staining (dark centre with lighter halo); periodic acid–Schiff (PAS) positive.

Axillary skin biopsy: PGB may be seen in myoepithelial cells of apocrine glands.

Brain biopsy: PGB seen in astrocytes.

Neurogenetics: adult PGB disease with diffuse peripheral and central involvement is allelic with Andersen disease (glycogen-storage disease type IV) with mutations in the gene encoding the glycogen branching enzyme.

Differential diagnosis Broad: other causes of degenerative dementia.

Treatment and prognosis No specific treatment.

References Robertson NP, Wharton S, Anderson J, Scolding NJ. Adult polyglucosan body disease associated with an extrapyramidal syndrome. *Journal of Neurology, Neurosugery and Psychiatry* 1998; **65**: 788–790.

Robitaille Y, Carpenter S, Karpati G *et al*. A distinct form of polyglucosan disease with massive involvement of central and peripheral neuronal processes and astrocytes. *Brain* 1980; **103**: 316–336.

Ziemssen F, Sindern E, Schroder JM *et al*. Novel missense mutations in the glycogen-branching enzyme gene in adult polyglucosan body disease. *Annals of Neurology* 2000; **47**: 536–540.

Other relevant entry Dementia: an overview.

▪ Polyglutamine disease, polyQ disease – see Trinucleotide repeat diseases

▪ Polymyalgia arteritica – see Giant cell arteritis

■ Polymyalgia rheumatica

Pathophysiology A late-onset, acute illness, probably inflammatory in nature, producing usually symmetrical muscular pain and stiffness around the shoulder girdle, without true weakness, and which responds to adequate doses of steroids. Polymyalgia rheumatica (PMR) is strongly associated with giant cell arteritis (GCA).

Clinical features: history and examination

- History of morning stiffness of >1 hour, symmetrical shoulder and upper arm pain; illness <2 weeks in duration.
- Age usually >65 years.
- Systemic features (weight loss, sweating, malaise) may be present.
- Response to steroids may be included amongst the diagnostic criteria.
- Examination discloses no true weakness of the shoulder girdle (*cf.* polymyositis) although this may be difficult to ascertain with the concurrent pain.

Investigations and diagnosis *Bloods*: raised ESR (>40 mm/hour), CRP, blood viscosity; may have elevated alkaline phosphatase (transaminases usually normal). Normal creatine kinase, rheumatoid factor, auto-antibodies, protein electrophoresis and thyroid function tests may be helpful in excluding other diagnoses.

Temporal artery biopsy is not considered helpful in pure PMR.

Differential diagnosis

Late-onset rheumatoid arthritis.
Osteoarthritis.
Rotator cuff disease.
Myeloma.
Hypothyroidism.
Polymyositis.
Proximal myopathy.
Connective tissue disorders.

Treatment and prognosis More than 80% of patients improve with prednisolone 15–20 mg/day. This is given for about 1 month and then weaned slowly. The majority of patients require a small maintenance dose of steroids. Prognosis is generally very good. Relapses may occur if the steroids are weaned too quickly. Steroid-induced adverse effects may emerge if large doses are required to keep the disorder in check (e.g. steroid myopathy). Prophylactic bisphosphonates may be indicated to prevent osteoporosis. There is a risk of subsequently developing GCA.

References Kyle V. Polymyalgia rheumatica. *Prescribers' Journal* 1997; **37**: 138–144.

Turnbull J. Temporal arteritis and polymyalgia rheumatica: nosographic and nosologic considerations. *Neurology* 1996; **46**: 901–906.

Other relevant entry Giant cell arteritis.

■ Polymyoclonus – see Myoclonus

■ Polymyositis

Pathophysiology An idiopathic, probably autoimmune, inflammatory myopathy, most usually affecting proximal limb musculature, and occurring between ages 30 and 60 years, although there is a smaller peak during adolescence; females predominate.

Clinical features: history and examination

- Weakness:
    Proximal limb muscles, trunk, limb girdles (may be asymmetrical)
    +/− neck ("dropped head syndrome")
    +/− bulbar (dysphonia, dysphagia)
    +/− respiratory muscles (rarely causes dyspnoea)
    extraocular muscles not involved.
- Mild atrophy.
- Painless in majority; pain, aching in *ca.* 15% of cases.
- Hyporeflexia.
- +/− cardiac arrhythmias.
- +/− lung fibrosis.
- May be concurrent connective tissue or autoimmune disease, for example myasthenia gravis, scleroderma, Hashimoto's thyroiditis.

Investigations and diagnosis *Bloods*: creatine kinase, ESR may be elevated; +/− ANA, anti-Jo1 auto-antibodies; check TFTs, AChRAb, other auto-antibodies for concurrent autoimmune disease.

ECG: may be abnormal.

Neurophysiology: EMG: myopathic: brief low voltage action potentials, fibrillation potentials, positive sharp waves, polyphasic units.

Muscle biopsy: scattered muscle-fibre necrosis and phagocytosis (macrophages); lymphocytic infiltration with predominantly CD8 T-cells (*cf.* dermatomyositis); evidence of regeneration (proliferating sarcolemmal nuclei, new myofibrils, small fibres in clusters). No perifascicular atrophy (*cf.* dermatomyositis).

Differential diagnosis

Dermatomyositis.

Inclusion body myositis.

Myasthenia gravis (may be present concurrently).

Eosinophilic myositis (may occur in context of hypereosinophilic syndrome).

Treatment and prognosis Untreated patients develop muscle atrophy, fibrosis, and contracture.

Treatment is with steroids (60–80 mg/day of prednisolone), slowly weaned as clinical and biochemical improvement progresses; azathioprine may be used as a steroid sparing agent; methotrexate, ciclosporin, and plasma exchange have been used. The majority of patients improve with steroid treatment, although there may be some residual weakness. Long-term steroid therapy mandates osteoporosis prophylaxis. Most patients require treatment for 2 years, many for 5 years, and some indefinitely.

Treatment of cardiac dysrhythmias as appropriate.

Small risk of underlying malignancy (*cf.* dermatomyositis).

Reference Mastaglia FL (ed.). *Inflammatory Myopathies*. London: Baillière Tindall, 1993.

Other relevant entries Dermatomyositis; Eosinophilic myopathy; Inclusion body myositis; Myositis; Proximal weakness.

Polyneuropathy – see Neuropathies: an overview

Pompe's disease – see Acid-maltase deficiency; Glycogen-storage disorders: an overview

Pontobulbar palsy with deafness – see Brown–Vialetto–Van Laere syndrome

Pontocerebellar hypoplasia

A rare disorder of autosomal-recessive inheritance, in which there is impaired maturation of infratentorial structures. Two types have been characterized:

- Type 1: spinal anterior horn cell degeneration, similar to infantile spinal muscular atrophy (SMA), with congenital contractures, neurogenic hypoventilation, and severe muscular hypotonia; pathology also involves degeneration of anterior horns and other grey matter structures.
- Type 2: severe chorea/dystonia which may sometimes respond to levodopa; no spinal anterior horn cell pathology, but reduced size of ventral pons, inferior lobe, dentate nucleus and thinning of cerebellar cortex.

References Barth PG. Pontocerebellar hypoplasias – an overview of a group of inherited neurodegenerative disorders with fetal onset. *Brain and Development* 1993; **15**: 411–422.

Grosso S, Mostadini R, Cioni M, Galluzzi P, Morgese G, Balestri P. Pontocerebellar hypoplasia type 2. Further clinical characterization and evidence of positive response of dyskinesia to levodopa. *Journal of Neurology* 2002; **249**: 596–600.

PORN syndrome

Progressive *o*uter *r*etinal *n*ecrosis (PORN) syndrome is a variant of necrotizing herpetic retinopathy, the majority of cases occurring in the context of AIDS, although it may be associated with other causes of immunocompromise. Most cases result from varicella zoster virus (VZV) retinitis, but occasional cases may be linked to HSV-1 infection. Treatment with ganciclovir, aciclovir, foscarnet, or combinations thereof may be tried, but generally the prognosis for vision is poor, with optic atrophy the end stage.

Other relevant entries HIV/AIDS and the nervous system; Optic atrophy; Varicella zoster virus and the nervous system.

■ Porphyria

Pathophysiology Inborn or acquired errors of porphyrin metabolism may cause visceral, dermatological, neurological, psychiatric, or mixed disorders. Those affecting the nervous system are the autosomal-dominant conditions of:

- acute intermittent porphyria (AIP);
- variegate porphyria (VP);
- hereditary coproporphyria (HCP);
- plumboporphyria (*q.v.*).

Gastrointestinal and peripheral nervous system features are thought to result from neuronal dysfunction, whereas cerebral manifestations may result from metabolic compromise, ischaemia, demyelination, or oxidative stress.

Clinical features: history and examination

Highly variable:

- Abdominal pain, cramping
- Psychosis
- Delirium
- Autonomic instability
- Peripheral neuropathy: motor; proximal weakness in arms > legs (especially wrist drop); patients may become quadriparetic; flaccidity, areflexia or hyporeflexia
- Cranial nerve palsies (III, VII, X)
- Seizures
- Sensory loss
- +/− Dermatological features: bullae, erythema (VP, HCP).

History of fasting, infection, drugs, lead exposure.

Investigations and diagnosis Need to demonstrate porphyrin precursor accumulation at the time of symptoms (*cf.* asymptomatic carriers) in either urine (AIP) or faeces (HCP, VP). Light sensitivity of porphyrins mandates storage of samples in dark and prompt transmission to the laboratory for analysis.

Urine porphobilinogen (PBG): a screening test, but with high frequency of false-positive and false-negative results; if clinical suspicion is high, the test should be repeated if initially negative.

Faecal PBG.

Skin biopsy (VP, HCP): homogeneous periodic acid–Schiff (PAS) positive thickening and IgG deposition in vessel walls.

Liaise with specialist laboratory familiar with diagnosis of porphyria for further tests.

Neurophysiology: EMG/NCS: denervation of muscles, consistent with axonal neuropathy.

CSF: usually normal, may be raised protein (non-specific).

Differential diagnosis

Lead poisoning (plumbism).

Tyrosinaemia (fumaryl-acetoacetate hydrolase deficiency).

Hexachlorobenzene poisoning.

Guillain–Barré syndrome, other acute axonal neuropathies.

Treatment and prognosis *Of acute attack*:

Increase carbohydrate intake

Treat intercurrent infection

Withdraw precipitants, especially drugs

Haem arginate may be useful (compensates for haem breakdown).

Acute attacks can be fatal despite supportive therapy, possibly due to cardiac arrhythmias.

Prevention:

Avoidance of porphyrinogenic agents (drugs, alcohol).

Adequate carbohydrate intake, avoid dieting.

Reference Crimlisk HL. The little imitator – porphyria: a neuropsychiatric disorder. *Journal of Neurology, Neurosugery and Psychiatry* 1997; **62**: 319–328.

Other relevant entries Autonomic failure; Guillain–Barré syndrome; Lead and the nervous system; Neuropathies: an overview; Plumboporphyria; Tyrosinaemia.

▧ Portal-systemic encephalopathy – see Hepatic encephalopathy

▧ Post-anoxic (action) myoclonus – see Lance–Adams syndrome

▧ Postconcussion syndrome – see Concussion

▧ Posterior cortical atrophy – see Alzheimer's disease

▧ Posterior inferior cerebellar artery syndrome – see Cerebellar disease: an overview; Lateral medullary syndrome

▧ Posterior interosseous syndrome

The posterior interosseous nerve is the purely motor terminal branch of the radial nerve in the forearm which supplies the supinator muscle, wrist and finger extensors. Posterior interosseous mononeuropathy as a consequence of entrapment, usually at the level of the supinator, is rare, produces weakness of wrist and finger extensors but with sparing of extensor carpi radialis (which receives a more proximal branch of the radial nerve), hence causing a wrist drop with radial deviation. There are no sensory signs but pain in the elbow or dorsal forearm may occur. Diagnosis is by clinical history and EMG/NCS.

Other relevant entry Radial neuropathy.

■ Posterior ischaemic optic neuropathy – see Ischaemic optic neuropathy

■ Posterior leukoencephalopathy syndrome

Pathophysiology A syndrome of rapidly evolving neurological dysfunction associated with rapidly increasing blood pressure, with marked white matter changes on brain imaging. Situations in which posterior leukoencephalopathy syndrome has been described include:

- Eclampsia
- Renal disease
- Hypertensive encephalopathy
- Cytotoxic/immunosuppressive drug therapy, for example ciclosporin, tacrolimus.

Clinical features: history and examination

- Headache, nausea and vomiting, seizures, visual disturbances, altered sensorium, +/− focal neurological deficits.
- Rapidly increasing blood pressure.

Investigations and diagnosis *Imaging*: MR brain shows oedematous lesions in posterior parietal and occipital white matter, occasionally extending to basal ganglia, brainstem and cerebellum. Grey matter sometimes involved.

Differential diagnosis Other causes of encephalopathy; encephalitis.

Treatment and prognosis Prompt control of blood pressure; control precipitating factors (drugs). With early treatment the condition is completely reversible, but delay may be associated with permanent neurological deficits.

> **Reference** Garg RK. Posterior leukoencephalopathy syndrome. *Postgraduate Medical Journal* 2001; **77**: 24–28.

> **Other relevant entries** Eclampsia; Encephalopathies: an overview; Hypertension and the nervous system; Immunosuppressive therapy and diseases of the nervous system; Renal disease and the nervous system.

■ Posterior spinal artery syndrome – see Spinal cord vascular diseases

■ Postherpetic neuralgia – see Herpes zoster and postherpetic neuralgia

■ Posthypoxic syndromes

Pathophysiology Posthypoxic syndromes are a consequence of reduced oxygen supply to the brain due to reduced perfusion (ischaemia), for example following a myocardial infarction, ventricular fibrillation, haemorrhage or "shock", or a reduced

■ Postural hypotension – see Autonomic failure

■ Postvaccinial encephalomyelitis – see Acute disseminated encephalomyelitis

■ Potassium-aggravated myotonia

Pathophysiology This autosomal-dominant disorder is linked to mutations in the α-subunit of the sodium channel gene SCN4A, hence is a sodium-channelopathy-like hyperkalaemic periodic paralysis and paramyotonia congenita.

Clinical features: history and examination
- Painful cramps, stiffness without weakness; fluctuation of symptoms, cold sensitivity is usual.
- A rare form, myotonia permanens, is characterized by severe persistent myotonia.

Investigations and diagnosis *Neurophysiology*: reduced compound muscle action potential (CMAP) amplitude with muscle cooling or exposure to K^+.
Neurogenetics: mutations in SCN4A gene (e.g. V1589M).

Differential diagnosis Other causes of muscle cramp, stiffness, for example autosomal-dominant myotonia congenita (Thomsen's disease).

Treatment and prognosis Mexilitene is the drug of choice for myotonia; may be required lifelong in myotonia permanens.

> **Reference** Orrell RW, Jurkat-Rott K, Lehmann-Horn F, Lane RJ. Familial cramp due to potassium-aggravated myotonia. *Journal of Neurology, Neurosurgery and Psychiatry* 1998; **65**: 569–572.

> **Other relevant entries** Channelopathies: an overview; Cramps; Episodic ataxias; Myotonia and myotonic disorders; Paramyotonia; Periodic paralysis.

■ Pott's disease
Pott's paraplegia

Pathophysiology Tuberculous infection of vertebra(e) (osteitis) may cause vertebral collapse and spinal deformity, with or without spinal cord compression. Tracking of pus into the epidural space may also cause spinal cord compression.

Clinical features: history and examination
- Kyphosis of spine due to collapsed infected vertebra(e).
- +/− Paraplegia.

Investigations and diagnosis
Imaging: spine and spinal cord: plain radiology and MRI.
Search for TB elsewhere: chest radiograph, early morning urine.
Consider HIV testing.

Differential diagnosis Other causes of cord compression; hydatid disease of the spine.

Treatment and prognosis Surgical exploration and excision of infective focus if possible; intervertebral grafting may be required; anti-tuberculous therapy.

Reference Shaw BA. Pott's disease with paraparesis. *New England Journal of Medicine* 1996; **334**: 958–959.

Other relevant entries Paraparesis: acute management and differential diagnosis; Tuberculosis and the nervous system.

■ Pourfour du Petit syndrome

Mydriasis, widening of the palpebral fissure, exophthalmos, hyperhidrosis (i.e. inverse Horner's syndrome, sympathetic overactivity), flushing and increased intraocular pressure due to irritation of the sympathetic chain in the neck.

Other relevant entry Horner's syndrome.

■ Prader–Willi syndrome
HHHO syndrome

Pathophysiology A syndrome of mental retardation (hypomentia), hypothalamic hypogonadism, hypotonia, obesity (HHHO syndrome), and diabetes mellitus, resulting from loss or abnormality of paternally derived chromosome 15q11–q13.

Clinical features: history and examination
- Neonatal hypotonia, feeding difficulties; gavage feeding often required.
- Mental retardation (IQ 50–70).
- Short stature, small hands and feet.
- Strabismus.
- Childhood obesity, hyperphagia.
- Non-insulin-dependent diabetes mellitus.
- Behavioural disorders.
- Hypothalamic hypogonadism; hypothermia.
- High-pitched nasal voice ("Donald Duck").
- Sleep apnoea, cor pulmonale (adulthood).

Investigations and diagnosis *Genetics*: loss or abnormality of paternally derived chromosome 15q11–q13:

Paternally derived interstitial deletion: 60%

Genomic imprinting with both abnormal genes maternally derived (maternal disomy): 30%

Microdeletions, point mutations: 10%

(both imprinting centres paternally derived leads to Angelman syndrome).

Differential diagnosis Not usually confused with other syndromes; may resemble Froehlich's syndrome.

Treatment and prognosis

Fluoxetine may be helpful to reduce food intake, obsessional behaviours.

Growth hormone may promote growth, coordination, muscle strength.

Obstructive sleep apnoea, nocturnal hypoventilation, cor pulmonale merit treatment.

References Cassidy SB, Schwartz S. Prader–Willi and Angelman syndromes. *Medicine* 1998; **77**: 140–151.

Couper RTL, Couper JJ. Prader–Willi syndrome. *Lancet* 2000; **356**: 673–675.

Holm VA, Cassidy SB, Butler MG *et al*. Prader–Willi syndrome: consensus diagnostic criteria. *Pediatrics* 1993; **91**: 398–402.

Khan NL, Wood NW. Prader–Willi and Angelman syndromes: update on genetic mechanisms and diagnostic complexities. *Current Opinion in Neurology* 1999; **12**: 149–154.

Other relevant entries Angelman syndrome; Froehlich's syndrome; Kleine–Levin syndrome.

■ Pre-eclampsia – see Eclampsia

■ Pregnancy and the nervous system: an overview

Pathophysiology Pregnancy and the puerperium may have an effect on a variety of chronic neurological conditions, such as epilepsy, migraine, and multiple sclerosis. It may also increase the risk of developing *de novo* neurological illness (cerebrovascular disease), the effects of which may continue after pregnancy. Eclampsia is a disease encountered only during pregnancy and the puerperium which may have neurological effects.

Clinical features: history and examination

- Neurological conditions during pregnancy

    Cerebrovascular disease:

    Increased incidence of stroke, probably multifactorial; increased risk of cerebral aneurysm rupture leading to intracerebral haemorrhage; increased risk of bleeding from arteriovenous malformations (especially spinal); increased risk of sinus and cortical venous thrombosis. Postpartum cardiomyopathy increases the risk of ischaemic stroke.

    Epilepsy:

    Control of pre-existing seizures may deteriorate, especially in the first trimester and in patients with poorly controlled epilepsy and/or poor compliance (altered metabolism of drugs, vomiting, impaired intake). *De novo* epilepsy may occur (oestrogens may lower seizure threshold); epilepsy confined to pregnancy ("gestational epilepsy") is described but rare. Anti-epileptic drug dosages may need to be increased during pregnancy to ensure optimal seizure control; monitoring of drug levels may be helpful in judging appropriate increases in dosage. Risk of teratogenicity with many anti-epileptic drugs, hence need for pre-conceptual counselling and prophylactic folic acid for those planning pregnancy. Carbamazepine has been the favoured drug for control of epilepsy during pregnancy, but some authors now favour lamotrigine. Risks to unborn child of uncontrolled epileptic seizures in the mother outweigh small risk of teratogenicity, so other anti-epileptic medications should not be stopped once pregnancy has occurred.

Idiopathic ("benign") intracranial hypertension:

May present in first trimester or puerperium (differential diagnosis = sinus thrombosis).

Migraine:

Tends to improve, although sometimes worsens or presents *de novo*.

Multiple sclerosis:

Decreased relapse rate during pregnancy; increased relapse rate during the puerperium.

Neuropathy:

Carpal tunnel syndrome, meralgia paraesthetica, Bell's palsy are said to be more common in pregnancy; femoral, obturator, and common peroneal palsies may occur as a consequence of delivery procedures. Neuropathies associated with porphyria and chronic inflammatory demyelinating polyneuropathy (CIDP) may be exacerbated.

Neuromuscular disease:

Myasthenia gravis: no clear effect: may improve, stay stable, or deteriorate.

Systemic lupus erythematosus:

May be exacerbated during puerperium.

- Conditions unique to pregnancy, puerperium:

Eclampsia (*q.v.*): hypertension, proteinuria, hyperreflexia, seizures.

Chorea gravidarum (rare).

Wernicke-type syndrome in patients with hyperemesis gravidarum.

Sheehan's syndrome (postpartum hypopituitarism, due to infarction of pituitary, usually associated with peripartum haemorrhage).

Investigations and diagnosis See individual entries.

Shielding of fetus necessary if procedures involving X-rays are undertaken.

Differential diagnosis See individual entries.

Treatment and prognosis Eclampsia necessitates urgent control of blood pressure and seizures; the condition is terminated by delivery of the infant.

References Aminoff MJ. Pregnancy and disorders of the nervous system. In: Aminoff MJ (ed.). *Neurology and General Medicine*. New York: Churchill Livingstone, 1989: 487–503.

Confavreux C, Hutchinson M, Hours MM, Cortinovis-Tourniaire P, Moreau T. Rate of pregnancy-related relapse in multiple sclerosis. Pregnancy in Multiple Sclerosis Group. *New England Journal of Medicine* 1998; **339**: 285–291.

Donaldson JO. *Neurology of Pregnancy* (2nd edition). London: Saunders, 1989.

Sawle GV, Ramsay MM. The neurology of pregnancy. *Journal of Neurology, Neurosurgery and Psychiatry* 1998; **64**: 711–725.

Other relevant entries Bell's palsy; Cerebrovascular disease: arterial; Cerebrovascular disease: venous; Chorea; Eclampsia; Epilepsy: an overview; Idiopathic intracranial hypertension; Myasthenia gravis; Neuropathies: an overview; Pituitary disease and apoplexy.

■ Presbyastasis

Disequilibrium of ageing

A condition of elderly patients who present with imbalance and disequilibrium that cannot be ascribed to a particular disease state or single causative factor (e.g. vestibular disease, visual impairment, peripheral neuropathy). It is thought that abnormal sensory input, abnormal central nervous system (CNS) sensory processing, abnormal control mechanisms for balance, a decreased range of movement and strength, may all contribute to symptoms. White matter changes on brain MRI have been associated with the condition. Vestibular rehabilitation therapy and avoidance of vestibular suppressant medications may be helpful.

> **Reference** Belal A, Glorig A. Disequilibrium of ageing (presbyastasis). *Journal of Laryngology and Otology* 1986; **100**: 1037–1041.
>
> **Other relevant entry** Gait disorders.

■ Presyncope – see Autonomic failure; Syncope

■ Pretectal syndrome – see Parinaud's syndrome

■ Pretibial syndrome

Muscle swelling within the pretibial compartment, due to trauma or excessive activity, may lead to ischaemic muscle necrosis and myoglobinuria. Clinically there is muscle pain, with swelling in pretibial compartment, often with a history of trauma or excessive activity (e.g. marching). Bloods may show elevated creatine kinase (rhabdomyolysis) and there may be myoglobinuria.

The condition may be mild, necessitating only supportive treatment. In more serious cases, incision of the pretibial fascia should relieve the syndrome. Prognosis is good if appropriate treatment is initiated early enough.

> **Other relevant entries** Compartment syndromes; Rhabdomyolysis.

■ Primary amoebic meningoencephalitis – see Acanthamoeba; Amoebic infection; Naegleria

■ Primary angiitis of the central nervous system – see Isolated angiitis of the central nervous system

■ Primary intracerebral haemorrhage – see Cerebrovascular disease: arterial; Intracerebral haemorrhage

■ Primary lateral sclerosis

Pathophysiology A rare syndrome of progressive, usually symmetrical, spinobulbar spasticity without lower motor neurone features, starting in adulthood, thought to be due to selective dysfunction or loss of the descending motor tracts, hence a motor neurone disease with exclusively upper motor neurone features.

Clinical features: history and examination
- Slowly progressive spastic quadriparesis, usually symmetrical.
- Pseudobulbar affect.
- Spastic dysarthria.
- Hyperreflexia, extensor plantar responses.
- Normal cognition.
- Bladder function preserved.
- No lower motor neurone features.

Investigations and diagnosis
Bloods: normal.

Imaging: MRI shows no alternative pathology (e.g. cord compression, multiple sclerosis); focal atrophy of the precentral gyrus may be evident. PET scan may show reduced metabolism in precentral gyrus.

CSF: normal.

Neurophysiology: EMG: normal, although may show occasional (asymptomatic) fibrillation potentials.

Few pathological reports, but those published suggest heavy loss of Betz cells from motor cortex of the precentral gyrus.

Differential diagnosis Other causes of exclusively upper motor neurone signs, for example multiple sclerosis (in which abdominal reflexes are said to be lost early, unlike the situation in motor neurone disease). MRI excludes the other likely diagnoses.

Treatment and prognosis No specific treatment. Symptomatic treatment of spasticity. Disease is slowly progressive.

> **Reference** Pringle CE, Hudson AJ, Munoz DG, Kiernan JA, Brown WF, Ebers GC. Primary lateral sclerosis: clinical features, neuropathology and diagnostic criteria. *Brain* 1992; **115**: 495–520.
>
> Le Forestier N, Maisonobe T, Piquard A *et al*. Does primary lateral sclerosis exist? A study of 20 patients and a review of the literature. *Brain* 2001; **124**(10): 1989–1999.
>
> **Other relevant entries** Mills' syndrome, Mills' variant; Motor neurone diseases: an overview.

■ Primary orthostatic tremor
Shaky legs syndrome

Pathophysiology A disorder characterized by tremor, predominantly of the lower limbs, present on standing and which disappears on sitting, walking, leaning, or when the patient is lifted off the ground. The 14–18-Hz oscillation is unique, approximately twice that of essential tremor, and is thought to be generated by a central oscillator (peripheral loading does not alter tremor frequency).

Clinical features: history and examination

- A feeling of unsteadiness, shakiness, or "like jelly" when standing still.
- Rapid rhythmic synchronized contractions of the leg muscles on standing causing knee tremor.
- Auscultation (with the diaphragm) over lower limb muscles: regular thumping sound (likened to hearing a helicopter rotors in the distance).
- Arm tremor much less frequent; a jaw tremor with features of primary orthostatic tremor (POT) has been described.

Investigations and diagnosis *Neurophysiology*: EMG: pathognomonic synchronous activity in leg muscles on standing, frequency of 14–18 Hz.

Differential diagnosis Very characteristic, unlikely to be mistaken for other types of tremor.

Treatment and prognosis A number of drugs may be helpful in POT, including phenobarbitone, primidone, clonazepam, and levodopa, but not propranolol or alcohol (*cf.* essential tremor).

References Heilman KM. Orthostatic tremor. *Archives of Neurology* 1984; **41**: 880–881.

Thompson PD. Orthostatic tremor. *Journal of Neurology, Neurosurgery and Psychiatry* 1999; **66**: 278.

Other relevant entry Tremor: an overview.

▓ Primary progressive aphasia
Progressive non-fluent aphasia

Pathophysiology A syndrome of dissolution of language to the point of mutism due to focal cerebral cortical degeneration involving the left perisylvian region, in the total or relative absence for two or more years of other neuropsychological deficits, for example of memory or visuospatial abilities. The term primary progressive aphasia (PPA) may also encompass a syndrome of progressive loss of speech output with dysarthria and orofacial dyspraxia. Suggested diagnostic criteria also require no disturbance of consciousness, or the presence of systemic disorders or brain disease which could account for the clinical findings. Functional imaging and pathological studies confirm the focal nature of the process. The neuropathological substrate is variable.

Clinical features: history and examination

- Impaired language output: aphasia (may be fluent or non-fluent); calculation, perception, and spatial abilities are preserved; verbal memory may be poor but non-verbal memory is preserved.
- +/− frontal lobe signs.
- +/− orofacial dyspraxia.

Investigations and diagnosis
Sequential neuropsychology.

Imaging:

Structural (CT/MRI) may show left perisylvian atrophy (low specificity and sensitivity).

Functional (SPECT/PET) shows early defects in left temporal and perisylvian area, extending later to left parietal and frontal lobes.

EEG: usually normal.

CSF: usually normal.

Pathology: variable: non-specific neuronal loss with gliosis and some spongiform changes ("dementia lacking distinctive histology"), Alzheimer's disease (AD), Pick's.

Neurogenetics: some familial cases have been reported with mutations in the τ-gene.

Differential diagnosis Other dementias presenting in a focal way, for example AD, Creutzfeldt–Jakob disease, but other deficits evolve.

Treatment and prognosis No specific treatment. Input from a speech and language therapist may be helpful to explore other avenues for communication. Patients usually remain independent despite their deficits, and are often able to continue at work despite mutism. Gradual progression to mutism, sometimes dementia and death (median duration of illness about 8 years).

References Duffy JR, Petersen RC. Primary progressive aphasia. *Aphasiology* 1992; **6**: 1–15.

Mesulam MM. Primary progressive aphasia. *Annals of Neurology* 2001; **49**: 425–432.

Mesulam M-M, Weintraub S. Spectrum of primary progressive aphasia. In: Rossor MN (ed.) *Unusual Dementias*. London: Bailliere Tindall, 1992: 583–609.

Other relevant entries Dementia: an overview; Frontotemporal dementia; Pick's disease.

■ Primary torsion dystonia

Dystonia musculorum deformans • Idiopathic torsion dystonia

Pathophysiology This is a pure dystonic syndrome, not a symptomatic or secondary dystonia. The identification of the genetic cause means that it is no longer appropriately labelled "idiopathic". The condition is commoner in Ashkenazi Jews, and is inherited as an autosomal-dominant condition with 40% penetrance.

Clinical features: history and examination

- Normal birth: no hypoxic–ischaemic birth injury, no kernicterus.
- Normal early developmental milestones.
- Variable phenotype: spectrum ranges from mild focal dystonia to disabling generalized dystonia.
- Variable age at onset:
    Childhood: majority will develop generalized dystonia; usually limb onset (leg > arm), with toe-walking, bizarre dystonic gait, falls.
    Adult: may present with writer's cramp, cranial dystonia.
- Cognition, sphincters, vision, hearing, sensory function all normal; no seizures.

- Stable once generalized dystonia present; relentless progression suggests secondary dystonia.
- Examine relatives for evidence of an inherited disorder.

Investigations and diagnosis *Investigations*: as outlined in the entry on Dystonia may be undertaken; all are negative. Particularly important to exclude Wilson's disease, since treatable.

Neurogenetics: linkage to chromosome 9q34 (DYT 1 locus) encoding ATP-binding protein torsin A is commonest identified genetic cause, especially found in childhood onset cases; other loci have been implicated in other families, viz. DYT6 (8p21–q22), DYT7 (18p31).

Differential diagnosis Odd gait and falls in childhood may be labelled "psychiatric".

Generalized dystonia in childhood may be misdiagnosed as cerebral palsy (importance of normal birth and early developmental milestones in diagnosis).

Adult (>20 years): very rare to develop generalized dystonia; usually onset in axial or cranial muscles.

Treatment and prognosis Prognosis linked to age at onset (see above).

A trial of levodopa is strongly recommended to exclude the diagnosis of dopa-responsive dystonia (DRD). In the event of no response to levodopa, the options are:

Anticholinergic therapy: benzhexol; large doses may be required
Tetrabenazine
Pimozide
Baclofen.

Focal dystonia best treated with botulinum toxin injections.

Reference Valente EM, Warner TT, Jarman PR *et al*. The role of DYT1 in primary torsion dystonia in Europe. *Brain* 1998; **121**: 2335–2339.

Other relevant entries Botulinum toxin therapy; Dopa-responsive dystonia; Dystonia: an overview.

▮ Primary writing tremor – see Writing tremor

▮ Primitive neuroectodermal tumours

These tumours occur predominantly in children and have a high rate of malignancy. They may occur in:

- Central nervous system (CNS)
  Neural
      Medulloblastoma
      Neuroblastoma
      Pineoblastoma

Glial
    Spongioblastoma
    Ependymoblastoma
- Non-CNS
    Retinoblastoma
    Adrenal neuroblastoma
    ?Ewing's sarcoma.

Histologically these tumours are composed of primitive, undifferentiated cells devoid of distinctive architecture; generally there are abundant mitoses. It is thought likely that primitive neuroectodermal tumours (PNETs) originate from multipotential stem cells. They often show extensive leptomeningeal spread.

Other relevant entries Medulloblastoma; Neuroblastoma; Pineal tumours; Retinoblastoma.

Primrose syndrome

This rare disorder is characterized by:

Mental retardation
Progressive muscle wasting
Ossification of the pinnae
Cystic changes in humeral and femoral heads
Paracentral posterior cataract
Hearing loss.

Other cases with late-onset progressive gait ataxia, pyramidal signs and cerebral calcification have been reported.

Reference Primrose DA. A slowly progressive degenerative condition characterized by mental deficiency, wasting of limb musculature and bone abnormalities, including ossification of the pinnae. *Journal of Mental Deficiency Research* 1982; **26**: 101–106.

Prion disease: an overview
Transmissible spongiform encephalopathy (TSE)

Pathophysiology Prion diseases result from accumulation of abnormal isoforms (PrP^{Sc}) of the cellular prion protein (PrP^{C}) within the brain, which have greater β-sheet conformation than the normal protein. The clinical phenotype is heterogeneous, partly influenced by polymorphisms within codon 129 of the PrP gene. Prion diseases may be classified aetiologically as:

Sporadic:
    Creutzfeldt–Jakob disease (CJD).

Inherited:

    Familial CJD (fCJD)

    Gerstmann–Sträussler–Scheinker disease (GSS)

    Fatal Familial Insomnia (FFI).

Acquired:

    Kuru

    Variant CJD (vCJD; "Human BSE").

Iatrogenic:

    Corneal transplantation

    Dura mater grafts

    Intracranial electrodes

    Human pituitary-derived hormones (growth hormone, gonadotrophins).

Clinical features: history and examination

- History requires informant interview regarding cognitive features.

Whilst the various prion diseases mentioned above often have distinctive clinical phenotypes, the following features are common to many:

- Dementia
- Cerebellar syndrome [kuru, GSS, Brownell–Oppenheimer (ataxic) variant of CJD]
- Myoclonus
- Encephalopathy (Nevin–Jones syndrome of CJD)
- Extrapyramidal syndrome
- Pyramidal signs
- Psychiatric disturbance
- Cortical blindness (Heidenhain variant of CJD)
- Sensory symptoms and signs (especially vCJD: hyperpathia)
- Amyotrophy (muscle wasting)
- Chorea (may be seen in vCJD)
- Akinetic mutism.

Investigations and diagnosis *Bloods*: no specific abnormalities known, other than abnormalities in PrP gene in inherited cases (missense mutations, deletions, insertions).

Imaging: CT/MRI: brain atrophy may be evident; high signal in posterior thalamus may be seen on MRI in vCJD (pulvinar sign).

CSF: moderately elevated protein may be seen in CJD; protein markers of neuronal injury (neurone-specific enolase, 14-3-3) and glial activation (S100β) may be elevated in vCJD but this finding is non-specific.

Neurophysiology: EEG: periodic complexes at a frequency of 2/sec in a markedly abnormal background are the classical changes in CJD, although they may not develop until late in the disease (hence repeated EEGs may be needed); atypical changes (focal changes, periodic lateralized epileptiform discharges) sometimes reminiscent of complex partial status epilepticus may also be seen. EEG is typically normal in vCJD.

Brain biopsy: typical features are:

spongiform vacuolation affecting any part of the cerebral grey matter (but cases
   without spongiform change have also been described);
astrocytic proliferation, gliosis;
neuronal loss, synaptic degeneration;
PrP-immunopositive amyloid plaques.

Tonsil biopsy: may be helpful in diagnosis of vCJD if PrP-immunopositive staining
is present.

Differential diagnosis
Paraneoplastic encephalitis.
Complex partial status epilepticus.
Cerebrovascular disease with multi-infarct dementia.
Lithium intoxication.
Vasculitis.
Hashimoto's encephalopathy.

Treatment and prognosis No specific treatment currently known; uniformly fatal,
often within weeks to months; vCJD may be more than a year; some inherited forms
may continue for many years.

References Collinge J, Palmer MS (eds). *Prion Diseases*. Oxford: OUP, 1997.

Larner AJ, Doran M. Prion diseases: update on therapeutic patents, 1999–2002.
   Expert Opinion on Therapeutic Patents 2003; **13**: 67–78.

Other relevant entries Creutzfeldt–Jakob disease; Dementia: an overview; Fatal
   familial insomnia; Gerstmann–Sträussler–Scheinker disease; Kuru; Variant
   Creutzfeldt–Jakob disease.

■ Progeria
Hutchinson–Gilford syndrome

A rare condition of uncertain aetiology characterized by premature ageing.
Common features, developing within the first few years of life, include short
stature, alopecia, reduced subcutaneous fat, and joint restriction. Thinning of the
bones, facial hypoplasia and micrognathia may also be features. Premature
atherosclerosis develops leading to coronary artery disease and stroke, the former
being the chief cause of death, usually during the second decade. Cognition is
conspicuously preserved.

References Eriksson M, Brown WT, Gordon LB *et al.* Recurrent de novo point
   mutations in lamin A cause Hutchinson–Gilford progeria. *Nature* 2003; **423**:
   293–298.

Matsuo S, Takeuchi Y, Hayashi S *et al.* Patient with unusual Hutchinson–Gilford
   syndrome (progeria). *Pediatric Neurology* 1994; **10**: 237–240.

Other relevant entry Werner's syndrome.

■ Progressive bulbar palsy – see Motor neurone disease

■ Progressive encephalomyelitis with rigidity and myoclonus

This condition may be a variant of stiff man/person syndrome. Like the latter, it is characterized by axial muscle stiffness, rigidity, and painful muscle spasms, but in contrast to stiff man syndrome there are often preceding or accompanying sensory symptoms or brainstem signs (ataxia, vertigo, ocular motility disorders, dysarthria). Autonomic features and myoclonus may be prominent in some cases. CSF may show a lymphocytic pleocytosis and elevated protein; EMG may show continuous motor activity. Pathology shows perivascular lymphocyte cuffing, neuronal loss in brainstem and cervical cord, especially spinal interneurones in some cases.

The course is progressive but highly variable, some rapidly deteriorating to death, others being protracted.

In some cases it appears to be a paraneoplastic condition.

Other relevant entry Stiff people: an overview.

■ Progressive external ophthalmoplegia – see Chronic progressive external ophthalmoplegia

■ Progressive fluent aphasia – see Primary progressive aphasia; Semantic dementia

■ Progressive loss of speech output

A syndrome of speech production impairment in association with orofacial dyspraxia (progressive orofacial dyspraxia) with loss of speech output, described in association with lesions in the region of the anterior Sylvian fissure on functional imaging. The exact relationship of this syndrome to primary progressive aphasia is uncertain. Some of these patients may have focal atrophy, perhaps with Pick-type or non-specific pathological change.

Reference Tyrrell PJ, Kartsounis LD, Frackowiak RSJ, Findley LJ, Rossor MN. Progressive loss of speech output and orofacial dyspraxia associated with frontal lobe hypometabolism. *Journal of Neurology, Neurosurgery and Psychiatry* 1991; **54**: 351–357.

Other relevant entry Primary progressive aphasia.

■ Progressive multifocal leukoencephalopathy

Pathophysiology A demyelinating disorder due to reactivated infection of oligodendroglia with the JC papovavirus, a double-stranded DNA virus, most often seen in the setting of immunocompromise, particularly AIDS, but also Hodgkin's disease, lymphoma, leukaemia, carcinoma, sarcoidosis, tuberculosis, organ transplantation, and other situations requiring therapeutic immunosuppression. Primary infection with JC virus is asymptomatic.

Clinical features: history and examination Focal or multifocal signs related to lesion location:

- Hemiparesis; quadriparesis
- Aphasia
- Visual field defects, especially hemianopia; cortical blindness
- Ataxia
- Cranial nerve palsies
- Cognitive disturbance, dementia in later stages
- Sensory abnormalities
- Clear consciousness; headache, seizures rare.

In one series, progressive multifocal leukoencephalopathy (PML) heralded AIDS in around one-fourth of patients.

Investigations and diagnosis *Bloods*: HIV status if not already known; CD4 count usually $< 200/mm^3$.

Imaging: CT: diffuse or multiple hypodensities; MRI: T_2-weighted hyperintensities extending right into the gyral cores, without mass effect or enhancement.

CSF: standard indices usually normal; PCR for JC virus (supersedes attempts at virus culture).

Neurophysiology: EEG: non-specific diffuse or focal slowing.

Brain biopsy: multifocal demyelination in subcortical white matter, with foamy macrophages; loss of oligodendroglia with sparing of axons; enlarged nuclei in remaining oligodendroglia. Electron microscopy shows oligodendroglial inclusions composed of papovavirus particles.

Differential diagnosis Other causes of central nervous system (CNS) mass lesion; in the context of HIV, consider particularly lymphoma and toxoplasmosis.

Treatment and prognosis No effective treatment currently known. Dismal prognosis, large majority of patients (>80%) dead within 1 year. Survival improved in patients receiving highly active antiretroviral therapy (HAART), a combination of nucleoside and non-nucleoside reverse transcriptase inhibitors and protease inhibitors, which reduces "virus load" (HIV RNA). However, such regimes have problematic side-effects and are difficult to adhere to.

Therapeutic success has been reported in one sarcoidosis-related case using cytarabine and α-interferon. Occasional spontaneous remissions have also been reported.

References Berger JR, Pall L, Lanska D, Whiteman M. Progressive multifocal leukoencephalopathy in patients with HIV infection. *Journal of Neurovirology* 1998; **4**: 59–68.

Berger JR, Major EO. Progressive multifocal leukoencephalopathy. *Seminars in Neurology* 1999; **19**: 193–200.

Greenlee JE. Progressive multifocal leukoencephalopathy: progress made and lessons relearned. *New England Journal of Medicine* 1998; **338**: 1378–1380.

Harrison MJG, McArthur JC. *AIDS and Neurology*. Edinburgh: Churchill
Livingstone, 1995: 141–148.
Other relevant entries Encephalitis: an overview; HIV/AIDS and the nervous system; Immunosuppressive therapy and diseases of the nervous system; Sarcoidosis; Tuberculosis and the nervous system.

▓ Progressive muscular atrophy – see Motor neurone disease

▓ Progressive myoclonic epilepsy

Pathophysiology The term "progressive myoclonic epilepsy (PME)" refers to a group of rare conditions which cause a progressive syndrome of myoclonus and epilepsy; cognitive impairment may also be present. PME is distinguished from other causes of myoclonus associated with epilepsy (e.g. idiopathic generalized epilepsies with prominent myoclonus) in consequence of the myoclonus being the predominant and initial symptom, hence also differentiating PME from progressive encephalopathies and ataxias.

The myoclonus in PME is generalized, multifocal, asymmetric, erratic, continuous for long periods of time, such that it may render the patient bed-bound and severely disabled.

Investigation and diagnosis *EEG*: usually shows generalized spike and slow-wave discharges, +/− photosensitivity, with slowing of background rhythms. EEG does not help distinguish individual disorders.

Differential diagnosis The differential diagnosis, including many inborn errors of metabolism, encompasses:

Unverricht–Lundborg disease (Baltic myoclonus)
Lafora body disease
Mitochondrial disorders (e.g. MERRF)
Sialidoses
Neuronal ceroid lipofuscinoses: Kufs' disease
Gangliosidoses (GM1, GM2)
Gaucher's disease: type III
Hallervorden–Spatz disease
Dentatorubral–pallidoluysian atrophy (DRPLA)
Alpers disease
Biotin-responsive encephalopathy
Action-myoclonus–renal failure syndrome (Andermann's syndrome)
FENIB.

Doose syndrome is an idiopathic generalized epilepsy syndrome with myoclonic-astatic and other seizure types.

Treatment and prognosis/other relevant entries See individual entries, including Andermann's syndrome (2).

References Berkovic SF, Andermann F, Carpenter S *et al*. Progressive myoclonus epilepsies: specific causes and diagnosis. *New England Journal of Medicine* 1986; **315**: 296–305.

Conry JA. Progressive myoclonus epilepsies. *Journal of Child Neurology* 2002; **17(suppl 1)**: S80–S84.

▪ Progressive neuronal degeneration of childhood with liver disease – see Alpers disease

▪ Progressive non-fluent aphasia – see Frontotemporal dementia; Primary progressive aphasia

▪ Progressive rubella panencephalitis – see Rubella

▪ Progressive subcortical gliosis (of Neumann)
Progressive subcortical glial dystrophy

Pathophysiology A rare dementing illness, sometimes familial, in which frontotemporal atrophy with extensive subcortical gliosis occurs. The diagnosis is based on pathology; the clinical features vary, sometimes suggesting frontotemporal dementia/Pick's disease (indeed Neumann originally thought this a form of Pick's disease, but later distinguished it as a separate entity) or Alzheimer's disease (AD). Mutation in the τ-protein gene on chromosome 17 has been demonstrated in familial progressive subcortical gliosis (of Neumann) (PSG).

Clinical features: history and examination
- Personality change (e.g. disinhibition), psychosis, dementia, parkinsonism, aphasia.
- Late pyramidal signs.
- Supranuclear gaze palsy has been reported.
- No amyotrophic lateral sclerosis (ALS).

Investigations and diagnosis *Imaging*: may show frontotemporal atrophy $+/-$ extensive subcortical white matter change, sometimes extending to basal ganglia.

Pathology:

Subcortical white matter gliosis/astrocytosis, including basal ganglia and thalamus, midbrain, medulla, ventral horns of spinal cord.
Neuronal loss; diffuse symmetrical atrophy of cortex.
Neuronal τ-positive inclusions but Pick bodies absent.
No Lewy bodies, AD senile plaques.

Differential diagnosis Frontotemporal dementia/Pick's disease.

AD.

Progressive supranuclear palsy (PSP).

Frontotemporal dementia (FTD)/motor neurone disease (MND) (pathology).

Treatment and prognosis No specific treatment. Disease may follow a prolonged course.

References Goedert M, Spillantini MG, Crowther RA *et al*. Tau gene mutation in familial progressive subcortical gliosis. *Nature Medicine* 1999; **5**: 454–457.

Neumann MA. Pick's disease. *Journal of Neuropathology and Experimental Neurology* 1949; **8**: 252–282.

Neumann MA, Cohn R. Progressive subcortical gliosis, a rare form of presenile dementia. *Brain* 1967; **90**: 405–418.

Other relevant entries Dementia: an overview; Frontotemporal dementia; Pick's disease; Progressive supranuclear palsy; Tauopathy.

▓ Progressive supranuclear palsy

Steele–Richardson–Olszewski (SRO) syndrome

Pathophysiology An akinetic rigid syndrome of unknown aetiology with a characteristic eye movement abnormality (although not all pathologically confirmed cases have the latter). Some prefer to retain the eponymous name, since there are various causes of the clinical syndrome of progressive supranuclear palsy.

Clinical features: history and examination

- Extrapyramidal syndrome: bradykinesia, axial rigidity, no tremor.
- Postural instability leading to early falls; *en bloc* sitting, "rocket man sign", extensor rigidity (retrocollis) associated with falls backwards.
- Vertical gaze failure corrected with vestibulo-ocular responses (i.e. supranuclear gaze palsy).
- Broken pursuit eye movements; saccades reduced in velocity and amplitude.
- Paucity of blinking; levator inhibition/eyelid apraxia.
- Bulbar symptoms: dysphagia, dysarthria; often prominent.
- Poor, unsustained response to anti-parkinsonian medications.
- Neuropsychological deficits, especially frontal executive functions: slow information processing, deficits in focused and divided attention, impaired initiation, memory impairment (active recall > recognition).

Investigations and diagnosis No diagnostic test available; diagnosis remains clinical.

Neuro-ophthalmology: eye movements; saccade error rate.

Neuropsychology: cognitive profile (subcortical dementia) may be suggestive in clinical context.

CSF/brain tissue: τ-protein profile: gel electrophoresis of τ reveals major bands of 64 and 68 kDa, and a minor band of 72 kDa (all derived from four C-terminal repeat τ-isoforms; hence tauopathy; *cf*. Alzheimer's disease).

Pathology: neuronal loss with neurofibrillary tangles, inclusions and gliosis in basal ganglai, brainstem, cerebellar nuclei, usually sparing cortex.

Differential diagnosis

Atypical Parkinson's disease.

Multiple system atrophy.

Corticobasal degeneration (overlap).

Dementia with Lewy bodies.

Pick's disease.

Vascular syndromes.

Supranuclear gaze palsy also reported in Creutzfeldt–Jakob disease (CJD), progressive subcortical gliosis (of Neumann) (PSG).

Treatment and prognosis Some patients may show L-dopa responsiveness. Deep brain stimulation yet to be systematically assessed, but unlikely to be helpful in light of lack of response to levodopa.

References Bak TH, Hodges JR. The neuropsychology of progressive supranuclear palsy. *Neurocase* 1998; **4**: 89–98.

Lees AJ. The Steele–Richardson–Olszewski syndrome (progressive supranuclear palsy). In: Marsden CD, Fahn S (eds). *Movement Disorders 2*. London: Butterworth, 1987: 272–287.

Litvan I, Agid Y, Calne D *et al*. Clinical research criteria for the diagnosis of progressive supranuclear palsy (Steele–Richardson–Olszewski syndrome): report of the NINDS-SPSP international workshop. *Neurology* 1996; **47**: 1–9.

Rehman HU. Progressive supranuclear palsy. *Postgraduate Medical Journal* 2000; **76**: 333–336.

Steele JC, Richardson JC, Olszewski J. Progressive supranuclear palsy: a heterogeneous degeneration involving the brainstem, basal ganglia and cerebellum with vertical gaze and pseudobulbar palsy, nuchal dystonia and dementia. *Archives of Neurology* 1964; **10**: 333–358.

Other relevant entries Dementia: an overview; Parkinsonian syndromes, parkinsonism; Parkinson's disease; Tauopathy.

■ Prolactinoma – see Pituitary disease and apoplexy

■ Prolonged QT syndromes

Pathophysiology Syndromes in which there is prolongation of the QT interval of the electrocardiogram may present as epileptic seizures, consequent upon impaired cerebral perfusion. Correction of the arrhythmia may abolish the seizures.

Causes include:

Inherited:

Jervell–Lange–Nielsen syndrome: autosomal-recessive, deafness

Romano–Ward syndrome: autosomal-dominant, no hearing deficit

Andersen's syndrome (*q.v.*).

Acquired:

Coronary artery disease

Cardiomyopathy
Drugs (tricyclic antidepressants, anti-arrhythmics)
Metabolic (hypocalcaemia, hypomagnesaemia, hypokalaemia).

At least five genes have been linked to the inherited long QT syndrome of Romano–Ward type:

LQT1 locus = KCNQ1 K^+ channel gene
LQT2 locus = KCNH2 K^+ channel gene
LQT3 locus = SCN5A Na^+ channel gene.

Andersen's syndrome also results from mutations in a skeletal muscle potassium channel gene (KCNJ2).

Clinical features: history and examination
- Ventricular tachy-arrhythmias.
- Family history of sudden death, deafness.
- Seizures: may be preceded by syncopal symptoms or palpitations.
- Periodic paralysis (Andersen's syndrome).

Investigations and diagnosis
ECG: prolonged QT interval after correction for heart rate (QTc).
Neurophysiology: EEG: typically normal.
Imaging: typically normal.

Differential diagnosis Other aetiologies of seizure.
Certain drugs may produce a prolongation of QT interval on ECG (e.g. pimozide).

Treatment and prognosis Untreated, there is a risk of sudden death due to malignant ventricular arrhythmias. Treatment with β-blockers, or with a pacemaker or implantable defibrillator, reduces risks and should abolish seizures.

Reference Pacia SV, Devinsky O, Luciano DJ, Vazquez B. The prolonged QT syndrome presenting as epilepsy: a report of two cases and literature review. *Neurology* 1994; **44**: 1408–1410.

Other relevant entries Andersen's syndrome; Channelopathies: an overview; Epilepsy: an overview; Syncope.

▓ Pronator teres syndrome
High median neuropathy

Entrapment of the median nerve between the heads of the pronator teres muscle produces the following features:
- Pain along the flexor side of the proximal forearm.
- Paraesthesia in median nerve distribution in the hand.
- Weakness in one or more hand muscles innervated by the median nerve (abductor pollicis brevis, flexor pollicis longus, opponens pollicis, flexor digitorum profundus).

Pressure over pronator teres may produce pain or paraesthesia.

It may be difficult on clinical grounds to distinguish pronator teres syndrome from anterior interosseous nerve syndrome.

Needle EMG may confirm median nerve involvement in the forearm and hand.

Other relevant entries Anterior interosseous syndrome; Entrapment neuropathies; Median neuropathy.

■ Propionic acidaemia

A disorder of organic acid metabolism, due to an autosomal-recessive defect in propionyl-CoA carboxylase (PCC), often presenting in the first few weeks of life with:

- Vomiting, failure to feed, lethargy
- Encephalopathy + metabolic acidosis
- Seizures: clonic, myoclonic, tonic–clonic
- Oral, perineal candidiasis
- Muscle tone usually reduced (*cf.* isovaleric acidaemia, methymalonic acidaemia)
- Extrapyramidal signs: choreoathetosis, dystonia
- Hyperammonaemia, reduced plasma carnitine, increased glycine
- Neutropenia, thrombocytopenia
- Ketonuria
- Urine organic acid analysis shows a typical, diagnostic, pattern: 3-hydroxypropionic acid, propionylglycine, methylcitrate.

Later presentation with mild mental retardation, episodic headache, and metabolic acidosis, may also occur.

PCC activity may be measured in leukocytes and cultured fibroblasts.

Clinically the condition may be indistinguishable from other disorders of organic acid metabolism such as methylmalonic aciduria and isovaleric aciduria.

Acute crisis should be treated with bicarbonate, glucose, and carnitine supplementation; sepsis should be treated. Ondansetron may be used for vomiting. Severe thrombocytopenia may require platelet transfusion. Once stable, treatment is with dietary restriction of isoleucine, valine, methionine and threonine, with supplemental carnitine. Prognosis remains poor: early death, mental retardation. Liver transplantation has been undertaken.

Other relevant entries Isovaleric acidaemia; Methymalonic acidaemia; Organic acidopathies.

■ Propriospinal myoclonus – see Myoclonus

■ Prosopagnosia

In this form of agnosia, there is a relatively selective impairment of facial recognition; equivalent stimuli such as animals ("zooagnosia") or cars may also be affected.

The disorder may be characterized as apperceptive, due to faulty perceptual analysis of faces; or associative, a semantic defect in recognition. Familiar individuals may be recognized by their voices or clothing.

Prosopagnosia may have various aetiologies:

- Cerebrovascular disease: right occipitotemporal lesions, often with concurrent left homonymous superior quadrantanopia, $+/-$ alexia, achromatopsia;
- Tumour, for example glioma: extending from one hemisphere to the other via the splenium of the corpus callosum;
- Epilepsy (paroxysmal prosopagnosia): due to bilateral foci or spread from one occipital focus to the contralateral hemisphere;
- Focal lobar atrophy, affecting the right temporal lobe (progressive prosopagnosia);
- Developmental/congenital.

The developmental syndrome suggests that facial recognition is a separate neuropsychological function (the acquired pathologies do not respect functional boundaries).

References Evans JJ, Heggs AJ, Antoun N, Hodges JR. Progressive prosopagnosia associated with selective right temporal lobe atrophy. A new syndrome? *Brain* 1995; **118**: 1–13.

Nunn JA, Postma P, Pearson R. Developmental prosopagnosia: should it be taken at face value? *Neurocase* 2001; **7**: 15–27.

Other relevant entries Achromatopsia; Agnosia; Alexia.

Proteinopathy

An increasingly widely accepted approach to the classification of degenerative neuromuscular disease is to label the aberrant protein.

See individual entries for:

Amyloid and the nervous system: an overview
Dysferlinopathy
Dystrophinopathy
Neuroferritinopathy
Prion diseases: an overview
Sarcoglycanopathy
Synucleinopathy
Tauopathy

Proteus syndrome

An autosomal-dominant syndrome characterized by:

Macrocephaly; thick calvarium
Exostoses
Asymmetrical, hypertrophic, limbs

Plantar hyperplasia: "moccasin feet"
Skin lesions: lipoma, hemangioma, epidermal naevi
+/− seizures.

The "Elephant man", Joseph Merrick, studied by the surgeon Sir Frederick Treves, may have suffered from Proteus syndrome (rather than neurofibromatosis, as previously thought).

Reference Tibbles JAR, Cohen Jr MM. The proteus syndrome: the Elephant man diagnosed. *British Medical Journal* 1986; **293**: 683.

Other relevant entries Gigantism; Neurofibromatosis.

■ Proximal myotonic myopathy
Myotonic dystrophy type 2 (DM2) • Ricker's disease • Thornton–Griggs–Moxley disease

Pathophysiology A recently described autosomal-dominant disorder characterized by myotonia, proximal myopathy, and cataracts, with onset between age 20 and 40 years. Clinically it seems to be more benign than classical dystrophia myotonica (myotonic dystrophy type 1, DM1). It has been linked to chromosome 3q and is associated with a CCTG repeat expansion in intron 1 of the zinc finger protein 9 (ZFN-9) gene, with repeats of unprecedented size, up to 5000.

Clinical features: history and examination
- Myotonia: intermittent, affecting hands, proximal legs.
- Proximal (not distal) limb weakness: mild, slowly progressive, without atrophy; normal face; muscle pain is prominent.
- +/− calf hypertrophy.
- Cataracts.
- ? cardiac arrhythmias (rare).

Investigations and diagnosis *Bloods*: creatine kinase normal.
Neurophysiology: EMG/NCS: myotonic discharges.
Muscle biopsy.
Neurogenetics: expansion of nucleotide quadruplet $[CCTG]_n$ repeats in gene encoding ZNF-9 on chromosome 3q.

Differential diagnosis Dystrophia myotonica: but no distal weakness, facial weakness, ptosis.

Treatment and prognosis No specific treatment.

References Day JW, Ricker K, Jacobsen JF *et al*. Myotonic dystrophy type 2. Molecular, diagnostic and clinical spectrum. *Neurology* 2003; **60**: 657–664.

Ricker J. Myotonic dystrophy and proximal myotonic myopathy. *Journal of Neurology* 1999; **246**: 334–338.

Other relevant entries Dystrophia myotonica; Myotonia and myotonic syndromes; Trinucleotide repeat diseases.

▓ Proximal weakness

Pathophysiology Weakness affecting predominantly the proximal musculature (shoulder abductors and hip flexors) is a pattern frequently observed in myopathic and dystrophic muscle disorders and neuromuscular junction transmission disorders, much more so than predominantly distal weakness (the differential diagnosis of which encompasses dystrophica myotonia, distal myopathy of Miyoshi type, desmin myopathy, and, rarely, myasthenia gravis). Some neuropathic disorders may also cause a predominantly proximal weakness (e.g. Guillain–Barré syndrome). Age of onset and other clinical features may help to narrow the differential diagnosis, but muscle biopsy may be required as the final arbiter.

Clinical features: history and examination
- Weakness +/− wasting of shoulder abductors and hip flexors > other muscle groups.
- Painful muscles may suggest inflammatory cause.
- Fatigue may suggest myasthenia gravis (although lesser degrees of fatigue may be seen in myopathic disorders).
- Weakness elsewhere may suggest diagnosis [e.g. face in facioscapulohumeral (FSH) dystrophy, diaphragm in acid-maltase deficiency].
- Calf pseudohypertrophy in Duchenne, Becker muscular dystrophy.
- Autonomic features, post-tetanic potentiation of reflexes in Lambert–Eaton myasthenic syndrome.
- Cachexia (malignant disease).

Investigations and diagnosis *Bloods*: creatine kinase: significant elevation may suggest inflammatory disorder or dystrophinopathy.

Neurophysiology: EMG/NCS: may indicate presence of myopathy, neuromuscular junction transmission disorder, or neuropathy.

Muscle biopsy: may be required to establish definitive diagnosis of myopathic disorder.

Differential diagnosis
Myopathies:

Inflammatory: polymyositis, dermatomyositis;
Progressive muscular dystrophies: Duchenne, Becker, limb-girdle, FSH;
Metabolic: acid-maltase deficiency; thyroid dysfunction, Cushing's syndrome;
Non-metastatic feature of malignant disease.

Neuromuscular junction transmission disorders:

Myasthenia gravis
Lambert–Eaton myasthenic syndrome.

Neuropathy:

Guillain–Barré syndrome.

Treatment and prognosis Of cause where identified.

Other relevant entries Acid-maltase deficiency; Dermatomyositis; Lambert–Eaton myasthenic syndrome; Muscular dystrophies: an overview; Myasthenia gravis; Myopathy: an overview; Polymyositis; Proximal myotonic myopathy.

■ Pseudobulbar palsy – see Dysarthria

■ Pseudochoreoathetosis – see Déjerine–Roussy syndrome

■ Pseudoclaudication – see Spinal stenosis

■ Pseudo-Foster–Kennedy syndrome – see Foster–Kennedy syndrome

■ Pseudo-Hurler's syndrome
Mucolipidosis type III (ML type III)

This condition results from deficiency or dysfunction of N-acetylglucosamine phosphotransferase, as in mucolipidosis type II (I-cell disease), but the phenotype is less severe: intelligence is normal or borderline, onset is later in childhood and progression slower. Corneal clouding and aortic regurgitation are common.

Other relevant entry Mucolipidoses.

■ Pseudohypertrophic muscular dystrophy – see Duchenne muscular dystrophy

■ Pseudomitochondrial disease

Occasional cases with the typical clinical phenotype of mitochondrial disease but without abnormalities on electromyography, aerobic exercise test, muscle biopsy, or mitochondrial DNA studies have been reported.

Reference Larner AJ, Williamson C, Ward NS, Acheson JF, Robinson S, Farmer SF. Isolated familial hypomagnesaemia with novel neurological features: causal link or chance concurrence? *European Journal of Neurology* 2001; **8**: 495–499.

Other relevant entry Mitochondrial disease: an overview.

■ Pseudoseizures
Non-epileptic attack disorder (NEAD) • Non-epileptic seizures • Psychogenic seizures

Pathophysiology Pseudoseizures are seizure-like attacks which arise for reasons other than epilepsy, often as a sign of emotional difficulties such as anxiety or depression. There is often a prior history of physical or sexual abuse. Pseudoseizures may coexist with true epileptic seizures. They are commoner in women.

Clinical features: history and examination
- Convulsive movements, often not typical of epileptic attacks, for example head shaking from side to side; resistance to eye opening, no deviation of eyes,

increased amplitude of movements with time and audience, "thrashing". Forced eye closure, distractibility, other evidence of responsiveness may be present. Pelvic thrusting is a common manifestation (although may be seen in epileptic seizures). Attacks may be prolonged: pseudostatus is described, often in individuals with a history of pseudoseizures, multiple episodes of "status", unexplained illness, and deliberate self-poisoning.

- No cyanosis, post-ictal confusion; urinary incontinence, tongue-biting rare.
- Self-injury absent or minimal (e.g. confined to carpet burns).
- No focal neurological signs, no pathological reflexes.
- No elevation in serum prolactin post-event.

Investigations and diagnosis Ideally investigations should be kept to a minimum.
Witness attack, video if possible (need patient's permission beforehand).
Neurophysiology: Telemetry: absence of EEG changes during attack is highly suggestive.
Imaging: CT/MRI normal, unless concurrent or incidental pathology.
Differential diagnosis Epileptic seizures.
Treatment and prognosis
Patient education with appropriate literature, counselling.
Cognitive behaviour therapy.
Withdraw inappropriate anti-epileptic medication if possible.
Treat any underlying anxiety or depression.

References Devinsky O, Sanchez Villasenor F, Vazquez B *et al*. Clinical profile of patients with epileptic and nonepileptic seizures. *Neurology* 1996; **47**: 621–625.

Howell SJ, Owen L, Chadwick DW. Pseudostatus epilepticus. *Quarterly Journal of Medicine* 1989; **71**: 507–519.

Thomas L, Trimble MR. *A Patient's Guide to Non-epileptic Seizures*. Petersfield: Wrightson Biomedical Publishing, 1995.

Other relevant entry Epilepsy: an overview.

▓ Pseudosyringomyelia – see Amyloid and the nervous system: an overview; Syringomyelia and syringobulbia; Tangier disease

▓ Pseudotabes – see Alcohol and the nervous system: an overview; Diabetes mellitus and the nervous system; Diphtheria

▓ Pseudothalamic syndrome – see Déjerine–Mouzon syndrome

▓ Pseudotumor cerebri – see Idiopathic intracranial hypertension

▓ Pseudoxanthoma elasticum

Pathophysiology An hereditary disorder of elastic tissue, of which both autosomal-dominant and recessive types have been described. The principal manifestations are dermatological, but elastic tissue in coronary and cerebral arteries may also be affected, the latter resulting in a vasculopathy with aneurysm formation which may cause multiple strokes or subarachnoid haemorrhage in a young person. The candidate gene underlying the majority of pseudoxanthoma elasticum (PXE) cases is ABCC6, an ATP-binding-cassette subfamily C member 6 transporter, encoded at chromosome 16p13.1, also known as multidrug-resistance-associated protein 6.

Clinical features: history and examination

- Dermatological: flexural plaques, "chicken-skin", cutis laxa.
- Ophthalmic: angioid streaks (degeneration of Bruch's membrane) leading to visual impairment, blindness.
- Coronary artery disease.
- Intermittent claudication.
- Gastrointestinal bleeding.
- Strokes.

Investigations and diagnosis

Diagnosis usually obvious from skin findings.

Imaging: for vascular disease, aneurysms.

Differential diagnosis Other causes of stroke in the young.

Treatment and prognosis As for other forms of stroke, aneurysm.

References Iqbal A, Alter M, Lee SH. Pseudoxanthoma elasticum: a review of neurological complications. *Annals of Neurology* 1978; **4**: 18–20.

Ringpfeil F, Lebwohl MG, Christiano AM, Uitto J. Pseudoxanthoma elasticum: mutations in the MRP6 gene encoding a transmembrane ATP-binding cassette (ABC) transporter. *Proceedings of the National Academy of Sciences of the USA* 2000; **97**: 6001–6006.

Other relevant entries Cerebrovascular disease: arterial; Phakomatosis; Subarachnoid haemorrhage.

■ Pseudo-Zellweger syndrome – see Peroxisomal disorders: an overview; Zellweger syndrome

■ Psittacosis
Ornithosis

Pathophysiology *Chlamydia psittaci*, the causative organism of psittacosis, is transmitted from birds to humans by inhalation.

Clinical features: history and examination

- History of exposure to birds.
- Symptoms:
    Respiratory: cough, often non-productive.
    Systemic: fever, myalgia.
    Neurological: infrequent; encephalitic or meningoencephalitic illness; raised intracranial pressure has also been described.

Investigations and diagnosis *Bloods*: leukocytosis, raised ESR; positive serology for *C. psittaci*.

Imaging:

CXR: pneumonia.
CT/MRI: normal.

CSF: may show elevated pressure.

Differential diagnosis Other causes of pneumonia with associated neurological features. Other causes of meningoencephalitis.

Treatment and prognosis Tetracycline 0.5 mg qds.
Recovery usually complete.

> **References** Hughes P, Chidley K, Cowie J. Neurological complications in psittacosis: a case report and literature review. *Respiratory Medicine* 1995; **89**: 637–638.
>
> Prevett M, Harding AE. Intracranial hypertension following psittacosis. *Journal of Neurology, Neurosurgery and Psychiatry* 1993; **56**: 425–426.
>
> **Other relevant entries** "Atypical pneumonias" and the nervous system; Mycoplasma; Q fever.

■ Psychiatric disorders and neurological disease

Pathophysiology Disorders labelled either psychiatric or neurological in origin are likewise disorders of the nervous system, and it is therefore not surprising that there should be overlap between them, that is, psychiatric features in neurological disease ("behavioural neurology") and a neurological origin for psychiatric symptoms (sometimes with neurological signs), often implicating the limbic system ("neuropsychiatry" or "biological psychiatry"). Close liaison between neurologists and psychiatrists may be required for the optimal management of "psychiatric" features in "neurological" disease, and to determine "neurological" causes for "psychiatric" symptoms.

Many patients presenting to the neurology clinic may have primarily psychiatric disease, particularly those with headache, pain syndromes, complaints of poor memory, and sleep disorders. Recognition of this fact is an important first step in appropriate management.

Clinical features: history and examination

- Frontal lobe pathology: impaired attention, distractibility, perseveration; personality changes: either apathy, indifference, self-neglect (abulia); or euphoria, disinhibition (may be labelled "mania" or "manic-depressive psychosis").
- Temporal lobe pathology: interictal psychosis, schizophreniform features may develop with dominant medial temporal focus. Geschwind's syndrome (hypergraphia, hyposexuality, hyperreligiosity).

Also see various disorders which may have prominent psychiatric features, for example epilepsy, multiple sclerosis, systemic lupus erythematosus, cerebrovascular disease.

Investigations and diagnosis *Imaging*: CT/MRI may show focal brain lesions to account for psychiatric symptoms (e.g. frontal meningioma).

Neurophysiology: EEG: seizure activity of temporal lobe origin may account for psychiatric symptoms.

Differential diagnosis Abulia: psychomotor retardation of depression, catatonia. Disinhibition: mania, bipolar disorder.

Psychiatric features may be seen in:

Neurodegenerative disease: Frontotemporal dementia (Pick's disease), Alzheimer's disease.

Cerebrovascular disease.

Inflammatory disease: multiple sclerosis, systemic lupus erythematosus.

Metabolic disease: adrenoleukodystrophy, porphyria, thyroid disease, Wilson's disease.

Neoplasia: frontal lobe tumours.

Treatment and prognosis Of individual condition where possible. Treatments aimed at psychiatric features *per se* may be required (e.g. antidepressants).

References Cummings JL, Mega MS. *Neuropsychiatry and Behavioral Neuroscience*. Oxford: OUP, 2003.

Feinstein A. *The Clinical Neuropsychiatry of Multiple Sclerosis*. Cambridge: Cambridge University Press, 1999.

Robinson RG. *The Clinical Neuropsychiatry of Stroke: Cognitive, Behavioral and Emotional Disorders Following Vascular Brain Injury*. Cambridge: Cambridge University Press, 1998.

Trimble MR. *Biological Psychiatry* (2nd edition). Chichester: Wiley, 1996.

Other relevant entries Adrenoleukodystrophy; Alzheimer's disease; Epilepsy: an overview; Multiple sclerosis; Pick's disease; Porphyria; Prion disease: an overview; Schizophrenia; Sleep disorders: an overview; Somatization disorders; Systemic lupus erythematosus and the nervous system; Thyroid disease and the nervous system; Wilson's disease.

■ Puerperium – see Pregnancy and the nervous system: an overview

■ Pugilistic encephalopathy – see Dementia pugilistica

■ Punch drunk syndrome – see Dementia pugilistica

■ Pure autonomic failure

Bradbury–Eggleston syndrome • Idiopathic autonomic failure • Idiopathic orthostatic hypotension

Pathophysiology This rare condition is characterized by an idiopathic degeneration of the postganglionic sympathetic fibres of the autonomic nervous system, with relative preservation of the parasympathetic nervous system. It is not associated with degeneration in any other neurological systems [*cf.* multiple system atrophy (MSA), autonomic failure associated with Parkinson's disease]. Some cases of MSA present with pure autonomic failure (PAF) before other features develop, and this has also been described in dementia with Lewy bodies.

Clinical features: history and examination Diagnosis is essentially clinical.

- Postural hypotension:

    Gradual fading of consciousness while patient is standing, walking.

    Neck ache, backache in "coathanger" distribution.

    Symptoms worse in morning, hot weather, after meals and exercise.

    Recumbent/supine hypertension, reversal of diurnal blood pressure pattern (may have adverse neurological consequences).

- Visual disturbances:

    Transient scotomata, hallucinations, tunnel vision (occipital lobe ischaemia).

- Defective sweating sexual dysfunction:

    Erectile failure, followed by disturbance of ejaculation.

- Gastrointestinal:

    Swallowing difficulty, laryngeal paresis.

Investigations and diagnosis *Bloods*: Plasma noradrenaline level low in resting state, no elevation with tilting or standing.

Pathology (postmortem): Lewy bodies in the sympathetic ganglia, with or without neuronal loss.

Differential diagnosis Autonomic failure due to other neurodegenerative disease: MSA, dementia with Lewy bodies (DLB): neurological, neuropsychological features emerge.

Dopamine b-hydroxylase deficiency: earlier onset than PAF, virtually absent plasma noradrenaline.

Autonomic dysfunction/postural hypotension due to other conditions: diabetes mellitus, phaeochromocytoma, amyloidosis.

Treatment and prognosis Management of postural hypotension:

Non-pharmacological: increased salt intake, head-up bed tilt, wearing a G-suit.
Pharmacological: fludrocortisone, ephedrine, midodrine.

Management of erectile dysfunction.

Outlook relatively good in PAF with management of postural hypotension, life expectancy only a little reduced.

References Consensus statement on the definition of orthostatic hypotension, pure autonomic failure and multiple system atrophy. *Clincal Autonomic Research* 1996; **6**: 125–126.

Mathias C, Kimber JR. Treatment of postural hypotension. *Journal of Neurology, Neurosurgery and Psychiatry* 1998; **65**: 285–289.

Pure motor stroke, pure motor hemiplegia – see Lacunar syndromes

Pure sensory stroke – see Lacunar syndromes

Pure word blindness – see Alexia; Aphasia

Pure word deafness – see Aphasia; Disconnection syndromes

Pyknolepsy – see Absence epilepsy; Epilepsy: an overview

Pyomyositis – see Myositis: an overview

Pyramidal decussation syndrome

A crossed hemiplegia syndrome, with weakness of one arm and the contralateral leg without involvement of the face, due to a lesion within the pyramid below the decussation of corticospinal fibres destined for the arm but above that for fibres destined for the leg.

Pyridoxine-dependent seizures

This syndrome typically presents in the newborn period with intractable seizures, of tonic–clonic type, which respond dramatically to pyridoxine (vitamin B_6, 100 mg intravenously). Atypical forms have also been described which respond only after a longer therapeutic trial of pyridoxine (50 mg/kg/day).

Other relevant entry Epilepsy: an overview.

Pyruvate carboxylase deficiency

Pyruvate carboxylase (PC) is a biotin-dependent enzyme, dependent on acetyl-CoA for its activity, that catalyses the carboxylation of pyruvate to form oxaloacetate. This fuels the tricarboxylic acid (Krebs) cycle and also the first step in gluconeogenesis. Lactic acidosis is a prominent feature of PC deficiency.

Two types of PC deficiency, both rare, are recognized:

- Type A: first few months of life: psychomotor retardation, intermittent acute metabolic acidosis; normal lactate/pyruvate (L/P) ratio.
- Type B: severe form, present in newborn with severe lactic acidosis, death within months; increased lactate/pyruvate (L/P) ratio, reduced 3-hydroxybutyrate or acetoacetate ratio; hyperammonaemia, increased plasma levels of citrulline, lysine, and proline.

Measurement of enzyme activities in leukocytes or fibroblasts is the diagnostic test.

Other relevant entry Lactic acidosis.

▨ Pyruvate dehydrogenase deficiency

Pathophysiology Pyruvate dehydrogenase (PDH) is a large multicomponent enzyme complex, composed of multiple subunits. Most patients with PDH deficiency have mutations of the X-linked E_1 subunit of the pyruvate decarboxylase component, despite which males and females are equally represented.

Clinical features: history and examination PDH deficiency is clinically heterogeneous:

- Newborn: characterized by persistent lactic acidosis; death within weeks, months; may be associated agenesis of the corpus callosum.
- Late infancy (common): psychomotor retardation, hypotonia, failure to thrive, seizures, $+/-$ bouts of severe lactic acidosis; subtle dysmorphic facial features; presentation may be as Leigh's disease.
- Benign disease: intermittent ataxia.

PDH deficiency may be the inborn error of metabolism underpinning the clinical syndrome of Alpers disease or other cases of chronic progressive encephalopathy with lactic acidosis.

Investigations and diagnosis Plasma lactate persistently elevated; acidosis, worse with carbohydrate intake.

Plasma or CSF lactate/pyruvate ratio is normal in this condition, since the accumulation of lactate is a result of defective pyruvate metabolism.

Enzyme deficiency demonstrated in cultured fibroblasts.

Differential diagnosis Other causes of persistent lactic acidosis: inborn errors of metabolism include pyruvate carboxylase deficiency, mitochondrial electron transport chain defects, disorders of gluconeogenesis [e.g. phosphoenolpyruvate carboxykinase (PEPCK) deficiency], fatty acid oxidation defects.

Treatment and prognosis No effective treatment.

Other relevant entries Agenesis of the corpus callosum; Fatty acid oxidation disorders; Lactic acidosis; Leigh's disease, Leigh's syndrome; Mitochondrial disease: an overview; Phosphoenolpyruvate carboxykinase deficiency; Pyruvate carboxylase deficiency.

▨ Pyruvate kinase deficiency – see Kernicterus

Qq

■ Q fever

Q fever is a zoonotic infection caused by the obligate intracellular organism *Coxiella burnetti*, belonging to the Rickettsiae family. A self-limiting coryzal illness is the commonest manifestation, but pneumonia and endocarditis may occur. Neurological complications are rare: meningoencephalitis is the commonest neurological feature, acute transverse myelitis has also been described. Culture-negative endocarditis is also a feature of *Coxiella* infection, which may result in embolic neurological sequelae.

The diagnosis is based on serological evidence of infection. Differential diagnosis encompasses other causes of pneumonia with associated neurological features and other causes of meningoencephalitis. Treatment is with doxycycline.

Reference Maurin M, Raoult D. Q fever. *Clinical Microbiology Reviews* 1999; **12**: 518–553.

Other relevant entries "Atypical pneumonias" and the nervous system; Endocarditis and the nervous system; Rickettsial diseases.

■ Quadriplegia: an overview

Pathophysiology Quadriplegia is weakness affecting all four limbs; quadriparesis refers to a lesser degree of weakness of similar distribution. This may result from upper motor neurone lesions, affecting the corticospinal pathways anywhere from motor cortex to cervical cord via the brainstem, but is most commonly seen with brainstem and upper cervical cord lesions. Lower motor neurone pathologies may also produce quadriplegia (acute neuropathies, anterior horn cell disease). Respiration may also be affected, necessitating careful clinical monitoring.

Clinical features: history and examination

- Lower motor neurone, and some acute upper motor neurone, pathologies produce a flaccid quadriparesis/quadriplegia with areflexia; urinary retention may be present.
- Upper motor neurone lesions, particularly if chronic, produce a spastic quadriparesis with hypertonia, sustained clonus, hyperreflexia, loss of abdominal and cremasteric reflexes, and bilateral Babinski's sign. There may also be enhanced flexion defence reflexes ("flexor spasms") which may develop over time into a fixed flexion deformity with secondary contractures ("paraplegia in flexion"). Incomplete or high spinal cord lesions may evolve to "paraplegia in extension", with extension at the hip and knee.

Investigations and diagnosis

Imaging: MRI brain, cervical spinal cord for upper motor neurone picture.
CSF: if inflammatory process suspected.
Neurophysiology: EMG/NCS: if acute neuropathic process suspected.

Differential diagnosis *Upper motor neurone lesions*: brainstem and upper cervical cord lesions, for example trauma, infarction (basilar artery occlusion, locked-in syndrome), inflammation.

Lower motor neurone lesions: Guillain–Barré syndrome, borreliosis (Lyme disease), porphyria, acute motor axonal neuropathy (AMAN), acute motor and sensory axonal neuropathy (AMSAN), critical illness polyneuropathy.

Treatment and prognosis Treatment of cause where possible. Full supportive care with particular attention to respiration (monitor vital capacity) and elective ventilation if necessary. In Guillain–Barré syndrome, cardiac monitoring for arrhythmias may be advisable; pacing for heart block may be necessary.

Attention to posture, skin hygiene, bladder, and bowel function are crucial to prevent infection and the development of flexor spasms, contractures.

Other relevant entries Cervical cord and root disease; Guillain–Barré syndrome; Locked-in syndrome; Paraparesis: acute management and differential diagnosis; Respiratory failure; Spinal cord trauma.

■ Quail eater's myopathy
Quail poisoning myoglobinuria

A myopathic syndrome characterized by muscle cramps, myalgia, rhabdomyolysis, and proximal weakness, often with nausea and vomiting, following consumption of quail meat. It is commonest in the Mediterranean basin, for example in Greece in the Spring following the migration of quails from North Africa. The pathogenesis is unknown, but it has been suggested to reflect poisoning with hemlock or laudanum since the birds eat seeds of these plants. It is said to be the earliest myopathy to have been described, in the Bible (Numbers 11: 31–34).

Other relevant entries Myopathy: an overview; Rhabdomyolysis.

Rr

■ Rabbit syndrome

The rabbit syndrome is a rest tremor of perioral and nasal muscles. It has been associated with both anti-psychotic drug therapy and idiopathic Parkinson's disease and is therefore presumably related to dopamine deficiency, although response to anticholinergic agents is reported. No specific investigations are required, but a drug history, including over the counter medication, is crucial. The condition may be confused with edentulous dyskinesia if there is accompanying tremor of the jaw and/or lip. Drug-induced rabbit syndrome may remit with drug withdrawal but not always. Appropriate treatment of Parkinson's disease may also improve the involuntary movements. Anticholinergics may be tried.

References Decina P, Caracci G, Scapicchio PL. The rabbit syndrome. *Movement Disorders* 1990; **5**: 263.

Deshmukh DK, Joshi VS, Agarwal MR. Rabbit syndrome – a rare complication of long-term neuroleptic medication. *British Journal of Psychiatry* 1990; **157**: 293.
Other relevant entries Drug-induced movement disorders; Parkinson's disease.

■ Rabies

Pathophysiology The rabies virus is transmitted to man from the saliva of affected mammals through skin bites or abrasions. The virus reaches the central nervous system (CNS) via the peripheral nerves by means of retrograde axoplasmic flow. There is a predilection for the brainstem and grey matter. The condition is almost uniformly fatal once neurological features occur. Post-exposure prophylaxis is available.

Clinical features: history and examination

- Incubation period very variable: days to months or even years.
- Fever, malaise, headache, sore throat; pain/paraesthesia at site of bite.
- Anxiety, depression, agitation, insomnia.
- Neurological features:

    "Furious": hyperacusis, hydrophobia, pharyngeal/laryngeal spasms leading to salivary drooling, respiratory arrest, opisthotonos; episodes of hallucination, profound agitation requiring restraint, sympathetic overactivity, but fully conscious and terrified in period between attacks; seizures; coma, flaccid paralysis, death.

    "Paralytic" or "dumb": flaccid paralysis only, leading to death.

    History of animal bite is not always forthcoming.

Investigations and diagnosis *Bloods*: serology for rabies virus.

Saliva: viral culture.

CSF: non-specific pleocytosis; antibodies to the rabies virus.

Pathology: primary encephalomyelitis with mononuclear cell infiltrate; characteristic Negri bodies (eosinophilic cytoplasmic inclusion body) seen in the majority of cases.

Differential diagnosis The "furious" syndrome is characteristic; flaccid paralysis may be mistaken for Guillain–Barré syndrome.

Tetanus.

Treatment and prognosis A combination of early passive (rabies immune serum) and active (rabies vaccine) immunization may be protective after exposure. Very rare reports of survival with full recovery mandate full intensive care support of patients with neurological disease.

References Warrell M. Rabies encephalitis and its prophylaxis. *Practical Neurology* 2001; **1**: 14–29.

Wilkinson L. Rabies. In: Cox FEG (ed.). *The Wellcome Trust Illustrated History of Tropical Diseases*. London: Wellcome Trust, 1996: 132–141.

Wood M, Anderson M. *Neurological Infections*. London: WB Saunders, 1988: 503–516.
Other relevant entries Encephalitis: an overview; Tetanus.

■ Rachischisis – see Spina bifida

■ Radial neuropathy

Pathophysiology The radial nerve may be compressed or damaged in the axilla, in the spiral groove of the humerus ("Saturday night palsy"), or more distally (posterior interosseous, superficial sensory branches). Some authors suggest the radial nerve is the most commonly injured peripheral nerve.

Clinical features: history and examination

- Motor: Weakness of triceps (axillary injury only), brachioradialis, supinator, wrist and finger extensors (hence wrist drop, finger drop); triceps reflex may be depressed or lost with axillary lesions.
- Sensory: Loss on dorsal aspect of hand, thumb, index, and middle fingers. No sensory loss with posterior interosseous lesions. Purely sensory findings with injury to superficial sensory branches, for example with handcuffs (cheiralgia paraesthetica).

Investigations and diagnosis *EMG/NCS*: may identify reduced amplitude compound muscle action potential (CMAP) in radial innervated muscles and reduced or absent SNAPs. Fibrillations in triceps suggest injury at axillary level. Abnormalities beyond radial nerve territory may refute a diagnosis of mononeuropathy.

Differential diagnosis Radiculopathy, brachial plexopathy: clinical features unlikely to be mistaken.

> **Reference** Staal A, Van Gijn J, Spaans F. *Mononeuropathies: Examination, Diagnosis and Treatment.* London: WB Saunders, 1999: 35–48.

> **Other relevant entries** Cheiralgia paraesthetica; Median neuropathy; Neuropathies: an overview; Posterior interosseous syndrome; Ulnar neuropathy.

■ Radiation injury – see Chemotherapy- and radiotherapy-induced neurological disorders

■ Radiculopathies: an overview

Pathophysiology Radiculopathies are disorders of nerve roots which may cause sensory and motor features in the corresponding dermatome and myotome, respectively. They may be single or multiple (polyradiculopathy, e.g. cauda equina syndrome), and may occur in conjunction with spinal cord disease (radiculo-myelopathy). Causes of radiculopathy include compression, trauma (root avulsion), diabetes, neoplasia, infection/inflammation (radiculitis), and demyelination.

Clinical features: history and examination

- Sensory: pain, paraesthesia, sensory diminution or loss, in a radicular distribution.
- Motor: lower motor neurone-type weakness; hyporeflexia or areflexia.

(For details on specific roots, see Cervical cord and root disease, Lumbar cord and root disease.)

Investigations and diagnosis *Neurophysiology*: EMG/NCS: may differentiate radiculopathy from neuropathy or plexopathy: sensory nerve action potentials are normal for intrathecal root lesions, and EMG shows involvement of paraspinal muscles; neurophysiology may also be used to localize levels of radiculopathy.

Imaging: MRI may demonstrate compression from prolapsed intervertebral disc, metastases, spondylolisthesis; fracture; infection.

Bloods: fasting glucose (to exclude diabetes); inflammatory markers; serology (if appropriate) for HIV (cytomegalovirus, CMV late in the course), Borrelia, syphilis (tabes dorsalis), herpes zoster.

CSF: protein, cell count, cytology (may need to be repeated if clinical suspicion of malignant infiltration high), oligoclonal bands.

Differential diagnosis Plexopathies; mononeuropathies, polyneuropathies.

Treatment and prognosis Of cause where identified (e.g. surgery for compressive lesions). Symptomatic treatment with drugs for neuropathic pain may be appropriate (e.g. amitriptyline, carbamazepine, gabapentin).

> **Reference** Chad DF. Nerve root and plexus disorders. In: Bogousslavsky J, Fisher M (eds). *Textbook of Neurology*. Boston: Butterworth-Heinemann, 1998: 491–506.

> **Other relevant entries** Arachnoiditis; Cervical cord and root disease; Failed back syndrome; Lumbar cord and root disease; Sciatica.

■ Raeder's paratrigeminal syndrome
Paratrigeminal syndrome of Raeder

Pathophysiology This is a rare facial pain syndrome, with unilateral oculosympathetic paralysis (Horner's syndrome) and ipsilateral head, face, or retro-orbital pain. It has been likened to cluster headache (CH) but with constant pain. The syndrome may on occasion be due to a parasellar (middle cranial fossa) mass lesion (tumour, aneurysm), although trauma (head injury) and infection have also been reported. "Idiopathic" cases have been reported, but there is a strong suspicion that such cases are in fact due to carotid artery dissection undetected by imaging techniques. Hence, the value of this eponym has been questioned.

Clinical features: history and examination
- Persistent pain in first and second divisions of the trigeminal nerve (V1 and V2): persistent, burning, throbbing, unilateral; may wake the patient at night, pain likened to that of tic douloureux.
- Oculosympathetic dysfunction (Horner's syndrome): ptosis, miosis, but preserved sweating (no anhidrosis).
- +/− trigeminal sensory loss.
- +/− weakness of trigeminal innervated muscles.
- +/− other cranial nerve lesions (II, III, IV, VI).

Investigations and diagnosis *Imaging*: MRI to exclude parasellar (trigeminal ganglion) lesion; MRI/MRA and/or angiography to exclude carotid artery dissection.

Differential diagnosis Differential diagnosis as for a painful Horner's syndrome, viz.

Carotid artery dissection
Cavernous sinus lesion (e.g. aneurysm)
CH (lacks oculomotor or trigeminal nerve dysfunction)
Orbital pseudotumour/"Tolosa–Hunt syndrome"
Syringomyelia.

Treatment and prognosis No specific treatment; symptomatic treatment of pain. The most important issue is to exclude other treatable causes for painful Horner's syndrome, especially carotid artery dissection.

References Mokri B. Raeder's paratrigeminal syndrome – original concept and subsequent deviations. *Archives of Neurology* 1982; **39**: 395–399.

Raeder JG. "Paratrigeminal" paralysis of oculo-pupillary sympathetic. *Brain* 1924; **47**: 149–158.

Solomon S, Lustig JP. Benign Raeder's syndrome is probably a manifestation of carotid artery disease. *Cephalalgia* 2001; **21**: 1–11.

Other relevant entries Carotid artery disease; Cluster headache; Horner's syndrome; Trigeminal neuralgia.

▓ Raised intracranial pressure – see Idiopathic intracranial hypertension; Traumatic brain injury; Tumours: an overview

▓ Ramsay Hunt syndrome (1) – see Unverricht–Lundborg disease

▓ Ramsay Hunt syndrome (2)
Geniculate herpes zoster • Herpes zoster oticus

Pathophysiology Facial palsy with herpetic eruption at the external auditory meatus was attributed to reactivation of herpes infection within the geniculate ganglion by Ramsay Hunt, although there is little evidence to confirm this; the infection may actually be within the brainstem. Adjacent cranial nerves (especially VIII) may also be affected.

Clinical features: history and examination
- Ear pain radiating to the tonsillar region.
- Lower motor neurone facial weakness.
- Herpetic eruption in external auditory meatus (otic zoster); occasionally in throat.
- Hyperacusis (lesion proximal to nerve to stapedius).
- +/− loss of taste, anterior two-third of tongue (lesion proximal to chorda tympani).
- +/− tinnitus, vertigo, deafness (VIII nerve involvement).

Investigations and diagnosis History and examination. No specific investigations.

Differential diagnosis Other causes of unilateral facial palsy (e.g. idiopathic Bell's palsy, sarcoidosis, Lyme disease).

Treatment and prognosis Appropriate analgesia. Aciclovir in the acute stage. Steroids contraindicated. Spontaneous recovery occurs but is said to be less complete than in idiopathic Bell's palsy (i.e. prognosis poorer).

> **Reference** Sweeney CJ, Gilden DH. Ramsay Hunt syndrome. *Journal of Neurology, Neurosurgery and Psychiatry* 2001; **71**: 149–154.

> **Other relevant entries** Bell's palsy; Borreliosis; Herpes zoster and postherpetic neuralgia; Vertigo.

■ Ramsay Hunt syndrome (3)

Pathophysiology This name is sometimes given to one of the syndromes of compression of the ulnar nerve in the wrist and palm, viz. compression of the proximal part of the deep terminal branch at the level of the pisiform bone, distal to Guyon's canal. The commonest cause is prolonged external pressure, for example by the handlebars of a bicycle (hence "cyclists' palsy", or "handlebar palsy").

Clinical features: history and examination

- Weak adductor policis, abductor digiti minimi, interossei muscles.
- No sensory loss (*cf.* superficial terminal branch of the ulnar nerve which supplies sensation to medial distal half of palm and the palmar surfaces of the ring and little fingers).
- Normal function in palmaris brevis (*cf.* superficial terminal branch).

Investigations and diagnosis *EMG/NCS:* may indicate level of the lesion.

Differential diagnosis Other forms of ulnar neuropathy in wrist and hand.

Treatment and prognosis No specific treatment; avoid precipitating causes. May recover gradually.

> **Reference** Hunt JR. Occupation neuritis of the deep palmar branch of the ulnar nerve. A well defined clinical type of professional palsy of the hand. *Journal of Nervous and Mental Disease* 1908; **35**: 673–689.

> **Other relevant entries** Entrapment neuropathies: an overview; Neuropathies: an overview; Ulnar neuropathy.

■ Rasmussen's encephalitis, Rasmussen's syndrome

Chronic encephalitis and epilepsy • Kojewnikoff's syndrome, Kozhevnikov syndrome

Pathophysiology Rasmussen and colleagues described a syndrome of chronic partial epilepsy with progressive focal neurological deficits and cognitive decline, associated with neuropathological features of a focal chronic encephalitis, in 1958. Onset is usually in childhood, with a relentlessly progressive course for several years until the disease process may appear to "burn out". Partial forms with pathology confined to the temporal lobes and presenting as intractable temporal lobe epilepsy have been reported. The condition may be related to viral infection, particularly with cytomegalovirus which has been identified in brain tissue in some cases, using the polymerase chain reaction.

Clinical features: history and examination

- Seizures: focal, secondary generalized, epilepsia partialis continua; often poorly controlled despite multiple anti-epileptic drugs.
- Focal signs: hemiparesis/hemiplegia, hemianopia, hemisensory loss, and occasionally movement disorders.
- Cognitive decline.

Investigations and diagnosis *Bloods*: auto-antibodies to the glutamate-receptor 3 (GluR3) have been found in some patients, but specificity and sensitivity remain to be established and thus probably not helpful.

Imaging: atrophy may be evident on CT/MRI.

Neurophysiology: EEG: epileptiform and non-epileptiform lateralized abnormalities; multiple independent interictal epileptiform abnormalities.

CSF: no specific abnormalities known; pleocytosis, oligoclonal bands in some.

Neuropsychology: cognitive deficits appropriate to affected hemisphere.

Brain biopsy: classical features are inflammation with microglial nodules, neuronophagia, perivascular lymphocyte cuffing, and glial scarring. However, findings may be non-specific later in the disease when the inflammatory process may have "burned out".

Differential diagnosis Space-occupying lesion, slow-growing neoplasm. Neuronal migration disorder, cortical dysplasia.

Treatment and prognosis Seizures are usually only partially responsive to standard anti-epileptic medications. Two other treatment options which have been tried and may be useful are:

- antivirals: ganciclovir, zidovudine
- immunomodulation: high-dose steroids, intravenous immunoglobulins, plasma exchange, interferon-α.

Hemispherectomy will stop the seizures but is only recommended when the patient is already hemiplegic.

References Andermann F (ed.). *Chronic Encephalitis and Epilepsy: Rasmussen's Syndrome*. Boston: Butterworth-Heinemann, 1991.

Larner AJ, Anderson M. Rasmussen's syndrome: pathogenetic theories and therapeutic strategies. *Journal of Neurology* 1995; **242**: 355–358.

Leach JP, Chadwick DW, Miles JB, Hart IK. Improvement in adult-onset Rasmussen's encephalitis with long-term immunomodulatory therapy. *Neurology* 1999; **52**: 738–742.

Other relevant entries Encephalitis: an overview; Epilepsy: an overview.

■ Raymond syndrome, Raymond–Céstan syndrome
Alternating abducens hemiplegia

Pathophysiology Raymond's name is associated with two pontine vascular syndromes causing crossed paralysis, affecting the ventral and dorsal pons, first described in 1895.

Clinical features: history and examination

- Raymond syndrome: a rare ventral medial pontine syndrome, causing lateral rectus paralysis (involvement of abducens [VI] cranial nerve fascicles) with contralateral hemiplegia sparing the face (pyramidal tract involvement); also known as alternating abducens hemiplegia.
- Raymond–Céstan syndrome: a rostral lesion of the dorsal pons causing cerebellar ataxia, contralateral hypoaesthesia to all modalities (medial lemniscus and spinothalamic tract involvement), + / − contralateral hemiparesis (ventral extension involving corticospinal tract).

Investigations and diagnosis MRI to confirm diagnosis of brainstem stroke.

Differential diagnosis Raymond syndrome: Millard–Gubler syndrome (additional ipsilateral facial paresis), Foville syndrome.

Treatment and prognosis Acute care on a stroke unit. Early aspirin. Secondary prophylaxis (control of risk factors: hypertension, hypercholesterolaemia).

> **Reference** Silverman IE, Lui GT, Galetta SL. The crossed paralyses. The original brain-stem syndromes of Millard–Gubler, Foville, Weber and Raymond–Céstan. *Archives of Neurology* 1995; **52**: 635–638.

> **Other relevant entries** Brainstem vascular syndromes; Cerebrovascular disease: arterial; Céstan syndrome; Foville's syndrome; Millard–Gubler syndrome.

◼ Raynaud's disease, Raynaud's phenomenon, Raynaud's syndrome

Pathophysiology Raynaud's phenomenon may occur in Raynaud's disease (idiopathic, primary) or Raynaud's syndrome (secondary, symptomatic). Recognized causes include connective tissue disease, especially systemic sclerosis: cervical rib or thoracic outlet syndromes; vibration white finger; hypothyroidism; and uraemia.

Clinical features: history and examination Raynaud's phenomenon consists of intermittent pallor or cyanosis, with or without suffusion and pain, of the fingers, toes, nose, ears, or jaw, in response to cold or stress. Commoner in females.

Investigations and diagnosis The phenomenon may be diagnosed on history alone. It may be observed by asking the patient to put their hands in cold water.

Associated symptoms should be sought to ascertain whether there is an underlying connective tissue disorder (e.g. rash, arthralgia, myalgia, calcium deposits in the skin, dysphagia). History of use of power tools should be sought (vibration white finger).

Bloods: thyroid function tests, auto-antibodies.

Differential diagnosis

Causalgia.

Erythromelalgia: "inverse Raynaud's".

Treatment and prognosis For Raynaud's syndrome, the treatment is that of the underlying cause where possible. For Raynaud's disease, and Raynaud's syndrome where there is no effective treatment of the underlying cause, the following approaches may be tried:

Non-drug: life style adjustment to avoid precipitants; heated gloves.

Drug therapy: oral vasodilators [calcium channel blockers, angiotensin converting enzyme (ACE) inhibitors], antioxidants (probucol), prostacyclin analogues (bolus, infusions). β-blockers should be avoided.

Surgery: sympathectomy.

Reference Bowling JCR, David PM. Raynaud's disease. *Lancet* 2003; **361**: 2078–2080.

Coffman JD. *Raynaud's Phenomenon*. New York: OUP, 1989.

Other relevant entries Collagen vascular disorders and the nervous system: an overview; Cryoglobulinaemia, cryoglobulinaemic neuropathy; Erythromelalgia; Systemic sclerosis; Thoracic outlet syndromes.

■ Red ear syndrome

Irritation of the C3 nerve root may cause pain, burning and redness of the pinna. This may also occur with temporomandibular joint dysfunction and thalamic lesions.

Reference Lance JW. The red ear syndrome. *Neurology* 1996; **47**: 617–620.

■ Reflex epilepsies

Reflex, or evoked, epilepsies are those in which seizures are precipitated in response to discrete or specific stimuli.

Examples include:
- In response to simple stimuli

  Photosensitive epilepsy (e.g. television, ? computer/video games); idiopathic photosensitive occipital lobe epilepsy; Jeavons syndrome (eyelid myoclonia with absences)

  Hot water/hot bath epilepsy

  Startle epilepsy

  Eating epilepsy.
- In response to complex stimuli

  Reading epilepsy

  Musicogenic epilepsy.

  Reference Panayiotopoulos CP. *A Clinical Guide to Epileptic Syndromes and Their Treatment: Based on The New ILAE Diagnostic Scheme*. Chipping Norton: Bladon, 2002: 214–239.

  Other relevant entry Epilepsy: an overview.

■ Reflex sympathetic dystrophy – see Complex regional pain syndromes

■ Refsum's disease

Hereditary motor and sensory neuropathy (HMSN) type IV of Dyck • Heredopathia atactica polyneuritiformis • Phytanic acid-storage disease

Pathophysiology An autosomal-recessive disorder of peroxisome function, with deficiency of phytanic acid α-hydroxylase, leading to the accumulation of phytanic acid, a branched-chain fatty acid, in the nervous system and elsewhere. The majority of cases present in the first or second decade of life with the classic triad of ataxia, retinitis pigmentosa, and polyneuropathy.

Clinical features: history and examination

- Night blindness (nyctalopia) due to retinal pigmentary degeneration (retinitis pigmentosa); early concentric field defect.
- Hypertrophic polyneuropathy, affecting the legs first; pes cavus, wasting, weakness, areflexia, distal sensory disturbance (especially proprioception) leading to gait disturbance.
- +/− cerebellar ataxia (slurred speech, intention tremor).
- Sensorineural hearing loss.
- Short fourth metatarsals leading to overriding toes.
- Anosmia.
- Ichythyosis (especially of shins).
- Cardiac conduction abnormalities.
- Cognition normal.
- Cataracts.
- Growth retardation.
- Hepatomegaly.

Investigations and diagnosis *Bloods*: raised phytanic acid.

Urine: raised phytanic acid.

CSF: raised protein.

Neurophysiology:

> EMG/NCS: reduced motor conduction velocities, reduced or absent sensory nerve action potentials
>
> ERG: may be absent.

ECG: may show cardiac conduction abnormalities.

Imaging: MRI may show thickening of affected nerves.

Differential diagnosis

> Nerve thickening
>
> > Charcot–Marie–Tooth type of hereditary motor and sensory neuropathy (HMSN)
> >
> > Déjerine–Sottas (HMSN type III).

Relapsing–remitting course
  Inflammatory polyneuropathy.
Hereditary pigmentary retinal degenerations
  Alström's syndrome
  Cockayne's syndrome
  Usher's syndrome.

Mitochondrial disease can cause potentially misleading increase in phytanic acid levels.

Treatment and prognosis All phytanic acid is of dietary origin; hence dietary restriction reduces levels. Plasma exchange has been tried. Exacerbations and remissions of the neuropathy are recognized. Survival may be for decades, but sudden unexpected death, perhaps related to cardiac conduction defects, is reported.

References Refsum S. Heredopathia atactica polyneuritiformis: a familial syndrome not hitherto described. A contribution to the clinical study of the hereditary diseases of the nervous system. *Acta Psychiatrica Scandinavica Supplement* 1946; **38**: 1–303.

Wills AJ, Manning NJ, Reilly MM. Refsum's disease. *Quarterly Journal of Medicine* 2001; **94**: 403–406.

Other relevant entries Alström's syndrome; Cockayne's syndrome; Hereditary motor and sensory neuropathy; Peroxisomal disorders: an overview; Retinitis pigmentosa; Usher's syndrome.

▇ Reinhold's syndrome – see Babinski-Nageotte syndrome

▇ Reiter's disease
Reactive arthritis

Pathophysiology The core features of Reiter's disease are the clinical triad of:
- seronegative arthropathy,
- non-specific urethritis,
- conjunctivitis

occurring 3–30 days after infection at a distant site (venereal or dysenteric, whence "reactive arthritis"). There may be other clinical features but the nervous system is rarely affected. The condition is related to HLA B27.

Clinical features: history and examination
- Sterile synovitis: oligoarticular, lower limbs, asymmetric, +/− lower back, buttock, heel pain.
- Urethritis.
- Conjunctivitis.
- +/− balanitis, uveitis, nail dystrophy, fever, oral ulceration.

- Neurological
    - Peripheral neuropathy, radiculopathy
    - Aseptic meningoencephalits, $+/-$ epilepsy
    - Psychosis
    - Cranial nerve palsies
    - Pyramidal signs
    - Myelopathy.

Investigations and diagnosis *Bloods*: raised ESR, acute phase reactants, $+/-$ mild anaemia; raised IgA in active disease; HLA B27 status. Serology/culture for Chlamydia, Salmonella, Yersinia, Shigella, Campylobacter.

Differential diagnosis Behçet's disease, systemic lupus erythematosus.

Treatment and prognosis Symptomatic treatment with analgesia. Prognosis generally very good, although recurrences may occur.

> **Reference** Scolding N. Neurological complications of rheumatological and connective tissue disorders. In: Scolding N (ed.). *Immunological and Inflammatory Disorders of The Central Nervous System*. Oxford: Butterworth-Heinemann, 1999: 147–180 [at 170–171].

> **Other relevant entries** Ankylosing spondylitis and the nervous system; Behçet's disease; Systemic lupus erythematosus and the nervous system.

■ Relapsing polychondritis

This very rare condition characterized by recurrent inflammatory episodes affecting the cartilage of the ear, nose, trachea, and larynx may be complicated by systemic and cerebral vasculitis, which may manifest as aseptic meningitis, encephalopathy, epileptic seizures, stroke or transient ischaemic attacks, ischaemic optic neuropathy, and cranial nerve palsies.

> **Reference** Stewart SS, Ashizawa T, Dudley AW *et al*. Cerebral vasculitis in relapsing polychondritis. *Neurology* 1988; **38**: 150–152.

> **Other relevant entry** Vasculitis.

■ REM sleep behaviour disorder

A syndrome of stereotypic behaviour with increased muscle tone occurring during REM sleep; bizarre behaviours may represent the acting out of dreams (the patient has recollection of the dreams the following day; *cf*. pavor nocturnus or night terrors). In older individuals, there is a link with parkinsonian syndromes such as dementia with Lewy bodies.

> **Other relevant entries** Dementia with Lewy bodies; Parasomnias; Pavor nocturnus; Sleep disorders: an overview.

▒ Renal disease and the nervous system

Pathophysiology A number of multisystem conditions affect both the renal and nervous systems. Uraemia, dialysis, and renal transplantation may all be associated with neurological syndromes.

Clinical features: history and examination

- Conditions affecting both the kidneys and the nervous system
  - Vasculitides
      primary: polyarteritis nodosa, Churg–Strauss syndrome, Wegener's granulomatosis
      secondary: infection (hepatitis B), toxins, neoplasia (lymphoid malignancy).
  - Connective tissue diseases: rheumatoid arthritis, systemic lupus erythematosus, Sjögren's syndrome
  - Plasma cell dyscrasias: myeloma, POEMS syndrome, MGUS, Waldenström's macroglobulinaemia
  - Genetically determined disease: Von Hippel–Lindau disease, polycystic kidney disease, Wilson's disease, Fabry's disease, Alport's syndrome, mitochondrial disease
  - Renal disease leading to vitamin D (1,25-dihydroxycholecalciferol) deficiency may lead to apparent limb weakness from osteomalacia.
- Conditions affecting both renal system and muscle
    Rhabdomyolysis
- Uraemia and the nervous system
    Central nervous system (CNS)
      Encephalopathy with myoclonus and asterixis; probably multifactorial aetiology
      Aseptic meningitis.
    Peripheral nervous system (PNS)
      Distal sensorimotor axonal neuropathy, affecting especially large myelinated axons, with secondary demyelination
      Isolated mononeuropathies (e.g. carpal tunnel syndrome)
      Vestibulocochlear (VIII) nerve: (exclude drug toxicity, hereditary conditions causing hearing loss and nephropathy)
      Myopathy: proximal wasting and weakness (exclude primary hyperparathyroidism and osteomalacia).
- Dialysis
  - Dialysis disequilibrium syndrome: restlessness, nausea, headache, cramps, progressing to delirium, myoclonus, seizures, raised intracranial pressure, cardiac arrhythmias; now very rare, and a diagnosis of exclusion
  - Wernicke's syndrome: may be atypical, without ophthalmoplegia
  - Subdural haematoma (SDH)
  - Dialysis dementia.

- Complications of renal transplantation.

   <u>Intraoperative</u>: compression of femoral nerve, lateral cutaneous nerve of thigh; conus medullaris syndrome (spinal cord ischaemia from iliac artery manipulation).

   <u>Postoperative</u>
   - Side-effects of immunosuppressive drugs
      Steroids: hypertension
      Ciclosporin A: tremor, seizures, posterior leukoencephalopathy syndrome
      FK506: posterior leukoencephalopathy syndrome.
   - Opportunistic infection: for example
      viral: cytomegalovirus (CMV), Epstein–Barr virus (EBV), JC virus causing progressive multifocal leukoencephalopathy
      fungal: aspergillus, cryptococcus
      bacterial: Nocardia, Listeria.
   - Lymphoproliferative disease: primary CNS lymphoma, possibly related to EBV infection of B lymphocytes
   - Rejection encephalopathy.

Investigations and diagnosis

Monitor renal function:

Blood: urea, creatinine, creatinine clearance; markers of inflammation, auto-antibodies, serology for infection (e.g. hepatitis B).

Urine: examine urine for cells, casts.

Imaging: CT/MRI: look for evidence of inflammation, infarction; SDH; MRA or catheter angiography in patients with polycystic kidney disease and family history of subarachnoid (and/or intracerebral) haemorrhage.

Neurophysiology:

EEG: slowing, especially frontally, with excess δ and θ in uraemic encephalopathy

EMG/NCS: slowing of proximal nerve conduction is the earliest finding in uraemic neuropathy, followed by reduced conduction velocity and action potential amplitudes.

CSF: raised protein, lymphocyte count in uraemic aseptic meningitis; organisms in immunosuppression-related opportunistic infection; Indian ink stain for fungi, polymerase chain reaction (PCR) for viruses, culture.

(For conditions affecting both kidney and nervous system, see under specific entries for investigation.)

Differential diagnosis As the aforegoing lists show, differential diagnosis is broad and requires a high index of clinical suspicion.

Treatment and prognosis Many of the features associated with uraemia improve with dialysis and may resolve entirely following successful renal transplantation.

   Reference Burn DJ, Bates D. Neurology and the kidney. *Journal of Neurology, Neurosurgery and Psychiatry* 1998; **65**: 810–821.

Other relevant entries Alport's syndrome; Carpal tunnel syndrome; Cerebrovascular disease: arterial; Churg–Strauss syndrome; Cranial nerve disease: VIII: Vestibulocochlear nerve; Dementia: an overview; Encephalopathies: an overview; Fabry's disease; Femoral neuropathy; Immunosuppressive therapy and diseases of the nervous system; Lymphoma; Neuropathies: an overview; Osteomalacia; POEMS syndrome; Polyarteritis nodosa; Posterior leukoencephalopathy syndrome; Progressive multifocal leukoencephalopathy; Rhabdomyolysis; Rheumatoid arthritis; Sjögren's syndrome; Subarachnoid haemorrhage; Subdural haematoma; Systemic lupus erythematosus and the nervous system; Vasculitis; Vitamin deficiencies and the nervous system; Von Hippel–Lindau disease; Wegener's granulomatosis; Wernicke–Korsakoff's syndrome; Wilson's disease.

▦ Rendu–Osler–Weber syndrome – see Osler–Weber–Rendu syndrome

▦ Renpenning's syndrome – see Fragile X syndrome

▦ Respiratory failure
Neurogenic respiratory failure

Pathophysiology Respiratory failure may result from a variety of neurological disorders as well as primary respiratory disease. Recognized neurological causes include:

Myopathy: acid-maltase deficiency (AMD); nemaline, centronuclear myopathies
Neuromuscular disease: myasthenia gravis
Neuropathy: Guillain–Barré syndrome
Neuronopathy: motor neurone disease; poliomyelitis
Myelopathy: high cervical cord lesions (involving C3–C5): structural, inflammatory (e.g. multiple sclerosis)
Primary central hypoventilation: Wolfram syndrome.

Clinical features: history and examination
- Symptoms and signs may be minimal prior to the development of respiratory failure.
- Paradoxical diaphragm movement.
- Metabolic encephalopathy, $+/-$ asterixis, papilloedema.
- Respiratory arrest.

Investigations and diagnosis (See individual entries for investigation of specific neurological disorders.)

In patients with conditions which might lead to respiratory failure, monitoring of respiratory parameters and intervention before the development of respiratory failure is required:

Forced vital capacity: may be difficult if weak facial muscles preclude good lip seal around vitalograph/spirometer, so need to use face mask for measurement.

Arterial blood gases

Chest radiograph; X-ray screening of diaphragm movement.

Differential diagnosis Other causes of encephalopathy.

In those already ventilated who prove difficult to wean, critical illness polyneuropathy may contribute.

Treatment and prognosis

Prevention if possible.

Recumbent position may further compromise respiration with diaphragm weakness. Avoid respiratory depressant drugs.

If required, ventilation.

In some chronic stable disorders, patients may compensate for respiratory failure, but also may require intermittent positive-pressure ventilation, now most easily delivered by means of nocturnal CPAP or NIPPY.

Reference Howard RS, El Kabir D, Williams AJ. Neurogenic respiratory failure. In: Greenwood RJ, Barnes MP, McMillan TM, Ward CD (eds). *Handbook of Neurological Rehabilitation* (2nd edition). Hove: Psychology Press, 2003: 313–325.

Other relevant entry Encephalopathies: an overview.

■ Restless legs syndrome

Anxietas tibiarum • Ekbom's syndrome

Pathophysiology A syndrome characterized by intense discomfort within the legs associated with a desire to move them; movement temporarily relieves the discomfort. Restless legs syndrome (RLS) is frequently associated with periodic limb movement disorder (PLMD, or periodic limb movements of sleep, PLMS). The pathogenesis is not understood but may relate to a central imbalance of serotoninergic and dopaminergic pathways, possibly at the level of the basal ganglia.

Clinical features: history and examination Diagnostic criteria have been proposed by the International Restless Legs Syndrome Study group (IRLSSG):

- History of compulsion to move legs due to deep discomfort; often worse at night; eased by activity, hot baths. May be a positive family history for the condition.
- History of leg movements during sleep (periodic movements of sleep, "nocturnal myoclonus"): brief slow periodic movements varying from dorsiflexion of big toe to triple flexion; bed partner may report being kicked at night.
- Secondary insomnia, depression.
- Normal neurological examination, unless accompanied by concurrent neurological disease (e.g. essential tremor).

The condition may be:

- Primary or idiopathic: in up to one-third of cases the condition is hereditary with evidence for autosomal-dominant transmission with variable penetrance.
- Secondary or symptomatic: need to exclude concurrent peripheral neuropathy, uraemia, and iron deficiency, and can be part of an extrapyramidal disorder (e.g. PD).

Investigations and diagnosis

Diagnosis is essentially clinical.

Bloods: biochemistry, iron status (looking for secondary causes).

Sleep studies: may record PLMS.

Consider EMG/NCS looking for a neuropathy.

Differential diagnosis Akathisia (associated with neuroleptic drug use).

Painful legs and moving toes.

PLMD may be confused with hypnic jerks, rapid eye movement (REM) sleep behaviour disorder, nocturnal epilepsy, abnormal movements secondary to associated obstructive sleep apnoea syndrome.

Treatment and prognosis Many agents have been tried for idiopathic disease, but evidence of efficacy from controlled trials versus placebo is lacking for all but a few drugs:

- Benzodiazepines: clonazepam
- Dopaminergic drugs: levodopa + dopa-decarboxylase inhibitor; dopamine agonists; latter may be preferred due to longer half-life (e.g. cabergoline); dyskinesias do not develop with long-term levodopa use for RLS (*cf.* Parkinson's disease)
- Anti-epileptic drugs: carbamazepine, gabapentin
- Opioids: oxycodone, dextropropoxyphene
- Chlorpromazine.

Drugs reported to exacerbate symptoms include amitriptyline and promethazine. Symptoms generally persist.

References Aldrich MS, Allen R, Ancoli-Israel S *et al.* Toward a better definition of the restless legs syndrome. *Movement Disorders* 1995; **10**: 634–642.

Ekbom KA. Restless legs syndrome. *Neurology* 1960; **10**: 868–873.

Sachdev P. *Akathisia and Restless Legs*. Cambridge: CUP, 1995: 295–341.

Other relevant entries Akathisia; Obstructive sleep apnoea syndrome; Painful legs and moving toes; Parasomnias; Parkinson's disease; REM sleep behaviour disorder; Sleep disorders: an overview.

■ Retinal migraine – see Migraine

■ Retinitis pigmentosa

Tapetoretinal degeneration

Pathophysiology Retinitis pigmentosa (RP) is a generic name for a group of inherited diseases characterized by retinal abiotrophy of both neuroepithelium and pigment epithelium. Despite the name, there is no inflammation; the pathogenetic mechanism may be apoptotic death of photoreceptors. The typical "bone spicule" appearance results from clumping of epithelial cells. These conditions may be autosomal recessive (linked to chromosome 1q), X-linked (Xp11, Xp21), or autosomal dominant (3q, 6p, 8); males are affected twice as often as females. At least some of these are related to mutations in the gene for the rod cell protein rhodopsin.

In most cases of RP there are no associated systemic or extraocular features, although RP is well recognized as a feature of several multisystem disorders including:

abetalipoproteinaemia (Bassen–Kornzweig syndrome; HARP syndrome);
Alström's syndrome;
Cockayne syndrome;
Friedreich's ataxia;
Laurence–Moon–Bardet–Biedl syndrome;
mitochondrial disorders (e.g. Kearns–Sayre syndrome and NARP);
neuronal ceroid lipofuscinosis;
peroxisomal disorders;
Refsum's disease;
Usher's disease.

(See individual entries for clinical features.)

Clinical features: history and examination

- Night blindness (nyctalopia), usually in the second decade; colour vision relatively preserved.
- Constricted visual fields.
- Peripheral "bone spicule" pigmentation in retina; arteriolar attenuation, with eventual unmasking of choroid blood vessels (retinal thinning); in some cases the pigment changes are not prominent but the other changes help to establish the diagnosis.
- Optic disc pallor ("waxy"; late).
- Maculopathy.

Investigations and diagnosis

Neurophysiology: ERG: eventually lost; diagnostic.
Neurogenetics: if positive family history.
Investigation for other systemic disorders as appropriate (see individual entries).

Differential diagnosis The funduscopic appearances are unlikely to be mistaken for anything else (e.g. tigroid fundus). Similar symptoms and signs may occur in paraneoplastic (cancer-associated) retinopathy, but this is rapidly progressive. Vitamin A deficiency may cause nyctalopia.

Treatment and prognosis No specific treatment; low vision aids; eventual blindness.

References Chapple P, Cheetham M. Looking at protein misfolding neurodegenerative disease through retinitis pigmentosa. *Advances in Clinical Neuroscience and Rehabilitation* 2003; **3(1)**: 12–13.

Dryja TP. Retinitis pigmentosa. In: Scriver CR, Beaudet AL, Sly WS, Valle D (eds). *The Metabolic and Molecular Basis of Inherited Disease.* New York: McGraw-Hill, 1995: 4297–4309.

Other relevant entries Abetalipoproteinaemia; Alström's syndrome; Bardet–Biedl syndrome; Cockayne's syndrome; Friedreich's ataxia; Laurence–Moon syndrome; Mitochondrial disease: an overview; Neuronal ceroid lipofuscinosis; Peroxisomal disorders: an overview; Refsum's disease; Usher's syndrome; Vitamin deficiencies and the nervous system.

◼ Retinoblastoma

This tumour of neuroretinal tissue may be hereditary, in young infants with bilateral tumours, or sporadic, in older children with unilateral tumours. Visual impairment and loss of the red reflex are typical clinical findings. The responsible gene, *RB*, on chromosome 13q14.1, is a tumour suppressor gene, encoding a nuclear phosphoprotein. Loss of RB function has also been implicated in the initiation or progression of osteosarcoma, soft tissue sarcoma, and prostate, breast and lung cancers.

Other relevant entries Neuroblastoma; Primitive neuroectodermal tumours.

◼ Retinocochleocerebral vasculopathy – see Susac syndrome

◼ Retrobulbar neuritis – see Optic neuritis

◼ Retroparotid space syndrome – see Collet–Sicard syndrome; Jugular foramen syndrome; Lannois – Jouty syndrome; Mackenzie syndrome; Villaret's syndrome

◼ Rett's syndrome

Pathophysiology A sporadic condition, exclusive to young girls, and causing mental and motor deterioration. Some cases have been linked to mutations in the gene encoding methyl-CpG-binding protein 2.

Clinical features: history and examination

Normal development to 6–18 months of age.

- Acquired microcephaly.
- Motor retardation.
- Manual stereotypies (washing, rubbing movements).
- Dementia.
- Hyperventilation, breath holding, air swallowing.
- Seizures.
- Truncal ataxia (late).
- Spasticity (late).

Investigations and diagnosis No specific investigations, the diagnosis is made on clinical grounds. The initial report by Rett of hyperammonaemia was not confirmed in later studies.

Differential diagnosis Autism.

Treatment and prognosis No specific treatment known. Symptomatic treatment for seizures and spasticity as necessary. After initial regression the condition stabilizes and patients usually survive into adulthood.

References Amir RE, Van den Veyver IB, Wan M, Tran CQ, Francke U, Zoghbi HY. Rett syndrome is caused by mutations in X-linked *MECP2*, encoding methyl-CpG-binding protein 2. *Nature Genetics* 1999; **23**: 185–188.

Hagberg B. Aicardi J, Dias K, Ramos O. A progressive syndrome of autism, dementia, ataxia, and loss of purposeful hand use in girls: Rett's syndrome: report of
35 cases. *Annals of Neurology* 1983; **14**: 471–479.

Rett A. *Uber ein cerebral-atrophisches Syndrome bei Hyperammonemie.* Vienna:
Bruder Hollinek, 1966.

The Rett Syndrome Diagnostic Criteria Work Group. Diagnostic criteria for Rett
syndrome. *Annals of Neurology* 1988; **23**: 425–428.

Other relevant entries Autism, Autistic disorder; Dementia: an overview.

■ Reversible ischaemic neurological deficit – see Cerebrovascular disease: arterial; Transient ischaemic attack

■ Reye's syndrome
Reye–Johnson syndrome

Pathophysiology An encephalopathy characterized by acute brain swelling and fatty
infiltration of the viscera, particularly the liver (non-icteric). The condition is of
uncertain aetiology, but mitochondrial dysfunction may be relevant. It predominantly affects young children following viral infections, especially if treated with
salicylates. It tends to occur in epidemics, but its incidence has declined dramatically
following public health initiatives to avoid salicylates in viral infection in children.
Other metabolic disorders presenting with encephalopathy, especially fatty acid
oxidation disorders, may previously have been included under the umbrella term
of Reye's syndrome.

Clinical features: history and examination
- Fever, upper respiratory tract infection, vomiting.
- Progression to drowsiness, stupor, and coma.
- Focal, generalized seizures.
- Sympathetic activation (tachycardia, mydriasis).
- Respiratory distress.
- Hepatomegaly.
- Progression to decorticate, decerebrate posture; death.

Investigations and diagnosis
Bloods:

Venous: raised transaminases, ammonia, prolonged prothrombin time;
hypoglycaemia

Arterial blood gases: metabolic acidosis, followed by respiratory alkalosis

Virology: may be positive for influenza B, varicella; less commonly influenza A,
Epstein–Barr virus (EBV), echovirus, rubella

Toxicology: salicylate levels.

Imaging: no specific abnormality.

CSF: raised pressure.

Neurophysiology: EEG: diffuse arrhythmic δ-activity, progressing to silence.

Differential diagnosis Other causes of childhood encephalopathy, acute liver failure; encephalitis, meningitis.

Hyperammonaemia: urea cycle enzyme disorders.

A Reye-like syndrome has been observed in children, usually under 3 years of age, with medium chain acyl-CoA dehydrogenase (MCAD) deficiency: encephalopathy, seizures; hypoglycaemia, mildly raised ammonia, creatine kinase, low carnitine and acyl carnitine; low urinary ketones but raised urinary organic acids (adipic, suberic).

Treatment and prognosis

High mortality untreated (60%); few survive once coma intervenes.

Treatment: correct metabolic abnormalities: ventilation, IV glucose.

Monitor intracranial pressure, treat high pressure (hypertonic solutions).

Full recovery may occur; severe deficits if cerebral perfusion pressure falls.

References Belay ED, Bresee JS, Holman RC, Khan AS, Shahriari A, Schonberger LB. Reye's syndrome in the United States from 1981 through 1997. *New England Journal of Medicine* 1999; **340**: 1377–1382.

Reye RDK, Morgan G, Baral J. Encephalopathy and fatty degeneration of the viscera: a disease entity in childhood. *Lancet* 1963; **2**: 749–752.

Other relevant entries Alpers disease; Encephalopathies: an overview; Medium-chain acyl-CoA dehydrogenase deficiency; Urea cycle enzyme defects.

■ Rhabdomyolysis

Crush syndrome • Necrotizing polymyopathy

Pathophysiology Rhabdomyolysis is a syndrome of necrotizing myopathy causing muscle pain, tenderness, weakness, and areflexia, which develops over about 24–48 hours. Muscle swelling may cause secondary ischaemic injury due to the development of a compartment syndrome. Release of intracellular contents may lead to myoglobinuria, acute renal failure, and death.

There are many recognized causes of rhabdomyolysis, including:

crush injury (e.g. earthquake survivors)

alcohol intoxication, drug use and prolonged drug-induced coma

electrolyte disturbances (hypernatraemia, hyperglycaemia, hypokalaemia, hypophosphataemia, hyperosmolality)

certain infections

metabolic myopathies.

Some cases remain idiopathic, and may recur (Meyer–Betz disease).

Clinical features: history and examination

• Muscle pain, tenderness, weakness, and areflexia.

• Oliguria, dark urine.

• History of trauma, alcohol intoxication, drug use.

Investigations and diagnosis *Bloods*: raised creatine kinase (usually >1000 U/l, sometimes >100 000 U/l).

Urine: myoglobinuria (dipstick positive for haemoglobin but no haematuria or haemoglobinuria on examination of urine).

Neurophysiology: EMG/NCS: severe myopathic picture.

Differential diagnosis Other acute and/or painful myopathies, such as dermatomyositis.

Treatment and prognosis Remove the cause of muscle necrosis if identified. Full supportive care with particularly careful monitoring of electrolytes and renal function, with dialysis if required. Ultimate prognosis is very good if the acute complications are appropriately managed.

> **References** Bywaters EGL, Beall D. Crush injuries with impairment of renal function. *British Medical Journal* 1941; **i**: 427–432.
>
> Gabow PA, Kaehny WD, Kelleher SP. The spectrum of rhabdomyolysis. *Medicine (Baltimore)* 1982; **61**: 141–152.
>
> Warren JD, Blumbergs PC, Thompson PD. Rhabdomyolysis: a review. *Muscle and Nerve* 2002; **25**: 332–347.
>
> **Other relevant entries** Alcohol and the nervous system: an overview; Compartment syndromes; Drug-induced myopathies; Meyer–Betz disease; Myopathy: an overview; Pretibial syndrome; Renal disease and the nervous system; Status dystonicus.

▪ Rheumatoid arthritis

Pathophysiology A multisystem chronic inflammatory disorder, classified with the connective tissue disorders, characterized by a symmetrical polyarthritis; lung and heart may also be affected. Neurological features may be due to direct involvement by rheumatoid nodules, vasculitis, or a consequence of bone disease.

Clinical features: history and examination

- Neurological:

    Central nervous system (CNS)

    Rheumatoid nodules: meningeal: often asymptomatic; parenchymal (very rare) may cause seizures

    Vasculitis (very rare, in context of multisystem rheumatoid vasculitis): seizures, hemiparesis, cranial nerve palsy, dementia

    Spinal cord compression: most commonly due to atlanto-axial subluxation (may also rarely cause vertebral artery compression); occasionally due to rheumatoid nodules.

    Peripheral nervous system (PNS)

    Entrapment/compression neuropathies (e.g. carpal tunnel syndrome, ulnar nerve) due to inflamed synovial joints

    Distal sensorimotor polyneuropathy (segmental demyelination + lesser axonal changes, ? vasculitic): mild, vibration sense particularly affected

Mononeuritis multiplex (axonal sensorimotor; vasculitic)
Autonomic neuropathy is reported.

- Rheumatological: oligoarticular arthritis, usually symmetrical; rheumatoid nodules.
- Pulmonary: pleurisy, pneumonitis, interstitial fibrosis (Caplan's syndrome).
- Eyes: sicca syndrome; Sjögren's syndrome may coexist.
- Haematology: anaemia; iron deficiency; splenomegaly, hypersplenism (Felty's syndrome).
- Cardiac: pericarditis (causing a rub), pericardial effusion.
- Kidney: amyloidosis.
- Drug therapy complications: e.g. myasthenia gravis with penicillamine.

Investigations and diagnosis *Bloods*: serology for rheumatoid factor (seropositivity).
Imaging:

plain radiology for typical articular changes
MRI cervical spine in cases of myelopathy.

CSF: raised protein (non-specific).
Neurophysiology: EMG/NCS: to elucidate peripheral nervous system involvement: entrapment, mononeuropathy multiplex, symmetrical polyneuropathy.

Differential diagnosis Other, seronegative, arthritides.
Neurology: other connective tissue diseases: systemic lupus erythematosus, Sjögren's syndrome, systemic sclerosis; vasculitis.

Treatment and prognosis Vasculitis: as for any vasculitis (immunosuppression).
Cervical subluxation: conservative: analgesia, protection from trauma (e.g. at intubation); majority remain stable or improve; deterioration may necessitate surgical stabilization.
Neuropathy: if mild, conservative treatment reasonable; if severe and/or progressive, immunosuppression as for systemic vasculitis may be tried.

References Keersmaeker A, Truyen L, Ramon F, Cras P, De Clerck L, Martin JJ. Cervical myelopathy due to rheumatoid arthritis: case report and review of the literature. *Acta Neurologica Belgica* 1998; **98**: 284–288.

Nadeau S. Neurologic Manifestations of connective tissue disease. *Neurologic Clinics* 2002; **20**: 151–178.

Other relevant entries Atlantoaxial dislocation, subluxation; Carpal tunnel syndrome; Collagen vascular disorders and the nervous system: an overview; Costen syndrome; Myasthenia gravis; Sjögren's syndrome; Systemic lupus erythematosus and the nervous system; Vasculitis.

■ Rhombencephalitis

Inflammation of the brainstem, as may occur with infection by Listeria, or in the context of Bickerstaff's brainstem encephalitis.

■ Richards-Rundle syndrome
Ataxia–hypogonadism–deafness

Pathophysiology An autosomal-recessive hereditary syndrome of hearing loss and ataxia with onset in early childhood or infancy.

Clinical features: history and examination
- Hearing loss: may be rapid; due to degeneration of cochlear spiral ganglion cells.
- Ataxia +/− generalized weakness (distal > proximal), loss of distal reflexes.
- Hypogonadism.
- Mental deficiency: slowly progressive.
- +/− horizontal nystagmus.
- +/− finger contractures.
- No obesity or retinitis pigmentosa.
- Family history for similar conditions.

Investigations and diagnosis Audiometry.

Differential diagnosis Laurence–Moon–Bardet–Biedl syndrome.

Treatment and prognosis No specific treatment; may progress to eventual deafness and inability to stand without support.

> **Reference** Richards BW, Rundle AT. A familial hormonal disorder associated with mental deficiency, deaf mutism and ataxia. *Journal of Mental Deficiency Research* 1959; **3**: 33–55.

> **Other relevant entries** Hearing loss: differential diagnosis; Jeune–Tommasi syndrome; Lichtenstein–Knorr syndrome; Rosenberg–Bergstrom syndrome; Telfer's syndrome.

■ Richner–Hanhart disease – see Tyrosinaemia

■ Rickettsial diseases

Pathophysiology Rickettsia are obligate intracellular parasites (Gram-negative coccobacilli) which have a life cycle involving an animal reservoir, an insect vector (lice, fleas, ticks, mites), and man. Diseases falling into this category, their causative agents, and insect vectors, include:
- Epidemic typhus (*Rickettsia prowazekii*; human body louse)
- Endemic (or murine) typhus (*Rickettsia typhi*, *R. mooseri*; fleas)
- Scrub typhus or tsutsugamushi fever (*Rickettsia orientalis* recently renamed as a new genus with only one species, *Orientia tsutsugamushi*; trombiculid mites, chiggers)
- Q fever (*Coxiella burnetii*; no necessary insect vector)
- Rocky Mountain spotted fever (*Rickettsia rickettsii*; various ticks).

Exposure to wildlife or livestock may be an important clue to diagnosis. Although uncommon in the developed world, about one-third of cases are said to develop neurological features. Severity of disease is variable.

Clinical features: history and examination
- Bacteraemic illness: fever, headache, prostration.
- Delirium, stupor, coma.
- +/− focal neurological signs.
- Meningitis, encephalitis, myelitis.
- Macular rash (not in Q fever): necrotic ulcer and eschar in scrub typhus.
- Lymphadenopathy: local, general.
- +/− disseminated intravascular coagulation.
- Q fever: atypical pneumonia, culture negative endocarditis.

Investigations and diagnosis *Bloods*: Weil–Felix test: for the presence of heterophile antibodies to strains of *Proteus mirabilis*; may be negative in up to 50% of cases. Serology: species specific ELISA, immunofluorescent antibody tests (IFAT), polymerase chain reaction (PCR).

CSF: normal, or modest lymphocytic pleocytosis.

Differential diagnosis Other causes of acute infective or inflammatory central nervous system (CNS) disease (e.g. viral meningitis).

Treatment and prognosis Antibiotics (tetracycline, chloramphenicol) +/− supportive care as appropriate. Early appropriate treatment is associated with good prognosis, neurological sequelae are rare.

> **Reference** Cowan G. Rickettsial diseases: the typhus group of fevers – a review. *Postgraduate Medical Journal* 2000; **76**: 269–272.

> **Other relevant entries** "Atypical pneumonias" and the nervous system; Ehrlichiosis; Q fever; Typhus.

▪ Rift valley fever – see Arbovirus disease

▪ Rigid spine syndrome

The rigid spine syndrome is a congenital muscular dystrophy, presenting with motor delay and axial rigidity, predominantly of the spine causing limitation of neck and trunk flexion. There may also be scoliosis, proximal myopathy, respiratory disturbance, and cardiac changes. Blood creatine kinase may be elevated, EMG is myopathic, and muscle biopsy shows a non-specific merosin-positive dystrophy. The differential diagnosis encompasses Duchenne, Becker, and Emery–Dreifuss dystrophies, and ankylosing spondylitis. The condition is linked to chromosome 1p and deficiency in the protein selenoprotein N1. Botulinum toxin injections may help the axial rigidity.

> **Reference** Sastre-Garriga J, Tintoré M, Montalban X, Bagó J, Ferrer I. Response to botulinum toxin in a case of rigid spine syndrome. *Journal of Neurology, Neurosurgery and Psychiatry* 2001; **71**: 564–565.

Other relevant entries Ankylosing spondylitis and the nervous system; Botulinum toxin therapy; Congenital muscular dystrophy; Emery–Dreifuss muscular dystrophy (EMD); Muscular dystrophies: an overview.

■ Riley–Day syndrome

Familial dysautonomia • Hereditary sensory and autonomic neuropathy (HSAN) III

Pathophysiology An autosomal-recessive neuropathy, now classified as hereditary sensory and autonomic neuropathy (HSAN) type III, occurring principally in Ashkenazi Jewish kindreds. It affects peripheral autonomic, sensory, and motor neurones and causes predominantly autonomic symptoms. Linked to chromosome 9q31–q33, a candidate gene (inhibitor of kappa light polypeptide gene, IKBKAP) has been identified.

Clinical features: history and examination

- Vasomotor
    - Orthostatic hypotension
    - Hyperhidrosis
    - Blotchy skin.
- Neurological
    - Decreased tendon reflexes
    - Decreased pain and temperature sensation
    - Relatively preserved tactile sense; reduced vibration sensation from teenage years
    - Progressive ataxia (adult years)
    - Below average IQ in *ca.* one-third; otherwise normal intelligence.
- Ocular
    - Lack of overflow tears
    - Corneal analgesia.
- Orthopaedic
    - Kyphoscoliosis.
- Gastrointestinal
    - Swallowing difficulties, oesophageal dilatation, reduced gastric motility
    - Absence of fungiform papillae on the tongue.
- Respiratory
    - Apnoeic episodes; risk of pneumonia.

Family history of similar disorder.

Investigations and diagnosis *Neurophysiology*: EMG/NCS: reduced conduction velocities, CMAP amplitude; raised thermal thresholds.

Bloods: normal or elevated supine plasma noradrenaline levels, but no increase on standing.

Neurogenetics: over 90% of patients have the same splice-site mutation in the IKBKAP gene.

Nerve biopsy: reduced unmyelinated fibres and small myelinated fibres.

Pathology: hypoplastic sympathetic ganglia; loss of neurones in dorsal roots, Lissauer's tracts and intermediolateral grey column of spinal cord.

Differential diagnosis Other causes of orthostatic hypotension (autonomic neuropathies, autonomic failure).

Other causes of hereditary sensory neuropathy.

Treatment and prognosis No specific treatment; symptomatic therapy for orthostatic hypotension, gastrointestinal symptoms; careful attention to posture when swallowing to avoid aspiration. Perhaps only 20% of patients survive to adulthood; pneumonia is the commonest cause of death.

Reference Axelrod FB. Familial dysautonomia. In: Mathias CJ, Bannister R (eds). *Autonomic Failure. A Textbook of Clinical Disorders of The Autonomic Nervous System* (4th edition). Oxford: OUP, 1999: 402–409.

Other relevant entries Autonomic failure; Hereditary sensory and autonomic neuropathy; Neuropathies: an overview; Pure autonomic failure.

▓ Rippling muscle disease

This condition is a benign myopathy with symptoms and signs of muscular hyperexcitability; it may be autosomal dominant or sporadic. Clinically, the complaint is often of muscle stiffness, and muscle contraction, visible from the surface and propagated in a rolling manner, may be elicited by percussion. Myoedema, or muscle mounding, is a feature, representing electrically silent muscle contractions provoked by mechanical stimuli or stretch.

Rippling muscle disease has been linked with mutations in the gene encoding caveolin 3 (CAV3), and hence is allelic with limb-girdle muscular dystrophy type 1c and some cases of idiopathic hyperCKaemia; it is not a channelopathy.

References Betz RC, Schoser BGH, Kasper D *et al*. Mutations in CAV3 cause mechanical hyper-irritability of skeletal muscle in rippling muscle disease. *Nature Genetics* 2001; **28**: 218–219.

Ricker K, Moxley RT, Rohkamm R. Rippling muscle disease. *Archives of Neurology* 1989; **46**: 405–408.

Torbergsen T. Rippling muscle disease: a review. *Muscle and Nerve* 2002; **suppl 11**: S103–S107.

Other relevant entries Channelopathies: an overview; Idiopathic hyperCKaemia; Limb-girdle muscular dystrophy.

▓ River blindness – see Onchocerciasis

▓ Rocky mountain spotted fever – see Rickettsial diseases

■ Rolandic epilepsy

Benign childhood epilepsy with centrotemporal spikes • Benign partial epilepsy • Benign rolandic epilepsy • Sylvian seizures

Pathophysiology Rolandic epilepsy, the commonest partial epilepsy of childhood, is genetically determined, with onset occurring between 2 and 13 years of age (usually 5–10 years). The typical EEG is often found in asymptomatic children. The prognosis is excellent, hence benign.

Clinical features: history and examination
- Focal EEG epileptiform discharges: usually clinically silent.
- Seizures: occur in <10% of children with rolandic spikes: typically simple partial, mainly motor (e.g. face, oropharyngeal musculature, with salivation or speech arrest); brief (30–60 seconds), often occurring when asleep or when awakening; secondary generalized seizures may occur in sleep.
- Normal examination.

Investigations and diagnosis *EEG*: focal epileptiform (spiking) discharges in lower rolandic, mid-temporal region.

Differential diagnosis Simple partial seizures due to focal brain lesion (injury, tumour, arteriovenous malformations, AVM).

Treatment and prognosis Excellent response to anti-epileptic drugs. Virtually all patients remit by early teenage; mild cognitive deficits persist in some patients.

> **Reference** Loiseau P, Duche B, Cordova S, Dartigues JF, Cohadon S. Prognosis of benign childhood epilepsy with centrotemporal spikes: a follow up study of 168 patients. *Epilepsia* 1988; **29**: 229–235.

> **Other relevant entries** Benign epilepsy syndromes; Epilepsy: an overview.

■ Romano–Ward syndrome – see Prolonged QT syndromes

■ Rosai–Dorfman disease

Sinus histiocytosis with massive lymphadenopathy

Pathophysiology An idiopathic histioproliferative disease usually affecting systemic lymph nodes, although extranodal and, very rarely, central nervous system (CNS) involvement is also described. The condition is more common in Afro-Caribbeans.

Clinical features: history and examination
- Bilateral painless lymphadenopathy, especially cervical.
- Fever, weight loss.
- Focal neurological signs, seizures if intracranial involvement.

Investigations and diagnosis *Bloods*: Polyclonal hypergammaglobulinaemia.

Imaging: brain CT/MRI may show multiple well-circumscribed mass lesions with dural attachment and homogenous enhancement with contrast.

Biopsy: proliferation of histiocytes, infiltration with plasma cells; lymphophago-cytosis (emperipolesis) is characteristic. S100 protein staining of cytoplasm.

Differential diagnosis Clinically and radiologically it may be impossible to distinguish Rosai–Dorfman disease from multiple meningioma. Multifocal CNS lymphoma may present a similar picture. Multiple metastases and sarcoidosis must also be considered.

Treatment and prognosis The condition usually resolves spontaneously. Hence the importance of making a pathological diagnosis and avoiding inappropriate and potentially toxic therapies.

References Petzold A, Thom M, Powell M, Plant GT. Relapsing intracranial Rosai–Dorfman disease. *Journal of Neurology, Neurosurgery and Psychiatry* 2001; **71**: 538–541.

Udono H, Fukuyama K, Okamoto H, Tabuchi K. Rosai–Dorfman disease presenting multiple intracranial lesions with unique findings on magnetic resonance imaging. Case report. *Journal of Neurosurgery* 1999; **91**: 335–339.

Other relevant entries Lymphoma; Meningioma; Sarcoidosis; Tumours: an overview.

■ Rosenberg–Bergstrom syndrome

Pathophysiology An autosomal-dominant hereditary syndrome of hearing loss and ataxia with onset in the second to third decade of life.

Clinical features: history and examination

- Sensorineural hearing loss: second to third decade.
- Ataxia: second to third decade.
- Hyperuricaemia $+/-$ abnormal renal function, rarely gout.
- $+/-$ proximal muscle wasting, weakness.
- No self-mutilation, telangiectasia.
- Family history for similar conditions.

Investigations and diagnosis *Bloods*: renal function, urate. Erythrocyte HGPRT is normal (*cf.* Lesch–Nyhan syndrome).

Differential diagnosis

Lesch–Nyhan syndrome.

Ataxia telangiectasia.

Treatment and prognosis No specific treatment.

Reference Rosenberg AL, Bergstrom L, Troost BT, Bartholomew BA. Hyperuricemia and neurologic deficits: a family study. *New England Journal of Medicine* 1970; **282**: 991–997.

Other relevant entries Ataxia telangiectasia; Hearing loss: differential diagnosis; Jeune–Tommasi syndrome; Lesch–Nyhan disease; Lichtenstein–Knorr syndrome; Richards–Rundle syndrome; Telfer's syndrome.

Rosenberg–Chutorian syndrome

Pathophysiology An autosomal-recessive hereditary syndrome of hearing loss and optic atrophy.

Clinical features: history and examination
- Progressive sensorineural hearing loss from infancy/childhood.
- Nyctalopia, progressive visual loss from second decade; optic atrophy.
- Progressive polyneuropathy: weakness, hyporeflexia, sensory loss.
- Normal extraocular movements.
- Family history for similar conditions.

Investigations and diagnosis *Neurophysiology*: EMG/NCS: reduced nerve conduction velocity + evidence of denervation.
Nerve biopsy: hypertrophy with onion bulb formation.

Differential diagnosis Hereditary motor and sensory neuropathy (HMSN).

Treatment and prognosis No specific treatment.

> **Reference** Rosenberg RN, Chutorian A. Familial opticoacoustic nerve degeneration and polyneuropathy. *Neurology* 1967; **17**: 827–832.

> **Other relevant entries** Hearing loss: differential diagnosis; Nyssen–van Bogaert syndrome; Sylvester disease; Tunbridge–Paley syndrome.

Ross syndrome

Ross syndrome consists of a combination of:
- progressive segmental hyperhidrosis with widespread hypohidrosis or anhidrosis
- a tonic (Holmes–Adie) pupil.
- hyporeflexia or areflexia.

There is phenotypic overlap between Ross syndrome and Holmes–Adie syndrome and Harlequin syndrome (isolated progressive segmental hypohidrosis).

Evidence from clinical studies and skin biopsies of reduced cholinergic sweat gland innervation supports the concept of a selective degenerative process affecting cholinergic sudomotor neurones in Ross syndrome.

> **References** Ross AT. Progressive selective sudomotor denervation. *Neurology* 1958; **8**: 809–817.

> Sommer C, Lindenlaub T, Zillikens D, Toyka KV, Naumann M. Selective loss of cholinergic sudomotor fibers causes anhidrosis in Ross syndrome. *Annals of Neurology* 2002; **52**: 247–250.

> Weller M, Wilhelm H, Sommer N *et al.* Tonic pupil, areflexia, and segmental anhidrosis. Two cases of Ross syndrome and review of the literature. *Journal of Neurology* 1992; **239**: 231–234.

> **Other relevant entries** Harlequin syndrome; Holmes–Adie syndrome.

Rostral vermis syndrome – see Cerebellar disease

■ Rothmund–Thomson syndrome
Poikiloderma congenitale

Pathophysiology A very rare autosomal-recessive syndrome of neurocutaneous anomalies with mental retardation. *In vitro* studies of cultured fibroblasts have suggested chromosomal instability.

Clinical features: history and examination
- Mental retardation.
- Short stature, abnormally small hands and feet, soft tissue contractures.
- Hypogonadism.
- Juvenile (4–7 years) zonular cataracts.
- Skin: mottled skin (poikiloderma): patchy atrophy, erythema, pigmentation, telangiectasia (at birth or within 6 months); alopecia; pink cheeks, ears, buttocks; skin malignancy; hypodontia.
- Absent eyebrows.
- Anaemia.
- Osteogenic sarcoma.

Investigations and diagnosis Diagnosis is on clinical grounds. Chromosomal studies may be undertaken.

Differential diagnosis Bloom syndrome.

Treatment and prognosis Protection from sunlight from birth may reduce risk of malignancy. Ophthalmological surveillance for cataract development is prudent. Prognosis is good unless skin malignancies develop.

> **Reference** Starr DG, McClure JP, Connor JM. Non-dermatological complications and genetic aspects of the Rothmund–Thomson syndrome. *Clinical Genetics* 1985; **27**: 102–104.
>
> **Other relevant entries** Phakomatosis; Werner syndrome (1).

■ Roussy–Déjerine syndrome – see Déjerine–Roussy syndrome

■ Roussy–Lévy syndrome
Hereditary areflexic dystasia

Pathophysiology Roussy–Lévy syndrome is an hereditary sensory ataxia with onset in infancy. Its nosological position was for many years controversial due to its similarities to Friedreich's ataxia and Charcot–Marie–Tooth (CMT) syndrome: some authorities included it in the peroneal muscular atrophy/hereditary motor and sensory neuropathy (HMSN) group as a variant of CMT-1; others regarded it as an entirely separate entity. Recently, tissue from the original family was shown to have a novel missense mutation in the P_0 gene, indicating that Roussy–Lévy syndrome is a subtype of CMT-1B.

Clinical features: history and examination
- Pes cavus, areflexia, atrophy (legs > hands).

- Sensory impairment: vibration, position sense causing sensory ataxia.
- Kyphoscoliosis.
- $+/-$ extensor plantar response(s).
- $+/-$ action tremor.
- No cerebellar ataxia, autonomic dysfunction, or nerve thickening.

Investigations and diagnosis *Neurophysiology*: EMG/NCS: denervation changes.
Pathology: similar findings were claimed in one patient with the Richards–Rundle syndrome.

Differential diagnosis
Friedreich's ataxia.
HMSN.

Treatment and prognosis Follow-up of four of the original seven cases of Roussy and Lévy after 30 years found little change in the condition.

References Lapresle J, Salisachs P. Roussy–Levy syndrome. In: Vinken PJ, Bruyn GW, De Jong JMBV (eds). *Handbook of Clinical Neurology: Volume 21: System Disorders and Atrophies Part I*. Amsterdam: North-Holland, 1975: 171–179.

Planté-Bordeneuve V, Guiochon-Mantel A, Lacroix C, Lapresle J, Said G. The Roussy–Lévy family: from the original description to the gene. *Annals of Neurology* 1999; **46**: 770–773.

Roussy G, Lévy G. Sept cas d'une maladie familiale particulière: troubles de la marche, pieds bots et aréflexie tendineuse généralisée avec, accessoirement, légère maladresse des mains. *Revue Neurologique* 1926; **1**: 427–450.

Other relevant entries Charcot–Marie–Tooth disease; Friedreich's ataxia; Hereditary motor and sensory neuropathy; Neuropathies: an overview; Richards–Rundle syndrome.

▪ Rowland–Payne syndrome – see Payne syndrome

▪ Rubella

Infection with the rubella virus, a RNA virus of the Togaviridae family, may have various consequences for the nervous system. Of these, congenital rubella syndrome (CRS) is the most common, despite the availability of vaccination, and the only one associated with direct viral invasion and replication within brain.

- Postinfectious encephalitis
  Follows acute infection with rubella virus. Pathogenesis unknown.
- CRS, Gregg syndrome
  Primary rubella infection in the mother during the first 20 weeks of pregnancy may infect the fetus, leading to CRS. The affected child has low birth weight, hepatosplenomegaly, congenital heart disease, sensorineural deafness, cataracts,

bone lesions, thrombocytopenia, microcephaly, and failure to thrive. Less severely affected children may have deafness, cataracts, and heart defects. Panencephalitis may cause a progressive cerebellar syndrome with dementia and optic atrophy. Diabetes mellitus may develop in later childhood.

Diagnosis is by viral culture (throat swab, urine) and assay for rubella-specific IgM in plasma. Periventricular calcification or lucencies may be seen on brain imaging. There is no specific treatment, but prevention through immunization has reduced the incidence of this condition.

- Progressive rubella panencephalitis (PRP)

    This extremely rare condition is thought to represent either a reactivation of latent viral infection causing a subacute or chronic viral illness, or an autoimmune reaction. Patients may have features of CRS, but then develop decline of intellect and behaviour with seizures, ataxia, and progressive dementia. Oligoclonal bands and raised rubella-specific antibody titres are found in the CSF. Pathologically there is white matter destruction but no inclusion bodies are seen. There is no specific treatment and death occurs within a few years, although spontaneous remissions have been reported.

Reference Frey TK. Neurological aspects of rubella virus infection. *Intervirology* 1997; **40**: 167–175.

Other relevant entries Encephalitis: an overview; Progressive multifocal leuko-encephalopathy; Subacute sclerosing panencephalitis.

■ Rubinstein–Taybi syndrome

Pathophysiology A dysmorphologic syndrome with mental retardation, probably aetiologically heterogeneous.

Clinical features: history and examination

- Morphology:
    Microcephaly
    Beaked nose, nasal septum extending below alae, downward slanting palpebral fissures, maxillary hypoplasia, strabismus, epicanthic folds
    Broad distal phalanges in thumbs and halluces, short stature
    Cryptorchidism in boys.
- Neurology:
    Mental retardation
    Spastic gait, hyperreflexia
    Seizures (*ca.* 25%)
    +/− absent corpus callosum.

Investigations and diagnosis No specific investigations.

Differential diagnosis Characteristic phenotype; Saethre–Chotzen syndrome, Silver–Russell syndrome may appear similar.

Treatment and prognosis No specific treatment; symptomatic treatment of seizures. Probably associated with reduced life expectancy; quality of life related to degree of mental retardation.

> **Reference** Rubinstein JH, Taybi H. Broad thumbs and toes and facial abnormalities. A possible mental retardation syndrome. *American Journal of Diseases of Childhood* 1963; **105**: 588–608.

> **Other relevant entries** Saethre–Chotzen syndrome; Silver–Russell syndrome.

■ Rucksack Paralysis

Carrying a heavy backpack may be followed by a disorder of the brachial plexus or isolated long thoracic nerve dysfunction. This may be due to direct nerve trauma or, in the case of neurlagic amyotrophy, to exercise-induced inflammatory disease.

> **Other relevant entries** Brachial plexopathies; Long thoracic nerve palsy; Neuralgic amyotrophy.

■ Russell–Silver syndrome – see Silver–Russell syndrome

■ Russell's syndrome – see Diencephalic syndrome

Ss

■ Sacral radiculopathy – see Lumbar cord and root disease

■ Saethre–Chotzen syndrome
Acrocephalosyndactyly III

Pathophysiology An autosomal-dominant syndrome of premature closure of cranial sutures, with fused digits; linked to chromosome 7p21.

Clinical features: history and examination

- Various craniostenoses; asymmetrical cranial (plagiocephalic) and facial deformities.
- Dysmorphism: low frontal hairline, beaked nose, hypertelorism, ptosis, prognathism, + / − low set ears.
- Mental retardation moderate or absent.
- Cryptorchidism.
- Heart / renal anomalies.

Investigations and diagnosis *Imaging*: shows cranial deformity.

Differential diagnosis Other acrocephalosyndactyly syndromes; Rubinstein–Taybi syndrome.

Treatment and prognosis No specific treatment.

> **Reference** Friedman JM, Hanson JW, Graham CB, Smith DW. Saethre–Chotzen syndrome: a broad and variable pattern of skeletal malformations. *Journal of Pediatrics* 1977; **91**: 929–933.

> **Other relevant entries** Apert syndrome; Craniostenosis; Crouzon syndrome; Carpenter syndrome; Pfeiffer syndrome.

Sagittal sinus thrombosis – see Cerebrovascular disease: venous

St Anthony's fire – see Ergotism

St Louis encephalitis – see Arbovirus disease; Encephalitis: an overview

St Vitus' dance – see Sydenham's chorea

Salaam seizures – see West's syndrome

Salla disease

This condition, which may be categorized as one of the sialidoses or mucolipidoses, has its onset in the first months of life with hypotonia, developmental delay, ataxia, motor and mental retardation. Short stature, thickened calvaria and strabismus are common features. There is a predilection for individuals of Finnish descent. Abnormal lysosomal morphology is seen in blood lymphocytes, skin, and liver. Urinary free sialic acid is increased.

> **Other relevant entries** Lysosomal-storage disorders: an overview; Sialidoses: an overview.

Sandhoff's disease

β-hexosaminidase A and B deficiency • GM2 gangliosidosis

Pathophysiology A rare form of late-infantile gangliosidosis, clinically almost indistinguishable from Tay–Sachs disease.

Clinical features: history and examination

- Onset 6–12 months of age.
- Developmental arrest, hypotonia.
- Exaggerated startle reflex.
- Macrocephaly.
- Seizures: difficult to control.
- Visual failure: macular cherry-red spot.

- +mild hepatomegaly (*cf*. Tay–Sachs).
- +mild dysostosis multiplex evident radiographically (*cf*. Tay–Sachs).
- Juvenile form: progressive ataxic dementia.
- Adult-onset cases: spinocerebellar degeneration.

Investigations and diagnosis *Bloods*: enzyme activity (total; HexA, HexB) can be measured in plasma, leukocytes, or fibroblasts.
Urine: oligosaccharides (*cf*. Tay–Sachs).
Imaging: CT/MRI brain may show typical bright thalami; cerebellar atrophy.
Neurogenetics: sequencing of hexosaminidase A and B genes.
Biopsy: rectal mucosa may show periodic acid–Schiff (PAS) positive foamy macrophages.
Differential diagnosis Tay–Sachs disease.
Treatment and prognosis No specific treatment.

> **Reference** Hara A, Uyama E, Uchino M *et al*. Adult Sandhoff's disease: R505Q and I207V substitutions in the HEXB gene of the first Japanese case. *Journal of the Neurological Sciences* 1998; **155**: 86–91.
>
> **Other relevant entries** Gangliosidoses: an overview; Tay–Sachs disease.

■ Sandifer's syndrome
Dyspeptic dystonia

Pathophysiology An involuntary movement disorder of childhood characterized by spasmodic posturing of the head and neck as a consequence of gastro-oesophageal reflux.
Clinical features: history and examination Spasmodic posturing of the head and neck; movements may increase at meal times; video recording may assist diagnosis.
Investigations and diagnosis Oesophageal pH monitoring to diagnose reflux.
Differential diagnosis Paroxysmal dystonia, paroxysmal torticollis, hyperekplexia.
Treatment and prognosis Successful treatment of gastro-oesophageal acid reflux, either medically (histamine H_2-receptor antagonists, proton pump inhibitors) or surgically (fundoplication) leads to resolution of the movements.

> **Reference** Mandel H, Tirosh E, Berant M. Sandifer syndrome reconsidered. *Acta Paediatrica Scandinavica* 1989; **78**: 797–799.
>
> **Other relevant entries** Dystonia; Paroxysmal dyskinesias.

■ Sanfilippo's disease
Mucopolysaccharidosis type III (MPS III)

A lysosomal-storage disorder characterized by developmental delay and extreme behavioural problems. Four biochemical and genetic variants, types A–D, all autosomal recessive, are recognized. All have excessive urinary excretion of heparan sulphate.

Clinical features: history and examination

- Clinical expression is heterogeneous, even within families.
- Presentation is usually in 2nd or 3rd year of life:
- Developmental slowing, particularly affecting speech, followed by developmental regression.
- Behavioural problems: impulsivity, aggression, hyperactivity, stereotyped motor automatisms, disturbed sleep.
- Relentlessly progressive dementia.
- Spastic quadriplegia.
- Non-neurological features:
    - Coarse facial features, short neck, stiff joints.
    - Hepatosplenomegaly: mild.
    - No corneal changes (*cf.* other mucopolysaccharidoses).

Investigations and diagnosis *Urine*: thin layer chromatography of urinary mucopolysaccharides shows increased excretion of heparan sulphate.

Enzyme analysis in cultured fibroblasts is the only way to distinguish the four types:

Type A: heparan-*N*-sulphatase deficiency
Type B: *N*-Acetyl-α-D-glucosaminidase deficiency
Type C: Acetyl-CoA: α-glucosaminide deficiency
Type D: *N*-Acetyl-α-D-glucosaminide-6-sulphatase deficiency (chromosome 12q14).

Imaging: radiographic dysostosis multiplex is subtle.

Treatment and prognosis No specific treatment; symptomatic treatment of behavioural problems. Death usual before age 20 years.

> **Reference** Barone R, Nigro F, Triulzi F, Musumeci S, Fiumara A, Pavone L. Clinical and neuroradiological follow-up in mucopolysaccharidosis type III (Sanfilippo syndrome). *Neuropediatrics* 1999; **30**: 270–274.

> **Other relevant entries** Lysosomal-storage disorders: an overview; Mucopolysaccharidoses.

▓ Santavuori–Haltia disease – see Neuronal ceroid lipofuscinosis

▓ Santavuori muscle–eye–brain syndrome – see Muscle–eye–brain disease

▓ Saphenous neuropathy

The saphenous nerve is a cutaneous branch of the femoral nerve which emerges from the parent trunk distal to Hunter's canal and medial and superior to the knee. It accompanies the saphenous vein in the medial part of the leg to the medial aspect of the foot supplying sensory innervation to these areas. Saphenous neuropathy, resulting in sensory loss to these areas, most commonly follows surgical injury to the nerve (e.g. saphenous vein removal, knee surgery).

Other relevant entries Femoral neuropathy; Neuropathies: an overview.

■ Sarcoglycanopathy

Sarcoglycans are a group of five distinct, dystrophin-associated, transmembrane proteins, deficiency of which results in autosomal-recessive limb-girdle muscular dystrophy (LGMD), often the severe childhood variants previously known as SCARMD (*severe childhood autosomal-recessive muscular dystrophy*). These conditions may be confused clinically with Duchenne muscular dystrophy but are genetically distinct. The hip abduction sign, abduction of the thighs when rising from the ground due to the relative weakness of hip adductors with relatively preserved strength in hip abductors, seems to be a sensitive and specific sign in sarcoglycanopathies. Since sarcoglycans are expressed in cardiac as well as skeletal muscle, the possibility of concurrent cardiomyopathy must not be forgotten. Abnormalities of these proteins have also been associated with the myoclonus–dystonia syndrome, *viz.*:

α-sarcoglycan (adhalin): LGMD type 2D, linkage to chromosome 17q
β-sarcoglycan: LGMD type 2E, linkage to chromosome 4q
γ-sarcoglycan: LGMD type 2C, linkage to chromosome 13q
δ-sarcoglycan: LGMD type 2F, linkage to chromosome 5q
ε-sarcoglycan: myoclonus–dystonia syndrome (MDS).

Other relevant entries Duchenne muscular dystrophy; Dystrophinopathy; Limb-girdle muscular dystrophy; Myoclonus–dystonia syndrome.

■ Sarcoidosis
Besnier–Boeck–Schaumann disease

Pathophysiology A sporadic systemic disease characterized pathologically by non-caseating epithelioid cell granulomata. Prevalence rates vary but the condition is much commoner in Afro-Caribbeans compared to whites, and slightly commoner in women. The cause remains unknown, although the condition is clearly immunologically mediated; whether or not cryptic infection underlies the disorder is not clear. The organs most commonly affected are the lymph nodes, lungs, liver, spleen, skin and eyes, but no system is exempt (with the possible exception of the adrenal glands), including the nervous system in approximately 5% of cases: the majority of these patients are known to have systemic sarcoidosis and then develop neurological signs; a small group have systemic disease presenting with neurological signs; very rarely, sarcoidosis may be confined exclusively to the nervous system.

Clinical features: history and examination *Neurological: (neurosarcoidosis).*

- Meningeal infiltration (granulomatous):
  - Cranial nerve palsies: especially VII, but optic neuritis and VIII lesions are also well recognized; Heerfordt syndrome is a facial nerve palsy of sarcoid origin with parotid enlargement and uveitis (uveoparotid fever).
  - Hypothalamo-pituitary effects: diabetes insipidus, hypopituitarism, hypothalamic sarcoid (hypersomnia, obesity, personality change), $+/-$ optic chiasm involvement causing visual disturbances.
- Vasculitis may occur (uncommon).
- Peripheral nerve involvement: mononeuropathy multiplex; plexopathy; polyneuropathy, cauda equina syndrome (rare).
- Muscle: sarcoid myopathy: proximal muscle atrophy, palpable nodules in muscle, may be present.
- Spinal cord: inflammatory (sarcoid) myelopathy.
- Intraparenchymal (hemisphere) mass lesions of brain and spinal cord ("sarcoid tumour").
- Intracerebral/intraretinal haemorrhage due to sarcoid-related thrombocytopenia (rare).
- Infarction? (reported in some series).

Almost any other organ system can be affected, but the commonest presentations are with:

Reticuloendothelial: lymphadenopathy; epitrochlear nodes said to be particularly suggestive of diagnosis.

Respiratory: bilateral hilar lymphadenopathy (asymptomatic); restrictive lung disease.

Gastrointestinal: hepatosplenomegaly.

Dermatological: erythema nodosum; lupus pernio.

Ophthalmological: uveitis (anterior > posterior); optic neuritis (occasionally bilateral).

Haematological: lymphopenia, thrombocytopenia.

- Progressive multifocal leukoencephalopathy (PML) can develop in patients with neurosarcoidosis.
- $+/-$ systemic features: fever, weight loss, lethargy.

Investigations and diagnosis _Bloods_: lymphopenia, thrombocytopenia, hypercalcaemia, polyclonal hypergammaglobulinaemia, raised serum angiotensin converting enzyme (ACE).

CSF: may find increased protein, pleocytosis; oligoclonal bands in acute disease, but not in stable chronic disease (_cf._ multiple sclerosis), raised ACE (non-specific); glucose may be low.

Imaging:

Chest X-ray: bilateral hilar lymphadenopathy; fine cut CT thorax is more sensitive.

Gallium scan: may show typical uptake in lymphoid tissues of nasopharynx (Waldeyer's ring), + lacrimal, salivary glands, mediastinum.

Neurosarcoidosis: MRI with gadolinium particularly helpful showing widespread meningeal enhancement and focal uptake in hypothalamic region; intraparenchymal mass lesions may be indistinguishable from tumours (glioma, meningioma).

Tissue: bone marrow aspirate, liver biopsy, bronchial biopsy, lymph node biopsy, muscle biopsy, may show characteristic epithelioid non-caseating granulomata if relevant organ is involved. Occasionally diagnosed on brain biopsy with changes in meninges or, less commonly, mass lesion.

Kveim test: no longer in use.

Differential diagnosis

Multiple sclerosis.

Vasculitides, especially Wegener's granulomatosis.

Other autoimmune/inflammatory conditions: SLE, rheumatoid arthritis, Behçet's.

Syphilis.

Tuberculosis.

Brain tumours, lymphoma (sarcoid tumour).

Treatment and prognosis There are no randomized-controlled trials of treatment options in sarcoidosis. The mainstay of treatment, when required, is with tapering doses of steroids and, if needed, steroid-sparing immunosuppressive agents such as azathioprine, methotrexate, or cyclophosphamide. Prolonged treatment may be required; early cessation may lead to relapse. Ciclosporin has been used in patients intolerant of or unresponsive to these treatments. Total body irradiation has been used as a last resort.

There are no longitudinal studies examining course of disease and prognosis in neurosarcoidosis. It seems likely that around 65% of patients have an acute and monophasic illness, the remainder have a chronic relapsing condition (especially those with hemisphere and cord lesions).

References Larner AJ, Ball JA, Howard RS. Sarcoid tumour: continuing diagnostic problems in the MRI era. *Journal of Neurology, Neurosurgery and Psychiatry* 1999; **66**: 510–512.

Newman LS, Rose CS, Maier LA. Sarcoidosis. *New England Journal of Medicine* 1997; **336**: 1224–1234.

Nowak DA, Widenka DC. Neurosarcoidosis: a review of its intracranial manifestation. *Journal of Neurology* 2001; **248**: 363–372.

Scadding JG, Mitchell DN. *Sarcoidosis* (2nd edition). London: Chapman & Hall, 1985.

Zajicek JP, Scolding NJ, Foster O *et al*. Central nervous system sarcoidosis – diagnosis and management. *Quarterly Journal of Medicine* 1999; **92**: 103–117.

Other relevant entries Cauda equina syndrome and conus medullaris disease; Multiple sclerosis; Myopathy: an overview; Neuropathies: an overview; Progressive multifocal leukoencephalopathy; Syphilis; Tuberculosis and the nervous system; Tumours: an overview; Vasculitis.

■ Satoyoshi syndrome

Komuragaeri disease • Myospasm gravis

A progressive syndrome of painful intermittent generalized muscle spasms, alopecia, diarrhoea, with secondary skeletal abnormalities and endocrinopathy with amenorrhoea. It is believed to be an autoimmune condition because of the frequent presence of auto-antibodies directed against acetylcholine receptors (in the absence of myasthenia gravis or thymoma) and the response to steroids, intravenous immunoglobulin, and tacrolimus.

Reference Satoyoshi E. A syndrome of progressive muscle spasm, alopecia, and diarrhea. *Neurology* 1978; **28**: 458–471.

■ Saturday night palsy – see Radial neuropathy

■ Savant syndrome

Idiot savant syndrome

Savant syndrome refers to individuals with developmental disability yet displaying skills at a level inconsistent with their general intellectual functioning. The outstanding ability may be feats of memory (recalling names), calculation (especially calendar calculation), music, or artistic skills, often in the context of autism or a pervasive developmental disorder.

Occasionally, skills such as artistic ability may emerge in the context of neurodegenerative disease (Alzheimer's disease, frontotemporal dementia).

Reference Miller LK. The savant syndrome: intellectual impairment and exceptional skill. *Psychological Bulletin* 1999; **125**: 31–46.

Other relevant entry Autism, autistic disorder.

■ SCA – see Spinocerebellar ataxia

■ Scalenus syndrome – see Thoracic outlet syndromes

■ Scapuloperoneal syndrome

Scapuloperoneal syndrome, as its name implies, describes periscapular wasting and weakness with associated scapular winging, and wasting and weakness of tibialis anterior causing weak ankle dorsiflexion or foot drop. This phenotype may be:
• Myogenic:
  Facioscapulohumeral (FSH) dystrophy: "forme fruste" without the facial weakness in some cases.
  Emery–Dreifuss syndrome (consider this if cardiomyopathy present, contractures).

- Neurogenic:
    Scapuloperoneal spinal muscular atrophy (rare; genetically heterogeneous).
    Dawidenkow syndrome (may be additional sensory findings).

Despite electrophysiological studies and muscle biopsy, it can be difficult to differentiate myogenic and neurogenic syndromes.

Reference Tawil R, Myers GJ, Weiffenbach B *et al*. Scapuloperoneal syndromes: absence of linkage to the 4q35 FSHD locus. *Archives of Neurology* 1995; **52**: 1069–1072.

Other relevant entries Dawidenkow syndrome; Emery–Dreifuss muscular dystrophy; Facioscapulohumeral dystrophy; Foot drop: differential diagnosis; Muscular dystrophies: an overview.

■ SCARMD – see Sarcoglycanopathy

■ Schaltenbrand's syndrome – see Spontaneous intracranial hypotension

■ Scheie's syndrome
Mucopolysaccharidosis type I-S (MPS I-S)

This condition, resulting from deficiency of the lysosomal enzyme L-iduronidase, is allelic with Hurler's syndrome; before this was discovered, it was also known as MPS type V. The clinical features are similar to Hurler's disease, but milder; carpal tunnel syndrome is common. Life expectancy is greater than Hurler's disease.

Other relevant entries Hurler's disease; Mucopolysaccharidoses.

■ Scheuermann's disease
Juvenile kyphosis

Thoracic or thoracolumbar kyphosis in adolescents causing low back pain with exercise; the syndrome is usually benign. However, occasionally spinal cord compression from thoracic disc herniation or severe kyphosis may occur.

Other relevant entries Scoliosis; Thoracic disc prolapse.

■ Schilder's disease
Diffuse sclerosis • Encephalitis periaxalis diffusa • Myelinoclastic diffuse sclerosis

Pathophysiology A rare, non-familial, acute or subacute demyelinating disorder of children or young adults, of unknown cause. It may be a devastating monophasic illness, or a relapsing–remitting disorder without full recovery. Schilder's disease may be a variant of multiple sclerosis (some authors regard it as a "transitional" form); clinical manifestations are similar although cortical features (dementia, hemiplegia, cortical blindness, and deafness) are more prominent. One of the original cases reported resembled adrenoleukodystrophy.

Clinical features: history and examination

- Hemiplegia.
- Visual field defects; cortical blindness.
- Pseudobulbar palsy.
- Deafness.
- Dementia.
- Intracranial hypertension.
- Psychiatric features.

Investigations and diagnosis There is no diagnostic test, but diagnostic criteria (pre-MRI era) have been suggested:

Subacute or chronic demyelinating disorder with one or two symmetric bilateral lesions involving the centrum semiovale (at least 3×2 cm);

No other lesions demonstrable clinically or by imaging;

No involvement of adrenal glands, peripheral nervous system;

Histological findings identical to multiple sclerosis, but large sharply demarcated foci, may involve whole lobe.

Investigations aiming to exclude other disorders:

Bloods: lactate, amino acids, arylsulphatase A, C26/C22 very long-chain fatty acid ratio: all normal.

CSF: lactate normal; oligoclonal bands usually negative; myelin basic protein elevated.

MRI: confluent or multifocal areas of high signal on T_2-weighted images, confined to white matter; may show mass effect during acute deteriorations.

Brain biopsy: inflammatory perivascular infiltrate with demyelination; cystic lesions in severe cases; axonal damage.

Differential diagnosis

Multiple sclerosis.

Encephalomyelitides [e.g. acute disseminated encephalomyelitis (ADEM)].

Other leukodystrophy [e.g. X-linked adrenoleukodystrophy (X-ALD), metachromatic leukodystrophy (MLD)].

Diffuse cerebral neoplasm.

Mitochondrial disease.

Isolated central nervous system (CNS) angiitis.

Treatment and prognosis Corticosteroids may improve the outcome of single episodes, but their effect, if any, on the course of the disease is unknown.

References Afifi AK, Bell WE, Menezes AH, Moore SA. Myelinoclastic diffuse sclerosis (Schilder's disease): report of a case and review of the literature. *Journal of Child Neurology* 1994; **9**: 398–403.

Poser CM, Goutières F, Carpentier M-A, Aicardi J. Schilder's myelinoclastic diffuse sclerosis. *Pediatrics* 1986; **77**: 107–112.

Schilder P. Zur Kenntnis der sogenannten diffusen Sklerose. *Zeitschrift für die Gesamte Neurologie und Psychiatrie* 1912; **10**: 1–60.

Other relevant entries Adrenoleukodystrophy; Leukodystrophies: an overview; Multiple sclerosis.

■ Schimmelpenning's syndrome – see Epidermal naevus syndrome

■ Schindler's disease
α-N-acetylgalactosaminidase deficiency

Pathophysiology An autosomal-recessive disease due to deficiency of the lysosomal enzyme α-N-acetylgalactosaminidase, causing developmental regression with features of a neuroaxonal dystrophy. The abnormal gene is located on chromosome 22q.

Clinical features: history and examination
- Loss of milestones.
- Optic atrophy, nystagmus, strabismus; eventually blindness.
- Limb hypotonia, hyperreflexia; eventual spastic quadriplegia.
- Seizures, may be myoclonic.
- Deafness (late).
- No visceral involvement.

Investigations and diagnosis
Bloods: normal.
Urine: increased oligosaccharide excretion (non-specific).
CSF: normal.
Evoked potentials: low amplitude, delayed.
MRI: atrophic cortex, cerebellum and brainstem.
ERG: normal.
Tissue (brain, cutaneous nerves, fibroblasts, leukocytes): heterogeneous inclusions, tubulovesicular and granular; enzyme analysis (diagnostic).

Differential diagnosis Other causes of neuroaxonal dystrophy (Seitelberger disease), developmental regression.

Treatment and prognosis No specific treatment, supportive therapy only. Patients bedridden by age 5 years.

Reference Schindler D, Bishop DF, Wolfe DE *et al*. Neuroaxonal dystrophy due to lysosomal α-N-acetylgalactosaminidase deficiency. *New England Journal of Medicine* 1989; **320**: 1735–1740.

Other relevant entry Neuroaxonal dystrophy.

■ Schistosomiasis
Bilharziasis

Pathophysiology Trematode *Schistosoma* parasites gain access to the human body via larvae (cercariae) shed by the intermediate snail host in water. They may affect spinal cord and brain.

Clinical features: history and examination

Cerebral (S. japonicum)

- acute
    meningoencephalitis
    focal signs (hemiplegia, spasticity, cranial nerve palsy)
    seizures (part of Katayama fever).
- chronic
    raised intracranial pressure
    seizures
    mass lesion
    cerebral vasculitis.

Spinal (S. mansoni in South America, S. haematobium in Africa).

- cauda equina and conus medullaris syndromes.
- paraplegia: transverse myelitis, cord infarct, granulomatous cord compression.

Investigations and diagnosis

Blood: eosinophilia. Serology for Schistosoma.

Stool: ova (often not helpful).

CSF: eosinophilia.

Imaging:

brain CT/MRI: dense multinodular lesions with enhancement, oedema (non-specific);
spinal cord MRI: swelling, arachnoiditis, granuloma.

Tissue: Rectal/liver/bladder biopsy.

Differential diagnosis Very broad! Other causes of meningoencephalitis, seizures, paraplegia, conus medullaris, and cauda equina syndrome. Travel history may be key to focusing differential diagnosis.

Treatment and prognosis Antischistosomal treatment: praziquantel, metrifonate, oxamniquine.

Corticosteroids.

Surgical decompression.

> **Reference** Bill PLA. Schistosomiasis. In: Shakir RA, Newman PK, Poser CM (eds). *Tropical Neurology* London: Saunders, 1996: 295–316.

> **Other relevant entries** Cauda equina and conus medullaris disease; Helminthic disease; Myelopathy: an overview.

▓ Schizophrenia

Pathophysiology A common mental disorder, characterized by psychotic features. There is evidence to suggest it is best classified as a neurodevelopmental disorder, although ultimately the aetiology and pathogenesis remain unknown.

Clinical features: history and examination The presence of Schneider's first rank symptoms is suggestive, although not pathognomonic, of the disease.

- Hallucinations:
  Audible thoughts.
  Voices commenting, in the third person, on what the patient does.
  Voices arguing with each other.
- Delusions:
  Delusions of passivity, control or influence.
  Thought withdrawal, thought insertion, thought broadcasting.
- Disturbance of language: flattening of expression, concrete thinking, schizophasia.
- Absence of mood disorder; clear consciousness.
- $+/-$ mannerisms.
- Clustering of signs is noted:
  Positive features: abnormal thought and behaviour:
    Reality distortion: delusions, hallucinations.
    Disorganization: incoherent speech, inappropriate emotional responses.
  Negative features:
    Psychomotor poverty: poverty of speech, action; blunted emotional responses.

Investigations and diagnosis Diagnosis is essentially clinical. Use of a detailed standardized interview scheme, such as the Present State Examination, may assist diagnosis.

Imaging: CT/MRI: in cohort studies, brain size is reduced in schizophrenia (enlarged ventricles, medial temporal lobe atrophy).

Neuropsychology: may show low IQ; impairments of memory, attention and executive function have been recorded.

Pathology: no specific neuropathological changes yet identified.

Differential diagnosis Schneiderian first rank symptoms ("schizophreniform psychoses") may also occur in:

Schizoaffective disorder
Mania
Depression (rare)
Amphetamine intoxication
Partial seizures
Cushing's syndrome
Variant Creutzfeldt–Jakob disease
Subacute sclerosing panencephalitis
Adrenoleukodystrophy
Huntington's disease.

Treatment and prognosis Neuroleptic medications are the mainstay of treatment, either traditional or classical medications such as chlorpromazine or haloperidol, or newer atypicals, such as clozapine, olanzapine, risperidone. Management is probably best supervised by a psychiatrist with monitoring (e.g. of compliance) by a community psychiatric nurse.

Post-psychotic depression is recognized.

Prognosis is variable, including a waxing–waning disorder, or partial remission with static or slowly worsening course. Chronic disability is the norm, and it is doubtful if full and complete remission ever occurs.

References Frith C, Johnstone E. *Schizophrenia. A Very Short Introduction*. Oxford: OUP, 2003.

Mellors CS. First-rank symptoms of schizophrenia. *British Journal of Psychiatry* 1970; **117**: 15–23.

Other relevant entry Psychiatric disorders and neurological disease.

▦ Schmidt's syndrome

Pathophysiology This syndrome of the lower cranial nerves is variously described in the literature, but most frequently refers to involvement of X and XI, due to an extramedullary lesion affecting the roots before they leave the skull (*cf.* Vernet's syndrome).

(NB. Endocrinologists recognize a different Schmidt's syndrome, of adrenal insufficiency and lymphocytic thyroiditis with hypothyroidism).

Clinical features: history and examination
- Weak ipsilateral soft palate, pharynx, larynx.
- Weak ipsilateral trapezius, sternocleidomastoid.

Investigations and diagnosis *Imaging*: MRI is modality of choice for examination of the brainstem.

Differential diagnosis Other syndromes of the lower cranial nerves: Vernet's syndrome, Tapia's syndrome, Jackson's syndrome, Collet–Sicard syndrome, Villaret's syndrome.

Treatment and prognosis Of cause if identified.

Other relevant entries Jugular foramen syndrome; Vernet's syndrome; Villaret's syndrome.

▦ Scholz's disease – see Metachromatic leukodystrophy

▦ Schwartz–Jampel syndrome
Chondrodystrophic myotonia

Pathophysiology A congenital (autosomal-recessive) condition with neurological and morphological features, the former characterized clinically by myotonia and continuous EMG activity which originates at the level of the muscle membrane and most likely represents a channelopathy. A candidate locus has been identified on chromosome 1p.

Clinical features: history and examination

- Neurological: Muscle stiffness, myotonia (action and percussion); blepharospasm, blepharophimosis; high-pitched voice.
- Morphological: Short stature, oculo-facial abnormalities, bone and joint deformities.

Investigations and diagnosis *Neurophysiology*: NCS: normal, including repetitive nerve stimulation and neuromuscular junction transmission. EMG: persistent spontaneous activity, myotonic discharges.

Differential diagnosis Other myotonic syndromes, but morphological features render confusion unlikely.

Treatment and prognosis No specific treatment.

References Schwartz O, Jampel RS. Congenital blepharophimosis associated with a unique generalized myopathy. *Archives of Ophthalmology* 1962; **68**: 52–57.

Spaans F, Theunissen P, Reekers AD, Smit L, Veldman H. Schwartz–Jampel syndrome: I. Clinical, electromyographic and histologic studies. *Muscle and Nerve* 1990; **13**: 516–527.

Other relevant entries Channelopathies: an overview; Myotonia and myotonic syndromes.

■ Sciatic neuropathy

Pathophysiology Containing fibres from the L4 to S3 roots, the sciatic nerve exits the pelvis via the sciatic notch, runs under the piriformis muscle, descends into the posterior thigh and divides above the knee into peroneal and tibial branches. This division is reflected more proximally by two trunks, lateral and medial, and lateral sciatic nerve trunk injury may produce a picture identical to that with isolated peroneal nerve involvement. Most cases of sciatic neuropathy relate to trauma: pelvic injury, hip injury, compression by tumour, haematoma, and, possibly, the piriformis muscle.

Clinical features: history and examination

- Motor: complete lesions cause weakness of all muscles below the knee as well as hamstrings (biceps femoris, semitendinosus, semimembranosus) with loss or depression of ankle and hamstring reflexes.

  However, lateral trunk injury is more common, producing foot drop as in a peroneal nerve palsy (weak tibialis anterior, extensor hallucis longus and extensor digitorum longus).
- Sensory: in the distribution of the peroneal and tibial nerves, hence whole foot, lateral calf.
- Pelvic examination for mass lesions may be indicated.

Investigations and diagnosis *EMG/NCS*: help to distinguish sciatic mononeuropathy from radiculopathy, lumbosacral plexopathy.

Differential diagnosis Lumbar radiculopathy, especially L5–S1.

Lumbosacral plexopathy.
Peroneal neuropathy, tibial neuropathy.

Reference Staal A, Van Gijn J, Spaans F. *Mononeuropathies: Examination, Diagnosis and Treatment.* London: WB Saunders, 1999: 117–123.

Other relevant entries Entrapment neuropathies; Foot drop: differential diagnosis; Neuropathies: an overview; Obturator neuropathy; Peroneal neuropathy; Piriformis syndrome; Tibial neuropathy.

■ Sciatica

Pathophysiology Sciatica is a clinical syndrome of radicular pain, involving the spinal roots L4, L5 or S1, from which the sciatic nerve takes its origin. Patients may also use the term to refer to more chronic back, buttock and leg pain which is consequent on an acute event or due to other pathologies, including musculoskeletal problems.

A rare catamenial variant is described, due to implantation of endometriosis in the sciatic nerve.

Clinical features: history and examination

- Pain: radiating from lower back to buttock, posterior thigh, posterolateral or anterolateral foot. If due to intervertebral disc prolapse, pain may develop acutely when bending or lifting a heavy object. Pain is exacerbated by manoeuvres which raise intracranial pressure (coughing, sneezing, straining, jugular vein compression), and by local stretching (straight leg raising, Lasègue's sign).
- Motor signs: loss of ankle jerk (L5, S1); weakness, atrophy, +/− fasciculation if anterior roots involved.

Investigations and diagnosis *Neurophysiology*: EMG/NCS: evidence of radiculopathy. *Imaging*: MRI, to look for root compression (e.g. disc).

CSF: may be required if no compressive lesion found on imaging, especially if malignant infiltration suspected.

Differential diagnosis History not likely to be mistaken for plexopathy, neuropathy.

Treatment and prognosis Pain usually settles with rest and adequate analgesia. If not, or if neurological signs develop (wasting, weakness), investigation should be pursued. Surgical decompression may be required.

Other relevant entries Failed back syndrome; Intervertebral disc prolapse; Lumbar cord and root disease; Radiculopathies: an overview; Sciatic neuropathy; Tarlov cyst.

■ Sciwora

Sciwora is an acronym for *s*pinal *c*ord *i*njury *w*ith*o*ut *r*adiologic *a*bnormality, most often seen in children, perhaps due to the laxity of spinal ligaments permitting self-reducing subluxation of the vertebrae, but sometimes in elderly patients with degenerative joint disease. The condition should be treated with immobilization, and avoidance of precipitating activities such as sports, since there is a high risk of delayed neurological dysfunction.

Other relevant entry Paraparesis: acute management and differential diagnosis.

■ Scleroderma – see Systemic sclerosis

■ Sclerodermatomyositis – see Dermatomyositis; Overlap syndrome; Systemic sclerosis

■ Scoliosis
Kyphoscoliosis

Scoliosis is abnormal curvature of the spine in the lateral plane; kyphosis is abnormal curvature anteroposteriorly; kyphoscoliosis is a combination of both.

Although perhaps 70% of childhood scoliosis is idiopathic, particularly in girls (F : M = 8 : 1), scoliosis may reflect an underlying neurological or muscular disorder. Certainly neurological investigation is appropriate if in addition to scoliosis there are neurological signs such as back pain, bowel and/or bladder problems, leg or foot weakness, or a midline patch of hair, pigmentation, or a mass over the spinal column. If so, in addition to plain radiographs of the spine, other neurological investigations such as MRI may be indicated. Kyphoscoliosis may contribute to respiratory compromise.

The differential diagnosis of scoliosis includes:
- Upper motor neurone disorders
    Cerebral palsy (spastic, quadriparetic, athetoid, dystonia)
    Torsion dystonia
    Spinocerebellar ataxia; Friedreich's ataxia
    Spinal cord tumour
    Syringomyelia
    Neurofibromatosis.
- Lower motor neurone disorders
    Neuropathies, for example Charcot–Marie–Tooth (peroneal muscular
        atrophy).
- Myopathies, for example nemaline.
- Abnormalities of bone:
    Congenital
        Hemivertebra
        Diastematomyelia.
    Acquired
        Pott's disease of the spine.
- Idiopathic scoliosis.
    Other relevant entries Respiratory failure; Scheuermann's disease.

■ Segawa syndrome – see Dopa-responsive dystonia; Dystonia: an overview

■ Seitelberger disease – see Neuroaxonal dystrophy; Schindler's disease

■ Seizures – see Epilepsy: an overview

■ Semantic dementia
Progressive fluent aphasia

Pathophysiology Semantic dementia (SD) is one of the variants of focal lobar degeneration of the brain, characterized by a loss of word meaning. Atrophy of the left anterior medial and inferior temporal gyri may be of particular importance as the anatomical substrate of semantic memory, either alone or as part of a functional network.

Clinical features: history and examination

- Progressive fluent aphasia with preserved syntax; impaired naming, loss of word meaning; with or without surface dyslexia and dysgraphia.
- Semantic memory impairment with relative preservation of episodic memory (*cf.* episodic memory disturbance in Alzheimer's disease); new learning (recognition memory) preserved early in disease.

Investigations and diagnosis *Neuropsychological profile.*

Imaging: volumetric MR brain imaging shows asymmetric atrophy (L > R) affecting all anterior temporal lobe structures (especially entorhinal cortex, amygdala, anterior medial and inferior temporal gyri, and anterior fusiform gyrus) with an anteroposterior gradient of atrophy (*cf.* Alzheimer's disease: symmetrical atrophy, especially medial temporal lobe structures including hippocampus; with no anteroposterior gradient).

Differential diagnosis

Alzheimer's disease.

Primary progressive aphasia (PPA): different language disorder.

Treatment and prognosis No specific treatment; no response to cholinesterase inhibitors.

> **References** Chan D, Fox NC, Scahill RI *et al.* Patterns of temporal lobe atrophy in semantic dementia and Alzheimer's disease. *Annals of Neurology* 2001: **49**: 433–442.
>
> Garrard P, Hodges JR. Semantic dementia: clinical, radiological and pathological perspectives. *Journal of Neurology* 2000; **247**: 409–422.
>
> **Other relevant entries** Alzheimer's disease; Dementia: an overview; Frontotemporal dementia; Memory; Pick's disease; Primary progressive aphasia.

■ Sengers syndrome

First described in 1975, this is a very rare syndrome, possibly inherited as an autosomal-recessive condition, comprising congenital cataracts, hypertrophic cardiomyopathy, mitochondrial myopathy, and lactic acidosis. Pathologically, muscle biopsy shows abnormal arrangement and loss of mitochondrial cristae, crystals within the mitochondrial matrix, and lipid and glycogen deposits. Despite this clinical and histopathological evidence for mitochondrial dysfunction, there is no evidence from biochemical studies for abnormal function of the mitochondrial respiratory chain. Evidence for deficiency of adenine nucleotide translocator 1 (ANT1), a transmembrane transport protein, in muscle tissue from Sengers syndrome patients has been presented, but there is no genetic mutation suggesting the deficiency results from transcriptional, translational, or post-translational events.

Reference Jordens EZ, Palmieri L, Huizing M *et al.* Adenine nucleotide translocator 1 deficiency associated with Sengers syndrome. *Annals of Neurology* 2002; **52**: 95–99.

Other relevant entry Mitochondrial disease: an overview.

■ Senior–Loken syndrome

An autosomal-recessive syndrome characterized by:

Pigmentary retinal degeneration, visual failure
Psychomotor retardation
Anaemia
Renal impairment leading to renal failure.

■ Sensorineural hearing loss – see Hearing loss: differential diagnosis

■ Sensory neuropathies – see Neuropathies: an overview

■ Sentinel headache – see Subarachnoid haemorrhage

■ Septic encephalopathy – see Encephalopathies: an overview

■ Septo-optic dysplasia
De Morsier's syndrome

Septo-optic dysplasia, or De Morsier's syndrome, is a developmental disorder of the nervous system characterized by bilateral optic nerve and chiasmal hypoplasia with reduced visual acuity, small optic discs, and an absent septum pellucidum. Hypothalamic–pituitary axis disturbances also occur, ranging from isolated growth hormone deficiency to panhypopituitarism.

▪ Serotonin syndrome

Serotonin syndrome refers to symptoms associated with a state of increasing central intrasynaptic serotonin release. The clinical features include:

- Mental status change, agitation.
- Myoclonus, shivering, tremor, incoordination, hyperreflexia.
- Diaphoresis, fever, diarrhoea.

Clinically it resembles the neuroleptic malignant syndrome, and some authors classify it as a form of "malignant catatonia".

Serotonin syndrome was initially reported in the context of an interaction between monoamine oxidase inhibitors and selective serotinin reuptake inhibitors (SSRIs), but may also occur with combinations of selegeline and SSRIs or tricyclic antidepressants. The syndrome is usually brief, but may persist despite drug withdrawal, mandating full supportive care.

References Bodner RA, Lynch T, Lewis L *et al*. Serotonin syndrome. *Neurology* 1995; **45**: 219–223.

Sternbach H. The serotonin syndrome. *American Journal of Psychiatry* 1991; **148**: 705–713.

Other relevant entries Catatonia; Neuroleptic malignant syndrome.

▪ Sex-linked forms of inherited metabolic diseases

Pathophysiology Mutations in genes located on the X-chromosome may be carried by heterozygous females who are usually asymptomatic, and manifested by hemizygous males. For X-linked-recessive disorders, female offspring of affected males have a 100% risk of being carriers, automatically inheriting their father's affected X-chromosome, whereas male offspring of affected males are normal, inheriting their X-chromosome from their mother. Sons of carrier females have a 50% chance of being affected; daughters of carrier females have a 50% chance of being carriers. X-linked recessive diseases thus show exclusively affected males in multiple generations with no male-to-male transmission.

Heterozygous female carriers may occasionally have clinical manifestations due to random inactivation of the X-chromosome (lyonization) resulting in mosaicism. Examples of such X-linked-recessive disorders include:

X-linked Adrenoleukodystrophy (X-ALD)
Becker and Duchenne-type muscular dystrophies (BMD, DMD)
Fragile X syndrome
Kennedy's syndrome (X-linked bulbospinal neuronopathy)
Lesch–Nyhan disease
Menkes' disease
Ornithine transcarbamoylase (OTC) deficiency
Pelizaeus–Merzbacher disease (PMD).

Clinical features/investigations and diagnosis/differential diagnosis/treatment and prognosis/references/other relevant entries See individual entries.

▓ Shaky legs syndrome – see Primary orthostatic tremor

▓ Shapiro syndrome

Shapiro syndrome is the rare concurrence of agenesis of the corpus callosum with a hypothalamic disturbance of thermoregulation producing a syndrome akin to spontaneous periodic hypothermia, with episodic hyperhidrosis and hypothermia. Early speculations that these phenomena might be epileptiform, so-called "diencephalic epilepsy", have not been confirmed: anti-epileptic medications are helpful in only a minority of cases. Clonidine has been reported to be beneficial.

References Noel P, Hubert JP, Ectors M *et al.* Agenesis of the corpus callosum associated with relapsing hypothermia. A clinico-pathological report. *Brain* 1973; **96**: 359–368.

Shapiro WR, Williams GH, Plum F. Spontaneous recurrent hypothermia accompanying agenesis of the corpus callosum. *Brain* 1969; **92**: 423–436.

Walker BR, Anderson JAM, Edwards CRW. Clonidine therapy for Shapiro's syndrome. *Quarterly Journal of Medicine* 1992; **82**: 235–245.

Other relevant entries Agenesis of the corpus callosum; Spontaneous periodic hypothermia.

▓ Sharp's syndrome – see Mixed connective tissue disease

▓ Sheehan's syndrome

Sheehan's syndrome is ischaemic necrosis of the pituitary gland, occurring most often in the postpartum period, which may result in panhypopituitarism.

Reference Kovacs K. Sheehan syndrome. *Lancet* 2003; **361**: 520–522.

Other relevant entry Pituitary disease and apoplexy.

▓ Shingles – see Herpes zoster and postherpetic neuralgia; Varicella zoster virus and the nervous system

▓ Short-lasting unilateral neuralgiform headache with conjunctival injection and tearing – see SUNCT syndrome

▓ Shoulder–hand syndrome

Pain in the shoulder and arm with secondary vasomotor changes in the hand may occur in an immobile arm following a stroke or myocardial infarction, with osteoporosis and atrophy of cutaneous and subcutaneous tissues (of Sudeck type). This condition probably falls within the rubric of complex regional pain syndromes.

Other relevant entry Complex regional pain syndromes.

▓ Shy–Drager syndrome – see Multiple system atrophy; Parkinsonian syndromes, parkinsonism

▓ Sialidoses: an overview

A number of conditions may be characterized as sialidoses or mucolipidoses, all with excess tissue accumulation of glycoproteins, glycolipids and oligosaccharides containing sialic acid and excess urinary excretion of sialo-oligosaccharides. Lysosomal dysfunction is common to all these disorders.

- Sialidoses with isolated deficiency of α-neuraminidase/sialidase:
    - Sialidosis (*q.v.*):
        - congenital
        - severe infantile
        - nephrosialidosis
        - mucolipidosis type I
        - cherry-red spot-myoclonus syndrome.
- Sialidoses with combined deficiency of α-neuraminidase/sialidase and β-galactosidase:
    - Galactosialidosis:
        - infantile (GM1-gangliosidosis phenotype)
        - Goldberg syndrome
    - Others:
        - Salla disease
        - Fucosidosis
        - Mannosidosis
        - Aspartylglycosaminuria
        - Mucolipidoses (types II–IV).

Reference Mancini GMS, Verheijen FW, Beerens CMT *et al*. Sialic acid storage disorders: observations on clinical and biochemical variation. *Developmental Neuroscience* 1991; **13**: 327–330.

Other relevant entries Aspartylglycosaminuria; Fucosidosis; Lysosomal-storage diseases: an overview; Mannosidosis; Mucolipidoses; Salla disease; Sialidosis.

▓ Sialidosis

α-neuraminidase deficiency ● Mucolipidosis type I (ML type I)

Pathophysiology Sialidosis is related to deficiency in lysosomal acid α-neuraminidase (or N-acetyl neuraminidase, sialidase), related to mutations in the sialidase gene on chromosome 6p, with resulting excretion of large quantities of sialyl oligosaccharides. The clinical syndromes are heterogeneous, encompassing cortical myoclonus, visual loss, and cognitive features.

Clinical features: history and examination

- Type I (cherry-red spot–myoclonus syndrome):
    Autosomal-recessive disorder due to isolated α-neuraminidase deficiency.
    Onset in late childhood, adolescence.
    Progressive visual loss, polymyoclonus, seizures (tonic–clonic), macular cherry red spot, optic atrophy, intellectual deterioration, $+/-$ cerebellar ataxia, painful peripheral neuropathy. No dysmorphism.
- Type II:
    Congenital, infantile, and juvenile forms recognized.
    Autosomal-recessive congenital form; often stillborn.
    Early infantile; hepatosplenomegaly.
    Dysmorphism: depressed nasal bridge.
    Macular cherry red spot.
    Severe psychomotor retardation.
    Myoclonus, seizures with longer survival.
    $+/-$ nephrosialidosis (secondary renal dysfunction, proteinuria).
    Angiokeratoma corporis diffusum may be prominent.

Investigations and diagnosis

- Types I and II:
    Urine: thin layer chromatography shows increased sialic acid-containing oligosaccharides.
    α-neuraminidase enzyme assay in fibroblasts, leukocytes.
    Bone marrow: foamy histiocytes.
- Type I:
    Imaging: cerebral/cerebellar atrophy.
    Blood film: vacuolated lymphocytes.

Differential diagnosis

- Type I:
    Myoclonic epilepsy with ragged red fibres (MERRF).
    Unverricht–Lundborg syndrome.
    Lafora body disease.
    Lipofuscinosis (neuronal ceroid lipofuscinosis type II).
    Late-onset GM2 gangliosidosis.
    Dentatorubral-pallidoluysian atrophy (DRPLA).
    Benign essential familial myoclonus.
    Andermann syndrome: action-myoclonus–renal failure syndrome.
- Type II:
    GM1 gangliosidosis.
    Hurler syndrome: similar dysmorphism, but no corneal clouding.
    Angiokeratoma corporis diffusum: Fabry's disease, fucosidosis.

Treatment and prognosis No specific treatment available; prenatal diagnosis possible. Symptomatic treatment for myoclonus, seizures. Early infantile form usually leads to death in the 2nd year.

> **Reference** Rapin I, Goldfischer S, Katzman R *et al*. The cherry-red spot–myoclonus syndrome. *Annals of Neurology* 1978; **3**: 234–242.

> **Other relevant entries** Andermann syndrome (2); Dentatorubral-pallidoluysian atrophy; Gangliosidoses: an overview; Lafora body disease; Lysosomal-storage diseases: an overview; Mitochondrial disease: an overview; Mucolipidoses; Myoclonus; Neuronal ceroid lipofuscinosis; Sialidoses: an overview; Unverricht–Lundborg syndrome.

Sicca syndrome – see Sjögren's syndrome

Sickle-cell disease

Stroke syndromes and epileptic seizures may complicate this haemoglobinopathy which may lead to occlusion of small intracerebral vessels.

> **Reference** Prengler M, Pavlakis SG, Prohovnik I *et al*. Sickle cell diseae: the neurological complications. *Annals of Neurology* 2002; **51**: 543–552.

> **Other relevant entry** Cerebrovascular disease: arterial.

Siderosis – see Superficial siderosis of the central nervous system

Siebenmann's syndrome – see Jugular foramen syndrome

Siemerling–Creutzfeldt disease – see Adrenoleukodystrophy

Silver–Russell syndrome

Russell–Silver syndrome

Pathophysiology A developmental syndrome characterized by a disproportionately large head, facial dysmorphism and sometimes hemiatrophy, short stature, with or without learning disability. There is considerable phenotypic variability. Raised urinary gonadotrophins, sometimes with precocious puberty, may aid diagnosis.

Clinical features: history and examination

- Intrauterine growth retardation.
- Normal head circumference, short stature, head seems disproportionately large ("pseudohydrocephalus"); lean body habitus; hemiatrophy.

- Facial dysmorphism, $+/-$ asymmetry; micrognathia, high hair line.
- High squeaky voice, heavy sweating.
- Generalized camptodactyly, distal arthrogryposis.
- Hypospadias, inguinal hernia.
- Learning disability.
- $+/-$ precocious puberty.

Investigations and diagnosis Raised urinary gonadotrophins.

Maternal uniparental disomy of chromosome 7 has been reported in some cases.

Differential diagnosis Parry–Romberg syndrome.

Rubinstein–Taybi syndrome.

Treatment and prognosis The prognosis is generally favourable. Growth hormone has been used to treat the short stature.

> **Reference** Patton MA. Russell–Silver syndrome. *Journal of Medical Genetics* 1988; **25**: 557–560.

> **Other relevant entries** Dwarfism; Hydrocephalus; Parry–Romberg syndrome; Rubinstein–Taybi syndrome.

◼ Simmonds syndrome – see Pituitary disease and apoplexy

◼ Sinus thrombosis – see Cerebrovascular disease: venous

◼ Sjögren's syndrome

Pathophysiology An autoimmune disorder of exocrine glands, occurring either as a primary disorder or secondary to another connective tissue disorder (e.g. rheumatoid arthritis); it more often affects women than men. Neurological complications may be both peripheral and central. Their pathogenesis is uncertain; small vessel vasculitis may be relevant in some cases.

Clinical features: history and examination
- Non-neurological
    Sicca syndrome: salivary glands (xerostomia), lacrimal glands (xerophthalmia): 50%
    Features of connective tissue disease (e.g. rheumatoid arthritis)
    Vasculitic skin rash
    Interstitial nephritis
    Lymphadenopathy
    Interstitial pneumonitis (rare).
- Neurological
    Peripheral (10–30%):
        distal symmetrical sensory neuropathy
        sensorimotor neuropathy

polyradiculopathy

mononeuropathy multiplex

trigeminal sensory neuropathy

sensory ataxic neuronopathy or ganglionopathy (rare, but pathognomonic).

Central:

aseptic meningitis, meningoencephalitis, encephalopathy

strokes, transient ischaemic attack (TIA); focal neurological deficits (hemisphere, brainstem)

seizures

acute transverse myelitis/chronic myelopathy

psychiatric disturbance

dementia (rare)

parkinsonism (rare)

dystonia (rare)

MS-like syndrome: optic neuropathy, cerebellar ataxia, internuclear ophthalmoplegia (significance debated).

Investigations and diagnosis *Bloods*: positive ANA (speckled), anti-Ro (SSA), anti-La (SSB) (75–80%).

Schirmer's test of tear production: (<5 mm wetness in 5 minutes).

Tissue: Salivary gland (lip) biopsy; destruction/fibrosis of glandular tissue with lymphocytic infiltrate.

With neurological features, the following investigations may be indicated:

Neurophysiology: EMG/NCS: if peripheral nerve disease.

Imaging: MRI brain: multifocal white matter lesions, mostly subcortical.

CSF: may show raised protein, white cell count, pressure, and oligoclonal bands in encephalopathy.

Differential diagnosis Broad: other causes of peripheral neuropathy, stroke; MS.

Treatment and prognosis Immunosuppression: prednisolone +/− cyclophosphamide. No controlled trials.

References Alexander E. Central nervous system disease in Sjögren's syndrome. New insights into immunopathogenesis. *Rheumatic Diseases Clinics of North America* 1992; **18**: 637–672.

Rosenbaum R. Neuromuscular complications of connective tissue disease. *Muscle and Nerve* 2001; **24**: 154–169.

Other relevant entries Collagen vascular disorders and the nervous system: an overview; Neuropathies: an overview; Rheumatoid arthritis; Systemic lupus erythematosus and the nervous system; Vasculitis.

■ Sjögren–Larsson syndrome

Pathophysiology A rare autosomal-recessive condition with infantile onset of neurological and dermatological features (hence a neurocutaneous syndrome), due to mutations in the gene for fatty aldehyde dehydrogenase (FALDH) which oxidizes long-chain aliphatic aldehydes to fatty acids. Accumulation of lipids may contribute to the pathogenesis of disease features. It may also be classified with the hereditary spastic parapareses (HSP).

Clinical features: history and examination
- Neurological:
  - Mental retardation
  - Spasticity with hyperreflexia: usually diplegia but sometimes tetraplegia
  - Seizures (40%)
  - Pseudobulbar dysarthria
  - Delayed speech
  - Glistening white dots surrounding the macula (pathognomonic) +/− reduced visual acuity.
- Dermatological:
  - Generalized ichthyosis with pruritus.

Investigations and diagnosis
Ophthalmoscopy: for macular white dots.
Imaging: brain MRI shows dysmyelination or delayed myelination.
Enzyme activity: cultured skin fibroblasts (=diagnostic test).

Differential diagnosis Additional features generally make distinction from other types of HSP.

Treatment and prognosis No specific treatment. Most affected individuals survive to adulthood.

References Sjögren T, Larsson T. Oligophrenia in combination with congenital ichthyosis and spastic disorders. *Acta Psychiatrica Neurologica Scandinavica* 1957; **32(suppl 113)**: 1–113.

Van Domburg PHMF, Willemsen MAAP, Rotteveel JJ *et al*. Sjögren–Larsson syndrome: clinical and MRI/MRS findings in FALDH-deficient patients. *Neurology* 1999; **52**: 1345–1352.

Other relevant entries Hereditary spastic paraparesis; Phakomatosis.

■ Skew deviation – see Hertwig–Magendie syndrome

■ Sleep apnoea syndromes

Sleep apnoea refers to a temporary cessation or absence of breathing during sleep. Sleep apnoea syndromes may be broadly divided into three categories, obstructive, central and mixed:
- *Obstructive*: cessation of airflow through nose and mouth with persistence of respiratory effort, diaphragmatic and intercostal muscle activity. Upper airway resistance may lead to paradoxical breathing, with thorax and abdomen

moving in opposite directions. The obstructive pattern may be seen in obstructive sleep apnoea syndrome (OSAS; *q.v.*) or sleep apnoea/hypopnoea syndrome (SAHS), and in upper airway resistance syndrome (UARS). Partial obstruction of nocturnal breathing, with or without snoring, may also occur as a consequence of obesity or neuromuscular disorder affecting pharyngeal muscles.

- *Central*: cessation of airflow through nose and mouth with no respiratory effort, diaphragmatic and intercostal muscle activity is absent. Central sleep apnoea (CSA) may occur with lower brainstem lesions (infarction, poliomyelitis, syringobulbia) with loss of automatic breathing, especially during sleep (primary hypoventilation, Ondine's curse). Cheyne–Stokes breathing, a waxing and waning depth of respiration, is a special type of central apnoea, characterized by a crescendo–decrescendo sequence separated by central apnoeas; it may be seen with neurological disorders and congestive heart failure.

- *Mixed*: initial cessation of airflow with no respiratory effort (i.e. central apnoea) is followed by a period of upper airway obstructive sleep apnoea.

Other relevant entries Obstructive sleep apnoea syndrome; Sleep disorders: an overview.

■ Sleep apnoea/hypopnoea syndrome – see Obstructive sleep apnoea syndrome

■ Sleep disorders: an overview

Pathophysiology Sleep disorders may be broadly classified into:

Insomnias: inability to sleep despite adequate opportunity
Parasomnias (*q.v.*)
Hypersomnias: excessive daytime somnolence (EDS).

The *International Classification of Sleep Disorders* (ICSD), the definitive work for sleep specialists, lists 84 disorders in all.

Clinical features: history and examination *Insomnia may be*:

- Primary: no other medical or psychiatric explanation for sleep disorder.
- Secondary: to pain, depression, other medical condition (e.g. restless legs syndrome; fatal familial insomnia).
  Some individuals feel that they do not get enough sleep yet polysomnographic studies fail to confirm this ("pseudo-insomnia").

EDS, hypersomnia may be caused by:

- Sleep apnoea syndromes:
  - Obstructive sleep apnoea syndrome (OSAS): as a consequence of obesity or neuromuscular disorder affecting pharyngeal muscles, nocturnal breathing is

partially obstructed leading to snoring and, in extremes, cessation of breathing with increasing respiratory efforts and brief arousals from sleep. These patients may complain of early morning headache, resolving as the day progresses; on examination they may have bounding pulses (hyperdynamic circulation) and asterixis. There may be clinical evidence of an underlying neurological disorder (e.g. motor neurone disease), obesity, and/or a narrow anteroposterior pharyngeal diameter; high alcohol intake may contribute to the syndrome. Heart failure may develop.

- Central sleep apnoea (CSA): associated with lower brainstem lesions (infarction, poliomyelitis, syringobulbia) with loss of automatic breathing, especially during sleep (primary hypoventilation, Ondine's curse).
- Narcolepsy, narcoleptic syndrome
- Nocturnal hypoventilation, for example as a consequence of neuromuscular disorders (poliomyelitis, Duchenne muscular dystrophy, motor neurone disease, dystrophia myotonica) or chest wall anomalies (kyphoscoliosis).
- Periodic hypersomnia: Kleine–Levin syndrome.
- Trypanosomiasis (African sleeping sickness).
- Encephalitis lethargica (Von Economo's disease).
- Idiopathic hypersomnia [essential central nervous system (CNS) hypersomnolence].

See individual entries for further details.

Investigations and diagnosis For insomnia, the history may be the most important route to diagnosis, particularly probing for evidence of depression.

Polysomnographic sleep studies (video, pulse oximetry, ECG) may be helpful in characterizing the cause of hypersomnolence. In obstructive sleep apnoea syndrome, snoring and repeated apnoeic episodes with oxygen desaturation and sinus bradycardia may be seen. Haematocrit may be raised.

Differential diagnosis Need to differentiate somnolence from fatigue, a major symptom in postviral fatigue syndromes, multiple sclerosis.

Treatment and prognosis Referral to designated Sleep Centre, or a physician with a special interest in sleep disorders, is appropriate.

Advice on appropriate "sleep hygiene" may assist with primary insomnia; specific treatment of underlying causes is appropriate for secondary insomnia.

Pharmacotherapy may be helpful in narcolepsy.

Treat any underlying neurological disorder where possible.

Nocturnal intermittent positive-pressure ventilation (NIPPV) is helpful in OSAS. Sometimes pharyngeal surgery to enlarge the diameter, $+/-$ adenotonsillectomy, may be appropriate.

Reduce alcohol intake, lose weight.

Avoid sedative drugs.

References Aldrich MS. *Sleep Medicine*. Oxford: OUP, 1999.

Chadwick D. Sleep and sleep disorders. In: Donaghy M (ed.). *Brain's Diseases of the Nervous System* (11th edition). Oxford: OUP, 2001: 711–716.

Chokroverty S. Sleep disorders. In: Bradley WG, Daroff RB, Fenichel GM, Marsden CD (eds). *Neurology in Clinical Practice* (3rd edition). Boston: Butterworth-Heinemann, 2000: 1781–1827.

Douglas NJ. *Clinicians' Guide to Sleep Medicine*. London: Arnold, 2002.

International Classification of Sleep Disorders (revised). Diagnostic and Coding Manual. Rochester: American Sleep Disorders Association, 1997.

Kryger MH, Roth T, Dement WC. *Principles and Practice of Sleep Medicine* (3rd edition). London: WB Saunders, 2000.

Shneerson JM. *Handbook of Sleep Medicine*. Oxford: Blackwell Science, 2000.

Other relevant entries Encephalitis lethargica; Fatal familial insomnia; Hypothalamic disease: an overview; Kleine–Levin syndrome; Motor neurone disease; Narcolepsy, narcoleptic syndrome; Obstructive sleep apnoea syndrome; Parasomnias; Pickwickian syndrome; Restless legs syndrome; Sleep apnoea syndromes; Trypanosomiasis; Williams syndrome.

Sleep paralysis – see Narcolepsy, narcoleptic syndrome

Sleeping sickness – see Trypanosomiasis

Slow channel syndrome – see Myasthenia gravis

Sluder's neuralgia – see Sphenopalatine (ganglion) neuralgia

Sly disease

Mucopolysaccharidosis type VII (MPS VII)

Deficiency of β-glucuronidase, transmitted as an autosomal-recessive trait linked to chromosome 7q21.1–q22, leads to excess dermatan sulphate and heparan sulphate in the urine. Clinically there is a variable phenotype, ranging from mild to complete Hurler phenotype (corneal clouding, hepatosplenomegaly, skeletal anomalies).

Other relevant entries Hurler's disease; Mucopolysaccharidoses.

Small's disease

Pathophysiology An inherited, probably autosomal-recessive, condition characterized by hearing loss and retinal disease.

Clinical features: history and examination

- Hearing deficit: moderate to severe.
- Visual impairment: tortuous retinal vessels, telangiectasias, retinal detachment, exudative retinitis.
- Low IQ.

- Progressive muscle weakness of face, limbs, trunk.
- No microphthalmia (*cf.* Norrie's disease).

Investigations and diagnosis Family history for similar conditions.

Differential diagnosis Norrie's disease.

Treatment and prognosis No specific treatment.

> **Reference** Small RG. Coats' disease and muscular dystrophy. *Transactions of the American Academy of Ophthalmology and Otolaryngology* 1968; **72**: 225–231.

> **Other relevant entries** Coats' disease; Hearing loss: differential diagnosis; Norrie disease.

■ Smith–Lemli–Opitz syndrome

Pathophysiology A common, autosomal-recessive, malformative syndrome involving many systems including the brain, related to a defect in 7-dehydrocholesterol Δ^7 reductase, which catalyses the conversion of 7-dehydrocholesterol to cholesterol (the last reaction in the cholesterol synthesis pathway), resulting in deficiency of cholesterol. Hence this may be viewed as a cholesterol-storage disease.

Clinical features: history and examination
- Neurological:
    Microcephaly; holoprosencephaly
    Mental retardation
    Behavioural problems
    Paraparesis, hyperreflexia, Babinski sign.
- Morphological:
    Facial: broad nasal tip, anteverted nares, hypertelorism, ptosis, low set ears, epicanthal folds.
    Limbs: syndactyly of second and third toes (commonest malformation), short stature, dislocated hips.
    Viscera: cardiac malformations, renal dysplasia, pyloric stenosis, Hirschsprung's disease.

Investigations and diagnosis *Bloods*: Cholesterol: low in plasma; elevated 7-dehydrocholesterol; normal amino acids, immunoglobulins, karyotype.
Tissue: Deficient 7-dehydrocholesterol Δ^7 reductase activity in fibroblasts.
Imaging: CT/MRI: may show holoprosencephaly.

Differential diagnosis Characteristic dysmorphology.
Low plasma cholesterol is also a feature in Tangier disease, cerebrotendinous xanthomatosis.

Treatment and prognosis High cholesterol diet.

> **Reference** Cunniff C, Kratz LE, Moser A *et al*. Clinical and biochemical spectrum of patients with RSH/Smith–Lemli–Opitz syndrome and abnormal cholesterol metabolism. *American Journal of Medical Genetics* 1997; **68**: 263–269.

> **Other relevant entries** Cerebrotendinous xanthomatosis; Holoprosencephaly; Niemann-Pick disease; Tangier disease; Wolman's disease.

■ Smith's disease – see Acid-maltase deficiency; Glycogen-storage disorders: an overview

■ Sneddon's syndrome

Pathophysiology A non-inflammatory thrombo-occlusive arteriolar vasculopathy, affecting skin and brain and often (but not always) associated with antiphospholipid antibodies. The disorder occurs primarily in young patients, with a female preponderance.

Clinical features: history and examination
- Livedo reticularis.
- Recurrent strokes in the absence of obvious risk factors.
- Focal neurological signs.
- Seizures: more common in antibody positive patients.
- Cognitive decline.
- Thrombocytopenia.
- Mitral regurgitation.

Investigations and diagnosis *Bloods*: antiphospholipid antibodies, thrombocytopenia. *Imaging*: brain CT/MRI for ischaemic infarcts in middle cerebral artery territory. *Neurophysiology*: EEG: non-specific changes. *Neuropsychology*.

Differential diagnosis Skin lesions usually make the diagnosis obvious. Other vasculopathies and vasculitides must be considered, for example collagen vascular diseases (systemic lupus erythematosus, Sjögren's syndrome), cerebral vasculitis, isolated central nervous system (CNS) angiitis, Susac's syndrome, fibromuscular dysplasia.

Treatment and prognosis Anticoagulation is recommended if antiphospholipid antibodies are present. Aspirin and immunosuppressive therapy have been tried but their place remains to be defined; they may be of more use in antibody-negative patients. Existing cognitive impairment does not reverse; the aim is to prevent further decline.

> **Reference** Frances C, Papo T, Wechsler B, Laporte JL, Biousse V, Piette JC. Sneddon syndrome with or without antiphospholipid antibodies: a comparative study in 46 patients. *Medicine (Baltimore)* 1999; **78**: 209–219.

> **Other relevant entries** Antiphospholipid (antibody) syndrome; Cerebrovascular disease: arterial; Vascular dementia

■ Solomon's syndrome – see Hypnic headache

■ Solvent exposure

Exposure to organic solvents, either accidentally or recreationally (e.g. glue sniffing), may occasionally be associated with neurological problems, especially if exposure is acute and occurs in poorly ventilated locations:
- Acute cerebellar ataxia, for example with toluene, carbon tetrachloride.
- Psychosis, cognitive impairment, pyramidal signs: toluene.

- Encephalopathy + behavioural disturbances with acute inhalation of carbon disulphide; chronic exposure may lead to extrapyramidal signs, retinopathy, peripheral neuropathy.
- Neuropathy, predominantly motor +/− dysautonomia with acute use of/exposure to hexacarbon solvents; with long-term exposure a chronic demyelinating sensori-motor neuropathy develops.

Whether low level chronic exposure to solvents over prolonged periods leads to adverse effects, such as "painter's encephalopathy", is less certain. A review of 40 studies found no reliable conclusions as to brain atrophy and deficits in neurophysiological studies.

> **Reference** Ridgway P, Nixon TE, Leach JP. Occupational exposure to organic solvents and long-term nervous system damage detectable by brain imaging, neurophysiology or histopathology. *Food and Chemical Toxicology* 2003; **41**: 153–187.

■ Somatization disorder – see Briquet syndrome; Somatoform disorders

■ Somatoform disorders

Classifications of mental disorders recognize a number of somatoform disorders which may often be seen in neurological clinics. Many of these patients would in the past have been given a label of hysteria (or conversion hysteria) but this is now seldom helpful, at least in part because of the pejorative overtones of this term.

The somatoform disorders include:
- Somatization disorder, Briquet's syndrome
  Multiple physical complaints, onset before age 30, usually female.
- Conversion disorder
  One or more symptoms affecting motor or sensory function, not fully explicable by a medical condition (e.g. monosymptomatic pseudoparalysis).
- Hypochondriasis
  Preoccupation with, or fear of, having a serious disease in spite of previous (negative) investigations and reassurance.
- Body dysmorphic disorder
  Preoccupation with an imagined defect in appearance (may also be classified amongst the obsessive–compulsive disorders).
- Pain disorder
  Pain is predominant symptom, and psychological factors are judged to have an important role in pathogenesis and maintenance.

Diagnosis is often difficult. Many patients have been repeatedly investigated and remain unreassured despite normal findings. Clues to the diagnosis include discrepancy between extent of symptoms and paucity or absence of findings on neurological examination, hemianaesthesia (more often on the left) with clear demarcation at the midline, patches of anaesthesia.

Identification of present or past psychopathology, including personality disorder and previous episodes of conversion, may also assist in diagnosis. Management is often very difficult.

Previous reports of a high rate of organic diagnoses emerging in patients previously labelled "hysterical" have not been borne out by more recent studies; psychiatric co-morbidity, either psychiatric disease or personality disorder, was, however, high.

Reference Crimlisk HL, Bhatia K, Cope H, David A, Marsden CD, Ron MA. Slater revisited: 6 year follow up study of patients with medically unexplained motor symptoms. *British Medical Journal* 1998; **316**: 582–586.

Other relevant entries Obsessive–compulsive disorder; Psychiatric disorders and neurological disease.

Somnambulism – see Parasomnias

Somniloquy – see Parasomnias

Sotos syndrome
Cerebral gigantism

This rare growth disorder is characterized by macrocephaly, somatic overgrowth, and psychomotor delay. It has been linked to chromosome 5q35 and study of sporadic cases suggests that haploinsufficiency of the NSD1 gene is the cause.

Reference Kurotaki N, Imaizumi K, Harada N *et al*. Haploinsufficiency of NSD1 causes Sotos syndrome. *Nature Genetics* 2002; **30**: 365–366.

Other relevant entry Gigantism.

Souques disease – see Camptocormia

Spanish toxic oil syndrome – see Eosinophilia–myalgia syndrome

Sparganosis

Infection with the larval tapeworm of the genus *Spirometra*, from drinking contaminated water or eating infected fish or snakes, is the cause of sparganosis, a disease most often seen in the east of Asia and Africa. The mobile worm causes subcutaneous swellings on chest and legs, and may penetrate the central nervous system (CNS) to cause seizures or focal signs (cysts, infarcts). Serial brain imaging may reveal parasite mobility. Investigations reveal eosinophilia and serological evidence of infection, but histology is required for definitive diagnosis. Treatment is by excision; anti-helminthic medications are not effective.

Other relevant entries Diphyllobothriasis; Helminthic diseases.

■ Spasmodic dysphonia

Spasmodic dysphonia is a dystonia of the vocal cords, of which two types are described:

- Adductor type: causing speech to sound strangled, strained, or fading away to nothing, accompanied by a complaint of tightness in the throat.
- Abductor type: if the cords are abducted, a breathy whispering speech results, sometimes likened to that of Marilyn Monroe.

There may often be a superimposed tremulous component.

Men and women are equally affected, usually in the 30–50-year-age range.

Spasmodic dysphonia may be treated with botulinum toxin injections into the vocal cords under direct visualization, by a practitioner experienced with these injections.

Other relevant entries Aphonia; Botulinum toxin therapy; Dystonia: an overview.

■ Spasmodic torticollis
Cervical dystonia • Nuchal dystonia • Wryneck

Pathophysiology Spasmodic torticollis is a focal dystonic syndrome which is usually idiopathic but may follow neck or head trauma, and occasionally has been associated with brainstem and basal ganglia lesions. It typically presents between the ages of 30–50 years of age and there is a female preponderance. In about one-third of patients dystonia spreads to other sites (e.g. face, arm, as a segmental dystonia) and in another third the disease spontaneously remits, usually in the first 5 years of the illness, although this is often transient.

Clinical features: history and examination

- In spasmodic torticollis, the head is twisted around one or several planes of the neck, often with an element of jerking +/− "no–no" head tremor and shoulder elevation, due to involuntary contraction of neck muscles, most usually sternocleido-mastoid, trapezius, and splenius capitis, although other muscles can be involved in more complex cases, such as levator scapulae.
- Patients sometimes discover that the dystonic movements may be overcome by a "sensory trick" or *geste antagoniste* such as placing a finger lightly on the face or back of the neck.
- There may be associated dystonic features elsewhere, as in a cranial segmental dystonia such as Meige's syndrome.

Investigations and diagnosis Diagnosis is clinical, no specific investigations required.

Differential diagnosis Unlikely to be mistaken; acute dystonic reactions may produce a similar picture.

Treatment and prognosis Treatment is with botulinum toxin, giving relief in *ca.* 80% of cases, although repeated injections, usually every 3 months, are required indefinitely.

Other treatments that have been tried include ventral rhizotomy of upper cervical roots and section of the spinal accessory nerve with denervation of the sternocleido-mastoid. Bilateral thalamotomy has been tried but surgical treatment has no benefit over botulinum toxin injections, and may be associated with significant side-effects.

Uncontrolled movements may result in premature degenerative disease of the cervical spine which may become clinically apparent, for example compressive myelopathy/radiculopathy from disc disease.

Reference Dauer WT, Burke RE, Greene P, Fahn S. Current concepts on the clinical features, aetiology and management of idiopathic cervical dystonia. *Brain* 1998; **121**: 547–560.

Other relevant entries Botulinum toxin therapy; Drug-induced movement disorders; Dystonia: an overview.

▓ Spasmus nutans

Spasmus nutans is a childhood syndrome comprising head nodding, pendular nystagmus, and torticollis, with onset usually between 4 and 12 months. The syndrome is usually benign, remitting after a few months or 2–3 years, but occasionally such movements reflect a chiasmal or third ventricular tumour. The differential diagnosis encompasses Pelizaeus–Merzbacher disease and the bobble head doll syndrome.

Other relevant entries Bobble head doll syndrome; Pelizaeus–Merzbacher disease.

▓ Spatz–Lindenberg disease – see Von Winiwarter–Buerger's disease

▓ Sphenopalatine (ganglion) neuralgia
Greater superficial petrosal neuralgia • Lower-half headache • Sluder's neuralgia • (Vail's) vidian neuralgia.

These various terms have been used to describe recurrent self-limited (2–4 hours) unilateral attacks of pain in the head and face, variously involving the orbit, mouth, nose, and posterior mastoid area. In addition to pain, there may be vasomotor activity, ipsilateral nasal discharge, eye irritation, and lacrimation.

The pain is thought to be of "vascular" origin; certainly there are similarities with cluster headache. Various treatments have been tried (no controlled trials), including injection of the sphenopalatine ganglion (which has also been reported to improve some cases of trigeminal neuralgia), for example with phenol; acupuncture; and stereotactic radiosurgery.

Other relevant entries Cluster headache; Facial pain: differential diagnosis; Migraine; Trigeminal neuralgia.

■ Sphingomyelinase deficiency, sphingomyelinoses – see Niemann–Pick disease

■ Spielmeyer–Sjögren disease – see Neuronal ceroid lipofuscinosis

■ Spielmeyer–Vogt–Batten disease – see Neuronal ceroid lipofuscinosis

■ Spinal atrophic paralysis – see Electrical injuries and the nervous system

■ Spina bifida
Spinal dysraphism

Pathophysiology Incomplete closure of the caudal neural tube during development may produce various deformities, ranging from the mild and entirely incidental spina bifida occulta, to the severe, with exposure of neural tissue to the surface (rachischisis). These defects may be associated with abnormal neurological function of the lower limbs, with or without sphincter involvement. Associated tethering of the spinal cord (*q.v.*) may lead to development of neurological problems in later life. Spina bifida may be a teratogenic consequence of drug therapy (e.g. certain anti-epileptic drugs).

Clinical features: history and examination
- Open spinal dysraphism (OSD)
    - Rachischisis: exposure of neural tissue to surface; evident at birth; severe disability.
    - Meningomyelocoele: commonest variant; sac of dura, arachnoid and neural tissue, evident at birth; severe disability likely.
    - Meningocoele: protruding sac of dura and arachnoid only; seldom neurological consequences.
    - All OSD associated with Chiari II malformation.
- Closed spinal dysraphism (CSD) = skin covered:
    - With spinal mass: lipoma, dural defect, meningocoele.
    - Without spinal mass:
        - Simple: tight filum terminale, intradural lipoma.

Spina bifida occulta: incomplete closure of the vertebral laminae; may be evident only as dimpling of the skin or a hairy patch over the lumbar spine, or only seen radiologically. May be asymptomatic or may present with progressive lower limb sensorimotor and sphincter dysfunction in later life due to cord tethering.

Complex: split cord malformation (diastematomyelia); caudal regression.

Investigations and diagnosis Imaging to assess extent of deformity may help in planning surgery.

Differential diagnosis Severe degrees of dysraphism are unlikely to be mistaken, but the progressive paraparesis of cord tethering has a broad differential, including structural and inflammatory disease of the cord.

Treatment and prognosis Surgical intervention for more severe deficits; cord tethering seldom amenable to surgery. Symptomatic treatment for deficits.

> **Reference** Tortori-Donati P, Rossi A, Cama A. Spinal dysraphism: a review of neuroradiological features with embryological correlations and proposal for a new classification. *Neuroradiology* 2000; **42**: 471–491.

> **Other relevant entries** Chiari malformations; Diastematomyelia; Paraparesis: acute management and differential diagnosis; Tethered cord syndrome.

▉ Spinal cord disease: an overview

Pathophysiology Spinal cord diseases may produce:

- Myelopathy (*q.v.*) which may be intramedullary or extramedullary; the latter may be intradural or extradural in origin. Although clinical features may give pointers to these subtypes, imaging is more certain in defining the locus of pathology. Certain pathologies have a predilection for certain parts of the cord, which may help in defining the cause of a myelopathy, along with the temporal pattern of disease.
- $+/-$ segmental radiculopathy: especially with extradural lesions.

Common causes of spinal cord disease and dysfunction include:

Structural anomalies: Spina bifida, syringomyelia.

Trauma.

Compression: spondylotic myelopathy, extradural tumours, atlanto-axial compression in rheumatoid arthritis.

Inflammation: demyelination, myelitis, arachnoiditis.

Neoplasia: intramedullary tumours (primary, metastatic); extramedullary tumours.

Vascular disease: anterior spinal artery occlusion, spinal arteriovenous malformation, angioma.

Metabolic: subacute combined degeneration of the cord (vitamin B_{12} deficiency).

Infection: syphilis, HIV-related vacuolar myelopathy.

Radiation myelopathy.

Neurodegeneration: spinocerebellar ataxias.

Clinical features: history and examination See Myelopathy, individual disease entries.

Investigations and diagnosis *Imaging* of the cord, preferably with MRI, is the most reliable way of localizing spinal cord disease and may give clues to diagnosis (tumour, inflammation, compression).

CSF examination: may also be indicated.

See individual entries for specific investigations.

Differential diagnosis Very occasionally, compressive spinal cord disease may be mimicked by Guillain–Barré syndrome.

Treatment and prognosis See individual entries.

> **Reference** Critchley E, Eisen A. *Diseases of the Spinal Cord.* London: Springer-Verlag, 1992.

> **Other relevant entries** Arachnoiditis; Brown–Séquard syndrome; Cauda equina syndrome and conus medullaris disease; Cerebellar disease: an overview; Cervical cord and root disease; Chemotherapy and radiotherapy and the nervous system; HIV/AIDS and the nervous system; Multiple sclerosis; Myelitis; Myelopathy: an overview; Paraparesis: acute management and differential diagnosis; Rheumatoid arthritis; Spina bifida; Spinal cord trauma; Spinal cord vascular diseases; Syringomyelia and syringobulbia; Tethered cord syndrome; Tumours: an overview; Vitamin B_{12} deficiency.

■ Spinal cord trauma

Pathophysiology Traumatic injury to the spinal cord is most likely to occur in the cervical and upper lumbar regions.

Clinical features: history and examination Acutely there may be "spinal shock", a flaccid quadriparesis. With time the signs may evolve, the clinical features defining the level of the lesion, and whether it is complete or incomplete:

- Sensorimotor deficit: often flaccid areflexic quadriplegia if above C6; the pattern varies with the nature of the injury, for example complete transection, anterior cord injury, central cord contusion (upper limbs especially affected), Brown–Séquard syndrome (hemisection), cauda equina syndrome.
- Sphincter dysfunction: often flaccid bladder; anal reflex should be tested.
- Respiratory dysfunction; likely if C3–C5 lesion.

Investigations and diagnosis

Monitor ventilation: supplementary oxygen, intubation and mechanical ventilation if necessary.

Monitor circulation: appropriate support if hypotension, bradycardia.

Collar to splint cervical spine if instability suspected.

High index of suspicion for associated trauma elsewhere (abdomen, head, thorax).

Urinary catheter: monitor fluid balance.

Imaging: Cervical spine X-ray to assess instability; MR preferred for extent of cord lesion.

Differential diagnosis Traumatic origin of dysfunction is usually obvious, but acute onset of paraparesis or quadriparesis may occasionally occur in spinal cord vascular disease (especially haemorrhage from a spinal arteriovenous malformation), Guillain–Barré syndrome, demyelination.

Treatment and prognosis Surgery for fixation of unstable fractures.

Steroids: role debated, but one meta-analysis suggests benefit.

Peptic ulcer prophylaxis: histamine H_2-receptor antagonists, proton pump inhibitors. DVT prophylaxis.

Nursing care appropriate for quadriplegic/paraplegic patient.

Skin integrity: close attention to pressure areas.

$+/-$ diaphragm/phrenic nerve stimulators for diaphragm weakness which leads to respiratory compromise.

Flaccid areflexic paralysis of >24 hours duration is unlikely to recover. Early motor recovery is an indicator of better prognosis. Partial cord injury does better than complete cord injury; central lesions, Brown–Séquard syndrome have better outcome than anterior lesions.

Some patients develop a post-traumatic syrinx which merits treatment in its own right.

Evolution to a chronic spastic quadriplegia/paraplegia is common.

References Alderson P, Roberts I. Corticosteroids in acute traumatic brain injury: systematic review of randomised controlled trials. *British Medical Journal* 1997; **314**: 1855–1859.

Chiles III BW, Cooper PR. Acute spinal injury. *New England Journal of Medicine* 1996; **334**: 514–520.

Grundy D, Swain A. *ABC of Spinal Cord Injury* (2nd edition). London: BMJ Publishing, 1993.

Other relevant entries Brown–Séquard syndrome; Cauda equina syndrome and conus medullaris disease; Myelopathy: an overview; Paraparesis: acute management and differential diagnosis; Quadriplegia: an overview; Spinal cord vascular diseases; Syringomyelia and syringobulbia.

▓ Spinal cord vascular diseases

Pathophysiology Vascular damage to the spinal cord most commonly results from:

- Infarction, secondary to anterior spinal artery occlusion (this may be iatrogenic, e.g. during thoraco-abdominal aneurysm repair). Both posterior spinal artery syndrome and venous infarction are uncommon.

- Haemorrhage within the cord (haematomyelia) and/or venous hypertension due to spinal angiomas: broadly these may be divided into dural arteriovenous fistulas (AVF), usually acquired, and arteriovenous malformations (AVMs), usually developmental.

Clinical features: history and examination.

- Anterior spinal artery syndrome (ASAS; *q.v.*):

    Anterior two-thirds of the cord may be infarcted with loss of descending motor and ascending sensory pathway integrity; posterior column function is preserved.

- Posterior spinal artery syndrome: Posterior one-third of the cord damaged, causing global sensory loss at level of lesion, loss of proprioception/vibration below the level, normal temperature/pain sensation, motor function preserved, reflexes lost below lesion; much less common than ASAS.

- Spinal dural arteriovenous fistula (DAVF): Present in middle age and beyond, most commonly in men, with a progressive painful myelopathy; venous hypertension causes hypoxia of the cord, which may progress to irreversible necrosis (Foix–Alajouanine syndrome; subacute necrotizing myelopathy). Stepwise progression may occur.

- Spinal AVMs: Tend to present earlier than DAVF, on average in the third decade but sometimes in childhood; may be at any level, on the surface of the cord, within the parenchyma, or both. High flow lesions which may have arterial aneurysms on the supplying vessels. Spinal haemorrhage is predominant manifestation, presenting with acute painful paraplegia, back pain, sciatica, with or without meningism and disturbance of consciousness; blood may track intracranially, simulating subarachnoid haemorrhage. Progressive neurological dysfunction less consistent than with DAVF. The presence of a spinal bruit (*ca.* 10%) and/or segmentally related cutaneous malformations may give a clue to the presence of an intradural AVM.

- Metameric vascular malformations: Spinal angioma in association with AVM of other organs or cutaneous angiomas: neurofibromatosis, haemangioblastomas, cerebral aneurysms; Cobb syndrome, Klippel–Trénaunay–Weber syndrome.

- Cavernous malformations.

Investigations and diagnosis

Imaging: MR of cord preferred; however, AVF/AVMs may not be seen in some cases, and if index of suspicion is high then myelography may be undertaken; spinal MRA is available in some centres.

Angiography: to define feeding vessels is helpful in planning treatment.

CSF: blood staining and/or xanthochromia may confirm spinal SAH.

Differential diagnosis

ASAS: unlikely to be mistaken for other causes of myelopathy.

DAVF: other causes of progressive myelopathy.

AVM haemorrhage: intracerebral subarachnoid haemorrhage (intracranial angiography negative).

Treatment and prognosis ASAS: supportive care and rehabilitation. Some authorities recommend a trial of steroids on the basis of their apparent utility in spinal trauma. Anticoagulation or antiplatelet therapy may be considered if there is an embolic cause.

Spinal AVF/AVM: some are amenable to surgical resection, other to embolization by interventional radiology.

References Aminoff MJ. *Spinal Angiomas*. Oxford: Blackwell Scientific, 1976.

Kendall BE, Valentine AR. Vascular malformation of the spine. In: Byrne JV (ed.). *Interventional Neuroradiology. Theory and Practice*. Oxford: OUP, 2002: 179–195.

Lamin S, Bhattacharya JJ. Vascular anatomy of the spinal cord and cord ischaemia. *Practical Neurology* 2003; **3**: 92–95.

Love BB. Spinal cord vascular syndromes. In: Noseworthy JH (ed.). *Neurological Therapeutics: Principles and Practice*. London: Dunitz, 2003: 558–562.

Other relevant entries Caisson disease; Cerebrovascular disease: arterial; Cerebrovascular disease: venous; Cobb syndrome; Foix–Alajouanine syndrome; Klippel–Trénaunay–Weber syndrome; Myelopathy: an overview; Paraparesis: acute management and differential diagnosis; Sciatica; Spinal cord disease: an overview; Von Hippel–Lindau disease.

▪ Spinal dysraphism – see Spina bifida

▪ Spinal interneuronitis – see Progressive encephalomyelitis with rigidity and myoclonus; Stiff people: an overview

▪ Spinal muscular atrophy
Hereditary motor neuropathy (HMN)

Pathophysiology The spinal muscular atrophies are a heterogeneous group of inherited disorders affecting motor neurones (hence "hereditary motor neuropathies"), principally the anterior horn cells (α-motor neurones) of the spinal cord but also those of the bulbar motor nuclei, resulting in neurogenic muscle atrophy. Current clinical classification of these conditions, based on age of onset, pattern of weakness, and mode of inheritance, reflects ignorance of the basic biochemical defect(s):

Childhood onset, proximal

Type I (Werdnig–Hoffmann disease; infantile)	autosomal recessive
Type II (intermediate)	autosomal recessive
Type III (Kugelberg–Welander; juvenile)	autosomal recessive
Chronic proximal-dominant spinal muscular atrophy (SMA)	autosomal dominant

Childhood onset, others

Distal SMA	autosomal recessive/autosomal dominant
Bulbar SMA (Fazio–Londe)	autosomal recessive/autosomal dominant

Bulbar SMA + deafness
(Brown Vialetto Van Laere)
SMA + external ophthalmoplegia autosomal recessive

Adult onset
Proximal SMA autosomal recessive / autosomal dominant
Kennedy's syndrome (X-linked X-linked
bulbospinal neuronopathy, XLBSN)
Distal SMA (O'Sullivan– autosomal recessive / autosomal dominant
McLeod syndrome)
Chronic asymmetric SMA ?not genetic
(CASMA, monomelic SMA)

Progress in genetic characterization is being made: childhood onset proximal SMA types I, II, and III have all been linked to chromosome 5q, and two unrelated genes in this region have been identified as responsible for SMA: survival motor neurone (SMN) and neuronal apoptosis inhibitory protein (NAIP).

Clinical features: history and examination Weakness, wasting, fasciculation of limb +/− bulbar muscles; +/− ophthalmoplegia; no sensory findings.

Investigations and diagnosis *Bloods*: creatine kinase normal in SMA type I, but elevated in SMA type III.

Neurophysiology: EMG: active and chronic denervation, fasciculations; polyphasic motor unit potentials indicative of reinnervation in SMA type III.

Neurogenetics: look for deletions in SMN and NAIP genes on chromosme 5.

Differential diagnosis Motor neurone disease and multifocal motor neuropathy with conduction block in adults.

Treatment and prognosis Varies with syndrome; death by age 2 years in Werdnig–Hoffmann disease; normal life expectancy in others.

References Lefebvre S, Burglen S, Reboullet S *et al*. Identification and characterization of a spinal muscular atrophy-determining gene. *Cell* 1995; **80**: 155–165.

Roy N, Mahadevan MS, McLean M *et al*. The gene for neuronal apoptosis inhibitory protein is partially deleted in individuals with spinal muscular atrophy. *Cell* 1995; **80**: 167–178.

Other relevant entries Fazio–Londe disease; Kennedy's syndrome; Monomelic amyotrophy; Motor neurone disease; Motor neurone diseases: an overview; Werdnig–Hoffmann disease.

■ **"Spinal shock" – see Paraparesis: acute management and differential diagnosis; Spinal cord trauma**

■ Spinal stenosis

Lumbar canal stenosis ● Neurogenic claudication ● Pseudoclaudication

Pathophysiology A syndrome of exertional back and leg pain, usually asymmetric, due to narrowing of the spinal canal. Pain is thought to be a consequence of the failure to meet or respond to the exercise-induced increase in metabolic rate of nervous tissue (cauda equina) within a stenosed lumbar canal. It is most common in the third to fifth decades of life. Spinal stenosis must be differentiated from arterial insufficiency of the legs (claudication).

Clinical features: history and examination The history is the most important part of evaluation.

- Leg pain induced by walking or standing, relieved by rest within minutes (*cf.* seconds for vascular claudication); sitting with flexed posture may ease pain (*cf.* standing in vascular claudication). Bicycling typically does not induce pain. Ambulatory distance before onset of pain may be variable (*cf.* fixed distance in vascular claudication).
- Numbness, paraesthesia, weakness, heaviness in legs may also be evident.
- Spinal movements may be limited; back pain is common.
- Neurological examination may be unremarkable at rest; mild nerve root dysfunction (e.g. L5) may be found.
- Peripheral pulses should be intact.

Investigations and diagnosis *Imaging*: Lumbar region CT/MRI may show canal stenosis, most often at L4/5 and L3/4, as a consequence of: hypertrophic facet joints; bulging of intervertebral discs; posterior osteophytes; hypertrophic ligamentum flavum; vertebral subluxations; or any combination thereof. In addition, there may be "redundancy", buckling, or kinking of nerve roots of the cauda equina above the canal stenosis. All these changes are, however, non-specific, and may be seen in the absence of any history of exercise-induced pain, hence, it is the conjunction of history, examination and radiological changes which establishes the diagnosis.
Neurophysiology: EMG/NCS: may show mild root dysfunction.

Differential diagnosis Arterial insufficiency (claudication).
Metabolic muscle disease, for example myophosphorylase deficiency, phosphofructokinase deficiency, carnitine palmityl transferase deficiency (often associated with cramps).
Spinal cord disease, for example multiple sclerosis.
Degenerative hip disease.

Treatment and prognosis In appropriately selected patients, surgical decompression may improve symptoms. Otherwise, conservative treatment involves living within walking limits.

> **Reference** Nelson PB. Approach to the patient with low back pain, lumbosacral radiculopathy, and lumbar stenosis. In: Biller J (ed.). *Practical Neurology* (2nd edition). Philadelphia: Lippincott Williams & Wilkins, 2002: 282–288.

■ Spinocerebellar ataxia

The classification of autosomal-dominant cerebellar ataxias (ADCAs), which are usually of late-onset (>25 years), is to some extent becoming clearer as the genes for these conditions are discovered. Many of these conditions are trinucleotide repeat diseases, with the number of repeats correlating with the severity of the disease; the greater the number, the younger the onset and the greater disease severity. In addition, these disorders show anticipation, with increasing severity of the condition in succeeding generations due to the increased expansion of the triplet repeat especially if inherited from an affected father. The disorders are characterized by a progressive cerebellar syndrome often in conjunction with signs of other neurological dysfunction, such as parkinsonism, dystonia, peripheral neuropathy, ophthalmoplegia, pigmentary retinopathy, optic atrophy and dementia. Although genetically distinct many of the diseases are phenotypically similar, hence a place remains for the phenotypic classification of ADCAs.

Gene	Locus	Mutation	Clinical classification	Protein
Spinocerebellar ataxia (SCA) 1	6p23–p24	CAG expansion	ADCA type I (*ca.* 13–35%)	ataxin-1
SCA2	12q23–q24	CAG expansion	ADCA type I (*ca.* 21–40%)	ataxin-2
SCA3	14q32	CAG expansion	ADCA type I (*ca.* 17–40%), including Machado–Joseph disease + ADCA type III	ataxin-3
SCA4	16q22	Unknown	Ataxia with sensory neuropathy (Biemond's ataxia)	
SCA5	11 centro-meric	Unknown	ADCA type III	
SCA6	19p13	CAG expansion	ADCA type III; allelic with episodic ataxia type 2 and familial hemiplegic migraine	
SCA7	3p12	CAG expansion	ADCA type II	ataxin-7
SCA8	13q21	CTG expansion	ADCA type I	
SCA9: Not categorized				
SCA10	22q13	ATTCT expansion	ADCA type III	
SCA11	15q14–q21	Unknown	ADCA type III	
SCA12	5q31	CAG expansion	ADCA type I	

(Continued)

SCA13	19q	Unknown	ADCA type I
SCA14	19q	Unknown	ADCA type III
SCA15	?	Unknown	ADCA type I
SCA16	8q	Unknown	ADCA type I
SCA17		polyglutamine	
SCA 18–21: Registered but not yet published			
SCA22	1p21–q23	Unknown	ADCA type III

Differential diagnosis A spinocerebellar syndrome may also occur in:

Multiple sclerosis

Vitamin E deficiency.

GM2 gangliosidoses may present with a spinocerebellar syndrome.

Reference Klockgether T. Ataxias. In: Goetz CG (ed.). *Textbook of Clinical Neurology* (2nd edition). Philadelphia: Saunders, 2003: 741–757.

Other relevant entries Autosomal-dominant cerebellar ataxia; Cerebellar disease: an overview; Dentatorubral–pallidoluysian atrophy; Episodic ataxia; Migraine; Trinucleotide repeat diseases.

▧ Splenio-occipital syndrome – see Alexia

▧ Spongiform encephalopathies – see Prion disease: an overview

▧ Spongy degeneration of infancy – see Canavan's disease

▧ Spontaneous intracranial hypotension

Essential aliquorrhoea ● Low pressure headache ● Schaltenbrand's syndrome

Pathophysiology Spontaneous intracranial hypotension is a rare syndrome characterized by postural headache and low CSF opening pressure. Leakage of CSF is thought to be the cause: most often this is idiopathic, but it may follow rupture of a spinal arachnoid cyst (e.g. in Marfan's syndrome). Low-pressure headache is, of course, more commonly iatrogenic, as a consequence of a lumbar puncture or neurosurgery; head trauma is also a cause. Acute subdural haematoma has been reported as a complication of spontaneous intracranial hypotension.

Clinical features: history and examination

- Low-pressure headache: worse with erect posture (*cf.* raised intracranial pressure).
- +/− nausea, vomiting, and vertigo.

- +/− tinnitus.
- +/− abducens nerve palsy (unilateral, bilateral).
- If increasing headache, focal signs, and impaired level of consciousness, consider subdural haematoma.
- Hyperacute onset may occur (secondary thunderclap headache).

Investigations and diagnosis

Imaging:

MRI: thin subdural effusions (hygroma) without mass effect; dural enhancement; venous sinus dilatation; +/− subdural haematoma.

Radioisotope studies: may demonstrate the leak.

CSF: low opening pressure.

Differential diagnosis Meningeal infiltration.

Treatment and prognosis It may be impossible to identify the site of CSF leakage. Headache may take months to resolve spontaneously; an epidural blood patch may help (also used for iatrogenic low-pressure headache).

Reference Davenport RJ, Chataway SJ, Warlow CP. Spontaneous intracranial hypotension from a CSF leak in a patient with Marfan's syndrome. *Journal of Neurology, Neurosurgery and Psychiatry* 1995; **59**: 516–519.

Other relevant entries Subdural haematoma; Thunderclap headache.

■ Spontaneous periodic hypothermia

A rare syndrome characterized by episodes, lasting minutes to hours, of hypothermia (rectal temperature <30°C), bradycardia, salivation, nausea, vomiting, vasodilatation, sweating and lacrimation, suggesting autonomic dysfunction. Seizures may occur (so-called "diencephalic seizures"). Between attacks there are no abnormal neurological signs. The syndrome has been described in association with cholesteatoma of the third ventricle, but is often idiopathic. A posterior hypothalamic lesion is suspected.

References Mooradian AD, Morley GK, McGeachie R *et al*. Spontaneous periodic hypothermia. *Neurology* 1984; **34**: 79–82.

Thomas DJ, Green ID. Periodic hypothermia. *British Medical Journal* 1973; **ii**: 696–697.

Other relevant entries Hypothalamic disease: an overview; Shapiro syndrome.

■ Sporadic fatal insomnia – see Fatal familial insomnia; Prion disease: an overview

■ Sprengel's shoulder
Sprengel's anomaly • Sprengel's deformity

Congenital undescended scapula or high scapula, is manifest by elevation, with or without hypoplasia, of the shoulder. An accessory ossicle, the omovertebral bone, may articulate the medial border of the scapula with one or more cervical vertebrae. The condition is unlikely to be confused with winging of the scapula due to weakness of serratus anterior seen with long thoracic nerve palsy or certain muscular dystrophies (facioscapulohumeral, scapuloperoneal). Surgical correction may be undertaken, at which time care must be taken not to injure the dorsal scapular nerve.

Other relevant entries Facioscapulohumeral dystrophy; Long thoracic nerve palsy; Scapuloperoneal syndromes.

Stargardt disease

Fundus flavimaculatus

Pathophysiology An hereditary (usually autosomal recessive) tapetoretinal degeneration or dystrophy with onset in the first two decades of life. A loss of central vision reflects a slowly progressive symmetric macular degeneration due to a selective loss of cones (*cf.* retinitis pigmentosa).

Clinical features: history and examination
- Progressive central visual loss; central scotomata.
- Fundoscopy: grey or yellow–brown macula, $+/-$ dystrophic retinal periphery.

Investigations and diagnosis
Neurophysiology: ERG: reduced or abolished.
Fluorescein angiogram.

Differential diagnosis Leber's hereditary optic neuropathy.
Fundal appearances may be confused with those of Kjellin's syndrome, a form of hereditary spastic paraparesis.

Treatment and prognosis No specific treatment; low vision aids.

Reference Bither PP, Berns LA. Stargardt's disease: a review of the literature. *Journal of the American Optometric Association* 1988; **59**: 106–111.

Other relevant entries Hereditary spastic paraparesis; Leber's hereditary optic neuropathy; Retinitis pigmentosa.

Startle syndromes

Pathophysiology The physiological startle reflex is a rapid, generalized motor response to a sudden, unexpected, surprise stimulus (usually auditory, but also tactile and visual) which may be followed by behavioural phenomena such as laughter. The reflex habituates markedly and is heightened by fear. Exaggerated startle responses, in which the motor response is too violent, and/or the triggering stimuli would not affect a normal individual, or there are atypical behavioural phenomena, occur in a variety of circumstances:
- Hyperekplexia (*q.v.*): hereditary, symptomatic.
- Startle epilepsy.
- A syndrome variously known in different parts of the world as latah, myriachit, Jumping Frenchmen of Maine, Ragin' Cajuns of Louisiana.
- Stiffman syndromes.
- Reticular reflex myoclonus.

Clinical features: history and examination

- Exaggerated startle: shock-like movement, with eye blink, grimace, abduction of arms, flexion of neck, trunk, elbows, hips, knees; patient may fall; there may be urinary incontinence.
- Behavioural features: echolalia, coprolalia, echopraxia, striking posture, automatic obedience (response to commands such as "jump", "throw").

Investigations and diagnosis Diagnosis is essentially clinical, from history and observation of the response. Laboratory testing of such phenomena has not proven easy. EEG may be undertaken to look for evidence of epilepsy.

Differential diagnosis The excessive features usually make differentiation from physiological startle responses easy.

Treatment and prognosis Symptomatic treatment with clonazepam or diazepam may be tried. Condition does not remit.

References Lajonchere C, Nortz M, Finger S. Gilles de la Tourette and the discovery of Tourette syndrome. Includes a translation of his 1884 article. *Archives of Neurology* 1996; **53**: 567–574.

Manford MR, Fish DR, Shorvon SD. Startle provoked epileptic seizures: features in 19 patients. *Journal of Neurology, Neurosurgery and Psychiatry* 1996; **61**: 151–156.

Matsumoto J, Hallett M. Startle syndromes. In: Marsden CD, Fahn S (eds). *Movement Disorders 3*. Boston: Butterworth, 1994: 418–433.

Other relevant entries Hyperekplexia; Reflex epilepsies; Sandhoff's disease.

■ Status cataplecticus – see Cataplexy

■ Status dystonicus

Status dystonicus is an unusual syndrome of increasingly frequent and relentless episodes of generalized dystonia. It may be precipitated by infection or drugs. Owing to bulbar and respiratory complications patients may need ventilation and sedation; rhabdomyolysis may occur. Medication with benzhexol, tetrabenazine, and pimozide may help. Outcome may vary from return to prior clinical situation, worsened clinical features, or death.

Reference Manji H, Howard RS, Miller DH *et al*. Status dystonicus: the syndrome and its management. *Brain* 1998; **121**: 243–252.

Other relevant entries Dystonia: an overview; Rhabdomyolysis.

■ Status epilepticus

Pathophysiology Status epilepticus has been described as the maximum expression of epilepsy, and may be defined as a condition in which epileptic activity persists for 30 minutes or more, without full recovery of consciousness between seizures. Status epilepticus may manifest as a wide range of clinical symptoms, with highly variable pathophysiological, anatomical and aetiological basis. The commonest forms are:

- Generalized convulsive status epilepticus.
- Non-convulsive status epilepticus (NCSE): includes absence status and complex partial status.
- Simple partial status epilepticus: repeated focal motor seizures, focal impairment of function (e.g. aphasia), epilepsia partialis continua (EPC).

Clinical features: history and examination

- Previous history of seizure disorder (although status may emerge *de novo*); change in anti-epileptic drug therapy.
- Acute cerebral insult: meningitis, encephalitis, head trauma, hypoxia, hypoglycaemia, drug intoxication.
- Encephalopathy, $+/-$ convulsive motor seizures.
- Non-convulsive status may manifest as a behavioural change.

Investigations and diagnosis *Neurophysiology*: EEG may be helpful in diagnosing non-convulsive status, and differentiating epileptic from non-epileptic (pseudo) status. Search for a precipitating event which mandates treatment in its own right, although treatment of generalized convulsive status epilepticus takes precedence over investigation.

Bloods: metabolic derangements: hypoxia, hypoglycaemia; toxicology screen; leukocytosis, raised ESR, CRP (signs of infection).

Urine: infection.

Imaging: CT, MRI brain.

CSF: look for evidence of meningitis, encephalitis.

Differential diagnosis Convulsive status: pseudostatus epilepticus.
Non-convulsive status: other encephalopathies.

Treatment and prognosis Generalized convulsive status epilepticus: this is an acute medical emergency, with a substantial mortality and neurological morbidity; prognosis is better if there is a previous history of epilepsy or there is a benign reversible cause. Inadequate seizure control can lead to multiple organ failure (e.g. rhabdomyolysis, acute tubular necrosis, disseminated intravascular coagulation).

Once diagnosed, the following standardized treatment plan is recommended:

- Maintain airway, adequate oxygenation.
- Maintain blood pressure.
- Establish intravenous access (preferably two lines): one for normal saline.
- Give: Intravenous benzodiazepine: lorazepam preferred to diazepam.
    Intravenous phenytoin (or fos-phenytoin) infusion, monitoring blood pressure, ECG.
    Intravenous phenobarbitone or, less often, chlormethiazole may also be used.
- If seizures continue for 60–90 minutes despite these interventions, the next step is anaesthesia, endotracheal intubation and ventilation; intravenous thiopentone or propofol are the most commonly used agents. Full ITU monitoring, including EEG monitoring, and supportive care are required.

- Increasingly frequent seizures may precede the development of generalized convulsive status epilepticus: lorazepam at this stage may abort deterioration into full blown status.
- Non-convulsive status and simple partial status: the urgency is less, since neurones are not dying as a consequence of this seizure activity. Complex partial status may be controlled with intravenous benzodiazepines and phenytoin. Absence status may be terminated with intravenous benzodiazepines. Simple partial status may be controlled with intravenous phenytoin.

References Anonymous. Stopping status epilepticus. *Drugs and Therapeutics Bulletin* 1996; **34**: 73–75.

Scholtes FB, Renier WO, Meinardi H. Non-convulsive status epilepticus: causes, treatment, and outcome in 65 patients. *Journal of Neurology, Neurosurgery and Psychiatry* 1996; **61**: 93–95.

Shorvon S. *Status Epilepticus: Its Clinical Features and Treatment in Children and Adults*. Cambridge: CUP, 1994.

Other relevant entries Encephalopathies: an overview; Epilepsy: an overview; Pseudoseizures; Rasmussen's encephalitis, Rasmussen's syndrome.

■ Status migrainosus – see Migraine

■ Steele–Richardson–Olszewski syndrome – see Progressive supranuclear palsy

■ Steinert's disease – see Dystrophia myotonica

■ Stellate ganglion syndrome

Pathophysiology Lesions of the stellate (superior cervical) ganglion are one of the many causes of Horner's syndrome (it may result from pathology in locations extending from the brainstem to the spinal cord to the internal carotid artery). In the stellate ganglion syndrome, the presence of additional clinical features may allow more precise clinical localization, namely sympathetic dysfunction in the ipsilateral arm. The stellate ganglion syndrome is most usually due to compression from an adjacent tumour of the superior sulcus of the lung.

Clinical features: history and examination
- Horner's syndrome:
    miosis (anisocoria)
    partial ptosis
    apparent enophthalmos
    anhidrosis over the side of the face.
- + warm and dry ipsilateral hand (impaired sympathetic reflexes in arm).
- (+wasted hand = Pancoast's syndrome).

Investigations and diagnosis Imaging of chest and/or bronchoscopy to identify lung tumour.

Differential diagnosis Other causes of Horner's syndrome.

Treatment and prognosis Of the underlying cause where possible; this also determines prognosis.

Other relevant entries Horner's syndrome; Pancoast's syndrome.

■ Stickler's syndrome
Hereditary arthro-ophthalmopathy

A multisystem disorder characterized by the following clinical features:

Ocular: retinal detachment, myopia, vitreoretinal degeneration.

Skeletal: craniofacial dysmorphology, such as midfacial hypoplasia, micrognathia, cleft palate.

Cardiac: mitral valve prolapse.

Stickler's syndrome enters the differential diagnosis of Marfan's syndrome.

Reference Stickler GB, Belau PG, Farel FJ *et al*. Hereditary progressive arthroophthalmopathy. *Mayo Clinic Proceedings* 1965; **40**: 433–455.

Other relevant entry Marfan syndrome.

■ Stiff people: an overview

Pathophysiology Stiff man syndrome was first described by Moersch and Woltman in 1956. This condition is presumed to be an autoimmune disorder associated with increased motor unit activity in the lower limbs and paraspinal/abdominal muscles. It presents with slowly increasing stiffness of the legs with jerking and falls, usually in the fourth to fifth decades, with equal sex incidence. It is associated with other autoimmune disorders and many patients have antibodies to glutamic acid decarboxylase (GAD) and concurrent insulin-dependent diabetes mellitus (IDDM). The pathophysiology is unknown: it is thought that anti-GAD antibodies may interfere with spinal inhibitory interneurones ("spinal interneuronitis"), and since GAD is also found in islet cells they may be important in development of the IDDM. The role of immunosuppressive therapy is debated; baclofen and benzodiazepines may be used. Stiffness is also a feature of a syndrome of progressive encephalomyelitis with rigidity and myoclonus (PERM), which is probably related.

Clinical features: history and examination

- Complaint of tightness and/or stiffness of axial and lower limb musculature; on examination there is increased stiffness of the lower limbs, often made worse by sensory stimuli; hyperlordosis of the lumbar spine with increased tone in the paraspinal muscles.

- Often there are associated intermittent painful spasms precipitated by voluntary movement, fright, sounds. Such stimulus-sensitive jerks ("jerking stiff man syndrome") are believed to be of brainstem origin.

- May be associated with excessive startle response, which coupled to the above features leads to falls.
- No sphincter abnormalities; upper limb involvement rare.
- No sensory abnormalities.
- Reflexes may be brisk, plantars flexor.

Associations:

IDDM (30–60%)
Epilepsy (10–15%)
Autoimmune thyroid disease, vitiligo and pernicious anaemia.

Investigations and diagnosis *Bloods*: may be diabetic; 60% of patients have positive anti-GAD antibodies, there may be other associated auto-antibodies including pancreatic islet cell, gastric parietal cell and thyroid microsomal antibodies.

Imaging: normal brain, cord; plain radiology may confirm lumbar hyperlordosis.

Neurophysiology: EMG/NCS: normal NCS, but continuous motor unit activity in paraspinal and lower limb muscles.

CSF: often difficult to obtain because of hyperlordosis. Oligoclonal bands are found in about 50% of patients. Normal protein, no cells.

Differential diagnosis

Progressive encephalomyelitis with rigidity ($+/-$ myoclonus; PERM).

Neuromyotonia (Isaacs syndrome).

Stiff limb syndrome.

Schwartz–Jampel syndrome.

Strychnine poisoning.

Tetanus.

Non-organic.

Treatment and prognosis

Symptomatic:

Benzodiazepines: usually diazepam, high doses (>30 mg/day).

Baclofen: usually at high dose (90 mg/day).

Other medications with anecdotal evidence of benefit include clonazepam, sodium valproate, tizanidine, and vigabatrin.

Baclofen pumps have been tried with variable success.

Immunosuppression:

Prednisolone, azathioprine and plasma exchange have all been tried with variable success.

IVIg (0.4 g/kg/day) has met with some success in this condition.

Prognosis is relatively benign, most patients remain ambulant. Major cause of death is from complications of IDDM.

References Barker R, Revesz T, Thom M, Marsden CD, Brown P. Review of 23 patients affected by the stiff man syndrome: clinical subdivision into stiff trunk (man) syndrome, stiff limb syndrome, and progressive encephalomyelitis with rigidity. *Journal of Neurology, Neurosurgery and Psychiatry* 1998; **65**: 633–640.

Meinck H-M, Thompson PD. Stiff man syndrome and related conditions. *Movement Disorders* 2002; **17**: 853–866.

Other relevant entries Diabetes mellitus and the nervous system; Immuno-suppressive therapy and diseases of the nervous system; Neuromyotonia; Progressive encephalomyelitis with rigidity and myoclonus; Schwartz–Jampel syndrome.

■ Strachan's syndrome
Jamaican neuritis • Jamaican neuropathy

Pathophysiology A syndrome affecting peripheral and optic nerves, probably of nutritional origin, originally described by Strachan (1897) amongst Jamaican sugar-cane workers but subsequently described in epidemic outbreaks elsewhere. The syndrome is associated with dietary deprivation and may reflect deficiency in vitamins of the B group, sharing some features with beriberi and pellagra.

Clinical features: history and examination
- Pain, numbness, paraesthesia of extremities (acroparaesthesia).
- Sensory ataxia, wasting, weakness, hyporeflexia.
- Reduced sensation: vibration, position sense.
- Subacute visual failure ("amblyopia"); optic disc pallor.
- $+/-$ hearing loss, tinnitus.
- $+/-$ mucocutaneous lesions: stomatoglossitis, corneal degeneration, genital dermatitis.
- $+/-$ myelopathic features reported in some cases (whether these cases represent a separate condition, tropical spastic paraparesis, is uncertain).
- Dietary history of nutritional depletion: deficient in meat, vegetables; rich in sugar (i.e. vitamin B deficient); alcohol consumption, smoking, are risk factors.

Investigations and diagnosis *EMG/NCS*: predominantly sensory neuropathy.

Differential diagnosis Beriberi, pellagra.

Treatment and prognosis Improvement with vitamin B supplements was reported in the Cuban epidemic of 1992–1993.

References Roman GC. An epidemic in Cuba of optic neuropathy, sensorineural deafness, peripheral sensory neuropathy and dorsolateral myeloneuropathy. *Journal of the Neurological Sciences* 1994; **127**: 11–28.

Strachan H. On a form of multiple neuritis prevalent in the West Indies. *Practitioner* 1897; **59**: 477–484.

Other relevant entries Beriberi; Neuropathies: an overview; Pellagra; Vitamin deficiencies and the nervous system.

■ Striatonigral degeneration – see Multiple system atrophy; Parkinsonian syndromes, parkinsonism

■ Stroke – see Brainstem vascular syndromes; Cerebrovascular disease: arterial; Cerebrovascular disease: venous; Lacunar syndromes; Spinal cord vascular diseases

■ Strongyloidiasis

Pathophysiology Infection with the nematode *Strongyloides stercoralis*, a parasite endemic to many tropical and subtropical regions, is the cause of strongyloidiasis. Infectious filariform larvae may develop many decades after initial infection, most often in the context of chronic illness or immunosuppression, leading to overwhelming autoinfection ("hyperinfection"). There is a risk of concurrent bacterial superinfection.

Clinical features: history and examination
- Initial infection may be entirely asymptomatic.
- Disseminated strongyloidiasis may cause:
    Abdominal pain, jaundice.
    Asthma-like symptoms.
    Acute pyogenic meningitis, progressing to coma; or subacute meningoencephalitis.

Investigations and diagnosis
Bloods: eosinophilia.
Stool: for larvae.
CSF: eosinophilic pleocytosis.

Differential diagnosis
Meningitis.
Vasculitis.

Treatment and prognosis Supportive therapy, treatment of bacterial superinfection. Anti-helminthics: Thiabendazole, mebendazole; efficacy may be improved if immunosuppression can be suspended or reduced.
Steroids contraindicated because they facilitate autoinfection.

> **Reference** Cook GC. Strongyloides stercoralis hyperinfection syndrome: how often is it missed? *Quarterly Journal of Medicine* 1987; **64(244)**: 625–629.

> **Other relevant entries** Helminthic disease; Trichinosis.

■ Strümpell–Lorrain disease – see Hereditary spastic paraparesis

■ Strychnine poisoning

Pathophysiology Strychnine is a potent alkaloid from the seeds of the *Strychnos nux-vomica* plant, which antagonizes the action of the inhibitory neurotransmitter glycine at its receptors in the spinal cord interneurones and Renshaw cells, so facilitating synaptic transmission. Cases of strychnine poisoning now only result from exposure to the drug when used as a rodenticide: <100 mg may prove fatal in an adult (less in a child).

Clinical features: history and examination

- Stiffness and spasms of limb, face (causing risus sardonicus), neck muscles, reflex excitability.
- Heightened awareness (hyperalert), visual hallucinations.
- Tetanic convulsions with opisthotonos, lasting 30 seconds to 2 minutes.
- No clouding of consciousness.
- During convulsions: respiratory arrest, rhabdomyolysis, myoglobinuria, lactic acidosis; death.

Investigations and diagnosis No specific investigations.

Differential diagnosis Tetanus (including risus sardonicus). Other causes of stiffness, for example stiff man/stiff person syndrome, stiff limb syndrome, progressive encephalomyelitis with rigidity, neuromyotonia, Schwartz–Jampel syndrome.

Treatment and prognosis Nursing in darkened room, minimize external stimuli. Diazepam or phenobarbital (GABA agonists) for convulsions; neuromuscular blockade (e.g. pancuronium) + ventilation may be required.

Empty stomach (gastric lavage) + charcoal instillation.

Monitor for renal failure and hepatic necrosis; appropriate fluid support.

The drug is rapidly metabolized, so support may only be required for a short period of time.

> **Reference** Scully RE, Mark EJ, McNeely WF *et al.* Case records of the Massachusetts General Hospital (Case 12-2001). *New England Journal of Medicine* 2001; **344**: 1232–1239.

> **Other relevant entries** Schwartz–Jampel syndrome; Stiff people: an overview; Tetanus.

■ Sturge–Weber syndrome

Encephalotrigeminal angiomatosis • Krabbe–Weber–Dimitri disease • Meningofacial angiomatosis

Pathophysiology Sturge–Weber syndrome describes angiomatous malformations of the face and parieto-occipital cortex; the latter may lead to epilepsy, progressive ischaemia of the cortex, and focal signs. The ultimate cause of this syndrome is unknown. Although classified with the phakomatoses there is no evidence of a genetic basis and no predisposition to neoplasia.

Clinical features: history and examination

- Neurological:
  - angioma of meninges, brain, especially parieto-occipital cortex;
  - focal epilepsy;
  - focal signs: hemiparesis, hemianopia, hemiatrophy, hemisensory deficits;
  - learning disability;
  - Onset of ipsilateral limb neurological symptoms and signs after trauma has been labelled Fegeler syndrome.

- Dermatological:
  - vascular naevus (naevus flammeus, port-wine naevus) covering large part of face and cranium (ophthalmic division of V most often affected) and sometimes trunk; present at birth; unilateral more often than bilateral.
- Ocular:
  - haemagioma of choroid, episclera, iris, ciliary body;
  - glaucoma, buphthalmos, blindness.

Investigations and diagnosis

Imaging:

Skull X-ray: tramline calcification outlining parieto-occipital cortical convolutions from 2nd year.

Brain imaging (MRI): abnormalities of cortex; atrophy.

Angiography: abnormal meningeal vessels usually not well seen (*cf.* arteriovenous malformations).

Differential diagnosis Other haemangiomatous conditions with neurological features, for example Von Hippel–Lindau disease, ataxia telangiectasia (Louis–Bar syndrome), Fabry's disease, and Osler–Weber–Rendu syndrome, are unlikely to be confused with Sturge–Weber syndrome.

Treatment and prognosis No specific treatment. Symptomatic treatment of epilepsy, spasticity. Early onset seizures are associated with a poor cognitive prognosis.

References Adamsbaum C, Pinton F, Rolland Y *et al*. Accelerated myelination in early Sturge–Weber syndrome: MRI–SPECT correlations. *Paediatric Radiology* 1996; **26**: 759–762.

Griffiths PD. Sturge–Weber syndrome revisited: the role of neuroradiology. *Neuropediatrics* 1996; **17**: 284–294.

Other relevant entry Phakomatosis.

■ Stylomastoid foramen syndrome – see Cranial nerve disease: VII: Facial nerve

■ Suarez–Kelly syndrome – see Dropped head syndrome

■ Subacute combined degeneration of the spinal cord

Subacute combined degeneration of the spinal cord (SACDOC) is one of the neurological consequences of vitamin B$_{12}$ deficiency. The dorsal and lateral parts of the spinal cord (i.e. dorsal columns, spinocerebellar and pyramidal tracts) are principally affected, especially in the cervical region although changes may extend to the thoracic and even lumbar regions. This produces a syndrome of sensory ataxia (especially if there is superadded peripheral neuropathy as a consequence of vitamin B$_{12}$ deficiency): loss of vibration or joint position sense in the legs is the most consistent abnormality. In addition there may be mild spasticity, with or without Lhermitte's sign, and sphincter involvement; reflexes may be brisk, or there may be a combination of brisk knee jerks, absent ankle jerks, and upgoing plantars.

MR scanning of the cervical cord may show increased signal on T$_2$-weighted images in the dorsal cord extending over several or many segments ("longitudinal myelitis"). EMG/NCS may show a peripheral neuropathy, usually of axonal type.

Overuse of nitrous oxide analgesia may produce a very similar clinical and neuroradiological syndrome.

The clinical and radiological changes may resolve with repletion therapy, but there is an inverse correlation between delay to diagnosis and treatment and extent of recovery.

References Hemmer B, Glocker FX, Schumacher M, Deuschl G, Lücking CH. Subacute combined degeneration: clinical, electrophysiological, and magnetic resonance imaging findings. *Journal of Neurology, Neurosurgery and Psychiatry* 1998; **65**: 822–827.

Larner AJ, Zeman AZJ, Antoun NM, Allen CMC. MRI appearances in subacute combined degeneration of the spinal cord due to vitamin B$_{12}$ deficiency. *Journal of Neurology, Neurosurgery and Psychiatry* 1997; **62**: 99–100.

Other relevant entries Common variable immunodeficiency; Myelopathy: an overview; Vitamin B$_{12}$ deficiency.

Subacute motor neuronopathy

Subacute, progressive, painless, asymmetrical lower motor neurone type weakness, affecting arms more than legs, may be seen in the context of an underlying lymphoma, and known as subacute motor neuronopathy. There may be associated monoclonal gammopathy, raised CSF protein and oligoclonal bands. The disease may simulate motor neurone disease. The course of the neurological syndrome may not reflect that of the underlying lymphoma, and is often benign with spontaneous remission.

Other relevant entries Lymphoma; Monoclonal gammopathies; Motor neurone disease.

Subacute myelo-optic neuropathy

This syndrome was seen as a complication of consumption of the anti-diarrhoeal agent clioquinol (iodochlorhydroxyquinoline) in Japan in the 1960s. Since withdrawal of the drug, the syndrome seems to have disappeared. Cases of transient global amnesia following clioquinol consumption have been reported.

Reference Baumgartner G, Gawel MJ, Kaeser HE *et al*. Neurotoxicity of halogenated hydroxyquinolones: clinical analysis of cases reported outside Japan. *Journal of Neurology, Neurosurgery and Psychiatry* 1979; **42**: 1073–1083.

■ Subacute necrotizing encephalomyelopathy – see Leigh's disease, Leigh's syndrome

■ Subacute necrotizing myelopathy – see Foix–Alajouanine syndrome; Spinal cord vascular diseases

■ Subacute sclerosing panencephalitis

Pathophysiology Subacute sclerosing panencephalitis (SSPE) is a chronic reactivation of latent measles virus infection causing progressive inflammation and gliosis of the brain. Defective maturation of virus in neural cells follows primary infection, usually in the first 2 years of life. Symptoms then emerge from around age 14 years, although occasional adult cases are reported.

In some children and adults another form of subacute measles encephalitis has been described that develops months (not years) after the primary infection and which leads to death within days or weeks. The illness is characterized by focal neurological signs, intractable focal seizures, stupor and coma. It is thought to occur in immunocompromised people, unlike SSPE, but has histological features similar to SSPE.

Clinical features: history and examination
- Change in behaviour; decline in intellect, personality.
- Myoclonus.
- Seizures.
- Progressive dementia.
- Ataxia.
- Progressive rigidity.
- Autonomic dysfunction.
- Late stages: pyramidal signs, stupor, decorticate posture, coma.

Investigations and diagnosis *Bloods*: normal.

Imaging: CT/MRI shows involvement of periventricular and subcortical white matter.

Neurophysiology: EEG: characteristic (pathognomonic) periodic complexes, bursts of two to three per second high voltage waves, with background slowing (i.e. burst suppression).

CSF: no cells, normal glucose, high protein with oligoclonal bands (CSF only); detection of measles virus-specific antibodies is diagnostic.

Pathology: nerve cell destruction in all sites except cerebellum; lymphocytic and mononuclear infiltrates. Eosinophilic inclusions in cytoplasm and nuclei of both neurones and glial cells.

Differential diagnosis

Metabolic disorders.

Prion disease (vCJD).

Treatment and prognosis Course is slowly progressive with death usually occurring in 1–3 years. No specific treatment available, although oral isoprinosine and intrathecal α-interferon has been reported to prolong survival.

Reference Frings M, Blaeser I, Kastrup O. Adult-onset subacute sclerosing panencephalitis presenting as a degenerative dementia syndrome. *Journal of Neurology* 2002; **249**: 942–943.

Other relevant entries Encephalitis: an overview; Progressive multifocal leukoencephalopathy; Rubella.

■ Subarachnoid haemorrhage

Pathophysiology Bleeding into the subarachnoid space usually originates from a ruptured aneurysm or arteriovenous malformation (intracranial, spinal). Both lesions are usually clinically silent prior to rupture although some patients give a (usually retrospective) history of events suggestive of "sentinel" or "warning" bleeds. Recognized risk factors for subarachnoid haemorrhage (SAH) include:

Smoking

Hypertension

positive family history of SAH, especially if associated with polycystic kidney disease, neurofibromatosis-1 (NF-1), Marfan's syndrome, Ehlers–Danlos syndrome type IV, fibromuscular dysplasia.

Clinical features: history and examination

- Sudden (instantaneous) onset of severe pain, especially occipital in location ("hit on the back of the head"), often during stress or exercise, with nausea, vomiting, sometimes brief loss of consciousness.
- Nuchal rigidity (secondary to chemical meningitis).
- Subhyaloid (venous) haemorrhage 25%, $+/-$ vitreal haemorrhage (Terson's syndrome).
- Focal signs, for example oculomotor nerve palsy, may occur secondary to raised intracranial pressure and mass effect; may be a consequence of arterial vasospasm, occurring in up to 25% of patients 4–12 days following the original bleed, or due to embolism from intra-aneurysmal thrombus.

Clinical grading scales for the classification of SAH have been devised, such as that of Hunt and Hess:

I   Asymptomatic, or mild headache, slight nuchal rigidity.

II   Moderate to severe headache, nuchal rigidity, no neurological deficit other than cranial nerve palsy.

III   Mild focal neurological deficit, drowsiness or confusion.

IV   Stupor, moderate to severe hemiparesis, possible early decerebrate rigidity.

V   Deep coma, decerebrate rigidity, moribund appearance.

Though widely used, this system is neither reliable nor valid. Another classification, based around the Glasgow Coma Scale, itself highly reliable and valid, is the World Federation of Neurological Surgeons scale:

I   GCS 15, focal deficit absent

II   GCS 14–13, focal deficit absent

III   GCS 14–13, focal deficit present

IV   GCS 12–7, focal deficit present or absent

V   GCS 6–3, focal deficit present or absent.

Investigations and diagnosis *Imaging*: CT is modality of choice for imaging sub-arachnoid blood in the acute phase; scans may be normal in a small percentage of patients with SAH, particularly if scanned very early (<12 hours) after onset.

If imaging is negative but clinical suspicion is high, lumbar puncture for CSF is mandatory to look for blood staining and xanthochromia, ideally using spectrophotometry rather than the naked eye; these changes are present up to 10–14 days following an acute bleed, but may not be found if LP is performed within 12 hours of onset.

If SAH is confirmed, angiography to look for aneurysmal bleeding source is indicated: catheter angiography remains the investigation of choice currently, rather than MRA.

Perimesencephalic bleeds (i.e. blood confined to the cisterns around the midbrain, ventral to the pons; =10% of SAH, two-thirds of angiogram-negative SAH) may not require angiography, because of the lack of association with an underlying aneurysm.

In patients presenting >2 weeks after event, appropriate investigation is uncertain; MRA is often deployed.

Differential diagnosis

Broad (*cf.* intracerebral haemorrhage):

Headache:
Migraine
Tension type headache
Coital headache
Ice-pick headache, idiopathic thunderclap headache
Meningitis:
Bacterial
Viral
Injury:
Head
Cervical spine
Intoxication: drug, alcohol
Hypertension: hypertensive encephalopathy, eclampsia
Cervial disc herniation
Pituitary apoplexy.

Treatment and prognosis Acute medical management includes monitoring of neurological status, fluid balance (central line recommended); there is some evidence to support the use of nimodipine to reduce the risk of vasospasm.

Surgical clipping of an aneurysm (if one is found) reduces the risk of re-bleeding, which carries a significant mortality. This has been the standard treatment, but in recent years endovascular coiling techniques with detachable platinum coils have been increasingly used, initially in patients with high surgical risk and with aneurysms of the posterior cerebral circulation, particularly those arising from the basilar artery. Recent evidence suggests that coiling is better than surgery for the majority of patients.

Prognosis correlates with the clinical grading on admission. Up to 30% of survivors have persisting sensorimotor and/or neuropsychological deficits and as SAH affects younger people there is a considerable impact on long-term mortality.

Perimesencephalic bleeds have an excellent prognosis and no risk of re-bleeding. Superficial siderosis of the CNS may be a consequence of SAH.

Screening of asymptomatic family members has been suggested in the past, but is of doubtful value unless there is a history of polycystic kidney disease.

Small aneurysms (<10 mm diameter) have a very low rupture rate, less than the risk associated with surgery, suggesting they should be managed conservatively.

References Chicoine MR, Dacey Jr RG. Clinical aspects of subarachnoid hemorrhage. In: Welch KMA, Caplan LR, Reis DJ *et al.* (eds) *Primer on Cerebrovascular Diseases*. San Diego: Academic, 1997: 425–432.

Hütter BO. *Neuropsychological Sequelae of Subarachnoid Hemorrhage and Its Treatment*. Berlin: Springer, 2000.

International Subarachnoid Aneurysm Trial (ISAT) Collaborative Group. International Subarachnoid Aneurysm Trial (ISAT) of neurosurgical clipping versus endovascular coiling in 2143 patients with ruptured aneurysms: a randomised trial. *Lancet* 2002; **360**: 1267–1274.

Johnston SR, Hammond A, Griffiths L, Greenwood R, Clarke CR. Subarachnoid haemorrhage – can we do better? *Journal of the Royal Society of Medicine* 1989; **82**: 721–724.

Pickard JD, Murray GD, Illingworth R *et al.* Effect of oral nimodipine on cerebral infarction and outcome after subarachnoid haemorrhage: British aneurysm nimodipine trial. *British Medical Journal* 1989; **298**: 636–642.

Van Gijn J, Rinkel GJE. Sub-arachnoid haemorrhage: diagnosis, causes and management. *Brain* 2001; **124**: 249–278.

Other relevant entries Aneurysm; Cerebrovascular disease: arterial; Coital cephalalgia, coital headache; Ehlers–Danlos syndrome; Glasgow Coma Scale; Headache: an overview; Fibromuscular dysplasia; Marfan syndrome; Neurofibromatosis; Pituitary disease and apoplexy; Spinal cord vascular diseases; Superficial siderosis of the central nervous system; Terson's syndrome; Thunderclap headache.

■ Subclavian steal syndrome

A haemodynamically significant stenosis of the subclavian artery located proximal to the origin of the vertebral artery may lead to reversal of blood flow in the vertebral artery, towards the axillary artery, sometimes provoked by ipsilateral arm exercise. This may cause neurological signs (vertebrobasilar transient ischaemic attacks), accompanied by typical signs (asymmetric blood pressure in the arms, supraclavicular bruit). However, asymptomatic steal, demonstrated at ultrasonography or angiographically, is much more common than symptomatic, perhaps because of collateral brainstem blood flow. Symptomatic subclavian steal may be treated surgically (endarterectomy, angioplasty).

Reference Hennerici M, Klemm C, Rautenberg W. The subclavian steal phenomenon: a common vascular disorder with rare neurological deficits. *Neurology* 1988; **38**: 669–673.

Other relevant entry Transient ischaemic attacks.

▥ Subcortical arteriosclerotic encephalopathy – see Binswanger's disease

▥ Subcortical band heterotopia – see Heterotopia

▥ Subcortical dementia, subcortical syndrome – see Dementia: an overview

▥ Subdural empyema

Pathophysiology Subdural empyema is purulent bacterial infection between the dura and pia mater which may spread over the hemispheres to lie in the parafalcine region (*cf.* cerebral abscess). Raised intracranial pressure and seizures may result. It occurs most commonly after trauma (including neurosurgery), although non-traumatic cases are well recognized, for example in association with severe middle ear and paranasal sinus disease. Other infective processes, such as meningitis (10%), cerebral abscess (20–25%) and cerebral venous thrombosis (20–40%) may also be present. It typically affects men between the ages of 10 and 30 years, and may be extremely difficult to diagnose in the early stages.

Clinical features: history and examination
- Headache: frontal, generalized.
- Fever, malaise, meningism.
- Drowsiness (rapid decline).
- Focal neurological deficits: hemiparesis, aphasia, cranial nerve lesions.
- +/− papilloedema, raised intracranial pressure.
- +/− seizures: focal, generalized (especially post-operative).
- A past history of sinus disease is common.

Investigations and diagnosis *Imaging*: CT may be normal initially, needing to be repeated if clinical suspicion is high or there is no access to MRI. Subdural collection, hemisphere swelling may be evident. The patient may require sedation if restless to ensure adequate scan quality.

Skull/sinus X-rays: sinus opacification (frontal > ethmoid > maxillary).

CSF: mild to moderate pleocytosis, raised protein, normal glucose; Gram stain (may be normal).

Differential diagnosis

Cerebral abscess.

Bacterial meningitis.

Treatment and prognosis Surgery (formal exploration preferred to burr holes) to aspirate pus + appropriate antibiotic therapy.

Microbiology: common organisms are *Streptococcus milleri, Staphylococcus aureus,* and *Escherichia coli*; appropriate antibiotics include penicillin, metronidazole.

Control of seizures: may be difficult; prophylaxis may be indicated.

Complete recovery may occur, but residual disability and seizures are possible. There remains an appreciable mortality rate.

References Hodges J, Anslow P, Gillett G. Subdural empyema – continuing diagnostic problems in the CT scan era. *Quarterly Journal of Medicine* 1986; **59**: 387–393.

Kubik CS, Adams RD. Subdural empyema. *Brain* 1943; **66**: 18–42.

Other relevant entries Abscess: an overview; Infection and the nervous system: an overview.

■ Subdural haematoma

Pathophysiology Collections of blood in the subdural space are more often cranial than spinal. Cranial subdural haematoma (SDH) may be acute (occurring within 72 hours of head injury), subacute, or chronic. The latter condition presents a particular diagnostic challenge as no history of head trauma may be forthcoming. Furthermore, SDH may mimic other neurological syndromes; the presenting features may be non-localizing, and imaging apparently normal. A high index of clinical suspicion is therefore necessary, particularly in elderly patients with altered behaviour. Besides head trauma (often in the context of alcohol overindulgence), other recognized risk factors for SDH include anticoagulation, chronic renal failure/haemodialysis, and, although rare, spontaneous intracranial hypotension.

Clinical features: history and examination

Cranial:

- Headache
- Cognitive impairment; fluctuating state of arousal
- Neurological signs may be absent, but sometimes there is accompanying papilloedema, pyramidal signs, brainstem compression, aphasia.

Spinal: acute spinal cord compression.

Investigations and diagnosis *Bloods*: clotting studies, especially INR in a patient receiving therapeutic anticoagulation with warfarin.

Imaging: CT may show subdural collection, effacement of cortical sulci, midline shift. However, isodense collections may be missed; bilateral lesions may not be accompanied by midline shift. MRI is more sensitive in such cases; it is the imaging modality of choice for spinal haematoma.

Differential diagnosis

Cranial:

Acute confusional states.

Evolving mass lesions, for example tumour, cerebral abscess.

Spinal:

spinal epidural or intramedullary haemorrhage, abscess; tumour; acute inflammatory myelopathy.

Treatment and prognosis Evacuation of clot; through burr holes for cranial SDH, especially if acute (if patient is anticoagulated this will need to be reversed before surgery). In chronic cases, conservative management may be preferable. Reaccumulation of cranial subdural collections may occur.

References Davenport RJ, Statham PFX, Warlow CP. Detection of bilateral isodense subdural haematomas. *British Medical Journal* 1994; **309**: 792–794.

McKissock W, Richardson A, Bloom WH. Subdural haematoma – a review of 389 cases. *Lancet* 1960; **1**: 1365–1369.

Other relevant entries Alcohol and the nervous system: an overview; Arachnoid cyst; Encephalopathies: an overview; Haematoma: an overview; Renal disease and the nervous system; Spontaneous intracranial hypotension.

■ Subependymoma – see Ependymoma

■ Submedullary syndrome – see Opalski's syndrome

■ Sudanophilic leukodystrophy – see Leukodystrophies: an overview; Pelizaeus–Merzbacher disease

■ Sudden unexplained death in epilepsy

The increased mortality in patients with epilepsy may be in part attributable to both the underlying disease and to epileptic seizures. At least part of this excess mortality is ascribed to sudden unexplained death in epilepsy (SUDEP), which may be defined as sudden unexpected non-traumatic and non-drowning death in an individual with epilepsy with or without evidence for a seizure, and excluding documented status epilepticus, where postmortem does not reveal a cause for death. It is believed likely that SUDEP is a seizure-related phenomenon whose prevention rests on optimization of seizure control.

Reference Langan Y, Nashef L. Sudden unexpected death in epilepsy (SUDEP). *Advances in Clinical Neuroscience and Rehabilitation* 2003; **2(6)**: 6–8.

Other relevant entry Epilepsy: an overview.

■ Sudeck's atrophy, Sudeck–Leriche syndrome – see Complex regional pain syndromes

▪ SUNCT syndrome

Pathophysiology *S*hort-lasting *u*nilateral *n*euralgiform headache with *c*onjunctival injection and *t*earing (SUNCT) syndrome is a paroxysmal disorder, attacks lasting seconds to minutes (rarely up to 2 hours) and occurring five to six times per hour, sometimes precipitated by neck movement. Men are more commonly affected than women. The duration of attacks distinguishes SUNCT from trigeminal neuralgia and episodic hemicrania.

Clinical features: history and examination
- Conjunctival injection, tearing.
- Other autonomic phenomena: sweating on the forehead, rhinorrhoea.

Investigations and diagnosis Diagnosis is by history. Imaging to look for secondary causes [e.g. cerebellopontine angle arteriovenous malformation (AVM)] is recommended.

Differential diagnosis
Cluster headache.
Trigeminal neuralgia.
Chronic paroxysmal (episodic) hemicrania.

Treatment and prognosis Verapamil may help; indomethacin does not (*cf.* episodic hemicrania).

> **Reference** Goadsby PJ, Lipton RB. A review of paroxysmal hemicranias, SUNCT syndrome and other short-lasting headaches with autonomic features, including new cases. *Brain* 1997; **120**: 193–209.

> **Other relevant entries** Chronic paroxysmal hemicrania; Cluster headache; Headache: an overview; Trigeminal neuralgia.

▪ Superficial siderosis of the central nervous system

Pathophysiology Siderosis is deposition of haemosiderin in the superficial layers of the central nervous system (CNS) close to CSF (i.e. subpial, subependymal deposition) as a consequence of chronic subarachnoid haemorrhage, with associated gliosis, neuronal loss, and demyelination.

Clinical features: history and examination
- Sensorineural deafness.
- Cerebellar ataxia.
- Pyramidal signs.
- Dementia.
- Bladder disturbance.
- Anosmia.

Investigations and diagnosis Pure tone audiometry to confirm sensorineural hearing loss; speech audiogram is much worse than expected on the basis of pure tone audiometry.

Imaging:

> MRI: T_2-weighted scans show signal void around affected areas of brain, corresponding to haemosiderin.
> Angiography: may identify a bleeding source.

CSF: elevated protein, ferritin.

Differential diagnosis Meningeal infiltration (inflammation, infection, tumour). Intrinsic brain stem lesion.

Treatment and prognosis

Treatment of bleeding source if found (ideally by surgical ablation).

Cochlear implants to help speech appreciation.

Iron-chelating agents (e.g. trientine): value not proven.

If no bleeding point identified, there is usually relentless progression of neurological signs with a grave prognosis.

> **Reference** Fearnley JM, Stevens JM, Rudge P. Superficial siderosis of the central nervous system. *Brain* 1995; **118**: 1051–1066.

> **Other relevant entry** Subarachnoid haemorrhage.

■ Superior oblique myokymia

Pathophysiology A syndrome of intermittent uniocular oscillopsia due to involuntary eye movements, usually following a superior oblique (trochlear nerve) palsy. It has been suggested that some cases result from vascular compression of the trochlear nerve.

Clinical features: history and examination

- Uniocular oscillopsia (i.e. illusion of movement or oscillation of the environment).
- Episodic involuntary eye movements, vertical, torsional, or oblique. May be precipitated by tiredness, reading.

Investigations and diagnosis Slit-lamp examination: best way to observe eye movements.

Differential diagnosis Other causes of oscillopsia: vestibular failure, upbeat nystagmus (usually bilateral).

Treatment and prognosis Carbamazepine may help. In the event of failure, surgical interventions may be tried.

> **Reference** Brazis PW, Miller NR, Henderer JD, Lee AG. The natural history and results of treatment of superior oblique myokymia. *Archives of Ophthalmology* 1994; **112**: 1063–1067.

> **Other relevant entries** Cranial nerve disease: IV: Trochlear nerve; Myokymia; Neurovascular compression syndromes; Oscillopsia.

■ Superior oblique tendon sheath syndrome – see Brown's syndrome

■ Superior orbital fissure syndrome – see Cranial nerve disease: III: Oculomotor nerve

■ Susac syndrome
Retinocochleocerebral vasculopathy

Pathophysiology A rare, idiopathic, non-inflammatory vasculopathy affecting principally young women, usually following a monophasic but fluctuating course, and causing small infarcts in the cochlea, retina, and brain.

Clinical features: history and examination

- Sensorineural deafness.
- Branch retinal arteriolar occlusions.
- Encephalopathy, +/− acute psychiatric features.
- Upper motor neurone limb signs (spasticity, hyperreflexia, Babinski sign).
- Cranial nerve palsies (III, VI, VII).
- Cognitive dysfunction (impaired short-term memory).
- Seizures.

Investigations and diagnosis *Imaging*: MRI: multifocal high intensity lesions on T_2-weighted scans, affecting white and (to a lesser extent) grey matter; lesions (infarcts) show enhancement with gadolinium during attacks.

Neurophysiology: EEG: diffuse slowing, +/− seizure activity.

CSF: raised protein, lymphocytic pleocytosis.

Pure tone audiometry: bilateral sensorineural hearing loss, especially at low frequencies.

Bloods: ANA negative.

Neurogenetics: Factor V Leiden mutation reported in one case, of uncertain significance.

Differential diagnosis

Multiple sclerosis.

Systemic vasculitides/vasculopathies.

Mitochondrial disease.

Adrenoleukodystrophy.

Treatment and prognosis Difficult to assess because of rarity of condition and variable natural history. The following have been tried:

Immunosuppression: prednisolone, cyclophosphamide, IVIg

Antiplatelet treatment: aspirin

Anticoagulation: warfarin.

Illness is usually monophasic.

References Papo T, Biousse V, Lehoang P *et al*. Susac syndrome. *Medicine (Baltimore)* 1998; **77**: 3–11.

Petty GW, Engel AG, Younge BR *et al*. Retinocochleocerebral vasculopathy. *Medicine (Baltimore)* 1998; **77**: 12–40.

Susac JO, Hardman JM, Selhorst JB. Microangiopathy of the brain and retina. *Neurology* 1979; **29**: 313–316.

Other relevant entries Cerebrovascular disease: arterial; Vasculitis.

■ Sweet's syndrome
Acute febrile neutrophilic dermatosis

This syndrome consists of acute multiple asymmetric erythematous oedematous mucocutaneous plaques with dense neutrophil infiltration; there may also be blood neutrophilia. In some cases a relapsing–remitting encephalitis has been noted, producing a clinical picture which may be mistaken for Behçet's disease. However, unlike Behçet's, there is a strong association with HLAB54. Drug-induced Sweet's syndrome has been reported. Sweet's syndrome is an exquisitely steroid-sensitive disease.

References Hisanaga K, Hosokawa M, Sato N, Mochizuki H, Itoyama Y, Iwasaki Y. "Neuro-sweet disease": benign recurrent encephalitis with neutrophilic dermatosis. *Archives of Neurology* 1999; **56**: 1010–1013.

Stenzel W, Frosch PJ, Schwarz M. Sweet's syndrome associated with acute benign encephalitis. A drug induced aetiology. *Journal of Neurology* 2003; **250**: 770–771.

Other relevant entries Behçet's disease; Encephalitis: an overview.

■ Sydenham's chorea
Rheumatic chorea ● St Vitus' dance

Pathophysiology A choreiform movement disorder related to group A streptococcal infection. The condition usually occurs in childhood and early-adult life, and is commoner in females. It is usually self-limiting but more persistent neurobehavioural features sometimes occur. An association with rheumatic heart disease was noted more than a century ago. Chorea may occur several months after infection. There may be an analogy with paediatric autoimmune neuropsychiatric disorders associated with streptococcal infection (PANDAS). Sydenham's chorea is now uncommon in developed countries.

Clinical features: history and examination

- Chorea: generalized > hemichorea; insidious onset, progressive course, gradual spontaneous resolution.
- +/− psychiatric symptoms, for example obsessive–compulsive behaviour.
- No cognitive deterioration (except possibly some slight frontal dysexecutive difficulties).

Investigations and diagnosis No diagnostic test; many investigations seek to rule out other causes of chorea:

Bloods: ASO titres; ANA, anti-cardiolipin antibodies, anti-basal ganglia antibodies; glucose, osmolality, thyroid function tests, haematocrit, haemoglobin.

Imaging:

CT usually normal;

MRI may show diffuse enlargement of basal ganglia (caudate, putamen, globus pallidus);

PET scan: striatal hypermetabolism.

Neurophysiology:

EEG: diffuse slowing;

Somatosensory evoked potential (SSEP): normal.

CSF: usually normal.

Differential diagnosis Other causes of chorea: Huntington's disease, neuroacanthocytosis, thyroid disorders, SLE, hyperosmolar non-ketotic syndrome (HONKS), polycythaemia rubra vera, drug induced (OC pill, phenytoin).

Treatment and prognosis May or may not require treatment: valproate, dopamine antagonists (e.g. haloperidol) have been used. In severe cases IVIg, plasmapheresis, and immunosuppression have been tried. Generally resolves spontaneously, but may recur within 2 years.

> **Reference** Giedd JN, Rapoport JL, Kruesi MJP *et al.* Sydenham's chorea: magnetic resonance imaging of the basal ganglia. *Neurology* 1995; **45**: 2199–2202.

> **Other relevant entries** Chorea; Huntington's disease; PANDAS syndrome; Systemic lupus erythematosus and the nervous system, Thyroid disease and the nervous system.

■ Sylvester disease

Pathophysiology An autosomal-dominant hereditary disease characterized by optic atrophy and visual loss, progressive hearing loss and ataxia. Its nosology is uncertain: it may perhaps represent a form of spinocerebellar ataxia (autosomal-dominant cerebellar ataxia) or of Friedreich's ataxia.

Clinical features: history and examination

- Progressive visual loss; peripheral constriction of visual fields, optic atrophy.
- Progressive hearing loss: moderate to severe.
- Ataxia.
- Muscle wasting: weak shoulder girdle, hands.
- Mentally "dull".
- +/− nystagmus.
- No diabetes.
- Family history of similar conditions.

Investigations and diagnosis In view of the similarity of the phenotype to that seen in Friedreich's ataxia, it may be worth looking at the frataxin gene in patients with suspected Sylvester disease.

Differential diagnosis

Friedreich's ataxia.

Spinocerebellar ataxia.

Treatment and prognosis No specific treatment. Prognosis variable dependent on age of onset: death may occur within months in childhood onset, or the disease may last many years.

> **Reference** Sylvester PE. Some unusual findings in a family with Friedreich's ataxia. *Archives of Disease in Childhood* 1958; **33**: 217–221.

> **Other relevant entries** Friedreich's ataxia; Nyssen–van Bogaert syndrome; Rosenberg–Chutorian syndrome; Spinocerebellar ataxia; Tunbridge–Paley syndrome.

■ Sylvian aqueduct syndrome – see Parinaud's syndrome

■ Syncope
Neurally mediated syncope • Vasovagal syncope

Pathophysiology Syncope is a sudden, transient (>30 minutes) loss of consciousness and postural tone, leading to collapse. It is often associated with reduced cerebral blood flow. Syncope may be classified as:

Neurally mediated:
Peripheral vascular reflex (vasovagal) syncope
Orthostatic (postural) syncope (as in autonomic failure).
Idiopathic ("syncope of unknown origin").

Cardiac:
Arrhythmia: bradycardia, tachy-arrhythmia
Valvular disease: aortic stenosis, hypertrophic subaortic stenosis.

Situational:
Cough/post-tusive
Micturition
Swallow/deglutition.

Metabolic:
Hypoglycaemia.
Psychogenic.

Syncopal attacks may provoke secondary (anoxic) epileptic seizures which may confuse the diagnosis.

Clinical features: history and examination

• Peripheral vascular reflex mechanisms (vasovagal syncope; common): premonitory symptoms (presyncope) include light-headedness (often described as "dizziness"), weakness, feeling of distance, blacking of vision, nausea, and sweating (useful to exclude seizure); gradual slump to ground; pallor; there may be some twitching movements at the periphery, or even marked and repeated myoclonic jerks, but not tonic–clonic movements (unless there is a secondary anoxic seizure); nonetheless an untrained observer may mistake these for a "convulsion" or "seizure"; urinary incontinence may occur even in the absence of epileptic seizure (some studies do not find incontinence a useful discriminator between seizure and syncope). A slow pulse may be detected. Rapid recovery, no prolonged postictal confusion; prolonged disorientation (more than few minutes) after a blackout increases the likelihood that it was a seizure (as does increasing age).

- Provoking features: cough syncope, micturition syncope: valsalva manoeuvre associated with these activities may trigger an attack. In swallow syncope, associated with metastatic disease of the glossopharyngeal or vagus nerves, or glossopharyn-geal neuralgia, swallowing stimulates baroreceptor nerves causing profound bradycardia.
- Orthostatic (postural) syncope: events similar to above associated with change in posture from lying or sitting to standing.
- Cardiac (rare): may be triggered by exercise. There may be signs of aortic stenosis, sick sinus syndrome, prolonged QT syndromes (Romano–Ward syndrome, Jervell–Lange–Nielsen syndrome), cardiac dysrhythmia.

Investigations and diagnosis Neural: diagnosis is largely by history alone; eyewitness account may be helpful (but see caveat above concerning twitching/convulsive movements).

Standing/lying blood pressure: if orthostatic syncope suspected (of no value in vaso-vagal syncope); may need to wait a few minutes after standing before drop occurs.

Bloods: to exclude anaemia and hyponatraemia, may be appropriate.

ECG: to exclude short PR interval, prolonged QT interval; +/− echocardiogram to exclude aortic stenosis, hypertrophic obstructive cardiomyopathy.

Tilt table testing: to exclude orthostatic syncope.

Neurophysiology: EEG: may be indicated if seizure seems more likely than syncope as cause of loss of consciousness.

Differential diagnosis

Epileptic seizure (atonic).

Drop attacks.

Transient ischaemic attack (TIA) (rarely associated with loss of consciousness).

Treatment and prognosis Reassurance is often all that is required for vasovagal attacks. Syncope of unknown origin is a useful diagnosis since it has an excellent prognosis. Drugs such as fludrocortisone, β-blockers, and serotonin reuptake inhibitors are sometimes used. For cardiogenic syncope, specific treatment (from cardiologists!) may be available, for example for arrhythmias.

References Arthur W, Kaye GC. Current investigations used to assess syncope. *Postgraduate Medical Journal* 2001; **77**: 20–23.

Brignole M, Alboni P, Benditt D *et al.* Guidelines on management (diagnosis and treatment) of syncope. *European Heart Journal* 2001; **22**: 1256–1306.

Hoefnagels WAJ, Padberg GW, Overweg J, van der Welde EA, Roos RAC. Transient loss of consciousness: the value of the history for distinguishing seizure from syncope. *Journal of Neurology* 1991; **238**: 39–43.

Lempert T, Bauer MS, Schmidt D. Syncope: a videometric analysis of 56 episodes of transient cerebral hypoxia. *Annals of Neurology* 1994; **36**: 233–237.

Martin GJ, Arron MJ. Approach to the patient with syncope. In: Biller J (ed.). *Practical Neurology* (2nd edition). Philadelphia: Lippincott Williams & Wilkins, 2002: 76–83.

Other relevant entries Autonomic failure; Drop attacks; Epilepsy: an overview; Glossopharyngeal neuralgia; Prolonged QT syndromes.

■ Syndrome of inappropriate ADH secretion

Pathophysiology Inappropriate (autonomous) production of antidiuretic hormone (ADH) leads to "water intoxication" with hyponatraemia and inappropriate antidiuresis; thirst is also abnormal. The resulting hyponatraemia may have neurological consequences, but only if severe (plasma sodium concentration <120 mmol/l). Treatment should be aimed at the underlying cause where possible, rather than to the electrolyte disturbance itself.

Various causes of SIADH are described including:

Ectopic ADH production, most commonly by oat cell carcinoma of the lung
Drug induced, for example carbamazepine, vincristine, cis-platinum
Non-specific effect of intracranial tumour
Following subarachnoid haemorrhage (SAH), especially anterior communicating artery aneurysm rupture (although low sodium may be due to cerebral salt wasting in some SAH patients)
Following bacterial meningitis, viral encephalitis, tuberculous meningitis
Head injury
Diabetic ketoacidosis
Porphyria (acute attacks).

Clinical features: history and examination
• Confusional state, lethargy, disorientation (encephalopathy).
• Muscle weakness, ataxia, tremulousness.
• Seizures.
• Focal signs.
• Coma.

Investigations and diagnosis Normal renal and adrenal function are *sine qua non* for the diagnosis of SIADH.

Concurrent studies of blood and urine which show:

Hyponatraemia (Na^+ <128 mmol/l) and reduced plasma osmolality
Increased urinary sodium excretion, urine osmolality >300 mosmol/l
Normal renal, hepatic, adrenal, thyroid function
No volume depletion/dehydration
No diuretic usage.

Cause may be obvious (SAH, meningitis, head injury); if not, chest radiography/ CT/MRI to look for lung tumour; review all drug therapy.

Differential diagnosis Other causes of encephalopathy, coma; hyponatraemia (e.g. cerebral salt wasting syndrome).

Treatment and prognosis Identify and treat primary cause where possible.

Specific treatment of SIADH: Restrict fluid intake to 0.5–1.5 l/day (dependent on the severity of hyponatraemia); in some circumstances care is needed as restriction itself may be hazardous, for example bacterial meningitis, SAH, increasing the risk of cerebral infarction.

Agents to induce nephrogenic diabetes insipidus have occasionally been used, for example demethylchlortetracycline (demeclocycline), lithium, phenytoin.

Occasionally sodium replacement may be indicated (2 N NaCl); however, rapid correction is best avoided since it increases the risk of "osmotic demyelination syndrome" or central pontine myelinolysis.

Reference Robertson GL. Syndrome of inappropriate antidiuresis. *New England Journal of Medicine* 1989; **321**: 538–539.

Other relevant entries Central pontine myelinolysis; Cerebral salt wasting syndrome; Chemotherapy- and radiotherapy-induced neurological disorders; Coma; Encephalopathies: an overview; Porphyria; Subarachnoid haemorrhage, Tuberculosis and the nervous system.

■ Synucleinopathy

A large kindred of autosomal-dominant Parkinson's disease (PD), the Contersi family, was linked to a substitution mutation in the gene encoding α-synuclein (labelled PD1) in 1997. The mutation occurs in a position which may disrupt protein α-helical structure in favour of β-sheet; it is possible that self-aggregation of the mutant protein might be the result. A number of other autosomal-dominant PD kindreds do not show genetic linkage to PD1, nor mutations in the α-synuclein gene: other genetic mutations underpinning PD have been described, for example in the parkin gene.

α-synuclein immunohistochemistry has shown this protein to be the major filamentous component of Lewy bodies in both PD and dementia with Lewy bodies (DLB), hence the use of "synucleinopathy" as a generic term. α-synuclein is also present in Alzheimer's disease cases with Lewy bodies. The glial cytoplasmic inclusions of multiple system atrophy also contain α-synuclein, although Lewy bodies are not seen.

References Polymeropoulos MH, Lavedan C, Leroy E *et al.* Mutation in the α-synuclein gene identified in families with Parkinson's disease. *Science* 1997; **276**: 2045–2047.

Spillantini MG, Crowther RA, Jakes R, Hasegawa M, Goedert M. α-synuclein in filamentous inclusions of Lewy bodies from Parkinson's disease and dementia with Lewy bodies. *Proceedings of the National Academy of Sciences of the USA* 1998; **95**: 6469–6473.

Other relevant entries Alzheimer's disease; Dementia with Lewy bodies; Lewy body disease: an overview; Multiple system atrophy; Parkinson's disease.

■ Syphilis

Pathophysiology Following infection, the spirochaete *Treponema pallidum* may invade the nervous system (neurosyphilis), usually within 18 months of inoculation, producing a meningitic picture (asymptomatic or clinically apparent) which may regress spontaneously or progress to parenchymal disease, which also involves the blood vessels. The clinical syndromes often show more widespread pathological evidence of chronic meningitis. In meningovascular syphilis, inflammation and fibrosis of arteries may be found (Heubner's arteritis). There has been a recent resurgence of neurosyphilis cases, partly in the context of HIV/AIDS.

Clinical features: history and examination Neurological features of treponemal infection include:

- Asymptomatic meningitis (based entirely on CSF findings)
- Meningeal: headache, stiff neck, cranial nerve palsies, no fever; $+/-$ raised intracranial pressure.
- Parenchymal:
  - Meningovascular: cerebrovascular events (e.g. in a young person) causing hemiplegia, aphasia, visual disturbances, sensory loss.
  - Tabes dorsalis, tabetic neurosyphilis: sensory (locomotor) ataxia, absent lower limb tendon reflexes, lightning pains in the legs, Charcot joints, urinary incontinence, Argyll Robertson pupils, ptosis, ophthalmoplegia, optic atrophy; pathologically there is degeneration of the posterior columns of the spinal cord.
  - General paralysis/paresis of the insane (GPI), dementia paralytica: dementia, myoclonus, seizures, hyperreflexia, Argyll Robertson pupils.
  - Syphilitic optic atrophy: often coexists with tabes dorsalis.
  - Spinal syphilis (other than tabes): meningomyelitis, meningovascular.
  - Syphilitic nerve deafness.
- Gummatous.
- Osteitis of skull and spine.

Investigations and diagnosis

Serology:

Venereal Disease Research Laboratory (VDRL) test: flocculation technique: may be negative in neurosyphilis.

Fluorescent treponemal antibody absorption (FTA-ABS) test: for antibodies specifically directed against treponemal antigens.

CSF: the key investigation in suspected neurosyphilis: raised cell count, mostly lymphocytes; raised protein; increased gammaglobulins with oligoclonal bands; normal glucose; positive serology.

Consider checking HIV status.

Imaging: may show consequences; brain atrophy, cerebrovascular changes.

Differential diagnosis Other causes of:

chronic meningitides: TB, neurobrucellosis, fungal;

stroke in the young: vasculitis, dissection;

sensory ataxia;

cognitive decline.

Other causes of positive VDRL: yaws, systemic lupus erythematosus (SLE) (false positive).

Treatment and prognosis Penicillin or erythromycin or tetracycline. Monitor CSF after 6 months to see if alterations have reversed (positive VDRL may persist); if not further courses of antibiotics may be given.

> **Reference** Wood M, Anderson M. *Neurological Infections*. London: WB Saunders, 1988: 517–537.

> **Other relevant entries** Argyll Robertson pupil; Ataxia; Autonomic failure; Brucellosis; HIV/AIDS and the nervous system; Radiculopathies: an overview; Sarcoidosis; Spinal cord disease: an overview; Systemic lupus erythematosus and the nervous system; Tuberculosis and the nervous system; Vasculitis; Vogt–Koyanagi–Harada syndrome.

■ Syringomyelia and syringobulbia

Pathophysiology Syringomyelia, or syringohydromyelia, is an expanding fluid-filled cavity within the spinal cord, which gradually impinges on nervous tissue, initially the crossing spinothalamic fibres of the ventral funiculus of the cord producing a suspended (vest-like, "cuirasse") and dissociated sensory loss (pain and temperature), but eventually involving descending motor pathways causing a paraparesis, and anterior horn cells causing localized lower motor neurone signs. The cavity may extend into the brainstem, where it is known as syringobulbia, causing cranial nerve signs. The cause of such cavities is uncertain but may relate to disordered CSF hydrodynamics. Syringomyelia is often associated with structural anomalies of the foramen magnum (Chiari malformations) and hydrocephalus, but there are other recognized causes and associations. A simple classification is as follows:

> Developmental
> Acquired
>> Sequel to:
>>> spinal cord trauma
>>> spinal cord tumours
>>> arachnoiditis
>>> intrinsic spinal cord inflammation (rare).
> Idiopathic.

Clinical features: history and examination

- Early: dissociated sensory loss (spinothalamic) in suspended pattern; may be asymmetrical; painless trauma to fingers, hands may occur.
- Late: upper limb radicular features; Charcot joints in upper limb; lower limb upper motor neurone features.
- Very late: dorsal column loss.
- +/− autonomic features.

Investigations and diagnosis *Imaging*: MRI is the examination of choice, including views of the foramen magnum for Chiari malformations, and the brain for hydrocephalus.

Neurophysiology: EMG/NCS: denervation changes with fibrillation potentials may be found, causing confusion with motor neurone disease (MND) if sensory signs are minimal.

Differential diagnosis Other intrinsic spinal cord pathology, such as tumour, trauma, inflammation. A selective loss of pain and temperature modalities with relative preservation of vibration and position sense (pseudosyringomyelia) may also be seen in amyloid polyneuropathy and Tangier disease (small fibre sensory neuropathy). Predominance of motor signs may lead to suspicion of MND.

Treatment and prognosis Where possible treatment is of the cause, for example foramen magnum decompression, tumour resection. In idiopathic cases, the judgement as to whether some form of surgical intervention will be beneficial is difficult. Some cavities are slowly but relentlessly progressive and lead to significant disability.

References Anson JA, Benzel EC, Awad IA (eds). *Syringomyelia and the Chiari Malformations*. Park Ridge, Illinois: American Association of Neurological Surgeons, 1997.

Barnett HJM, Foster JB, Hudgson P. *Syringomyelia*. London: WB Saunders, 1973.

Larner AJ, Muqit MMK, Glickman S. Concurrent syrinx and inflammatory CNS disease detected by magnetic resonance imaging: an illustrative case and review of the literature. *Medicine (Baltimore)* 2002; **81**: 41–50.

Other relevant entries Amyloid and the nervous system: an overview; Arachnoiditis; Chiari malformations; Hydrocephalus; Myelopathy: an overview; Spinal cord disease: an overview; Tangier disease.

■ Systemic lupus erythematosus and the nervous system

Pathophysiology Systemic lupus erythematosus (SLE) is a multisystem autoimmune disorder of the collagen vascular disease group; very rarely there may be a true vasculitis. It is commoner in women and Afro-Caribbeans. Diagnostic criteria are available.

Clinical features: history and examination

- Non-neurological
    Systemic: fever, malaise.
    Rheumatological: symmetrical non-erosive arthritis of large and small joints.
    Dermatological: malar (butterfly) rash, maculopapular rash, livedo reticularis, photosensitivity.
    Renal: glomerulonephritis.
    Pulmonary: pleurisy, pneumonitis.
    Cardiac: pericarditis, Libman–Sacks endocarditis.
    Haematological: anaemia, thrombocytopenia, lupus anticoagulant (predisposing to arterial and venous thromboses).
- Neurological: 25–75% of patients affected in different series; uncommon as a presenting sign of SLE

Central nervous system (CNS):

  Headache: migraine, venous sinus thrombosis, "idiopathic" intracranial hypertension, aseptic meningitis.

  Psychiatric: hallucinations, delusions, schizophreniform psychosis, depression.

  Delirium: "lupus encephalopathy".

  Arterial strokes, repeated transient ischaemic attacks (TIAs): associated with anti-cardiolipin antibodies (secondary antiphospholipid antibody syndrome); cerebral embolism secondary to endocarditis; venous sinus thrombosis; may cause focal signs, hemiparesis, aphasia.

  Cognitive impairment, dementia: may be reversible (not if due to multiple infarcts).

  Chorea, choreoathetosis, ballism, parkinsonism, tremor (rare).

  Myelopathy: acute or subacute (rare).

  Cranial nerve palsy (III, IV, V, VI) (rare).

  Optic neuropathy (rare).

  Cerebellar ataxia (rare).

Peripheral nervous system (PNS):

  Peripheral neuropathy:

    Acute or subacute symmetrical demyelinating polyneuropathy

    Guillain–Barré syndrome-like illness

    Mononeuropathy, single or multiple

  + iatrogenic neurological problems (e.g. opportunistic infection in immunosuppressed patient).

Investigations and diagnosis *Bloods*: anaemia, leucopenia, thrombocytopenia; lupus anticoagulant (prolonged activated partial thromboplastin time and Russell Viper Venom time).

  Serology: ANA (usually >1/160), anti-ds DNA (50%), anti-Ro (30%), anti-La (15%), anti-Sm (75%), anti-RNP (30%), anti-cardiolipin (IgG, IgM, IgA antiphospholipid); false positive Venereal Disease Research Laboratory (VDRL).

  Imaging: CT/MRI brain: infarcts, haemorrhage; multiple subcortical lesions more prevalent than periventricular lesions; MRI cord to exclude compression in cases of myelopathy.

  CSF: raised protein, pleocytosis; positive oligoclonal bands in around 50%; low glucose may be found in association with myelopathy.

  Hunt for secondary/iatrogenic problems, for example complications of immunosuppression.

Differential diagnosis Broad! Other multisystem disorders: Behçet's, vasculitic syndromes; multiple sclerosis.

Treatment and prognosis No randomized-controlled trial data available.

Inflammation: steroids +/− azathioprine, cyclophosphamide (oral, IV pulsed); plasma exchange for acute fulminant cases; IVIg.

Stroke with anti-cardiolipin antibodies (NB positive in 25% of normal population): warfarin (aim for INR >3).

Symptomatic treatment of epilepsy, psychosis, chorea.

Treatment of opportunistic infection.

Prognosis: reasonable, but neurological involvement is second only to renal disease as a cause of death.

References Scolding N. Neurological complications of rheumatological and connective tissue disorders. In: Scolding N (ed.). *Immunological and Inflammatory Disorders of the Central Nervous System.* Oxford: Butterworth-Heinemann, 1999: 147–180.

Scolding NJ, Joseph FG. The neuropathology and pathogenesis of systemic lupus erythematosus. *Neuropathology and Applied Neurobiology* 2002; **28**: 173–189.

Shapiro HS. Psychopathology in the patient with lupus. In: Wallace DJ, Hahn BH (eds). *Dubois' Lupus Erythematosus* (5th edition). Baltimore: Williams & Wilkins, 1997: 755–782.

Tan EM, Cohen AS, Fries JF *et al.* The 1982 revised criteria for the classification of systemic lupus erythematosus. *Arthritis Rheumatism* 1982; **25**: 1271–1277.

Wallace DJ, Metzger AL. Systemic lupus erythematosus and the nervous system. In: Wallace DJ, Hahn BH (eds). *Dubois' Lupus Erythematosus* (5th edition). Baltimore: Williams & Wilkins, 1997: 723–754.

Other relevant entries Antiphospholipid (antibody) syndrome; Cerebrovascular disease: arterial; Cerebrovascular disease: venous; Chorea; Collagen vascular disorders and the nervous system; Vasculitis.

▇ Systemic panniculitis – see Weber–Christian disease

▇ Systemic sclerosis

Progressive systemic sclerosis • Scleroderma

Pathophysiology A disorder of excess collagen deposition in blood vessels (hence "collagen vascular disease") affecting particularly the skin, but also other organs. Nervous system involvement is rare.

Clinical features: history and examination

- Non-neurological
    Dermatological: scleroderma: calcinosis, Raynaud's phenomenon, telangiectasia (=CREST syndrome when combined with oesophageal strictures); limited forms of cutaneous scleroderma occur (morphoea, some cases of Parry–Romberg syndrome, *coup de sabre*).
    Pleura, pericardia, kidney (glomerulonephritis) and eye may be involved.
- Neurological
    Peripheral nervous system (PNS):
        Trigeminal sensory neuropathy +/− pain

Peripheral neuropathy (sensorimotor axonopathy)

Myopathy, dermatomyositis (overlap syndrome, sclerodermatomyositis).

Central nervous system (CNS):

Cerebral angiopathy

Focal hemisphere/brainstem signs, extrapyramidal signs

Myelopathy

Cognitive decline, dementia (rare, but potentially reversible).

Investigations and diagnosis *Serology*: anti-centromere (85%); anti-SCL70 (50%); raised creatine kinase with muscle involvement.

CSF: raised protein.

Differential diagnosis Other collagen vascular disorders; eosinophilic fasciitis may mimic skin lesions.

Treatment and prognosis Very difficult: no disease modifying drugs known; symptomatic treatment of trigeminal sensory neuropathy (e.g. carbamazepine, gabapentin). Prognosis reasonable, renal and cardiac involvement being the principal causes of death.

References Black CM. The aetiopathogenesis of systemic sclerosis: thick skin – thin hypotheses. *Journal of the Royal College of Physicians of London* 1995; **29**: 119–130.

Scolding N. Neurological complications of rheumatological and connective tissue disorders. In: Scolding NJ (ed.). *Immunological and Inflammatory Disorders of the Central Nervous System*. Oxford: Butterworth-Heinemann, 1999: 147–180.

Other relevant entries Collagen vascular disorders and the nervous system; Dermatomyositis; Parry–Romberg syndrome; Raynaud's disease. Raynaud's phenomenon, Raynaud's syndrome; Systemic lupus erythematosus and the nervous system; Trigeminal sensory neuropathy.

Tt

■ Tabes dorsalis – see Syphilis

■ Takayasu's disease

Aortic arch/branch disease • Pulseless disease • Takayasu's arteritis

Pathophysiology A vasculitic disease affecting large blood vessels, especially the aorta and the proximal portions of its major branches, particularly affecting young women.

Clinical features: history and examination

- Absence of peripheral pulses, different blood pressure in two arms, bruits.
- Acute limb ischaemia.
- Hypertension, angina, heart murmurs (valvular incompetence).

- Visceral infarctions.
- Neurological:
    Syncope, especially related to exercise
    Headache
    Transient ischaemic attack (TIA) (carotid territory)
    Completed stroke (hemiparesis)
    +/− seizures
    +/− myelopathy.

Investigations and diagnosis *Bloods*: anaemia, raised ESR, hypergammaglobulinaemia.

Imaging: angiography (MRA, catheter) is first line investigation if diagnosis is suspected.

Pathology: similar to giant cell arteritis; vasa vasorum are involved. Cellular infiltrate is in the adventitia and outer media (*cf.* elastic lamina in giant cell arteritis).

Differential diagnosis Other vasculitides affecting large vessels (e.g. giant cell arteritis), although these tend not to affect the aorta and its major branches.
Occlusive atheromatous vascular disease.

Treatment and prognosis Steroids, +/− methotrexate, cyclophosphamide. Surgery for some stenoses.

References Kerr GS. Takayasu's arteritis. *Rheumatologic Disease Clinics of North America* 1995; **21**: 1041–1058.

Nadeau SE. Neurologic manifestations of systemic vasculitis. *Neurologic Clinics* 2002; **20**: 123–150.

Other relevant entries Giant cell arteritis; Isolated angiitis of the central nervous system; Polymyalgia rheumatica; Vasculitis.

▪ Tangier disease

Analphalipoproteinaemia • Familial high-density lipoprotein deficiency

Pathophysiology A very rare autosomal-recessive disorder affecting the reticuloendothelial system and peripheral nerves, with onset in childhood, resulting from severe deficiency of plasma high-density lipoproteins (HDL) leading to cholesterol ester deposition in many tissues. The condition was originally described in individuals originating from Tangier Island, Virginia. Mutations in a gene on chromosome 9q31 encoding the ATP-binding-cassette transporter 1 (ABCA1) protein are responsible.

Clinical features: history and examination
- Two neuropathic variants are described:
    Progressive symmetrical neuropathy: faciobrachial muscle wasting and weakness with dissociated pain and temperature loss.
    Relapsing multifocal mononeuropathies (cranial, trunk, limb nerves).
- Other features:
    Enlarged yellow–orange tonsils (cholesterol laden).
    Early atherosclerosis.

Investigations and diagnosis *Bloods*: low HDL and serum cholesterol; raised or normal triglycerides; the lipid profile is diagnostic.

Neurophysiology: EMG/NCS: reduced motor conduction velocities; reduced amplitude sensory nerve action potentials.

Nerve biopsy:

> multifocal mononeuropathy variant: segmental demyelination/remyelination; symmetrical variant; loss of small myelinated and unmyelinated fibres; lipid vacuoles in Schwann cells.

Bone marrow: fat-laden macrophages.

Neurogenetics: mutation, insertion, and deletion of the ABCA1 gene have been reported.

Differential diagnosis Progressive symmetrical neuropathy may be mistaken for syringomyelia; multifocal mononeuropathy variant may be confused with vasculitic neuropathies and hereditary neuropathy with liability to pressure palsies.

Treatment and prognosis No specific treatment known.

References Brousseau ME, Schaefer EJ, Dupuis J *et al*. Novel mutations in the gene encoding ATP-binding cassette 1 in four Tangier disease kindreds. *Journal of Lipid Research* 2000; **41**: 433–441.

Frederickson DS, Altrocchi PH, Avioli LV, Goodman DS, Goodman HL. Tangier disease. *Annals of Internal Medicine* 1961; **55**: 1016–1031.

Kocen RS, King RHM, Thomas PK, Haas LF. Nerve biopsy findings in two cases of Tangier disease. *Acta Neuropathologica (Berlin)* 1973; **26**: 317–327.

Other relevant entries Autonomic failure; Neuropathies: an overview; Syringomyelia and syringobulbia.

■ Tapia's syndrome

A lower cranial nerve syndrome involving the extramedullary vagus (X) and hypoglossal (XII) nerves, characterized clinically by:

> Unilateral weakness of pharynx and larynx
> Unilateral weakness and atrophy of tongue
> Accessory nerve may or may not be involved (*cf.* Jackson's syndrome)
> +/− cervical sympathetic involvement.

The differential diagnosis encompasses the syndromes described by Jackson, Collet–Sicard, and Villaret in which the X and XII cranial nerves are involved, along with other lower cranial nerves.

Imaging with MRI may indicate the nature of the extramedullary brainstem pathology, and hence determine the appropriate treatment.

Other relevant entries Collet–Sicard syndrome; Jackson's syndrome; Jugular foramen syndrome; Schmidt's syndrome; Vernet's syndrome; Villaret's syndrome.

■ Tardive syndromes (akathisia, dyskinesia, dystonia, tic) – see Drug-induced movement disorders

■ Tarlov cyst
Sacral nerve root cyst

These cysts of the sacral nerve roots are sufficiently common to be regarded as normal variants. Often asymmetrical, with density as for CSF, they may enlarge the nerve root/sheath complex and cause benign expansion of the sacral nerve root canal. They may sometimes be associated with sciatica-like pain.

Other relevant entries Cysts: an overview; Sciatica.

■ Tarsal tunnel syndrome – see Tibial neuropathy

■ Tarui disease
Glycogen-storage disease (GSD) type VII • Muscle phosphofructokinase (PFK) deficiency

Pathophysiology Deficiency of the glycolytic pathway enzyme phosphofructokinase (PFK), inherited as an autosomal-recessive condition, leads to failure to convert glucose-6-phosphate to glucose-1-phosphate. Exercising (anaerobic) muscles are therefore unable to produce lactate; they become painful, cramped, and unable to relax. The muscle PFK isoenzyme is normally composed of four identical (M) subunits which are absent in Tarui disease. Mutations in the PFK M subunit gene on chromosome 1 have been reported. The disease is commoner in Ashkenazi Jews and Japanese than in other ethnic groups.

Clinical features: history and examination As for type V glycogen-storage disease, (GSD) McArdle's disease:
- Cramps, pain, and weakness of muscles with exercise; "second wind phenomenon" with subsequent moderate exercise
- +/− myoglobinuria, rhabdomyolysis
- +/− haemolytic anaemia.

Investigations and diagnosis *Bloods*: elevated creatine kinase during cramping attacks; compensated haemolytic anaemia +/− hyperuricaemia.
Ischaemic lactate test: no rise in blood lactate (not produced in contracted muscles).
Neurophysiology: EMG: electrical silence in contracted muscle.
Muscle biopsy: PFK histochemistry negative.

Differential diagnosis Type V GSD (McArdle's disease); in Tarui disease onset is earlier, attacks of cramps more severe, and aggravated by high-carbohydrate meals.

Treatment and prognosis No specific treatment. Avoid strenuous (anaerobic) exercise.

References Tarui S. Phosphofructokinase deficiency in skeletal muscle: a new type of glycogenosis. *Biochemistry and Biophysics Research Communications* 1965; **19**: 517–523.

Tsujino S, Servidei S, Tonin P *et al*. Identification of three novel mutations in non-Ashkenazi Italian patients with muscle phosphofructokinase deficiency. *American Journal of Human Genetics* 1994; **54**: 812–819.

Other relevant entries Glycogen-storage disorders: an overview; McArdle's disease.

Tauopathy

Tauopathy is the generic name for conditions resulting from abnormal processing of the microtubule-associated protein τ which is an important component of the neuronal cytoskeleton. These conditions may result from mutations within the gene encoding τ on chromosome 17. Various phenotypes have been described, including:

- Frontotemporal dementia with parkinsonism linked to chromosome 17 (FTDP-17).
- Disinhibition–dementia–parkinsonism–amyotrophy complex (DDPAC).
- Pallido-ponto-nigral degeneration (PPND).
- Familial progressive subcortical gliosis of Neumann (PSG).

A number of other neurodegenerative conditions may be described as tauopathies, even though they are not linked to τ gene mutations, but there is abnormal τ-protein processing, manifested as intraneuronal neurofibrillary tangles and neuropil threads, or abnormal τ-protein isoform profiles. Some are associated with τ-gene polymorphisms which seem to be risk factors for disease development:

Alzheimer's disease (AD)

Corticobasal degeneration (CBD)

Pick's disease

Progressive supranuclear palsy (PSP).

References Lee VM, Goedert M, Trojanowski JQ. Neurodegenerative tauopathies. *Annual Review of Neuroscience* 2001; **24**: 1121–1159.

Spillantini MG, Goedert M. Tau protein pathology in neurodegenerative diseases. *Trends in Neurosciences* 1998; **21**: 428–433.

Other relevant entries Alzheimer's disease; Corticobasal degeneration; Dementia: an overview; Progressive subcortical gliosis (of Neumann); Progressive supranuclear palsy.

Tay–Sachs disease

β-hexosaminidase A deficiency • GM2 gangliosidosis

Pathophysiology The commonest form of the severe late-infantile variant of GM2 gangliosidosis. Formerly common amongst Ashkenazi Jews, the incidence has dropped as a result of carrier screening and prenatal diagnosis. Unlike GM1 gangliosidosis, visceromegaly and bone involvement are not features of GM2 gangliosidosis, with the exception of Sandhoff disease (*q.v.*).

Clinical features: history and examination

- Type 1: Infantile; Tay–Sachs disease, Familial amaurotic idiocy

    Total hexosaminadase A deficiency: mutations in α-subunit, chromosome 15q23

    Onset in first 3–6 months of life

    Developmental delay and then regression

    Progressive irritability with exaggerated startle response (auditory myoclonus)

    Macrocephaly

    Hypotonia which then develops into spasticity

    Myoclonic seizures: difficult to control

    Visual failure: macular cherry-red spot (Tay sign)

    Deafness.

- Type 2: Juvenile:

    Reduced hexosaminidase A activity

    Onset from 2 to 6 years of age

    Gait difficulty with ataxia initially

    Spastic paraplegia and decerebrate rigidity

    Intellectual decline, dementia

    Polymyoclonus

    Seizures

    Dystonia

    Visual loss is late feature.

- Type 3: Adult:

    Partial hexosaminidase A deficiency

    Onset over 15 years of age

    Variable phenotype:

        Either: slowly progressive muscular atrophy or spinocerebellar syndrome

        Or: speech loss, dysarthria, spastic paraparesis, cerebellar ataxia, dystonia, choreoathetosis.

Investigations and diagnosis *Bloods*: vacuolated leukocytes may be seen; enzyme deficiency may be measured in plasma, leukocytes, or fibroblasts.

Urine: oligosaccharides not found.

Imaging: CT/MRI brain may show typical bright thalami.

Neurophysiology: abnormal EEG, abnormal ERG/VEP.

Neurogenetics: mutations in hexosaminidase α-subunit (chromosome 15q23), β-subunit (chromosome 5), or GM2 glycoprotein activator gene (chromosome 5q32–q33).

Differential diagnosis Sandhoff disease.

Treatment and prognosis

No specific treatment

Type 1: Infantile: typically die before the age of 3 years old
Type 2: Juvenile: typically die in second decade of life
Type 3: may survive to middle adulthood.

References Lyon G, Adams RD, Kolodny EH. *Neurology of Hereditary Metabolic Diseases of Children* (2nd edition). New York: McGraw-Hill, 1996: 49–52, 141, 235–237.

Maertens P, Dyken PR. Storage diseases: neuronal ceroid-lipofuscinoses, lipidoses, glycogenoses, and leukodystrophies. In: Goetz CG (ed.). *Textbook of Clinical Neurology* (2nd edition). Philadelphia: Saunders, 2003: 601–628.

Other relevant entries Gangliosidoses: an overview; Sandhoff disease.

◼ Telfer's syndrome

This rare autosomal-dominant hereditary syndrome is characterized clinically by:

Neural hearing loss of variable severity (80% of cases)
Ataxia (80%)
Congenital piebaldism, especially pubic hair, white forelock, variable involvement of face, trunk, limbs
Mental retardation/low IQ (80%).

There may be a family history of similar conditions.
The differential diagnosis encompasses Waardenburg syndrome.

Reference Telfer MA, Sugar M, Jaeger EA, Mulcahy J. Dominant piebald trait (white forelock and leucoderma) with neurological impairment. *American Journal of Human Genetics* 1971; **23**: 383–389.

Other relevant entries Hearing loss: differential diagnosis; Jeune–Tommasi syndrome; Lichtenstein–Knorr syndrome; Richards–Rundle syndrome; Rosenberg–Bergstrom syndrome; Waardenburg syndrome.

◼ Temporal arteritis – see Giant cell arteritis

◼ Tension-type headache – see Headache: an overview

◼ Teratoma

A germ-cell tumour, often occurring in the pineal gland, radiologically and histologically heterogeneous with multiloculated cysts. There may be raised serum and CSF levels of α-fetoprotein.

Other relevant entries Germ-cell tumours; Pineal tumours.

■ Terson's syndrome

This name is given to preretinal haemorrhages associated with subarachnoid haemorrhage which break into the vitreous cavity, as occurs in perhaps half of cases. Vitreal haemorrhages related to trauma may also be described as Terson's syndrome.

Other relevant entry Subarachnoid haemorrhage.

■ Tetanus

Pathophysiology Infection with the Gram-negative anaerobic bacillus *Clostridium tetani*, particularly in necrotic wounds or septic abortion, may result in tetanus due to release of the bacterial exotoxin. Tetanus is now very rare in industrialized nations due to the widespread availability of immunization with tetanus toxoid.

Clinical features: history and examination

- Stiffness, pain, rigidity in voluntary muscles, leading to involuntary spasms, for example in the jaw (trismus), and dystonic movements in the face (risus sardonicus), back (opisthotonos), abdomen, neck, pharynx and larynx causing dysphagia, and respiratory failure.
- Minimal fever.
- Ophthalmoplegia, facial weakness rare.
- History and/or signs of responsible wound, trauma.

Investigations and diagnosis Diagnosis is usually clinically obvious (infected wound). CSF is normal (*cf.* Rabies).

Differential diagnosis

Drug-induced dystonia.

Rabies.

Strychnine poisoning.

Treatment and prognosis Debridement of the wound clearing all necrotic tissue. Intravenous antibiotics (benzylpenicillin); antitetanus immunoglobulin. Supportive nursing including sedation, paralysis/intubation/ventilation if respiration threatened. Recovery occurs over several months; 10% case fatality. Prevention: tetanus toxoid immunization.

> **References** Farrar JJ, Yen LM, Cook T *et al.* Tetanus. *Journal of Neurology, Neurosurgery and Psychiatry* 2000; **69**: 292–301.
>
> Thwaites CL. Tetanus. *Practical Neurology* 2002; **2**: 130–137.
>
> **Other relevant entries** Drug-induced movement disorders; Dystonia: an overview; Rabies; Stiff people: an overview; Strychnine poisoning.

■ Tethered cord syndrome
Low conus syndrome

Pathophysiology Malascent of the conus medullaris of the spinal cord during development may have various causes: intradural fibrous adhesions, intradural lipomas, diastematomyelia, tight filum terminale. These result in a syndrome characterized by lower limb sensorimotor dysfunction, and pain which may present at any time between birth and the second or third decade of life.

Clinical features: history and examination

- Progressive lower limb sensorimotor segmental deficits.
- Intense pain in perineo-gluteal region.
- Non-dermatomal leg pain.
- Cutaneous stigmata of spinal dysraphism (e.g. subcutaneous lipoma, midline hypertrichosis, sacral naevus).
- Bladder or bowel dysfunction.
- Mild lower limb upper motor neurone signs, ascribed to longitudinal stresses transmitted within the spinal cord.

Investigations and diagnosis

Imaging:

Plain spinal radiography: spina bifida in >95%
MRI.

Differential diagnosis Multiple lumbosacral radiculopathy.
Cauda equina syndrome.

Treatment and prognosis Some causes of tethered cord syndrome may be amenable to surgical correction.

> **Reference** Pang D, Wilberger JE. Tethered cord syndrome in adults. *Journal of Neurosurgery* 1982; **57**: 32–47.
>
> **Other relevant entries** Cauda equina syndrome and conus medullaris disease; Diastematomyelia; Radiculopathies: an overview; Spina bifida.

■ Thalamic syndromes
Déjerine–Roussy syndrome

Pathophysiology A variety of clinical syndromes may result from damage to the thalamus. That described by Déjerine and Roussy in 1906 is characterized by contralateral hemisensory loss; there may be associated hemiparesis if the internal capsule is also involved (capsular–thalamic lesion). Delayed onset pain syndrome, various movement disorders (dystonia, chorea, tremor, myoclonus), and dementia have also been described. Stroke (haemorrhage or infarct) and tumour are the commonest causes of thalamic syndromes.

Clinical features: history and examination

- Acute: Hemisensory loss (dissociated pain and temperature or light touch and vibration; proprioceptive loss usual, often with astereognosis); cheiro-oral syndrome (*q.v.*) hemiparesis, often transient; hemiataxia–hypaesthesia (lateral thalamic syndrome).

- Delayed: Pain (thalamic pain): spontaneous or evoked by stimulation; unpleasant, persistent; complex involuntary movements: dystonia, athetosis, chorea associated with position sensory loss ("pseudochoreoathetosis"), with or without intention/action tremor and jerky myoclonus associated with cerebellar ataxia.

Investigations and diagnosis

Bloods: appropriate for stroke.

Imaging: MRI is modality of choice.

Differential diagnosis A similar clinical picture can sometimes be produced by lesions of the parietal lobe (Verger–Déjerine syndrome, Déjerine–Mouzon syndrome), medial lemniscus, or dorsolateral medulla.

Treatment and prognosis Pain may be resistant to many analgesics and electrical stimulation.

References Kim JS. Delayed onset mixed involuntary movements after thalamic stroke. Clinical, radiological and pathophysiological findings. *Brain* 2001; **124**: 299–309.

Melo TP, Bogousslavsky J. Hemiataxia–hypesthesia: a thalamic stroke. *Journal of Neurology, Neurosurgery and Psychiatry* 1992; **55**: 581–584.

Nasreddine ZS, Saver JL. Pain after thalamic stroke: right diencephalic predominance and clincal features in 180 patients. *Neurology* 1997; **48**: 1196–1199.

Other relevant entries Cerebrovascular disease: arterial; Cheiro-oral syndrome; Creutzfeldt–Jakob disease; Déjerine–Mouzon syndrome; Top of the basilar syndrome; Verger–Déjerine syndrome.

■ Thalassaemia

These congenital haemolytic anaemias may be complicated by neurological features including transient neurological features (possibly related to anaemia), headache, seizures, and occasionally stroke. Extramedullary haematopoiesis in the spinal epidural space may cause a compressive myelopathy. Bone marrow hypertrophy causing facial deformity may cause cranial nerve root compression (e.g. deafness).

■ Thallium poisoning – see Heavy metal poisoning

■ Thévenard's syndrome

Acropathie ulcéro-mutilante of Thévenard

Neurogenic plantar ulceration, with bone resorption, following repeated trauma and infection in insensitive feet. Some use this term in the context of alcoholic neuropathy, for others it is a familial autosomal-dominant condition (perhaps a hereditary sensory and autonomic neuropathy). Similar changes may sometimes be seen in the context of syphilis, syringomyelia.

■ Thiamine deficiency – see Alcohol and the nervous system: an overview; Beriberi; Wernicke–Korsakoff's syndrome

■ Thomsen disease – see Myotonia and myotonic syndromes; Myotonia congenita

■ Thoracic disc prolapse

As compared to the lumbar and cervical spine, thoracic spinal dic protrusion is extremely rare, principally because the thoracic spine is more rigid. However, the small capacity of the thoracic spinal cord makes compression more critical, and operation more difficult. Concurrence with Scheuermann's disease may be noted.

Other relevant entries Intervertebral disc prolapse; Scheuermann's disease.

■ Thoracic outlet syndromes

Cervical rib syndrome • Cervicobrachial neurovascular compression syndrome • Naffziger's syndrome • Neurogenic outlet syndrome • Scalenus syndrome.

Pathophysiology Angulation of the fibres from C8 and T1 roots entering the brachial plexus over an abnormal cervical rib or, more commonly, a fibrous band extending from C7 to the first rib can cause wasting and weakness in the hand and medial forearm with paraesthesia (neurogenic thoracic outlet syndrome). Angulation of the subclavian artery may cause Raynaud's phenomenon, aneurysmal dilatation, and emboli (vascular thoracic outlet syndrome). The neurogenic and vascular syndromes seldom occur concurrently. Division of the band or rib may improve symptoms, but careful case selection is required, since these abnormal structures may be incidental to sensory hand and arm symptoms. Unambiguous cases of thoracic outlet syndrome are rare. Most cervical ribs or bands are asymptomatic.

Clinical features: history and examination
- Motor:
    Wasting, weakness of intrinsic hand muscles, medial forearm wrist and finger
        flexors (i.e. muscles innervated by both the median and ulnar nerves).
- Sensory:
    Numbness, paraesthesiae, medial border of forearm, hand +/− pain
    +/− Horner's syndrome.

Investigations and diagnosis
Imaging:

Cervical spine plain films: cervical rib, elongated C7 transverse process.

MRI of the thoracic outlet has been reported useful in some centres for identifying angulation of the lower cords of the brachial plexus.

Neurophysiology:

EMG/NCS to exclude radiculopathy, neuropathy. Typically shows reduced amplitude ulnar sensory potentials with normal median sensory potential, +/− reduced amplitude of median and ulnar compound motor action potentials; fibrillation potentials in muscles innervated by the lower trunk of the brachial plexus.

SSEP: found helpful by some investigators.

Differential diagnosis

C8, T1 radiculopathies.

Carpal tunnel syndrome (thenar wasting).

Ulnar/median neuropathies.

Treatment and prognosis In carefully selected cases, removal of the rib or band leads to improvement, sensory symptoms showing greater benefit than motor.

> **References** Gilliatt RW, Willison RG, Dietz V, Williams IR. Peripheral nerve conduction in patients with a cervical rib and band. *Annals of Neurology* 1978; **4**: 124–129.
>
> Panegyres PK, Moore N, Gibson R, Rushworth G, Donaghy M. Thoracic outlet syndromes and magnetic resonance imaging. *Brain* 1993; **116**: 823–841.
>
> Wilbourn AJ. The thoracic outlet syndrome is overdiagnosed. *Archives of Neurology* 1990; **47**: 328–330.
>
> Yiannikas C, Walsh JC. Somatosensory evoked responses in the diagnosis of thoracic outlet syndrome. *Journal of Neurology, Neurosurgery and Psychiatry* 1983; **46**: 234–240.

> **Other relevant entries** Brachial plexopathies; Horner's syndrome; Raynaud's disease, Raynaud's phenomenon, Raynaud's syndrome.

■ Thornton–Griggs–Moxley disease – see Proximal myotonic myopathy

■ Thromboangiitis obliterans – see Von Winiwarter–Buerger's disease

■ Thrombotic thrombocytopenic purpura

Moschowitz syndrome

This occlusive disorder of arterioles and capillaries may affect any organ, including the brain. Systemic platelet aggregation in the microcirculation is secondary to multimeric von Willebrand factor (vWF), itself a consequence of defective vWF-cleaving metalloproteinase. The syndrome may be acute, idiopathic, recurrent, and associated with the use of drugs such as ticlopidine and clopidogrel.

Neurological features are almost always present, as a consequence of microscopic ischaemic lesions, and include delirium, altered consciousness, and seizures, but gross infarction is rare. Thrombocytopenia may give rise to haemorrhagic complications, in addition to the symptoms of fever, anaemia, renal, and hepatic dysfunction.

Treatment is by means of plasma exchange, which both removes multimeric vWF and replaces vWF-cleaving metalloproteinase, but the effect may be short lived and require repetition.

References Bakshi R, Shaikh ZA, Bates VE *et al*. Thrombotic thrombocytopenic purpura: brain CT and MRI findings in 12 patients. *Neurology* 1999; **52**: 1285–1288.

Moake JL. Thrombotic thrombocytopenic purpura: the systemic clumping "plague". *Annual Review of Medicine* 2002; **53**: 75–88.

Other relevant entry Cerebrovascular disease: arterial.

▪ Thunderclap headache

Pathophysiology Severe explosive headache, sudden, and unexpected like a clap of thunder, mandates urgent investigation to exclude subarachnoid haemorrhage. However, many such headaches are idiopathic, benign, and recurrent, presumably a variant of migraine. Other symptomatic causes may also be identified. Whether thunderclap headache is a marker for unruptured intracranial aneurysm, as originally claimed, is now thought doubtful, and extensive investigation to exclude aneurysm is not recommended.

Clinical features: history and examination
- Instantaneous or hyperacute onset of head pain (<30 seconds).
- Very severe pain intensity.
- Headache may occur spontaneously or be precipitated by Valsalva manoeuvre, sexual activity or exercise.
- Duration usually 1 hour to 10 days; may be up to 4 weeks.
- Headache may recur over a 7-day period but not regularly over subsequent weeks and months.

Investigations and diagnosis Investigation is always required to rule out secondary causes (see Differential diagnosis).

Imaging: CT to exclude subarachnoid haemorrhage; if negative, procede to CSF examination.

CSF: to look for blood, xanthochromia; opening pressure.

If CT, CSF are normal, then additional investigations to look for an unruptured intracranial aneurysm are unwarranted. Other secondary causes may be disclosed with MRI.

Angiography: may show segmental vasoconstriction, reversible.

Differential diagnosis Secondary causes of thunderclap headache include:

Subarachnoid haemorrhage
Cerebral venous sinus thrombosis
Pituitary apoplexy

Spontaneous intracranial hypotension
Acute hypertensive crisis.

Treatment and prognosis Prognosis of idiopathic thunderclap headache is excellent, although headaches may be recurrent.

> **Reference** Dodick DW. Thunderclap headache. *Journal of Neurology, Neurosurgery and Psychiatry* 2002; **72**: 6–11.

> **Other relevant entries** Aneurysm; Cerebrovascular disease: venous; Coital cephalalgia, coital headache; Headache: an overview; Migraine; Pituitary disease and apoplexy; Spontaneous intracranial hypotension; Subarachnoid haemorrhage.

▓ Thymoma – see Myasthenia gravis

▓ Thyroid disease and the nervous system

Pathophysiology A broad spectrum of clinical neurological disorders may be associated with thyroid gland dysfunction, both over- and underactivity. Since thyroid dysfunction is often treatable, thyroid disease should be frequently considered in the differential diagnosis of neurological syndromes.

Clinical features: history and examination
- Hyperthyroidism: Thyrotoxicosis
    Neuromuscular symptoms (67%): myopathy, polyneuropathy (distal sensorimotor)
    Tremor (enhanced physiological tremor)
    Cognitive and mental changes: insomnia, poor concentration, reduced attention span; delirium (rare)
    Seizures (rare); exacerbation of underlying seizure disorder; Hashimoto's encephalopathy
    Headache: migraine or tension type
    Thyroid ophthalmopathy, dysthyroid eye disease, Graves' disease: eyelid retraction, exophthalmos, restrictive ophthalmopathy due to oedema of intraorbital tissues, $+/-$ optic neuropathy (rare)
    Chorea (rare)
    Parkinsonism? (may be chance concurrence of two common conditions)
    Acute neuropathy (Basedow's paraplegia; rare)
    Association with other neurological disorders, for example myasthenia gravis, periodic paralysis (Kitamura syndrome).
- Hypothyroidism:
    Cognitive slowing; dementia, coma
    Neuropsychiatric syndromes: psychosis ("myxoedema madness"), delirium
    Neuromuscular symptoms (75%): myopathy, mononeuropathy, sensorimotor axonal polyneuropathy, carpal tunnel syndrome, slow-relaxing ("hung-up") tendon reflexes (pseudomyotonia; Woltman's sign)

Seizures; Hashimoto's encephalopathy.

Cerebellar ataxia (controversial: one case reported as such was later shown to have pathology of multiple system atrophy)

Hearing loss, vestibular dysfunction (congenital): Pendred's syndrome.

Investigations and diagnosis *Bloods*: measurement of thyroid function tests, *viz.* thyroid stimulating hormone (TSH), thyroxine (T4) $+/-$ tri-iodothyronine (T3). Thyroid auto-antibodies (thyroglobulin, microsomal): may be present in high titre despite normal thyroid function tests in Hashimoto's encephalopathy.

CSF: may show raised protein in Hashimoto's encephalopathy.

Imaging, EEG to exclude other disorders.

Differential diagnosis Of individual features: see entries on chorea, coma, encephalopathy, tremor. Cognitive impairment in hypothyroidism needs to be distinguished from depression.

Treatment and prognosis Many features resolve with adequate treatment of the thyroid disorder.

References Abend WK, Tyler HR. Thyroid disease and the nervous system. In: Aminoff MJ (ed.). *Neurology and General Medicine: The Neurological Aspects of Medical Disorders* (2nd edition). New York: Churchill Livingstone, 1995: 333–347.

Duyff RF, van den Bosch J, Laman DM, Potter van Loon B-J, Linssen WHJP. Neuromuscular findings in thyroid dysfunction: a prospective clinical and electrodiagnostic study. *Journal of Neurology, Neurosurgery and Psychiatry* 2000; **68**: 750–755.

Swanson JW, Kelly JJ, McConahey WM. Neurologic aspects of thyroid dysfunction. *Mayo Clinic Proceedings* 1981; **56**: 504–512.

Other relevant entries Basedow's paraplegia; Carpal tunnel syndrome; Chorea; Coma; Dementia: an overview; Encephalopathy: an overview; Endocrinology and the nervous system; Hashimoto's encephalopathy; Hoffman's syndrome; Kocher–Débre–Sémélaigne syndrome; Myasthenia gravis; Myopathy; Myotonia and myotonic syndromes; Pendred's syndrome; Periodic paralysis; Tremor: an overview.

■ Tibial neuropathy

Pathophysiology The tibial nerve emerges from the medial trunk of the sciatic nerve, carrying fibres from L5–S2 roots, to supply gastrocnemius, soleus, tibialis posterior, flexor digitorum, hallucis longus, and all intrinsic foot flexor muscles. At the ankle, the nerve runs posterior to the medial malleolus under the flexor retinaculum which forms the tarsal tunnel, wherein the tibial nerve may be compressed (analogous to the carpal tunnel in the wrist, but a very much rarer entity). Tibial neuropathy is much less frequent than peroneal neuropathy.

Clinical Features: history and examination

- Motor: Weak ankle plantar flexion and inversion may be evident; more distal lesions may cause weakness of intrinsic toe flexors only; no reflex loss.
- Sensory: Loss on sole of foot.

- Tarsal tunnel syndrome: perimalleolar pain, pain +/− paraesthesia in the foot, wasting of intrinsic foot muscles.

Investigations and diagnosis *EMG/NCS* may confirm or refute diagnosis, distinguishing isolated tibial neuropathy from radiculopathy or sciatic neuropathy. Slowing of distal tibial motor conduction may be observed in tarsal tunnel syndrome.

Differential diagnosis

Lumbar radiculopathy.

Lumbosacral plexopathy.

Sciatic neuropathy.

> **References** McNamara B. The tibial nerve and tarsal tunnel syndrome. *Advances in Clinical Neuroscience and Rehabilitation* 2003; **3**(4): 18.
>
> Staal A, Van Gijn J, Spaans F. *Mononeuropathies: Examination, Diagnosis and Treatment*. London: WB Saunders, 1999: 125–132.
>
> **Other relevant entries** Neuropathies: an overview; Peroneal neuropathy; Sciatic neuropathy.

▓ Tic convulsif

Tic convulsif is a name that has been given to the combination of trigeminal neuralgia (tic douloureux) with hemifacial spasm. Both may be characterized as neurovascular compression syndromes.

> **Reference** Maurice-Williams RS. Tic convulsif: the association of trigeminal neuralgia and hemifacial spasm. *Postgraduate Medical Journal* 1973; **49**: 742–745.
>
> **Other relevant entries** Hemifacial spasm; Trigeminal neuralgia.

▓ Tic douloureux – see Trigeminal neuralgia

▓ Tics

Habit spasms

Pathophysiology Tics are abrupt, jerky, repetitive movements of variable intensity which may be temporarily suppressed by an effort of will. The pathophysiology of tics is uncertain. Once thought to be a reflection of basal ganglia dysfunction, evidence has recently emerged of dysfunction within the cingulate and orbitofrontal cortex which may be related to excessive endorphin release. Recognized causes/associations of tic include Gilles de la Tourette syndrome, obsessive–compulsive disorder (OCD), and structural brain damage, but many tics are idiopathic, or induced by certain drugs.

Clinical features: history and examination

- Abrupt, jerky, repetitive movements of variable intensity, involving discrete muscle groups (=tics); mostly involve face and neck.

- Often accompanied by sensory urge ("itchy") in palms, shoulder blades.
- Temporary suppression of the movements by effort of will, associated with growing inner tension relieved by further performance of the movement.
- Alcohol may improve movements.
- History of brain injury, drug use (neuroleptics).
- History of other obsessive and/or compulsive features, suggestive of an underlying diagnosis of obsessive–compulsive disorder.

Investigations and diagnosis To look for symptomatic/secondary causes.

Bloods: films to exclude acanthocytes; copper, caeruloplasmin to exclude Wilson's disease.

Imaging:

CT/MRI: no diagnostic features may be evident, but secondary causes may be identified.

Functional imaging (SPECT, PET): increased cingulate activity in OCD.

Neurophysiology: EEG: no diagnostic changes; no *bereitschaftpotential*, unlike the same movements mimicked by the patient.

Neurogenetics: to exclude Huntington's disease.

Differential diagnosis

Transient tic disorder of childhood/transient motor tic: benign condition, $M:F = 4:1$.

Chorea (e.g. Huntington's disease, neuroacanthocytosis).

Dystonia (e.g. Wilson's disease).

Myoclonus.

Stereotypy.

Restless legs syndrome.

Treatment and prognosis Dopamine antagonists (haloperidol, sulpiride, pimozide): risk of sedation, tardive dyskinesia.

Opioid antagonists (naltrexone).

Clonidine (central α_2-adrenergic-receptor antagonist).

Tetrabenazine (dopamine-depleting agent).

References Lees AJ. *Tics and Related Disorders*. Edinburgh: Churchill Livingstone, 1985.

Lennox G. Tics and related disorders. In: Sawle G (ed.). *Movement Disorders in Clinical Practice*. Oxford: Isis Medical Media, 1999: 135–146 [with CD ROM].

Other relevant entries Drug-induced movement disorders; Huntington's disease; Neuroacanthocytosis; Obsessive–compulsive disorder; Tourette syndrome; Wilson's disease.

▓ Tinnitus – see Vestibular disorders: an overview

▓ Tobacco–alcohol amblyopia – see Alcohol and the nervous system: an overview

■ Todd's paralysis see – Epilepsy: an overview

■ Tolosa–Hunt syndrome
Orbital pseudotumour

Originally described in the 1950s, this is a clinical syndrome occurring most often in the fourth to sixth decades, comprising severe periorbital pain with any combination of ophthalmoplegia, diplopia, and facial sensory symptoms reflecting multiple cranial nerve palsies (III, IV, VI, V), and responsive to treatment with systemic corticosteroids. It is now known to reflect granulomatous inflammation in the cavernous sinus and/or superior orbital fissure, and may be known as orbital pseudotumour, for which reason some authorities prefer to abandon completely the term "Tolosa–Hunt syndrome". Wegener's granulomatosis, sarcoidosis, and lymphoma enter the differential diagnosis.

Ophthalmoplegic migraine enters the differential diagnosis, as do other pathologies in the cavernous sinus and superior orbital fissure. Imaging of this area, preferably with MRI, is therefore mandatory in any patient presenting with these clinical features.

Other relevant entries Cavernous sinus disease; Ophthalmoplegic migraine; Orbital tumour.

■ Toluene
Glue sniffers' encephalopathy

Found in paints and glues, inhalation of toluene can produce an euphoric effect. In addition it may cause an acute cerebellar ataxia, psychosis, cognitive impairment, and signs of pyramidal tract, brainstem and cranial nerve dysfunction.

Other relevant entries Cerebellar disease: an overview; Solvent exposure.

■ Tomaculous neuropathy – see Hereditary neuropathy with liability to pressure palsies

■ Tonin's disease – see Glycogen-storage disorders: an overview; Phosphoglycerate mutase deficiency

■ Top of the basilar syndrome
Rostral basilar artery syndrome

Pathophysiology "Top of the basilar" syndrome is the result of infarction of midbrain, thalamus, and portions of the occipital and temporal lobes due to occlusion of the rostral basilar artery, usually due to an embolus, resulting in severe visual, oculomotor, and behavioural features without prominent motor or sensory features.

Clinical features: history and examination

Myriad

Behavioural features: acute confusional state invariable, +/− drowsiness, coma

- Posterior hemisphere:
    Visual agnosia
    Anosognosia
    Klüver–Bucy syndrome
    Colour anomia, amnesia
    Topographic disorientation
    Anton's syndrome
    Balint's syndrome
    Charcot–Wilbrand syndrome
- Brainstem/diencephalon:
    Peduncular hallucinosis
    Change in sleep–wake cycle
    Pathological crying

Ophthalmic/visual features:

- Posterior hemisphere:
    Homonymous hemianopia
    Visual hallucinations
    Visual illusory phenomena (allesthesia, palinopsia)
- Brainstem/diencephalon:
    Internuclear ophthalmoplegia
    Vertical gaze paresis
    Parinaud's syndrome
    Weber syndrome
    Benedikt syndrome
    Nothnagel syndrome

Motor features:

    Cerebellar ataxia.

Investigations and diagnosis *Bloods*: look for evidence of vasculitis.

Imaging: MRI preferable, to show extent of infarction, any abnormalities in basilar artery (occlusion).

CSF: no diagnostic changes.

Echocardiography: to look for embolic source.

Differential diagnosis Other causes of acute confusional state.

Treatment and prognosis Secondary prevention: appropriate treatment of any embolic source.

The outlook is poor if there is a previous history of hypertension and vertebrobasilar ischaemic episodes; in the absence of these features the syndrome may be reversible with a good prognosis.

References Caplan LR. "Top of the basilar" syndrome. *Neurology* 1980; **30**: 72–79.

Mehler MF. The rostral basilar artery syndrome: diagnosis, etiology, prognosis. *Neurology* 1989; **39**: 9–16.

Other relevant entries Brainstem vascular syndromes; Cerebrovascular disease: arterial; Encephalopathies: an overview; Parinaud's syndrome; Weber's syndrome.

■ Torticollis – see Dystonia: an overview; Spasmodic torticollis; Spasmus nutans

■ Toruloma, torulosis – see Cryptococcosis

■ Tourette syndrome
Gilles de la Tourette syndrome

Pathophysiology A condition of multiple vocal and motor tics of variable severity, commoner in males (M : F = 4 : 1) sometimes in conjunction with an obsessive–compulsive disorder (OCD). The condition typically develops in adolescence. Twin studies show greater concordance in monozygotic as compared to dizygotic twins, suggesting a genetic component. The patho-anatomical substrate was thought to be in the basal ganglia, since drugs that interfere with dopaminergic neurotransmission have been tried with some success, but more recently functional imaging studies have implicated the cingulate and orbitofrontal cortex. Other neurotransmitters, such as serotonin and opioids, may also be involved. The condition persists despite therapy in the majority of cases, although periods of long remission are not uncommon.

Although the name derives from the French neurologist who described the condition in 1885, previous accounts may be detected in earlier medical and non-medical literature: Dr Samuel Johnson was a noted sufferer.

Clinical features: history and examination
- Motor tics: multiple and multifocal; present for >12 months.
- Vocal tics: including animal noises and, in some cases, coprolalia; palilalia (repeating one own's words), echolalia and echopraxia may occur.
- OCD is relatively common; less frequently attention deficit hyperactivity is seen.
- Often the tics wax and wane in time and change in their nature and location.
- Self-injurious compulsions may occur.

Investigations and diagnosis *Bloods*: all normal.

Imaging: structural imaging (CT, MRI) is normal; functional imaging (SPECT, PET) may show increased activity in cingulate and orbitofrontal cortex.

CSF: normal.

Neurophysiology: usually non-contributory although non-specific EEG abnormalities are not uncommon; no *bereitschaftpotential*, unlike the same movements mimicked by the patient.

Psychometry: may reveal deficits, especially in attentional domains.

Differential diagnosis

Simple tics.

Startle syndromes.

Treatment and prognosis The course of the illness is unpredictable, but the majority of patients have lifelong disease. However the condition often varies with time and often improves after puberty, which means that drug therapy should be initiated and monitored with care.

A number of agents have been tried, including:

Haloperidol (0.25 mg/day increasing to 2–10 mg a day)
Pimozide
Sulpiride
Clonidine
Tetrabenazine.

Concurrent OCD should be treated with serotonin reuptake inhibitors (clomipramine, SSRIs).

References Goetz CG, Klawans HL. Gilles de la Tourette on Tourette syndrome. *Advances in Neurology* 1982; **35**: 1–16.

Robertson MM. Tourette syndrome, associated conditions and the complexities of treatment. *Brain* 2000; **123**: 425–462.

Other relevant entries Obsessive–compulsive disorder; Startle syndromes; Tics.

Toxic oil syndrome – see Eosinophilia–Myalgia syndrome

Toxocariasis

Visceral larva migrans

Nematode larvae of the dog and cat ascarids, *Toxoplasma canis* and *Toxoplasma cati*, may infect children playing with infected animals or in contact with contaminated soil. A pulmonary syndrome with hepatomegaly and eosinophilia is the commonest clinical manifestation. Neurological features, though rare, include focal deficits (hemiparesis), encephalopathy, seizures, and a retinal inflammatory mass (ocular larva migrans). Diagnosis may be confirmed by ELISA. Treatment is with anti-helminthic drugs such as thiabendazole or mebendazole, supplemented with steroids to reduce inflammatory complications of infection.

Other relevant entry Helminthic diseases.

Toxoplasmosis

Pathophysiology *Toxoplasma gondii*, an obligate intracellular protozoan parasite, causes congenital or acquired infection, the latter most usually due to contact with cat faeces. Most of these infections are asymptomatic but may become manifest (opportunistic infection) in the context of immunosuppression, particularly HIV related, in which toxoplasmosis is top of the differential diagnosis for multiple enhancing brain lesions.

Clinical features: history and examination

- Rash, lymphadenopathy.
- Meningoencephalitis.
- Inflammatory myopathy.
- Focal cerebral mass lesions.

Investigations and diagnosis

Bloods: raised creatine kinase; serology (may be negative in AIDS).

Imaging: CT/MRI: multiple (>single) nodular brain lesions.

CSF: lymphocytic pleocytosis, increased protein; organisms in sediment.

+/− investigation for underlying immunodeficiency (HIV test, CD4 count).

Differential diagnosis In immunocompetent: other causes of brain abscess. In context of HIV/AIDS, immunocompromise: other causes of brain abscess; cerebral lymphoma, TB, cryptococcal meningitis, progressive multifocal leukoencephalopathy (PML).

Treatment and prognosis Sulphadiazine, pyrimethamine: 4 weeks in immunocompetent patients, lifelong in immunodeficient. Regression of lesions is typical in HIV; cerebral biopsy may be considered if no improvement occurs, but since treatment for the treatable alternatives (TB, cryptococcal meningitis) is likely to have been instituted, and the other conditions (cerebral lymphoma, PML) are essentially untreatable, not all would procede to biopsy.

> **Reference** Porter SB, Sande MA. Toxoplasmosis of the central nervous system. *New England Journal of Medicine* 1992; **327**: 1643–1648.

> **Other relevant entries** Abscess: an overview; Cryptococcosis; HIV/AIDS disease and the nervous system; Lymphoma; Progressive multifocal leukoencephalopathy; Tuberculosis and the nervous system.

■ Transcortical aphasia – see Aphasia

■ Transient epileptic amnesia

Pathophysiology A syndrome of episodic transient amnesia of epileptic origin.

Clinical features: history and examination

- Recurrent, witnessed episodes of transient amnesia, often manifested by recurrent questioning; attacks are usually brief (1 hour or less); attacks often occur on waking.
- Co-occurrence of other seizure types (not in all patients).
- Persistent interictal defects in autobiographical memory have been observed in some patients.

Investigations and diagnosis *Neurophysiology*: EEG: epileptiform abnormalities of temporal lobe origin; more evident on sleep EEG.

Imaging: usually normal.

Neuropsychology: may show persistent interictal defects in autobiographical memory.

Differential diagnosis Transient global amnesia.

Treatment and prognosis Generally responds favourably to standard anti-epileptic medications (valproate, carbamazepine).

References Kapur N. Transient epileptic amnesia: a clinical update and a reformulation. *Journal of Neurology, Neurosurgery and Psychiatry* 1993; **56**: 1184–1190.

Zeman AZJ, Boniface SJ, Hodges JR. Transient epileptic amnesia: a description of the clinical and neuropsychological features in 10 cases and a review of the literature. *Journal of Neurology, Neurosurgery and Psychiatry* 1998; **64**: 435–443.

Other relevant entries Amnesia, amnesic syndrome; Epilepsy: an overview; Transient global amnesia.

■ Transient global amnesia

Pathophysiology A syndrome consisting of an abrupt attack of impaired anterograde memory of brief duration (<24 hours) without clouding of consciousness or focal neurological signs. The aetiology of this temporary deactivation of mesial temporal and thalamic structures is unknown, but may be triggered by physical or emotional stressors (e.g. sea bathing, pain, sexual intercourse). A previous history of migraine may be found. A reported association between transient global amnesia (TGA) and patent foramen ovale (PFO) remains to be confirmed. Drug-induced cases (e.g. clioquinol) are also reported.

Clinical features: history and examination

- Abrupt onset of repeated questioning; implicit memory functions are usually intact (e.g. driving).
- Absence of other neurological symptoms and signs.
- Resolution within 24 hours with no recollection of amnesic period.
- Informant interview may be helpful, particularly if the patient is seen after resolution of the episode (as is usual).

Investigations and diagnosis

Neuropsychology:

During attack:
  dense, severe, anterograde amnesia;
  variably severe retrograde amnesia;
  working memory intact;
  semantic memory intact;
  non-declarative/procedural/implicit memory intact.
After attack:
  often normal,
  may be subtle impairment of anterograde verbal memory.

Imaging: structural imaging usually normal; functional imaging (e.g. SPECT scan) during attack may show hypoperfusion of medial temporal lobe +/− thalamus.

Neurophysiology: EEG: normal.

Echocardiography for PFO: not currently a standard investigation.

Differential diagnosis

Transient epileptic amnesia.

Migraine.

Head injury.

Vertebrobasilar circulation transient ischaemic attack (usually accompanied by other neurological symptoms and signs).

Drug toxicity.

Psychogenic amnesia.

Treatment and prognosis No specific treatment. Majority of attacks occur in isolation and quoted recurrence rate is low (3% per year).

References Fisher CM, Adams RD. Transient global amnesia. *Acta Neurologica Scandinavica* 1964; **40**(**Suppl 9**): 1–81.

Hodges JR. *Transient Amnesia: Clinical and Neuropsychological Aspects*. London: Saunders, 1991.

Zeman AZJ, Hodges JR. Transient global amnesia. *British Journal of Hospital Medicine* 1997; **58**: 257–260.

Other relevant entries Amnesia, amnesic syndrome; Cerebrovascular disease: arterial; Migraine; Patent foramen ovale; Transient epileptic amnesia; Transient ischaemic attack; Transient semantic amnesia.

▪ Transient ischaemic attack

Pathophysiology Transient ischaemic attacks (TIAs) are temporary focal neurological deficits, presumed due to ischaemia of nervous tissue; most last <30 minutes, although by definition they may last up to 24 hours (longer reversible events may be labelled "reversible ischaemic neurological deficits" (RIND)). A distinction may be drawn between embolic TIAs, usually reflecting a source in the ipsilateral carotid artery or heart, and haemodynamic TIA, where inadequate perfusion pressure is causal. Embolic events are more common.

Clinical features: history and examination

- Embolic TIAs

    Anterior/Carotid circulation TIA:

        Ocular TIA/amaurosis fugax/transient monocular blindness: brief episode unilateral visual loss.

        Hemisphere TIA/transient hemispheral attacks: contralateral motor or sensory dysfunction, aphasia, homonymous hemianopia or combination thereof.

    Vertebrobasilar circulation TIA:

        Bilateral or shifting motor/sensory dysfunction, complete or partial loss of vision in homonymous fields, combination thereof; subclavian steal syndrome (*q.v.*).

Previous TIA is a risk factor for stroke. Increasing frequency of TIA ("crescendo TIA"), particularly hemisphere TIA or combination of hemisphere and ocular TIA, is thought particularly ominous.

May be an ipsilateral carotid artery bruit, reflecting turbulent blood flow; but carotid bruits may be asymptomatic, in which case probably best left alone; moreover some critically stenosed carotid arteries may not have a bruit.

Look for evidence of concurrent coronary artery disease: may influence decisions regarding surgery for symptomatic carotid artery stenosis.

Look for hypertension, stigmata of hypercholesterolaemia (modifiable risk factors for TIA).

Smoking history.

- Haemodynamic TIAs

  Carotid territory: "Limb shaking": recurrent, involuntary, irregular movements described as shaking, trembling, twitching, flapping; associated with severely stenosed or occluded carotid, exhausted cerebral vasomotor reactivity.

Investigations and diagnosis *Bloods*: cholesterol.

Imaging:

Of the carotid artery for stenotic change: Doppler ultrasonography in skilled hands, MRA, digital subtraction angiography. Degree of stenosis is important for deciding on most appropriate management (medical or surgical), criteria exist for determination.

Of the brain (CT/MRI) for ischaemic damage ipsilateral to a stenotic artery (suggestive of symptomatic effect).

Of the heart: echocardiography (transthoracic, transoesophageal) to look for embolic source if carotids clear.

Differential diagnosis TIA and minor stroke are overdiagnosed: 27% of those referred with this diagnosis were "undone" in a neurovascular clinic, the revised diagnoses for transient neurological symptoms including:

Migraine
Epilepsy
Hyperventilation
Multiple sclerosis
Unclassified (the largest group).

Treatment and prognosis Modify the modifiable risk factors: treat hypertension, hypercholesterolaemia.

Medical: antiplatelet agents (aspirin, clopidogrel) reduce risk of ischaemic stroke; probably ticlopidine, dipyridamole, also. Warfarin may be indicated for mild stenosis which continues to be symptomatic despite antiplatelet therapy and is not suitable for surgery.

Surgery: symptomatic stenosis of >70% is best managed with surgery (carotid endarterectomy).

References Albers GW, Hart RG, Lutsep HL *et al.* Supplement to the guidelines for
the management of transient ischemic attacks: a statement from the Ad Hoc
Committee on Guidelines for the Management of Transient Ischemic Attacks,
Stroke Council, American Heart Association. *Stroke* 1999; **30**: 2502–2511.

Martin PJ, Young G, Enevoldson TP, Humphrey PRD. Overdiagnosis of TIA and
minor stroke: experience at a regional neurovascular clinic. *Quarterly Journal of
Medicine* 1997; **90**: 759–763.

Other relevant entries Cerebrovascular disease: arterial; Limb shaking; Migraine;
Subclavian steal syndrome.

■ Transient semantic amnesia

Whereas in transient global amnesia (*q.v.*), semantic memory is intact, an analogous
syndrome of transient amnesia in which semantic memory was impaired has been
described.

Reference Hodges JR. Transient semantic amnesia. *Journal of Neurology,
Neurosurgery and Psychiatry* 1997; **63**: 548–549.

Other relevant entry Transient global amnesia.

■ Transient unresponsiveness of the elderly

Idiopathic recurrent stupor • Psychogenic unresponsiveness

This ill-understood condition of the elderly is characterized by recurrent self-limited
episodes of unresponsiveness with no obvious structural, toxic, metabolic, convulsive, or
psychiatric disorder, and no specific imaging or EEG signature. Flumazenil may reverse
some of these episodes. It is self-evidently a diagnosis of exclusion (if not desperation).

References Haimovic JC, Beresford HR. Transient unresponsiveness in the elderly.
Archives of Neurology 1992; **49**: 35–37.

Tinuper P, Montagna P, Plazzi G *et al.* Idiopathic recurring stupor. *Neurology* 1994;
44: 621–625.

■ Transmissible spongiform encephalopathies (TSE) – see Prion disease: an overview

■ Transverse myelitis, transverse myelopathy

Pathophysiology An acute or subacute spinal cord syndrome, usually complete. The
condition is aetiologically heterogeneous; primary or idiopathic cases occur, but
most are secondary, with an inflammatory or immunopathogenic basis, with a wide
variety of underlying diagnoses:

Post-infectious (varicella, Epstein-Barr virus (EBV), mycoplasma, herpes zoster):
may be a localized form of post-infectious encephalomyelitis

Post-vaccination (e.g. influenza)

Multiple sclerosis (MS), neuromyelitis optica (Devic's syndrome)

Sarcoidosis

Collagen vascular disease: Systemic lupus erythematosus (SLE), Sjögren's syndrome, antiphospholipid antibody syndrome, giant cell arteritis

Idiopathic; clincally isolated syndrome.

Clinical features: history and examination

- Lower limb weakness, paraesthesia.
- Urinary retention, incontinence.
- +/− pain in the spine.
- Symptoms usually evolve rapidly, may extend cranially.
- Usually a monophasic illness, involving a complete spinal cord segment. Recurrent cases are described.
- Phenotype differs in idiopathic versus MS transverse myelitis: latter is usually partial, whereas idiopathic is usually complete.

Investigations and diagnosis *Imaging*: spinal cord MRI may show swelling of and signal change within the spinal cord; this may involve part of or the whole anteroposterior diameter of the cord, and single, multiple, or several contiguous cord segments ("longitudinal myelitis"). There may be patchy enhancement with gadolinium in the acute stage. Longitudinal myelitis is not typical of multiple sclerosis, which tends to affect single segments; inflammatory lesions on brain MRI may support a diagnosis of multiple sclerosis.

CSF: moderate pleocytosis, raised protein; +/− oligoclonal bands.

Bloods: serology for infective agents; auto-antibodies for certain collagen vascular diseases.

Neurophysiology: central motor conduction time (CMCT) to tibialis anterior abnormal in 90% in one series, CMCT to abductor digiti minimi in 30%; tibial somatosensory evoked potential (SEP) abnormal in 77%, median SEP in 15%; EMG evidence of denervation in 51%; suggests pronounced involvement of dorsal region of spinal cord.

Differential diagnosis Spinal cord vascular disease: infarction, subarachnoid haemorrhage.

Treatment and prognosis Of cause where established: intravenous steroids for MS, post-infectious, post-vaccination; immunosuppression for SLE; anticoagulation for antiphospholipid antibody syndrome.

Partial syndromes are more likely to improve; complete syndromes less so.

Isolated transverse myelitis, particularly if partial, may be the harbinger of more widespread inflammation, that is, a clinically isolated syndrome heralding MS.

References Al-Deeb SM, Yaqub BA, Bruyn GW, Biary NM. Acute transverse myelitis. A localized form of postinfectious encephalomyelitis. *Brain* 1997; **120**: 1115–1122.

Ford B, Tampieri D, Francis G. Long-term follow-up of acute partial transverse myelitis. *Neurology* 1992; **42**: 250–252.

Kalita J, Misra UK. Neurophysiological studies in acute transverse myelitis. *Journal of Neurology* 2000; **247**: 943–948.

Larner AJ, Farmer SF. Myelopathy following influenza vaccination in inflammatory CNS disorder treated with chronic immunosuppression. *European Journal of Neurology* 2000; **7**: 731–733.

Pandit L, Rao S. Recurrent myelitis. *Journal of Neurology, Neurosurgery and Psychiatry* 1996; **60**: 336–338.

Transverse Myelitis Consortium Working Group. Proposed diagnostic criteria and nosology of acute transverse myelitis. *Neurology* 2002; **59**: 499–505.

Other relevant entries Acute disseminated encephalomyelitis; Antiphospholipid (antibody) syndrome; Clinically isolated syndromes; Devic's disease, Devic's syndrome; Epstein–Barr virus infection and the nervous system; Herpes zoster and postherpetic neuralgia; Multiple sclerosis; Myelitis: an overview; Sarcoidosis; Sjögren's syndrome; Spinal cord diseases: an overview; Spinal cord vascular diseases; Systemic lupus erythematosus and the nervous system.

■ Traumatic brain injury

Pathophysiology Traumatic brain injury (TBI) may be classified as:

- Primary: related to the impact, the severity of injury *per se*.
- Secondary: evolving after the primary impact, for anything up to 1 week.

Although preventive (epidemiological) measures may reduce the severity and frequency of primary brain injury, secondary injury is potentially amenable to medical intervention. Timely (i.e. early) transfer to a trauma centre with neurosurgical facilities is probably the optimum management, in order to monitor and treat brain swelling, raised intracranial pressure, falling cerebral perfusion pressure, hypotension, and hypoxaemia, recognized causes of secondary injury due to brain ischaemia.

Clinical features: history and examination TBI may be graded according to Glasgow Coma Scale (GCS) score at presentation:

- Mild: GCS 13–15; often no more than concussion; loss of consciousness or amnesia <30 minutes.
- Moderate: GCS 9–13; patient lethargic, stuporous; loss of consciousness or amnesia 30 minutes to 24 hours; may be accompanying skull fracture;
- Severe: GCS 3–8; loss of consciousness >24 hours; may be accompanying subdural haematoma, brain contusion.

Investigations and diagnosis *Imaging*: CT crucial to identify lesions which may be amenable to neurosurgical intervention, for example subdural/extradural haematoma, parenchymal haematoma (temporal, frontal).

Differential diagnosis Usually TBI is obvious, but occasionally there may be difficulty, for example someone suffering a subarachnoid haemorrhage when driving leading to an accident or falling downstairs.

Treatment and prognosis Treatment at the scene of any accident may be crucial, because of the time factor in preventing secondary injury. Intubation and hand ventilation may be required to prevent hypoxaemia, as well as intravenous access for fluids to prevent hypotension (both recognized to increase the risk of secondary injury). Once the patient is stabilized, transfer to a trauma centre is recommended; some would advocate helicopter transfer if the distances involved are large.

Following imaging, if immediate neurosurgical intervention is not required, arrangements for ICP monitoring should be made (ventricular catheter preferred to a bolt); normal ICP = 0–10 mmHg; intervention probably appropriate if ICP > 15–20 mmHg, by means of:

> Ventricular drainage of CSF
> Hyperventilation (but may risk hypocapnic vasoconstriction and brain ischaemia)
> Diuretics (but may risk hypovolaemia and brain ischaemia)
> Mannitol (but may only be given intermittently).

Repeat imaging may be appropriate to define cause of rising ICP.

Monitoring of central venous pressure may assist in decisions regarding hypotension, fluid balance.

The place of prophylactic steroids and anti-epileptic medications in TBI remains uncertain; clearly any seizures should be treated as they may be associated with worsening of brain ischaemia.

Prognosis is dependent on severity of TBI:
- Mild: full recovery usual, may be residual concentration or short-term memory problems.
- Moderate, Severe: linear correlation between GCS score 3–9 and outcome of death, vegetative state, and severe neurological disability.

Post-traumatic seizures may be described as:
- Early: within 7 days of TBI.
- Late: >7 days after TBI.

Mild and moderate TBI are associated with a small increased risk of epilepsy; severe TBI with a substantial increase in risk. There is currently no strong evidence that prophylactic anti-epileptic medication alters these risks, that is, they relate to primary rather than secondary brain injury.

References Chadwick D. Seizures and epilepsy after traumatic brain injury. *Lancet* 2000; **355**: 334–336.

Ghajar J. Traumatic brain injury. *Lancet* 2000; **356**: 923–929.

Mendelow D. Head injury. In: Donaghy M (ed.). *Brain's diseases of the Nervous System* (11th edition). Oxford: OUP, 2001: 507–525.

Other relevant entries Amnesia, amnesic syndrome; Concussion; Epilepsy: an overview; Glasgow Coma Scale; Vegetative states.

■ Treacher Collins syndrome

First pharyngeal arch syndrome • Franceschetti–Zwahlen–Klein syndrome • Mandibulofacial dysostosis

Pathophysiology An autosomal-dominant syndrome with characteristic oculo-auriculocephalic anomalies, due to disappearance or abnormal development of the various components of the embryological first pharyngeal arch; insufficient migration of neural crest cells may be relevant. Mental retardation may occur.

Clinical features: history and examination

- Characteristic facial dysmorphism: "fish" or "bird-like" facies (mandibulofacial dysostosis), usually symmetrical, occasionally asymmetric, or even unilateral:

    Antimongoloid slant of palpebral fissures; coloboma, lateral half of lower eyelid

    Flat frontonasal angle

    Hypoplastic zygomata, upper and lower jaws, sunken cheeks

    Macrostomia, cleft palate

    External ear malformation, +/− middle and inner ear anomalies, leading to conductive hearing impairment.

- +/− cardiac anomalies.
- Intelligence generally normal.

Investigations and diagnosis Diagnosis at birth. Assessment of cardiac status and hearing function are appropriate in order to initiate treatment if required.
Neurogenetics: TCOF1 locus at chromosome 5q31.3–q32 encodes a 1411 amino acid protein named treacle; mutations include insertions and deletions.

Differential diagnosis

Goldenhar syndrome.

Hallermann–Streiff syndrome.

Pierre Robin syndrome.

Treatment and prognosis Symptomatic treatment of hearing impairment with hearing aids; plastic +/− orthodontic surgery. Life expectancy good.

References Marsh KL, Dixon MJ. Treacher Collins syndrome. *Advances in Otorhinolaryngology* 2000; **56**: 53–59.

Marszalek B, Wojcicki P, Kobus K, Trzeciak WH. Clinical features, treatment and genetic background of Treacher Collins syndrome. *Journal of Applied Genetics* 2002; **43**: 223–233.

Other relevant entries Goldenhar syndrome, Goldenhar–Gorlin syndrome; Hallermann–Streiff syndrome; Pierre Robin syndrome.

■ Tremor: an overview

Pathophysiology Tremor is an involuntary movement, roughly rhythmic and sinusoidal, although some tremors (e.g. dystonic) are irregular in amplitude and periodicity. Many types of tremor are recognized.

Clinical features: history and examination

- Physiological tremor: normal; exacerbated by anxiety states, hyperthyroidism, drugs (especially β_2-agonists).
- Rest tremor: present when limb supported against gravity and no voluntary muscle activation, for example 4–6 Hz "pill-rolling" hand tremor of Parkinson's disease (PD); Holmes's/midbrain/rubral tremor due to lesions interrupting cerebellothalamic and/or cerebello-olivary projections (most commonly seen in multiple sclerosis).
- Action tremor: present during any voluntary muscle contraction; various subdivisions:

    Postural tremor: present during voluntary maintenance of posture opposed by gravity, for example arm tremor of essential tremor (ET); 6 Hz postural tremor sometimes seen in PD, may predate emergence of akinesia/rigidity/rest tremor; modest postural tremor of cerebellar disease; some drug-induced tremors; tremor of IgM paraproteinaemic neuropathy.

    Kinetic tremor: present with movement, often with an exacerbation at the end of a goal-directed movement (intention tremor), for example cerebellar/midbrain tremor (3–5 Hz).

    Task-specific tremor: evident during the performance of a highly skilled activity, for example primary writing tremor.

    Isometric tremor: present when voluntary muscle contraction is opposed by a stationary object, for example primary orthostatic tremor (POT) (14–16 Hz).

- Psychogenic tremors: difficult to classify, with changing characteristics; the frequency with which such tremors are observed varies greatly between different clinics.

    Diagnosis is usually clinical, based on the appearance of the tremor and the circumstances in which it occurs. Other neurological features may also help, for example bradykinesia and rigidity in PD, ataxia in cerebellar disease, peripheral sensory deficits in neuropathy. Family history may help (ET). Drug history is also crucial.

Investigations and diagnosis *Bloods*: thyroid function tests to exclude hyperthyroidism and immunoglobulins to exclude a paraprotein.

Neurophysiology: EMG: may be useful for determining tremor frequency, and diagnostic in POT.

Imaging: if other neurological features suggest an underlying disorder.

Differential diagnosis Tremor is unlikely to be mistaken for dystonia or myoclonus.

Treatment and prognosis See individual entries; in brief:

ET: alcohol, propranolol, primidone, alprazolam, flunarizine, nicardipine, ? topiramate

PD: levodopa, anticholinergics (e.g. benzhexol), dopamine agonists

POT: clonazepam, primidone, levodopa

Cerebellar: isoniazid, ondansetron, carbamazepine, clonazepam, primidone, propranolol (but most pharmacotherapy ineffectual); limb weights, stereotactic surgery.

Reference Deuschl G, Bain P, Brin M and an Ad Hoc Scientific Committee. Consensus statement of the Movement Disorder Society on tremor. *Movement Disorders* 1998; **13(suppl 3)**: 2–23.

Other relevant entries Cerebellar disease: an overview; Drug-induced movement disorders; Essential tremor; Multiple sclerosis; Paraproteinaemic neuropathies; Parkinson's disease; Primary orthostatic tremor; Thyroid disease and the nervous system.

■ Trichinosis
Trichinellosis

Pathophysiology Trichinosis is infection with the nematode worm *Trichinella spiralis*, due to ingestion of undercooked pork containing encysted *T. spiralis* larvae (hence Ambrose Bierce's definition of trichinosis as "the pig's reply to proponents of porcophagy"). Gastric juices free the larvae which then develop in the duodenum and jejunum to form new larvae which spread via the lymphatics and the bloodstream to all tissues. They survive only in muscle to encyst and calcify.

Clinical features: history and examination

- Acute (1–2 days): mild gastroenteritis.
- Subacute (1–6 weeks): fever, painful tender muscles, oedematous eyelids, +/− headache, stiff neck, confusional state.
- Chronic (months): myalgia of inflammatory myopathy, affecting extraocular muscles, tongue, proximal limb muscles, diaphragm, myocardium (emboli may lead to brain infarction).
- Central nervous system (CNS) disease (from larval invasion): meningoencephalitis, cranial vessel thrombosis.

Investigations and diagnosis *Bloods*: eosinophilia; mild increase in creatine kinase.
Imaging: CT/MRI: may show multiple infarcts or haemorrhagic lesions.
CSF: may show lymphocytosis, + (rarely) parasites.
ECG: tachycardia.
Serology: ELISA positive by 3rd week.
Neurophysiology: EMG: fibrillation potentials (disconnection of muscle fibres from end-plates).
Muscle biopsy: inflammatory myopathy; segmental necrosis of muscle fibres with eosinophil infiltrate; observation of *Trichinella* larvae is diagnostic.

Differential diagnosis Other causes of inflammatory myopathy (polymyositis).

Treatment and prognosis Often asymptomatic.

Thiabendazole or albendazole (anti-helminthics), +/− prednisolone (anti-inflammatory). The value of steroids is not definitively established, and may theoretically enhance larval dissemination. Recovery is usual.

Reference Bundy DAP, Michael E. Trichinosis. In: Cox FEG (ed.). *The Wellcome Trust Illustrated History of Tropical Diseases*. London: Wellcome Trust, 1996: 310–317.

Other relevant entries Helminthic disease; Myopathy: an overview.

Trichopoliodystrophy – see Menkes' disease

Trichothiodystrophy – see Xeroderma pigmentosum and related conditions

Trigeminal neuralgia
Fothergill's disease • Tic douloureux

Pathophysiology A syndrome of neuropathic pain in the distribution of the sensory branches of the trigeminal nerve, especially mandibular and maxillary divisions (rarely ophthalmic), occurring in middle to late life and slightly commoner in women. Although most cases are idiopathic/primary, symptomatic/secondary causes are recognized.

Clinical features: history and examination History usually typical and diagnostic:

- Brief, severe, paroxysmal, lancinating, unilateral, facial pain, causing patient to wince or even cry.
- Frequently recurrent.
- May be initiated by stimulation of specific facial "trigger zones", for example by washing, shaving, chewing, wind on the face (hence may be a form of allodynia).
- Sensory/motor cranial nerve deficit usually absent (may not be so in symptomatic group).

Investigations and diagnosis *Imaging*: MRI preferred: to exclude secondary/symptomatic causes, for example multiple sclerosis, basilar artery aneurysm, acoustic/trigeminal neuroma, tortuous blood vessel(s) (usually posterior cerebellar artery) impinging on trigeminal nerve. Normal in idiopathic cases.

Differential diagnosis

Postherpetic neuralgia.

Cluster headache.

Chronic paroxysmal (episodic) hemicrania (CPH).

Short-lasting *u*nilateral *n*euralgiform headache with *c*onjunctival injection and *t*earing (SUNCT) syndome.

Atypical facial pain.

Treatment and prognosis Medical: Anticonvulsants are beneficial in most cases, especially carbamazepine (commence with low doses, increase slowly to avoid toxicity, up to doses of 600–1200 mg/day) > phenytoin; +/− baclofen. Gabapentin, lamotrigine may be tried if these fail or are inadequate. Lidocaine-like anti-arrhythmics may also be tried.

Surgical: (Percutaneous) Radiofrequency thermocoagulation; microvascular decompression (requires posterior fossa craniotomy), especially if there is radiological evidence of a vascular loop contacting the dorsal root entry zone of the symptomatic trigeminal nerve. May be followed by anaesthesia dolorosa.

References Fields HL. Treatment of trigeminal neuralgia. *New England Journal of Medicine* 1996; **334**: 1125–1126.

Love S, Coakham HB. Trigeminal neuralgia: pathology and pathogenesis. *Brain* 2001; **124**: 2347–2360.

Stookey B, Ransohoff J. *Trigeminal Neuralgia: Its History and Treatment.* Springfield: Charles C Thomas, 1959.

Zakrzewska JM. *Trigeminal Neuralgia.* London: WB Saunders, 1995.

Other relevant entries Atypical facial pain; Chronic paroxysmal hemicrania; Cluster headache; Cranial nerve disease: V: Trigeminal nerve; Facial pain: differential diagnosis; Glossopharyngeal neuralgia; SUNCT syndrome.

■ Trigeminal neuropathy – see Cranial nerve disease: V: Trigeminal nerve

■ Trigeminal sensory neuropathy

Trigeminal sensory neuropathy (TSN) is usually a slowly evolving, unilateral or bilateral, facial numbness, with or without pain, paraesthesia, and disturbed taste sensation. Electrophysiological testing of the blink reflex may show a modest prolongation of latency suggesting an afferent defect, consistent with a lesion in the trigeminal ganglion or proximal part of the main trigeminal divisions. Systemic sclerosis (scleroderma), Sjögren's syndrome and mixed connective tissue disease are frequent causes, but infiltrating skull base tumours and other inflammatory disorders enter the differential diagnosis; some cases remain idiopathic.

Reference Lecky BR, Hughes RA, Murray NM. Trigeminal sensory neuropathy. A study of 22 cases. *Brain* 1987; **110**: 1463–1485.

Other relevant entries Cranial nerve disease: V: Trigeminal nerve; Sjögren's syndrome; Systemic sclerosis.

■ Trinucleotide repeat diseases
Polyglutamine disease • PolyQ disease • Triplet repeat disease

Pathophysiology A number of inherited neurodegenerative conditions have been linked to expansions of a trinucleotide repeat sequence in a gene co-segregating with the disease. Since these repeats are potentially unstable during meiosis, increasing in size in successive generations, this may explain the clinical observation of anticipation in many of these conditions (i.e. increasing phenotypic severity across generations). The biochemical mechanism by which expansions cause disease is uncertain, but many of the repeats encode polyglutamine, proteins containing which may aggregate into insoluble fibrils which may manifest as pathological inclusions ("aggregopathies"); this would represent a toxic gain of function rather than a loss of function. However, not all trinucleotide repeats are in coding sequences so this cannot be the only mechanism. Moreover, genotype/phenotype correlation is not perfect, some disease-free individuals harbouring pathological repeats, some affected individuals having "normal" numbers of repeats.

Disorders shown to be trinucleotide repeat diseases are as follows:

Kennedy's syndrome (X-linked bulbospinal neuronopathy, XLBSN)
Huntington's disease (HD)
Dentatorubral-pallidoluysian atrophy (DRPLA)
Spinocerebellar ataxia (SCA), types 1, 2, 3 (Machado–Joseph disease), 6, 7, 17
Friedreich's ataxia (FA)
Dystrophia myotonica (DyM)
Fragile X syndrome (FRAX)
Oculopharyngeal muscular dystrophy (OPMD).

Trinucleotide repeat diseases

Disease	Gene	Triplet	Location	Protein	Normal	Abnormal
XLBSN	Androgen receptor	CAG	Exon	Polyglutamine	9–34	38–75
HD	Huntingtin	CAG	Exon	Polyglutamine	9–34	36–125
SCA1	Ataxin	CAG	Exon	Polyglutamine	6–36	39–81
SCA2		CAG	Exon	Polyglutamine	15–34	34–64
SCA3 (MJD)		CAG	Exon	Polyglutamine	12–40	60–84
SCA6		CAG	Exon	Polyglutamine	4–16	21–27
SCA7		CAG	Exon	Polyglutamine	6–17	34–130
DRPLA		CAG	Exon	Polyglutamine	3–36	49–88
FRAX	FMR1	CGG	5′	Untranslated	7–50	50–1500
DyM	DMPK	CTG	3′	Untranslated	5–40	40–3000
FA	Frataxin	GAA	Intron	Untranslated	6–30	90–1700
OPMD	PAB2	GCG	Exon	Polyalanine	6–7	8–13

Quadruplet expansions have also been described, for example in proximal myotonic myopathy (PROMM; myotonic dystrophy type 2; CCTG), and SCA 10 results from an expansion of tandem repeats of five nucleotides (ATTCT).

Clinical features: history and examination See individual entries.

Investigations and diagnosis Trinucleotide repeats form the basis for rapid diagnostic tests for the associated diseases using PCR technology, but care is needed in interpreting results because of the imperfect genotype/phenotype correlations (see above).

Genetic counselling is generally required before gene testing.

Treatment and prognosis Most of these conditons are progressive and lack specific treatment. However, if they have a shared pathogenesis related to the intraneuronal accumulation of pathological proteins, generic therapy to block protein aggregation might theoretically be applicable to many of the diseases in this category.

References Paulson HL, Fishbeck KH. Trinucleotide repeats in neurogenetic disorders. *Annual Review of Neuroscience* 1996; **19**: 79–107.

Perutz MF. Glutamine repeats and neurodegenerative diseases: molecular aspects. *Trends in Biochemical Sciences* 1999; **24**: 58–63.

Rosenberg RN. DNA-triplet repeats and neurologic disease. *New England Journal of Medicine* 1996; **335**: 1222–1224.

Other relevant entries Dentatorubral-pallidoluysian atrophy; Fragile X syndrome; Friedreich's ataxia; Huntington's disease; Kennedy's syndrome; Myotonia and myotonic syndromes; Oculopharyngeal muscular dystrophy; Proximal myotonic myopathy; Spinocerebellar ataxia; Wolf–Hirschhorn syndrome.

■ Triple A syndrome – see Allgrove's syndrome

■ Trisomy 13 – see Patau syndrome

■ Trisomy 21 – see Down's syndrome

■ Trochlear nerve palsy – see Cranial nerve disease: IV: Trochlear nerve

■ Tropical neurology

The notion that various dieases of the nervous system are in some way peculiar to tropical latitudes and their indigenous populations has found less support in recent years, partly due to the increasing mobility of populations. Hence this categorization is regarded as redundant by some authors. Nonetheless, some conditions are more prevalent in tropical latitudes, and hence unfamiliar in Western practice. Travel history should not be forgotten in patients presenting with neurological symptoms and signs of uncertain aetiology.

Reference Shakir RA, Newman PK, Poser CM (eds). *Tropical Neurology*. London: Saunders, 1996.

Spillane JD (ed). *Tropical Neurology*. Oxford: OUP, 1973.

Other relevant entries Konzo; Lathyrism; Leprosy; Malaria; Schistosomiasis; Trypanosomiasis.

■ Tropical spastic paraparesis – see HTLV-1 myelopathy

■ Troyer syndrome

Troyer syndrome is an autosomal recessive, complicated hereditary spastic paraparesis, seen in high frequency amongst the Old Order Amish community. In addition to lower limb spasticity, the additional features are short stature, mental retardation, dysarthria, and marked atrophy of small hand muscles. The condition maps to chromosome 13q12.3 and has been associated with frameshift mutations in the SPG20 gene, encoding the protein spartin.

Reference Patel H, Cross H, Proukakis C *et al*. SPG20 is mutated in Troyer syndrome, an hereditary spastic paraplegia. *Nature Genetics* 2002; **31**: 347–348.

Other relevant entries Charlevoix–Saguenay syndrome; Hereditary spastic paraparesis.

■ Trypanosomiasis
African sleeping sickness

Pathophysiology African trypanosomiasis results from infection with the protozoan *Trypanosoma brucei gambiense* in West Africa or *Trypanosoma brucei rhodesiense* in East Africa, transmitted to humans by tsetse flies (*Glossina* species). These produce either a chronic illness (Gambian, West African), which may not become clinically apparent for up to 1 year after infection, or a more acute progressive illness (Rhodesian, East African). Both are characterized by daytime hypersomnia with nocturnal insomnia (African sleeping sickness).

South American trypanosomiasis (Chagas' disease) results from infection with *Trypanosoma cruzi*, transmitted to humans by the bite of reduviid bugs. As with the African disease, the sequence of local lymphadenopathy, haematogenous spread and chronic meningoenecephalitis is seen.

Clinical features: history and examination

- African:

   Local: chancre (trypanoma) at site of bite: hard, painful

   Dissemination: headache, fever, tachycardia

   Systemic: recurrent episodes lasting several days with asymptomatic periods of weeks in between

   Gambian:

      Lymphadenopathy, non-tender, especially posterior cervical location with consistency likened to ripe plums (Winterbottom's sign)

      Subtle neurological changes: indifference, reversal of sleep–wake cycle, tremor

      Somnolence and insomnia, tremor, incoordination, thermoregulatory dysfunction, hyperreflexia

      Stupor, coma, death

   East African: onset within days of bite

      Lymphadenopathy unusual

      Other symptoms similar to Gambian but more acute; early central nervous system (CNS) invasion, death rapid (cardiac failure)

- South American:

   Acute flu-like illness; inoculation chagoma may be seen; Romana's sign (unilateral conjunctivitis and oedema from ocular contamination by bug faeces)

   Asymptomatic phase

Chronic phase: destruction of cardiac and gastrointestinal autonomic nerves: postural hypotension, arrhythmias; oesophageal achalasia. Chronic meningoencephalitis; a predominantly sensory peripheral neuropathy may occur.

Investigations and diagnosis *Bloods*: anaemia, monocytosis, raised IgM (nonspecific); indirect fluorescent antibody test for trypanosomes.

Tissue: blood smears, CSF examination, bone marrow aspirate, to look for trypanosomes: diagnostic.

CSF: raised protein, pleocytosis (with morular cells), raised IgM.

Differential diagnosis Disturbance of sleep–wake cycle with systemic illness following time in Africa unlikely to be mistaken for anything else.

Other causes of autonomic neuropathy should be considered with Chagas' disease

Treatment and prognosis Suramin (East African): may cause albuminuria, $+/-$ shock, febrile reactions, rash.

Pentamidine (West African): may cause hypotension, fever, rash.

Organic arsenicals for CSF penetration: melarsopol, may cause optic atrophy, rash, encephalopathy.

Despite these, deaths still occur.

References Miles MA. New World trypanosomiasis. In: Cox FEG (ed.). *The Wellcome Trust Illustrated History of Tropical Diseases*. London: Wellcome Trust, 1996: 192–205.

Sanner BM, Büchner N, Kotterba S, Zidek W. Polysomnography in acute African trypanosomiasis. *Journal of Neurology* 2000; **247**: 878–879.

Williams BI. African trypanosomiasis. In: Cox FEG (ed.). *The Wellcome Trust Illustrated History of Tropical Diseases*. London: Wellcome Trust, 1996: 178–191.

Other relevant entries Leprosy; Neuropathies: an overview; Sleep disorders: an overview; Tuberculosis and the nervous system.

■ Tsujino's disease – see Glycogen-storage disorders: an overview; Lactate dehydrogenase deficiency

■ Tuberculosis and the nervous system

Pathophysiology Infection with *Mycobacterium* species (most usually *M. tuberculosis*) may produce a number of neurological syndromes, ranging from meningitis (tuberculous meningitis) to a cerebral mass lesion (tuberculoma). Disease of bone, for example in the vertebral column, may also produce neurological dysfunction (Pott's paraplegia). Tuberculous infection has increased in recent years, mainly related to concurrent HIV infection. Most patients have evidence of active tuberculosis (TB) elsewhere, but on occasion the infection is confined to the nervous system.

Clinical features: history and examination _Tuberculous meningitis (TBM)_: basal meninges particularly affected, $+/-$ hydrocephalus. Pathological process (tubercles with central caseation surrounded by epithelioid cells) may invade the underlying brain to produce a meningoencephalitis.

- Fever, headache, irritability, lethargy, vomiting
- Meningeal irritation (nuchal rigidity: Kernig's sign, Brudzinski's sign)
- Seizures: may be due to meningitis _per se_, hydrocephalus, hyponatraemia
- Altered level of consciousness: may be staged as I (fully responsive), II (drowsy, often with cranial nerve palsies), III (unconscious)
- Focal signs: cranial nerve palsies (inflammatory exudates in subarachnoid space): III, IV, VI > VII > VIII; hemiparesis (inflammation of arteries leading to infarction); gaze palsies, internuclear ophthalmoplegia
- Ischaemia: cortex, brainstem
- Hydrocephalus, raised intracranial pressure, papilloedema
- Stupor, coma, death (if untreated)

Tuberculoma: may occur concurrently with TBM; may be asymptomatic, depending on precise location:

- Focal signs
- Seizures.

Spinal cord syndrome: arachnoiditis, paraplegia, with or without involvement of the vertebral column (Pott's disease).

Investigations and diagnosis

Tuberculous meningitis (TBM):

Bloods: usually unremarkable but may show low sodium if there is associated syndrome of inappropriate ADH secretion.

Imaging: in case of raised intracranial pressure, focal signs: MRI shows enhancement of basal meninges; hydrocephalus; infarction; chest radiograph may give evidence of TB elsewhere.

CSF: raised pressure, protein, cell count (increasing proportion of lymphocytes with increasing duration of illness); low glucose versus serum (hypoglycorrhacia); PCR may be used to demonstrate _M. tuberculosis_ but its sensitivity is not as high as was hoped; therefore traditional culture methods are still required although slow (weeks). In many cases of suspected TB of the nervous system, the diagnosis is not proven, yet the patient improves with anti-TB therapy.

Tuberculoma:

Brain imaging for mass lesion(s).

CSF: because of proximity of mass lesion to meninges, CSF may contain raised protein, lymphocytes.

$+/-$ stereotactic biopsy.

Evidence for tuberculous disease elsewhere (e.g. chest X-ray, sputum, bronchial washings: early morning urine samples; bone marrow aspirate; look for acid-fast bacilli: Ziehl–Nielsen stain).

Consider checking HIV status.

Differential diagnosis *TBM*: other meningitides:

Bacterial: *Listeria*, partially treated bacterial meningitis, focal parameningeal infection (subdural empyema), neurosyphilis.

Fungal: cryptococcosis; coccidioidomycosis, histoplasmosis, candidiasis.

Viral: HSV, HIV, Japanese encephalitis.

Others: toxoplasmosis, sarcoidosis, neoplastic meningitis, venous sinus thrombosis.

Focal features of acute onset may prompt consideration of cerebrovascular disease.

In context of HIV, also need to consider toxoplasmosis, cerebral lymphoma, PML.

Tuberculoma: other mass lesions: bacterial abscess, tumour.

Treatment and prognosis Anti-tuberculous chemotherapy: intravenous triple therapy probably required:

isoniazid (+prophylactic pyridoxine to prevent neuropathy);

pyrizinamide;

rifampicin;

+/− ethambutol, streptomycin (cross inflamed meninges, so worth using in first 3 months).

Monitor liver function tests, abnormality may necessitate cessation of isoniazid; monitor visual acuity and colour vision, deterioration may require ethambutol to be stopped. Resistance to drugs is evident in some cases. No need for intrathecal therapy. Duration of treatment uncertain; may need to switch to oral therapy for up to 1 year. If risk of non-compliance, directly observed therapy (DOT) regimens may be used.

TBM:

Steroids often recommended in conjunction with anti-tuberculous therapy to prevent subarachnoid blockage.

Shunting may be undertaken if CSF pathways are blocked, but revision for shunt blockage is often necessary.

Tuberculoma: If unresponsive to anti-tuberculous therapy, surgical excision may be attempted.

Complete recovery is possible if the diagnosis is made early and appropriate therapy instituted. Poor prognostic features are increasing age (>60 years), prolonged duration of illness before diagnosis (>2 months), impaired consciousness at presentation. Delayed diagnosis is associated with a high fatality rate, especially among infants, HIV-positive patients, although the treatment and prognosis of TBM is similar in HIV-positive and -negative patients.

Neurological sequelae are common (25–40%): seizures, cranial nerve palsies, hemiplegia, paraplegia.

References Leonard JM, Des Prez RM. Tuberculosis and the central nervous system. In: Aminoff MJ (ed.). *Neurology and General Medicine: the Neurological Aspects of Medical Disorders* (2nd edition). New York: Churchill Livingstone, 1995: 703–716.

Parsons M. *Tuberculous meningitis. A Handbook for Clinicians.* Oxford: OUP, 1979.

Thwaites G, Chau TTH, Mai NTH, Drobniewski F, McAdam K, Farrar J. Tuberculous meningitis. *Journal of Neurology, Neurosurgery and Psychiatry* 2000; **68**: 289–299.

Other relevant entries Arachnoiditis; Brucellosis; HIV/AIDS and the nervous system; Hydrocephalus; Meningitis: an overview; Pott's disease; Sarcoidosis; Syndrome of inappropriate ADH secretion; Syphilis.

■ Tuberculous meningitis – see Tuberculosis and the nervous system

■ Tuberous sclerosis

Bourneville disease • Epiloia • Pringle disease • Tuberose sclerosis

Pathophysiology An autosomal-dominant condition characterized by multiple hamartomas of ectodermal structures (hence a phakomatosis). New mutations account for 70% of cases. The condition is clinically and genetically heterogeneous; chromosomal linkage to two loci has been established, at 9q34 (TSC1) encoding "hamartin", and at 16p13 (TSC2) encoding "tuberin". These may be tumour suppressor genes.

Clinical features: history and examination

- Neurological:
    Epilepsy (75%): often early onset
    Mental retardation (50%)
    Astrocytomas (5–10%)
    Raised intracranial pressure (rare).
- Dermatological:
    Hypopigmented "ash leaf" patches (80–90%)
    Adenoma sebaceum (facial angiofibromas) (40–90%)
    Shagreen patches (subepidermal fibrosis) (20–40%)
    Forehead fibrous plaque (25%)
    Ungual fibromas (15–50%).
- Ocular:
    Optic nerve/retina hamartoma (phakoma) (50%)
- Renal:
    Angiomyolipoma (60%)
    Renal cysts (20%)
    Renal cell carcinoma
    Cardiac rhabdomyoma
    Rectal polyps
    Lung fibrosis.

Investigations and diagnosis *Imaging*: CT/MRI: intracranial mass lesions; CT better for detecting calcification. Renal imaging (ultrasound/CT) for cysts, tumours. Woods (UV) lamp examination of the skin. Echocardiography for rhabdomyoma. *Neurophysiology*: EEG.

Differential diagnosis Other early onset epilepsy syndromes unlikely to be mistaken if typical dermatological features looked for.

Treatment and prognosis Morbidity most usually due to central nervous system (CNS) complications, for example status epilepticus; occasionally renal (e.g. bleed from angiomyolipoma, development of renal cell carcinoma).

Symptomatic treatment of epilepsy, skin lesions (dermabrasion), raised intracranial pressure (shunting); resection of brain/renal tumours sometimes possible.

Progressive course.

Genetic counselling for family.

References Curatolo P. *Tuberous Sclerosis Complex. From Basic Science to Clinical Phenotypes.* Cambridge: MacKeith Press, 2003.

Gomez MR, Sampson JR, Whittemore VH (eds). *Tuberous Sclerosis Complex* (3rd edition). New York: Oxford University Press, 1999.

O'Callaghan FJK. Tuberous sclerosis. *British Medical Journal* 1999; **318**: 1019–1020.

Other relevant entry Phakomatosis.

■ Tumarkin's otolithic crisis
Otolithic catastrophe of Tumarkin

Drop attacks, or Tumarkin's otolithic crisis, are episodes of sudden loss of balance in patients with Ménière's disease, with or without falls (patients may report a sensation of being pushed or knocked) but with preserved consciousness. There may be a sensation of movement or environmental tilt just before falling, but not true vertigo. These episodes, which are common in advanced disease, are thought to be due to changes in otolith function.

If there is true loss of consciousness, syncope is the more likely diagnosis.

Other relevant entries Drop attacks; Ménière's disease; Syncope.

■ Tumours: an overview

Pathophysiology Tumours affecting the nervous system may arise from:
- Glia: glioma, oligodendroglioma, ependymoma, Schwannoma (e.g. VIIIth nerve: vestibular Schwannoma/acoustic neuroma; spinal roots: neurofibroma)
- Meninges: meningioma
- Extraneous sites:
    Proximate (e.g. nasopharyngeal carcinoma, choroid plexus papilloma);
    Distant: metastases from bronchus, breast, melanoma.
- Lymphoid cells: lymphoma; angioendotheliomatosis
- Pituitary gland: pituitary adenoma

- Primitive germ cells : teratoma, germinoma, epidermoid/dermoid
- Neural elements (rare in adults): primitive neuroectodermal tumours (PNET, e.g. medulloblastoma); central neurocytoma; ganglioglioma
- Developmental residua: (e.g. notochordal elements: chordoma; Rathke's pouch: craniopharyngioma)
- Vascular endothelia: haemangioblastoma
- Hamartoma: tuberous sclerosis.

Of these, the commonest in adults are glioma, meningioma, and distant metastases. Tumours in children have a different frequency and distribution (more infratentorial lesions in children).

Tumours can also have distant, non-metastatic effects on the nervous system (paraneoplastic syndromes).

Clinical features: history and examination

- Consequences of raised intracranial pressure:
  Headache, with postural features (worse on lying, bending, straining); may cause nocturnal waking
  Transient visual obscurations, papilloedema
  "False-localizing signs", especially VIth nerve palsy, sometimes IIIrd nerve palsy with transtentorial temporal lobe herniation; Kernohan's (notch) syndrome
  Cushing reflex, Cushing response: hypertension, bradycardia
- Focal effects (legion): these signs are usually gradually progressive, but spontaneous "remissions" may occur, erroneously suggesting an inflammatory aetiology:
  Hemiparesis/monoparesis/paraparesis
  Visual field defects: homonymous hemianopia, bitemporal hemianopia
  Epileptic seizures: focal, secondary generalized
  Personality change, cognitive decline (e.g. focal meningioma, subfrontal lesions; primary (CNS) lymphoma)
  Stroke-like episodes (especially meningioma; bleed into a tumour)
  Anosmia (olfactory groove meningioma)
  Tumours of the spinal cord can be primary or secondary and present with local +/− radicular pain with a compressive spinal cord syndrome.
- Endocrine effects (functioning pituitary tumours):
  Somnolence, galactorrhoea, reduced facial hair growth and need for shaving: prolactinoma
  Cushingoid appearance
  Acromegaly
- Certain tumours have a predilection for certain sites:
  Meningioma: olfactory groove, petrous apex, falx
  Chordoma: skull base, spinal column.

Investigations and diagnosis
Imaging: CT/MRI +/− contrast medium: may be diagnostic or highly suggestive of diagnosis: mass lesion (meningioma, glioma, lymphoma, pituitary lesion) +/− mass effect, midline shift, vasogenic oedema.

Biopsy: Stereotactic: for diagnosis.

Open: for diagnosis, debulking, resection (if possible).

May need to investigate for primary tumour if metastases suspected.

Differential diagnosis

Very broad:

> Other mass lesions: cyst, haematoma, abscess; occasionally an inflammatory mass (multiple sclerosis (MS), sarcoidosis)
>
> Cord compression: degenerative bone disease, Paget's disease
>
> Stroke-like episodes: cerebrovascular disease, mitochondrial disease (MELAS)
>
> Cognitive/personality changes: neurodegenerative disease, depression/affective disorder.

Treatment and prognosis Some tumour types are amenable to complete surgical resection (certain meningiomas).

Radiotherapy, either external or internal from implanted rods or seeds, is required for radiosensitive tumours (glioma, lymphoma).

Symptomatic treatment includes steroids (dexamethasone) to reduce cerebral oedema, analgesia for headache, other pain syndromes from nerve compression.

Prognosis very variable dependent on tumour type and location, ranging from a life expectancy of only weeks (glioblastoma multiforme) to complete recovery.

References Behin A, Hoang-Xuan K, Carpentier AF, Delattre J-Y. Primary brain tumours in adults. *Lancet* 2003; **361**: 323–331.

De Angelis LM. Brain tumors. *New England Journal of Medicine* 2001; **344**: 114–123.

North B, Reilly P. *Raised Intracranial Pressure: A Clinical Guide.* Oxford: Heinemann, 1990.

Rees J. Neurological manifestations of malignant disease. *Hospital Medicine* 2000; **61**: 319–325.

Short SC, Brada M. The treatment of malignant cerebral tumours. *Hospital Medicine* 2000; **61**: 772–777.

Other relevant entries Abscess: an overview; Cushing reflex, Cushing response; Cysts: an overview; Haematoma: an overview; Hydrocephalus; Glioma; Lymphoma; Meningioma; Myelopathy: an overview; Neurofibromatosis; Oligodendroglioma; Paget's disease; Paraneoplastic syndromes; Paraparesis: acute management and differential diagnosis; Pituitary disease and apoplexy; Primitive neuroectodermal tumours; Radiculopathies: an overview; Spinal cord disease: an overview; Tuberous sclerosis; Von Hippel–Lindau syndrome.

■ Tunbridge–Paley syndrome

Pathophysiology An autosomal-recessive hereditary syndrome of progressive hearing loss, optic atrophy with visual loss, and diabetes mellitus. It is possible that this syndrome should now be reclassified, possibly as a mitochondrial disorder or as Wolfram syndrome.

Clinical features: history and examination

- Progressive hearing loss, variable severity, from first decade.
- Progressive visual loss, optic atrophy, from first decade.
- Juvenile diabetes mellitus, usually mild, from first or second decade.
- No ataxia, hypogonadism, retinitis pigmentosa.

Investigations and diagnosis Family history for similar conditions.

In view of the similarity of the phenotype to that seen in some mitochondrial disorders, it may be worth looking at mitochondrial DNA for point mutations in patients with the Tunbridge–Paley syndrome.

Differential diagnosis

Alström's syndrome.

Wolfram syndrome.

Treatment and prognosis No specific treatment; control diabetes with diet and medication (oral hypoglycaemics, insulin) if needed.

> **Reference** Tunbridge RE, Paley RG. Primary optic atrophy in diabetes mellitus. *Diabetes* 1956; **5**: 295–296.

> **Other relevant entries** Alström's syndrome; Diabetes mellitus and the nervous system; Mitochondrial disease: an overview; Nyssen–van Bogaert syndrome; Rosenberg–Chutorian syndrome; Sylvester disease; Wolfram syndrome.

■ Turcot syndrome

A familial polyposis coli syndrome, associated with malignant neuroepithelial tumours such as glioblastoma and medulloblastoma. May be dominantly or recessively inherited.

> **Reference** Foulkes WG. A tale of four syndromes: familial adenomatous polyposis, Gardner syndrome, attenuated APC and Turcot syndrome. *Quarterly Journal of Medicine* 1995; **88**: 853–863.

> **Other relevant entry** Gardner's syndrome.

■ Turner's syndrome

Pathophysiology A clinical syndrome produced by absence of one X-chromosome (XO), causing characteristic dysmorphic features. X-linked-recessive conditions normally seen only in boys may rarely occur in girls with Turner's syndrome (e.g. Duchenne muscular dystrophy).

Clinical features: history and examination

- Dysmorphism:
    Short stature
    Webbed neck

Cubitus valgus

Shield-shaped chest, widely spaced nipples.

- Streak gonads, primary amenorrhoea, infertility.
- Coarctation of the aorta, hypertension (+/− cardiovascular, cerebrovascular consequences thereof).
- Normal IQ.
- Increased susceptibility to:

Autoimmune thyroiditis

Osteoporosis

Renal disease

Inflammatory bowel disease.

Investigations and diagnosis Diagnosis clinical, usually evident at birth.

Chromosome studies to confirm XO. Absence of Barr bodies in cultured cells.

Differential diagnosis Unlikely to be mistaken.

Treatment and prognosis

Monitoring of cardiac, renal function. Control risk factors (hypertension).

Life expectancy is reduced as a consequence of cardiovascular disease.

> **Reference** Elsheikh M, Conway GS, Wass JA. Medical problems in adult women with Turner's syndrome. *Annals of Medicine* 1999; **31**: 99–105.

> **Other relevant entry** Coarctation of the aorta.

■ Typhus

Pathophysiology A number of different types of typhus are described, caused by various *Rickettsia*, Gram-negative coccobacilli which have a life cycle involving an animal reservoir, an insect vector (lice, fleas, ticks, mites), and man:

- Epidemic or louse-borne typhus (*Rickettsia prowazekii*; human body louse): jail fever, ship fever, camp fever, famine fever.
- Endemic (or murine) typhus (*Rickettsia typhi*, *Rickettesia mooseri*; fleas).
- Scrub typhus or tsutsugamushi fever (*Rickettsia orientalis* recently renamed as a new genus with only one species, *Orientia tsutsugamushi*; trombiculid mites, chiggers).

Exposure to wildlife or livestock may be an important clue to diagnosis. Although uncommon in the developed world, about one-third of cases are said to develop neurological features. Severity of disease is variable.

Clinical features: history and examination

- Bacteraemic illness: fever, headache, prostration.
- Deliruim, stupor, coma.
- +/− focal neurological signs.
- Meningitis, encephalitis, myelitis.
- Macular rash: necrotic ulcer and eschar in scrub typhus.
- Lymphadenopathy: local, general.
- +/− Disseminated intravascular coagulation.

Investigations and diagnosis

Bloods:

  Weil–Felix test: for the presence of heterophile antibodies to strains of *Proteus mirabilis*; may be negative in up to 50% of cases.
  Serology: species-specific ELISA, immunofluorescent antibody tests (IFAT), PCR.

CSF: normal, or modest lymphocytic pleocytosis.

Differential diagnosis Other causes of acute infective or inflammatory central nervous system (CNS) disease (e.g. viral meningitis).

Treatment and prognosis Although a cause of catastrophic epidemics in the past, associated with conditions of filth and poverty, and which may have influenced the course of history, early treatment with antibiotics (tetracycline, chloramphenicol) $+/-$ supportive care as appropriate means the condition is now associated with good prognosis; neurological sequelae are rare. Untreated, the condition may be fatal.

  Reference Cowan G. Rickettsial diseases: the typhus group of fevers – a review. *Postgraduate Medical Journal* 2000; **76**: 269–272.

  Other relevant entry Meningitis; Rickettsial diseases.

■ Tyrosinaemia

Pathophysiology An aminoacidopathy presenting in childhood, due to deficiency of various enzymes. Three types are recognized:

- Hereditary tyrosinaemia type I: hepatorenal tyrosinaemia, fumaryl-acetoacetate hydrolase deficiency.
- Hereditary tyrosinaemia type II: oculocutaneous tyrosinaemia, tyrosine aminotransferases deficiency, Richner–Hanhart disease.
- Hereditary tyrosinaemia type III: 4-hydroxyphenylpyruvate bisoxygenase/dioxygenase deficiency.

Clinical features: history and examination

Hereditary tyrosinaemia type I: hepatorenal tyrosinaemia:

- Severe progressive hepatocellular dysfunction: may present as acute liver failure in infancy or at a few months of age with failure to thrive
- Renal tubular dysfunction
- Porphyric crises
- Hepatomegaly: modest enlargement with hard irregular edge (cirrhosis)
- Hypotonia, depressed tendon reflexes (peripheral neuropathy)
- $+/-$ rickets
- $+/-$ cardiomyopathy sufficient to cause congestive heart failure.

Hereditary tyrosinaemia type II: oculocutaneous tyrosinaemia:

- Mild to moderate mental retardation with language deficits
- Incoordination of limbs, self-mutilation

- Corneal herpetiform erosions, causing lacrimation, photophobia, red eyes
- Palmar and plantar hyperkeratosis, hyperhidrosis.

Hereditary tyrosinaemia type III:
- Benign transient neonatal tyrosinaemia.

Investigations and diagnosis Hereditary tyrosinaemia type I: hepatorenal tyrosinaemia.

Bloods: anaemia, thrombocytopenia, hyperbilirubinaemia, mild elevation of transaminases, severe coagulopathy, hypoglycaemia, mild hyperammonaemia; elevated levels of tyrosine are non-specific (other causes of liver disease); renal tubular acidosis; α-fetoprotein levels extremely high.

Urine: elevated levels of tyrosine, not particularly helpful; urinary organic acid analysis of oxime derivatives more helpful, since may show succinylacetone, derived from accumulating fumaryl-acetoacetate, which is disease specific (may need to repeat urinary organic acid analysis if clinical suspicion is high). Succinylacetone inhibits δ-aminolaevulinic acid dehydratase, causing the episodic features of acute intermittent porphyria.

Enzyme levels in leukocytes, erythrocytes, fibroblasts, or liver tissue taken at biopsy is definitive diagnostic test.

Differential diagnosis

Hereditary tyrosinaemia type I: Other causes of hepatic failure

Neuropathy:

Lead poisoning (plumbism)

Guillain–Barré syndrome

Porphyria

Hexachlorobenzene poisoning.

Hereditary tyrosinaemia type II:

Chédiak–Higashi syndrome.

Treatment and prognosis Hereditary tyrosinaemia type I: hepatorenal tyrosinaemia.

Infantile acute liver failure is usually fatal; liver transplantation may be considered.

Childhood disease: a diet low in tyrosine and phenylalanine improves symptoms if started early. 4-hydroxyphenylpyruvate bisoxygenase inhibitors have also been suggested. Liver failure, hepatocellular carcinoma and early death occur without treatment.

Reference Holme E, Lindstedt S. Diagnosis and management of tyrosinemia type I. *Current Opinion in Pediatrics* 1995; **7**: 726–732.

Other relevant entries Aminoacidopathies: an overview; Chédiak–Higashi syndrome; Guillain–Barré syndrome; Lead and the nervous system; Porphyria.

Uu

■ Ulcerative colitis – see Gastrointestinal disease and the nervous system

■ Ullrich's disease

An autosomal-recessive condition, also known as hypotonic–sclerotic muscular dystrophy, Ullrich's disease was first described in 1930. It is characterized by generalized muscle weakness and wasting, contractures of proximal joints, hyperflexibility of distal joints, and a progressive course. Intellect and sensory function are normal. Creatine kinase is normal but muscle biopsy shows dystrophic features. Deficiency of collagen VI and mutations within the gene encoding collagen VI have been reported.

Reference Higuchi I, Shiraishi T, Hashiguchi T *et al*. Frameshift mutation in the collagen VI gene causes Ullrich's disease. *Annals of Neurology* 2001; **50**: 261–265.

Other relevant entry Muscular dystrophies: an overview.

■ Ulnar neuropathy
Ulnar nerve palsy

Pathophysiology The ulnar nerve carries fibres from spinal roots C7, C8, and T1. It supplies most of the small muscles of the hand (with the exception of those supplied by the median nerve), the long flexors of the ring and little finger, and the flexor of the ulnar side of the wrist (flexor carpi ulnaris). In perhaps 2% of individuals all small hand muscles are supplied by the ulnar nerve ("all ulnar hand"). Lesions of the ulnar nerve may occur at the elbow, wrist, and in the hand, each producing a slightly different pattern of deficits which may be of localizing value. The common causes of ulnar neuropathy are trauma, fracture/dislocation of surrounding bones, and compression (e.g. in the cubital tunnel, Guyon's canal).

Clinical features: history and examination

- Motor: wasting of the small hand muscles supplied by the ulnar nerve, especially evident in the first dorsal interosseous muscle (DIO), abductor digiti minimi (ADM), but eventually evident in all interossei and medial lumbricals producing dorsal guttering. With ulnar nerve lesions above the elbow an abnormal posture of the hand, claw hand or *main en griffe*, is seen, with hyperextension at the metacarpophalangeal joints (fifth, fourth, and, to a lesser extent, third finger) and flexion at the interphalangeal joints caused by the unopposed action of long finger extensors and flexors. Froment's prehensile thumb sign may be observed.
- Sensory: pain along inner forearm; paraesthesia/sensory impairment in little finger and medial half of ring finger, ulnar side of palm.

More restricted weakness and sensory loss in more distal lesions, that is, in wrist or palm (see Ramsay Hunt syndrome (3)).

- There may be a prior history of elbow trauma (with or without fracture), sometimes years before, hence "tardy ulnar palsy".
  Sites of ulnar nerve entrapment are:
- cubital tunnel (_q.v._);
- wrist, Guyon's canal: deep or superficial terminal branches.

Investigations and diagnosis _EMG/NCS_: reduced amplitude and delay of ulnar sensory nerve action potential from little finger; reduced motor nerve conduction velocity across lesion (e.g. at medial epicondyle); reduced compound muscle action potential; increased distal motor latency to ADM, DIO.

Differential diagnosis Radiculopathy: C8/T1 root lesions; no splitting of sensory loss in ring finger.

Plexopathy: lower part of brachial plexus (Déjerine–Klumpke type); no splitting of ring finger sensory loss.

Non-neurogenic causes of clawing: Dupuytren's contracture, camptodactyly.

Treatment and prognosis For lesions at the elbow, avoid pressure, repetitive flexion/extension; surgical decompression and/or transposition is an option. For lesions in the wrist or hand, removal of a compressing lesion may be possible.

References _Aids to the Examination of the Peripheral Nervous System_. London: HMSO, 1976.

Capitani D, Beer S. Handlebar palsy – a compression syndrome of the deep terminal (motor) branch of the ulnar nerve in biking. _Journal of Neurology_ 2002; **249**: 1441–1445.

Staal A, Van Gijn J, Spaans F. _Mononeuropathies: Examination, Diagnosis and Treatment_. London: WB Saunders, 1999: 69–84.

Other relevant entries Cubital tunnel syndrome; Entrapment neuropathies; Froment's (prehensile thumb) sign; Neuropathies: an overview; Ramsay Hunt syndrome (3).

■ Unverricht–Lundborg disease

Baltic myoclonus (epilepsy) • Dyssynergia cerebellaris myoclonica • Ramsay Hunt syndrome

Pathophysiology An autosomal-recessive condition with onset between age 6 and 15 years, equal sex incidence, but variable geographical distribution. It presents with myoclonus which is progressively more difficult to control. Ataxia and tremor develop; tonic–clonic seizures may occur but are not usually a serious problem. There is slow intellectual decline. Unverricht–Lundborg disease is the commonest cause of progressive myoclonic epilepsy (PME).

Clinical features: history and examination
- Polymyoclonus of cortical origin: spon-taneous, action induced, stimulus sensitive; progressive.
- Cerebellar ataxia, tremor, dementia (mild, slowly progressive), seizures.

Investigations and diagnosis *Bloods*: no diagnostic biochemical or pathological abnormality yet demonstrated.
Imaging: CT/MRI: atrophy may occur, not specific.
Neurophysiology:

  EEG: potentials time-locked to myoclonus; generalized spike and slow-wave. discharges, slow background activity, +/− photosensitivity.
  SSEP: giant cortical potentials, not specific.

Neurogenetics: mutations in EPM1 gene encoding cystatin B on chromosome 21q22.3; pathogenetic mechanism not understood.

Differential diagnosis Differential diagnosis of progressive myoclonus epilepsy (PME):

  Lafora body disease
  Sialidosis (types I and II)
  Myoclonic epilepsy with ragged red fibres (MERRF)
  Neuronal ceroid lipofuscinosis (NCL)
  Gaucher's disease
  Neuroaxonal dystrophy
  Dentatorubral–pallidoluysian atrophy (DRPLA)
  Biotin-responsive encephalopathy.

Treatment and prognosis Symptomatic therapy for myoclonus, epilepsy: sodium valproate, benzodiazepines (e.g. clonazepam), piracetam; ? zonisamide. Anecdotal evidence suggests that phenytoin may exacerbate situation, so best avoided.

References Lalioti MD, Scott HS, Buresi C *et al*. Dodecamer repeat expansion in cystatin B gene in progressive myoclonus epilepsy. *Nature* 1997;
  386: 847–851.
Pennacchio LA, Lehesjoki AE, Stone NE *et al*. Mutations in the gene encoding cystatin B in progressive myoclonus epilepsy (EPM1). *Science* 1996;
  271: 1731–1734.

Other relevant entries Cerebellar disease: an overview; Myoclonus; Progressive myoclonic epilepsy.

▓ Upper airway resistance syndrome – see Obstructive sleep apnoea syndrome

▓ Uraemia – see Renal disease and the nervous system

▓ Urea cycle enzyme defects

Pathophysiology Deficiencies of any of the six enzymes which comprise the urea (Krebs–Henseleit) cycle which converts ammonia to urea can result in a hyperammonaemic syndrome, leading to coma and death, usually in the neonatal period. Partial defects may have a delayed onset until adolescence or even adulthood. In addition to hyperammonaemia, there may be concurrent respiratory alkalosis, citrullinaemia, and increases in urinary orotic acid. Ornithine transcarbamoylase (OTC) deficiency, probably the commonest of the urea cycle disorders, is X-linked; carrier mothers may show signs of mild neurological dysfunction.

The urea cycle pathway involves the following reactions:

- Carbamoylphosphate synthase I (CPS-I) catalyses the condensation of ammonium with bicarbonate to form carbamoylphosphate; N-acetylglutamate (NAG) is an obligatory effector (not substrate) for this reaction, itself produced by N-acetylglutamate synthetase (NAGS).
- OTC condenses carbamoylphosphate with ornithine to produce citrulline.
- Argininosuccinic acid (ASA) synthase catalyses condensation of citrulline with aspartate to form ASA.
- ASA lyase cleaves ASA to produce arginine and fumarate.
- Arginase cleaves arginine to urea and ornithine.
- A transport system returns ornithine to the intramitochondrial compartment. The following UCED are recognized:
- CPS-I deficiency: low or undetectable plasma citrulline levels; absence of urinary orotic acid.
- NAGS deficiency: low or undetectable plasma citrulline levels; absence of urinary orotic acid.
- OTC deficiency: low or undetectable plasma citrulline levels, normal plasma ornithine; raised urinary orotic acid.
- ASA synthase deficiency: markedly elevated citrulline levels ($>1000\,\mu mol/l$) = citrullinaemia.
- ASA lyase deficiency: normal or modestly elevated plasma citrulline; argininosuccinic aciduria; arginine deficiency, secondary deficiency of ornithine within mitochondria.
- Arginase deficiency: normal or modestly elevated plasma citrulline, raised plasma arginine; argininosuccinic aciduria.

Clinical features: history and examination

- Neonatal failure to thrive; poor feeding, vomiting.
- Rigidity, opisthotonos; severe hypertonia.
- Seizures: usually myoclonic.
- Hyperpnoea.
- Hepatomegaly.
- Coma, atonia, death.
- No dysmorphism.
- Arginase deficiency presents in later infancy and early childhood with "cerebral palsy".

Investigations and diagnosis
Bloods: hyperammonaemia (*ca.* 1000 μM, NR 15–45); respiratory alkalosis; no ketoacidosis. Urea may be normal or reduced; normal

glucose. Liver-related blood tests are normal or near normal (*cf*. hepatic failure as a cause of hyperammonaemia), with the exception of OTC deficiency. Citrulline, ornithine may be raised in plasma in some defects.

Urine: orotic acid elevated in OTC deficiency.

CSF: raised ammonia.

Imaging: MRI brain may show diffuse, partly reversible, high signal change.

Neurogenetics: DNA analysis for specific genes in some cases.

Other: specific enzyme assays on liver biopsy.

The key parameters in interpretation of UCED are:

> Plasma citrulline: elevated in ASA synthase deficiency.
> Urinary orotic acid: elevated in OTC deficiency; absent in CPS-I deficiency, NAGS deficiency.

Differential diagnosis Severe hepatocellular dysfunction: viral infection, intoxication, inborn errors of metabolism.

Organic acidaemias (e.g. methylmalonic acidaemia, proprionic acidaemia).

Reye's syndrome.

Mitochondrial disorders.

Toxic disorders.

Treatment and prognosis Reduce blood ammonia concentration: haemodialysis, intravenous sodium benzoate, intravenous sodium phenylacetate.

High-calorie, low-protein diet (increase protein intake may precipitate exacerbations).

Argininosuccinic acid (ASA) lyase deficiency causing arginine deficiency: therapeutic response to arginine (4 mmol/kg intravenously) is dramatic.

Liver transplantation corrects enzyme deficiency.

If appropriate treatment is not instituted early, then death results. Survivors may also have neurological sequelae. Intermittent episodes of hyperammonaemia with clinical deterioration may be provoked by excess protein intake or infection.

Valproate should be avoided as it may cause liver failure.

References Batshaw ML. Inborn errors of urea synthesis. *Annals of Neurology* 1994; **35**: 133–141.

Steiner RD, Cederbaum SD. Laboratory evaluation of urea cycle disorders. *Journal of Pediatrics* 2001; **138** (**suppl 1**): S21–S29.

Other relevant entries Ornithine transcarbamoylase deficiency; Reye's syndrome.

■ Urinary system

Neurogenic bladder dysfunction

Pathophysiology The neurological pathways subserving micturition extend from the medial frontal lobes via a micturition centre in the dorsal tegmentum of the pons, to spinal cord pathways, to Onuf's nucleus in spinal cord segments S2–S4, the cauda equina, and hence to the pudendal nerves. Damage in any of these areas may produce urinary dysfunction, which may include:

- Urinary incontinence with urgency (frequency/urgency/urge incontinence): spastic bladder;
- Overflow incontinence with atonic bladder;
- Detrusor sphincter dyssynergia.

Many pathological processes may be responsible, including multiple sclerosis, epilepsy, frontal lobe degeneration, normal pressure hydrocephalus.

Clinical features: history and examination History should assess:

- Urinary habits: frequency of micturition, urgency, episodes of incontinence;
- Awareness of desire to micturate, ability to initiate and terminate urination, force of stream, urinary volume;
- Sensation/awareness of bladder fullness: sensation may be preserved but volitional voiding compromised with cauda equina lesions (motor paralytic bladder);
- + sexual function;
- + bowel function.

Urinary dysfunction of neurological origin is most often accompanied by other neurological signs, for example:

- *Frontal lobe*: frontal-type dementia; primitive reflexes (frontal-release signs), extrapyramidal signs
- *Brainstem* (pontine micturition centre): internuclear ophthalmoplegia
- *Spinal cord*: myelopathy, conus medullaris or cauda equina syndrome.

Investigations and diagnosis Clinical features may point to the likely location of abnormality in CNS, but imaging of whole neuraxis may be necessary to establish locus of pathology.

Urine: exclude infection.

In–out catheterization/ultrasonography: for post-micturition residual volume: high with incomplete bladder emptying.

Urodynamics: cystometry, +/− micturating cystourethrography, cystourethroscopy, retrograde urethrography:

Spastic bladder: decreased capacity, reduced compliance, uninhibited detrusor contractions.

Atonic bladder: increased capacity, increased compliance, low voiding pressure and flow rate.

Sphincter dyssynergia: fluctuating voiding pressure, intermittent flow rate.

Neurophysiology: EMG/NCS: of pelvic floor, especially anal sphincter (S4) for evidence of denervation; pudendal nerve conduction velocity abnormal in neuropathic causes.

Imaging: cauda equina, conus, spinal cord, brain (as appropriate).

Differential diagnosis Urological causes of dysfunction, especially urinary tract infection and prostatic enlargement, should also be considered in the differential diagnosis.

Treatment and prognosis Treatment of underlying cause is sometimes possible with resolution of symptoms (e.g. normal pressure hydrocephalus).

Urgency due to detrusor hyperreflexia causing abrupt increases in detrusor pressure (e.g. in multiple sclerosis) may be helped by anticholinergic medications (e.g. oxybutynin); intravesical capsaicin.

Incomplete bladder emptying due to detrusor sphincter dyssynergia, with a post-micturition residual volume of >100 ml is best treated by clean intermittent self-catheterization or, if this is not possible, permanent suprapubic catheterization.

Overflow incontinence/atonic bladder (e.g. spinal shock, conus medullaris and cauda equina lesions, neuropathy, multiple system atrophy): clean intermittent self-catheterization.

References Fowler CJ. Neurological disorders of micturition and their treatment. *Brain* 1999; **122**: 1213–1231.

Garg BP. Approach to the patient with bladder, bowel, or sexual dysfunction and other autonomic disorders. In: Biller J (ed.). *Practical Neurology* (2nd edition). Philadelphia: Lippincott Williams & Wilkins, 2002: 366–376.

Other relevant entries Cauda equina syndrome and conus medullaris disease; Dementia: an overview; Epilepsy: an overview; Multiple sclerosis; Multiple system atrophy; Myelopathy: an overview; Normal pressure hydrocephalus.

■ Usher's syndrome

Pathophysiology A clinically and genetically heterogeneous autosomal-recessive disorder characterized by hereditary hearing loss and slowly progressive retinitis pigmentosa. Various subtypes have been defined, for example Type I (severe hearing loss, abnormal vestibular function) accounting for 50–70% of cases, and Type II (moderate hearing loss, normal vestibular function) accounting for most of the rest.

Clinical features: history and examination
- Sensorineural hearing loss, probably of cochlear origin; mutism.
- Retinitis pigmentosa: presenting with nyctalopia in late childhood or adolescence.
- Vestibular hypofunction in some patients.
- Mental deficiency.
- Psychosis.
- +/− cataracts, glaucoma.
- Ataxia.
- Nystagmus (rare).
- Male infertility.
- No obesity, diabetes mellitus, peripheral neuropathy, skin or skeletal involvement.

Investigations and diagnosis Genetics: several loci now identified.

Differential diagnosis Alström's syndrome, Cockayne's syndrome, Refsum's syndrome.

Treatment and prognosis No specific treatment.

References Hallgren B. Retinitis pigmentosa combined with congenital deafness; with vestibulo-cerebellar ataxia and mental abnormality in a proportion of cases. A clinical and genetico-statistical study. *Acta Psychiatrica et Neurologica Scandinavica* 1959; **34**(suppl 138): 1–101.

Smith RJH, Berlin CI, Hejtmancik JF *et al*. Clinical diagnosis of the Usher syndrome. *American Journal of Human Genetics* 1994; **50**: 32–38.

Other relevant entries Alström's syndrome; Cockayne's syndrome; Refsum's syndrome; Retinitis pigmentosa.

■ Uveitis

Inflammation of the uvea may be classified as:
- Anterior: iris and/or ciliary body (iritis, cyclitis, iridocyclitis).
- Posterior: choroid (choroiditis).

These syndromes may occur in isolation or as part of a multisystem disease which may have other neurological features, for example in sarcoidosis or Vogt–Koyanagi–Harada (VKH) syndrome.

Other relevant entries Cranial nerve disease: II: Optic nerve; Glaucoma; Reiter's disease; Sarcoidosis; Vogt–Koyanagi–Harada syndrome.

■ Uveoretinal meningoencephalitic syndromes – see Vogt–Koyanagi–Harada syndrome

Vv

■ Vagus nerve disease – see Cranial nerve disease: X: Vagus nerve

■ Van Buchem's syndrome

Hyperostosis cranialis generalisata • Sclerosteosis

This autosomal-recessive syndrome of osteosclerosis affects the ribs, clavicles, long bones and pelvis as well as the skull (*cf.* hyperostosis cranialis interna), causing a prominent jaw and hypertelorism. About half of cases develop involvement of the facial (VII) and vestibulocochlear (VIII) nerve, but optic nerve involvement and raised intracranial pressure is rare.

Reference Van Buchem FS. Hyperostosis cranialis generalisata: eight new cases. *Acta Medica Scandinavica* 1971; **189**: 257–267.

Other relevant entries Hyperostosis cranialis interna; Paget's disease.

■ Vanishing white matter disease

Childhood ataxia with central nervous system hypomyelination (CACH) • Cree leukoencephalopathy • Fatal infantile leukodystrophy • Myelinolysis centralis diffusa • Ovarioleukodystrophy

There are a number of rare conditions characterized by an orthochromatic leukodystrophy with striking cavitary lesions (= vanishing white matter). They may present from the age of a few months up to the third decade, and have a spectrum of severity ranging from acute onset with death in weeks (as in Cree leukoencephalopathy) to a mild variant lasting many years. The clinical picture encompasses a non-specific progressive mental deterioration, spasticity, cerebellar ataxia, and epilepsy. Ovarian pathology and glaucoma have also been noted as associations. Onset may follow cranial trauma or fever. MRI of brain shows diffuse symmetrical white matter change and cerebellar vermian atrophy, with cavitary lesions. MR spectroscopy suggests an axonopathy rather than demyelination. Neuropathology shows a cavitary leuko-encephalopathy. Some cases are associated with mutations in the gene encoding eukaryotic initiation factor 2B (eIF2B).

Reference Fogli A, Rodriguez D, Eymard-Pierre E *et al.* The large clinical spectrum of eIF2B mutations: from infant to adult white matter disorders. *Journal of Neurology* 2003; **250**(suppl II): II34 (abstract 104).

■ Variant Creutzfeldt–Jakob disease

"Human BSE"

Pathophysiology Although <200 cases of variant Creutzfeldt–Jakob disease (vCJD) have been described, most in the UK, the condition has attracted huge attention and research effort since it is believed to be an iatrogenic disease, caused by the transmission of the prion agent which causes bovine spongiform encephalopathy (BSE) into the human food chain and across the species barrier.

Clinical features: history and examination

- Psychiatric features predominate in early stages, including dysphoria, withdrawal, anxiety, insomnia, and loss of interest.
- Neurological features precede (15%) or coincide with (22%) psychiatric features; these include poor memory, pain (hyperpathia), sensory symptoms, unsteadiness of gait, and dysarthria. Chorea is also described.

Investigations and diagnosis *Bloods*: no specific abnormalities.

Imaging: high signal in posterior thalamus (pulvinar sign).

CSF: protein markers of neuronal injury (Neurone-Specific Enolase, 14-3-3) and glial activation (S100β) may be elevated in vCJD but this finding is non-specific.

Neurophysiology: EEG: typically normal in vCJD (*cf.* sporadic CJD in which periodic complexes may be seen).

Tonsil biopsy: may be helpful if PrP-immunopositive staining is present.

Brain biopsy: features as for sporadic CJD but kuru-type PrP-immunopositive amyloid plaques are abundant.

Neurogenetics: no mutations in PrP gene; all cases of vCJD described thus far have had the MM genotype at codon 129 of the PrP gene.

Differential diagnosis

Sporadic, iatrogenic, or inherited CJD.

Wilson's disease.

Limbic encephalitis.

Cerebral vasculitis.

Diagnosis may be very difficult in the early stages if psychiatric features occur in isolation.

Treatment and prognosis No specific treatment. Some laboratory evidence in favour of quinacrine; trial underway. Pentosan polyphosphate has been given in one case after appeal to the High Court (no clinical evidence in favour of use).

References Collinge J. Variant Creutzfeldt–Jakob disease. *Lancet* 1999; **354**: 317–323.

Lowman A, Knight R, Ironside J. Variant Creutzfeldt–Jakob disease. *Practical Neurology* 2001; **1**: 2–13.

Spencer MS, Knight RSG, Will RG. First hundred cases of variant Creutzfeldt–Jakob disease: retrospective case note review of early psychiatric and neurological features. *British Medical Journal* 2002; **324**: 1479–1482.

Other relevant entries Creutzfeldt–Jakob disease; Prion disease: an overview.

◼ Varicella zoster virus and the nervous system

Varicella zoster virus (VZV) may be associated with various neurological syndromes:

Peripheral nervous system (PNS)
  Herpes zoster (shingles)
  Radiculoneuropathy
  Ganglionitis
  Postherpetic neuralgia.
Central nervous system (CNS)
  Myelitis
  Encephalomyelitis
  Arteritis (large or small vessel)
  Ventriculitis, meningitis.

VZV has also been implicated in some cases of Reye's syndrome, Guillain–Barré syndrome, PORN syndrome.

Reference Gilden DH, Kleinschmidt-DeMasters BK, LaGuardia JJ, Mahalingam R, Cohrs RJ. Neurologic complications of the reactivation of varicella-zoster virus. *New England Journal of Medicine* 2000; **342**: 635–645.

Other relevant entries Encephalitis: an overview; Herpes zoster and postherpetic neuralgia; PORN syndrome; Ramsay Hunt syndrome (2); Reye's syndrome; Transverse myelitis, transverse myelopathy.

■ Variegate porphyria – see Porphyria

■ Vascular dementia

Multi-infarct dementia (MID) • Vascular cognitive impairment (VCI)

Pathophysiology That cerebrovascular disease may cause cognitive impairment, as well as sensory and motor dysfunction, is self-evident, but classifying vascular dementia or VCI has not proven straightforward. Vascular change may often coexist with Alzheimer's disease (there are shared risk factors). Although said to be the second most common cause of cognitive decline after AD, cases of pure vascular dementia are rare: witness the difficulty of recruiting sufficient patients for international therapeutic intervention trials.

Recognized varieties of VCI include:

- MID: multiple infarcts involving cortical and subcortical areas, usually from large vessel occlusions.
- Strategic infarct dementia: single or multiple infarcts affecting structures crucial for cognitive function (e.g. bilateral hippocampal infarcts, bilateral thalamic infarctions, paramedian–mesencephalic–diencephalic infarcts).
- Subcortical white matter disease = small vessel dementia (e.g. Binswanger's disease).
- Familial vascular encephalopathies (e.g. CADASIL).

Clinical features: history and examination

- Focal signs more likely than in other dementia syndromes, for example hemiparesis, aphasia, *marche à petit pas*.
- Cognitive syndrome: executive, subcortical, and frontal lobe dysfunction said to predominate over disorders of memory and language (*cf.* AD); behavioural features may also be prominent (e.g. emotional lability).
- The classical teaching that vascular dementia has a sudden onset and/or stepwise progression does not always hold true; a considerable proportion have a gradual progression.
- History of hypertension, other cardiovascular risk factors, common.

Investigations and diagnosis *Imaging*: the finding of vascular changes on CT/MRI may, or may not, correlate with cognitive/behavioural syndrome. Tightest correlation is in (rare) examples of strategic infarct dementia. Functional imaging (SPECT) may show multifocal, patchy deficits.

Bloods: check cholesterol; homocysteine may be a risk factor for cerebrovascular disease but what, if any, response may be made to an elevated level is currently unknown; Venereal Disease Research Laboratory (VDRL) test.

CSF: no specific findings.

Differential diagnosis

AD.

Frontotemporal dementia.

Dementia with Lewy bodies.

Treatment and prognosis There is no licenced treatment for vascular dementia currently. Trials of cholinesterase inhibitors have suggested symptomatic benefit greater than placebo, but this is less than seen in AD.

Control of risk factors for cerebrovascular disease (hypertension, hypercholesterolaemia) is appropriate.

References Amar K, Wilcock G. Vascular dementia. *British Medical Journal* 1996; **312**: 227–231.

Bowler JV, Hachinski V. Vascular cognitive impairment: a new approach to vascular dementia. In: Hachinski V (ed.). *Cerebrovascular Disease*. London: Baillière Tindall, 1995: 357–376.

Bowler JV, Hachinski V (eds). *Vascular Cognitive Impairment: Preventable Dementia*. Oxford: OUP, 2003.

Chiu E, Gustafson L, Ames D, Folstein MF (eds). *Cerebrovascular Disease and Dementia: Pathology, Neuropsychiatry and Management*. London: Martin Dunitz, 2000.

De Leeuw FE, van Gijn J. Vascular dementia. *Practical Neurology* 2003; **3**: 86–91.

Román GC, Tatemichi TK, Erkinjuntti T *et al.* Vascular dementia: diagnostic criteria for research studies. Report of the NINDS–AIREN international workshop. *Neurology* 1993; **43**: 250–260.

Other relevant entries Alzheimer's disease; Angioendotheliomatosis; Binswanger's disease; CADASIL; Cerebrovascular disease: arterial; Dementia with Lewy bodies; Frontotemporal dementia; Von Winiwarter–Buerger's disease.

▨ Vascular disease – see Brainstem vascular syndromes; Cerebrovascular disease: arterial; Cerebrovascular disease: venous; Lacunar syndromes

▨ Vasculitis

Pathophysiology The vasculitides are inflammatory disorders of blood vessels which may produce neurological symptoms and signs if intracerebral vessels or the vasa nervorum of the peripheral nervous system (PNS) are involved. The inflammation may be autoimmune in origin, for example associated with markers for lupus or with anti-neutrophil cytoplasmic antibodies (ANCA). This may occur in the context of a variety of disorders, typically affecting vessels of differing calibre:

- Large arteries: Giant cell arteritis, Kawasaki disease, classical polyarteritis nodosa, Takayasu's arteritis.
- Medium arteries: Churg–Strauss syndrome, microscopic polyangiitis, Wegener's granulomatosis.
- Small vessels: Cryoglobulinaemia.

Vasculits may also occur on occasion in a variety of other conditions, such as rheumatoid arthrits, Sjögren's syndrome, systemic lupus erythematosus (SLE), sarcoidosis, syphilis, other infections (hepatitis B, C), and following use of certain recreational drugs (e.g. amphetamines, cocaine).

Clinical features: history and examination
Very diverse.

- Central nervous system
  Acute/subacute encephalopathy
  "Multiple sclerosis (MS)-like" presentation (relapsing–remitting disorder + features atypical of MS, such as seizures) but often with headache
  Rapidly progressive space-occupying lesion.
- PNS
  Mononeuritis multiplex
  Mononeuropathies.

Investigations and diagnosis *Bloods*: may have raised ESR, CRP; auto-antibody profile: ANA, anti-ds DNA, ANCA, cryoglobulins; check hepatitis serology; drug screen.

Imaging:

MRI: may show periventricular white matter abnormalities akin to those of MS, or frank infarctions
SPECT: may show patchy focal ischaemic deficits
Cerebral angiography: although once used as the criterion for the diagnosis of vasculitis, this is not specific, nor is it sensitive; its main use is to exclude atheromatous disease as a cause of the neurological syndrome.

CSF: may find oligoclonal bands in central nervous system (CNS) vasculitis
Ophthalmology: slit-lamp examination of anterior segment may show inflammatory changes in CNS vasculitis; fluorescein angiogram may corroborate this.
Biopsy: histopathology is the gold standard for the diagnosis of vasculitis, but the procedure is not without risk and the false-negative rate must also be taken into consideration; biopsy may be helpful in ruling out other diagnoses.

Differential diagnosis Other causes of encephalopathy.
Inflammatory CNS/PNS disease (e.g. multiple sclerosis, sarcoidosis, SLE).
Tumour.
Mitochondrial disorders (e.g. MELAS).

Other vasculopathies (e.g. fibromuscular dysplasia, moyamoya disease, amyloid angiopathy, CADASIL, Marfan's syndrome, pseudoxanthoma elasticum, Fabry's disease, homocysteinuria, Ehlers–Danlos syndrome).

Infection.

Cholesterol embolization syndrome.

Treatment and prognosis Steroids may be adequate for localized disease, but for systemic or CNS disease, steroids in combination with cyclophosphamide are generally required. This treatment may need to be lifelong.

References Alrawi A, Trobe JD, Blaivas M, Musch DC. Brain biopsy in primary angiitis of the central nervous system. *Neurology* 1999; **53**: 858–860.

Ferro JM. Vasculitis of the central nervous system. *Journal of Neurology* 1998; **245**: 766–776.

Scolding N. Cerebral vasculitis. In: Scolding N (ed.). *Immunological and Inflammatory Disorders of the Central Nervous System*. Oxford: Butterworth-Heinemann, 1999: 210–257.

Scolding NJ, Jayne DRW, Zajicek JP, Meyer PAR, Wraight EP, Lockwood CM. Cerebral vasculitis – recognition, diagnosis and management. *Quarterly Journal of Medicine* 1997; **90**: 61–73.

Other relevant entries Behçet's disease; Cholesterol embolization syndrome; Churg–Strauss syndrome; Collagen vascular disorders and the nervous system: an overview; Cryoglobulinaemia, cryoglobulinaemic neuropathy; Giant cell arteritis; Herpes zoster and postherpetic neuralgia; Isolated angiitis of the central nervous system; Neuropathies: an overview; Polyarteritis nodosa; Polymyalgia rheumatica; Rheumatoid arthritis; Sarcoidosis; Sjögren's syndrome; Syphilis; Systemic lupus erythematosus and the nervous system; Takayasu's disease; Wegener's granulomatosis.

■ Vasovagal syncope – see Syncope

■ Vegetative states
Apallic syndrome • Coma vigil • Neocortical death

Pathophysiology Following head injury or extensive ischaemic–hypoxic brain injury, for example following resuscitation after prolonged cardiac arrest, cognitive brain function may be lost due to neocortical damage whilst vegetative functions are preserved due to intact brainstem centres. A persistent vegetative state (PVS) may be diagnosed if this persists for >12 months following trauma (UK; 6 months in USA) or for >6 months following anoxia (UK; 3 months in USA).

Clinical features: history and examination
- No awareness of self or environment, for example to noxious visual stimuli (visual threat), auditory, or tactile stimuli.
- Preserved autonomic, respiratory function.

- Primitive postural and reflex limb movements may be observed.
- Brainstem reflexes may be preserved.
- No reasonable prospect of improvement.
- Repeated and prolonged observations may be necessary to ensure the absence of awareness; other sources of information (nursing observations, relatives) should also be consulted.

Investigations and diagnosis Clinical observation is the key investigation. The suggestion that functional imaging (PET) may be helpful in establishing the diagnosis has been challenged.

No specific neuropathological correlate.

Differential diagnosis

Coma.

Abulia/akinetic mutism.

Locked-in syndrome.

Catatonia.

Treatment and prognosis In PVS the prognosis is poor; however, very occasional well-substantiated reports of very late recovery have appeared.

Withdrawal of medical treatment requires the approval of the High Court, which decides whether continued treatment is in the patient's best interests, though serious ethical questions remain.

Death usually occurs within 14 days of withdrawal of treatment.

References Jennett B. *The Vegetative State. Medical Facts, Ethical and Legal Dilemmas*. Cambridge: CUP, 2002.

Wade DT, Johnston C. The permanent vegetative state: practical guidelines on diagnosis and management. *British Medical Journal* 1999; **319**: 841–844.

Zeman A. The persistent vegetative state: conscious of nothing? *Practical Neurology* 2002; **2**: 214–217.

Other relevant entries Brain death, Brainstem death; Coma; Locked-in syndrome; Posthypoxic syndromes.

■ Venous sinus thrombosis – see Cerebrovascular disease: venous

■ Verger–Déjerine syndrome

An anterior parietal lobe syndrome characterized by contralateral impairment of discriminative sensory function (position sense, localization of touch and pain, two-point discrimination) but with relative sparing of primary sensory modalities (*cf*. Déjerine–Mouzon syndrome).

Other relevant entries Déjerine–Mouzon syndrome; Déjerine–Roussy syndrome; Thalamic syndromes.

■ Vernant's disease

Recurrent optic neuromyelitis with endocrinopathies

Pathophysiology In 1997, Vernant and colleagues described eight Antillean women with a syndrome of recurrent optic and spinal cord inflammation (with dissociated sensory loss, sometimes with syrinx formation), associated with various endocrine disturbances. Whether this is a unique disease, or simply a variant of Devic's disease (neuromyelitis optica), which it resembles in its neurological features, has yet to be determined.

Clinical features: history and examination

- Optic neuropathy: unilateral or bilateral, recurrent.
- Myelopathy: acute or subacute, recurrent; syringomyelia-like dissociated sensory loss.
- +/− amenorrhoea, galactorrhoea, diabetes insipidus, hypothyroidism, hyperphagia.

Investigations and diagnosis *Bloods*: thyroid function tests; FSH/LH; prolactin, may be abnormal.

Imaging: MR brain normal; spinal cord may show syrinx cavity.

CSF: raised white cell count (up to 200); oligoclonal bands negative.

Differential diagnosis

Devic's neuromyelitis optica.

Multiple sclerosis.

HTLV-1 myelopathy.

Treatment and prognosis Immunosuppression is without effect. Six of the original eight cases died within 5 years.

> **References** Román G. Tropical myeloneuropathies revisited. *Current Opinion in Neurology* 1998; **11**: 539–544.
>
> Vernant J-C, Cabre P, Smadja D *et al.* Recurrent optic neuromyelitis with endocrinopathies: a new syndrome. *Neurology* 1997; **48**: 58–64.
>
> **Other relevant entries** Devic's disease, Devic's syndrome; Multiple sclerosis; Syringomyelia and syringobulbia.

■ Vernet's syndrome

Pathophysiology A jugular foramen syndrome with simultaneous unilateral involvement of cranial nerves IX, X, and XI. It is mainly associated with tumours and inflammatory/infectious processes adjacent to the jugular foramen, but occasionally with trauma (as in Vernet's original case) or ischaemia.

Clinical features: history and examination

- Dysphonia.
- Dysphagia.
- Palatal paresis.
- Vocal cord paralysis.
- Sternocleidomastoid weakness.
- +/− temporal/retroparotid pain.

Investigations and diagnosis *Blood*: markers of infection/inflammation (leukocytosis, raised ESR).

Imaging: of skull base to exclude mass lesion, collection.

Differential diagnosis Other skull base/jugular foramen syndromes (e.g. Collet–Sicard syndrome and Villaret's syndrome).

Treatment and prognosis Of cause where possible (e.g. tumour resection).

References Gout O, Viala K, Lyon-Caen O. Giant cell arteritis and Vernet's syndrome. *Neurology* 1998; **50**: 1862–1864.

Vernet M. Syndrome du trou dechire posterieur. *Revue Neurologique* 1918; **2**: 117–154.

Other relevant entries Collet–Sicard's syndrome; Cranial polyneuropathy; Jugular foramen syndrome; Villaret's syndrome.

■ Vertebral artery dissection

Pathophysiology Dissection of the vertebral artery within the neck or extending into the skull may occur spontaneously or as a result of predisposing events such as neck trauma (possibly including osteopathic/chiropractic manipulation of the neck). Dissection *per se* may cause neck and/or occipital head pain or be asymptomatic, but neurological complications may result from thrombosis and artery-to-artery embolism from the dissected vessel wall.

Clinical features: history and examination

- Neck and/or occipital head pain, leading to TIA/stroke (especially lateral medullary syndrome) in hours to 2 weeks.
- Ophthalmic findings common: diplopia (45% of episodes), nystagmus (37%), ocular misalignment (cranial nerve palsy or skew; 33%), Horner's syndrome (27%), visual field defects (10%), internuclear ophthalmoplegia (4%).
- Vertebrobasilar ischaemia without pain.
- Vertebrobasilar ischaemia followed by head/neck pain.
- Subarachnoid haemorrhage.
- Isolated occipital headache.
- Asymptomatic.
- +/− history of neck trauma.

Investigations and diagnosis *Imaging*: intra-arterial angiography was formerly the investigation of choice, showing narrowing of the vertebral artery lumen ("string sign"). MRI may show an eccentric signal void surrounded by semilunar hyperintensity on spin echo images, characteristic of mural haematoma, but the shape may vary, sometimes being oval or circumferential. This approach has now largely superseded intra-arterial angiography.

Differential diagnosis The constellation of brainstem signs may be recognized as of vascular origin but ascribed to ischaemia without vertebral artery dissection being thought of. The signs may be mistaken for multiple sclerosis (MS), but the acute onset makes this unlikely.

Treatment and prognosis Anticoagulation, initially with heparin followed by oral warfarin, is recommended in those deemed at risk of further embolic events, although there is no randomized-controlled trial evidence currently available to support this policy.

References Blunt SB, Galton C. Cervical carotid or vertebral artery dissection: an underdiagnosed cause of stroke in the young. *British Medical Journal* 1997; **314**: 243.

Hicks PA, Leavitt JA, Mokri B. Ophthalmic manifestations of vertebral artery dissection. Patients seen at the Mayo Clinic from 1976 to 1992. *Ophthalmology* 1994; **101**: 1786–1792.

Mokri B, Houser OW, Sandok BA, Piepgras DG. Spontaneous dissections of the vertebral arteries. *Neurology* 1988; **38**: 880–885.

Other relevant entries Carotid artery disease; Cerebrovascular disease: arterial; Lateral medullary syndrome; Subarachnoid haemorrhage; Transient ischaemic attack.

■ Vertigo

Pathophysiology Vertigo is an illusion of movement (rotation which may be horizontal, vertical, or rotatory; or tilting) causing a feeling of imbalance or disequilibrium, often triggered by head movement; there may be associated autonomic features (sweating, pallor, nausea, vomiting). The pathophysiological basis of vertigo is an asymmetry of signalling anywhere in the central or peripheral vestibular pathways. Vertiginous dizziness needs to be differentiated from light-headed dizziness, if pos-sible, since the potential causes differ: in some patients, this remains a significant challenge.

Clinical features: history and examination Is it vertigo ("spinning") or non-specific light-headedness or giddiness?

If vertigo, determine
- timing
- triggering factors (especially posture)
- symptoms related to hearing (deafness, tinnitus, aural fullness)
- medication history: any ototoxins (e.g. gentamicin, anticonvulsants)
- family history.

Causes of vertigo: Peripheral versus Central:
- Peripheral:

    Acute onset

    Nystagmus

    +/− concurrent hearing loss, tinnitus (vestibulocochlear nerve involvement)

    +/− facial weakness and ipsilateral ataxia: suggest cerebellopontine angle lesion

    +/− autonomic features (sweating, pallor, nausea, vomiting)

    Usually compensates rapidly and completely, nystagmus disappears after a few days.

- Central:
  - Associated diplopia, bulbar dysfunction and long tract signs
  - $+/-$ autonomic features (sweating, pallor, nausea, vomiting)
  - Compensates slowly, nystagmus persists.

The clinical pattern (time course, provoking factors) may also be helpful in diagnosis.

- Acute: labyrinthitis or vestibular neur(on)itis (peripheral).
- Prolonged: otomastoiditis, vestibular neuritis, labyrinthine concussion, isolated labyrinthine infarct, vestibular nerve section, drug induced (peripheral); brain-stem/cerebellar haemorrhage, infarction, demyelination (central).
- Recurrent, episodic: benign paroxysmal positional vertigo (BPPV), Ménière's disease (vestibular-only form), isolated or systemic autoimmune inner ear disease, recurrent vestibular neuritis, perilymph fistula, rarely migraine or epilepsy (peripheral); vertebrobasilar ischaemia (central; rare).
- Positional: BPPV (peripheral); multiple sclerosis, Chiari malformation, brainstem/cerebellar tumours, spinocerebellar atrophy (central).
- Chronic: vestibular decompensation/failure (peripheral); neurological disorder, psychogenic (central).

Investigations and diagnosis Dix–Hallpike (positioning) manoeuvre is essential for the diagnosis of BPPV.

Imaging: in the presence of other neurological signs (ataxia, long tract signs) imaging of the brainstem (ideally MRI) is recommended. Not required for cases of BPPV.

Vestibular testing: if available, may greatly assist with diagnosis.

Audiometry: indicated if concurrent otological symptoms, for example for the diagnosis of Ménière's disease.

Differential diagnosis Other types of "dizziness", light-headedness: vasovagal attacks, presyncope, cardiac arrhythmias.

Treatment and prognosis Vestibular sedatives (e.g. cinnarizine, Serc) are appropriate in the acute phase, but exercises to "rehabilitate" the semicircular canals should be begun as soon as possible in peripheral causes.

In BPPV, most patients respond to the Epley (or particle repositioning) manoeuvre, to reposition the otoconia which are thought to cause the condition (canalolithiasis).

Cawthorne–Cooksey exercises are helpful in vestibular decompensation or failure.

References Baloh RW. Vertigo. *Lancet* 1998; **352**: 1841–1846.

Brandt T. *Vertigo: Its Multisensory Syndromes* (2nd edition). London: Springer, 1999.

Hain TC, Uddin MK. Approach to the patient with dizziness and vertigo. In: Biller J (ed.). *Practical Neurology* (2nd edition). Philadelphia: Lippincott Wiliams & Wilkins, 2002: 189–205.

Luxon LM. Vertigo: new approaches to diagnosis and management. *British Journal of Hospital Medicine* 1996; **56**: 519–520, 537–541.

Other relevant entries Benign paroxysmal positional vertigo; Cogan syndrome (2); Ménière's disease; Multiple sclerosis; Syncope; Vestibular disorders: an overview; Vestibular neuritis.

■ Vestibular disorders: an overview
Inner ear disease

Pathophysiology Vestibular dysfunction causing vertigo may be a symptom of various disease processes within the inner ear.

The differential diagnosis of vestibulopathy encompasses:

Vestibular neur(on)itis
Failed vestibular compensation following vestibular neuritis
Benign paroxysmal positional vertigo
Ménière's disease
Labyrinthine concussion
Drug ototoxicity: aminoglycoside antibiotics, chemotherapeutic agents, diuretics, erythromycin, salicylates
Vascular: acute cerebellar infarction (posterior or anterior inferior cerebellar artery territory); vertebrobasilar insufficiency (rare)
Migraine-associated dizziness; benign recurrent vertigo of childhood is probably a migraine equivalent
Multiple sclerosis
Epilepsy (rare).

Clinical features: history and examination Additional clinical features may be clues to diagnosis, for example tinnitus, hearing loss: Ménière's.
Drug history important.

Investigations and diagnosis/treatment and prognosis See individual entries.

Differential diagnosis See individual entries. Vestibular dysfunction needs to be distinguished from postural hypotension or presyncope.

References Baloh RW, Halmagyi GM (eds). *Disorders of the Vestibular System.* New York: OUP, 1996.
Furman JM, Cass SP. *Vestibular Disorders. A Case-Study Approach.* Oxford: OUP, 2003.
Other relevant entry Vertigo; Vestibular neuritis.

■ Vestibular neuritis
Labyrinthitis ● Vestibular neuronitis

Pathophysiology Vestibular neuritis, often known as labyrinthitis, reflects the acute loss of vestibular function unilaterally.

Clinical features: history and examination
- Vertigo, nausea, vomiting for several hours, blurred vision, disequilibrium; often very prostrated.
- No hearing loss, tinnitus, fullness in the ears (*cf.* Ménière's disease).
- May be prior history of viral infection.
- Horizontal–torsional nystagmus; increased in intensity with loss of fixation; abnormal head thrust test. Positive Unterberger's test.

Investigations and diagnosis Additional investigations seldom required if the history and examination are consistent with the diagnosis.

In centres with specialist interest, videonystagmography may be undertaken, showing spontaneous vestibular nystagmus that increases with loss of fixation; caloric testing shows absence of responses unilaterally.

MR brain normal.

Audiometry: normal in vestibular neuritis; may show high-frequency hearing loss with a more generalized labyrinthitis (*cf*. low-tone sensorineural hearing loss with Ménière's disease).

Differential diagnosis Other causes of an acute vestibular syndrome:

Endolymphatic hydrops: "vestibular-only" Ménière's disease
Demyelinating disorder: unlikely in absence of other neurological signs
Infarction of labyrinth, brainstem.

Treatment and prognosis Symptoms gradually settle spontaneously by a process of vestibular compensation in most patients. A course of steroids may decrease the duration of symptoms. Vestibular suppressants and anti-emetic medications may be given as needed.

Other relevant entries Nystagmus: an overview; Vertigo.

▓ Vestibular schwannoma
Acoustic neurinoma • *Acoustic neuroma*

Pathophysiology Vestibular schwannomas, also known as acoustic neuromas or neurinomas, are benign tumours arising from the Schwann cells of the vestibular component of the vestibulocochlear (VIII) cranial nerve in the region of the internal auditory meatus, first described pathologically by Leyden in 1776. Their rate of division is slow which means that they present insidiously and can grow to considerable size before the diagnosis is made, although occasionally intratumoral haemorrhage causes acute presentation. The typical presentation is with progressive sensorineural hearing loss with local involvment of the fifth and seventh cranial nerves and ipsilateral cerebellar signs. There may be associated brainstem compression with long tract signs and hydrocephalus. Vestibular schwannomas are a feature of neurofibromatosis (NF), particularly type II in which bilateral tumours may occur: increased division of Schwann cells may be due to loss of a tumour suppressor gene. The tumour is treated surgically, but because of the late presentation there is often a significant morbidity associated. Vestibular schwannomas account for 2–8% of all primary intracranial neoplasms, with an incidence of 1 : 100,000, female preponderance, usual presentation around 40–50 years of age. In contrast, NF type II nearly always presents before the age of 21 years.

Pathology usually shows an encapsulated oval tumour, 2–3.5 cm in diameter. Histologically the tumour may be classified as either:

Antoni A: whorls of elongated spindle cells; or
Antoni B: disorganized myxoid tissue with abundant ground substance and scattered stellate cells.

Occasionally tumors are cystic or haemorrhagic; it is rare to find evidence of many mitoses.

Clinical features: history and examination

- Sensorineural hearing loss: usually the earliest symptom; may be associated with tinnitus and vertigo. However the slow compression of the vestibular nerve allows for compensation and acute attacks of vertigo are rare.
- Local cranial nerve involvement
  Trigeminal (V) nerve: loss of sensation beginning with V1; loss of the corneal reflex may be the earliest sign, followed by facial dysaesthesia
  Facial (VII) nerve: lower motor neurone facial weakness
  Abducens (VI) nerve: diplopia, rare
  Glossopharyngeal (IX), vagal (X) nerves: occasionally dysphagia.
- Local pressure effects
  Cerebellar ataxia: ipsilateral to the lesion due to compression of cerebellum, although the patient may complain of unsteadiness before the ataxia is clinically apparent
  Headache: due to hydrocephalus from compression of fourth ventricle with raised intracranial pressure and papilloedema: late features
  Long tract signs: from compression of brainstem
  Ipsilateral horizontal gaze paresis: occasionally occurs from local brainstem compression.

Investigations and diagnosis *Bloods*: normal; neurogenetic tests for NF may be appropriate.

Imaging: MRI (>CT) brain with special views of the internal auditory meatus.

Audiogram.

Neurophysiology: brainstem auditory evoked potential (BSAEP): always abnormal, even in the absence of hearing loss.

CSF: usually not needed, and may be contraindicated with large tumours causing brainstem distortion; very high CSF protein may be found with large tumours.

Differential diagnosis Other tumours of the cerebellopontine angle, for example meningioma, dermoid cyst, cholesteatoma.

Ménière's disease.

Posterior fossa demyelination.

Posterior fossa stroke.

Occasionally a meningitic process (granulomatous or syphilitic) can mimic an acoustic neuroma.

Treatment and prognosis Surgical removal involves either a posterior fossa craniotomy or a translabyrinthine approach, in which case no attempt is made to save hearing. In such circumstances there is usually a combined approach involving both neurosurgical and ENT teams.

If the tumour is small (<2 cm in diameter) then there is a 50% chance of preserving hearing, but the likelihood falls with larger tumours. Furthermore with large tumours preservation of V–XII cranial nerves may prove difficult, and a significant morbidity from dysphagia may ensue.

References Frohlich AM, Sutherland GR. Epidemiology and clinical features of vestibular schwannoma in Manitoba, Canada. *Canadian Journal of Neurological Sciences* 1993; **20**: 126–130.

Ojemann RG. Management of acoustic neuromas (vestibular schwannomas). *Clinical Neurosurgery* 1993; **40**: 498–535.

Other relevant entries Cerebellopontine angle syndrome; Cranial nerve disease: VIII: Vestibulocochlear nerve; Ménière's disease; Neurofibromatosis; Tumours: an overview; Vertigo.

■ Vestibulocochlear nerve disease – see Cranial nerve disease: VIII: Vestibulocochlear nerve

■ Villaret's syndrome

Villaret's syndrome is one of the multiple lower cranial nerve palsy syndromes, involving cranial nerves IX, X, XI, XII and also the sympathetic chain and sometimes VII, due to lesions of the retroparotid or retropharyngeal space. The clinical features are dysphonia, dysphagia, palatal paresis, weakness of sterno-cleidomastoid, tongue deviation to affected side, Horner's syndrome, + / − ipsilateral lower motor neurone facial weakness. The investigation of choice is imaging of retropharyngeal space with MRI, specifically looking for tumour or infection.

Other relevant entries Collet–Sicard syndrome; Cranial polyneuropathy; Tapia's syndrome; Vernet's syndrome.

■ Visual anosognosia – see Anton's syndrome

■ Visual loss: differential diagnosis

- Transient visual loss
    - Monocular
        - Vascular
            - Ocular transient ischaemic attack (amaurosis fugax): embolic
            - Migraine: vasospasm
            - Hypoperfusion: hypotension, hyperviscosity (more usually bilateral)
            - Partial retinal vein occlusion
            - Vasculitis (e.g. giant cell arteritis).
        - Ocular
            - Angle-closure glaucoma

Inflammation
    Uhthoff's phenomenon
Psychogenic
Binocular:
    Transient visual obscurations, papilloedema
    Vascular
        Migraine
        Hypoperfusion: hypotension, hyperviscosity.
    Epilepsy
    Psychogenic.

- Sudden, non-progressive visual loss
  - Monocular
    - Central or branch retinal artery/vein occlusion
    - Anterior ischaemic optic neuropathy
    - Retinal detachment
    - Vitreous haemorrhage
    - Psychogenic.
  - Bilateral
    - Occipital lobe infarctions
    - Pituitary apoplexy
    - Leber's hereditary optic neuropathy (LHON)
    - Psychogenic.
- Progressive visual loss
  - Hereditary optic neuropathy
  - Anterior visual pathway compression: tumour, aneurysm, dysthyroid eye disease
  - Anterior visual pathway inflammation: optic neuritis, sarcoidosis, meningitis
  - Toxic and nutritional optic neuropathies
  - Drug-induced optic neuropathy
  - Paraneoplastic retinal degeneration
  - Low-tension glaucoma.

Other relevant entries Cranial nerve disease: II: Optic nerve; Glaucoma; Ischaemic optic neuropathy; Leber's hereditary optic neuropathy; Migraine; Multiple sclerosis; Paraneoplastic syndromes; Pituitary disease and apoplexy; Sarcoidosis; Transient ischaemic attacks; Vasculitis.

■ Vitamin B$_{12}$ deficiency
Cobalamin deficiency

Pathophysiology Vitamin B$_{12}$ or cobalamin is involved in DNA synthesis throughout the body as well as myelination in the nervous system. A deficiency of this vitamin may cause a megaloblastic anaemia, glossitis, and hypospermia (all due to impaired

peripheral DNA synthesis); and a variety of neurological disorders:
- peripheral neuropathy, usually of axonal type;
- subacute combined degeneration of the cord, affecting principally the dorsal and lateral columns;
- optic neuropathy: typically with centrocaecal scotoma;
- cognitive decline;
- leukoencephalopathy (rare);
- Imerslund–Grasbeck syndrome (rare).

It is well attested that the neurological manifestations of vitamin B_{12} deficiency can occur in the absence of a megaloblastic anaemia.

The commonest cause of vitamin B_{12} deficiency is pernicious anaemia, the autoimmune destruction of gastric parietal cells that produce the intrinsic factor (IF) which is essential for absorption of vitamin B_{12} in the terminal ileum. Correction of the vitamin deficiency in the early stages by parenteral vitamin B_{12} injections can reverse the neurological deficits, but there is a well recognized inverse relationship between duration of deficiency and extent of neurological recovery following repletion. Hence early recognition is important; cases are still missed.

Incidence of vitamin B_{12} deficiency is 1–3% in individuals over the age of 65 years in European populations and may be higher in populations from the Indian subcontinent.

Total body stores of vitamin B_{12} amount to 2–5 mg, of which 50% is stored in liver. The average Western diet contains 20 µg/day, but required daily intake is only 6 µg/day. It usually takes 2–5 years to develop deficiency by depleting body stores.

Recognized causes of vitamin B_{12} deficiency include:

Pernicious anaemia (usually ~60 years old, F : M = 1–2 : 1)
Gastric or ileal resection
Gastrointestinal (GI) disease: tropical sprue, Crohn's disease, diphyllobothriasis
Antibody deficiency: common variable immunodeficiency (CVID)
  syndrome

Cobalamin is a cofactor to two enzymes: methionine synthase and methylmalonyl-CoA mutase; the former seems most significant for the consequences of vitamin B_{12} deficiency, since it catalyses the transfer of a methyl group from methyltetrahydrofolate to homocysteine to form methionine; if this reaction is impaired it eventually leads to impaired DNA synthesis.

Clinical features: history and examination
- Inquire for
  Dietary history: vegan, vegetarian
  Previous surgery to GI tract, or disease thereof
  Family history.
- Systemic features
  Megaloblastic anaemia
  Glossitis

Hypospermia/azoospermia

Features of GI disease and/or other autoimmune disorders (e.g. grey hair, lemon tinge to skin in pernicious anaemia)

- Neurological features
  - Peripheral neuropathy: usually starts with symmetric paresthesiae involving the feet and fingers with loss of joint position sense and vibration perception. It is usually an axonal neuropathy although demyelinating features are sometimes found; there is occasional involvement of the autonomic nervous system.
  - Subacute combined degeneration of the spinal cord (SACDOC): affects dorsal and lateral parts of the spinal cord (i.e. dorsal columns, spinocerebellar, and pyramidal tracts). It presents with sensory ataxia (especially with superadded peripheral neuropathy) and mild spasticity +/− Lhermitte's sign and sphincter involvement.
  - Optic neuropathy: typically with centrocaecal scotoma
  - Cognitive decline; although often stated to be a cause of reversible dementia, this is in fact extremely rare
  - Leukoencephalopathy
  - Other non-specific complaints are common, including anosmia, reduced manual dexterity.

Investigations and diagnosis *Bloods*: FBC and blood film. A megaloblastic anaemia which is characterized by raised mean corpuscular volume (MCV), hypersegmented neutrophils and in some instances a pancytopenia. However, neurological features of vitamin B_{12} deficiency may develop in the absence of any haematological abnormalities.

Vitamin B_{12} and folate levels: usually low. However the assay is variable and so in the first instance, a low value should prompt a repeat assay. If the level is still low it maybe worthwhile measuring the levels of the metabolites homocysteine and methylmalonic acid and/or performing a Schilling test.

Routine biochemistry screen is usually normal. Auto-antibody screen can be abnormal: especially important are whether antibodies reactive with IF and gastric parietal cells are present, as in cases of pernicious anaemia.

Schilling test: an amount of radioactive vitamin B_{12} is given and the amount excreted in the urine over 24 hours calculated:

	Pernicious anaemia	Malabsorption
Part 1	Abnormal	Abnormal
Part 2 (+IF)	Corrected	Not corrected

Imaging: CT/MRI brain is usually normal. Occasionally a leukoencephalopathy is found. MR spinal cord may show a "longitudinal myelitis" of the posterior columns in SACDOC, especially in the cervical cord.

CSF: usually normal.

Neurophysiology:

EMG/NCS: sensorimotor neuropathy of axonal, demyelinating, or mixed axonal/demyelinating type

Evoked potentials: visual evoked potentials (VEPs) may be abnormal (even in absence of visual symptoms, likewise somatosensory evoked potentials (SSEPs), but brainstem auditory evoked potentials (BSAEPs) are rarely abnormal.

Neuropsychology: may reveal deficits in memory.

Other: investigation of haematology, gastroenterology may necessitate specific consults.

Differential diagnosis

Some leukodystrophies.

Coeliac disease.

Vitamin E deficiency.

Cerebellar degenerations.

Mitochondrial disease.

Multiple sclerosis.

Sarcoidosis.

Treatment and prognosis Once vitamin B_{12} deficiency is diagnosed, a cause should be sought.

The mainstay of treatment is vitamin B_{12} replacement: a typical regime for pernicious anaemia is 1 mg intramuscularly on five consecutive days, followed by 1 mg every month thereafter.

Occasionally neurological symptoms worsen with vitamin B_{12} treatment; folate therapy with vitamin B_{12} deficiency has been said to exacerbate neurological deficits, although this has been questioned.

In the early stages, a full clinical and haematological recovery may be expected. All patients make some improvement in the first 3 months of therapy, and it is rare to be left with a severe neurological deficit from pure vitamin B_{12} deficiency, although troubling dysaesthetic symptoms sometimes persist after SACDOC.

References Green R, Kinsella LJ. Current concepts in the diagnosis of cobalamin deficiency. *Neurology* 1995; **45**: 1435–1440.

Larner AJ. Missed diagnosis of vitamin B_{12} deficiency presenting with paraesthetic symptoms. *International Journal of Clinical Practice* 2002; **56**: 377–378.

Larner AJ, Janssen JC, Cipolotti L, Rossor MN. Cognitive profile in dementia associated with vitamin B_{12} deficiency due to pernicious anaemia. *Journal of Neurology* 1999; **246**: 317–319.

Other relevant entries Alcohol and the nervous system: an overview; Autonomic failure; Common variable immunodeficiency; Dementia: an overview; Diphyllobothriasis; Drug-induced neuropathies; Gastrointestinal disease and the nervous system; Glossodynia; Imerslund–Grasbeck syndrome; Methylmalonic acidaemia; Mitochondrial disease: an overview; Multiple sclerosis; Neuropathies: an overview; Subacute combined degeneration of the spinal cord; Vitamin deficiencies and the nervous system.

■ Vitamin deficiencies and the nervous system

Pathophysiology Nutritional deficiency of vitamins may have profound adverse effects on nervous system function. These conditions are usually seen in individuals with poor nutritional intake; alcohol abuse may lead to vitamin deficiency.

Clinical features: history and examination

- *Vitamin A (β-carotene)*: xerophthalmia, nyctalopia (night blindness).
- *Vitamin B complex (riboflavin, thiamine)*: beriberi, pellagra; nutritional polyneuropathy; nutritional amblyopia; Wernicke–Korsakoff syndrome; ? Strachan's syndrome.
- *Vitamin B$_6$ (pyridoxine)*: polyneuropathy.
- *Vitamin B$_{12}$ (cobalamin)*: subacute combined degeneration of the spinal cord (predominantly posterior column myelopathy + peripheral neuropathy), optic neuropathy, neurobehavioural disorder, reversible cognitive decline (rare), white matter lesions on MRI (significance uncertain).
- *Vitamin C*: scurvy.
- *Vitamin D (calciferol)*: rickets, osteomalacia, muscle weakness (? myopathy), tetany; deficiency may be induced by prolonged use of anti-epileptic medications (especially phenytoin, phenobarbitone).
- *Vitamin E (tocopherol)*: spinocerebellar ataxia (in context of intestinal malabsorption, e.g. cystic fibrosis, although an autosomal-recessive isolated vitamin E-deficiency syndrome, ataxia with vitamin E deficiency (AVED), does occur).
- *Vitamin K*: clotting disorders.

Investigations and diagnosis Assay of certain vitamins is possible, but usually the dietary status leads to clinical suspicion strong enough to suggest diagnosis and appropriate treatment.

Differential diagnosis

See individual entries.

Vitamin A: retinitis pigmentosa

Vitamin E: AVED, Bassen–Kornzweig syndrome.

Treatment and prognosis Restoration of adequate nutrition +/− vitamin supplements may reverse many neurological features.

> **Reference** Mancall EL. Nutritional disorders of the nervous system. In: Aminoff MJ (ed.). *Neurology and General Medicine: The Neurological Aspects of Medical Disorders* (2nd edition). New York: Churchill Livingstone, 1995: 323–339.

> **Other relevant entries** Abetalipoproteinaemia; Alcohol and the nervous system: an overview; Ataxia with vitamin E deficiency; Beriberi; Cerebellar disease: an overview; Cerebrotendinous xanthomatosis; Myopathy: an overview; Osteomalacia; Pellagra; Strachan's syndrome; Vitamin B$_{12}$ deficiency; Wernicke–Korsakoff syndrome.

■ Vogt–Koyanagi–Harada syndrome

Uveoretinal meningoencephalitic syndrome

Pathophysiology An inflammatory disorder, but not a true vasculitis, affecting predominantly the eyes and skin, and sometimes cranial nerves and brain parenchyma. There is some evidence for cellular and humoral immune responses to melanocytes.

Clinical features: history and examination

- Ophthalmological
    Uveitis
    Retinal haemorrhages.
- Dermatological
    Depigmentation of eyebrows, eyelashes, and scalp hair (vitiligo, poliosis).
- Neurological
    Aseptic meningitis
    Sensorineural hearing loss
    Headache
    Cranial nerve involvement (especially III, IV, VI)
    Hemiplegia
    Transverse myelitis
    Neuropsychiatric changes.

Investigations and diagnosis *Bloods*: unremarkable.

Imaging: MRI may show high intensity periventricular lesions, choroidal changes.

CSF: lymphocytic pleocytosis, raised protein.

Ophthalmic assessment: acutely hyperaemic disc with retinal haemorrhages and detachments; convalescent pale atrophic disc with orange–red discolouration of the fundus.

Differential diagnosis Uveoretinal meningoencephalitic syndromes: may be inflammatory for example sarcoidosis, systemic lupus erythematosus (SLE), vasculitis; infectious, for example syphilis, tuberculosis, herpes viruses (simplex or zoster); or malignant, for example lymphoma, leukaemia.

Treatment and prognosis High-dose intravenous steroids advocated. For refractory cases other immunosuppressive therapy may be used such as ciclosporin or intravenous immunoglobulin. The majority of patients retain moderate to good vision.

Reference Moorthy RS, Inomata H, Rao NA. Vogt–Koyanagi–Harada syndrome *Survey in Ophthalmology* 1995; **39**: 265–292.

Other relevant entry Vasculitis.

■ Vogt–Spielmeyer disease – see Neuronal ceroid lipofuscinosis

■ Volkman's ischaemic contracture – see Compartment syndromes

■ Von Bechterew's disease – see Ankylosing spondylitis and the nervous system

■ Von Economo's disease – see Encephalitis lethargica

■ Von Hippel–Lindau disease
Cerebello-retinal angiomatosis • Haemangioblastoma of the cerebellum

Pathophysiology An autosomal-dominant phakomatosis characterized by haemangio-blastomas of the cerebellum (60%), retina and optic nerve head (60%, often asympto-matic), spinal cord (13–44%) and brainstem (18%), and sometimes associated with renal cell carcinoma and phaeochromocytoma. It is usually diagnosed in the third decade. The condition may result from mutation(s) in a tumour suppressor gene; the disease gene has been mapped to chromosome 3p25.5, and encodes a 213 amino acid protein (pVHL), the exact biochemical function of which remains uncertain.

Clinical features: history and examination
- Cerebellar signs (gait, limb ataxia).
- Raised intracranial pressure.
- Cord compression, pain.
- Polycythaemia: secondary to renal cell carcinoma.
- Hypertension, orthostatic hypotension: due to phaeochromocytoma.
- Abdominal mass (renal cell carcinoma; pancreatic cyst, adenoma).
- Endolymphatic sac tumour.
- Cystadenoma of the epididymis or broad ligament.
- Family history of similar conditions.

Investigations and diagnosis *Bloods*: polycythaemia.
Urine: elevated VMA may be found.
Imaging:

MRI brain: cerebellar cyst with enhancing nodular lesion on wall
MRA/angiography: hypervascular nodule(s) with dilated draining veins
MRI cord: haemangioblastoma of cord, often multiple, often of posterior columns, causing compression +/− syrinx formation
CT/MRI/ultrasonography of kidneys, adrenals, pancreas

Ophthalmology opinion +/− fluorescein angiography.
Neurogenetics.

Differential diagnosis Isolated cerebellar, cord tumours. Wyburn–Mason disease (retinal angioma).

Treatment and prognosis Surgical resection of cerebellar/cord lesions may be possible; ataxia, paraplegia may persist.

Laser therapy of retinal lesions.

Debulking of renal tumours, partial nephrectomy; renal cell carcinoma is leading cause of death. Appropriate medical management of phaeochromocytoma followed by surgical resection.

Tumours have a tendency to recur, hence screening of patients as well as at-risk individuals is recommended.

References Latif F, Tory K, Gnarra J, Yao M, Duh F-M, Orcutt ML. Identification of the Von Hippel–Lindau disease tumor suppressor gene. *Science* 1993; **260**: 1317–1320.

Maher ER, Yates JRW, Harries R *et al.* Clinical features and natural history of Von Hippel–Lindau disease. *Quarterly Journal of Medicine* 1990; **77**: 1151–1163.

Sims KB. Von Hippel–Lindau disease: gene to bedside. *Current Opinion in Neurology* 2001; **14**: 695–703.

Singh AD, Shields CL, Shields JA. Von Hippel–Lindau disease. *Survey of Ophthalmology* 2001; **46**: 117–142.

Other relevant entries Phakomatosis; Spinal cord vascular diseases; Wyburn–Mason disease.

■ Von Recklinghausen's disease – see Neurofibromatosis; Vestibular schwannoma

■ Von Winiwarter–Buerger's disease
Cerebral thromboangiitis obliterans • Spatz–Lindenberg disease

Pathophysiology Von Winiwarter–Buerger's disease is an isolated cerebral form of thromboangiitis obliterans, a non-inflammatory occlusive vasculopathy which usually affects peripheral tissues. Cases were described in the late 1930s by Spatz and Lindenberg which, unlike Buerger's disease, occurred in the absence of vascular risk factors (hypertension, smoking). The condition usually presents with dementia and pyramidal signs; there are no specific clinical or histopathological features. Only a handful of cases with pathological verification have been published.

Clinical features: history and examination
- Dementia; informant interview required.
- Pyramidal signs.
- Focal and secondarily generalized epilepsy.

Investigations and diagnosis *Bloods*: no specific abnormalities known.

Imaging: subcortical leukoencephalopathy; atrophy may be evident.

CSF: no specific abnormalities known.

Brain biopsy: an occlusive arteriopathy affecting both leptomeningeal and intraparenchymal vessels, due to profound intimal thickening, with an intact and reduplicated internal elastic lamina, but no evidence of inflammation or infiltration of blood vessels. Cortex shows non-specific gliosis.

Differential diagnosis Other causes of vascular dementia with subcortical leukoencephalopathy, viz.

Multi-infarct dementia
Binswanger's disease/encephalopathy
CADASIL
Cerebral vasculitis.

Treatment and prognosis No specific treatment known; symptomatic control of seizures, spasticity; neurorehabilitation.

References Larner AJ, Kidd D, Elkington P, Rudge P, Scaravilli F. Spatz–Lindenberg disease: a rare cause of vascular dementia. *Stroke* 1999; **30**: 687–689.

Zhan S-S, Beyreuther K, Schmitt HP. Vascular dementia in Spatz–Lindenberg disease (SLD): cortical synaptophysin immunoreactivity as compared with dementia of Alzheimer type and non-demented controls. *Acta Neuropathologica (Berlin)* 1993; **86**: 259–264.

Other relevant entries Binswanger's disease; CADASIL; Dementia: an overview; Vascular dementia; Vasculitis.

■ Vulpian–Bernhart syndrome – see Flail arm syndrome; Motor neurone disease

Ww

■ Waardenburg syndrome

This may refer to either:
- a rare congenital syndrome classified with the acrocephalosyndactyly syndromes, characterized by the combination of craniosynostosis with genital, digital, and cardiac anomalies;

or:
- a syndrome of nerve deafness, heterochromia iridis, white forelock, abnormal skin pigmentation, synophrys.

Other relevant entries Acrocephalosyndactyly; Telfer's syndrome.

■ Waldenström's macroglobulinaemia – see Bing–Neel syndrome; Endocarditis and the nervous system; Paraproteinaemic neuropathies; Renal disease and the nervous system

▪ Walker–Warburg syndrome

Cerebro-ocular dysplasia (COD) • Chemke syndrome • Pagon syndrome

Pathophysiology Walker–Warburg syndrome (WWS) is a lethal congenital muscular dystrophy syndrome, probably autosomal recessive, of unknown aetiology, often presenting as a floppy infant with visual deficits, eye, facial, and limb abnormalities. Mental retardation is associated with the muscle weakness. It may be equivalent to the Finnish muscle–eye–brain syndrome.

Clinical features: history and examination "HARD + E syndrome":

- *H*ydrocephalus (usually aqueduct stenosis)
- *A*gyria (type II lissencephaly: neuronal migration defect)
- *R*etinal *d*ysplasia, microphthalmia (thought to be less severe and consistent than in muscle–eye–brain disease)
- *E*ncephalocoele
- +/− cerebellar malformations, severe developmental retardation.

Investigations and diagnosis Diagnosis usually evident at birth. Imaging confirms agyria.

Differential diagnosis Other congenital muscular dystrophies, especially Finnish muscle–eye–brain syndrome, but Fukuyama muscular dystrophy and merosin (α_2-laminin) deficiency also enter the differential diagnosis. Muscle involvement said to be less prominent in WWS compared to other congenital muscular dystrophies.

Treatment and prognosis No specific treatment. Prognosis poor, progressive course, average life expectancy is 9 months, although some survive a few years.

Reference Williams RS, Swisher CN, Jennings M, Ambler M, Caviness Jr VS. Cerebro-ocular dysgenesis (Walker–Warburg syndrome): neuropathologic and etiologic analysis. *Neurology* 1984; **34**: 1531–1541.

Other relevant entries Congenital muscular dystrophies; Fukuyama muscular dystrophy; Lissencephaly; Muscle–eye–brain disease.

▪ Wallenberg's syndrome – see Brainstem vascular syndromes; Cerebrovascular disease: arterial; Lateral medullary syndrome

▪ Wartenberg's neuropathy

Multifocal relapsing sensory neuropathy • Wartenberg's migrant sensory neuritis

Pathophysiology A disorder characterized by recurrent attacks of pain followed by sensory loss in the distribution of various cutaneous sensory nerves (hence "migrant"), with resolution of symptoms over a period of weeks. Onset is usually in the fourth or fifth decade. This may be a syndrome produced by more than one underlying condition rather than a single entity. A possible genetic influence is suggested by its coincidence with hereditary neuralgic amyotrophy.

Clinical features: history and examination

- Pain followed by sensory loss in the distribution of a cutaneous nerve; attacks may be precipitated by limb movement or stretching.
- Motor function not affected.
- Reflexes retained.

Investigations and diagnosis *Neurophysiology*: NCS may be able to confirm involvement of cutaneous sensory nerve(s); motor studies normal.

Nerve biopsy: only one report, showing loss of large myelinated fibres, fibrosis, axonal regeneration.

Differential diagnosis Other causes of sensory mononeuropathy, usually compression.

Treatment and prognosis No specific treatment known. Symptomatic treatment of pain if necessary. Sensory loss usually improves over a few weeks and often returns to normal.

References Matthews WB, Esiri M. The migrant sensory neuritis of Wartenberg. *Journal of Neurology, Neurosurgery and Psychiatry* 1983; **46**: 1–4.

Thomas PK, Ormerod IEC. Hereditary neuralgic amyotrophy associated with a relapsing multifocal sensory neuropathy. *Journal of Neurology, Neurosurgery and Psychiatry* 1993; **56**: 107–109.

Other relevant entries Neuralgic amyotrophy; Neuropathies: an overview.

■ Watanabe–Vigevano syndrome
Benign infantile seizures

This rare, idiopathic, localization-related seizure disorder of infancy may be familial or non-familial. Between the age of 3–20 months, focal seizures of short duration commence, characterized by arrest of movement, decreased responsiveness, staring, eye and head deviation, sometimes with automatisms. Clinically infants are normal, as is brain imaging. Interictal EEG is normal but ictal studies demonstrate focal discharges. Anti-epileptic drug therapy (carbamazepine, sodium valproate) may be used during the active seizure period but can be withdrawn after a year or two without relapse.

Reference Panayiotopoulos CP. *A Clinical Guide to Epileptic Syndromes and their Treatment: Based on the New ILAE Diagnostic Scheme.* Chipping Norton: Bladon, 2002: 53–54.

■ Waterhouse–Friederichsen syndrome – see Meningococcal disease

■ Watershed infarct – see Cerebrovascular disease: arterial

■ Weber–Christian disease
Systemic panniculitis

Pathophysiology An inflammatory condition of fatty tissue (*cf.* vasculitis) usually presenting with red tender nodules in the skin, recurrent or relapsing fevers, with myalgia and arthralgia; neurological features are rare. The condition may be associated with pancreatic or autoimmune pathology but is often idiopathic.

Clinical features: history and examination

- Meningeal xanthogranuloma, with brainstem or cerebellar signs.
- Myopathy.
- Intramedullary partial myelopathy.

Investigations and diagnosis *Bloods*: raised ESR, CRP, LFTs, ACE; hypergamma-globulinaemia, hypocomplementaemia (all non-specific).

CSF: no specific abnormalities; may have oligoclonal bands matched with serum.

Imaging: CT/MRI may show meningeal mass lesion; may be remarkably normal.

Biopsy of skin lesion: non-suppurative lobular panniculitis; mononuclear or pleomorphic cellular infiltrate with fat-laden macrophages.

Differential diagnosis Extra-axial/meningeal mass lesion.

Intramedullary inflammatory myelopathy (e.g. sarcoid).

Treatment and prognosis Empirical immunosuppressive treatment, with steroids and/or cyclophosphamide.

References Larner AJ, Marshall B, Ma RCW, Ball JA. Systemic Weber–Christian disease complicated by partial transverse myelopathy. *International Journal of Clinical Practice* 2000; **54**: 472–474.

Panush RS, Yonker RA, Dlesk A, Longley S, Caldwell JR. Weber–Christian disease. Analysis of 15 cases and review of literature. *Medicine* 1985; **64**: 181–191.

Other relevant entry Vasculitis.

■ Weber's syndrome

This brainstem vascular syndrome affecting the midbrain is characterized by:

- ipsilateral oculomotor (fascicular) nerve palsy with pupil involvement (involvement of parasympathetic fibres); with
- contralateral hemiplegia, including the face, due to involvement of corticospinal and corticobulbar fibres in the cerebral peduncle.

Weber's syndrome may be differentiated from other midbrain vascular syndromes (Benedikt's syndrome, Claude's syndrome, and Nothnagel's syndrome) on clinical grounds but whether this is helpful in management is doubtful. It often results from occlusion of a penetrating branch of the posterior cerebral artery to the midbrain, less commonly from basilar artery involvement. MRI may confirm midbrain infarction; occasionally other intrinsic or extrinsic lesions may be seen.

References Bogousslavsky J, Maeder P, Regli F, Meuli R. Pure midbrain infarction: clinical syndromes, MRI, and etiologic patterns. *Neurology* 1994; **44**: 2032–2040.

Liu GT, Crenner CW, Logigian EL *et al*. Midbrain syndromes of Benedikt, Claude and Nothnagel: setting the record straight. *Neurology* 1992; **42**: 1820–1822.

Silverman IE, Lui GT, Galetta SL. The crossed paralyses. The original brain-stem syndromes of Millard–Gubler, Foville, Weber and Raymond–Céstan. *Archives of Neurology* 1995; **52**: 635–638.

Benedikt's syndrome; Brainstem vascular syndromes;
Cerebrovascular disease: arterial; Claude's syndrome; Nothnagel's syndrome;
Top of the basilar syndrome.

■ Wegener's granulomatosis

Pathophysiology A vasculitic granulomatous condition predominantly affecting the respiratory tract with destructive cartilaginous change (e.g. saddle nose deformity). Renal disease is usual, ocular disease may occur. Neurological features are predominantly in the peripheral nervous system, and result from spread of granulomata, more frequently than is the case in vasculitis.

Clinical features: history and examination

- Neurological features, affecting either central of peripheral nervous system, are present in about one-third of cases.
- Peripheral neuropathy (10–20% of cases): mononeuropathy multiplex, distal symmetrical sensorimotor polyneuropathy.
- Cranial neuropathy, external ophthalmoplegia, cavernous sinus involvement; involvement of II, V, VI, VII, VIII; *ca.* 10% of cases: possibly due to granulomatous infiltration of orbit, cavernous sinus and ear.
- Cerebrovascular events.
- Seizures.
- Cerebritis.
- Hearing loss (VIII).
- Raised intracranial pressure (extravascular jugular vein compression).
- Orbital pseudotumour.
- + respiratory, renal (glomerulonephritis) involvement.
- Can present as a pachymeningitis.

Investigations and diagnosis *Bloods*: positive cANCA is a marker, although this may be persistently negative in the early stages of disease, becoming positive only with disease progression; may be eosinophilia. In localised meningeal disease it can also be negative.

Neurophysiology: EMG/NCS for peripheral neuropathic involvement.

Imaging: CT/MRI may be indicated, especially cavernous sinus, orbit.

CSF: raised protein, lymphocytosis; may be normal.

Nerve biopsy: confirmation of necrotizing granulomatous vasculitis.

Differential diagnosis Other intracranial vasculitides.

Treatment and prognosis Immunosuppression, usually involving a combination of prednisolone and oral cyclophosphamide (reported remission rate of 75%). Methotrexate has also been used. For acute disease, a course of intravenous methylprednisolone is recommended. Limited disease may respond to trimethoprim/sulphamethoxazole.

References Nadeau SE. Neurologic manifestations of systemic vasculitis. *Neurologic Clinics* 2002; **20**: 123–150.

Nishino H, Rubino FA, DeRemee R, Swanson JW, Parisi J. Neurological involvement in Wegener's granulomatosis: an analysis of 324 consecutive patients at the Mayo Clinic. *Annals of Neurology* 1993; **33**: 4–9.

Weinberger LM, Cohen ML, Remler BF *et al*. Intracranial Wegener's granulomatosis. *Neurology* 1993; **43**: 1831–1834.

Other relevant entries Cranial polyneuropathy; Vasculitis.

Weir Mitchell syndrome – see Erythromelalgia

Welander's myopathy

Late-adult-onset distal myopathy type 1 • Swedish-type distal myopathy

Weakness in the distal muscles of the upper extremities, usually commencing in the fifth decade, is typical of this condition, with spread to the distal lower extremities but seldom with proximal involvement; reflexes are preserved with the possible exception of ankle jerks. Creatine kinase is normal or slightly elevated; EMG shows myopathic or mixed myopathic–neurogenic features. Muscle biopsy shows a dystrophic pattern with central nuclei, fibre splitting, increased connective tissue, and sometimes rimmed vacuoles. The condition is linked to chromosome 2q.

Other relevant entries Distal muscular dystrophy, distal myopathy; Markesbery–Griggs/Udd myopathy.

Werdnig–Hoffmann disease

Acute infantile spinal muscular atrophy • Hereditary motor neuropathy type I • Severe spinal muscular atrophy • Type I spinal muscular atrophy

Pathophysiology An autosomal-recessive spinal muscular atrophy with childhood onset (always before 6 months) and dismal prognosis.

Clinical features: history and examination

- Hypotonia ("floppy baby"); severe limb weakness worse proximally; "frog's leg" posture; areflexia.
- Tongue fasciculation (50%); facial muscles little affected if at all.
- Bulbar, respiratory (intercostal, not diaphragm) involvement; weak cry.
- Failure to attain developmental motor milestones (i.e. sitting).
- (Decreased fetal movements in pregnancy, in perhaps one-third of cases.)

Investigations and diagnosis *Bloods*: creatine kinase normal (*cf*. SMA type III, Kugelberg–Welander disease).

Neurophysiology: EMG/NCS: reduced compound muscle action potential amplitude, acute denervation; sensory studies normal.

Muscle biopsy: types I/II muscle-fibre atrophy in fascicles or groups of fascicles, + hypertrophied type I fibres in other fascicles.

Neurogenetics: Survival motor neurone (SMN) deletions in *ca*. 95% (exons 7 and 8); neuronal apoptosis inhibitory protein (NAIP) deletions in 20–50% (exons 5 and 6), although genotype/phenotype studies suggest these may not be sufficient by themselves to produce disease.

Differential diagnosis

Infantile hypotonia

Pompe disease
Centronuclear myopathy
Nemaline myopathy
Congenital muscular dystrophy
Central core disease
Myotonic dystrophy.

Treatment and prognosis No specific treatment; supportive, respiratory care. Most die by age 2 years, from overwhelming respiratory infection; some survive into childhood.

Reference Le Febvre S, Bürglen L, Frézal J *et al*. The role of the SMN gene in proximal spinal muscular atrophy. *Human Molecular Genetics* 1998; **7**: 1531–1536.

Other relevant entries Motor neurone diseases: an overview; Spinal muscular atrophy.

■ Werner syndrome (1)

A rare autosomal-recessive disorder, also known as "progeria of the adult", first described by Werner in 1904. Clinically there is scleroderma-like thin tight skin, bilateral cataracts, and accelerated ageing, both *in vivo* and *in vitro*. The condition has been associated with mutations in the WRN locus which encodes a RecQ DNA helicase. DNA helicase mutations also underpin Rothmund–Thomson syndrome and Bloom syndrome.

Reference Nehlin JO, Skovgaard GL, Bohr VA. The Werner syndrome. A model for the study of human aging. *Annals of the New York Academy of Sciences* 2000; **908**: 167–179.

Other relevant entries Progeria; Rothmund–Thomson syndrome; Systemic sclerosis.

■ Werner syndrome (2)

Eaton–McKusick syndrome

A rare autosomal-dominant syndrome of variable expression, characterized by tibial hypoplasia or absence. Additional features include broad bowed thickened fibulae, club feet, five- to six-fingered hands without thumbs or with triphalangeal thumbs, absent thenar musculature, $+/-$ syndactyly, camptodactyly. Diagnosis is made at birth; no specific investigations are required. Imaging of the bones may be helpful in planning orthopaedic/orthotic interventions.

Other relevant entry Camptodactyly.

■ Wernicke–Korsakoff syndrome

Pathophysiology A neurological (Wernicke's disease) and neuropsychological (Korsakoff's psychosis) syndrome, the features of which may be seen in isolation or combination, most usually occurring in alcoholic, nutritionally deficient, individuals (chronic vomiting as in pregnancy is also a recognized cause). Thiamine deficiency may be of particular pathogenetic significance; thiamine preparations should be given to all patients in whom this diagnosis is suspected.

Clinical features: history and examination

- Wernicke's disease/encephalopathy

    Acute/subacute nystagmus (horizontal and vertical), ophthalmoplegia (horizontal > vertical, e.g. internuclear ophthalmoplegia), cerebellar ataxia of gait, + disturbance of consciousness/mentation: global confusional state, alcohol withdrawal, stupor and coma, amnesic state.

- Korsakoff's psychosis

    Amnesic disorder (anterograde and retrograde amnesia) due to mammillary body/medial temporal lobe involvement.

    Confabulation occurs, but is very rare (probably requires an additional frontal lobe lesion).

    Intact immediate memory, attention, language.

- Concurrent features
    + +/− peripheral neuropathy
    + +/− optic neuropathy
    + +/− impaired olfaction
    + +/− vestibular paresis (unilateral, bilateral).

Autopsy studies demonstrate a higher incidence of WKS than recognized in life, isolated delirium without eye signs, or ataxia being the most common feature in cases not diagnosed during life.

Conditions associated with WKS include: alcoholism, prolonged intravenous feeding, hyperemesis gravidarum, anorexia nervosa, prolonged fasting, refeeding after starvation, gastric plication surgery.

Investigations and diagnosis *Bloods*: low erythrocyte transketolase level (=index of thiamine deficiency); raised LFTs may indicate chronic alcohol abuse.
Imaging: MRI: medial thalamic, periaqueductal anomalies may be visualized.
CSF: usually normal, may be slightly increased protein.
Neurophysiology: EEG: may show diffuse mild to moderate slow activity.

Differential diagnosis Encephalopathy: delirium.
Acute ophthalmoplegia: Miller Fisher syndrome, Bickerstaff's brainstem encephalitis.
Internuclear ophthalmoplegia: MS, vascular disease.
Amnesic disorder: Alzheimer's disease, temporal lobe epilepsy, transient global amnesia, head injury, third ventricular tumour, herpes simplex encephalitis.

Treatment and prognosis Thiamine should be given as soon as diagnosis is considered and the diagnosis may be difficult in the confused alcoholic patient – but if in doubt treat. Features of Wernicke' encephalopathy are promptly reversed; neuropsychological deficits may persist.

References Harper CG, Giles M, Finlay-Jones R. Clinical signs in the Wernicke–Korsakoff complex. *Journal of Neurology, Neurosurgery and Psychiatry* 1986; **49**: 341–345.

Victor M, Adams RD, Collings GH. *The Wernicke–Korsakoff Syndrome and Related Neurologic Disorders due to Alcoholism and Malnutrition* (2nd edition). Philadelphia: Davis, 1989.

Other relevant entries Alcohol and the nervous system: an overview; Alzheimer's disease; Amnesia, amnesic syndrome; Beriberi; Dementia: an overview; Eating disorders; Encephalopathies: an overview; Herpes simplex encephalitis; Pregnancy and the nervous system: an overview; Transient global amnesia; Vitamin deficiencies and the nervous system.

■ Wernicke's aphasia – see Aphasia

■ Western equine encephalitis – see Arbovirus disease; Encephalitis: an overview

■ Westphal variant – see Huntington's disease

■ Westphal–Strümpell pseudosclerosis – see Wilson's disease

■ West's syndrome
Infantile spasms • Salaam seizures

Pathophysiology An epilepsy syndrome of infancy and early childhood, often with characteristic EEG findings, and associated with impaired mental development ("epileptic encephalopathy"). There are many recognized causes, including tuberous sclerosis, brain dysgenesis, acquired lesions, cerebral maldevelopment, metabolic and degenerative disorders. No cause is found in around 40%.

Clinical features: history and examination Classically a triad of:

- infantile seizures or "spasms" of Salaam or jack-knife type (brief flexion of trunk and limbs: *Blitznickundsalaamkrampf*);
- EEG with continuous multifocal spikes and slow waves of large amplitude (hypsarrhythmia);
- arrested mental development.

Peak onset 4–8 months of age.

Investigations and diagnosis *Neurophysiology*: EEG: disorganized, chaotic succession of high voltage slow waves with intermingled multifocal asynchronous spike and sharp waves: hypsarrhythmia; this pattern is not specific, it may be seen in other disorders.

Imaging: CT/MRI: often normal, but may show evidence of cortical dysplasia, neurocutaneous syndromes, hypoxic–ischaemic injury, metabolic disorders, post-infective change. Functional imaging (positron emission tomography, PET) may show diffuse or focal hypometabolism.

Pathology: cortical dysgenesis may be found.

Differential diagnosis Other infantile seizure disorders with impaired mental development: Ohtahara's syndrome.

Non-epileptic syndromes of infancy

benign myoclonus of early infancy (benign non-epileptic infantile spasms)
benign neonatal sleep myoclonus
Sandifer's syndrome.

Treatment and prognosis Underlying disorders are managed as appropriate. Various treatments have been suggested to ameliorate seizures

Steroids/ACTH
Sodium valproate
Benzodiazepines: clonazepam, nitrazepam, clobazam
Ketogenic diet
Vigabatrin
Levetiracetam
Excisional surgery of EEG-defined area of cortical abnormality.

Occasionally there is a dramatic effect on the seizures.

Intractable epileptic seizures is the norm; 25–50% of cases evolve into the Lennox–Gastaut syndrome.

Seizures may diminish spontaneously by the 5th or 6th year but the patient is usually left mentally impaired (>90%).

Idiopathic cases may achieve normality.

References Panayiotopoulos CP. *A Clinical Guide to Epileptic Syndromes and Their Treatment: Based on the New ILAE Diagnostic Scheme.* Chipping Norton: Bladon, 2002: 57–63.

Shorvon S. *Status Epilepticus: Its Clinical Features and Treatment in Children and Adults.* Cambridge, CUP, 1994: 42–45.

West WJ. On a peculiar form of infantile convulsions. *Lancet* 1841; **1**: 724–725.

Other relevant entries Epilepsy: an overview; Lennox–Gastaut syndrome; Tuberous sclerosis.

■ Whiplash injury
Neck sprain

Pathophysiology A collection of painful symptoms following injury to the neck, usually of hyperextension–flexion type, but sometimes torsional, without symptoms or signs of traumatic nerve root or spinal cord dysfunction.

The young and old (>60 years) seem largely spared, and there is a female predominance. Psychogenic factors may contribute to the chronicity of the syndrome.

Clinical features: history and examination

- Acute: painful stiff neck within 24 hours of injury; limitation of neck movement with spread of pain to shoulders, occiput.
- Chronic/late: still symptomatic after 6 months: neck ache, stiff neck, headache, anxiety, irritability, depression, concentration deficits. Marked disability in the absence of significant physical findings. Neurologically unexplained ("non-organic") signs are common (e.g. spurious weakness and non-anatomical sensory loss).

Investigations and diagnosis

Acute: radiology (plain X-ray, MRI) to exclude nerve root/spinal cord injury.
Chronic: MRI and EMG/NCS invariably normal.

Differential diagnosis Traumatic nerve root or spinal cord injury.

Treatment and prognosis Acute: most patients (one-third to half) better after 1 month. Chronic: majority recover by 6 months, hence overall prognosis is very good, but symptoms persist (and may be reported to worsen) in a small number who are not helped by analgesia, physiotherapy. Whether the prospect of litigation and/or compensation may contribute to these features is not clear.

Reference Pearce JMS. Post-traumatic and whiplash injuries. In: Kennard C (ed.). *Recent Advances in Clinical Neurology 8.* Edinburgh: Churchill Livingstone, 1995: 133–150.

Other relevant entry Radiculopathies: an overview.

■ Whipple's disease

Pathophysiology A multisystem granulomatous disorder caused by the organism *Tropheryma whippelii.* Gastrointestinal and systemic features usually predominate but neurological involvement, sometimes in isolation, occurs in perhaps 10% of cases. Although uncommon, Whipple's disease is treatable and hence the condition often figures in the differential diagnosis of multisystem disease.

Clinical features: history and examination

Systemic

- Weight loss, abdominal pain
- Diarrhoea, steatorrhoea
- Fever, malaise
- Arthropathy
- Anaemia
- Erythema nodosum
- Pigmentation
- Lymphadenopathy.

Neurological (in 10% of patients, presenting features in 5%)

- Dementia (>70%)
- Ophthalmoplegia (may be supranuclear; >50%)

- Seizures (*ca.* 20%)
- Ataxia (*ca.* 20%)
- Pyramidal signs (>30%)
- Myoclonus
- Oculo-facial or oculo-masticatory myorhythmia with vergence oscillations: said to be pathognomonic of Whipple's disease
- Hypothalamic features: somnolence, polydipsia, hypogonadism
- Eye disease: keratitis, uveitis, papilloedema, ptosis
- Cranial neuropathies
- Stroke-like episodes.

Investigations and diagnosis *Imaging*: CT/MRI: may be normal; may reveal mul-tiple high signal intensity areas on T_2-weigthed images, particularly in region of hypothalamus; enhancing mass lesions also reported.

CSF: elevated protein, pleiocytosis; periodic acid–Schiff (PAS) positive bacilli may be identified (*ca.* 30%).

Small bowel/mesenteric lymph node biopsy: PAS positive bacilli; electron microscopy is mandatory (diagnosis may otherwise be overlooked).

Polymerase chain reaction (PCR) amplification of *Tropheryma whippelii* DNA in CSF, *in situ* in brain tissue.

Differential diagnosis

Sarcoidosis.

Multiple sclerosis.

Treatment and prognosis Uniformly fatal without treatment. Responds to antibiotics (e.g. penicillin, streptomycin and co-trimoxazole). Relapse is not uncommon; PCR for *T. whippelii* may be useful to monitor treatment efficacy.

References Anderson M. Neurology of Whipple's disease. *Journal of Neurology, Neurosurgery and Psychiatry* 2000; **68**: 2–5.

Fleming JL, Wiesner RH, Shorter RG. Whipple's disease: clinical, biochemical, and histopathologic features and assessment of treatment in 29 patients. *Mayo Clinic Proceedings* 1990; **63**: 539–551.

Louis ED, Lynch T, Kaufmann P, Fahn S, Odel J. Diagnostic guidelines in central nervous system Whipple's disease. *Annals of Neurology* 1996; **40**: 561–568.

Peters G, du Plessis DG, Humphrey PR. Cerebral Whipple's disease with a stroke-like presentation and cerebrovascular pathology. *Journal of Neurology, Neurosurgery and Psychiatry* 2002; **73**: 336–339.

Other relevant entries Gastrointestinal disease and the nervous system; Sarcoidosis.

Williams syndrome

Fanconi–Schlesinger syndrome • Williams–Beuren syndrome

Pathophysiology A relatively common syndrome, usually sporadic but occasionally autosomal dominant, with typical facial dysmorphism ("elfin facies"), low IQ, and psychological features akin to autism.

Clinical features: history and examination

- Facial dysmorphism ("elfin facies"): broad forehead, suprapalpebral fullness, hyper/hypotelorism, large mouth.
- Short stature, microcephaly.
- Low IQ: friendly, lively disposition, sociable, "happy-go-lucky", talkative, good memory for faces, places, but underlying evidence for anxiety, sleep problems, features akin to autism.
- +/− supravalvular aortic stenosis, ventricular septal defect, atrial septal defect, pulmonary arterial stenosis.
- +/− renal anomalies.
- +/− infantile hypercalcaemia (?raised 1,25 dihydroxyvitamin D_2).
- +/− dental malformations.
- +/− epilepsy (50%).

Investigations and diagnosis Diagnosis usually evident at birth or shortly thereafter. Deletions of chromosome 7q11–q23 have been reported in some patients. Investigations for cardiac anomalies may be undertaken.

Differential diagnosis Autism.

Treatment and prognosis Symptomatic control of seizures if present. Clomipramine may be given for anxiety, sleep disorders. Treatment of hypertension if present, since this, along with cardiac anomalies, is a cause of early death.

> **Reference** Udwin O. A survey of adults with Williams syndrome and idiopathic infantile hypercalcaemia. *Developmental Medicine and Child Neurology* 1990; **32**: 129–141.

> **Other relevant entry** Autism, autistic disorder.

■ Wilson's disease
Hepatolenticular degeneration ● Westphal–Strümpell pseudosclerosis

Pathophysiology Wilson's disease is an autosomal-recessive disorder of copper metabolism, usually presenting in young adults with hepatic and/or neurological dysfunction, due to accumulation of copper in affected tissues.

Clinical features: history and examination

Hepatic (tend to be first features to manifest, in later childhood).

- Fulminant hepatic failure
- Chronic active hepatitis
- Cirrhosis.

Neurological (adolescence, early adulthood).

Early

- Abnormal behaviour, psychiatric symptoms
- Kayser–Fleischer rings (copper deposition in Descemet's membrane)
- Akinetic-rigid syndrome: dystonia, rigidity, grimacing, excessive salivation
- Cerebellar syndrome: ataxia, tremor (flapping, wing-beating), titubation, dysarthria.

Late
- Dystonia
- Spasticity
- Seizures
- Dementia
- Flexion contractures.

Investigations and diagnosis *Bloods*: elevated copper (although this is non-specific and may occur in cholestatic liver disease); reduced caeruloplasmin (<20 mg/dl) is more specific.

Urine: 24-hour copper excretion high (>100 μg).

Slit-lamp examination: for Kayser–Fleischer rings; sunflower cataracts.

Imaging: CT/MRI may show low attenuation/signal intensity lesions in basal ganglia.

Liver biospy: for hepatic copper content; may be required in cases lacking Kayser–Fleischer rings, neurological features and with a normal plasma caeruloplasmin.

Neurogenetics: linked to chromosome 13q14.3–q21.1; mutated gene encodes a copper transporting ATPase.

Differential diagnosis Other early onset parkinsonian syndromes. An acquired hepatocerebral degeneration occurring as a rare complication of chronic (usually alcoholic) liver disease has been described but its nosological status remains uncertain.

Treatment and prognosis Early and continued copper chelation therapy is mandatory to prevent the otherwise progressive and irreversible neurological sequelae. Options include:

D-penicillamine (250–500 mg qds) + prophylactic oral pyridoxine.

Trientine (triethylene tetramine).

Tetrathiomolybdate.

British anti-Lewisite (now rarely used).

Oral zinc reduces dietary copper absorption (i.e. it is not a chelating agent); its use is favoured in asymptomatic patients and during pregnancy.

Liver transplantation cures the condition and may reverse some neurological features.

Family screening.

References Walshe JM, Yealland M. Chelation treatment of neurological Wilson's disease. *Quarterly Journal of Medicine* 1993; **86**: 197–204.

Wilson SAK. Progressive lenticular degeneration: a familial nervous disease associated with cirrhosis of the liver. *Brain* 1912; **34**: 295–509.

Other relevant entries Acaeruloplasminaemia; Dystonia: an overview; Gastrointestinal disease and the nervous system; Menkes' disease; Non-Wilsonian hepatocerebral degeneration; Parkinsonian syndromes, parkinsonism.

■ Wiskott–Aldrich syndrome – see Lymphoma

■ Withdrawal–emergent syndrome – see Drug-induced movement disorders

■ Wolf–Hirschhorn syndrome
Chromosome 4p syndrome • Wolf syndrome

Pathophysiology A rare chromosomal disorder causing learning disability, associated with telomeric rearrangement on chromosome 4p, undetectable using traditional cytogenetic methods. Two-third of cases are girls. Loss of the tip of the short arm of chromosome 4 is usually of paternal origin. This also causes deletion of the huntingtin gene. Since the clinical syndrome bears no relation to Huntington's disease (HD), this is a strong argument for the trinucleotide (CAG) repeat which underpins HD producing a toxic gain of function rather than a loss of function.

Clinical features: history and examination
- Intrauterine growth retardation.
- Microcephaly.
- Hypertelorism, prominent glabella, divergent strabismus, low set dysplastic ears.
- Learning disability; severe psychomotor retardation.
- Epilepsy (*ca.* 80%).

Investigations and diagnosis Sequencing of chromosome 4p to identify telomeric rearrangement.

Differential diagnosis Other causes of learning disability.

Treatment and prognosis No specific treatment. Symptomatic control of seizures. About one-third of cases die in the first year of life, possibly due to increased susceptibility to infection.

> **Reference** Altherr MR, Bengtsson U, Elder FFB *et al*. Molecular confirmation of Wolf–Hirschhorn syndrome with a subtle translocation of chromsome 4. *American Journal of Human Genetics* 1991; **49**: 1235–1242.

> **Other relevant entries** Huntington's disease; Trinucleotide repeat diseases.

■ Wolfram syndrome
Diabetes insipidus, diabetes mellitus, optic atrophy, and deafness • DIDMOAD syndrome

Pathophysiology Wolfram syndrome is a hereditary neurodegenerative disorder (autosomal-recessive, linked to chromosome 4p) characterized by juvenile-onset diabetes mellitus and optic atrophy, with various other neurological features (including diabetes insipidus and deafness) related to brainstem atrophy and dysfunction. A disorder of mitochondrial function was suspected, even though mutations in mitochondrial DNA have been identified only very rarely in sporadic cases; mutations in a gene (WFS1) encoding a transmembrane protein have been reported.

Clinical features: history and examination

Diagnostic criteria have been suggested

- Juvenile-onset diabtes mellitus and optic atrophy (*sine qua non*).

Other features

- Positive family history
- Brainstem signs: dysarthria, dysphagia, nystagmus, gaze palsies (Parinaud's syndrome), primary respiratory failure
- Diabetes insipidus (50%)
- Sensorineural deafness (50%)
- Anosmia
- Seizures/myoclonus
- Truncal ataxia
- Axial rigidity
- Neuropsychiatric/cognitive abnormalities
- Neurogenic incontinence
- Hyporeflexia, areflexia
- Extensor plantar responses
- Renal tract abnoramlities, GI dysmotility, primary gonadal atrophy.

Investigations and diagnosis *Imaging*: MRI: brainstem atrophy, especially involving pons and midbrain.

Neurophysiology: NCS/EMG: may show mild axonal neuropathy (consistent with diabetes mellitus).

EEG: non-specific abnormalities (e.g. slowing).

Neurogenetics: Mitochondrial DNA analysis has occasionally been reported to show mutations.

Differential diagnosis The full DIDMOAD syndrome is characteristic, but in partial forms there may be confusion with inflammatory disorders (multiple sclerosis, Behçet's disease) or degenerative conditions (Tunbridge–Paley syndrome).

Treatment and prognosis No specific treatment known. Appropriate medical treatment of diabetes mellitus, diabetes insipidus. Low vision/hearing aids for visual failure/deafness. Respiratory support may be necessary in cases of primary respiratory failure/central apnoea. The median age of death is 30 years.

References Inoue H, Tanizawa Y, Wasson J *et al*. A gene encoding a transmembrane protein is mutated in patients with diabetes mellitus and optic atrophy (Wolfram syndrome). *Nature Genetics* 1998; **20**: 143–148.

Scolding NJ, Kellar-Wood HF, Shaw C, Shneerson JM, Antoun N. Wolfram syndrome: hereditary diabetes mellitus with brainstem and optic atrophy. *Annals of Neurology* 1996; **39**: 352–360.

Other relevant entries Mitochondrial disease: an overview; Tunbridge–Paley syndrome.

■ Wolman's disease
Acid lipase deficiency

Pathophysiology Deficiency of the enzyme acid lipase (cholesterol ester hydrolase) leads to the intralysosomal storage of triglycerides and cholesterol esters in the viscera (especially liver and spleen). The nervous system is occasionally affected. Wolman's disease is an autosomal-recessive disorder of acid lipase dysfunction; cholesterol ester-storage disease (CESD) is a milder variant due to greater residual enzyme activity.

Clinical features: history and examination
- Onset in infancy, usually first 3 months of life.
- Vomiting, failure to thrive.
- Digestive disorder, diarrhoea, steatorrhoea.
- Hepatosplenomegaly: massive.
- Developmental delay with marked hypotonia; may evolve to spasticity, clonus.
- +/− tapetoretinal degeneration.

Investigations and diagnosis *Bloods*: raised plasma cholesterol. Enzyme deficiency in lymphocytes or fibroblasts.
Imaging: plain radiography/ultrasonography of abdomen: adrenal calcification.
Tissue: vacuolated cells may be seen in bone marrow, intestinal cells.

Differential diagnosis The finding of adrenal calcification is virtually pathognomonic of the disease in young infants with the appropriate clinical picture.

Treatment and prognosis No specific treatment known; death usually within the 1st year. Bone marrow transplantation is being examined.

> **Other relevant entries** Cerebrotendinous xanthomatosis; Niemann–Pick disease; Smith–Lemli–Opitz syndrome.

■ Worster-Drought syndrome (1)
Familial British (presenile) dementia (FBD) ● Familial cerebral amyloid angiopathy

Pathophysiology This is an autosomal-dominant progressive dementia syndrome with associated cerebellar ataxia and spastic paraparesis, due to deposition of a novel cerebrovascular amyloid. The condition is linked to a mutation in the stop codon of the A-Bri gene on chromosome 13. The C-terminus of this enlarged protein forms the amyloidogenic peptide.

Clinical features: history and examination
- Family history of presenile dementia.
- Progresive dementia (presenting sign, onset age 40–57 years).
- Cerebellar ataxia (early).
- Spastic paraparesis (late).

Investigations and diagnosis *Imaging*: CT/MRI: mild ventricular dilatation; low attenuation/high signal intensity in frontoparietal white matter.

Pathology: severe cerebrovascular amyloid involving vessels of brain grey and white matter, spinal cord, and leptomeninges; non-neuritic plaques, perivascular plaques, some neurofibrillary tangles, and white matter changes with myelin loss and small cystic infarcts.

Neurogenetics: for mutations in A-Bri gene.

Differential diagnosis Other familial (autosomal-dominant) dementias, especially familial Alzheimer's disease, although the other signs largely rule this out (spastic paraparesis may be a feature in early-onset AD with exon 9 deletion mutations in the presenilin-1 gene). Inflammatory dementias, such as vasculitides, Sjögren's syndrome, may have spastic paraparesis but lack a family history; ditto von Winiwarter–Buerger's disease.

Treatment and prognosis Uniformly fatal prognosis, death occurring at age 50–66 years. Currently no specific treatment.

References Plant GT, Revesz T, Barnard RO, Harding AE, Gautier-Smith PC. Familial cerebral amyloid angiopathy with nonneuritic plaque formation. *Brain* 1990; **113**: 721–747.

Vidal R, Frangione B, Rostagno A *et al*. A stop-codon mutation in the *BRI* gene associated with familial British dementia. *Nature* 1999; **399**: 776–781.

Worster-Drought C, Hill TR, McMenemey WH. Familial presenile dementia with spastic paralysis. *Journal of Neurology and Psychopathology* 1933; **14**: 27–34.

Other relevant entries Alzheimer's disease; Cerebral amyloid angiopathy; Dementia: an overview; Familial Danish dementia; Von Winiwarter–Buerger's disease.

Worster-Drought syndrome (2)
Congenital childhood suprabulbar palsy

Pathophysiology A childhood disorder of isolated paresis/weakness of oral muscula-ture without major motor signs in the trunk or limbs. This condition often presents as a developmental dysarthria. It is thought to result from agenesis or hypogenesis of the corticobulbar fibres innervating the vagus (X) and hypoglossal (XII) nerve nuclei.

Clinical features: history and examination
- Dysarthria: hypernasality, misarticulation.
- +/− dysphagia.
- Weak lips, pharynx, palate, tongue.
- Brisk jaw jerk.
- No long tract (pyramidal) signs.

Investigations and diagnosis No specific investigations; condition described before advent of CT/MRI.

Differential diagnosis Congenital pseudobulbar palsy with cognitive deficits and seizures may result from ischaemic injury of the brain during prenatal development (perisylvian syndrome). Acquired suprabulbar palsy may occur secondary to encephalitis or head injury (may have additional facial rigidity). Facial weakness and swallowing difficulties in early childhood may occur in myotonic dystrophy and myasthenia gravis. In patients labelled as "cerebral palsy" in whom bulbar or oromotor dysfunction is prominent, this diagnosis needs to be considered.

Treatment and prognosis Speech therapy.

References Clark M, Carr L, Reilly S, Neville BG. Worster-Drought syndrome, a mild tetraplegic perisylvian cerebral palsy. Review of 47 cases. *Brain* 2000; **123**: 2160–2170.

Worster-Drought C. Suprabulbar paresis. *Developmental Medicine and Child Neurology* 1974; **16(suppl 30)**: 1–30.

Other relevant entries Cerebral palsy, cerebral palsy syndromes; Perisylvian syndrome.

■ Writer's cramp

Graphospasm • *La crampe des écrivains* • Scrivener's palsy

Writer's cramp is a focal dystonia involving the hand and/or arm muscles, causing abnormal posturing of the hand when writing; it is the commonest task-specific dystonia. When attempting to write, patients may find that they are involuntarily gripping the pen harder, and there may also be involuntary movement at the wrist or in the arm. A tremor may also develop, not to be confused with primary writing tremor in which there is no dystonia. Handwriting becomes illegible. Attempts to use the contralateral hand may be made, but this too may become affected with time. The problem may be exclusive to writing (simple writer's cramp) but some people develop difficulties with other activities as well (e.g. shaving; dystonic writer's cramp), reflecting a dystonia of the hand or arm.

There is some neurophysiological evidence that the condition is due to abnormalities within the spinal cord segmental motor programmes and muscle spindle afferent input to them.

Writer's cramp may be amenable to local botulinum toxin injections into the hand or arm muscles responsible for the involuntary movement. Other strategies which may be used include writing with a different grip (e.g. whole hand grip), using a fat-bodied pen, or using a word processor.

Reference Rivest J, Lees AJ, Marsden CD. Writer's cramp: treatment with botulinum toxin. *Movement Disorders* 1991; **6**: 55–59.

Other relevant entries Botulinum toxin therapy; Dystonia: an overview; Writing tremor.

■ Writing tremor

Primary writing tremor

Writing tremor is a task-specific tremor, evident as a pronation–supination movement of 5–7 Hz on attempting to write. It may be limited to writing or evident in other movements as well; some individuals also have a postural tremor.

The condition is much rarer than writer's cramp, a focal dystonia in which tremor may also occur. Whether the two conditions are separate or related remains uncertain;

cerebellar activation similar to that seen in essential tremor has been reported in positron emission tomography (PET) scan studies of primary writing tremor.

Treatment may be attempted with:

anticholinergic drugs (as for dystonias);
propranolol, primidone, alcohol (as for essential tremor);
stereotactic thalamotomy.

> **Reference** Bain PG, Findlay LJ, Britton TC *et al*. Primary writing tremor. *Brain* 1995; **118**: 1461–1472.

> **Other relevant entries** Dystonia: an overview; Essential tremor; Tremor: an overview; Writer's cramp.

■ Wyburn–Mason disease
Dechaume–Blanc–Bonnet syndrome

Pathophysiology A sporadic neurocutaneous syndrome characterized by retinal arteriovenous malformation (AVM), usually unilateral, and independent intracranial AVM which may extend along the visual pathway to the cerebral peduncle and cerebellar hemisphere. Facial (periorbital) involvement may also occur. Rupture may occur.

Clinical features: history and examination
- Usual onset in adulthood.
- Retinal AVM: proptosis; visual loss (acute, chronic); glaucoma, optic atrophy.
- Neurological features: seizures, headache, subarachnoid haemorrhage.
- Facial angiomas: unilateral, bilateral.

Investigations and diagnosis Fluorescein angiography may demonstrate the racemose angioma; MRI may demonstrate intracerebral AVM.

Differential diagnosis Von Hippel–Lindau disease (inherited); Sturge–Weber syndrome.

Treatment and prognosis
Surgical resection.
Embolization.
Radiosurgery.

> **Reference** Theron J, Newton TH, Hoyt WF. Unilateral retinocephalic vascular malformations. *Neuroradiology* 1974; **7**: 185–196.

> **Other relevant entries** Phakomatosis; Sturge–Weber syndrome; Von Hippel–Lindau disease.

Xx

■ Xanthomatosis – see Cerebrotendinous xanthomatosis

■ Xeroderma pigmentosum and related conditions
De Sanctis–Cacchione syndrome

Pathophysiology A rare, heterogeneous, group of autosomal-recessive disorders characterized by cutaneous lesions in childhood (dermatitis, skin cancer) due to the inability to repair DNA damaged by ultraviolet (UV) radiation (i.e. hypersensitivity to UV radiation). Various mutations underpin the reduced capacity for excision repair of UV-induced DNA damage. The De Sanctis–Cacchione syndrome forms a subgroup of xeroderma pigmentosum (XP) in which skin changes are associated with retarded growth and sexual development and neurological complications. In trichothiodystrophy, mental retardation is associated with ichthyosis, brittle hair and nails. Neurological manifestations are said to occur in about 20% of XP patients.

Clinical features: history and examination
Neurological (not all patients)

- motor/mental retardation,
- microcephaly,
- sensorineural deafness,
- cerebellar ataxia,
- choreoathetosis,
- axonal polyneuropathy,
- spastic quadriplegia.

Ocular

- keratitis, conjunctivitis.

Dermatological

- hyperpigmented macules, atrophy, telangiectasia; benign tumours (e.g. keratoma, fibroma and angiomyoma); malignant tumours (basal cell, squamous cell, melanoma).

Investigations and diagnosis
Neurophysiology:

EEG: generalized slowing; focal slow-wave and spike discharges may be seen.
EMG/NCS: axonal polyneuropathy.

Neurogenetics: heterogeneous, seven subtypes or complementation groups are recognized, caused by mutations in a number of genes which encode DNA repair proteins.

Differential diagnosis Cockayne's syndrome.

Treatment and prognosis Protection from sunlight; skin surveillance; early excision of tumours.

Death from disseminated tumours by second to third decade is usual.

Reference Mimaki T, Itoh N, Abe J *et al.* Neurological manifestations in xeroderma pigmentosum. *Annals of Neurology* 1986; **20**: 70–75.

Other relevant entry Phakomatosis

▓ Xerophthalmia – see Lambert–Eaton myasthenic syndrome; Vitamin deficiencies and the nervous system

▓ X-linked adrenoleukodsytrophy – see Adrenoleukodystrophy

▓ X-linked bulbospinal neuronopathy – see Kennedy's syndrome; Trinucleotide repeat diseases

▓ X-linked Dystonia–Parkinsonism syndrome

Lubag

This rare condition, manifest almost exclusively amongst men originating from the Philippine Islands, usually begins in midlife with axial and lower limb involvement, although upper limb involvement and cranial dystonia at onset are also recognized. The majority develop a generalized dystonia within the first few years, others have parkinsonism which does not respond to levodopa. The patients typically die of their disease after 5–10 years, and at post-mortem there is degeneration with a so-called mosaic pattern within the striatum. The condition is linked to the DYT3 locus at Xq13.

Reference Waters CH, Faust PL, Powers J *et al*. Neuropathology of lubag (X-linked dystonia parkinsonism). *Movement Disorders* 1993; **8**: 387–390.

Other relevant entries Dystonia: an overview; Parkinsonian syndromes, parkinsonism.

▓ X-linked myopathy with excessive autophagy

A rare hereditary myopathy of childhood onset, characterized by a slowly progressive proximal myopathy (especially of the lower limbs), with normal life expectancy. EMG shows polyphasic motor units with high mean amplitude and normal duration; abundant myotonic discharges occur in clinically affected and unaffected muscles. Muscle biopsy shows abundant sarcoplasmic vacuoles, immunopositive for dystrophin and laminin, containing debris and lysosomal enzymes. XMEA is distinct from the X-linked vacuolar myopathy with cardiomyopathy and mental retardation due to deficiency of lysosome-associated membrane protein 2 (LAMP-2), also known as Danon disease.

Reference Kalimo H, Savontaus M-L, Lang H *et al*. X-linked myopathy with excessive autophagy: a new hereditary muscle disease. *Annals of Neurology* 1988; **23**: 258–265.

Other relevant entries Danon disease; Myopathy: an overview.

Yy

■ **Yaws** – see Syphilis

■ **Yips** – see Occupational dystonias

■ **Yolk sac tumour** – see Germ-cell tumours

Zz

■ Zellweger syndrome
Cerebrohepatorenal disease

Pathophysiology An autosomal-recessive, multisystem disorder of infancy due to the virtual absence of peroxisomes. A Zellweger-like phenotype due to defective peroxisomal function also occurs. Mutations in a variety of PEX genes, encoding peroxin proteins, are responsible for these disorders of peroxisome biogenesis.

Clinical features: history and examination

- Hypotonia, areflexia.
- Absent psychomotor development.
- Visual impairment leading to pendular nystagmus; cataracts, corneal opacities, Brushfield spots.
- Hearing impairment.
- Seizures.
- Craniofacial dysmorphology: high and prominent forehead, hypoplastic supraorbital ridges, epicanthic folds, depressed and broad root of nose; patellar calcification said to be very characteristic.
- Hepatomegaly.
- Renal cysts.

Investigations and diagnosis Physical features may be sufficiently characteristic to allow diagnosis on inspection alone, but numerous non-classical variants of Zellweger exist, which may necessitate further investigation.

Plasma VLCFA: elevated C26 : 0/C22 : 0 ratio.

Neurophysiology:

ERG: absent due to retinal pigmentary degeneration.
BSAEP: absent or reduced.

Imaging:

Brain MRI: leukodystrophy, abnormal convolution pattern (pachygyria, poly-microgyria, neuronal heterotopia).

Renal ultrasound: cysts.

Liver biopsy: virtual absence of peroxisomes (EM, cytochemistry for catalase).
Slit lamp: cornea, lens abnormalities.
Neurogenetics: PEX gene mutations.
Differential diagnosis Down's syndrome
Zellweger-like syndromes:

Neonatal adrenoleukodystrophy
Infantile Refsum's disease
Hyperpipercolic aciduria

Lowe syndrome.
Treatment and prognosis No specific treatment known; death usually occurs within the first few months of life.

Reference Brosius U, Gärtner J. Cellular and molecular aspects of Zellweger syndrome and other peroxisome biogenesis disorders. *Cellular and Molecular Life Sciences* 2002; **59**: 1058–1069.

Other relevant entries Adrenoleukodystrophy; Peroxisomal disorders: an overview; Refsum's disease.

▧ Zinc deficiency
Acrodermatitis enteropathica

Pathophysiology There is an autosomal-recessive disorder of zinc metabolism and malabsorption usually presenting in the first year of life, following weaning from breast milk, with a characteristic skin disorder, with or without neurobehavioural features.

Whether disordered zinc metabolism may contribute to adult cognitive decline, specifically within the context of Alzheimer's disease (AD), remains contentious, with different groups advocating too much or too little zinc as important factors in the pathogenesis of the typical neuropathological lesions of AD. A poor diet will also result in biochemical zinc deficiency, not necessarily accompanied by neurological features.

Clinical features: history and examination
- Distinctive vesico-bullous skin disorder, especially around orifices (mouth, anus).
- Alopecia.
- Diarrhoea.
- Failure to thrive.
- Increased susceptibility to infection.
- +/− neurobehavioural features: lethargy, irritability, depression.

Investigations and diagnosis Reduced serum and urinary zinc; low alkaline phosphatase.

Differential diagnosis Skin rash is characteristic.

Treatment and prognosis Lifelong oral zinc sulphate supplementation is associated with a normal life expectancy. Untreated, patients progress and succumb to infection.

> **References** Nachev PC, Larner AJ. Zinc and Alzheimer's disease. *Trace Elements and Electrolytes* 1996; **13**: 55–59.
>
> Prasad A. Zinc deficiency. *British Medical Journal* 2003; **326**: 409–410.
>
> **Other relevant entry** Gastrointestinal diseases and the nervous system.

▣ Zoster – see Herpes zoster and postherpetic neuralgia

▣ Zygomycosis – see Mucormycosis